Ocular
Pathology

Commissioning Editor: Russell Gabbedy
Development Editor: Sharon Nash
Project Manager: Bryan Potter
Design: Charles Gray
Marketing Manager(s) (UK/USA): John Canelon/William Veltre

Ocular Pathology

SIXTH EDITION

MYRON YANOFF, MD

Professor and Chair
Department of Opthalmology
Drexel University College of Medicine
Philadelphia PA

JOSEPH W. SASSANI, MD MHA

Professor of Ophthalmology and Pathology
Pennsylvania State University
Hershey Medical Center
Hershey, PA

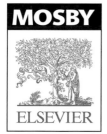

MOSBY

ELSEVIER

MOSBY
ELSEVIER

MOSBY an imprint of Elsevier Inc.

First edition 1975
Second edition 1982
Third edition 1989
Fourth edition 1996
Fifth edition 2002

ISBN: 978-0-323-04232-1

British Library Cataloguing in Publication Data
A catalogue record for this book is available from the British Library

Library of Congress Cataloging in Publication Data
A catalog record for this book is available from the Library of Congress

Notice
Medical knowledge is constantly changing. Standard safety precautions must be followed, but as new research and clinical experience broaden our knowledge, changes in treatment and drug therapy may become necessary or appropriate. Readers are advised to check the most current product information provided by the manufacturer of each drug to be administered to verify the recommended dose, the method and duration of administration, and contraindications. It is the responsibility of the practitioner, relying on experience and knowledge of the patient, to determine dosages and the best treatment for each individual patient. Neither the Publisher nor the author assume any liability for any injury and/or damage to persons or property arising from this publication.

The Publisher

ELSEVIER your source for books, journals and multimedia in the health sciences

www.elsevierhealth.com

Working together to grow libraries in developing countries

www.elsevier.com | www.bookaid.org | www.sabre.org

ELSEVIER   BOOK AID International   Sabre Foundation

The publisher's policy is to use paper manufactured from sustainable forests

Printed in China
Last digit is the print number: 9 8 7 6 5 4 3 2

Contents

Foreword

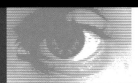

When I was invited to write the Foreword for this sixth edition of Yanoff and Fine's *Ocular Pathology*, by Myron Yanoff and Joseph W. Sassani, I felt honored considering that those who have authored the Foreword for the prior editions were amongst the "masters" of academic ophthalmology and ophthalmic pathology, namely Drs. Morton E. Smith, J. Donald M. Gass, Frederick A. Jakobiec, Paul Henkind, Harold G. Scheie, and Lorenz E. Zimmerman.

This textbook is one of the few in my 35 years of practice of ophthalmology and ophthalmic pathology that I have obtained from the immediate availability of each edition, since it first was published in 1975, both for my clinical office and for my ophthalmic pathology research laboratory that is inhabited by my fellows, residents, and medical students. Furthermore, the authors, originally Myron Yanoff and Ben Fine, and now including Joe Sassani, have been both career-long colleagues and very close friends of mine, mainly as a result of the frequent crossing of our paths at multiple annual academic meetings; these events almost always include our spouses, giving us a feeling of family with the elite in our field.

As expressed by the writers of the Foreword of the previous editions, Ocular Pathology is without a doubt the best current ophthalmic pathology textbook, being a combination of a well organized review text presented in point-like fashion and an atlas with an extensive number of color photographs of most of the described ophthalmic conditions. Furthermore, it is one of the few textbooks on this important subject that is consistently being updated with the latest clinical and pathologic information including more recent "avant-garde" disciplines associated with ophthalmic pathology such as the corresponding advances in molecular genetics.

The names, "Yanoff" and "Fine" as co-authors of major textbooks in academic ophthalmology are indicative of a fruitful "marriage" of two of the most outstanding contributors to our knowledge of ophthalmic pathology during the past four decades. These two individuals have shared their extensive experience involving two different approaches to this discipline, namely histopathology and electron microscopy respectively, in a continuous, composite fashion almost unmatched in academic ophthalmology.

Dedicating this sixth edition of *Ocular Pathology* as a tribute to the late Ben S. Fine is most appropriate. Ben, a fellow Canadian, was a pioneer of the electron microscopic examination of ocular tissues. It was my good fortune that Ben's academic office was directly across from my cubicle during my fellowship at the Armed Forces Institute of Pathology (AFIP) during the early 1970's. From Ben I learned not only the basics of electron microscopy, which I still practice today, but also his approach to ocular diseases utilizing uniquely clear thought processes. Ben was always available to share his expertise and gave the premier course on the ultrastructure of normal ocular tissues for several decades in addition to his publications on the electron microscopic findings of numerous pathologic ocular disease processes.

Myron Yanoff has demonstrated amazing energy, dedication and proficiency in the development of this text while serving both as director of ophthalmic pathology and as a most successful chair of the Department of Ophthalmology, currently at Drexel University in Philadelphia. During the past 4 decades, Myron has been a full professor of both ophthalmology and pathology; his distinguished career was culminated by his being the recipient of the American Academy of Ophthalmology's Zimmerman Gold Medal just prior to the onset of the 21st century. I take my hat off to his continuous productivity and to his seeing to it that this "jewel" in academic ophthalmology is being perpetuated.

The addition of Dr. Joe Sassani as a co-author is a masterful step forward to ensure the continuity of this most important textbook in ophthalmic pathology. Joe is a disciple of Myron Yanoff who has evolved to be one of the leaders in the field of ophthalmic pathology including having served as president of the American Association of Ophthalmic Pathologists. Joe is director of ophthalmic pathology and professor of ophthalmology and pathology at the Milton Hershey Medical Center in Hershey Pennsylvania. He also provides additional perspective in his fields of clinical expertise including glaucoma. Having this relatively youthful star participate in the authorship should ensure the continuation of this invaluable resource especially since Joe has broad academic shoulders with a strong reputation of responsibility and commitment.

Ocular Pathology is most highly recommended for all residents in ophthalmology and fellows in ophthalmic pathology and is an excellent resource for medical students, general pathologists who review ocular specimens, and ophthalmologists who desire to fulfill their academic curiosity. It provides very succinctly the basics of ophthalmic pathology and includes the key information on almost every described ophthalmological disease process with an extensive reference list to enable more elaborate further studies. I would like to express "Bravo" to the authors for providing this update of their masterpiece from which so many will benefit.

Seymour Brownstein, *MD FRCSC*
Les Amis Chair in Vision Science
Professor, Departments of Ophthalmology
and Laboratory Medicine (Pathology)
Director, Ophthalmic Pathology Laboratory
University of Ottawa Eye Institute
The Ottawa Hospital / University of Ottawa
Ottawa Health Research Institute
Ottawa, Ontario, Canada

Forewords

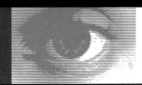

to the First Edition

During the year of the observance of the 100th anniversary (1874–1974) of the University of Pennsylvania's Department of Ophthalmology, it is exciting to have the publication of a volume whose coauthors have contributed significantly to the strides in ocular pathology taken by the Department in the past several years.

Myron Yanoff, a highly regarded member of our staff, began a residency in ophthalmology in 1962, upon graduating from the University's School of Medicine. The residency continued for the next five years, during the first two of which he also held a residency in the Department of Pathology. His keen interest and ability in ocular pathology were readily apparent, and I encouraged him to apply for a fellowship at the Armed Forces Institute of Pathology (AFIP), Washington, DC. From July, 1964, through June, 1965, he carried out exceptional research at the AFIP in both ophthalmology and pathology. He returned to our Department in July, 1965, where the caliber both of his clinical and research work was of the highest. When he completed his residency in June, 1967, I invited him to join the staff, and he has recently attained the rank of full professor. During the ensuing years he has contributed substantially to the literature, particularly in the fields of ophthalmic and experimental pathology. He is Board certified in ophthalmology and in pathology.

Ben Fine, noted for his work in electron microscopy at AFIP and at George Washington University, has shared his expertise in the field through lectures presented as part of the curriculum of the annual 16-week Basic Science Course in the Department's graduate program.

It can be said that 100 years ago ophthalmology was a specialty that had been gradually evolving during the preceding 100 years, dating from the time of the invention of bifocals by Benjamin Franklin in 1785. Few American physicians of that era, however, knew how to treat diseases of the eye, but as medical education became more specialized it was inevitable that ophthalmology would also become a specialty.

With the invention of the ophthalmoscope in 1851, great advances were made in the reaching and practice of ophthalmology. This contributed greatly, of course, to setting the scene for the establishment of the University's Department of Ophthalmology. It was on February 3, 1874, that Dr. William F. Norris was elected First Clinical Professor of Diseases of the Eye. Similar chairs had been established earlier in only three other institutions. The chair at the University of Pennsylvania later became known as the William F. Norris and George E. de Schweinitz Chair of Ophthalmology.

Both Dr. Norris and Dr. de Schweinitz actively engaged in the study of ocular pathology. Dr. Norris stressed the importance of the examination of the eye by microscopy and of the correlation of findings from pathology specimens with the clinical signs. Dr. de Schweinitz was instrumental in having a member of his staff accepted as ophthalmic pathologist with the Department of Pathology.

In the years that followed under succeeding chairmen of the Department, other aspects of ophthalmology were stressed. Then, in 1947, during the chairmanship of Dr. Francis Heed Adler, Dr. Larry L. Calkins was appointed to a residency. Dr. Calkins, like Dr. Yanoff, displayed a keen interest in ocular pathology. Accordingly, he was instrumental in its study being revitalized during the three years of his residency. Another resident, Dr. William C. Frayer, who came to the Department in 1949, joined Dr. Calkins in his interest in ocular pathology. Dr. Frayer received additional training in the Department of Pathology and then became the ophthalmic pathologist of the department.

The importance of ocular pathology was increasingly evident, but facilities for carrying out the work in the Department of Ophthalmology were unfortunately limited. Until 1964, the pathology laboratory had been confined to a small room in the outpatient area of the Department. Then we were able to acquire larger quarters in the Pathology Building of the Philadelphia General Hospital located next door to the Hospital of the University of Pennsylvania. Although the building was earmarked for eventual demolition, the space was fairly adequate for research and also for conducting weekly ophthalmic pathology teaching conferences. Despite the physical aspects, we saw to it that Dr. Yanoff and his team of workers had a well equipped laboratory.

During the next several years as I saw that my dream for an eye institute with facilities for patient care, reaching and research under one roof was to become a reality, I was delighted to be able to include prime space on the research floor for the ever enlarging scope of ocular pathology. In addition to all that Dr. Yanoff has had to build upon from the past tradition of our Department of Ophthalmology, I would like to think that the new facilities at the Institute have in some measure contributed to the contents of this excellent volume. With grateful appreciation, therefore, I look upon this book as the authors' birthday present to the Department. From these same facilities, as Dr. Yanoff and Dr. Fine continue to collaborate, I can hope will come insights and answers for which all of us are ever searching in the battle against eye disease.

Harold G. Scheie, MD
Chairman, Department of Ophthalmology
University of Pennsylvania
Director, Scheie Eye Institute

From their earliest days in ophthalmology Myron Yanoff and Ben Fine impressed me as exceptional students. As they have matured and progressed up the academic ladder, they have become equally dedicated and effective teachers. Their anatomical studies of normal and diseased tissues have always been oriented toward providing meaningful answers to practical as well as esoteric clinical questions. Their ability to draw upon their large personal experience in clinical ophthalmology, ocular pathology, and laboratory investigation for their lectures at the Armed Forces Institute of Pathology and at the University of Pennsylvania have contributed immeasurably to the success of those courses. Now they have used the same time-tested approach in assembling their material for this book. Beginning with their basic lecture outlines, then expanding these with just enough text to substitute for what would have been said verbally in lecture, adding a remarkable amount of illustrative material for the amount of space consumed, and then providing pertinent references to get the more ambitious student started in the pursuit of a subject, Drs. Yanoff and Fine have provided us with a sorely needed teaching aid for both the student and the teacher of ocular pathology. It should prove to be especially popular among medical students and residents in both ophthalmology and ocular pathology. With it one gets good orientation from the well-conceived outlines and fine clinicopathologic correlations from the selection of appropriate illustrations.

It is with considerable pride and admiration that I've watched the evolution of the authors' work and its fruition in the form of this latest book. I am proud that both authors launched their respective careers with periods of intensive study at the Armed Forces Institute of Pathology and that ever since, they have remained loyal, dedicated, and highly ethical colleagues. I admire their youthful energy, their patient, careful attitude, their friendly cooperative nature, and their ability to get important things accomplished. I'm appreciative of this opportunity to express my gratitude for the work they have been doing. If it is true that "by his pupils, a teacher will be judged," I could only wish to have had several dozen more like Drs. Yanoff and Fine.

Lorenz E. Zimmerman, MD
Chief, Ophthalmic Pathology Division
Armed Forces Institute of Pathology
Washington, DC

Preface

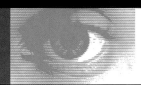

It has been 33 years since the first edition of OCULAR PATHOLOGY was published in 1975. At that time the book contained the basics of eye pathology, which still are very much current. New entities have appeared and have been incorporated into subsequent editions, as well as into this edition. The enormous recent explosion of information that has expanded our knowledge and understanding of ocular pathology has occurred mainly in the fields of genetics, immunohistochemistry, and molecular biology. Newer imaging techniques such ultrasound biomicroscopy and optical coherence tomography are bringing resolution approaching histopathologic techniques to the clinical setting. We have integrated the pertinent information from these fields into this sixth edition.

Among the numerous entities introduced into this sixth edition are De Barsy Syndrome; autoimmune polyendocrinopathy-candidiasis-ectodermal dystrophy, endothelial dystrophy, iris hypoplasia, congenital cataract, and stromal thinning (EDICT) syndrome; dentatorubropallidoluysian atrophy; microdot stromal degeneration; corneal fibrosis syndrome; toxic anterior segment syndrome; laryngo-onycho-cutaneous (LOC or Shabbir) syndrome; conjunctivochalasis; nevus lipomatosus (pedunculated nevus); Laugier-Hunziker syndrome; melanoma-associated spongiform scleropathy; Knobloch Syndrome; Maffuci's syndrome, malignant mesenchymoma; mantle cell lymphoma; congenital simple hamartoma of the retinal pigment epithelium; TNM (tumor, node, metastasis) classification; posterior microphthalmos; lymphedema–distichiasis syndrome; solitary spindle-cell xanthogranuloma; arteriovenous malformation of the iris; retinal angiomatous proliferation; complications of LASIK surgery; fibrous hamartoma of infancy, and others.

Additionally, numerous existing topics have been updated. They include the classification system for retinoblastoma, genetic features of persistent hyperplastic primary vitreous, pathobiology of Norrie's disease, multiple new insights into the pathology of incontinentia pigmenti, anatomic and pathologic correlates in the cornea, immunopathology of Herpes keratitis, updated genetics of corneal dystrophies, new features of Schnyder's corneal crystalline dystrophy (central stromal crystalline corneal dystrophy) and keratoconus, complications of retinal reattachment and glaucoma surgery, pathobiology of corneal abrasion; extensive revision of such topics as the anatomy of the conjunctiva, the pathobiology of vernal keratoconjunctivitis, and of graft-versus-host disease.

Other updated topics include the pathobiology of conjunctival and orbital lymphoma, squamous cell carcinoma of the conjunctiva, the genetics of pseudoexfoliation and uveal melanoma, and the inclusion of specific entities such as Fabry disease.

Particular attention has been directed at the pathobiology of diabetes mellitus. New and modified diabetes-related topics include the international clinical classification of diabetic retinopathy, diabetic, diabetic macular edema severity scales, and the role of VEGF and other factors in the pathobiology of diabetic complications.

Multiple changes and updates in Glaucoma include; syndromes associated with congenital glaucoma such as Hennekam syndrome, nail-patella syndrome, and familial amyloidotic polyneuropathy type I (Met 30). The pathobiology of myocilin/TIGR gene in the development of glaucoma has been revised and new clinical syndromes associated with angle-closure glaucoma have been added. The pathobiology of corticosteroid-induced glaucoma, and of glaucoma-associated damage to ocular tissues have been expanded. Latest features on the pathobiology of central corneal thickness as it relates to the development and diagnosis of glaucoma are discussed.

A unique feature, introduced in this 6th edition of OCULAR PATHOLOGY, is a DVD. It contains the contents of seven histopathology glass slides and the ImageScope™ software required to view them. The software permits the observation of these virtual microscope slides on the computer video monitor by varying magnification, field of observation, etc. just as could be done with an optical microscope. Also included on the DVD, are all of the images from the book, which are searchable and able to be exported to HTML/PowerPoint slide shows.

Finally, all illustrations have been digitally enhanced and color corrected. New tables and numerous updated references have been added.

This book could not have been completed without the understanding and patience of our wives Karin L. Yanoff, Ph.D. and Gloria Sassani, M.A. We also wish to acknowledge the help of our assistants, William F. Devers and Sharon Dunkle. Finally, the members of the Elsevier production and editorial team including Russell Gabbedy and Sharon Nash, and also Bryan Potter, Charles Gray and William Veltre have provided invaluable help and guidance in the production of this 6th edition of OCULAR PATHOLOGY.

Dedication

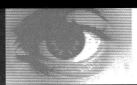

The fifth edition of this book was dedicated to the memory of Fruma I. Fine, the wife of Ben S. Fine, the long-time coauthor of this book. Now Ben is no longer with us but his memory, so vivid, lives on as an inspiration to the multitude of people trained by him, and also to those who have been educated by him through his seminal writings. Ben was one of the earliest pioneers in the field of ocular electron microscopy, first clarifying in exquisite detail the normal anatomy of the eye, then elucidating the mysteries of numerous ocular pathological entities. His groundbreaking discoveries remain unchallenged as some of the finest work done in the field, and we miss him always. We dedicate this sixth edition to his memory, for his spirit lives on in the pages of this book and in the minds and souls of his peers and students.

Basic Principles of Pathology

INFLAMMATION

Definition*

I. Inflammation is the response of a tissue or tissues to a noxious stimulus.

   A. The tissue may be predominantly cellular (e.g., retina), composed mainly of extracellular materials (e.g., cornea), or a mixture of both (e.g., uvea).

   B. The response may be localized or generalized, and the noxious stimulus infectious or noninfectious.

II. In a general way, inflammation is a response to a foreign stimulus that may involve specific (immunologic) or nonspecific reactions. Immune reactions arise in response to specific antigens, but may involve specific components (e.g., antibodies, T cells) or nonspecific components [e.g., natural killer (NK) cells, lymphokines].

Causes

I. Noninfectious causes.

   A. Exogenous causes: originate outside the eye and body, and include local ocular physical injury (e.g., penetrating perforating trauma, radiant energy), chemical injuries (e.g., alkali), or allergic reactions to external antigens (e.g., conjunctivitis secondary to pollen).

*Inflammation is not synonymous with infection. Inflammation may be caused by an infection (e.g., postoperative staphylococcal endophthalmitis), but it may also be caused by noninfectious agents, such as chemical burns. Conversely, infection is not always accompanied by significant inflammation. For example, in certain diseases of the immune system, widespread infection may be present, but the patient is incapable of mounting an inflammatory response.

   B. Endogenous causes: sources originating in the eye and body, such as inflammation secondary to cellular immunity [phacoanaphylactic endophthalmitis (phacoantigenic uveitis)]; spread from continuous structures (e.g., the sinuses); hematogenous spread (e.g., foreign particles); and conditions of unknown cause (e.g., sarcoidosis).

II. Infectious causes include viral, rickettsial, bacterial, fungal, and parasitic agents.

Phases of Inflammation

I. Acute (immediate or shock) phase (Fig. 1.1).

   A. Five cardinal signs: (1) redness (rubor) and (2) heat (calor)—both caused by increased rate and volume of blood flow; (3) mass (tumor)—caused by exudation of fluid (edema) and cells; (4) pain (dolor) and (5) loss of function (functio laesa)—both caused by outpouring of fluid and irritating chemicals.

   B. The acute phase is related to histamine release from mast cells and factors released from plasma (kinin, complement, and clotting systems).

Without a continuous stimulus the phase is transient, lasting from 3 to 5 hours. Chemical mediators,* whether directly or indirectly, cause smooth-muscle contraction (arteriolar constriction) and a local increase in vascular permeability. The chemical mediators seem to increase vascular permeability by causing the usually "tight" junctions between adjacent ocular vascular endothelial cells (especially in venules) to open, thereby allowing luminal fluid to leak into the surrounding tissue spaces.

*The chemical mediators include, but are not limited to, histamine, serotonin, kinins, plasmin, complement, prostaglandins, and peptide growth factors.

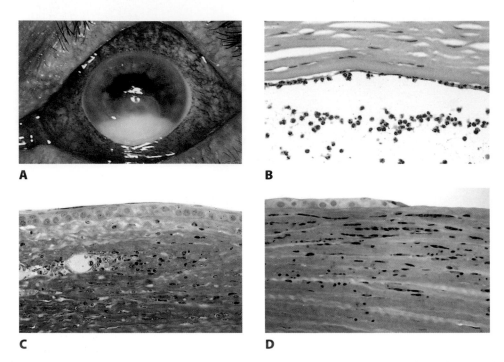

Fig. 1.1 Acute inflammation. **A,** Corneal ulcer with hypopyon (purulent exudate). Conjunctiva hyperemic. **B,** Polymorphonuclear leukocytes (PMNs) adhere to corneal endothelium and are present in the anterior chamber as a hypopyon (purulent exudate). **C,** Leukocytes adhere to limbal, dilated blood vessel wall (margination) and have emigrated through endothelial cell junctions into edematous surrounding tissue. **D,** PMNs in corneal stroma do not show characteristic morphology but are recognized by "bits and pieces" of nuclei lining up in a row. (**C** and **D** are thin sections from rabbit corneas 6 hours post corneal abrasion.)

1. *Histamine* is found in the granules of mast cells, where it is bound to a heparin–protein complex; it is also present in basophils and platelets.
2. The *kinins* are peptides formed by the enzymatic actin of kallikrein on the α_2-globulin kininogen. Kallikrein is activated by the coagulation factor XII, the *Hageman factor*, or by plasmin.
3. *Plasmin*, the proteolytic enzyme responsible for fibrinolysis, has the capacity to liberate kinins from their precursors and probably to activate kallikrein, which brings about the formation of plasmin from plasminogen.
4. The *complement system* consists of at least nine discrete protein substances. Complement achieves its effect through a cascade of the separate components working in special sequences (Fig. 1.2).

    At least two pathways exist for the activation of the complement system. The classic pathway is activated by immune complexes of the immunoglobulin M (IgM; macroglobulin) or IgG type. Another pathway is activated by aggregates of IgA, polysaccharides, lipopolysaccharides, or cell-bound IgG. The biologic functions of the complement components include histamine release, facilitation of phagocytosis of foreign protein, generation of anaphylatoxins (which leads to vasodilatation), immune adherence or fixation of an organism to a cell surface, polymorphonuclear leukocyte (PMN) chemotaxis, and lysis of bacteria, red cells, and so forth. Complement, therefore, plays a key role in the inflammatory process.

5. *Prostaglandins*, which have both inflammatory and anti-inflammatory effects, are 20-carbon, cyclical, unsaturated fatty acids with a 5-carbon ring and 2 aliphatic side chains.
6. *Major histocompatibility complex (MHC)*, called the *human leukocyte antigen (HLA) complex* in humans, is critical to the immune response.
    a. HLAs are present on most nucleated cells of the body.

    The HLA region is on autosomal chromosome 6. In practice, the blood lymphocytes are the cells tested for HLA.

    b. The five genetic loci belonging to HLA are designated by letters following HLA. Thus, HLA-A and HLA-B indicate loci A and B, and so forth (HLA-C, HLA-D, and HLA-DR).
    c. Individual alleles of each locus (and the corresponding specificities) are designated by numbers following the locus letter; thus HLA-B 35 indicates allele 35 on locus B.
    d. A tentatively identified specificity carries the additional letter "W" (workshop) and is inserted between the locus letter and the allele number, e.g., HLA-BW 15.
    e. The HLA system is the main human leukocyte isoantigen system and the major human histocompatibility system.

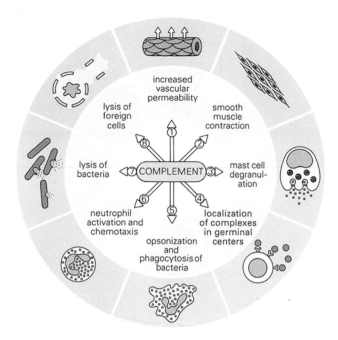

Fig. 1.2 Summary of the actions of complement and its role in the acute inflammatory reaction. Note how the elements of the reaction are induced: increased vascular permeability (1) due to the action of C3a and C5a on smooth muscle (2) and mast cells (3) allows exudation of plasma protein. C3 facilitates both the localization of complexes in germinal centers (4) and the opsonization and phagocytosis of bacteria (5). Neutrophils, which are attracted to the area of inflammation by chemotaxis (6), phagocytose the opsonized micro-organisms. The membrane attack complex, C5–9, is responsible for the lysis of bacteria (7) and other cells recognized as foreign (8). (Adapted with permission from Roitt IM, Brostoff J, Male DK: *Immunology*, 2nd edn. London, Gower Medical. Copyright Elsevier 1989.)

1) HLA-B 27 is positive in a high percentage of young women who have acute anterior uveitis and in young men who have ankylosing spondylitis or Reiter's disease.
2) HLA-B 5 is positive in a high percentage of patients who have Behçet's disease.
3) Factors (mainly unknown) other than HLA play an important role in the pathogenesis of ocular inflammation.

7. *Nonspecific soluble mediators* of the immune system include cytokines, such as interleukins, which are mediators that act between leukocytes, interferons (IFNs), colony-stimulating factors (CSFs), tumor necrosis factor (TNF), transforming growth factor-β, and lymphokines (produced by lymphocytes).
   a. The TNF ligand family encompasses a large group of secreted and cell surface proteins (e.g., TNF and lymphotoxin-α and -β) that may affect the regulation of inflammatory and immune responses.

Both are homotrimers and are soluble products of activated lymphocytes (e.g., CD4+ type 1 T-helper cells,

CD8+ lymphocytes, and certain B lymphoblastoid and monocytoid cell lines.

   b. The actions of the TNF ligand family are somewhat of a mixed blessing in that they can protect against infection, but they can also induce shock and inflammatory disease.
C. Immediately after an injury, the arterioles briefly contract (for approximately 5 minutes), and then gradually relax and dilate because of the chemical mediators discussed earlier and from antidromic axon reflexes.

After the transient arteriolar constriction terminates, blood flow increases above the normal rate for a variable time (up to a few hours), but then diminishes to below normal (or ceases) even though the vessels are still dilated. Part of the decrease in flow is caused by increased viscosity from fluid loss through the capillary and venular wall. The release of heparin by mast cells during this period probably helps to prevent widespread coagulation in the hyperviscous intravascular blood.

D. During the early period after injury, the leukocytes (predominantly the PMNs) stick to the vessel walls, at first momentarily, but then for a more prolonged time; this is an active process called margination (see Fig 1.1C).
   1. Ameboid activity then moves the PMNs through the vessel wall (intercellular passage) and through the endothelial cell junctions (usually taking 2 to 12 minutes); this is an active process called *emigration*.
   2. PMNs, small lymphocytes, macrophages, and immature erythrocytes may also pass actively across endothelium through an intracellular passage in a process called *emperipolesis*.
   3. Mature erythrocytes escape into the surrounding tissue, pushed out of the blood vessels through openings between the endothelial cells in a passive process called *diapedesis*.
E. *Chemotaxis*, a positive unidirectional response to a chemical gradient by inflammatory cells, may be initiated by lysosomal enzymes released by the complement system, thrombin, or the kinins.
   1. A family of low-molecular-weight proteins, the chemokines, may help control leukocyte chemotaxis.
   2. MIP-1α, a member of the β chemokine subfamily, induces chemotaxis of monocytes, CD8+ T cells, CD4+ T cells, and B cells *in vitro*, and is an important mediator of virus-induced inflammation *in vivo*.
   3. RANTES ("regulated on activation, normal T cell expressed and secreted") is a potent chemoattractant chemokine (cytokine) for monocytes and T cells of the memory phenotype.
   4. Mature erythrocytes escape into the surrounding tissue, pushed out of the blood vessels through openings between the endothelial cells in a passive process called *diapedesis*.

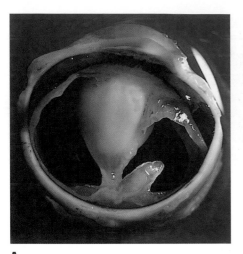

A

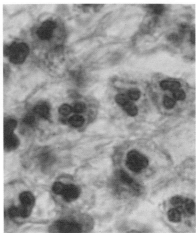

B

C

Fig. 1.3 Polymorphonuclear leukocyte (PMN). **A,** Macroscopic appearance of abscess, that is, a localized collection of pus (purulent exudate), in vitreous body. **B,** PMNs are recognized in abscesses by their segmented (usually three parts or trilobed) nucleus. **C,** Electron micrograph shows segmented nucleus of typical PMN, and its cytoplasmic spherical and oval granules (storage granules or primary lysosomes).

F. PMNs (neutrophils; Fig. 1.3) are the main inflammatory cells in the acute phase of inflammation.

> All blood cells originate from a small, common pool of multipotential hematopoietic stem cells. Regulation of the hematopoiesis requires locally specialized bone marrow stromal cells and a co-ordinated activity of a group of regulatory molecules—growth factors consisting of four distinct regulators known collectively as CSFs.

1. PMNs are born in the bone marrow and are considered "the first line of cellular defense."
2. CSFs (glycoproteins that have a variable content of carbohydrate and a molecular mass of 18 to 90 kD) control the production, maturation, and function of PMNs, macrophages, and eosinophils mainly, but also of megakaryocytes and dendritic cells.

> Interleukin-8 (IL-8) induces PMN shape change, chemotaxis, granule release, and respiratory burst by binding to receptors of the seven transmembrane segment class. The oxidative bursts of human PMNs, which are critical to the inflammatory response, are mediated by a multicomponent nicotinamide-adenine dinucleotide phosphate hydrogenase (NADPH) oxidase regulated by the small guanosine triphosphatase (GTPase) Rac2.

3. PMNs are the most numerous of the circulating leukocytes, making up 50% to 70% of the total.
4. PMNs function at an alkaline pH and are drawn to a particular area by chemotaxis (e.g., by neutrophilic chemotactic factor produced by human endothelial cells).
5. The PMNs remove noxious material and bacteria by phagocytosis and lysosomal digestion (e.g., by

lysozyme, superoxide anion, *N*-chloramines, alkaline phosphatase, collagenase, and acyloxyacyl hydrolysis).

> PMNs produce highly reactive metabolites, including hydrogen peroxide, which is metabolized to hypochlorous acid and then to chlorine, chloramines, and hydroxyl radicals, all important in killing microbes. Lysosomes are saclike cytoplasmic structures containing digestive enzymes and other polypeptides. Lysosomal dysfunction or lack of function has been associated with numerous heritable storage diseases: Pompe's disease (glycogen storage disease type 2) has been traced to a lack of the enzymes α-1,4-glucosidase in liver lysosomes (see p. 454 in Chapter 11); Gaucher's disease is caused by a deficiency of the lysosomal enzyme β-glucosidase (see p. 454, Table 11.5, in Chapter 11). Metachromatic leukodystrophy is caused by a deficiency of the lysosomal enzyme arylsulfatase-A (see p. 454, Table 11.5, in Chapter 11). Most of the common acid mucopolysaccharide, lipid, or polysaccharide storage diseases are caused by a deficiency of a lysosomal enzyme specific for the disease (see under appropriate diseases in Chapters 8 and 11). Chédiak–Higashi syndrome may be considered a general disorder of organelle formation (see section on congenital anomalies in Chapter 11) with abnormally large and fragile leukocyte lysosomes.

6. PMNs are end cells; they die after a few days and liberate proteolytic enzymes, which produce tissue necrosis.

G. Eosinophils and mast cells (basophils) may be involved in the acute phase of inflammation.

1. Eosinophils (Fig. 1.4) originate in bone marrow, constitute 1% to 2% of circulating leukocytes, increase in number in parasitic infestations and

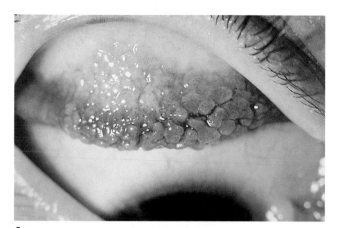

A

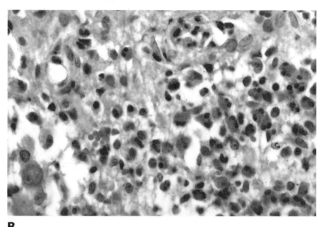

B

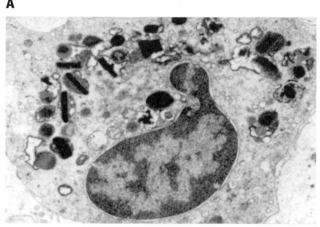

C

Fig. 1.4 A, Eosinophils are commonly seen in allergic conditions like this case of vernal catarrh. **B,** Eosinophils are characterized by bilobed nucleus and granular, pink cytoplasm. **C,** Electron micrograph shows segmentation of nucleus and dense cytoplasmic crystalloids in many cytoplasmic storage granules. Some granules appear degraded.

allergic reactions, and decrease in number after steroid administration or stress. They elaborate toxic lysosomal components (e.g., eosinophil peroxidase) and generate reactive oxygen metabolites.

2. Mast cells (basophils; Fig. 1.5) elaborate heparin, serotonin, and histamine, and are imperative for the initiation of the acute inflammatory reaction.

> Except for location, mast cells appear identical to basophils; mast cells are fixed-tissue cells, whereas basophils constitute approximately 1% of circulating leukocytes. Basophils are usually recognized by the presence of a segmented nucleus, whereas the nucleus of a mast cell is large and nonsegmented.

H. The acute phase is an exudative* phase (i.e., an outpouring of cells and fluid from the circulation) in which the nature of the exudate often determines and characterizes an acute inflammatory reaction.

1. Serous exudate is primarily composed of protein (e.g., seen clinically in the aqueous "flare" in the anterior chamber or under the neural retina in a rhegmatogenous neural retinal detachment).

2. Fibrinous exudate (Fig. 1.6) has high fibrin content (e.g., as seen clinically in a "plastic" aqueous).

3. Purulent exudate (see Figs 1.1 and 1.3) is composed primarily of PMNs and necrotic products (e.g., as seen in a hypopyon).

> The term "pus" as commonly used is synonymous with a purulent exudate.

4. Sanguineous exudate is composed primarily of erythrocytes (e.g., as in a hyphema).

II. Subacute (intermediate or reactive countershock and adaptive) phase.†

A. The subacute phase varies greatly and is concerned with healing and restoration of normal homeostasis (formation of granulation tissue and healing) or with the exhaustion of local defenses, resulting in necrosis, recurrence, or chronicity.

---

*Exudation implies the passage of protein-containing fluid (and cells) through the opened endothelial vascular junctions into the surrounding tissue (inflammatory exudate). Transudation implies the passage of fluid through an intact vessel wall into the surrounding tissue so that its protein content is low or nil (aqueous fluid).

†Although the immune reaction is described separately in this chapter, it is intimately related to inflammation, especially to this phase. Many of the processes described under the section on inflammation are a direct result of the immune process.

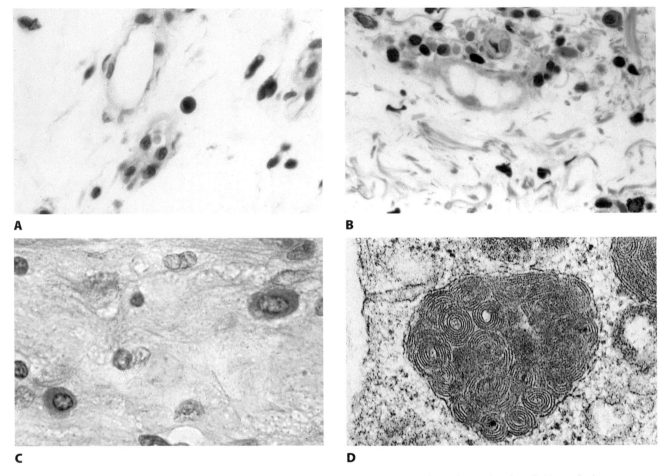

Fig. 1.5 A, Mast cell seen in center as round cell that contains slightly basophilic cytoplasm and round to oval nucleus. **B,** Mast cells shows metachromasia (purple) with toluidine blue (upper right and left and lower right) and **C,** positive (blue) staining for acid mucopolysaccharides with Alcian blue. **D,** Electron microscopy of granules in cytoplasm of mast cell often shows typical scroll appearance.

B. PMNs at the site of injury release lysosomal enzymes into the area.
  1. The enzymes directly increase capillary permeability and cause tissue destruction.
  2. Indirectly, they increase inflammation by stimulating mast cells to release histamine, by activating the kinin-generating system, and by inducing the chemotaxis of mononuclear (MN) phagocytes.

C. MN cells (Fig. 1.7) include lymphocytes and circulating monocytes.
  1. Monocytes constitute 3% to 7% of circulating leukocytes, are bone marrow-derived, and are the progenitor of a family of cells (monocyte–histiocyte–macrophage family) that have the same fundamental characteristics, including cell surface receptors for complement and the Fc portion of immunoglobulin, intracellular lysosomes, and specific enzymes; production of monokines; and phagocytic capacity.
  2. Circulating monocytes may subsequently become tissue residents and change into tissue histiocytes, macrophages, epithelioid histiocytes, and inflammatory giant cells.

  3. CSFs (glycoproteins that have a variable content of carbohydrate and a molecular mass of 18 to 90 kD) control the production, maturation, and function of MN cells.
  4. These cells are the "second line of cellular defense," arrive after the PMN, and depend on release of chemotactic factors by the PMN for their arrival.
    a. Once present, MN cells can live for weeks, and in some cases even months.
    b. MN cells cause much less tissue damage than do PMNs, are more efficient phagocytes, and produce IL-1, formerly called *lymphocyte-activating factor*.
  5. Monocytes have an enormous phagocytic capacity and are usually named for the phagocytosed material [e.g., blood-filled macrophages (erythrophagocytosis), lipid-laden macrophages (Fig. 1.8), lens-filled macrophages (as in phacolytic glaucoma), and so forth].

D. Lysosmal enzymes, including collagenase, are released by PMNs, MN cells, and other cells (e.g., epithelial cells and keratocytes in corneal ulcers) and result in considerable tissue destruction.

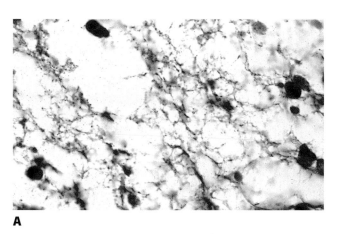

Fig. 1.6 A, Cobweb appearances of fibrinous exudate, stained with periodic acid–Schiff. Cells use fibrin as scaffold to move and to lay down reparative materials. **B,** Electron micrograph shows periodicity of fibrin cut in longitudinal section. **C,** Fibrin cut in cross-section.

A

B   **C**

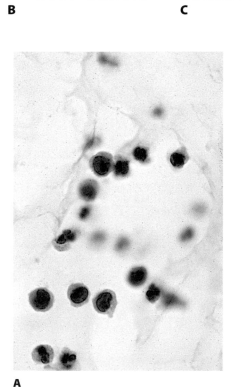

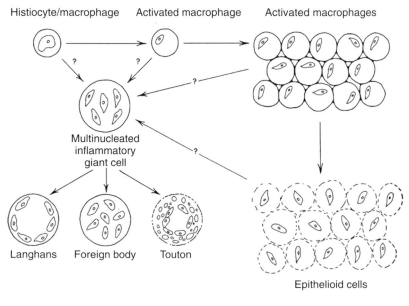

A   **B**

Fig. 1.7 A, Monocytes have lobulated, large, vesicular nuclei and moderate amounts of cytoplasm, and are larger than the segmented polymorphonuclear leukocytes and the lymphocytes, which have round nuclei and scant cytoplasm. **B,** Possible origins of multinucleated inflammatory giant cells and of epithelioid cells.

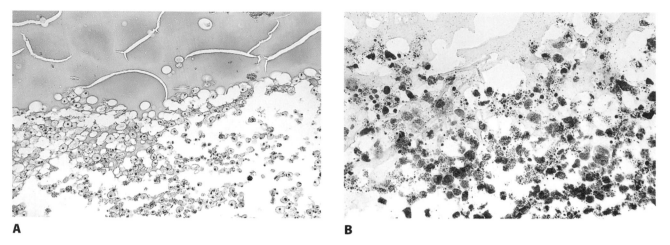

Fig. 1.8 A, Foamy and clear lipid-laden macrophages in subneural retinal space. **B,** Cytoplasm of macrophages stains positively for fat with oil red-O technique.

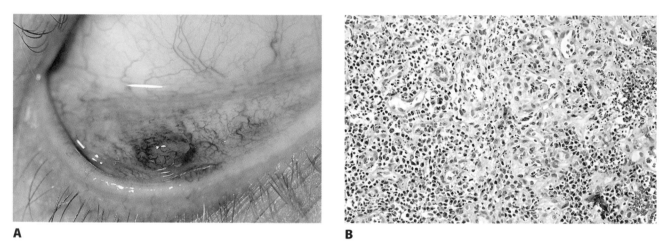

Fig. 1.9 Granulation tissue. **A,** Pyogenic granuloma, here in region of healing chalazion, is composed of granulation tissue. **B,** Three components of granulation tissue are capillaries, fibroblasts, and leukocytes.

In chronic inflammation, the major degradation of collagen may be caused by collagenase produced by lymphokine-activated macrophages.

E. If the area of injury is tiny, PMNs and MN cells alone can handle and "clean up" the area with resultant healing.

F. In larger injuries, *granulation tissue* is produced.

1. Granulation tissue (Fig. 1.9) is composed of leukocytes, proliferating blood vessels, and fibroblasts.

2. MN cells arrive after PMNs, followed by an ingrowth of capillaries that proliferate from the endothelium of pre-existing blood vessels.

The new blood vessels tend to leak fluid and leukocytes, especially PMNs.

---

3. Fibroblasts (see Fig. 1.9), which arise from fibrocytes and possibly from other cells (monocytes), proliferate, lay down collagen (Table 1.1), and elaborate ground substance.

4. With time, the blood vessels involute and disappear, the leukocytes disappear, and the fibroblasts return to their resting state (fibrocytes). This involutionary process results in shrinkage of the collagenous scar and a reorientation of the remaining cells into a parallel arrangement along the long axis of the scar.

5. If the noxious agent persists, the condition may not heal as described previously, but instead may become chronic.

6. If the noxious agent that caused the inflammation is immunogenic, a similar agent introduced at a future date can start the cycle anew (recurrence).

III. Chronic phase

A. The chronic phase results from a breakdown in the preceding two phases, or it may start initially as a chronic inflammation (e.g., when the resistance of the body and the inroads of an infecting agent, such as

TABLE 1.1 Heterogeneity of Collagens in the Cornea*

Type	Polypeptides	Monomer	Polymer
I	$[\alpha 1(I)]_2\alpha 2(I)$		
II	$[\alpha 1(II)]_3$		
III	$[\alpha 1(III)]_3$		
IV	$[\alpha 1(IV)]_2\alpha 2(IV)$		
V	$[\alpha 1(V)]_2\alpha 2(V)$		
VI	$[\alpha 1(VI)]_2\alpha 2(VI)\alpha 3(VI)$		
VII	$[\alpha 1(VII)]_3$?		
VIII	$[\alpha 1(VIII)]_2\alpha 2(VIII)$?		
IX	$[\alpha 1(IX)]_2\alpha 2(IX)\alpha 3(IX)$		
XII	$[\alpha 1(XII)]_3$		

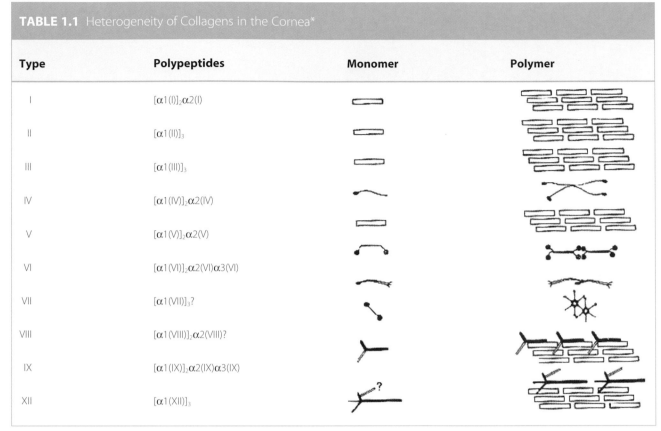

*At least 10 genetically distinct collagens have been described in the corneas of different animal species, ages, and pathologies. Types I, II, III, and V collagens are present as fibrils in tissues. Types IV, VI, VII, and VIII form filamentous structures. Types IX and XII are fibril-associated collagens. The sizes of the structures are not completely known. Type II collagen is only found in embryonic chick collagen associated with the primary stroma. Type III collagen is found in Descemet's membrane and in scar tissue. Types I and V form the heterotypic fibrils of lamellar stroma. Type VII has been identified with the anchoring fibrils, and type VIII is only present in Descemet's membrane. Type IX collagen, associated with type II fibrils in the primary stroma, and type XII collagen, associated with type I/V fibrils, are part of a family of fibril-associated collagens with interrupted triple helices. Both type IX and XII are covalently associated with a chondroitin sulfate chain.

(Reproduced from Cintron C: In Podos SM, Yanoff M, eds: Textbook of Ophthalmology, vol. 8. London, Mosby. Copyright Elsevier 1994.)

the organisms of tuberculosis or syphilis, nearly balance; or in conditions of unknown cause such as sarcoidosis).

B. *Chronic nongranulomatous inflammation* is a proliferative inflammation characterized by a cellular infiltrate of lymphocytes and plasma cells (and sometimes PMNs or eosinophils).

  1. The lymphocyte (Fig. 1.10) constitutes 15% to 30% of circulating leukocytes and represents the competent immunocyte.

    a. All lymphocytes probably have a common stem cell origin (perhaps in the bone marrow) from which they populate the lymphoid organs: the thymus, spleen, and lymph nodes.

    b. Two principal types of lymphocytes are recognized: (1) the bone marrow-dependent (or bursal equivalent) B lymphocyte is active in humoral immunity, is the source of immunoglobulin production (Fig. 1.11), and is identified by the presence of immunoglobulin on its surface; (2) the thymus-dependent T lymphocyte participates in cellular immunity, produces a variety of lymphokines, and is identified by various surface antigens (e.g., the antigen common to T cells, T3, and well as T4, T8, and particularly the antigen representing the erythrocyte-rosette receptor, T11).

  1) Helper-inducer T lymphocytes (T4-positive) initiate the immune response in conjunction with macrophages and interact with (helper) B lymphocytes.

T-helper 1 (T_H1) and T-helper 2 (T_H2) cells secrete a distinctive suite of cytokines: T_H1 produces predominantly cell-mediated immunity (e.g., cytotoxic T-cell response); T_H2 produces particular classes of immunoglobulin antibodies. For CD4 T cells to be activated, they need to receive signals from mature dendritic cells in peripherals lymphoid organize. T_H1 immunity protects against intracellular

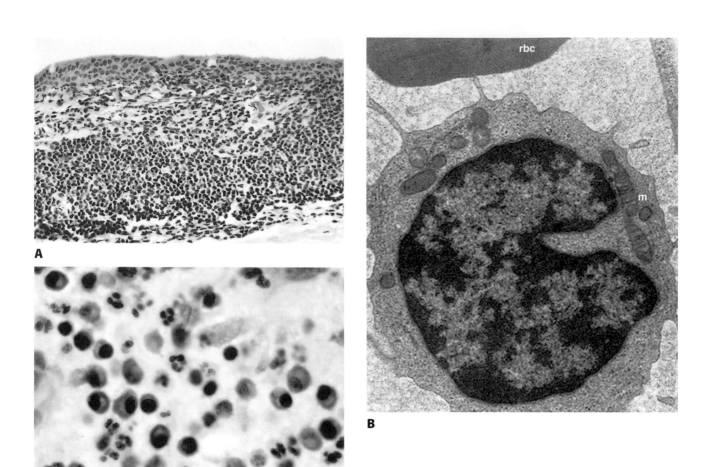

Fig. 1.10 Lymphocyte. **A,** Low magnification shows cluster of many lymphocytes appearing as a deep blue infiltrate. Cluster appears blue because cytoplasm is scant and mostly nuclei are seen. **B,** Electron micrograph shows lymphocyte nucleus surrounded by small cytoplasmic ring containing several mitochondria (m), diffusely arrayed ribonucleoprotein particles, and many surface protrusions or microvilli (rbc, red blood cell).
C, Lymphocytes seen as small, dark nuclei with relatively little cytoplasm. Compare with polymorphonuclear leukocytes (segmented nuclei) and with larger plasma cells (eccentric nucleus surrounded by halo and basophilic cytoplasm).

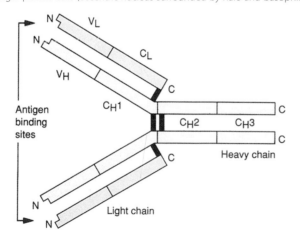

Fig. 1.11 The basic immunoglobulin structure. The unit consists of two identical light polypeptide chains linked together by disulfide bonds (black). The amino-terminal end (N) of each chain is characterized by sequence variability (V_L, V_H), whereas the remainder of the molecule has a relatively constant structure (C_L, C_H^1–C_H^3). The antigen-binding sites are located at the N-terminal end. (Adapted with permission from Roitt IM, Brostoff J, Male DK: *Immunology*, 2nd edn. London, Gower Medical. Copyright Elsevier 1989.)

parasites (e.g., *Leishmania*), and T_H2 immunity protects against extracellular parasites (e.g., nemotodes).

2) Suppressor-cytotoxic T lymphocytes (T8-positive) suppress the immune response and are capable of killing target cells (e.g., cancer cells) through cell-mediated cytotoxicity.

2. The plasma cell (Fig. 1.12) is produced by the bone marrow-derived B lymphocyte, elaborates immunoglobulins (antibodies), and occurs in certain modified forms in tissue sections.

After germinal center B cells undergo somatic mutation and antigen selection, they become either memory B cells or plasma cells. CD40 ligand directs the differentiation of germinal center B cells toward memory B cells rather than toward plasma cells.

a. *Plasmacytoid cell* (Fig. 1.13A and B): this has a single eccentric nucleus and slightly eosinophilic granular cytoplasm (instead of the normal basophilic cytoplasm of the plasma cell).

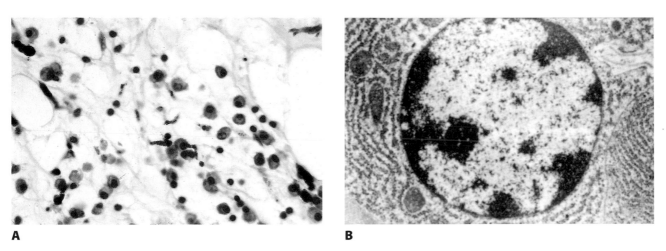

A　　　　　　　　　　　　　　　　　　　　　**B**

Fig. 1.12 Plasma cell. **A,** Plasma cells are identified by eccentrically located nucleus containing clumped chromatin and perinuclear halo in basophilic cytoplasm that attenuates opposite to nucleus. Plasma cells are larger than small lymphocytes, which contain deep blue nuclei and scant cytoplasm. **B,** Electron microscopy shows exceedingly prominent granular endoplasmic reticulum that accounts for cytoplasmic basophilia and surrounds nucleus. Mitochondria are also present in cytoplasm.

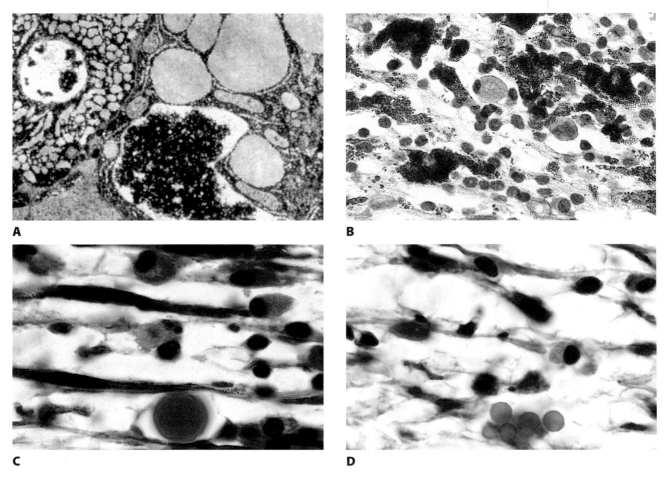

A　　　　　　　　　　　　　　　　　　　　　**B**

C　　　　　　　　　　　　　　　　　　　　　**D**

Fig. 1.13 Altered plasma cells. **A,** Electron micrograph shows that left plasmacytoid cell contains many small pockets of inspissated material (γ-globulin) in segments of rough endoplasmic reticulum; right cell contains large globules (γ-globulin), which would appear eosinophilic in light microscopy. **B,** Plasmacytoid cell in center has eosinophilic (instead of basophilic) cytoplasm that contains tiny pink globules (γ-globulin). **C,** Russell body appears as large anuclear sphere or **D,** multiple anuclear spheres.

b. *Russell body* (see Fig. 1.13C and D): this is an inclusion in a plasma cell whose cytoplasm is filled and enlarged with either eosinophilic grapelike clusters (morular form), with single eosinophilic globular structures, or with eosinophilic crystalline structures; usually the nucleus appears as an eccentric rim or has disappeared.

The eosinophilic material in plasmacytoid cells and in Russell bodies appears to be immunoglobulin that has become inspissated, as if the plasmacytoid cells can no longer release the material because of defective transport by the cells ("constipated" plasmacytoid cells). In addition, as has been shown in Russell bodies in B-cell lymphoma cells, other glycoprotein accumulations may be found (e.g., CD5, CD19, CD22, CD25, and Leu 8).

C. *Chronic granulomatous inflammation* is a proliferative inflammation characterized by a cellular infiltrate of lymphocytes and plasma cells (and sometimes PMNs or eosinophils).
1. Epithelioid cells (epithelioid histiocytes, Fig. 1.14) are bone marrow-derived cells in the monocyte–histiocyte–macrophage family (Fig. 1.15)
   a. In particular, epithelioid cells are tissue monocytes that have abundant eosinophilic cytoplasm, somewhat resembling epithelial cells.
   b. They are often found oriented around necrosis as large polygonal cells that contain pale nuclei

and abundant eosinophilic cytoplasm whose borders blend imperceptibly with those of their neighbors in a pseudosyncytium ("palisading" histiocytes in a granuloma).
c. All cells of this family interact with T lymphocytes, are capable of phagocytosis, and are identified by the presence of surface receptors for complement and the Fc portion of immunoglobulin.

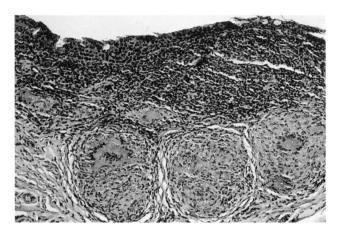

Fig. 1.14 Epithelioid cells in conjunctival, sarcoidal granuloma, here forming three nodules, which are identified by eosinophilic color resembling epithelium. Giant cells, simulating Langhans' giant cells, are seen in nodules.

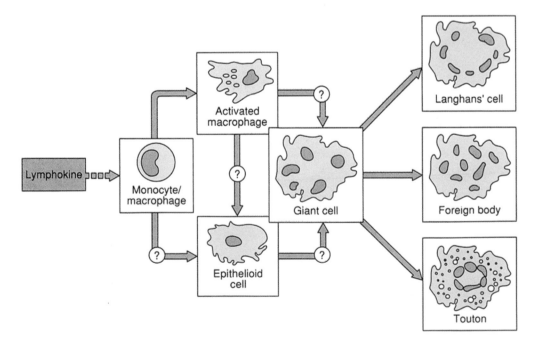

Fig. 1.15 Proposed scheme for the terminal differentiation of cells of the monocyte/macrophage system. The pathologic changes result from the inability of the macrophage to deal effectively with the pathogen. Lymphokines from active T cells induce monocytes and macrophages to become activated macrophages. Where prolonged antigenic stimulation exists, activated macrophages may differentiate into epithelioid cells and then into giant cells *in vivo*, in granulomatous tissue. The multinucleated giant cell may be derived from the fusion of several epithelioid cells. (Adapted with permission from Roitt IM, Brostoff J, Male DK: *Immunology*, 2nd edn. London, Gower Medical. Copyright Elsevier 1989.)

2. Inflammatory giant cells, probably formed by fusion of macrophages rather than by amitotic division, predominate in three forms:

a. *Langhans' giant cell* (Fig. 1.16; see Fig. 1.14): this is typically found in tuberculosis, but is also seen in many other granulomatous processes. When sectioned through its center, it shows a perfectly homogeneous, eosinophilic, central cytoplasm with a peripheral rim of nuclei.

> It is important to note that the central cytoplasm is perfectly homogeneous. If it is not, foreign material such as fungi may be present: the cell is then not a Langhans' giant cell but a foreign-body giant cell. When a Langhans' giant cell is sectioned through its periphery, it simulates a foreign-body giant cell.

b. *Foreign-body giant cell* (Fig. 1.17): this has its nuclei randomly distributed in its eosinophilic cytoplasm and contains foreign material.

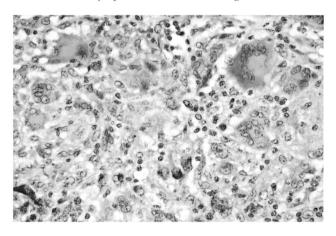

Fig. 1.16 Langhans' giant cells have homogeneous central cytoplasm surrounded by rim of nuclei.

c. *Touton giant cell* (Fig. 1.18): this is frequently associated with lipid disorders such as juvenile xanthogranuloma; it appears much like a Langhans' giant cell with the addition of a rim of foamy (fat-positive) cytoplasm peripheral to the rim of nuclei.

3. Three patterns of inflammatory reaction may be found in granulomatous inflammations:

a. *Diffuse type* (Fig. 1.19A): this typically occurs in sympathetic uveitis, disseminated histoplasmosis and other fungal infections, lepromatous leprosy, juvenile xanthogranuloma, Vogt–Koyanagi–Harada syndrome, cytomegalic inclusion disease, and toxoplasmosis. The epithelioid cells (sometimes with macrophages or inflammatory giant cells, or both) are distributed randomly against a background of lymphocytes and plasma cells.

b. *Discrete type* (sarcoidal or tuberculocidal; see Fig. 1.19B): this typically occurs in sarcoidosis, tuberculoid leprosy, and miliary tuberculosis. An accumulation of epithelioid cells (sometimes with inflammatory giant cells) forms nodules (tubercles) surrounded by a narrow rim of lymphocytes (and perhaps plasma cells).

c. *Zonal type* (see Fig 1.19C): this occurs in caseation tuberculosis, some fungal infections, rheumatoid scleritis, chalazion, phacoanaphylactic (phacoimmune) endophthalmitis, toxocara endophthalmitis, and cysticercosis.

   1) A central nidus (e.g., necrosis, lens, foreign body) is surrounded by palisaded epithelioid cells (sometimes with PMNs, inflammatory giant cells, and macrophages) that in turn are surrounded by lymphocytes and plasma cells.

   2) Granulation tissue often envelops the entire inflammatory reaction.

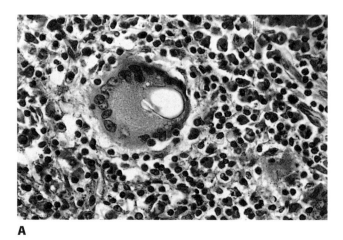

A

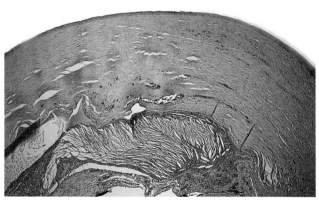

B

Fig. 1.17 A, Foreign-body giant cell (FBGC) simulating Langhans' giant cells, except that homogeneous cytoplasm is interrupted by large, circular foreign material. **B,** Anterior-chamber FBGCs, here surrounding clear clefts where cholesterol had been, have nuclei randomly distributed in cytoplasm.

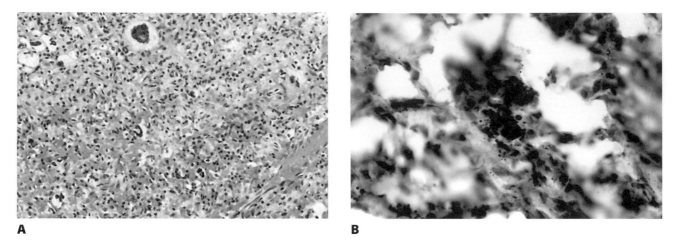

Fig. 1.18 A, Touton giant cells in juvenile xanthogranuloma closely resemble Langhans' giant cells except for the addition of peripheral rim of foamy (fat-positive) cytoplasm in the former. **B,** Increased magnification showing fat positivity of peripheral cytoplasm with oil red-O technique. (Case presented by Dr. M Yanoff to the Eastern Ophthalmic Pathology Society, 1993, and reported in *Arch Ophthalmol* 113:915, 1995.)

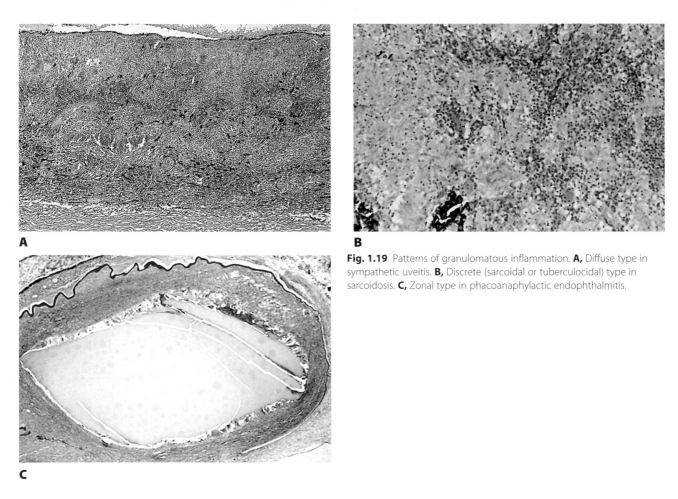

Fig. 1.19 Patterns of granulomatous inflammation. **A,** Diffuse type in sympathetic uveitis. **B,** Discrete (sarcoidal or tuberculocidal) type in sarcoidosis. **C,** Zonal type in phacoanaphylactic endophthalmitis.

Staining Patterns of Inflammation

I. Patterns of inflammation are best observed microscopically under the lowest (scanning) power.

II. With the hematoxylin and eosin (H&E) stain, an infiltrate of deep blue (basophilia) usually represents a chronic non-granulomatous inflammation. The basophilia is produced by lymphocytes that have blue nuclei with practically no cytoplasm, and by plasma cells that have blue nuclei and blue cytoplasm.

III. A deep blue infiltrate with scattered gray (pale pink) areas ("pepper and salt") usually represents a chronic

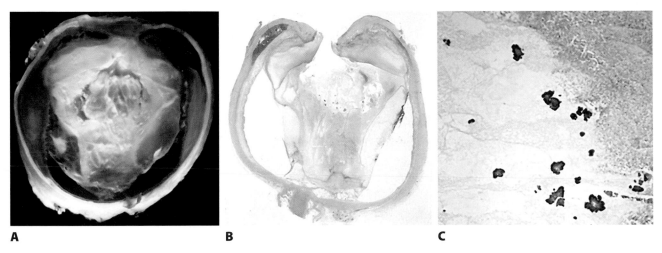

Fig. 1.20 Staining patterns of inflammation. **A,** Macroscopic appearance of diffuse vitreous abscess. **B,** Diffuse abscess, here filling vitreous, characteristic of bacterial infection. **C,** Special stain shows Gram-positivity of bacterial colonies in this vitreous abscess.

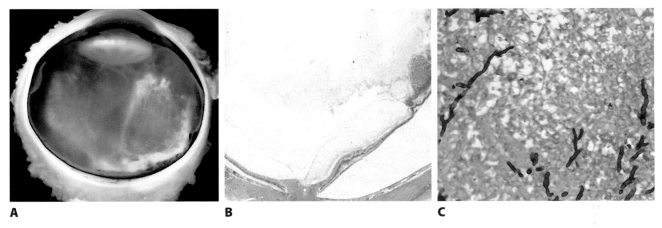

Fig. 1.21 Staining patterns of inflammation. **A,** Macroscopic appearance of multiple vitreous microabscesses, characteristic of fungal infection. **B,** One vitreous microabscess contiguous with detached retina. **C,** Septate fungal mycelia (presumably *Aspergillus*) from same case stained with Gomori's methenamine silver.

granulomatous inflammation, with the blue areas lymphocytes and plasma cells, and the gray areas islands of epithelioid cells.

IV. A "dirty" gray infiltrate usually represents a purulent reaction with PMNs and necrotic material.

    A. If the infiltrate is diffuse [Fig. 1.20; e.g., filling the vitreous (vitreous abscess)], the cause is probably bacterial.

    B. If the infiltrate is localized into two or more small areas (Fig. 1.21; i.e., multiple abscesses or microabscesses), the cause is probably fungal.

IMMUNOBIOLOGY

Background

I. Many reactions in cellular immunity are mediated by lymphocyte-derived soluble factors known collectively as *lymphokines*, which exert profound effects on inflammatory cells such as monocytes, neutrophils, and lymphocytes themselves. Such action falls into three main categories: (1) effects on cell motility (migration inhibition, chemotaxis, and chemokinesis); (2) effects on cell proliferation or cellular viability; and (3) effects on cellular activation for specific specialized functions.

The immune system provides the body with a mechanism to distinguish "self" from "nonself." The distinction, made after a complex, elaborate process, ultimately relies on receptors on the only immunologically specific cells of the immune system, the B and T lymphocytes.

II. All lymphocytes in mammalian lymph nodes and spleen have a remote origin in the bone marrow: those that have undergone an intermediate cycle of proliferation in the thymus (thymus-dependent, or T lymphocytes) mediate cellular immunity, whereas those that seed directly into lymphoid tissue (thymus-independent, or B lymphocytes) provide the precursors of cells that produce circulating antibodies.

The Janus family tyrosine kinase, Jak3, is essential for lymphoid development. B and T lymphocytes are quiescent until called on by a specific, unique antigen to proliferate into a clonal population. Once the antigen is eliminated, excess B and T cells are removed by apoptosis (programmed cell death), thereby keeping the total number of B and T cells in correct balance.

A. Thus, mediators of immune responses can be either specifically reactive lymphocytes (*cell-mediated immunity*) or freely diffusible antibody molecules (*humoral immunity*).
B. Antibody-producing B cells or killer T-type cells are only activated when turned on by a specific antigen.

When an antigen (immunogen) penetrates the body, it binds to an antibodylike receptor on the surface of its corresponding lymphocyte that proliferates and generates a clone of differentiated cells. Some of the cells (large B lymphocytes and plasma cells) secrete antibodies, T cells secrete lymphokines, and other lymphocytes circulate through blood, lymph, and tissues as an expanded reservoir of antigen-sensitive (memory) cells. When the immunogen encounters the memory cells months or years later, it evokes a more rapid and copious secondary anamnestic response. Other immune cells (e.g., NK) are less specific and eliminate a variety of infected or cancerous cells.

III. *T lymphocytes* derive from lymphoid stem cells in the bone marrow and mature under the influence of the thymus.

Interactions between immature thymocytes and thymic stromal cells expressing CD81 appear to be required for T-cell development.

A. T lymphocytes are identified by surface antigens (T3, T4, T8, T11).
   1. T lymphocytes are divided into two major subsets that express either CD4 or CD8 protein on their surface.
   2. ZAP-70, a 70-kD cytosolic T-cell tyrosine kinase, is essential for human T-cell function, and $CD4^+$ and $CD8^+$ T cells depend on different signaling pathways to support their development and survival.
B. T lymphocytes are the predominant lymphocytes in the peripheral blood and reside in well-defined interfollicular areas in lymph nodes and spleen.
C. The T-lymphocyte system is responsible for the recognition of antigens on cell surfaces and, thus, monitors self from nonself on live cells (Fig. 1.22).

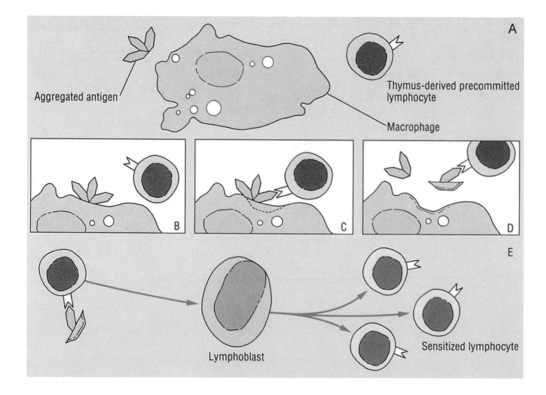

Fig. 1.22 Cellular immunity. **A,** The participants in the cellular immune response include the thymus-derived precommitted lymphocyte (T cell), bone marrow-derived monocyte (macrophage), and the aggregated antigens. **B,** Aggregated antigen is seen attaching to the surface of the macrophage. **C,** The T cell is shown as it attaches to the aggregated antigen. **D,** The substance originating in the macrophage passes into the T cell, which is attached to the antigen. **E,** The combined T-cell, antigen, and macrophagic material causes the T cell to enlarge into a lymphoblast. Sensitized or committed T lymphocytes arise from lymphoblasts. (From Yanoff M, Fine BS: *Ocular Pathology, A Color Atlas*, 2nd edn. New York, Gower Medical. Copyright Elsevier 1992.)

D. The MHC (HLA) allows T cells to recognize foreign antigen in cells and then, aided by macrophages, mobilizes helper T cells to make killer T cells to destroy the antigen-containing cells.

The chemokine RANTES can act as an antigen-independent activator of T cells *in vitro*.

E. T lymphocytes, therefore, initiate cellular immunity (delayed hypersensitivity), are responsible for graft-versus-host reactions, and initiate the reactions of the body against foreign grafts such as skin and kidneys (host-versus-graft reactions).

F. When activated (by an antigen), they liberate lymphokines such as macrophage inhibition factor (MIF), macrophage activation factor (MAF), IFN, and interleukins IL-2 (previously called *T-cell growth factor*), IL-3, and IL15 (Fig. 1.23).

1. Activation of peripheral T cells by an antigen-presenting cell is the result of the engagement of both the T-cell receptor and CD4 or CD8 coreceptors, and of receptor–ligand pairs, such as LFA-1–

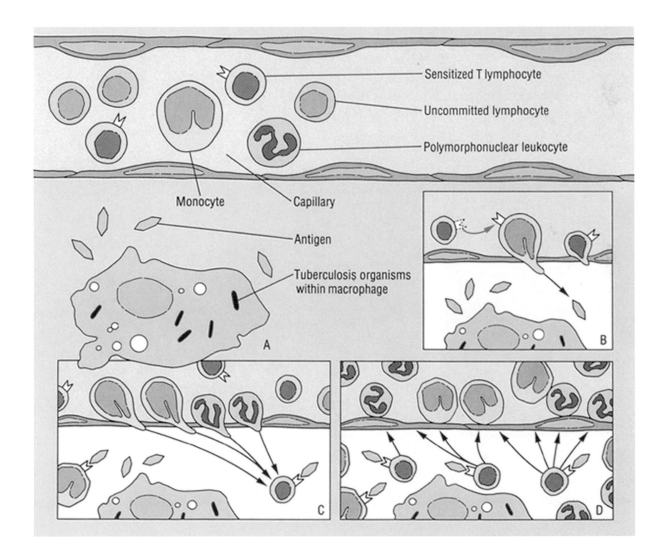

Fig. 1.23 Cellular immunity. **A,** Sensitized T lymphocytes (SL) are seen in a capillary. Along with the SL are other leukocytes, including monocytes, at an antigenic site. A macrophage, which contains tubercle bacilli and antigen may be seen in the surrounding tissue. **B,** Monocytes become sensitized when cytophilic antibody from SL is transferred to them. They migrate toward the antigenic stimulus. **C,** Biologically active molecules, which cause the monocytes and leukocytes to travel to the area, are released by SL when they have encountered a specific antigen. **D,** Monocytes arriving at the site are immobilized by migration inhibitory factor (MIF), which is released by SL, which also release cytotoxin and mitogenic factor. Cytotoxin causes tissue necrosis (caseation), and mitogenic factor causes proliferation of cells. Some of these cells undergo transformation, becoming epithelioid cells, causing the formation of a tuberculoma. (From Yanoff M, Fine BS: *Ocular Pathology, A Color Atlas,* 2nd edn. New York, Gower Medical. Copyright Elsevier 1992).

intracellular adhesion molecule, CD2–CD48, and CD28–CD80.

Cytokine Eta-1 (also called osteopontin), a gene product, may play an important role in the early development of cell-mediated (type 1) immunity.

---

2. When both the CD3 T-cell receptor and the CD28 receptor are occupied by their appropriate ligands, T cells are stimulated to proliferate and produce Il-2, whereas occupation of the T-cell receptor alone favors T-cell anergy or apoptosis.

The proliferation and differentiation of T lymphocytes are regulated by cytokines that act in combination with signals induced by the engagement of the T-cell antigen receptor. A principal cytokine is IL-2, itself a product of activated T cells. IL-2 also stimulates B cells, monocytes, lymphokine-activated killer cells, and glioma cells. Another growth factor that stimulates the proliferation of T lymphocytes, the cytokine IL-15, competes for binding with IL-2 and uses components of the IL-2 receptor. T lymphocytes will not go "into action" against an "enemy" unless they are triggered by several signals at once. When one of the signals needed is lacking, the T cell becomes "paralyzed" (anergy). The cause for the anergy may lie in a block early in the Ras signal pathway. For CD4 T cells to be acti-

vated, they need to receive signals from mature dendritic cells in peripheral lymphoid organs.

G. T lymphocytes also regulate B-cell responses to antigens by direct contact and by the release of diffusible factors that act as short-range stimulators of nearby B cells.

IV. The B *lymphocyte* also arises from lymphoid stem cells in the bone marrow, but is not influenced by the thymus.
   A. It resides in follicular areas in lymphoid organs distinct from the sites of the T lymphocyte.
   B. The B-lymphocyte system is characterized by an enormous variety of immunoglobulins having virtually all conceivable antigenic specificities that are capable of being recognized by at least a few B-lymphocyte clones.

After germinal center B cells undergo somatic mutation and antigen selection, they become either memory B cells or plasma cells. CD40 ligand directs the differentiation of germinal center B cells toward memory B cells rather than toward plasma cells.

   C. The system is well designed to deal with unpredictable and unforeseen microbial and toxic agents.
   D. The B lymphocyte can be stimulated by antigen to enlarge, divide, and differentiate to form antibody-secreting plasma cells (Fig. 1.24).

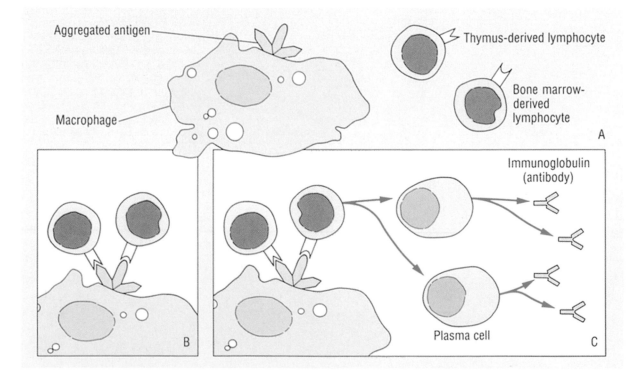

Fig. 1.24 Humoral immunity. **A** and **B,** Four prerequisites for immunoglobulin formation are demonstrated, including thymus-derived lymphocyte (T cell), thymus-independent bone marrow-derived lymphocyte (B cell), bone marrow-derived monocyte (macrophage), and aggregated antigen. In **A,** aggregated antigens are seen attached to macrophages. In **B,** T and B cells are seen attached to different determinants on the aggregated antigen. **C,** Co-operative interaction that occurs between T and B cells causes the B cells to differentiate into plasma cells. (From Yanoff M, Fine BS: *Ocular Pathology, A Color Atlas*, 2nd edn. New York, Gower Medical. Copyright Elsevier 1992.)

Under most circumstances, T lymphocytes collaborate with B lymphocytes during the induction of antibody-forming cells by the latter (see section on humoral immunoglobulin, later).

V. *Null lymphocytes*, which constitute approximately 5% of lymphocytes in peripheral blood, lack the surface markers used to identify T and B lymphocytes.
   A. Most mull cells carry a surface receptor for the Fc portion of the immunoglobulins, can function as killer cells in antibody-dependent cell-mediated cytotoxicity, and are called *NK cells*.
   B. NK cells are probably a separate lineage of cells.
VI. Initially, the sheep red blood cell resetting test (especially with fixed, embedded tissue) and the immunofluorescence or immunoperoxidase techniques that demonstrate surface immunoglobulins were the principal techniques for identification of T or B lymphocytes, respectively.
   A. Now, *monoclonal antibodies* (especially with fresh tissue) are used for the localization of lymphocyte subsets in tissue sections, and their use has revolutionized research in immunology, cell biology, molecular genetics, diagnosis of infectious diseases, tumor diagnosis, drug and hormone assays, and tumor therapy.
   B. A myriad of different types of monoclonal antibodies now exist, and new ones are continuously being created.
   C. Monoclonal antibodies can be obtained against B and T lymphocytes, monocytes, Langerhans' cells, keratins, type IV collagen, retinal proteins (e.g., human s-100), and tumor antigens (e.g., factor VIII, intermediate filaments—cytokeratins, vimentin, desmin, neurofilaments, and glial filaments—neuron-specific enolase, and glial fibrillary acidic protein; all may be found in tumors).

Cellular Immunity (Delayed Hypersensitivity)*

I. Two distinct cell types participate in cellular immunity: the T lymphocyte and the macrophage (histiocyte).
   A. Phagocytic cells of the monocytic line (monocytes, reticuloendothelial cells, macrophages, Langerhans' dendritic cells, epithelioid cells, and inflammatory giant cells—all are different forms of the same cell) are devoid of antibody and immunologic specificity.
      1. Macrophages, however, have the ability to process proteins (antigens) and activate the helper T cells.
      2. Macrophages also secrete proteases, complement proteins, growth-regulating factors (e.g., IL-1), and arachidonate derivatives.
   B. All lymphocytes seem to be precommitted to make only one type of antibody, which is cell-bound.
II. The delayed hypersensitivity reaction begins with perivenous accumulation of sensitized lymphocytes and other MN cells (i.e., monocytes, which constitute 80% to 90% of the cells mobilized to the lesion). The infiltrative lesions enlarge and multiply (e.g., in tuberculosis, where the lesions

*The terms **cellular immunity** and **hypersensitivity** are synonymous.*

take a granulomatous form), and cellular invasion and destruction of tissue occur.
III. Delayed hypersensitivity is involved in transplantation immunity, in the pathogenesis of various autoimmune diseases (e.g., sympathetic uveitis), and in defense against most viral, fungal, protozoal, and some bacterial diseases (e.g., tuberculosis and leprosy). Perhaps the most important role is to act as a natural defense against cancer, i.e., the immunologic rejection of vascularized tumors and immunologic surveillance of neoplastic cells.

Humoral Immunoglobulin (Antibody)

I. Four distinct cell types participate in humoral immunoglobulin (antibody) formation: the T lymphocyte, the B lymphocyte, the monocyte (macrophage), and the plasma cell.
   A. Macrophages process antigen in the early stage of the formation of cellular immunity and secrete IL-1.
   B. Specifically precommitted cells of both the T and B lymphocytes attach to different determinants of the antigen; T cells then secrete a B-cell growth factor (BCGF).
   C. BCGF and IL-1 evoke division of triggered B cells, which then differentiate and proliferate into plasma cells that elaborate specific immunoglobulins. All humoral immunoglobulins (antibodies) are made up of multiple polypeptide chains and are the predominant mediators of immunity in certain types of infection, such as acute bacterial infection (caused by streptococci and pneumococci) and viral diseases (hepatitis).
II. The B lymphocyte, once a specific antigen causes it to become committed (sensitized) to produce an immunoglobulin, makes that immunoglobulin and none other, as does its progeny. It, or its progeny, may produce immunoglobulin or become a resting memory cell to be reactivated at an accelerated rate (anamnestic response) if confronted again by the same antigen.

Immunohistochemistry

I. As stated previously, monoclonal antibodies can be obtained against B and T lymphocytes, monocytes, Langerhans' cells, keratins, type IV collagen, retinal proteins, and so forth (Figs 1.25 and 1.26).
   A. *Keratin* and *epithelial membrane antigen* are markers for epithelia.
   B. *Factor VIII* and Ulex europaeus-1 are markers for vascular endothelia.
   C. *Intermediate filaments*: *vimentin* is a marker for mesenchymal cells, including smooth muscle, Schwann cells, histiocytes, and fibrocytes; *desmin* is a marker for smooth and striated muscles; *cytokeratin* is a marker for epithelia; *neurofilament* is a marker for neurons; and *glial fibrillary acidic protein* is a marker for astrocytes and Schwann cells.
   D. *Neuron-specific enolase* is a marker for Schwann cells, neurons, smooth muscle, and neuroendocrine cells.

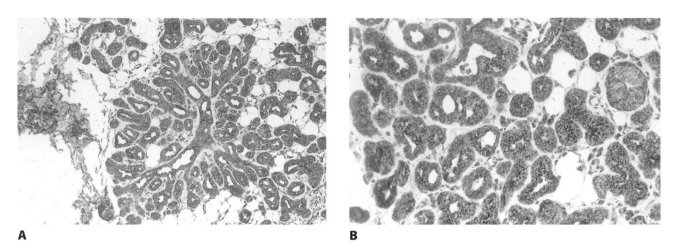

A

B

Fig. 1.25 Immunocytochemistry. **A,** Cathepsin-D, which here stains cytoplasm of conjunctival submucosal glands (shown under increased magnification in **B**), is an excellent stain for lipofuscin.

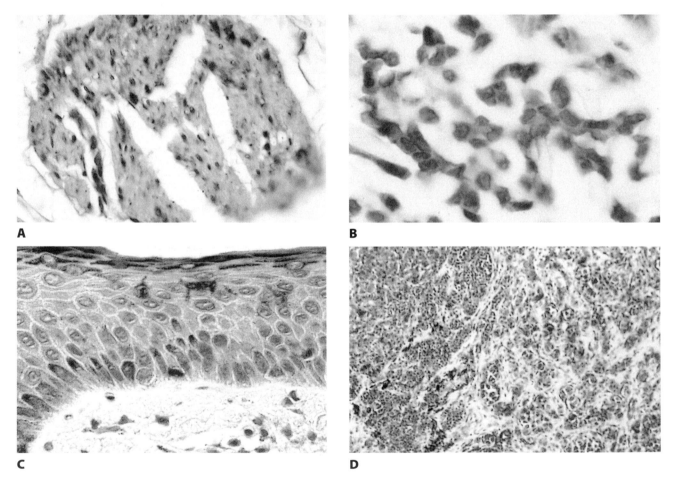

A

B

C

D

Fig. 1.26 Immunocytochemistry. **A,** Monoclonal antibody against desmin, one of the cytoskeletal filaments, reacts with both smooth and striated muscles, and helps to identify tumors of muscular origin. **B,** Monoclonal antibody against λ chains in plasma cells. **C** and **D,** Polyclonal antibody against S-100 protein in melanocytes and Langerhans' cells in epidermis (**C**) and in malignant melanoma cells (**D**). (From Schaumberg-Lever G, Lever WF: *Color Atlas of Pathology of the Skin.* Philadelphia, JB Lippincott, 1988, with permission).

E. *S-100* and *antimelanoma antigen* are markers for melanin-containing and neural tissue.

F. *Muscle actin* is a marker for smooth and striated muscles; *smooth-muscle actin* for smooth muscles.

G. *Ubiquitin* is a marker for lymphocyte-homing receptor.

H. Many antibodies are available for immunophenotyping of lymphomas and leukemias, both on fresh and paraffin-embedded tissue—the following are a few examples:

1. In non-Hodgkin's lymphoma, markers are available to diagnose both B-cell and T-cell lymphomas. In B-cell lymphoma, the determination of surface immunoglobulin light-chain restriction by either immunofluorescence microscopy or flow cytometry is most useful in distinguishing malignant lymphoma from reactive follicular hyperplasia.

Normally, κ light-chain expression is more prevalent and has a normal ratio of 3 to 4:1 over λ light chains. Any marked alteration from the normal ratio is strongly suggestive of malignancy.

---

2. In Hodgkin's lymphoma, CD15 is relatively specific in identifying Reed–Sternberg cells. CD30 and peanut agglutinin are also helpful.

3. In histiocytic proliferations, S-100 stain and peanut agglutinin are useful in identifying histiocytes (e.g., in Langerhans' histiocytosis).

4. In the acute leukemias, CD34 is helpful in the diagnosis. A polyclonal antibody for myeloperoxidase is now available to help diagnose acute myeloblastic leukemia.

5. In the plasma cell disorders κ and λ light-chain markers are most useful in making the diagnosis.

I. Many other markers are available, and new markers seem to appear almost weekly!

1. Useful websites for further information regarding immunohistochemical stains and techniques include the following:

   a. http://www.chemicon.com/resource/ANT101/a2D.asp

   b. http://www.ipox.org/login.cfm?IQMessage=1&RequestTimeout=200

2. Throughout this textbook, appropriate key immunohistochemical markers will be cited where appropriate for each histopathologic diagnosis.

3. Similarly, although genetics is not the focus of this textbook, critical genetic abnormalities will be highlighted as appropriate.

Immunodeficiency Diseases

I. More than 50 genetically determined immunodeficiency diseases occur; only a few that are of major ocular importance are discussed.

II. Wiskott–Aldrich syndrome (see p. 176 in Chapter 6).

III. Ataxia–telangiectasia (see p. 36 in Chapter 2).

IV. Chédiak–Higashi syndrome (see p. 396 in Chapter 11).

V. Severe combined immunodeficiencies (SCIDs)—heterogeneous group of inherited disorders characterized by profound deficiency of both T-cell and B-cell immunity.

Males who have X-linked SCID have defects in the common cytokine receipt γ chain (γc) gene that encodes a shared essential component of the receptors for IL-2, IL-4, IL-7, IL-9, and IL-15. The lack of Jak3 plays a role in the development of SCID and is essential for lymphoid development.

VI. Chronic granulomatous disease of childhood (see p. 98 in Chapter 4).

VII. Acquired immunodeficiency syndrome (AIDS).

A. From an ocular point of view, this is the most important immunodeficiency disease.

B. AIDS, first recognized in the 1980s, is caused by the highly lethal retrovirus, the human immunodeficiency virus (HIV).

1. HIV type 1 (HIV-1) causes almost all cases in the United States and HIV-2 in West Africa.

2. HIV-1 and HIV-2 have an affinity for the CD4 antigen on T lymphocytes, macrophages, and other cells (see Fig. 1.25).

HIV-1 consists of an electron-dense core surrounding a single-stranded RNA genome, both enveloped by a cell membrane. Retroviruses contain DNA polymerase (reverse transcriptase) complexed to the RNA in the viral core. Reverse transcriptase catalyzes the transcription of the RNA genome into DNA form (the provirus). The provirus migrates from the host cell's cytoplasm to the nucleus, assumes a double-stranded circular form, integrates into the host cell DNA, and may remain throughout the life of the host cell.

C. Patients are prone to life-threatening opportunistic infections, wasting, central nervous system dysfunction, generalized lymphadenopathy, and Kaposi's sarcoma.

Kawasaki's syndrome has been reported in association with HIV infection. Also, multifocal leukoencephalopathy may occur as a result of AIDS.

D. Cytomegalovirus is the most common opportunistic agent. The other agents include most of the viral, bacterial, fungal, and parasitic agents customarily associated with cellular immunodeficiency, with herpes simplex virus, *Mycobacterium tuberculosis* and *Myobacterium avium–intracellulare*, cat-scratch bacillus (*Bartonella henselae*), *Candida albicans*, *Cryptococcus neoformans*, *Pneumocystis carinii*, and *Toxoplasma gondii* heading the list.

E. The location and character of the retinal vascular changes in AIDs indicate an ischemic pathogenesis, most profound in cytomegalovirus retinitis.

F. The histologic appearance depends on the site of involvement and the causative agent (see under appropriate sections of this book).

Transplantation Terminology

  I. *Autograft*: transplantation of tissue excised from one place and grafted to another in the same individual.

  II. Syngraft (isograft): transplantation of tissue excised from one individual and grafted to another who is identical genetically.

  III. *Allograft (homograft)*: transplantation of tissue excised from one individual and grafted to another of the same species.

  IV. *Xenograft (heterograft)*: transplantation of tissue excised from one individual and grafted to another of a different species.

  V. *Orthotopic graft*: transplantation to an anatomically correct position in the recipient.

  VI. *Heterotopic graft*: transplantation to an unnatural position.

CELLULAR AND TISSUE REACTIONS

Hypertrophy

Hypertrophy is an increase in size of individual cells, fibers, or tissues without an increase in the number of individual elements [e.g., retinal pigment epithelium (RPE) in RPE hypertrophy].

Hyperplasia

Hyperplasia is an increase in the number of individual cells in a tissue; their size may or may not increase. Hyperplasia, therefore, is cellular proliferation in excess of normal, but the growth eventually reaches an equilibrium and is never indefinitely progressive (e.g., RPE hyperplasia secondary to trauma; see section on neoplasia, later).

Aplasia

Aplasia is the lack of development of a tissue during embryonic life (e.g., aplasia of the optic nerve).

Hypoplasia

Hypoplasia is the arrested development of a tissue during embryonic life [e.g., hypoplasia of the iris (aniridia)].

Metaplasia

Metaplasia is the transformation of one type of adult tissue into another type [e.g., fibrous metaplasia of lens epithelium (in anterior subcapsular cataract)].

Atrophy

Atrophy is a diminution of size, a shrinking of cells, fibers, or tissues that had previously reached their full development (e.g., retinal vascular atrophy in retinitis pigmentosa).

Dysplasia

Dysplasia is an abnormal growth of tissue during embryonic life (e.g., retinal dysplasia).

Neoplasia

  I. *Neoplasia* is a continuous increase in number of cells in a tissue, caused by unregulated proliferation and, in some cases, failure of mechanisms (e.g., apoptosis) that lead to cell death.

    A. The neoplastic proliferation is probably caused by either excessive or inappropriate activation of oncogenes or reduced activity of genes that downregulate growth (antioncogenes).

    B. It differs from hyperplasia in that its growth never attains equilibrium.

    C. The neoplasm* may be benign or malignant.

  II. A malignant neoplasm differs from a benign one in being *invasive* (it infiltrates and actively destroys surrounding tissue), in having the ability to *metastasize* (develop secondary centers of neoplastic growth at a distance from the primary focus), and in showing *anaplasia* [histologically, the features of a malignancy that include variation from the normal structure (Fig. 1.27) or behavior in the sense of a loss of specialized or "adult" characteristics of the cell or tissue, e.g., loss of cellular or tissue polarity, or inability to form photoreceptors].

Mutations in the *p53* tumor suppressor gene, located on the short arm of chromosome 17 at position 17p13.1, represent the most frequent genetic alteration detected in human solid malignancies. In approximately half of all cancer cases, *p53* is inactivated by mutations and other genomic alterations, and in many of the remaining cases the binding of the cellular MDM2 oncoprotein, a

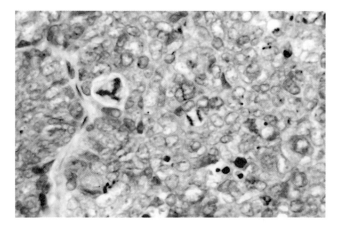

Fig. 1.27 Abnormal tripolar mitotic figure in a sebaceous gland carcinoma.

*A neoplasm is a tumor, but not all tumors are neoplasms. **Tumor** *simply means "mass" and may be secondary to neoplasia, inflammation, or edema.*

cellular inhibitor of the *p53* tumor suppressor, functionally inactivates *p53*. The *p53* gene encodes a 53-kD nucleophosphoprotein that binds DNA, is involved in the regulation of transcription and the induction of programmed cell death (apoptosis), and negatively regulates cell division, preventing progression from G to S phase. Approximately 25% of adult sarcomas of different types are associated with *p53* abnormalities. It also appears to be a marker of tumor progression (i.e., a direct correlation seems to exist between mutations at the *p53* locus and increasing histologic grade). The *ras* proto-oncogene initiates *p53*-independent apoptosis, but is suppressed through the activation of nuclear factor-κB.

Degeneration and Dystrophy

I. A dystrophy is a primary (bilateral), inherited disorder that has distinct clinicopathologic findings. The individual dystrophies are discussed elsewhere under their individual tissues.

II. A degeneration (monocular or binocular) is a secondary phenomenon resulting from previous disease. It occurs in a tissue that has reached its full growth.

 A. *Cloudy swelling* is a reversible change in cells secondary to relatively mild infections, intoxications, anemia, or circulatory disturbances. The cells are enlarged and filled with granules or fluid and probably represent an intracellular edema.

 B. *Hydropic degeneration* is a reversible change in cells also secondary to relatively mild infections, intoxications, anemia, or circulatory disturbances. The cells are enlarged and contain cytoplasmic vacuoles and probably represent an early stage of swelling of the endoplasmic reticulum.

 C. *Fatty change* results when fat accumulates in cells for unknown reasons or after damage by a variety of agents (e.g., chloroform and carbon tetrachloride).

 D. *Glycogen infiltration* results from diseases such as diabetes mellitus (e.g., lacy vacuolation of iris pigment epithelium; see p. 599 in Chapter 15) and from a lack of nutrition (e.g., in long-standing neural retinal detachment and in proliferating retinal pigment epithelial cells).

 E. *Amyloid* may be found in ocular tissues in primary amyloidosis (see p. 238 in Chapter 7 and p. 488 in Chapter 12), such as in primary familial amyloidosis and lattice corneal dystrophy (in which case it is a dystrophic change) or in secondary amyloidosis (see p. 238 in Chapter 7), in which case it is a degenerative change.

 F. *Hyaline* degeneration is quite common, consists of acellular, amorphous, eosinophilic material, and may be found in places such as the walls of arteriolosclerotic vessels or in the ciliary processes in elderly people.

Necrosis

I. Necrosis occurs when cells die an "accidental" death, such as from severe and sudden injury (e.g., ischemia), sustained hyperthermia, physical or chemical trauma, complement attack, or metabolic poisons.

Necrosis should be differentiated from apoptosis—see later.

Necrosis is accompanied by:
- Swelling of the cytoplasm and organelles (especially the mitochondria) and only mild changes in the nucleus.
- Organelle dissolution and rupture of the plasma membrane.
- Leakage of cellular contents into the extracellular space.
- Inflammatory response to the released cellular debris.

No inflammation occurs in apoptosis—see later.

II. *Coagulative necrosis*: this is a firm, dry necrosis generally formed in tissue that has been shut off from its blood supply.

 A. The gray, opaque clinical appearance of the retina after a central retinal artery occlusion is caused by coagulative necrosis (ischemic necrosis). As seen by electron microscopy, coagulative necrosis (e.g., after a laser burn) is produced by widespread focal densification of membranes in the necrotic cell.

 B. *Caseation*, characteristic of tuberculosis, is a combination of coagulative and liquefaction (see later) necrosis.

III. *Hemorrhagic necrosis*: this type is caused by occlusion of venous blood flow but with retention of arterial blood flow, as seen classically in central retinal vein thrombosis.

IV. *Liquefaction necrosis*: necrosis of this type results from autolytic (see section on autolysis and putrefaction, later) decomposition, usually in tissue that is rich in proteolytic enzymes (e.g., suppuration is a form of liquefaction necrosis in which rapid digestion is brought about by the proteolytic enzymes from the leukocytes, especially PMNs, present in the area). It also occurs from complete dissolution of all cell components, as in ultraviolet photocomposition.

V. *Fat necrosis*: necrosis causes liberation of free fatty acids and glycerol that results in a lipogranulomatous reaction.

Apoptosis

I. Apoptosis is "physiologic" or programmed cell death, unrelated to "accidental death" (necrosis)—see earlier.

 A. Apoptosis is a spontaneous death of cells that occurs in many different tissues under various conditions. *Bcl-2* oncogene acts mainly on the pathways of apoptosis (programmed death) and plays a crucial role in the control of cellular growth of lymphoid and nonlymphoid cells.

Two other types of oncogenes are recognized: oncogenes such as *myc, ras,* and *abl* act as growth and proliferative regulatory genes; and oncogenes such as *Rb* and *p53* inhibit growth and proliferation.

B. Two steps accompany apoptosis:
   1. First, the cell undergoes nuclear and cytoplasmic condensation, eventually breaking up into a number of membrane-bound fragments containing structurally intact organelles.

   Cells undergoing apoptosis demonstrate shrinkage, nuclear condensation associated with DNA fragmentation, a relatively intact cell membrane, loss of viability, and absence of inflammation.

   ---

   2. Second, the cell fragments, termed *apoptotic bodies*, are phagocytosed by neighboring cells and rapidly (within minutes) degraded.

   The apoptotic bodies are membrane-encapsulated, thus preventing exposure of cellular contents to the extracellular space and possible inflammatory reaction.

C. Apoptosis appears to play a major role in regulating cell populations.
D. Defective apoptosis may play a role in the genesis of cancer, AIDS, autoimmune diseases, degenerative and dystrophic diseases of the central nervous system (including the neural retina), and diabetic retinopathy.

Calcification

I. *Dystrophic (degenerative) calcification*: this occurs when calcium is deposited in dead or dying tissue (e.g., in long-standing cataracts, in band keratopathy, and in retinoblastoma).
II. *Metastatic calcification*: this type of calcification occurs when calcium is deposited in previously undamaged tissue [e.g., in the cornea of people with high serum calcium levels (hyperparathyroidism, vitamin D intoxication), where it shows as a horizontal band, and in the sclera, where it shows as a senile plaque].

An unusual cause of metastatic calcification is *Werner's syndrome*, a heredofamilial disorder characterized by premature graying and baldness, short stature, gracile build, and "bird face". Ocular findings include blue sclera, bullous keratopathy, presenile posterior subcapsular cataract, degenerative corneal changes post cataract surgery, retinitis pigmentosalike features, and paramacular degeneration.

Autolysis and Putrefaction

I. Autolysis is partly the self-digestion of cells using their own cellular digestive enzymes contained in lysosomes ("suicide bags"), and partly other unknown factors.
II. When certain bacteria (especially clostridia) invade necrotic (autolytic) tissue, the changes catalyzed by destructive bacterial enzymes are called *putrefaction*.

Pigmentation

I. In ocular histologic sections stained with H&E, some commonly found pigments may resemble each other closely: (1) melanin and lipofuscin; (2) hemosiderin; (3) exogenous iron; and (4) acid hematin.
II. *Melanin* is found in uveal melanocytes as fine, powdery, brown granules barely resolvable with the light microscope, and in pigment epithelial cells of the retina, ciliary body, and iris as rather large, black granules. *Lipofuscin* occurs in aged cells and in the RPE and may be difficult to identify by conventional light microscopy, but by electron microscopy differs considerably in structure and density from melanin.
III. *Hemosiderin* results from intraocular hemorrhage when hemoglobin is oxidized to hemosiderin.
   A. It occurs as an orange-brown pigment in macrophages and, when plentiful in the eye, is called *hemosiderosis bulbi*.
   B. Systemic *hemochromatosis* (see p. 188 in Chapter 6) consists of portal cirrhosis and elevated iron content in parenchymal cells of multiple organs. When increased amounts of iron are deposited in tissues of multiple organs but cirrhosis and its complications are lacking, systemic *hemosiderosis* is present.
   C. The distribution of iron in the eye differs in local ocular disease (hemosiderosis bulbi and siderosis bulbi) and systemic disease (Table 1.2).
IV. Exogenous iron results from an intraocular iron foreign body. The resultant ocular iron deposition is called *siderosis bulbi* (see Table 1.2).
V. Acid hematin is an artifact produced by action of acid fixatives, particularly formaldehyde, on hemoglobin.
VI. Differentiation of the pigments.
   A. Only acid hematin is birefringent to polarized light.

TABLE 1.2 Deposition of Iron in the Eye of Local* and Systemic (Hemo) Siderosis

Tissue	Local Siderosis and Hemosiderosis	Systemic Hemochromatosis
Corneal epithelium	Yes	No
Trabecular meshwork	Yes	No
Iris epithelium	Yes	No
Iris dilator and sphincter muscles	Yes	No
Ciliary epithelium	Yes	Yes
Lens epithelium	Yes	No
Vitreous body	Yes	No
Sclera	No	Yes
Blood vessels	Yes	No
Sensory retina	Yes	No
Retinal pigment epithelium	Yes	Yes

*With local iron foreign body, iron is usually deposited in all adjacent (contiguous) tissues.
(Modified from Roth AM, Foos RY: Arch Ophthalmol 87:507, 1972. © American Medical Association.)

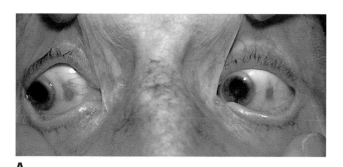

A

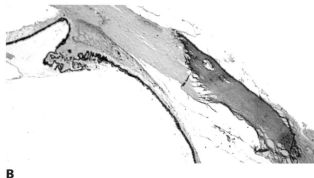

B

Fig. 1.28 A, Scleral calcium plaques present where horizontal rectus muscles insert. Plaques appear translucent gray. **B,** Calcium deposited through full thickness of sclera in region of insertion of rectus muscles.

B. Only melanin bleaches with oxidizing agents, such as hydrogen peroxide.

C. The cathepsin-D reaction is helpful in identifying lipofuscin.

D. Only iron stains positively with the common stains for iron.

> Hemosiderin and exogenous iron cannot be differentiated on their staining properties and sometimes may not be differentiated on structural grounds.

Growth and Aging

I. In general, ocular tissue in infants and young people is quite cellular. Cellularity decreases with aging as the collagenization of tissues increases.

II. The eye is at least two-thirds of its adult size at birth, and usually reaches full size by the end of the second decade of life.

> Although the eyeball reaches full size, the lens, an inverted epithelial structure, continues to grow throughout life. Nuclear cataract results from the increased density of the central (unclear) lens cells (and other factors) and can be considered an aging change.

III. Certain chemicals may be deposited in ocular tissues during the aging process, including calcium in the insertion of the rectus muscles (*senile plaque*; Fig. 1.28) and in Bruch's membrane (calcification of Bruch's membrane), and sorbitol in the lens.

IV. The important growth and aging changes of individual tissues are taken up in the appropriate sections in the remaining chapters.

BIBLIOGRAPHY

Inflammation

Arpin C, Déchanet J, van Kooten C *et al.*: Generation of memory B cells and plasma cells and plasma cells in vitro. *Science* 268:720, 1995

Bacon KB, Premack BA, Gardner P *et al.*: Activation of dual T cell signaling pathways by the chemokine RANTES. *Science* 269:1727, 1995

Cintron C: The molecular structure of the corneal stroma in health and disease. In Podos SM, Yanoff M, eds: *Textbook of Ophthalmology*, vol. 5. London, Mosby, 1994:5.6

Claman HN: The biology of the immune response. *JAMA* 268:2790, 1992

Cohen MC, Cohen S: Cytokine function: A study in biologic diversity. *J Clin Pathol* 105:589, 1996

Cook DN, Beck MA, Coffman TM *et al.*: Requirement of MIP-1α for an inflammatory response to viral infection. *Science* 269:1583, 1995

Elias JM, Margiotta M, Gaborc D: Sensitivity and detection efficiency of the peroxidase antiperoxidase (PAP), avidin-biotin peroxidase complex (ABC), and peroxidase-labeled avidin-biotin (LAB) methods. *Am J Clin Pathol* 92:62, 1989

El-Okada M, Ko YH, Xie S-S *et al.*: Russell bodies consist of heterogeneous glycoproteins in B-cell lymphoma cells. *Am J Clin Pathol* 97:866, 1992

Fine BS, Zimmerman LE: Exogenous intraocular fungus infections. *Am J Ophthalmol* 48:151, 1959

Gallagher R: Tagging T cells T$_H$1 or T$_H$2? *Science* 275:1615, 1997

Godfrey WA: Characterization of the choroidal mast cell. *Trans Am Ophthalmol Soc* 85:557, 1987

Gronenborn AM, Clore GM: Similarity of protein G and ubiquitin. *Science* 254:581, 1991

Henriquez AS, Kenyon KR, Allansmith MR: Mast cell ultra-structure: Comparison in contact lens-associated giant papillary conjunctivitis and vernal conjunctivitis. *Arch Ophthalmol* 99:1266, 1981

Hsu S-M, Hsu P-L, McMillan PN *et al.*: Russell bodies: A light and electron microscopic immunoperoxidase study. *Am J Clin Pathol* 77:26, 1982

Knaus UG, Morris S, Dong H-J *et al.*: Regulation of human leukocyte p21-activated kinases through G protein-coupled receptors. *Science* 269:221, 1995

Metcalf D: Control of granulocytes and macrophages: molecular, cellular, and clinical aspects. *Science* 254:529, 1991

Miller JK, Laycock KA, Nash MN *et al.*: Corneal Langerhans cell dynamics after herpes simplex virus reactivation. *Invest Ophthalmol Vis Sci* 34:2282, 1993

Ngan B-Y, Picker LJ, Medeiros LJ *et al.*: Immunophenotypic diagnosis of non-Hodgkin's lymphoma in paraffin sections. *Am J Clin Pathol* 91:579, 1989

Papadopoulos KP, Bagg A, Bezwoda WR *et al.*: The routine diagnostic utility of immunoglobulin and T-cell receptor gene rearrangements in lymphoproliferative disorders. *Am J Clin Pathol* 91:633, 1989

Perkins SL, Kjeldsberg CR: Immunophenotyping of lymphomas and leukemias in paraffin-embedded tissues. *Am J Clin Pathol* 99:362, 1993

Rao NA, Foster DJ: Basic principles. In Podos SM, Yanoff M, eds: *Textbook of Ophthalmology*, vol. 2. New York, Gower Medical Publishing, 1992:1.11, 1.15

Rissoan M-C, Soumelis V, Kadowaki N *et al.*: Reciprocal control of T helper cell and dendritic cell differentiation. *Science* 283:1183, 1999

Strieter RM, Kunkel SL, Showell DG *et al.*: Endothelial cell gene expression of a neutrophil chemotactic factor by TNF-α, LPS, and IL-1β. *Science* 243:1467, 1989

Tamura Y, Konomi H, Sawada H *et al.*: Tissue distribution of type VII collagen in human adult and fetal eyes. *Invest Ophthalmol Vis Sci* 32:2636, 1991

Trocme SD, Aldave AJ: The eye and the eosinophil. *Surv Ophtalmol* 39:241, 1994

Truong LD, Rangedaeng S, Cagle P *et al.*: The diagnostic utility of desmin: A study of 584 cases and review of the literature. *Am J Clin Pathol* 93:305, 1990

Yanoff M, Perry HD: Juvenile xanthogranuloma of the corneoscleral limbus. *Arch Ophthalmol* 113:915, 1995

Immunobiology

Arpin C, Déchanet J, van Kooten C *et al.*: Generation of memory B cells and plasma cells in vitro. *Science* 268:720, 1995

Ashkar S, Weber GF, Jansson M *et al.*: Eta-1 (osteopontin): an early component of type-1 (cell-mediated) immunity. *Science* 287:860, 2000

Bacon KB, Premack BA, Gardner P *et al.*: Activation of dual T cell signaling pathways by the chemokine RANTES. *Science* 269:1727, 1995

Bauer S, Groh V, Wu J *et al.*: Activation of NK cells and T cells by NKG2D, a receptor for stress-inducible MICA. *Science* 285:727, 1999

Blackman M, Kappler J, Marrack P: The role of the T cell receptor in positive and negative selection of developing T cells. *Science* 248:1335, 1990

von Boehmer H, Kisielow P: Self-nonself discrimination by T cells. *Science* 248:1369, 1990

Boise LH, Thompson CB: Hierarchical control of lymphocyte survival. *Science* 274:67, 1996

Boismenu R, Rhein M, Fischer WH *et al.*: A role for CD81 in early T cell development. *Science* 271:198, 1996

Buckley RH: Immunodeficiency diseases. *JAMA* 268:2797, 1992

Chan AC, Kadlecek TA, Elder ME *et al.*: ZAP-70 deficiency in an autosomal recessive form of severe combined immunodeficiency. *Science* 264:1596, 1994

Claman HN: The biology of the immune response. *JAMA* 268:2790, 1992

Cohen MC, Cohen S: Cytokine function: A study in biologic diversity. *J Clin Pathol* 105:589, 1996

Elder ME, Lin D, Clever J *et al.*: Human severe combined immunodeficiency due to a defect in ZAP-70, a T cell tyrosine kinase. *Science* 264:1599, 1994

Elenitoba-Johnson KSJ, Medeiros LJ, Khorsand J *et al.*: p53 expression in Reed–Sternberg cells does not correlate with gene mutations in Hodgkin's disease. *Am J Clin Pathol* 106:728, 1996

Glasgow BJ, Wiesberger AK: A quantitative and cartographic study of retinal microvasculopathy in acquired immunodeficiency syndrome. *Am J Ophthalmol* 118:46, 1994

Grabstein KH, Eisenman J, Shanebeck K *et al.*: Cloning of a T cell growth factor that interacts with the chain of the interleukin-2 receptor. *Science* 264:365, 1994

Goodnow CC, Adelstein S, Basten A: The need for central and peripheral tolerance in the B cell repertoire. *Science* 248:1373, 1990

Gorina S, Pavletich NP: Structure of the p53 tumor suppressor bound to the ankyrin and SH3 domains of 53BP2. *Science* 274:948, 1996

Grakoul A, Bromley SK, Sumen C *et al.*: The immunological synapse: a molecular machine controlling T cell activation. *Science* 285:21, 1999

Hagmann M: A trigger of natural (and others) killers. *Science* 285:645, 1999

Halling KC, Scheithauer BW, Halling AC *et al.*: p53 expression in neurofibroma and malignant peripheral nerve sheath tumors: An immunohistochemical study of sporadic and ND-1 associated tumors. *Am J Clin Pathol* 106:282, 1996

Hoffman M: Determining what immune cells see. *Science* 255, 1992

Ioachim HL: *Pathology of AIDS*. Philadelphia, JB Lippincott, 1989: 238

Jabs DA: Acquired immunodeficiency syndrome and the eye: 1996 (editorial). *Arch Ophthalmol* 114:863, 1996

Jabs DA, Green WR, Fox R *et al.*: Ocular manifestations of acquired immune deficiency syndrome. *Ophthalmology* 96:1092, 1989

Kronish JW, Johnson TE, Gilberg SM *et al.*: Orbital infections in patients with human immunodeficiency virus infections in patients with human immunodeficiency virus infection. *Ophthalmology* 103:1483, 1996

Kurumety UR, Lustbader JM: Kaposi's sarcoma of the bulbar conjunctiva as an initial clinical manifestation of acquired immunodeficiency syndrome. *Arch Ophthalmol* 113:978, 1995

Kussie PH, Gorina S, Marechal V *et al.*: Structure of the MDM2 oncoprotein bound to the p53 tumor suppressor transactivation domain. *Science* 274:948, 1996

Li L, YeeC, Beavo JA: CD3- and CD28-dependent induction of PDE7 required for T cell activation. *Science* 283:848, 1999

Malissen B: Dancing the immunological two-step. *Science* 285:207, 1999

Matsuno A, Nagashima T, Matsuura R *et al.*: Correlation between MIB-1 staining index and the immunoreactivity of p53 protein in recurrent and non-recurrent meningioma. *Am J Clin Pathol* 106:776, 1996

Musarella MA: Gene mapping of ocular diseases (review). *Surv Ophthalmol* 36:285, 1992

Ormerod LD, Rhodes RH, Gross SA *et al.*: Ophthalmologic manifestations of acquired immune deficiency syndrome-associated progressive multifocal leukoencephalopathy. *Ophthalmology* 103:899, 1996

Patel SS, Rutzen AR, Marx JL *et al.*: Cytomegalic papillitis in patients with acquired immune deficiency syndrome. *Ophthalmology* 103:1476, 1996

Perkins SL, Kjeldsberg CR: Immunophenotyping of lymphomas and leukemias in paraffin-embedded tissues. *Am J Clin Pathol* 99:362, 1993

Ramsdell F, Fowlkes BJ: Clonal deletion versus clonal anergy: the role of the thymus in inducing self tolerance. *Science* 248:1343, 1990

Ratech H: The use of molecular biology in hematopathology. *Am J Clin Pathol* 99:381, 1993

Rissoan M-C, Soumelis V, Kadowaki N *et al.*: Reciprocal control of the T helper cell and dendritic cell differentiation. *Science* 283:1183, 1999

van Rood JJ, Claas RJH: The influence of allogenic cells on the human T and b cell repertoire. *Science* 248:1388, 1990

Russell SM, Tayebi N, Nakajima H *et al.*: Mutation of Jak3 in a patient with SCID: essential role of Jak3 in lymphoid development. *Science* 270:797, 1995

Schaumburg-Lever G, Leven WF: *Color Atlas of Histopathology of the Skin*. Philadelphia, JB Lippincott, 1988:10–13

Schwartz RH: A cell culture model for T lymphocyte anergy. *Science* 248:1349, 1990

Sinha AA, Lopez MT, McDevitt HO: Autoimmune diseases: the failure of self tolerance. *Science* 248:1380, 1990

Sprent J, Gao E-K, Webb SR: T cell reactivity to MHC molecules: immunity versus tolerance. *Science* 248:1357, 1990

Weiss SW: p53 gene alterations in benign and malignant nerve sheath tumors. *Am J Clin Pathol* 106:271, 1996

Williams N: T cell inactivation linked to Ras block. *Science* 271:1234, 1996

Wolf CV II, Wolf JR, Parker JS: Kawasaki's syndrome in a man with the human immunodeficiency virus. *Am J Ophthalmol* 120:117, 1995

Wu J, Song Y, Bakker ABH *et al.*: An activating immunoreceptor complex formed by NKG2D and DAP10. *Science* 285:730, 1999

Cellular and Tissue Reactions

Carson DE, Ribeiro JM: Apoptosis and disease. *Lancet* 341:1251, 1993

Cheng EH-Y, Kirsch DG, Clem RJ *et al.*: Conversion of Bcl-2 to a bax-like death effector by caspases. *Science* 278:1966, 1997

Corbally N, Grogan L, Keane MM *et al.*: Bcl-2 rearrangement in Hodgkin's disease and reactive lymph nodes. *Am J Clin Pathol* 101:756, 1994

Fine BS, Yanoff M: *Ocular Histology: A Text and Atlas*, 2nd edn. New York, Harper & Row, 1979

Finkelstein EM, Boniuk M: Intraocular ossification and hematopoiesis. *Am J Ophthalmol* 68:683, 1969

Hetts SW: To die or not to die: An overview of apoptosis and its role in disease. *JAMA* 279:300, 1998

Inghirami G, Frizzera G: Role of the bcl-2 oncogene in Hodgkin's disease. *Am J Clin Pathol* 101:681, 1994

Lanza G Jr, Maestra I, Dubini A *et al.*: p53 expression in colorectal cancer: Relation to tumor type, DNA ploidy pattern, and short-term survival. *Am J Pathol* 105:604, 1996

Lazzaro DR, Lin K, Stevens JA: Corneal findings in hemochromatosis. *Arch Ophthalmol* 116:1531, 1998

Marx J: Oncogenes reach a milestone. *Science* 266:1942, 1994

Mayo MW, Wang C-Y, Cogswell PC *et al.*: Requirement of NF-KB activation to suppress p53-independent apoptosis induced by oncogenic ras. *Science* 278:1812, 1997

Norn MS: Scleral plaques: II. Follow up, cause. *Acta Ophthalmol (Copenh)* 52:512, 1974

Ross DW: Apoptosis. *Arch Pathol Lab Med* 121:83, 1997

Roth AM, Foos RY: Ocular pathologic changes in primary hemochromatosis. *Arch Ophthalmol* 87:507, 1972

Schwartzman RA, Cidlowski JA: Apoptosis: the biochemistry and molecular biology of programmed cell death. *Endocrinol Rev* 14:133, 1993

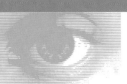

2

Congenital Anomalies

PHAKOMATOSES (DISSEMINATED HEREDITARY HAMARTOMAS)

General Information

I. The phakomatoses are a heredofamilial group of congenital tumors having disseminated, usually benign, hamartomas in common.

The term *phakomatosis* (Greek: *phakos* = "mother spot" or "birthmark") was introduced by van der Hoeve in 1923.

II. In each type of phakomatosis, the hamartomas tend to affect one type of tissue predominantly (e.g., blood vessels in angiomatosis retinae and neural tissue in neurofibromatosis).

A *hamartoma* is a congenital tumor composed of tissues normally found in the involved area, in contrast to a *choristoma*, which is a congenital tumor composed of tissues not normally present in the involved area.

Angiomatosis Retinae [von Hippel's Disease (VHL)]

I. General information
   A. The onset of ocular symptoms is usually in young adulthood.
   B. Retinal capillary hemangiomas (hemangioblastomas) occur in over 50% of patients (Fig. 2.1), and central nervous system lesions occur in 72% of patients.
   C. VHL disease is an inherited cancer syndrome (autosomal-dominant) characterized by a predisposition to development of multiple retinal angiomas, cer-

ebellar "hemangioblastomas," bilateral renal cysts and carcinomas, bilateral pheochromocytomas, pancreatic cysts, and epididymal cysts.

The combination of retinal and cerebellar capillary hemangiomas (and capillary hemangiomas of medulla and spinal cord) is called *von Hippel–Lindau* disease. The retinal component, *von Hippel's disease*, was the first to be described. The responsible *VHL* gene resides at human chromosome 3 (band 3p25.5–p26). Genetically, the disease gene behaves as a typical tumor suppressor, as defined in Knudson's theory of carcinogenesis.

II. Ocular findings
   A. A retinal capillary hemangioma (see p. 544 in Chapter 14), usually supplied by large feeder vessels, may occur in the optic nerve or in any part of the retina.

Unusual retinal hamartomas may be seen in the inner retina, usually adjacent to a retinal vein, and are characterized by small, moss fiberlike, relatively flat, vascular lesions with smooth or irregular margins but without enlarged afferent and efferent vessels.

   B. Retinal exudates, often in the macula even when the tumor is peripheral, result when serum leaks from the abnormal tumor blood vessels.
   C. Ultimately, organized fibroglial bands may form and neural retinal detachment may develop. Secondary closed-angle glaucoma may also be found.
III. Systemic findings
   A. A retinal capillary hemangioma may occur in the cerebellum, brainstem, and spinal cord.
   B. Cysts of pancreas and kidney are commonly found.
   C. Hypernephroma and pheochromocytoma (usually bilateral) occur infrequently.

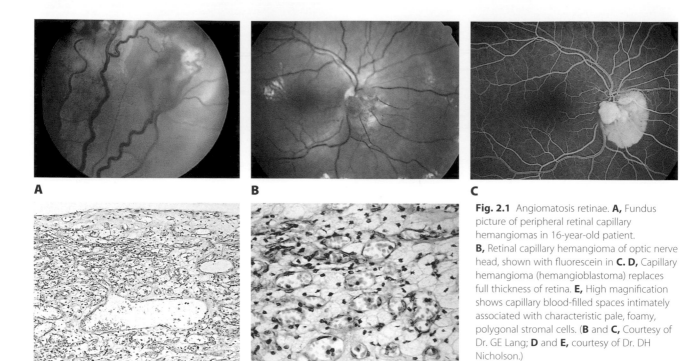

Fig. 2.1 Angiomatosis retinae. **A,** Fundus picture of peripheral retinal capillary hemangiomas in 16-year-old patient. **B,** Retinal capillary hemangioma of optic nerve head, shown with fluorescein in **C. D,** Capillary hemangioma (hemangioblastoma) replaces full thickness of retina. **E,** High magnification shows capillary blood-filled spaces intimately associated with characteristic pale, foamy, polygonal stromal cells. (**B** and **C,** Courtesy of Dr. GE Lang; **D** and **E,** courtesy of Dr. DH Nicholson.)

IV. Histology
  A. The basic lesion is a capillary hemangioma (hemangio-blastoma) (see p. 544 in Chapter 14).
    1. The tumor, a capillary hemangioma, is composed of endothelial cells and pericytes.
    2. Between the capillaries are foamy stromal cells that appear to be of glial origin.
      a. Immunohistochemical studies show that the foamy stromal cells stain positively for glial fibrillary acid protein and neuron-specific enolase.
      b. The *VHL* gene deletion may be restricted to the stromal cells, suggesting that the stromal cells are the neoplastic component in retinal hemangiomas and induce the accompanying neovascularization.
  B. Secondary complications may be found, such as retinal exudates and hemorrhages, fixed retinal folds and orga-nized fibroglial membranes, neural retinal detachment, iris neovascularization, peripheral anterior synechiae, and chronic closed-angle glaucoma.

Meningocutaneous Angiomatosis [Encephalotrigeminal Angiomatosis; Sturge–Weber Syndrome (SWS)]

I. General information
  A. SWS (Fig. 2.2) usually consists of unilateral (rarely bilateral) meningeal calcification, facial nevus flammeus (port-wine stain, phakomatosis pigmentovascularis), frequently along the distribution of the trigeminal nerve, and congenital glaucoma.

  B. The condition is congenital (heredity does not seem to be an important factor).
II. Ocular findings
  A. The most common intraocular finding is a cavernous hemangioma (see p. 544 in Chapter 14) of the choroid on the side of the facial nevus flammeus.

  > Extremely rarely, the choroidal nevus can be bilateral even with unilateral facial nevus flammeus.

  B. A cavernous hemangioma or telangiectasis (see pp. 544 and 545 in Chapter 14) of the lids on the side of the facial nevus flammeus is common.
  C. Congenital glaucoma is associated with ipsilateral hem-angioma of the facial skin in approximately 30% of patients.

  > When nevus flammeus and congenital oculodermal melano-cytosis occur together, especially when each extensively involves the globe, a strong predisposition exists for the devel-opment of congenital glaucoma.

    1. The lids, especially the upper, are usually involved.
    2. The cause of the glaucoma is unclear, but in most instances it is not related to the commonly found ipsilateral choroidal hemangioma.
III. Systemic findings
  A. Cavernous hemangioma or telangiectasis of the skin of the face ("birthmark" or port-wine stain) is the most common visible sign.
  B. Hemangioma of the meninges and brain on the side of the facial hemangioma is usually present.

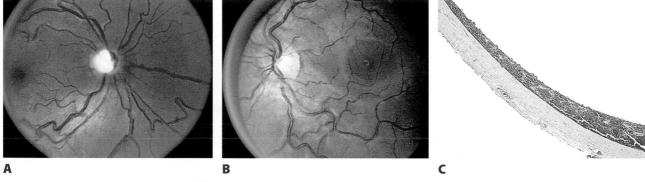

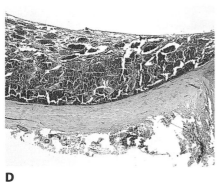

Fig. 2.2 Meningocutaneous angiomatosis. **A,** The fundus shows both the characteristic bright-red appearance, caused by the choroidal hemangioma, and an enlarged optic nerve cup, secondary to increased pressure. **B,** Left eye in same patient shows normal fundus for comparison. **C,** Choroid thickened posteriorly by cavernous hemangioma that blends imperceptibly into normal choroid. **D,** Cavernous hemangioma of choroid in same eye shows large, thin-walled, blood-filled spaces. (**A** and **B,** Courtesy of Dr. HG Scheie; **C** and **D,** courtesy of Dr. R Cordero-Moreno.)

Meningeal or intracranial calcification allows the area of the hemangioma to be located radiographically.

  C. Seizures and mental retardation are common.
IV. Histology
  A. The basic lesion in the skin of the face (including lids), the meninges, and the choroid is a cavernous hemangioma (see p. 544 in Chapter 14).

The vascular dermal lesion in the SWS differs, however, from a non-SWS, "garden-variety" cavernous hemangioma in that the vascular wall in the SWS lesion lacks a multilaminar smooth muscle. The vascular abnormality in SWS, therefore, as suggested by Lever, would be better termed a *vascular malformation* or *nevus telangiectaticus*, rather than *cavernous hemangioma*.

---

    1. In addition, telangiectasis (see p. 545 in Chapter 14) of the skin of the face may occur.
    2. The choroidal hemangiomas in SWS show a diffuse angiomatosis and involve at least half the choroid, often affecting the episcleral and intrascleral perilimbal plexuses.
    3. SWS hemangioma shows infiltrative margins, making it difficult to tell where hemangioma ends and normal choroid begins.

Hemangioma of the choroid unrelated to SWS, conversely, is usually well circumscribed, shows a sharply demarcated pushing margin, often compresses surrounding melanocytes and choroidal lamellae, and usually (in 70% of cases) occurs in the region of the posterior pole (area centralis).

  B. Congenital glaucoma may be present.
  C. Secondary complications such as microcystoid degeneration of the overlying retina (see p. 422 in Chapter 11) and leakage of serous fluid (see p. 422 in Chapter 11) are common.

Neurofibromatosis (Figs 2.3–2.5)

  I. Neurofibromatosis type 1 (NF-1: von Recklinghausen's disease or peripheral neurofibromatosis)
  A. General information
    1. Diagnosis of NF-1 is made if two or more of the following are found: six or more café-au-lait spots >5 mm in greatest diameter in prepubertal persons and 15 mm in postpubertal persons; two or more neurofibromas of any type or one plexiform neurofibroma; freckling in the axillary, inguinal, or other intertriginous region; optic nerve glioma; two or more Lisch nodules; a distinctive osseous lesion (e.g., sphenoid bone dysplasia); a first-degree relative who has NF-1.
    2. Multiple tumors are found that are derived from Schwann cells of peripheral and cranial nerves and glial cells of the central nervous system.
    3. A superimposed malignant change (fibrosarcoma, neurofibrosarcoma, malignant schwannoma) may occur.
    4. NF-1 is transmitted as an irregular autosomal-dominant trait (prevalence approximately 1 in 3000 to 4000). The responsible gene is located on chromosome 17 (band 17q11.2).
  B. Ocular findings
    1. Café-au-lait spots

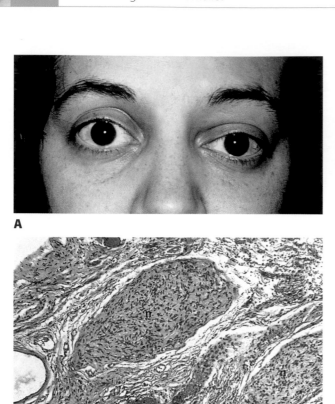

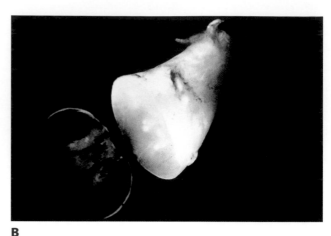

Fig. 2.3 Neurofibromatosis. **A,** A plexiform neurofibroma has enlarged the left upper lid; the neurofibroma was removed. **B,** The gross specimen shows a markedly expanded nerve. A thin slice of the nerve is present at the bottom left. **C,** In another similar case diffuse proliferation of Schwann cells within the nerve sheath enlarges the nerve (n, thickened abnormal nerves). (**A,** Courtesy of Dr. WC Frayer.)

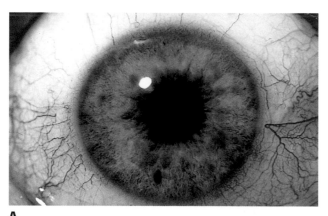

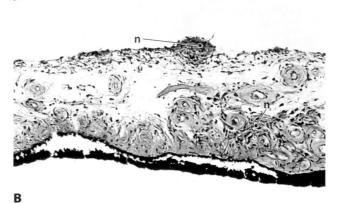

Fig. 2.4 Neurofibromatosis. **A,** Iris shows multiple, spider-like melanocytic nevi, characteristic of neurofibromatosis. **B,** (light microscope; n, nevi) and **C,** (scanning electron microscope): The iris nevi, also called *Lisch nodules,* are composed of collections of nevus cells. (**C,** Courtesy of Dr. RC Eagle, Jr.)

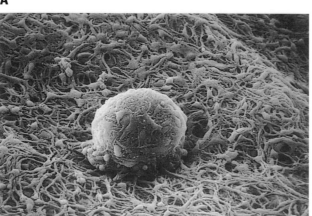

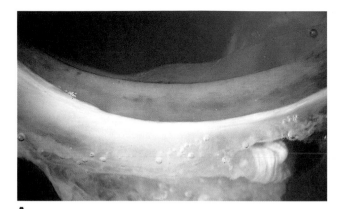

A

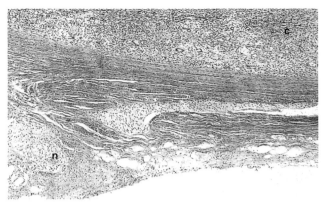

B

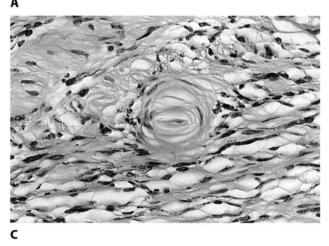

C

Fig. 2.5 Neurofibromatosis. **A** and **B,** Gross and microscopic appearance of hamartomatously, markedly thickened choroid (c). Sclera contains thickened, abnormal nerves (n). **C,** High magnification of diffuse choroidal hamartoma shows structures resembling tactile nerve endings and cells resembling nevus cells. (**A** and **C,** Courtesy of Dr. RC Eagle, Jr.; **B,** courtesy of Dr. L Calkins.)

2. Neurofibromas
   a. Fibroma molluscum, the common neurofibroma, results from proliferation of the distal end of a nerve and produces a small, localized skin tumor.
   b. Plexiform neurofibroma ("bag of worms") is a diffuse proliferation in the nerve sheath and produces a thickened and tortuous nerve.
   c. Elephantiasis neuromatosa is a diffuse proliferation outside the nerve sheath that produces a thickening and folding of the skin.
3. Thickening of corneal and conjunctival nerves and congenital glaucoma

---

If a plexiform neurofibroma of the eyelid is present (especially upper eyelid), 50% will have glaucoma.

---

4. Hamartomas in trabecular meshwork, uvea, neural retina, and optic nerve head
   a. Melanocytic nevi in trabecular meshwork and uvea

Clinically, the multiple, small, spider-like, melanocytic iris nevi (Lisch nodules) are the most common clinical feature of adult NF-1, found in 93% of adults. Rarely, Lisch nodules may be found in NF-2.

---

   b. Glial hamartomas in neural retina and optic nerve head
   c. Retinal capillary hemangiomas and combined pigment epithelial and retinal hamartomas
5. Sectoral neural retinal pigmentation (sector retinitis pigmentosa of Bietti)
6. Optic nerve glioma (juvenile pilocytic astrocytoma)

About 25% of patients who have optic nerve gliomas have neurofibromatosis, almost exclusively type 1. NF-1 patients who have negative neuroimaging studies of the optic pathways may later develop optic nerve gliomas.

---

7. Orbit: plexiform neurofibroma; neurilemmoma (schwannoma); absence of greater wing of sphenoid; enlarged optic foramen; pulsating exophthalmos

---

The pulsating exophthalmos may be associated with an orbital encephalocele.

C. Histology
1. In the skin and orbit, a diffuse, irregular proliferation of peripheral nerve elements (predominantly

Schwann cells) results in an unencapsulated neurofibroma.

2. The tumor is composed of numerous cells that contain elongated, basophilic nuclei and faintly granular cytoplasm associated with fine, wavy, "maiden-hair," immature collagen fibers.
   a. Special stains often show nerve fibers in the tumor.
   b. Vascularity is quite variable from tumor to tumor and in the same tumor.

   Histologically, neurofibromas are often confused with dermatofibromas, neurilemmomas, schwannomas (see p. 588 in Chapter 14), or leiomyomas (see p. 350 in Chapter 9).

   ---

3. In the eye, the lesion may be a melanocytic nevus (see p. 697 in Chapter 17), slight or massive involvement of the uvea (usually choroid) by a mixture of hamartomatous neural and nevus elements, or a glial hamartoma (see later).

   Rarely, a uveal melanoma may arise from the uveal nevus component, although this is probably a coincidental occurrence rather than cause and effect.

II. Neurofibromatosis type 2 (NF-2; central neurofibromatosis, bilateral acoustic neurofibromatosis)
   A. General information
      1. Diagnosis of NF-2 is made if a person has either bilateral eighth-nerve tumors or a first-degree relative who has NF-2; and either a unilateral eighth-nerve tumor or two or more of the following: neurofibroma; meningioma (especially primary nerve sheath meningioma); glioma; schwannoma; ependymoma; or juvenile posterior subcapsular lenticular opacity.
         a. NF-2 is transmitted as an irregular autosomal-dominant (prevalence about 1 in 40 000).
         b. The responsible gene is located on chromosome 22 (band 22q12).
      2. Combined pigment epithelial and retinal hamartomas may occur.

      The most common ocular abnormalities found in NF-2 are lens opacities (67%—mainly plaque-like posterior subcapsular or capsular, cortical, or mixed lens opacities) and retinal hamartomas (22%).

III. Because of the neuromas, café-au-lait spots, and prominent corneal nerves that may be found, the condition of *multiple endocrine neoplasia* (MEN) type IIB must be differentiated from neurofibromatosis.
   A. MEN, a familial disorder, is classified into three groups.
      1. Type I (autosomal-dominant inheritance) consists of multiple neoplasms of the pituitary, parathyroid, pancreas islets, and less often pheochromocytoma

(as a late feature) and neoplasms of the adrenal and thyroid glands.

The Zollinger–Ellison syndrome consists of gastric, duodenal, and jejunal ulcers associated with gastrin-secreting non-β islet cell tumors of the pancreas (gastrinomas). The tumors may arise in multiple sites in MEN type I.

---

2. Type IIA (autosomal-dominant inheritance; also called *Sipple syndrome*) consists of medullary thyroid carcinoma, pheochromocytoma (as an early feature), parathyroid hyperplasia, and prominent corneal nerves (less prominent than in type IIB).
3. Type IIB (Fig. 2.6; 50% autosomal-dominant and 50% sporadic inheritance; also called *type III*) consists of medullary thyroid carcinoma and, less often, pheochromocytoma.
   In addition, marfanoid habitus, skeletal abnormalities, prominent corneal nerves (more prominent than in IIA), multiple mucosal (including conjunctival, tongue, and intestinal) neuromas, café-au-lait spots, and cutaneous neuromas or neurofibromas may occur.
B. Linkage analysis shows:
   1. In MEN I, the predisposing genetic linkage is assigned to chromosome region 11q13.
   2. In MEN IIA and IIB, predisposing genetic linkage is assigned to chromosome region 10q11.2.

The mutation for MEN IIA and IIB occurs at the site of the human *RET* proto-oncogene at 10q11.2, the same site where a mutation also causes the autosomal-dominant Hirschsprung's disease. An oncogenic conversion (not a loss of suppressor function) converts *RET* into a dominant transforming gene.

Tuberous* Sclerosis (Bourneville's Disease; Pringle's Disease)

I. General information
   A. Symptoms usually appear during the first 3 years of life and consist of the triad of mental deficiency, seizures, and adenoma sebaceum (angiofibroma).
   B. The prognosis is poor (death occurs in 75% of patients by 20 years of age).
   C. The disease is transmitted as an irregular autosomal-dominant (prevalence approximately 1 in 10 000). Tuberous sclerosis complex (TSC)-determining loci have been mapped to chromosome 9q34 (*TSC1*) and 16p13.3 (*TSC2*)
II. Ocular findings (Fig. 2.7)
   A. Lids: adenoma sebaceum (angiofibroma)
   B. Eyeball
      1. Glial hamartoma of retina occurs in 53% of patients.

The name originates from the shape of the tumor (i.e., like a potato or tuber).

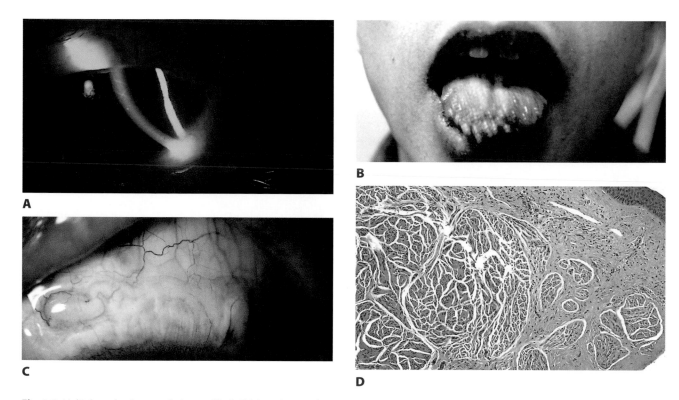

Fig. 2.6 Multiple endocrine neoplasia type IIB. **A,** Thickened corneal nerves are seen to criss-cross in the slit beam. **B,** Characteristic neurofibromatous submucosal nodules are seen along the front edge of the tongue. **C,** A large submucosal neurofibromatous nodule is present in the conjunctiva. **D,** Histologically, the conjunctival nodule consists of enlarged nerves in the conjunctival substantia propria.

2. Most retinal hamartomas remain stable over time, but some become calcified, and rarely some may show progressive growth.

> Hamartomas of the neural retina in infants have a smooth, spongy appearance with fuzzy borders, are gray-white, and may be mistaken for retinoblastoma. Older lesions may become condensed, with an irregular, white surface, resembling a *mulberry*. The whitened, wrinkled clinical appearance is caused by avascularity, not calcium deposition. The lesions are frequently multiple and vary in size from one-fifth to two disc diameters. New lesions may rarely develop from areas of previously normal-appearing retina.

3. Glial hamartoma of optic disc anterior to lamina cribrosa (*giant drusen*) may occur.

> The giant drusen of the optic nerve head may be mistaken for a swollen disc (i.e., pseudopapilledema). Most patients who have drusen of the optic nerve do not have tuberous sclerosis.

4. Neuroectodermal hamartomas of the iris pigment epithelium and ciliary body epithelium may occur rarely.

III. Systemic findings
   A. Glial hamartomas in the cerebrum occur commonly and result in epilepsy in 93% of patients, in mental deficiency in 62% of patients, and in intracranial calcification in 51% of patients.
   B. Adenoma sebaceum (really an angiofibroma) of the skin of the face occurs in 83% of patients.
   C. Hamartomas of lung, heart, and kidney, which may progress to renal cell carcinoma, may also be found.

IV. Histology
   A. Giant drusen of the optic disc occur anterior to the lamina cribrosa and are glial hamartomas (see p. 520 in Chapter 13).
   B. Adenoma sebaceum are not tumors of the sebaceous gland apparatus but are angiofibromas (see Fig. 6.34 in Chapter 6).
   C. Glial hamartomas in the cerebrum (usually in the walls of the lateral ventricles over the basal ganglia) and neural retina are composed of large, fusiform astrocytes separated by a coarse and nonfibrillated, or finer and fibrillated, matrix formed from the astrocytic cell processes.
      1. The cerebral tumors are usually well vascularized, but the neural retinal tumors tend to be sparsely vascularized or nonvascularized.
      2. Calcospherites may be prominent, especially in older lesions.

> Retinal tumors display the same spectrum of aberrant development and morphologic characteristics as other

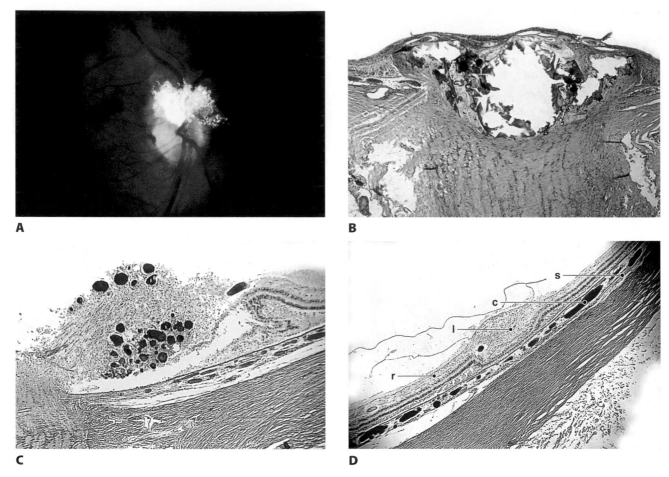

Fig. 2.7 Tuberous sclerosis. **A,** Fundus shows typical mulberry lesion involving the superior part of the optic nerve. **B,** Histologic section of another case shows a giant druse of the optic nerve. **C,** The lesion, as seen in the fundus of a young child before it grows into the mulberry configuration, is quite smooth and resembles a retinoblastoma. **D,** Histologic section of an early lesion shows no calcification but simply a proliferation of glial tissue (s, sclera; c, choroid; l, lesion; r, retina). (**C,** Courtesy of Dr. DB Schaffer.)

central nervous system lesions, including the occurrence of giant cell astrocytomas that stain positive for γ-enolase but negative for glial acid fibrillary protein and neural filament protein.

Other Phakomatoses

Numerous other phakomatoses occur. *Ataxia–telangiectasia* (Louis–Bar syndrome), an immunodeficient disorder, consists of an autosomal-recessive inheritance pattern (gene localized to chromosome 11q22), progressive cerebellar ataxia, oculocutaneous telangiectasia, and frequent pulmonary infections; *arteriovenous* communication of retina and brain (Wyburn–Mason syndrome) consists of a familial pattern, mental changes, and arteriovenous communication of the midbrain and retina (see p. 545 in Chapter 14) associated with facial nevi. Most other phakomatoses are extremely rare or do not have salient ocular findings.

CHROMOSOMAL ABERRATIONS

I. Normally, the human cell is *diploid* and contains 46 chromosomes: 44 autosomal chromosomes and two sex chromosomes (XX in a female and XY in a male).

  A. Individual chromosomes may be arranged in an array according to morphologic characteristics.

    1. The resultant array of chromosomes is called a *karyotype*.

    2. A karyotype is made by photographing a cell in metaphase, cutting out the individual chromosomes, and arranging them in pairs in chart form according to predetermined morphologic criteria (i.e., karyotype; Fig. 2.8).

    3. The paired chromosomes are designated by numbers.

    4. In genetic shorthand, 46(XX) means that 46 chromosomes occur and have a female pattern; 46(XY) means that 46 chromosomes occur and have a male pattern.

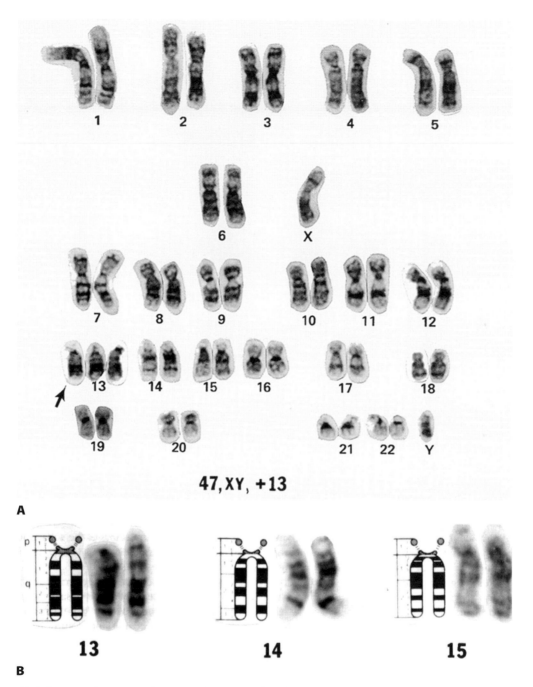

47, XY, +13

A

13   **14**   **15**

B

Fig. 2.8 Trisomy 13. **A,** Karyotype shows extra chromosome in 13 group (*arrow*). **B,** Karyotype shows banding in normal 13, 14, and 15 pairs of chromosomes. (**A** and **B,** Courtesy of Drs. BS Emanuel and WJ Mellman.)

B. To differentiate the chromosomes, special techniques are used, such as autoradiography or chromosomal band patterns, as shown with fluorescent quinacrine (see Fig. 2.8).

II. Chromosomes may be normal in total number (i.e., 46), but individual chromosomes may have structural alterations.

A. The genetic shorthand for structural alterations is as follows: p = short arm, q = long arm, + = increase in length, − = decrease in length, r = ring form, and t = translocation.

B. Therefore 46,18p− means a normal number of chromosomes, but one of the pair of chromosomes 18 has a deletion (decrease in length) of its short arms. Similarly, 46,18q− and 46,18r mean a normal number of chromosomes but a deletion of the long arms or a ring form, respectively, of one of the pair of chromosomes 18.

III. Chromosomes may also be abnormal in total number, either with too many or too few.

   A. For example, trisomy 13 has an extra chromosome in the 13 pair (three chromosomes instead of two) and may be written 47,13+, meaning 47 chromosomes with an extra chromosome (+) in the 13 group.

   B. Trisomy 18 may be written 47,18+, and trisomy 21 (Down's syndrome, or mongolism) may be written 47,21+.

   C. Finally, too few chromosomes may occur [e.g., in 45(X), Turner's syndrome, where only 45 chromosomes exist and one of the sex chromosomes is missing].

IV. A chromosomal abnormality has little to do with specific ocular malformations. In fact, except for the presence of cartilage in a ciliary-body coloboma in trisomy 13, no ocular malformations appear specific for any chromosomal abnormality.

Trisomy 8

See later, under *Mosaicism*.

Trisomy 13 (47,13+; Patau's Syndrome)

I. General information

   A. Trisomy 13 results from an extra chromosome in the 13 pair of autosomal chromosomes (i.e., one set of chromosomes exists in triplicate rather than as a pair; see Fig. 2.8).

     1. Caused by an accidental failure of disjunction of one pair of chromosomes during meiosis (meiotic nondisjunction).

     2. It has no sex predilection.

   B. The condition, present in 1 in 14000 live births, is usually lethal by age 6 months.

   C. Because the condition was described in the prekaryotype era, many names refer to the same entity: arhinencephaly, oculocerebral syndrome, encephalo-ophthalmic dysplasia, bilateral retinal dysplasia (Reese–Blodi–Straatsma syndrome), anophthalmia, and mesodermal dysplasia (cleft palate).

   D. Ocular anomalies, usually severe, occur in all cases (Fig. 2.9; see Fig. 2.15).

II. Systemic findings include mental retardation; low-set and malformed ears; cleft lip or palate or both; sloping forehead; facial angiomas; cryptorchidism; narrow, hyperconvex fingernails; fingers flexed or overlapping or both; polydactyly of hands or feet, or of both; posterior prominence of the heels ("rocker-bottom feet"); characteristic features of the dermal ridge pattern, including transverse palmar creases; cardiac and renal abnormalities; absence or hypoplasia of the olfactory lobes (arhinencephaly); bicornuate uterus; apneic spells; apparent deafness; minor motor seizures; and hypotonia.

III. Ocular findings

   A. Bilateral microphthalmos (<15 mm in greatest diameter) is common and may be extreme so as to mimic anophthalmos (i.e., clinical anophthalmos). In rare

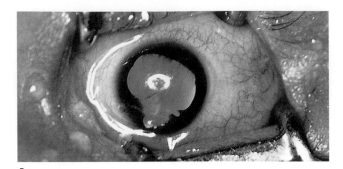

A

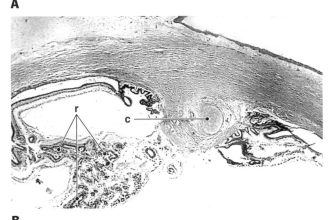

B

Fig. 2.9 Trisomy 13 (see also Fig. 2.15, synophthalmos). **A,** An inferior nasal iris coloboma and leukoria are present. **B,** A coloboma of the ciliary body is filled with mesenchymal tissue containing cartilage (c). Note the retinal dysplasia (r). In trisomy 13, cartilage is usually present in microphthalmic eyes smaller than 10 mm. (**A,** Courtesy of Dr. DB Shaffer; **B,** reported in Hoepner J, Yanoff M: *Am J Ophthalmol* 74:729, 1972. Copyright Elsevier 1972.)

instances, synophthalmos (cyclops, see later) or glaucoma can occur.

   B. Coloboma of the iris and ciliary body, cataract, and persistent hyperplastic primary vitreous are present in most (approximately 80%) of the eyes.

   C. Retinal dysplasia is found in at least 75% of eyes. Retinal folds and microcystoid degeneration of the neural retina are also common findings.

> When retinal dysplasia is unilateral and the other eye is normal, the condition is usually unassociated with trisomy 13 or other systemic anomalies.

   D. Central and peripheral dysgenesis of the cornea and iris (see pp. 260–263 in Chapter 8) is present in at least 60% of eyes.

IV. Histology

   A. The coloboma of the iris and ciliary body often contains a mesodermal connection between the sclera and the retrolental area. Cartilage is present in the mesodermal tissue in approximately 65% of eyes, most commonly when the eyes are small (i.e., <10 mm).

Ocular cartilage has also been reported in teratoid medulloepithelioma, in chromosome 18 deletion defect, in angiomatosis retinae, in synophthalmos, and in a unilateral anomalous eye in an otherwise healthy individual; however, in none of these conditions is the cartilage present in a coloboma of the ciliary body, as occurs in trisomy 13.

B. The cataract may be similar to that seen in rubella, Leigh's disease, and Lowe's syndrome, and shows retention of cell nuclei in the embryonic lens nucleus. Anterior subcapsular, anterior and posterior cortical, nuclear, and posterior subcapsular cataractous changes may also be seen.

Trisomy 18 (47,18+; Edwards' Syndrome)

I. General information
   A. Trisomy 18 has an extra chromosome in the 18 pair of autosomal chromosomes.
   B. The condition has approximately the same incidence as trisomy 13 (i.e., 1 in 14 000 live births) and similarly proves fatal at an early age. Girls are predominantly affected.
   C. Ocular malformations, usually minor, occur in approximately 50% of patients.
II. Systemic findings include mental retardation; low-set, malformed, and rotated ears; micrognathia; narrow palatal arch; head with prominent occiput, relatively flattened laterally; short sternum; narrow pelvis, often with luxation of hips; fingers flexed, with the index overlapping the third or the fifth overlapping the fourth; hallux short, dorsiflexed; characteristic features of the dermal ridge pattern, including an exceptionally high number of arches; cardiac and renal malformations; Meckel's diverticulum; heterotopic pancreatic tissue; severe debility; moderate hypertonicity.
III. Ocular findings tend to be minor and mainly involve the lids and bony orbit: narrow palpebral fissures, ptosis, epicanthus, hypoplastic supraorbital ridges, exophthalmos, hypertelorism or hypotelorism, and nystagmus.
   Rare ocular anomalies include nictitating membrane, corneal opacities, anisocoria, uveal and optic disc colobomas, cataract, microphthalmos, severe myopia, megalocornea, keratitis, scleral icterus, blue sclera, persistent hyaloid artery, increased or absent retinal pigmentation, and irregular retinal vascular pattern.
IV. Histology—especially related to hyperplasia, hypertrophy, and cellular abnormalities
   A. Corneal epithelium, mainly in the basal layer, may show cellular hypertrophy, swelling, disintegration, bizarre chromatin patterns, and atypical mitoses. Focal or diffuse hyperplasia of the corneal endothelium may be present.
   B. Posterior subcapsular cataracts, minor neural retinal changes (gliosis, hemorrhage), and optic atrophy may be seen.
      1. The retinal pigment epithelium (RPE) may show hypopigmented or hyperpigmented areas.

2. In addition, severe optic disc colobomas have been reported.

Trisomy 21 (47,21+; Down's Syndrome; Mongolism)

I. General information
   A. Trisomy 21 results from an extra chromosome in the 21 pair of autosomal chromosomes.
   B. The condition is the most common autosomal trisomy, with an incidence of 1 in 700 live births (in white populations). Major ocular malformations are rare.
II. Systemic findings include severe mental retardation; flat nasal bridge; an open mouth with a furrowed, protruding tongue and small, malformed teeth; prominent malformed ears with absent lobes; a flat occiput with a short, broad neck; loose skin at the back of the neck and over the shoulders (in early infancy); short, broad hands; short, curved little fingers with dysplastic middle phalanx; specific features of the dermal ridge, including a transverse palmar crease; cardiovascular defects; Apert's syndrome; and anomalous hematologic and biochemical traits.
III. Ocular findings include hypertelorism; oblique or arched palpebral fissures; epicanthus; ectropion; upper-eyelid eversion; speckled iris (*Brushfield spots*); esotropia, high myopia; rosy optic disc with excessive retinal vessels crossing its margin; generalized attenuation of fundus pigmentation regardless of iris coloration; peripapillary and patchy peripheral areas of pigment epithelial atrophy; choroidal vascular "sclerosis"; chronic blepharoconjunctivitis; keratoconus (sometimes acute hydrops); and lens opacities.
IV. Histology
   A. Brushfield spots consist of areas of relatively normal iris stroma that are surrounded by a ring of mild iris hypoplasia. They may also show focal stromal condensation or hyperplasia.
   B. A cataract may have abnormal anterior lens capsular excrescences similar to that seen in Lowe's and Miller's syndromes.
   C. Keratoconus may occur (see p. 302 in Chapter 8).

The aforementioned three trisomies are all autosomal chromosomal trisomies. An example of a sex chromosomal trisomy is *Klinefelter's syndrome* (47,XXY—a rare case of Klinefelter's syndrome associated with incontinentia pigmenti has been reported); the ocular pathologic process in this condition is not striking. In XYY syndrome (47,XYY), patients have normal height, psychological and social problems, gonadal atrophy, luxated lenses, and iris and choroid colobomas.

Triploidy

I. General information
   A. The anomaly of triploidy refers to that specific defect in which an individual's cells have 69 chromosomes (three of each autosome and three of each sex chromosome) instead of the normal component of 46 chromosomes (22 pairs of autosomes and two sex chromosomes).

B. Triploidy is common in spontaneous abortions but rare in live births.

Triploid mosaic individuals may survive to adult life. Survivors have some cell lines with 46 chromosomes and other cell lines with 69 chromosomes.

II. Systemic findings include triangular face; low-set ears; absent nose or nose with single nostril; cleft lip; cleft palate; single transverse palmar crease; talipes equinovarus; syndactyly; meningomyeloceles; cardiac abnormalities; genitourinary abnormalities; and adrenal hyperplasia.

III. Ocular findings include telecanthus; hypotelorism or hypertelorism; blepharophimosis; blepharoptosis; proptosis; microphthalmos; ectopic pupil; anophthalmos (unilateral); microcornea; and iris and cornea colobomas.

A. Normal eyes have also been reported.

IV. Histologic ocular findings include microcornea; iris and choroid colobomas; persistent hyaloid vasculature; retinal dysplasia; optic atrophy.

Chromosome 4 Deletion Defect

The chromosome 4 deletion defect (4p–) results from a partial deletion of the short arm of chromosome 14 (46,4p–). Also known as the *Wolf–Hirschhorn syndrome* (or *Wolf's syndrome*), it consists of profound mental retardation, antimongoloid slant, epicanthal folds, hypertelorism, ptosis, strabismus, nystagmus, cataract, and iris colobomas.

Chromosome 5 Deletion Defect (46,5p–; Cri du Chat Syndrome)

I. General information
A. Chromosome 5 deletion defect results from a deletion of part of the short arm of chromosome 5 (46,5p–). Only one of the chromosome 5 pair is affected.
B. Many newborn infants with the defect have an abnormal cry that sounds like a cat, hence the name *cri du chat syndrome*. The abnormal cry usually disappears as the child grows older.

Chromosome 4 deletion defect differs from cri du chat syndrome in not having the distinctive cry.

C. Affected patients usually live a normal lifespan.
II. Systemic findings include severe mental retardation; low-set ears; microcephaly; micrognathia; moon-shaped face; short neck; transverse palmar creases; scoliosis and kyphosis; curved fifth fingers; limitation of flexion or extension of fingers; and abnormalities of the cardiovascular system and kidneys.
III. Ocular findings include hypertelorism; epicanthus; mongoloid or antimongoloid eyelid fissures; exotropia; optic atrophy; tortuous retinal artery and veins; and pupils supersensitive to 2.5% methacholine.
IV. Significant histologic ocular findings have not been reported.

Chromosome 11 Deletion Defect

Deletion of chromosome 11p (aniridia–genitourinary–mental retardation syndrome—AGR triad) shows aniridia as its main ocular finding.

A. The chromosome band 11p13 has been associated with aniridia and *Wilms' tumor*.
B. Deletion of chromosome 11q results in trigonocephaly, broad nasal bridge and upturned nose, abnormal pinnae, carp mouth, and micrognathia; and numerous ocular abnormalities.

Chromosome 13 Deletion Defect

See pp. 734 and 735 in Chapter 18.

Chromosome 17 Deletion (17p11.2; Smith–Magenis Syndrome)

I. General information: the Smith–Magenis syndrome is a multiple-anomaly, mental retardation syndrome associated with deletions of a contiguous region of chromosome 17p11.2.
II. Systemic findings include dysmorphic facial features (brachycephaly, prominent forehead, synophrys, epicanthal folds, broad nasal bridge, ear anomalies, and prognathism), brachydactyly, self-injurious behaviors, autoamplexation (self-hugging) stereotypy, speech delay, sleep disturbances, mental and developmental retardation, and peripheral neuropathy.
III. Ocular findings include ptosis, telecanthus, strabismus, myopia, microcornea, iris abnormalities (Brushfield spots, colobomas), bilateral cataract, optic nerve hypoplasia, and retinal detachment.
IV. Significant histologic ocular findings have not been reported.

Chromosome 18 Deletion Defect (46,18p–; 46,18q–; or 46,18r; Partial 18 Monosomy) (Fig. 2.10)

I. General information
A. Chromosome 18 deletion defect results from a straight deletion of part of the short arm of chromosome 18 (46,18p–), part of the long arm (46,18q–), or parts or all of the long and short arms, resulting in a ring form (46,18r). Only one of the chromosome 18 pair is affected.
B. No specific ocular abnormalities relate to the different forms of deletion.
C. Affected patients usually live a normal lifespan.
II. Systemic findings include low-set ears; nasal abnormalities; external genital abnormalities; hepatosplenomegaly; cardiovascular abnormalities; and holoprosencephaly.
III. Ocular findings include hypertelorism; epicanthus; ptosis; strabismus; nystagmus; myopia; glaucoma; microphthalmos; microcornea; corneal opacities; posterior keratoconus; Brushfield spots; cataract; uveal colobomas, including

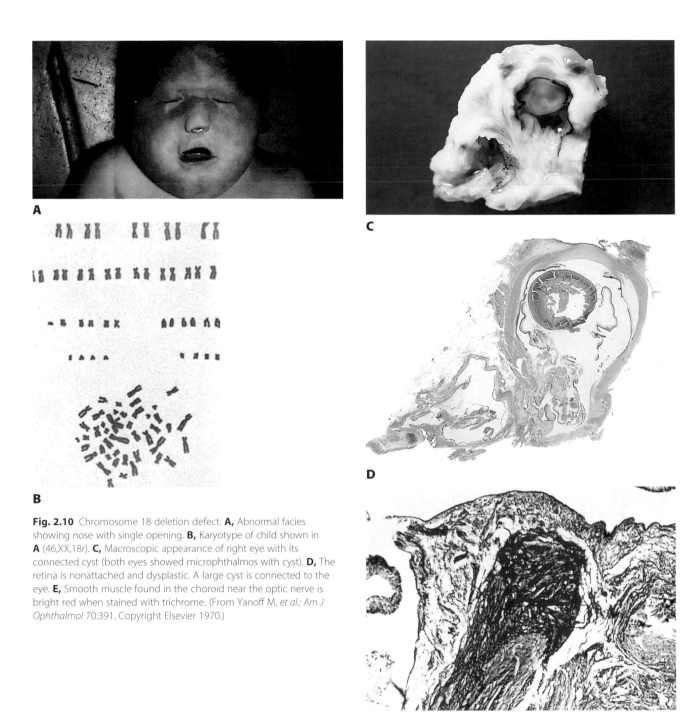

Fig. 2.10 Chromosome 18 deletion defect. **A,** Abnormal facies showing nose with single opening. **B,** Karyotype of child shown in **A** (46,XX,18r). **C,** Macroscopic appearance of right eye with its connected cyst (both eyes showed microphthalmos with cyst). **D,** The retina is nonattached and dysplastic. A large cyst is connected to the eye. **E,** Smooth muscle found in the choroid near the optic nerve is bright red when stained with trichrome. (From Yanoff M, *et al.: Am J Ophthalmol* 70:391. Copyright Elsevier 1970.)

microphthalmos with cyst; retinal abnormalities; optic atrophy; and "cyclops."

IV. Histology

    A. Microphthalmos with cyst (see p. 531 in Chapter 14) and uveal colobomas are discussed elsewhere (see p. 338 in Chapter 9).

    B. Intrascleral cartilage and intrachoroidal smooth muscle may be present anterior to and associated with a coloboma of the choroid.

    C. Other findings include hypoplasia of the iris, immature anterior-chamber angle, persistent tunica vasculosa lentis, cataract, retinal dysplasia, and neural retinal nonattachment.

Chromosome 47 Deletion Defect

I. Turner's syndrome (gonadal dysgenesis; Bonnevie–Ullrich syndrome; ovarian agenesis; and ovarian dysgenesis)

A. Turner's syndrome is usually caused by only one sex chromosome being present, the X chromosome (45,X), or is due to a mosaic (45,X;46,XY).

B. Some cases, however, are caused by an X long-arm isochromosome [46,X(Xqi)], X deletion defect of the short arm [46,X(Xp-)], or X deletion (partial or complete) of all arms, resulting in a ring chromosome [46,X(Xr)].

C. Ocular findings include epicanthus, blepharoptosis, myopia, strabismus, and nystagmus.

Noonan's syndrome (Bonnevie–Ullrich or Ullrich's syndrome; XX Turner phenotype or "female Turner"; and XY Turner phenotype or "male Turner") probably is an inherited condition in which the person (either male or female) phenotypically resembles Turner's syndrome but has a normal karyotype (46,XY or XX).

In Noonan's syndrome, ocular anomalies are even more frequent than in Turner's syndrome, and include antimongoloid slant of the palpebral fissures, hypertelorism, epicanthus, blepharoptosis, exophthalmos, keratoconus, high myopia, and posterior embryotoxon.

Mosaicism

I. General information

A. Chromosomal mosaicism refers to the presence of two or more populations of karyotypically distinct chromosomes in cells from a single individual.

Individuals with mixtures of cells derived from different zygotes are usually called *chimeras* (e.g., in a true hermaphrodite 46,XX; 46,XY), and the term *mosaic* is reserved for individuals who have cell mixtures arising from a single zygote.

B. Mosaicism may occur in most of the previously described chromosomal abnormalities.

II. Tetraploid–diploid mosaicism (92/46; Fig. 2.11)

A. In tetraploid–diploid mosaicism, two karyotypically distinct populations of cells exist: a large-size cell with increased DNA content containing 92 chromosomes (tetraploid), and a normal-size cell with a normal complement of 46 chromosomes (diploid). The condition is incompatible with longevity.

B. Systemic findings include micrognathia, horizontal palmar creases, deformities of the fingers and toes,

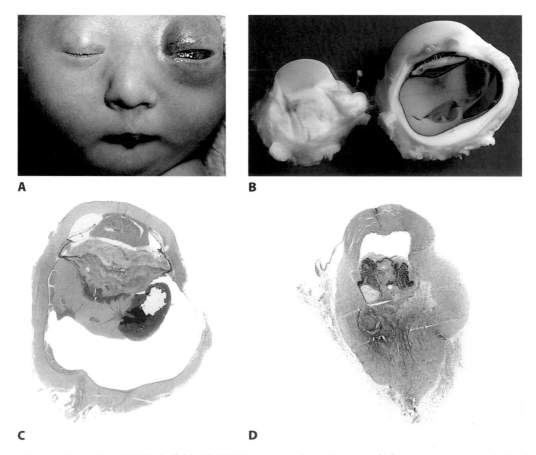

A

B

C

D

Fig. 2.11 Tetraploid–diploid mosaicism (92/46). **A,** Child with 92/46 had peculiar facies. Proptosis of left eye is secondary to orbital cellulitis and endophthalmitis. **B,** Gross appearance of opened, mildly microphthalmic right eye (on right) and markedly microphthalmic left eye (on left). **C** and **D,** Microscopic appearance of right (**C**) and left (**D**) eyes. Right eye shows peripheral anterior synechiae, ectropion uveae, cataract adherent to posterior cornea, and detached gliotic neural retina containing calcium. The left eye shows phthisis bulbi as a result of the endophthalmitis.

cardiovascular abnormalities, microcephalus, and fore-brain maturation arrest.

   C. Ocular anomalies include microphthalmos, corneal opacities, and leukokoria.

   D. Histologically, the eyes may show iris neovascularization, anterior peripheral synechiae, luxated and cataractous lens, nonattachment of the neural retina, and massive hyperplasia of the pigment epithelium.

  III. Most cases of trisomy 8(47,8+) are mosaics. The main ocular findings are strabismus and dense, geographic, stromal corneal opacities.

INFECTIOUS EMBRYOPATHY

Congenital Rubella Syndrome (Gregg's Syndrome)

   I. Congenital rubella syndrome consists of cataracts, cardiovascular defects, mental retardation, and deafness. The syndrome results from maternal rubella infection during pregnancy (50% of fetuses are affected if mother contracts rubella during first 4 weeks of pregnancy; 20% affected if contracted during first trimester).

Congenital varicella cataract has been reported in infants whose mothers had varicella during their pregnancies.

  II. Systemic findings include low birth weight; deafness; congenital heart defects (especially patent ductus arteriosus); central nervous system abnormalities; thrombocytopenic purpura; diabetes mellitus; osteomyelitis; dental abnormalities; pneumonitis; hepatomegaly; and genitourinary anomalies.

  III. Ocular findings include cataract; congenital glaucoma; iris abnormalities; and a secondary pigmentary retinopathy (Figs 2.12 and 2.13).

Rubella retinopathy is the most characteristic finding and, on rare occasions, may be progressive. Approximately 30% of patients with congenital rubella have cataracts and 9% have glaucoma. When rubella cataract is present, congenital glaucoma is present in 9% of cases; when congenital glaucoma is present, cataract is present in 33% of cases. Congenital rubella cataract and glaucoma therefore occur together at the frequency expected of coincidental events occurring independently. Subneural retinal neovascularization has been reported in patients between the ages of 10 and 18 years who have congenital rubella. Persistence of the rubella virus has been implicated in the delayed onset of Fuchs' heterochromic iridocyclitis.

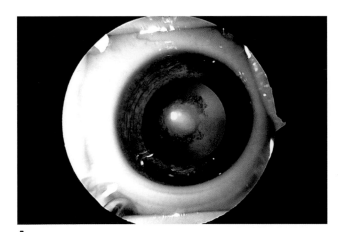

A

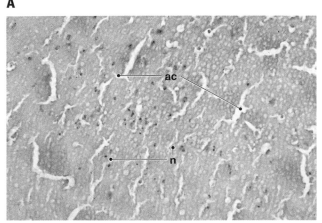

C

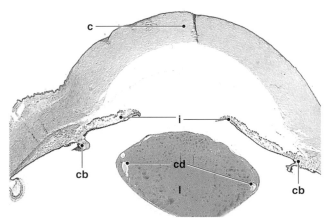

B

Fig. 2.12 Rubella. **A,** A dense nuclear cataract surrounded by a mild cortical cataract is seen in the red reflex. **B,** Cortical and nuclear cataract present. Note Lange's fold, which is an artifact of fixation, at the ora serrata on the left (c, cornea; i, iris; cb, ciliary body; l, lens; cd, cataractous degeneration). **C,** The dense nuclear cataract shows lens cell nuclei (n) retained in the embryonic nucleus (ac, artifactitious clefts in lens nucleus). (**A,** Courtesy of Dr. DB Schaffer; **B** and **C,** from Yanoff M, *et al.: Trans Am Acad Ophthalmol Otolaryngol* 72:896. Copyright Elsevier 1968.)

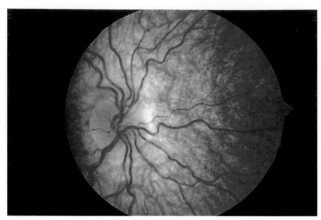

A

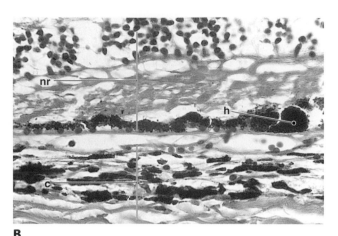

B

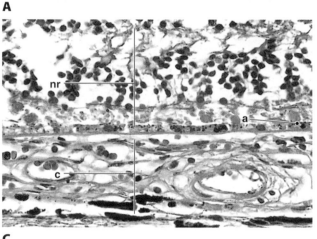

C

Fig. 2.13 Rubella. **A,** Fundus picture shows mottled "salt-and-pepper" appearance with both fine and coarse pigmentation. **B** and **C,** From same eye. Retinal pigment epithelium (RPE) shows areas of hyperpigmentation (**B**) (h, hypertrophied RPE) and hypopigmentation (**C**) (a, atrophy). The alternating areas of hyperpigmentation and hypopigmentation cause the salt-and-pepper appearance of the fundus (nr, neural retina; c, choroid). (Modified from Yanoff M: In Tasman W, ed: *Retinal Diseases in Children*, New York, Harper & Row, 1971:223–232. © Lippincott Williams & Wilkins.)

IV. The rubella virus can pass through the placenta, infect the fetus, and thereby cause abnormal embryogenesis.

> The rubella virus can survive in the lens for at least 3 years after birth. Surgery on rubella cataracts may release the virus into the interior of the eye and cause an endophthalmitis.

V. Histology
  A. Retention of lens cell nuclei in the embryonic lens nucleus is characteristic (but not pathognomonic, because it may also be seen in trisomy 13, Leigh's disease, and Lowe's syndrome) and posterior cortical lens degeneration and dysplastic lens changes may be seen.
  B. The iris shows a poorly developed dilator muscle and necrotic epithelium along with a chronic, nongranulomatous inflammatory reaction.

> The combination of the dilator muscle abnormality and chronic inflammation often causes the iris to dilate poorly and to appear leathery.

  C. The ciliary body shows pigment epithelium necrosis, macrophagic pigment phagocytosis, and a chronic non-granulomatous inflammatory reaction.

D. Atrophy and hypertrophy, frequently in alternating areas of RPE, are seen in most, if not all, cases, resulting in the clinically observed "salt-and-pepper" fundus of rubella retinopathy.
E. Other findings, such as Peters' anomaly and Axenfeld's anomaly, may occasionally be seen.
F. After cataract or iris surgery, complications caused by virus infection may cause a chronic nongranulomatous inflammatory reaction around lens remnants and secondary disruption of intraocular tissues with fibroblastic overgrowth, resulting in cyclitic membrane and neural retinal detachment.

Cytomegalic Inclusion Disease

See p. 77 in Chapter 4.

Congenital Syphilis

See p. 82 in Chapter 4 and p. 267 in Chapter 8.

Toxoplasmosis

See p. 88 in Chapter 4.

DRUG EMBRYOPATHY

Fetal Alcohol Syndrome (FAS) (Fig. 2.14)

I. FAS is a specific, recognizable pattern of malformations caused by alcohol's teratogenic effect secondary to maternal alcohol ingestion during pregnancy. The leading cause of mental retardation in the United States, FAS involves various neural crest-derived structures.
II. Systemic findings include developmental delay and retardation; midface hypoplasia (flattened nasal bridge and thin upper lip); smooth or long philtrum; and central nervous system manifestations, including microcephaly, hyperactivity, and seizures.
III. Ocular findings include narrow palpebral fissures, epicanthal folds, ptosis; blepharophimosis; strabismus; severe myopia; microcornea; Peters' anomaly (see Fig. 2.14); iris dysplasia; glaucoma; hypoplasia of the optic nerve head; and microphthalmia.
IV. Histology depends on the structures involved.

Thalidomide

I. Thalidomide ingestion during the first trimester of pregnancy may result in a condition known as *phocomelia*, the condition of having the limbs extremely shortened so that the feet or hands arise close to the trunk.
II. Ocular findings include ocular motility problems (e.g., Möbius' and Duane's syndromes), uveal colobomas, microphthalmos, and anophthalmos.
III. Histologically, hypoplasia of the iris and colobomas of the uvea and optic nerve may be seen.

Lysergic Acid Diethylamide (LSD)

I. LSD ingestion during the first trimester of pregnancy may result in multiple central nervous system and ocular abnormalities.
II. Central nervous system abnormalities: arhinencephaly; fusion of the frontal lobes; Arnold–Chiari malformation with hydrocephalus; and absence of the normal convolutional pattern in cerebral hemispheres and of foliar markings in the cerebellum.
III. Ocular findings include cataract and microphthalmia.
IV. Histologically, the lens may show anterior and posterior cortical degeneration and posterior migration of lens epithelial nuclei, and the neural retina may contain posterior retinal neovascularization and juvenile retinoschisis.

OTHER CONGENITAL ANOMALIES

Cyclopia and Synophthalmos

I. Cyclopia and synophthalmos (Fig. 2.15) are conditions in which anterior brain and midline mesodermal structures develop anomalously (holoprosencephaly—also called *arhinencephaly* and *holotelencephaly*).
A. The conditions are incompatible with life.
B. The prevalence is approximately 1 in 13 000 to 20 000 live births.

Chromosomal studies may show normal or abnormal chromosomes, usually trisomy 13, rarely 13q– and 18p– karyotypes. Embryologically, the gene, *ET*, acts as a transcription factor and causes the retina in the frog, *Xenopus laevis*, to emerge early as a single retinal field. A transcription factor is a DNA-binding protein that controls gene activity. A nearby piece of the embryo, the precordial mesoderm, suppresses retinal formation in the median region, resulting in the resolution of the single retinal field into two retinal primordia. The lack or deficiency of the splitting induction, as has been shown also with the *PAX6* gene in chick embryos, may result in either cyclops or synophthalmos in humans.

II. The prosencephalon fails to cleave, a large dorsal cyst develops, and midline structures such as the corpus callosum, septum pellucidum, olfactory lobes, and neurohypophysis are lacking.
III. The orbital region is grossly deformed from failure of the frontonasal bony processes to develop; the maxillary processes then fuse, resulting in an absent nasal cavity and a single central cavity or pseudo-orbit. The nose is usually present as a rudimentary proboscis above the pseudo-orbit.
IV. If only one eye is present (i.e., complete and total fusion of the two eyes) in the pseudo-orbit, the condition is called *cyclopia*.
A much more common situation is *synophthalmos*, wherein two eyes are present in differing degrees of fusion, but never complete fusion.

Even rarer is a supernumerary eye, called *diplophthalmos*.

V. Histology
A. In cyclopia, the one eye may be relatively normal, completely anomalous, or display all degrees of abnormality in between.
B. In synophthalmos, the partially fused two eyes may be relatively normal, totally anomalous, or display all degrees of abnormality in between.

Anencephaly

I. Anencephaly is the most serious congenital malformation occurring spontaneously in humans that is compatible with completion of pregnancy.
A. The condition is characterized by absence of the cranial vault.
B. The cerebral hemispheres are missing completely or reduced to small masses attached to the base of the skull.
C. The incidence is approximately 1 per 1000 in the general population.

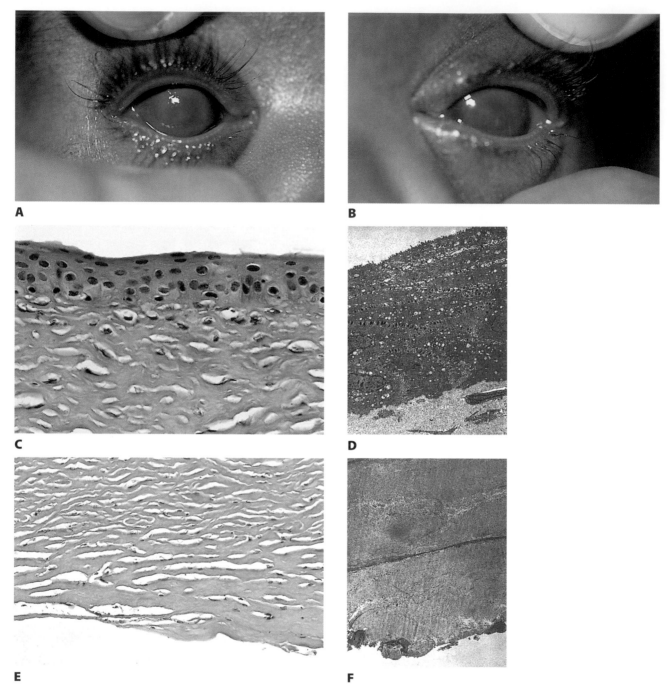

Fig. 2.14 Fetal alcohol syndrome. Child who was born with the fetal alcohol syndrome was seen because of cloudy corneas (**A** and **B**). Corneal grafts were performed. Light (**C**) and electron microscopy (**D**) of the anterior cornea show irregular epithelium and absence of Bowman's membrane. The epithelial cells project processes from their bases directly into anterior stroma. Light (**E**) and electron microscopy (**F**) of the posterior cornea show irregularity of stromal lamellae and absence of Descemet's membrane (Peters' anomaly). (From Sassani JW: Presented at the Eastern Ophthalmic Pathology Society meeting, 1991.)

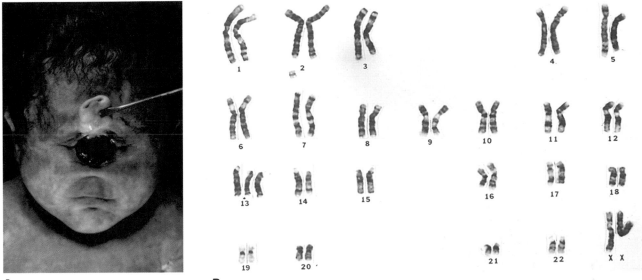

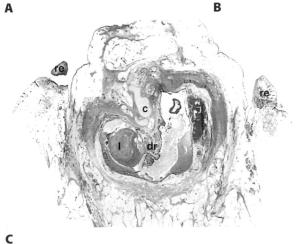

Fig. 2.15 Synophthalmos. **A,** The patient was born with clinical cyclops. When the proboscis is lifted, a single pseudo-orbit is seen clinically. Note the fairly well-formed eyelids under the proboscis. **B,** Karyotype from the same patient shows an extra chromosome (three instead of two) in the 13 group (trisomy 13). **C,** Histologic section shows that the condition is not true cyclops (a single eye), but the more commonly seen synophthalmos (partial fusion of the two eyes) (re, rudimentary eyelid; c, cartilage; l, lens; dr, dysplastic retina).

D. The condition appears to be caused by a defect in the development of the affected tissues at the fifth to 10th week of gestation, probably close to the fifth week.

II. Macroscopically, the eyes are normal.

A. Histologically, the main finding is hypoplasia (or atrophy) of the retinal ganglion cell and nerve fiber layers and of the optic nerve.

B. Uncommonly, uveal colobomas, retinal dysplasia, corneal dermoids, anterior-chamber angle anomalies, and vascular proliferative retinal changes may be seen.

Anophthalmos (Fig. 2.16)

I. The differentiation between anophthalmos (complete absence of the eye) and extreme microphthalmos (a rudimentary small eye) can be made only by the examination of serial histologic sections of the orbit. The differentiation cannot be made clinically.

The term *clinical anophthalmos* is applied to the condition where no eye can be found clinically.

II. Three types of anophthalmos are recognized:

A. Primary anophthalmos: caused by suppression of the optic anlage during the mosaic differentiation of the optic plate after formation of the rudiment of the forebrain (occurs before the 2-mm stage of embryonic development).

B. Secondary anophthalmos: caused by the complete suppression or grossly anomalous development of the entire anterior portion of the neural tube.

C. Consecutive or degenerative anophthalmos: caused by atrophy or degeneration of the optic vesicle after it has been formed initially.

Consecutive anophthalmos has been reported in the *focal dermal hypoplasia syndrome* (Goltz's syndrome, congenital cutis hypoplasia).

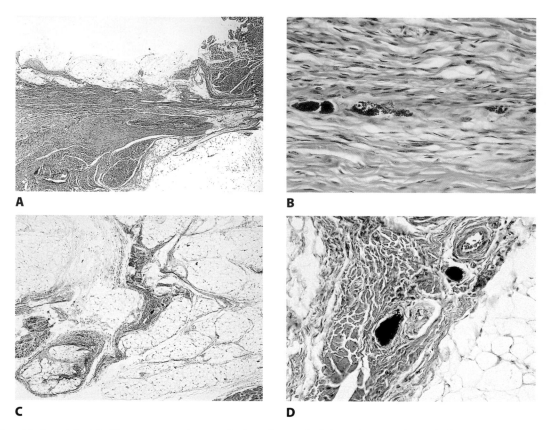

Fig. 2.16 Anophthalmos. Infant died from postoperative complications after repair of choanal atresia; other multiple systemic congenital anomalies were found. Apparent anophthalmos was present bilaterally. Serial sections of the orbital contents showed small nests of pigmented cells in each orbit (**A** and **B,** right orbit; **C** and **D,** left orbit) as only evidence of eyes. (From Sassani JW, Yanoff M: *Am J Ophthalmol* 83:43. Copyright Elsevier 1977.)

III. Histologically, serial sections of the orbit fail to show any ocular tissue.

Microphthalmos

I. Microphthalmos (see Figs 2.9–2.11) is a congenital condition in which the affected eye is smaller than normal at birth (<15 mm in greatest diameter; normal eye at birth varies between 16 and 19 mm).

> Microphthalmos, a congenital abnormality, should be differentiated from atrophia bulbi, an acquired condition wherein the eye is of normal size at birth but shrinks secondary to ocular disease. Rarely, the microphthalmos disproportionately affects the posterior ocular segment, called *posterior microphthalmos.*

II. Three types of microphthalmos are recognized:
  A. Pure microphthalmos alone (*nanophthalmos* or *simple microphthalmos*), wherein the eye is smaller than normal in size but has no other gross abnormalities except for a high lens/eye volume
    1. Such eyes are usually hypermetropic and may have macular hypoplasia.

    2. Nanophthalmic eyes may have thickened sclera and a tendency toward postoperative or spontaneous uveal effusion, secondary neural retinal, and choroidal detachments, and are susceptible to acute and chronic closed-angle glaucoma.

> A fraying or unraveling of the collagen fibril into its constituent 2- to 3-nm subunits may occur and may be related to an abnormality of glycosaminoglycan metabolism.

  B. Microphthalmos with cyst (see Fig. 2.10, p. 41 in Chapter 9, and p. 531 in Chapter 14).
  C. Microphthalmos associated with other systemic anomalies (e.g., in trisomy 13 and congenital rubella). This type of microphthalmos is discussed in the appropriate sections.
III. Histologically, the eye ranges from essentially normal in nanophthalmos to rudimentary in clinical anophthalmos, and all degrees of abnormality in between.

Walker–Warburg Syndrome

I. Walker–Warburg syndrome (Fig. 2.17) is a lethal, autosomal-recessive, oculocerebral disorder. The diagnosis is

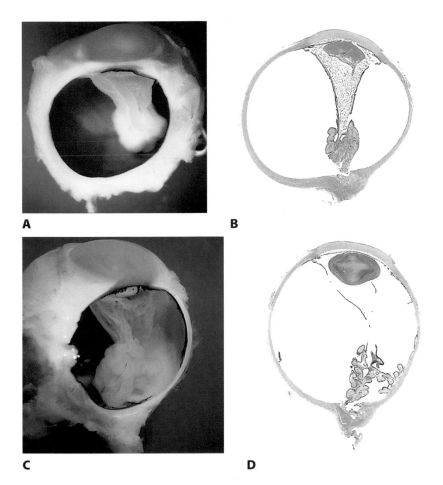

A

B

C

D

Fig. 2.17 Walker–Warburg syndrome. A 3890-g child at birth died at age 5 days. Autopsy showed type II lissencephaly ("smooth" brain), hydrocephalus, and occipital meningocele. Gross and microscopic examination of the right (**A** and **B**) and left (**C** and **D**) eyes showed bilateral Peters' anomaly, cataract, total neural retinal detachment, neural retinal dysplasia, and colobomatous malformation of the optic nerve. In addition, the right eye showed peripheral anterior synechiae, anterior displacement of the ciliary processes, and persistent hyperplastic primary vitreous. (From Yanoff M: Presented at the meeting of the Verhoeff Society, 1989.)

based on at least four abnormalities: type II lissencephaly; cerebellar malformation; retinal malformation; and congenital muscular dystrophy.

Type II lissencephaly (lissencephaly variant) consists of a smooth cerebral surface [agyria, polymicrogyria, and pachygyria (broad gyri)] and microscopic evidence of incomplete neuronal migration. Type I lissencephaly (classic lissencephaly) also consists of a smooth cerebral surface but excludes polymicrogyria. The most frequent cause of classical lissencephaly is deletions of the lissencephaly critical region in chromosome 17p13.3.

II. Previous names for Walker–Warburg syndrome include Warburg's syndrome, Walker's lissencephaly, Chemke's syndrome, cerebro-ocular–muscular syndrome, cerebro-ocular dysplasia muscular dystrophy, and cerebro-ocular dysgenesis.
III. Ocular findings include microphthalmia, microcornea, Peters' anomaly, anterior-chamber malformations, coloboma, cataracts, persistent hyperplastic primary vitreous, retinal detachment, retinal disorganization, and retinal dysplasia.

Oculocerebrorenal Syndrome of Miller

I. Miller's syndrome consists of Wilms' tumor, congenital nonfamilial aniridia* (Fig. 2.18), and genitourinary anomalies.
   A. Mental and growth retardation, microcephaly, and deformities of the pinna may be present.
   B. Aniridia and Wilms' tumor have been found in deletion of the short arm of chromosome 11 and are associated with the chromosome band 11p13.

Aniridia is caused by point mutations or deletions affecting the *PAX6* gene, located on chromosome 11p13. A rapid polymerase chain reaction-based DNA test can be performed to rule out chromosome 11p13 deletion and its high risk of Wilms' tumor in patients who have sporadic aniridia.

II. In patients without Wilms' tumor, the incidence of aniridia is 1 in 50 000; with Wilms' tumor, the incidence is 1 in 73; the cause of this association is not known.

---

*Aniridia *is a misnomer. The iris is not absent but is hypoplastic and rudimentary.*

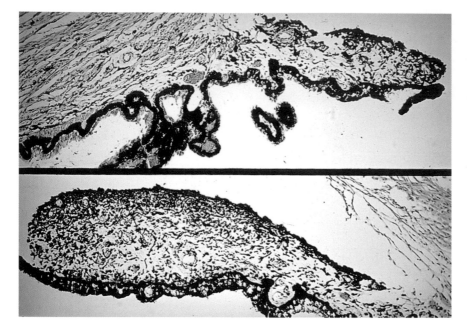

Fig. 2.18 Oculocerebrorenal syndrome of Miller. A 6½-month-old, mentally retarded, microcephalic child had clinical "aniridia" and congenital cortical and nuclear cataract in addition to bilateral Wilms' tumor. Top and bottom show different planes of section to demonstrate rudimentary iris having both uveal and neuroepithelial layers but lacking sphincter and dilator muscles. Almost all cases of clinical aniridia turn out to be iris hypoplasia. (From Zimmerman LE, Font RL: *JAMA* 196:684, 1966, with permission. © American Medical Association. All rights reserved.)

A case of two monozygous twins has been reported in which both had bilateral aniridia and cataracts, but only one had Wilms' tumor.

III. Histologically, the iris is hypoplastic. The cataract shows cortical degenerative changes and capsular excrescences similar to those seen in trisomy 21 and Lowe's syndrome.

Subacute Necrotizing Encephalomyelopathy (Leigh's Disease)

I. Leigh's disease is a mitochondrial enzymatic deficiency (point mutation at position 8993 in the adenosine triphosphatase subunit gene of mtDNA) that shares similar ocular findings to those seen in Kearns–Sayre syndrome, another mitochondrial disorder (see p. 539 in Chapter 14).
  A. Leigh's disease is a central nervous system disorder characterized by onset between 2 months and 6 years of age, feeding difficulties, failure to thrive, generalized weakness, hypotonia, and death in several weeks to 15 years.
  B. The disease has an autosomal-recessive inheritance pattern.
  C. The symptoms are nonspecific, and a familial history helps make the diagnosis.
II. The disorder is thought to result from inhibition of a thiamine-dependent enzymatic process and may be modified by increased thiamine intake.
III. Ocular findings include blepharoptosis, nystagmus, strabismus, Parinaud's syndrome, pupillary abnormalities, field defects, absent foveal retinal reflexes, ophthalmoplegia, and optic atrophy.

IV. Histologically, the eyes show glycogen-containing, lacy vacuolation of the iris pigment epithelium; no cataracts but persistence of lens cell nuclei in the deep cortex similar to that seen in congenital rubella, Lowe's syndrome, and trisomy 13 lenses; atrophy of neural retinal ganglion cell and nerve fiber layers; epineural retinal macular membranes; periodic acid–Schiff-positive macrophages; and optic atrophy.

Meckel's Syndrome (Dysencephalia Splanchnocystica; Gruber's Syndrome)

I. Meckel's syndrome consists of posterior encephalocele, polydactyly, and polycystic kidneys as the most important diagnostic features, but also includes sloping forehead, microcephaly, cleft lip and palate, and ambiguous genitalia. The condition has an autosomal-recessive inheritance pattern.
II. Ocular findings include cryptophthalmos, dysplasia of the palpebral fissure, hypertelorism or hypotelorism, clinical anophthalmos, microphthalmos (Fig. 2.19), Peters' anomaly, aniridia, retinal dysplasia, and cataract.
III. Histologically, microphthalmos, central and peripheral dysgenesis of cornea and iris, cataract, uveal colobomas, retinal dysplasia, and optic atrophy may be found.

The condition resembles trisomy 13, but the karyotype in Meckel's syndrome is normal.

Potter's Syndrome

I. Potter's syndrome is an idiopathic multisystem condition that includes bilateral agenesis or dysplasia of the kidneys, oligohydramnios, pulmonary hypoplasia, and a wizened facial appearance; 75% of cases occur in boys.

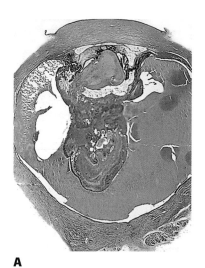
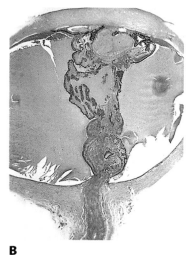

A **B**

Fig. 2.19 Meckel's syndrome. A 1460-g infant died an hour after birth. Both the right (**A**) and the left (**B**) eyes were microphthalmic and showed multiple congenital anomalies, including Peters' anomaly and retinal dysplasia. (From Daicker B: Presented at the meeting of the European Ophthalmic Pathology Society, 1982.)

II. Ocular findings include dilated intraocular blood vessels, sometimes simulating the vasoproliferative stage of retinopathy of prematurity.

Menkes' Kinky-Hair Disease

I. Menkes' kinky-hair disease is characterized by early, progressive psychomotor deterioration, seizures, spasticity, hypothermia, pili torti, bone changes resembling those of scurvy, tortuosity of cerebral arteries from fragmentation of the internal elastic lamina, and characteristic facies.
  A. The condition has an X-linked recessive inheritance pattern (defect on chromosome Xq12–13), but about one-third of cases are new mutations.
  B. Incidence is 1 in 100 000 to 25 000 live births
II. The disease is caused by a generalized copper deficiency in the body.
  A. Levels of serum copper, copper oxidase, and ceruloplasmin are abnormally low.
  B. A defect is present in the intracellular transport of copper in the gut epithelium and in the release of copper from these cells into the blood.
  C. The lower copper levels in cells and tissue fluid appear to interfere seriously with certain enzyme systems and the maintenance of neural cells and hair.
III. Ocular findings include aberrant lashes, iris anterior stromal hypoplasia, nystagmus, iris depigmentation, tortuosity of retinal vessels, and an abnormal electroretinogram that shows moderately decreased photopic β waves (measure of cone function) and almost no scotopic β waves (measure of rod function) or visually evoked response.
IV. Histologically, the main findings consist of diminished neural retinal ganglion cells and a thinned nerve fiber layer, decrease in and demyelination of optic nerve axons, loss of pigment from retinal and iris pigment epithelial cells, and microcysts of iris pigment epithelial cells (Fig. 2.20).

Aicardi's Syndrome

I. Aicardi's syndrome is characterized by infantile spasms, agenesis of the corpus callosum, severe mental retardation, and an X-linked inheritance pattern (a rare male 47,XXY has been reported).
II. Clinically, microphthalmia and a characteristic chorioretinopathy with lacunar defects are noted.
III. Histologically, hypoplasia of the optic nerves, coloboma of the juxtapapillary choroid and optic disc, neural retinal detachment, retinal dysplasia, chorioretinal lacunae with focal thinning, and atrophy of the RPE and choroid have been found.

Dwarfism

I. Ocular anomalies occur frequently in many different types of dwarfism.
  A. Dwarfism secondary to mucopolysaccharidoses (see p. 298 in Chapter 8)
  B. Dwarfism secondary to osteogenesis imperfecta (see p. 314 in Chapter 8)
  C. Dwarfism secondary to stippled epiphyses (Conradi's syndrome) with cataracts
  D. Dwarfism secondary to Cockayne's syndrome with retinal degeneration and optic atrophy (see p. 447 in Chapter 11)
  E. Dwarfism secondary to Lowe's syndrome (see p. 367 in Chapter 10)
  F. The syndrome of dwarfism, myotonia, diffuse bone disease, myopia, and blepharophimosis
  G. The syndrome of dwarfism with disproportionately short legs, reduced joint mobility, hyperopia, glaucoma, cataract, and retinal detachment
  H. The syndrome of dwarfism, congenital trichomegaly, mental retardation, and retinal pigmentary degeneration
  I. Achondroplastic dwarfism with mesodermal dysgenesis of cornea and iris

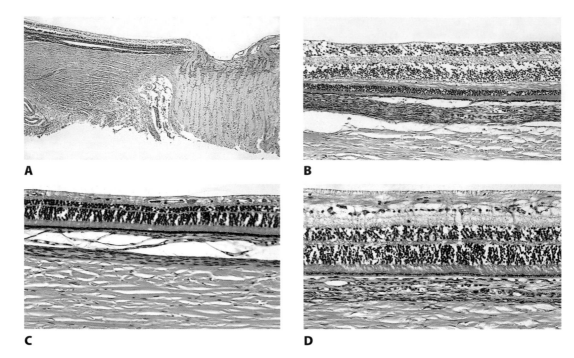

Fig. 2.20 Menkes' kinky-hair disease. **A,** Section of eye from child who died from Menkes' kinky-hair disease shows apparently normal optic nerve and temporal retina. **B,** Macular retina also appears normal. **C,** Neural retina temporal to macula shows loss of ganglion cells. **D,** Nasal neural retina shows near-normal number of ganglion cells but an increased cellularity of the nerve fiber layer. (Case courtesy of Prof. D Toussaint.)

J. Ateleiotic dwarfism with soft, wrinkled skin of lids
K. Diastrophic dwarfism with mild retinal pigment epithelial disturbance in macular and perimacular areas
L. Spondyloepiphyseal dysplastic dwarfism with retinal degeneration (including lattice degeneration), retinal detachment, myopia, and cataracts
M. Cartilage-hair hypoplastic dwarfism with fine, sparse hair of eyebrows and cilia and trichiasis
II. The histologic features are described in the appropriate sections under the individual tissues.

Other Syndromes

I. Other syndromes include *Williams syndrome* ("elfin" facies, congenital cardiac defects that may include supravalvular aortic stenosis, infantile idiopathic hypercalcemia, developmental delay, stellate anterior iris stromal pattern, retinal vessel abnormalities, and strabismus); *CHARGE syndrome* (coloboma of the uvea and optic nerve, heart defects, atresia of the choanae, retarded growth and development, genital hypoplasia, and ear anomalies); *Klippel–Trenaunay–Weber syndrome* (triad of port-wine hemangiomas or vascular nevi of skin, varicose veins, and soft-tissue and bony hypertrophy; also ocular vascular findings and glaucoma).
II. Many other congenital syndromes occur and are discussed in their appropriate sections.

BIBLIOGRAPHY

Angiomatosis Retinae

Akiyama H, Tanaka T, Itakura H *et al.*: Inhibition of ocular angiogenesis by an adenovirus carrying the human von Hippel–Lindau tumor-supressor gene in vivo. *Invest Ophthalmol Vis Sci* 45:1289, 2004

Chan C-C, Vortmeyer AO, Chew EY *et al.*: VHL gene deletion and enhanced VEGF gene expression detected in the stromal cells of retinal angioma. *Arch Ophthalmol* 117:625, 1999

Filling-Katz MR, Choyke PL, Oldfield E *et al.*: Central nervous system involvement in von Hippel–Lindau disease. *Neurology* 41:41, 1991

Grossniklaus HE, Thomas JW, Vigneswaran DMD *et al.*: Retinal hemangioblastoma: A histologic, immunohistochemical, and ultra-structural evaluation. *Ophthalmology* 99:140, 1992

Liang X, Shen D, Huang Y *et al.*: Molecular pathology and CXCR4 expression in surgically excised retinal hemangioblastomas associated with von Hippel–Lindau disease. Ophthalmology 114:147, 2007

McCabe CM, Flynn HW, Shields CL *et al.*: Juxtapapillary capillary hemangiomas: clinical features and visual acuity outcomes. *Ophthalmology* 107:2240, 2000

Patel RJ, Appukuttan B, Ott S *et al.*: DNA-based diagnosis of the von Hippel–Lindau syndrome. *Am J Ophthalmol* 258:166, 2000

Schmidt D, Neumann HPH: Retinal vascular hamartoma in von Hippel–Lindau disease. *Arch Ophthalmol* 113:1163, 1995

Singh AD, Nouri M., Shields CL *et al.*: Retinal capillary hemangiomas: A comparison of sporadic cases and cases associated with von Hippel–Lindau disease. *Ophthalmology* 108:1907, 2001

Singh AD, Shields CL, Shields JA: von Hippel–Lindau disease. *Surv Ophthalmol* 46:95, 2001

Singh AD, Shields JA, Shields CL: Hereditary retinal capillary hemangioma. Hereditary (von Hippel–Lindau disease) or nonhereditary? *Arch Ophthalmol* 119:232, 2001

Tse JYM, Wong JHC, Lo K-W *et al.*: Molecular genetic analysis of the von Hippel–Lindau disease tumor suppressor gene in familial and sporadic cerebellar hemangioblastomas. *Am J Clin Pathol* 107:459, 1997

Meningocutaneous Angiomatosis

Amirikia A, Scott IU, Murray TG: Bilateral diffuse choroidal hemangiomas with unilateral facial nevus flammeus in Sturge–Weber syndrome. *Am J Ophthalmol* 130:362, 2000

Lever WF, Schaumberg-Lever G: *Histopathology of the Skin*. Philadelphia, JB Lippincott, 1990:689–691

Shin GS, Demer JL: Retinal arteriovenous communications associated with features of the Sturge–Weber syndrome. *Am J Ophthalmol* 117:115, 1994

Teekhasaenee C, Ritch RF: Glaucoma in phakomatosis pigmentovascularis. *Ophthalmology* 104:150, 1997

Witschel H, Font RL: Hemangioma of the choroid: A clinicopathologic study of 71 cases and a review of the literature. *Surv Ophthalmol* 20:415, 1976

Neurofibromatosis

Bosch MM, Boltshauser E, Harpes P *et al.*: Ophthalmologic findings and long-term course in patients with neurofibromatosis type 2. *Am J Ophthalmol* 141:1068, 2006

Bosch MM, Wichmann WW, Boltshauser E *et al.*: Optic nerve sheath meningiomas in patients with neurofibromatosis type 2. *Arch Ophthalmol* 124:379, 2006

Bouzas EA, Parry DM, Eldridge R *et al.*: Familial occurrence of combined pigment epithelial and retinal hamartomas associated with neurofibromatosis 2. *Retina* 12:103, 1992

Brandi ML, Weber G, Svensson A *et al.*: Homozygotes for the autosomal dominant neoplasia syndrome (MEN1). *Am J Hum Genet* 53:1167, 1993

Charles SJ, Moore AT, Yates JRW *et al.*: Lisch nodules in neurofibromatosis type 2. *Arch Ophthalmol* 107:1571, 1989

Dennehy PJ, Feldman GL, Kambouris M *et al.*: Relationship of familial prominent corneal nerves and lesions of the tongue resembling neuromas to multiple endocrine neoplasia type 2B. *Am J Ophthalmol* 120:456, 1995

Destro M, D'Amico DJ, Gragoudas ES *et al.*: Retinal manifestations of neurofibromatosis: Diagnosis and management. *Arch Ophthalmol* 109:662, 1991

Eubanks PJ, Sawicki MP, Samara GJ *et al.*: Putative tumor-suppressor gene on chromosome 11 is important in sporadic endocrine tumor formation. *Am J Surg* 167:180, 1994

Fink A, Lapidot M, Spierer A: Ocular manifestations in multiple endocrine neoplasia type 2b. *Am J Ophthalmol* 126:305, 1998

Gutmann DH, Aylsworth A, Carey JC *et al.*: The diagnostic evaluation and multidisciplinary management of neurofibromatosis 1 and neurofibromatosis 2. *JAMA* 278:51, 1997

van Heyningen V: Genetics. One gene—four syndromes (news). *Nature* 367:319, 1994

Honavar SG, Singh AD, Shields CL *et al.*: Iris melanoma in a patient with neurofibromatosis. *Surv Ophthalmol* 45:231, 2000

Imes RK, Hoyt WF: Magnetic resonance imaging signs of optic nerve gliomas in neurofibromatosis 1. *Am J Ophthalmol* 111:729, 1991

Kalina PH, Bartley GB, Campbell RJ *et al.*: Isolated neurofibromas of the conjunctiva. *Am J Ophthalmol* 111:694, 1991

Kinoshita S, Tanaka F, Ohashi Y *et al.*: Incidence of prominent corneal nerves in multiple endocrine neoplasia type 2A. *Am J Ophthalmol* 111:307, 1991

Landau K, Dossetor FM, Hoyt WF *et al.*: Retinal hamartomas in neurofibromatosis 2. *Arch Ophthalmol* 108:328, 1990

Listernick R, Charrow J, Greenwald M *et al.*: Natural history of optic pathway tumors in children with neurofibromatosis type 1: A longitudinal study. *J Pediatr* 125:63, 1994

Liu GT, Brodsky MC, Phillips PC, *et al.*: Optic radiation involvement in optic pathway gliomas in neurofibromatosis. *Am J Ophthalmol* 137:407, 2004

Liu GT, Schatz NJ, Curtin VT *et al.*: Bilateral extraocular muscle metastases in Zollinger–Ellison syndrome. *Arch Ophthalmol* 112:451, 1994

Lubs M-LE, Bauer MS, Formas ME *et al.*: Lisch nodules in neurofibromatosis type 1. *N Engl J Med* 324:1264, 1991

Massry GG, Morgan CF, Chung SM: Evidence of optic pathway gliomas after previously negative neuroimaging. *Ophthalmology* 104:930, 1997

Meyer DR, Wobig JL: Bilateral localized orbital neurofibromas. *Ophthalmology* 99:1313, 1992

Moir DT, Dorman TE, Xue F *et al.*: Rapid identification of overlapping YACs in the MEN2 region of human chromosome 10 by hybridization with Alu element-mediated PCR products. *Gene* 136:177, 1993

Perry HD, Font RL: Iris nodules in von Recklinghausen's neurofibromatosis: Electron microscopic confirmation of their melanocytic origin. *Arch Ophthalmol* 100:1635, 1982

Pinna A, Demontis S, Maltese G *et al.*: Absence of the greater sphenoid wing in neurofibromatosis 1. *Arch Ophthalmol* 123:1454, 2005

Ragge NK, Baser ME, Klein J *et al.*: Ocular abnormalities in neurofibromatosis 2. *Am J Ophthalmol* 120:634, 1995

Rehany U, Rumeldt S: Iridocorneal melanoma associated with type 1 neurofibromatosis: A clinicopathologic study. *Ophthalmology* 106:614, 1999

Rettele GA, Brodsky MC, Merin LM *et al.*: Blindness, deafness, quadriparesis, and a retinal hamartoma: The ravages of neurofibromatosis 2. *Surv Ophthalmol* 41:135, 1996

Santoro M, Carlomagno F, Romano A *et al.*: Activation of RET as a dominant gene by germline mutations of MEN2A and MEN2B. *Science* 267:381, 1995

Sedun F, Hinton DR, Sedun AA: Rapid growth of an optic nerve ganglioglioma in a patient with neurofibromatosis 1. *Ophthalmology* 103:794, 1996

Shields JA, Shields CL, Perez N: Choroidal metastasis from medullary thyroid carcinoma in multiple endocrine neoplasia. *Am J Ophthalmol* 134, 607, 2002

Wiznia RA, Freedman JK, Mancini AD *et al.*: Malignant melanoma of the choroid in neurofibromatosis. *Am J Ophthalmol* 86:684, 1978

Yanoff M, Sharaby ML: Multiple endocrine neoplasia type IIB. *Arch Ophthalmol* 114:228, 1996

Yanoff M, Zimmerman LE: Histogenesis of malignant melanomas of the uvea: III. The relationship of congenital ocular melanocytosis and neurofibromatosis to uvea melanomas. *Arch Ophthalmol* 77:331, 1967

Zhu Y, Ghosh P, Charney P *et al.*: Neurofibromas in NF1: Schwann cell origin and role of tumor environment. *Science* 296:920, 2002

Tuberous Sclerosis

Eagle RC Jr, Shields JA, Shields CL *et al.*: Hamartomas of the iris and ciliary epithelium in tuberous sclerosis. *Arch Ophthalmol* 118:711, 2000

Gündüz K, Eagle RC Jr, Shields CL *et al.*: Invasive giant cell astrocytoma of the retina in a patient with tuberous sclerosis. *Ophthalmology* 106:639, 1999

Margo CE, Barletta JP, Staman JA: Giant cell astrocytoma of the retina in tuberous sclerosis. *Retina* 13:155, 1993

Milot J, Michaud J, Lemieux N et al.: Persistent hyperplastic primary vitreous with retinal tumor in tuberous sclerosis: Report of a case including tumoral immunuhistochemistry and cytogenetic analyses. *Ophthalmology* 106:614, 1999

Shields JA, Eagle RC Jr, Shields CL et al.: Aggressive retinal astrocytomas in 4 patients with tuberous sclerosis complex. *Arch Ophthalmol* 123:856, 2005

von Slegtenhorst M, de Hoogt R, Hermans C et al.: Identification of the tuberous sclerosis gene TSC1 on chromosome 9q34. *Science* 277:805, 1997

Zimmer-Galler IE, Robertson DM: Long-term observation of retinal lesions in tuberous sclerosis. *Am J Ophthalmol* 119:318, 1995

Other Phakomatoses

Buckley RH: Immunodeficiency diseases. *JAMA* 268:2797, 1992

Carbonari M, Cherchi M, Paganelli R et al.: Relative increase in T cells expressing the gamma/delta rather than the alpha/beta receptor in ataxia-telangiectasia. *N Engl J Med* 322:73, 1990

Danis R, Appen RE: Optic atrophy and the Wyburn–Mason syndrome. *J Clin Neuroophthalmol* 4:91, 1984

Effron L, Zakov ZN, Tomask RL: Neovascular glaucoma as a complication of the Wyburn–Mason syndrome. *J Clin Neuroophthalmol* 5:95, 1985

Farr AK, Shalev B, Crawford TO et al.: Ocular manifestations of ataxia-telangiectasia. *Am J Ophthalmol* 134:891, 2002

Font RL, Ferry AP: The phakomatoses. *Int Ophthalmol Clin* 12:1, 1972

Hopen G, Smith JL, Hoff JT et al.: The Wyburn–Mason syndrome: concomitant chiasmal and fundus vascular malformations. *J Clin Neuroophthalmol* 3:53, 1983

Mansour AM, Wells CG, Jampol LM et al.: Ocular complications of arteriovenous communication of the retina. *Arch Ophthalmol* 107:232, 1989

Shin GS, Demer JL: Retinal arteriovenous communications associated with features of the Sturge–Weber syndrome. *Am J Ophthalmol* 117:115, 1994

Wyburn-Mason R: Arteriovenous aneurysm of the midbrain and retina with facial naevus and mental changes. *Brain* 66:12, 1943

Chromosomal Trisomy Defects

Fowell SAM, Greenwald MJ, Prendiville JS et al.: Ocular findings of incontinentia pigmenti in a male infant with Klinefelter syndrome. *J Pediatr Ophthalmol Strabismus* 29:180, 1992

Frangoulis M, Taylor D: Corneal opacities: A diagnostic feature of the trisomy 8 mosaic syndrome. *Br J Ophthalmol* 67:619, 1983

Guterman C, Abboud E, Mets MB: Microphthalmos with cyst and Edward's syndrome. *Am J Ophthalmol* 109:228, 1990

Hoepner J, Yanoff M: Craniosynostosis and syndactylism (Apert's syndrome) associated with a trisomy 21 mosaic. *J Pediatr Ophthalmol* 8:107, 1971

Hoepner J, Yanoff M: Ocular anomalies in trisomy 13–15: An analysis of 13 eyes with two new findings. *Am J Ophthalmol* 74:729, 1972

Jacoby B, Reed JW, Cashwell LF: Malignant glaucoma in a patient with Down's syndrome and corneal hydrops. *Am J Ophthalmol* 110:434, 1990

Lueder GT: Clinical ocular abnormalities in infants with trisomy 13. *Am J Ophthalmol* 141:1057, 2006

McDermid HE, Duncan AMV, Brasch KR et al.: Characterization of the supernumerary chromosome in cat eye syndrome. *Science* 232:646, 1986

Robb RM, Marchevsky A: Pathology of the lens in Down's syndrome. *Arch Ophthalmol* 96:1039, 1978

Seiberth V, Kachel W, Knorz MC et al.: Ophthalmic findings in partial monosomy 4p (Wolf syndrome) in combination with partial trisomy 10p. *Am J Ophthalmol* 117:411, 1994

Traboulsi EI, Levine E, Mets MB et al.: Infantile glaucoma in Down's syndrome (trisomy 21). *Am J Ophthalmol* 105:389, 1988

Yanoff M, Font RL, Zimmerman LE: Intraocular cartilage in a microphthalmic eye of an otherwise healthy girl. *Arch Ophthalmol* 81:238, 1969

Yanoff M, Frayer WC, Scheie HG: Ocular findings in a patient with 13–15 trisomy. *Arch Ophthalmol* 70:372, 1963

Triploidy and Chromosomal Deletion Abnormalities

Bonetta L, Kuehn SE, Huang A et al.: Wilms tumor locus on 11p13 defined by multiple CpG island-associated transcripts. *Science* 250:994, 1990

Cameron JD, Yanoff M, Frayer WC: Turner's syndrome and Coats' disease. *Am J Ophthalmol* 78:852, 1974

Chen RM, Lupski JR, Greenberg F et al.: Ophthalmic manifestations of Emith–Magenis syndrome. *Ophthalmology* 103:1084, 1996

Chrousos GA, Ross JL, Chrousos G et al.: Ocular findings in Turner syndrome: A prospective study. *Ophthalmology* 91:926, 1984

Dowdy SF, Fasching CL, Araujo D et al.: Suppression of tumorigenicity in Wilms tumor by the p15.5–p14 region of chromosome 11. *Science* 254:293, 1991

Finger PT, Warren FA, Gelman YP et al.: Adult Wilms' tumor metastatic to the choroids of the eye. *Ophthalmology* 109:2134, 2002

Fulton AB, Howard RO, Albert DM et al.: Ocular findings in triploidy. *Am J Ophthalmol* 84:859, 1977

Chromosomal Deletion Defects

Gupta SK, deBecker I, Guernsey DL et al.: Polymerase chain-reaction based risk assessment for Wilms tumor in sporadic aniridia. *Am J Ophthalmol* 125:687, 1998

Gupta SK, deBecker I, Tremblay F et al.: Genotype/phenotype correlations in aniridia. *Arch Ophthalmol* 126:203, 1998

Huang A, Campbell CE, Bonetta L et al.: Tissue, developmental, and tumor-specific expression of divergent transcripts in Wilms tumor. *Science* 250:991, 1990

Küchle M, Kraus J, Rummelt C et al.: Synophthalmia and holoprosencephaly in chromosome 18p deletion defect. *Arch Ophthalmol* 109:136, 1991

Meyer DR, Selkin RP: Ophthalmic manifestations of the chromosome 11q deletion syndrome. *Am J Ophthalmol* 115:673, 1993

Rauscher FJ III, Morris JF, Tournay OE et al.: Wilms' tumor locus zinc finger protein to the ERG-1 consensus sequence. *Science* 250:1259, 1990

Schechter RJ: Ocular findings in a newborn with cri du chat syndrome. *Ann Ophthalmol* 10:339, 1978

Schwartz DE: Noonan's syndrome associated with ocular abnormalities. *Am J Ophthalmol* 73:955, 1972

Seiberth V, Kachel W, Knorz MC et al.: Ophthalmic findings in partial monosomy 4p (Wolf syndrome) in combination with partial trisomy 10p. *Am J Ophthalmol* 117:411, 1994

Wright LL, Schwartz MF, Schwartz S et al.: An unusual ocular finding associated with chromosome 1q deletion syndrome. *Pediatrics* 77:786, 1986

Yanoff M, Rorke LB, Niederer BS: Ocular and cerebral abnormalities in chromosome 18 deletion defect. *Am J Ophthalmol* 70:391, 1970

Mosaicism

Hoepner J, Yanoff M: Craniosynostosis and syndactylism (Apert's syndrome) associated with a trisomy 21 mosaic. *J Pediatr Ophthalmol* 8:107, 1971

Yanoff M, Rorke LB: Ocular and central nervous system findings in tetraploid-diploid mosaicism. *Am J Ophthalmol* 75:1036, 1973

Infectious Embryopathy

Arnold JJ, McIntosh EDG, Martin FJ et al.: A fifty-year follow-up of ocular defects in congenital rubella: Late ocular manifestations. *Aust N Z J Ophthalmol* 22:1, 1994

Cotlier E: Congenital varicella cataract. *Am J Ophthalmol* 86:627, 1978

Gregg NM: Congenital cataract following German measles in the mother. *Trans Ophthalmol Soc Aust* 3:35, 1941

Quentin CD, Reiber H: Fuchs heterochromi cyclitis: rubella virus antibodies and genome in aqueous humor. *Am J Ophthalmol* 138:45, 2004

Yanoff M, Schaffer DB, Scheie HG: Rubella ocular syndrome: Clinical significance of viral and pathologic studies. *Trans Am Acad Ophthalmol Otolaryngol* 72:896, 1968

Drug Embryopathy

Bogdanoff B, Rorke LB, Yanoff M et al.: Brain and eye abnormalities: Possible sequelae to prenatal use of multiple drugs including LSD. *Am J Dis Child* 123:145, 1972

Chan CC, Fishman M, Egbert PR: Multiple ocular anomalies associated with maternal LSD ingestion. *Arch Ophthalmol* 96:282, 1978

Edward DP, Li J, Sawaguchi S et al.: Diffuse corneal clouding in siblings with fetal alcohol syndrome. *Am J Ophthalmol* 115:484, 1993

Miller MT, Strömland K: Ocular motility in thalidomide embryopathy. *J Pediatr Ophthalmol Strabismus* 28:47, 1991

Streissguth AP, Aase JM, Clarren SK et al.: Fetal alcohol syndrome in adolescents and adults. *JAMA* 265:1961, 1991

Other Congenital Anomalies

Boynton JR, Pheasant TR, Johnson BL et al.: Ocular findings in Kenny's syndrome. *Arch Ophthalmol* 97:896, 1979

Brunquell PJ, Papale JH, Horton JC et al.: Sex-linked hereditary bilateral anophthalmos: Pathologic and radiologic correlation. *Arch Ophthalmol* 102:108, 1984

Chestler RJ, France TD: Ocular findings in CHARGE syndrome. *Ophthalmology* 95:1613, 1988

Cohen SM, Brown FR III, Martyn L et al.: Ocular histopathologic and biochemical studies of the cerebrohepatorenal syndrome (Zellweger's syndrome) and its relationship to neonatal adrenoleukodystrophy. *Am J Ophthalmol* 96:488, 1983

Dobyns WB, Pagon RA, Armstrong D et al.: Diagnostic criteria for Walker–Warburg syndrome. *Am J Med Genet* 32:195, 1989

Dobyns WB, Reiner O, Carrozo R et al.: Lissencephaly: A human brain malformation associated with deletion of the LIS1 gene located at chromosome 17p13. *JAMA* 270:2838, 1993

Dooling EC, Richardson EP: Ophthalmoplegia and Ondine's curse. *Arch Ophthalmol* 95:1790, 1977

Ferreira RC, Heckenlively JR, Menkes JH et al.: Menkes disease: New ocular and electroretinographic findings. *Ophthalmology* 105:1076, 1998

Font RL, Marines HM, Cartwright J Jr et al.: Aicardi syndrome: A clinicopathologic case report including electron microscopic observations. *Ophthalmology* 98:1727, 1991

Fries PD, Katowitz JA: Congenital craniofacial anomalies of ophthalmic importance. *Surv Ophthalmol* 35:87, 1990

Frydman M, Kauschansky A, Leshem I et al.: Oculo-palato-cerebral dwarfism: A new syndrome. *Clin Genet* 27:414, 1985

Gasch AT, Caruso RC, Kaler SG et al.: Menkes' syndrome. Ophthalmic findings. *Ophthalmology* 109:1477, 2002

Hayashi N, Geraghty MT, Green WR: Ocular histologic study of a patient with the T 8993-G point mutation in Leigh's syndrome. *Ophthalmology* 40:197, 2000

Heggie P, Grossniklaus HE, Roessmann U et al.: Cerebro-ocular dysplasia-muscular dystrophy syndrome: Report of two cases. *Arch Ophthalmol* 105:520, 1987

Howard MA, Thompson JT, Howard RO: Aplasia of the optic nerve. *Trans Am Ophthalmol Soc* 91:267, 1993

Kass MA, Howard RO, Silverman JP: Russell–Silver dwarfism. *Ann Ophthalmol* 8:1337, 1976

Khairallah M, Messaoud R, Zaouali S et al.: Posterior segment changes associated with posterior microphthalmos. *Ophthalmology* 109:569, 2002

Kremer I, Lerman-Sagie T, Mukamel M et al.: Light and electron microscopic findings in Leigh's disease. *Ophthalmologica* 199:106, 1989

Kretzer FL, Hittner HM, Mehta RS: Ocular manifestations of the Smith–Lemli–Opitz syndrome. *Arch Ophthalmol* 99:2000, 1981

Krohel GB, Wirth CR: Engelmann's disease. *Am J Ophthalmol* 84:520, 1977

Lewis RA, Crowder WE, Eierman LA et al.: The Gardner syndrome: Significance of ocular features. *Ophthalmology* 91:916, 1984

Lichtig C, Ludatscher RM, Mandel H et al.: Muscle involvement in Walker–Warburg syndrome: Clinicopathologic features of four cases. *J Clin Pathol* 100:493, 1993

MacRae DW, Howard RO, Albert DM et al.: Ocular manifestations of the Meckel syndrome. *Arch Ophthalmol* 88:106, 1972

Marcus DM, Shore JW, Albert DM: Anophthalmia in the focal dermal hypoplasia syndrome. *Arch Ophthalmol* 108:96, 1990

Millay RH, Weleber RG, Heckenlively JR: Ophthalmologic and systemic manifestations of Alström's disease. *Am J Ophthalmol* 102:482, 1986

Murata T, Ishibashi T, Ohnishi Y et al.: Cornea choristoma with microphthalmos. *Arch Ophthalmol* 109:1130, 1991

O'Rahilly R, Müller F: Interpretation of some median anomalies as illustrated by cyclopia and symmelia. *Teratology* 40:409, 1989

Reynolds JD, Johnson BL, Gloster S et al.: Glaucoma and Klippel-Traunay–Weber syndrome. *Am J Ophthalmol* 106:494, 1988

Rosenthal AR, Ryan SJ, Horowitz P: Ocular manifestations of dwarfism. *Trans Am Acad Ophthalmol Otolaryngol* 76:1500, 1972

Rotberg M, Klintworth GK, Crawford JB: Ocular vasodilation and angiogenesis in Potter's syndrome. *Am J Ophthalmol* 97:16, 1984

Sassani JW, Yanoff M: Anophthalmos in an infant with multiple congenital anomalies. *Am J Ophthalmol* 83:43, 1977

Sedwick LA, Burde RM, Hodges FJ III: Leigh's subacute necrotizing encephalomyelopathy manifesting as spasmus nutans. *Arch Ophthalmol* 102:1046, 1984

Stefani FH, Hausmann N, Lund O-E: Unilateral diplophthalmos. *Am J Ophthalmol* 112:581, 1991

Stewart DH, Streeten BW, Brockhurst RJ et al.: Abnormal scleral collagen in nanophthalmos: An ultrastructural study. *Arch Ophthalmol* 109:1017, 1991

Torczynski E, Jakobiec FA, Johnston MC et al.: Synophthalmia and cyclopia: A histopathologic, radiographic, and organogenetic analysis. *Doc Ophthalmol* 44:311, 1977

Toussaint D, Danis P: Dystrophie maculaire dans une maladie de Menkes: Etude histogogique oculaire. *J Fr Ophthalmol* 1:457, 1978

Weiss AH, Kousseff BJ, Ross EA *et al.*: Simple microphthalmos. *Arch Ophthalmol* 107:1625, 1989

Yamani A, Wood I, Sugino I *et al.*: Abnormal collagen fibrils in nanophthalmos: A clinical and histologic study. *Am J Ophthalmol* 127:106, 1999

Yanoff M: Walker–Warburg syndrome. Presented at the 1989 Verhoeff Society Meeting, Boston, MA

Yanoff M: In discussion of Howard MA, Thompson JT, Howard RO: Aplasia of the optic nerve. *Trans Am Ophthalmol Soc* 91:267–281, 1993

Yanoff M, Rorke LB, Allman MI: Bilateral optic system aplasia with relatively normal eyes. *Arch Ophthalmol* 96:97, 1978

Yue BYJT, Kurosawa A, Duvall J *et al.*: Nanophthalmic sclera: Fibronectin studies. *Ophthalmology* 95:56, 1988

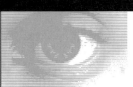
Nongranulomatous Inflammation: Uveitis, Endophthalmitis, Panophthalmitis, and Sequelae

DEFINITION

I. *Suppurative* nongranulomatous inflammation.

   A. This is an acute, nongranulomatous (no epithelioid or giant cells), purulent inflammatory reaction in which the predominant cell type is the polymorphonuclear leukocyte.

   B. The reaction usually has an acute onset and is characterized by suppuration (i.e., the formation of pus).

This type of inflammation is usually secondary to infection with bacteria that cause a purulent (pus) inflammatory reaction, such as *Staphylococcus aureus*.

II. *Nonsuppurative* nongranulomatous inflammation.

   A. This may be an acute (cellulitis secondary to *Streptococcus hemolyticus*) or chronic (the common type of uveitis) inflammation.

Streptococcal gangrene of the eyelids, caused by group A hemolytic *Streptococcus* (also called *flesh-eating disease*, *necrotizing fasciitis*, *necrotizing erysipelas*, and *gangrenous erysipelas*), although rare, appears to be increasing in prevalence.

   B. The predominant cell type in acute inflammation is the polymorphonuclear leukocyte, and in chronic inflammation it is the lymphocyte and the plasma cell.

Nongranulomatous inflammation may have an acute, sub-acute, or chronic course.

CLASSIFICATION

Terminology

I. If a single tissue is involved, the inflammation is classified according to involved tissue (e.g., cornea—keratitis; retina—retinitis; vitreous—vitritis; optic nerve—optic neuritis; sclera—scleritis; and uvea—uveitis).

If more than one tissue is involved but not an adjacent cavity (a most unusual occurrence), then the inflammation is classified by the tissues involved with the site of primary involvement first (e.g., retinochoroiditis in toxoplasmosis and chorioretinitis in tuberculosis).

II. Endophthalmitis (Fig. 3.1) is an inflammation of one or more coats of the eye and adjacent cavities.

By this definition, a corneal ulcer with a hypopyon or an iritis with aqueous cells and flare would be an endophthalmitis, but most clinicians require a vitritis before calling an ocular inflammation an endophthalmitis.

III. Panophthalmitis (Fig. 3.2) is an inflammation of all three coats of the eye (and adjacent cavities); it often starts as an endophthalmitis that then involves the sclera and spreads to orbital structures.

Sources of Inflammation

I. Exogenous: sources originate outside the eye and body [e.g., local ocular physical injury (surgical trauma, penetrating and perforating nonsurgical trauma, radiant

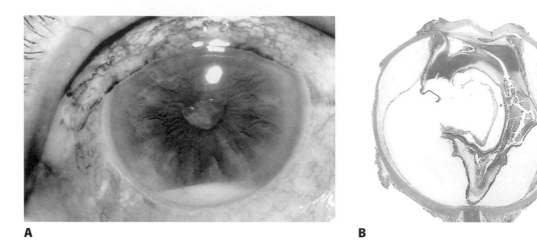

Fig. 3.1 Endophthalmitis. **A,** The patient contracted "sterile" endophthalmitis after undergoing extracapsular cataract extraction and a posterior-chamber lens implant. Note the hypopyon. **B,** Another patient contracted a suppurative bacterial endophthalmitis after intracapsular cataract extraction. The diffuse abscess seen filling the vitreous cavity is characteristic of bacterial infection (fungal infection usually causes multiple tiny abscesses). The neural retina and its adjacent cavity, the vitreous, are involved, but the choroid and sclera are not.

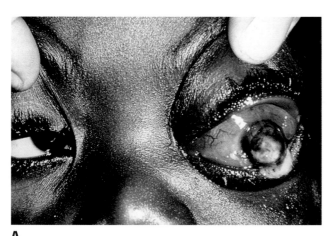

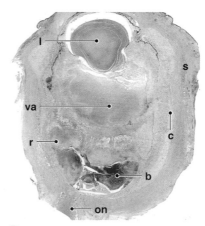

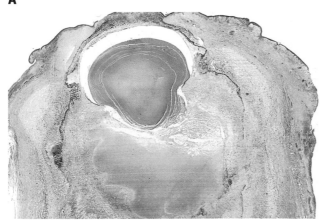

Fig. 3.2 Panophthalmitis. **A,** The patient had a regular measles infection; subsequently, pain and inflammation developed in the left eye that led to panophthalmitis and corneal perforation. **B,** Histologic section shows the vitreous body, adjacent retina, choroid, and sclera are all involved, and the inflammation extends through the coats of the eye into the episcleral tissue (l, lens; va, vitreous abscess; r, necrotic inflamed retina; c, inflamed choroid; b, fresh blood; on, optic nerve; s, thickened inflamed sclera and episclera). **C,** Increased magnification shows the corneal perforation and the inflammation involving all coats of the eye. (**A,** Courtesy of Dr. RE Shannon.)

energy); chemical injuries (acid and alkali); and allergic reactions to external antigens (conjunctivitis secondary to pollen)].

II. Endogenous: sources originate in the eye [e.g., inflammation secondary to cellular immunity (phacoanaphylactic endophthalmitis); spread from contiguous structures (the sinuses); hematogenous spread (virus, bacteria, fungus, foreign particle); and conditions of unknown cause (sarcoidosis)].

SUPPURATIVE ENDOPHTHALMITIS AND PANOPHTHALMITIS

Clinical Features

I. Severe ocular congestion, chemosis, and haziness of the cornea, aqueous, and vitreous are characteristic. A purulent exudate, frequently visible as a hypopyon, may be present in the anterior chamber.

II. Pain is prominent in both conditions, but especially in panophthalmitis.

III. Extension into orbital tissue often results in congestion and edema of the lids and even exophthalmos.

IV. The cause may be infectious or noninfectious.

Classification

I. Exogenous
 A. Infectious keratitis and corneal ulcers may cause a reflex sterile suppurative iridocyclitis and hypopyon.
 B. Nonsurgical penetrating or perforating trauma (or, rarely, surgical) may lead to the presence of a contaminated or sterile intraocular foreign body, producing a suppurative inflammation.
 C. Postoperative suppurative inflammation in the first day or two after surgery is usually purulent, fulminating (i.e., rapid), and caused by bacteria.
  1. Delayed (e.g., a month or two after intraocular surgery) endophthalmitis suggests a fungal infection.
  2. A bacterial infection is also a possible cause of delayed endophthalmitis, especially with less virulent bacteria such as *Staphylococcus epidermidis* and *Propionibacterium acnes* (see p. 121 in Chapter 5).

II. Endogenous
 A. Metastatic septic emboli, especially in children or debilitated persons, may occur in subacute bacterial endocarditis, meningococcemia, or other infections associated with a bacteremia, viremia, or fungemia.
 B. Necrosis of an intraocular neoplasm, particularly retinoblastoma, may rarely result in a suppurative endophthalmitis or even panophthalmitis.

Histologically, necrosis of a malignant melanoma is more likely to induce an inflammatory reaction (usually lymphocytes and plasma cells) than is necrosis of a retinoblastoma. Clinically, however, inflammation is seen more frequently in retinoblastoma than in melanoma. In fact, retinoblastoma may clinically simulate inflammation in approximately 8% of retinoblastoma eyes.

C. Inflammation of contiguous or nearby structures (e.g., orbital abscess or cellulitis, meningitis, or a nasal phycomycosis) may rarely spread into the eye.

Histology

Suppurative inflammation is characterized by polymorphonuclear leukocytic infiltration into the involved tissues (Figs 3.3 and 3.4). Marked tissue necrosis causes a suppurative or purulent exudate (pus).

Examples

I. Behçet's disease (see Fig. 3.3) is an example of a chronic endogenous endophthalmitis.
 A. It is a triple-symptom complex consisting of ocular inflammation (occurs in 70% to 80% of patients), oral ulceration (aphthous stomatitis), and genital ulceration (conjunctival ulcers may also occur).

Eating English walnuts can exacerbate Behçet's disease.

 B. The disease is most common in men between the ages of 20 and 30 years, has a male predominance, and men have a more severe involvement with a greater risk of vision loss than women.
 C. Arthritis or arthralgia, cutaneous lesions, thrombophlebitis, ulcerative colitis, encephalopathy, pancreatitis, central and peripheral neuropathy, vena caval obstruction, subungual infarctions, and malignant lymphomas may also be seen.
 D. Plasminogen activator levels may be decreased.
 E. A hypercoagulable or general vascular endothelial dysfunction is usually found.
 F. S-antigen-responsive lymphocytes are increased in the peripheral blood during episodes of ocular inflammation.
 G. To make the diagnosis of Behçet's disease, patients must have at least three episodes of aphthous or herpetiform ulcerations in 12 months and two of the following four findings: recurrent genital ulceration; ocular signs (e.g., anterior or posterior uveitis, vitritis, or retinal vasculitis); skin lesions (e.g., erythema nodosum, pseudofolliculitis, or papulopustules); and positive pathergy test (sterile pustule developing within 24 to 48 hours at site of a cuticular needle puncture).

Plasma exchange, by removing immune complexes from the circulation, may be an alternative treatment for severe cases of Behçet's disease.

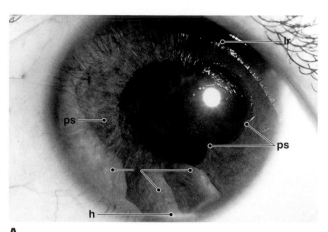

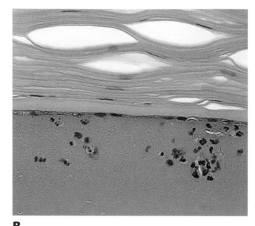

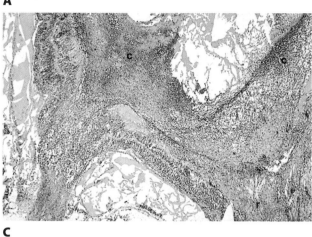

A

B

C

Fig. 3.3 Behçet's disease. **A,** The patient has a hypopyon (h). Note the posterior synechiae (ps), a sign of the recurrent iridocyclitis in this patient (l, light reflexes; lr, lid reflexes). **B,** Anterior chamber contains exudate and polymorphonuclear leukocytes (hypopyon). **C,** A histologic section shows necrosis and perivasculitis of the neural retina. An organizing cyclitic membrane (c) has caused a detachment of the inflamed neural retina (r, detached, necrotic, inflamed retina). (Case shown in **B** reported by Green WR, Koo BS: *Surv Ophthalmol* 12:324. Copyright Elsevier 1967; **C,** presented by Dr. TA Makley at the meeting of the Verhoeff Society, 1976.)

H. The ocular inflammation is characterized by recurrent iridocyclitis and hypopyon (often motile), usually involving both eyes but not necessarily simultaneously.
  1. In addition, macular edema, retinal pigmentary changes and periphlebitis, vitritis, periarteritis, and retinal and vitreal hemorrhages may occur (even when visual complaints are not present, fluorescein angiography shows leakage from superficial optic nerve capillaries and venules and peripheral retinal capillaries).
  2. The presence of small patches of retinal whitening is characteristic.
  3. Secondary posterior synechiae may lead to iris bombé, peripheral anterior synechiae, and secondary angle closure glaucoma.
  4. Rarely, a bilateral immune corneal ring (Wessely ring) may occur.
I. Biopsy of mucocutaneous lesions shows vasculitis.
J. The serum may show variable increases in polyclonal immunoglobulins and anticytoplasmic antibodies. Serum and aqueous humor sialic acid levels are elevated during the active and remission phases of Behçet's disease.
K. Human leukocyte antigen (HLA)-B51, which belongs to the HLA-B5, B35 cross-reacting group, is the most strongly associated genetic marker on Behçet's disease over many ethnic groups.
  1. The gene *HLA-B* appears to be responsible for, and determines the susceptibility to, Behçet's disease.
  2. Factor V Leiden mutations are a risk factor for the development of Behçet's disease.
L. Histologically, the main process appears to be a small or moderate-sized blood vessel vasculitis.
  1. Retinal perivasculitis, vasculitis, hemorrhagic infarction, and detachment, along with a chronic nongranulomatous uveitis, may be seen.
  2. An acute, suppurative inflammatory infiltrate with neutrophils occurs in the anterior chamber (hypopyon).
  3. A secondary chronic nongranulomatous inflammatory infiltrate is frequently noted in adjacent tissues (see Fig. 3.4).

The choroidal infiltrate is predominantly CD4$^+$ T lymphocyte, and some B lymphocytes and plasma cells.

---

  4. Spontaneous rupture of the lens can cause phaco-anoaphylactic endopthalmitis.

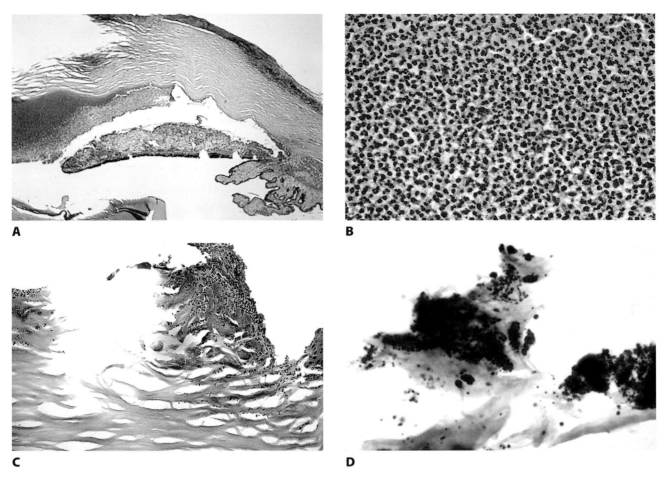

Fig. 3.4 Suppurative endophthalmitis (see also **Fig. 3.1**). **A,** Suppurative inflammation present in area of perforating corneal ulcer and in hypopyon in anterior chamber. Iris contains chronic nongranulomatous inflammatory infiltrate of lymphocytes and plasma cells. **B,** Polymorphonuclear leukocytes (PMNs) in hypopyon shown with increased magnification. **C,** Edge of corneal ulcer shown in **A** demonstrates corneal necrosis, PMNs seen as a lining-up of nuclear particles along stromal lamellae, and "smudgy" areas that represent bacterial colonies (seen as Gram-positive cocci with special stain in **D**).

NONSUPPURATIVE, CHRONIC NONGRANULOMATOUS UVEITIS AND ENDOPHTHALMITIS

Clinical Features

I. Anterior involvement often causes a severe, acute, "plastic" or exudative recurrent iridocyclitis, whereas posterior involvement produces a choroiditis or chorioretinitis.

II. A chronic nongranulomatous uveitis of unknown cause characterizes the "garden-variety" type of uveitis.

Classification

I. Exogenous: the inflammation is usually secondary to trauma.

A. The most common type is the iridocyclitis (*traumatic iridocyclitis*) that follows many injuries to the eye, particularly blunt trauma or intraocular surgery.

B. Penetrating or perforating injuries may produce a sterile, chronic nongranulomatous inflammation, resulting from multiple, tiny foreign bodies, degenerating blood, necrotic uvea, and so forth.

II. Endogenous (Fig. 3.5)

A. Idiopathic inflammation (i.e., "garden-variety" anterior uveitis) is the most common form of endogenous uveitis. The cause is unknown but may be related to cellular immunity.

Rhegmatogenous retinal detachment may occur in about 3% of cases of uveitis. A close association exists with the HLA-B27 antigen (also found in the rheumatoid group of diseases). In addition, the anterior uveitis may follow, and be related to, infection with a variety of Gram-negative bacteria (e.g., *Yersinia* species and *Chlamydia trachomatis*) or with Mollicutes (see discussion of Crohn's disease, later).

B. The inflammation may be associated with viral infections such as rubella and subacute sclerosing panencephalitis (SSPE); bacterial infections such as syphilis;

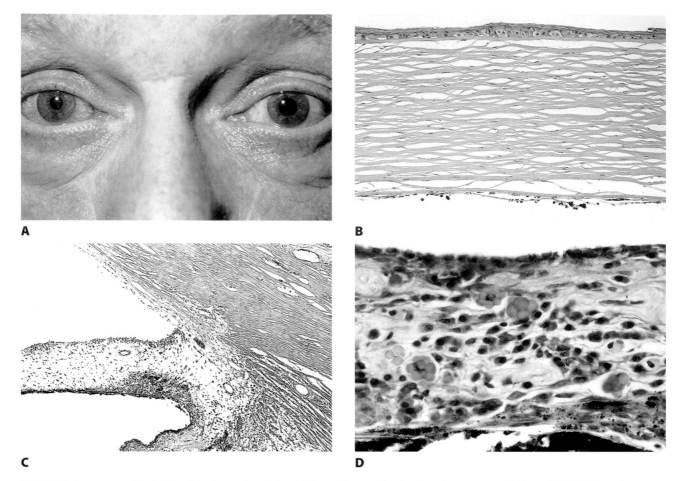

Fig. 3.5 Endogenous uveitis. **A,** Ciliary injection and constricted right pupil caused by chronic endogenous uveitis ("acute" iritis). **B,** Corneal epithelium shows edema of its basal layer. Lymphocytes, plasma cells, and pigment are seen on the posterior corneal surface (fine keratic precipitates). **C,** Chronic nongranulomatous inflammation of lymphocytes and plasma cells is present in iris root and ciliary body. Note early peripheral anterior synechia formation. **D,** Iris shows chronic nongranulomatous inflammation with lymphocytes, plasma cells, and Russell bodies (large, pink, globular structures).

local ocular (nonsystemic) entities such as pars planitis, Fuchs' heterochromic iridocyclitis (FHI), uveal effusion (see p. 355 in Chapter 9), and glaucomatocyclitic crisis (Posner–Schlossman syndrome; see p. 645 in Chapter 16); and systemic diseases such as Reiter's syndrome, Behçet's disease (see earlier), Kawasaki's disease (mucocutaneous lymph node syndrome), phacoanaphylactic endophthalmitis (the uvea usually shows a chronic, nongranulomatous uveitis; see p. 75 in Chapter 4), collagen vascular disease (including rheumatoid arthritis), Crohn's disease (regional enteritis; see p. 67 in this chapter), ulcerative colitis, and Whipple's disease (see p. 484 in Chapter 12); and atopy.

Examples

I. Viral infections such as herpes simplex and zoster, Epstein–Barr virus (EBV), SSPE, rubella (see p. 43 in Chapter 2), and rubeola may cause an endogenous nonsuppurative, chronic nongranulomatous uveitis.

A. Herpes simplex virus (HSV; Fig. 3.6)
  1. HSV consists of a linear, double-stranded DNA packaged in an icosahedral capsid and covered by a lipid-containing membrane.
    a. HSV-1 is usually responsible for initial infections in children and for most herpetic eye infections in all ages.
    b. HSV-2, usually responsible for genital herpes, may rarely cause ocular disease in neonates (contamination at birth by mother's genital herpes) or adults.
  2. Neonatal HSV most commonly causes a nonfollicular conjunctivitis followed by keratitis.
    a. Other ocular findings include retinochoroiditis (or chorioretinal scarring), iritis, cataracts, optic atrophy or neuritis, and microphthalmia.
    b. The differential diagnosis consists of the *TORCH syndrome* (toxoplasmosis, rubella, cytomegalovirus, and herpes simplex).

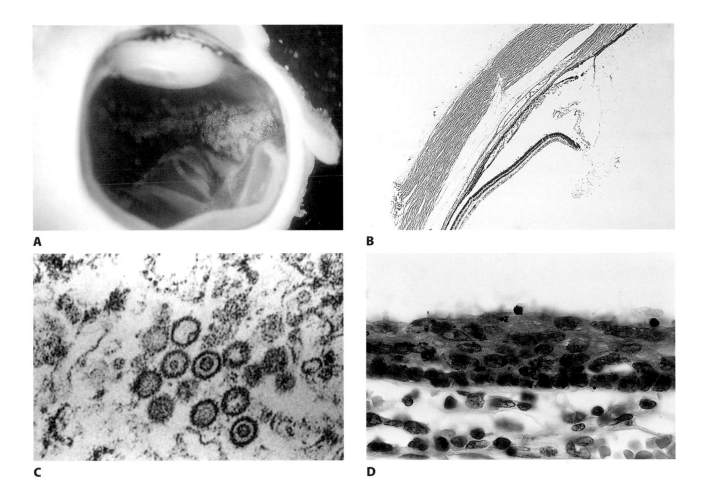

Fig. 3.6 Congenital herpes simplex type 2 endophthalmitis. Infant died from effects of disseminated herpes simplex. **A,** Gross appearance of necrotic peripheral neural retina. **B,** Necrotic peripheral neural retina sharply demarcated from relatively normal retina. **C,** Complete capsids containing nucleoids, along with empty capsids, present in necrotic neural retina. **D,** Retinal pigment epithelium forms hyperplastic plaque under peripheral neural retina in area of neural retinal necrosis. (Adapted from Yanoff M, Allman MI, Fine BS: *Trans Am Ophthalmol Soc* 75:325, 1977.)

Lymphocytic choriomeningitis virus can cause a congenital chorioretinitis and can be added to the TORCH list.

---

3. Acquired HSV in children and adults is similar to that in neonates.

Children who have HSV keratitis may have bilateral involvement and are at risk for recurrent keratitis and amblyopia.

---

   a. A mucocutaneous eruption is common.
   b. HSV retinitis (a cause of the acute retinal necrosis syndrome) may occur in immunocompetent or immunodeficient people (e.g., in acquired immunodeficiency syndrome).
   c. The most common ocular manifestation is keratitis (see p. 267 in Chapter 8).
4. Histologically, the infected area reveals both acute and chronic nongranulomatous inflammation.

   a. Intranuclear inclusions (Cowdry type A) may be seen.
   b. HSV can be detected by monoclonal antibodies, such as the avidin–biotin complex immunoperoxidase technique, and by *in situ* DNA hybridization method using viral genome segments.
B. Epstein-Barr virus (EBV)
   1. The EBV, a B-lymphotrophic virus, accounts for most cases of infectious mononucleosis, is associated with Burkitt's lymphoma (see p. 579 in Chapter 14), and is detected in up to 50% of B-cell malignancies encountered in immunosuppressed patients.

EBV, after infecting the host's cells, can hide from the immune system by producing a protein that inhibits its own synthesis, thereby minimizing the amount that appears on the cell surface.

2. Ocular manifestations, most commonly a follicular conjunctivitis, usually occur in association with infectious mononucleosis.
3. *X-linked lymphoproliferative syndrome* (XLP), one of the reactive histiocytic disorders, is a disease in which a primary EBV infection results in a fatal outcome from infectious mononucleosis, aplastic anemia, malignant lymphoma, and hypogammaglobulinemia in most male patients who have the *XLP* gene.

Epithelial keratitis, episcleritis, iritis, uveitis, dacryoadenitis, cranial nerve palsies, Sjögren's syndrome, and Parinaud's oculoglandular syndrome (see p. 232 in Chapter 7) may also occur. Also, the Fas (also known as Apo1 and CD95) antigen, a cell surface receptor involved in apoptotic cell death, may be defective (through a deletion) in XLP, resulting in incomplete elimination of peripheral autoreactive cells.

---

4. Histologically, a chronic nongranulomatous inflammation is seen.

C. SSPE (Fig. 3.7)
1. SSPE, caused by measles slow virus infection, is a chronic, progressive disease of the central nervous system in children and young adults, which produces an intracellular infection of brain, retina, and lymphoid tissue.
2. The disease usually emerges 5 to 7 years after the child has had an uneventful measles (rubeola) infection.

SSPE has been reported in a young (20 years of age) male intravenous drug abuser.

---

  a. Patients have high titers of measles antibody in their serum and cerebrospinal fluid.
  b. Measles antigen can be demonstrated in brain tissue by immunofluorescence.
3. The ocular findings consist mainly of macular degeneration, optic atrophy, and peripheral retinochoroidal lesions.

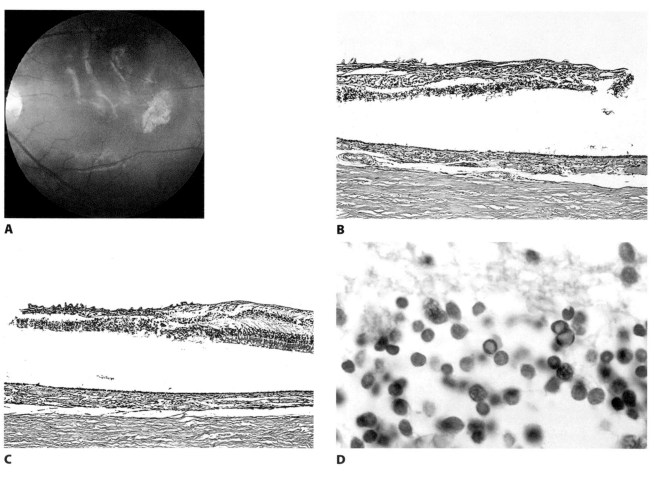

Fig. 3.7 Subacute sclerosing panencephalitis (SSPE). Clinical (**A**) and light microscopic (**B** and **C**) appearance of necrotic macula (acute retinitis with foveal hole formation) in patient who had SSPE. **D,** Many intranuclear inclusions (myxoviruses) are present in the inner nuclear layer of the foveomacular neural retina. The nuclear chromatin is clumped in the peripheral nucleus. (Modified from Nelson DA *et al.: Arch Ophthalmol* 84:613, 1970, with permission. © American Medical Association. All rights reserved.)

The ophthalmologic signs and symptoms may antedate those of the central nervous system by as long as 2 years.

4. Histologically, the neural retina is necrotic, is infiltrated by lymphocytes, and shows conglomerations of multinucleated cells. Intranuclear inclusion bodies in retinal cells can be seen with light and electron microscopy.

II. Local ocular (nonsystemic) syndromes such as pars planitis and FHI may cause a nonsuppurative, chronic nongranulomatous uveitis.
A. Pars planitis (intermediate uveitis, peripheral uveitis, chronic cyclitis)
1. Pars planitis is a chronic process, usually of children and young adults, that consists of vitreous opacities, exudation, and organization of the vitreous base ("snowbanking") in the region of the pars plana, and neural retinal edema, especially of the posterior pole (cystoid macular edema).

A 36-kD protein (p-36) is elevated in the blood of many patients with active pars planitis. A pars planitis-like picture may be seen in cat-scratch disease. A significant association also exists between pars planitis and serum HLA-DR15 (HLA-DR15 specificity has been associated with other entities such as multiple sclerosis, idiopathic optic neuritis, and narcolepsy).

Relative sparing of the anterior chamber occurs.

Cataract and cystoid macular edema are common complications. Uncommon complications include band keratopathy, glaucoma, neural retinal detachment, retinoschisis, vitreous hemorrhage, and neural retinal hemorrhage. A link may exist between pars planitis and multiple sclerosis, especially when retinal periphlebitis is present at the time of diagnosis of pars planitis (multiple sclerosis develops in perhaps 15% of patients with pars planitis when they are followed for at least 8 years).

2. Histologically, a chronic nongranulomatous inflammation of the vitreous base, retinal perivasculitis, and microcystoid degeneration of the macular retina are seen.
a. The snowbank noted clinically corresponds microscopically to a loose fibrovascular layer in a condensed vitreous, containing occasional fibrocyte-like cells and scattered mononuclear inflammatory cells adjacent to a hyperplastic, nonpigmented pars plana epithelium.
b. The layer appears continuous with similar pre-retinal fibroglial membranes.

B. Fuchs' heterochromic iridocyclitis (FHI) (Figs 3.8 and 3.9)
1. FHI, a condition of unknown cause (although persistence of the rubella virus has been implicated as the cause) consists of a unilateral, chronic, mild iridocyclitis with characteristic, translucent, stellate,

relatively unchanging keratic precipitates; heterochromia iridum with the involved iris becoming the lighter iris; and cataract and glaucoma development in the hypochromic eye.

The hypochromia of the involved eye is caused by iris stromal atrophy with loss of stromal pigment (the atrophy and depigmentation are not limited to the iris but are also found in the surrounding ocular wall). The iris stromal atrophy may become so severe that the iris pigment epithelium can be observed directly. The result is a *paradoxical heterochromia* with the involved eye becoming the darker eye. The glaucoma is probably caused by a combination of neovascularization of the anterior-chamber angle, a trabeculitis, and possibly an associated atrophy of the uveal portion of the drainage angle.

2. Characteristically, in spite of the chronic uveitis and iris neovascularization, anterior and posterior synechiae do not occur (even though a cataract forms), and intraocular surgery is tolerated well.

A subgroup of FHI has an association, which may be causal, with toxoplasmic retinochoroiditis, toxocariasis, and herpetic ocular infections.

3. White, opalescent iris nodules may develop in black patients.
4. Histologically, a chronic nongranulomatous inflammatory reaction is seen in the iris, ciliary body, and trabecular meshwork.

Plasma cells and Russell bodies are prominent in the iris stroma. The Russell bodies may be seen clinically with the slit lamp as subtle iris crystals.

a. Inflammatory membranes are common over the anterior surface of the iris and anterior face of the ciliary body.
b. A fine neovascularization of the anterior surface of the iris and anterior-chamber angle may be present.

The iris neovascularization is quite fine and just within the anterior-border layer of the iris. Anterior-segment perfusion defects and iris vasculature leakage may be seen. Chronic anterior-segment ischemia, therefore, may play a role in the development of iris neovascularization. Fine, translucent, stellate keratic precipitates, observed clinically, have their counterpart in small clumps of mononuclear cells, lymphocytes, and macrophages on the posterior surface of the cornea.

c. The iris stroma and the pigment epithelium show atrophy with loss of pigment, especially in the stroma and the posterior layer of pigment epithelium.
III. Systemic syndromes such as Reiter's syndrome, rheumatoid arthritis, and Crohn's disease
A. Reiter's syndrome

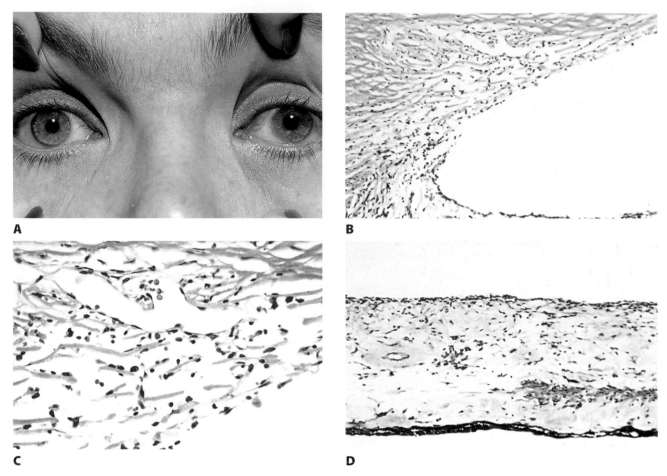

Fig. 3.8 Fuchs' heterochromic iridocyclitis. **A,** Blue-green uninvolved right eye is darker than light-blue involved left eye, which also contained a cataractous lens. **B,** Anterior face of ciliary body and trabecular meshwork contain chronic nongranulomatous inflammation. **C,** High magnification of trabecular meshwork demonstrates chronic trabeculitis with infiltration by lymphocytes and plasma cells. **D,** Iris shows loss of dilator muscle, stromal atrophy, nodular and diffuse infiltration by lymphocytes and plasma cells, and a fine iris surface neovascularization. (**B–D**, modified from Perry H *et al.: Arch Ophthalmol* 93:337, 1975, with permission. © American Medical Association. All rights reserved.)

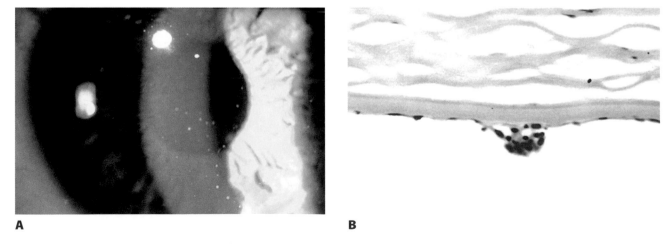

Fig. 3.9 Fuchs' heterochromic iridocyclitis. **A,** Slit-lamp examination shows typical stellate keratic precipitates (KPs), which tend to change very little over long periods. **B,** The KPs are composed of lymphocytes and histiocytes. (**B,** Modified from Perry H *et al.: Arch Ophthalmol* 93:337, 1975, with permission. © American Medical Association. All rights reserved.)

1. The classic triad of nonbacterial urethritis, conjunctivitis or iridocyclitis, and arthritis characterize Reiter's syndrome.
2. HLA-B27 is positive in a high percentage of patients.
3. Bilateral mucopurulent conjunctivitis is present in most cases, whereas iridocyclitis tends to be seen only in recurrent cases.

Rarely, a keratoconjunctivitis occurs. Epithelial erosions and pleomorphic infiltrates in the anterior stroma characterize the keratitis.

---

4. Histologically, edema and a lymphocytic and neutrophilic inflammatory infiltrate are noted in the conjunctiva.

B. Rheumatoid arthritis
1. Ankylosing spondylitis has a 10% to 15% prevalence of uveitis, and Still's disease has a 15% to 20% prevalence.
2. Juvenile rheumatoid arthritis (JR) is the most common specific childhood entity associated with uveitis in children.
   a. Risk factors for uveitis in children who have JR include female sex, pauciarticular onset of arthritis, circulating antinuclear antibodies, and HLA-DW5 and HLA-DPw2 antigens.
   b. Approximately 12% of patients with JR in whom uveitis develops eventually become blind.

C. Crohn's disease
1. Crohn's disease is an idiopathic, chronic, inflammatory bowel disease that shows frequent extra-bowel inflammation in the eyes, eyelids, orbits, lungs, joints, and skin.
   A Mollicute-like organism (i.e., a noncultivatable, cell wall-deficient bacterial pathogen) may cause Crohn's disease and the uveitis.

Bacteria can be classified as Firmicutes (Gram-positive), Gracilicutes (Gram-negative), or *Mollicutes* (lack a cell wall, enclosed only by a plasma membrane, and stain poorly with biologic stains). Obligate intracellular Mollicutes, previously called *mycoplasma-like organisms*, are prokaryotic (unicellular), have no cell wall or distinct nucleus, and are the smallest prokaryote capable of self-replication.

---

2. Ocular findings include, most commonly, acute episcleritis, scleritis, acute anterior uveitis, and marginal keratitis; less commonly, conjunctivitis, orbital inflammation, optic neuritis, ischemic optic neuropathy, and retinal vasculitis.

Similar ocular findings can occur in ulcerative colitis.

---

3. Histologically, a granulomatous process is most common, but a chronic nongranulomatous inflammation may also be found.

SEQUELAE OF UVEITIS, ENDOPHTHALMITIS, AND PANOPHTHALMITIS

Cornea

I. Corneal endothelial degeneration or glaucoma, or both, may result in chronic stromal and epithelial edema and ultimately in bullous keratopathy (Fig. 3.10).
   A. Pannus degenerativus may follow bullous keratopathy.
   B. Keratic precipitates of mononuclear cells (mainly lymphocytes and plasma cells) along with pigment (see Figs 3.5B and 3.9B) may be found on the endothelium.
II. Ruptured corneal bullae may become infected secondarily, leading to a corneal ulcer.

Corneal ulceration may lead to perforation. Perforation and the resultant abrupt decrease in intraocular pressure may cause a ciliary artery to rupture, producing an expulsive intraocular hemorrhage.

III. Band keratopathy (i.e., calcium deposition; see Figs 8.23 to 8.25) is common beneath the corneal epithelium in chronically inflamed eyes, especially in children who have Still's disease.
IV. Corneal vascularization (see Fig. 8.18)

Anterior Chamber

I. Products of inflammation or hemorrhage may become organized, resulting in cicatrization.
II. The cicatrization or iris neovascularization may obliterate the angle of the anterior chamber.

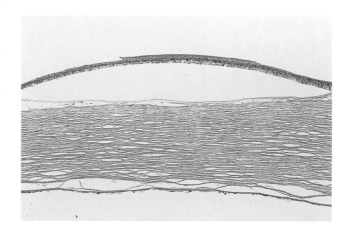

Fig. 3.10 Corneal edema. The cornea is edematous and shows large bullous formation. The corneal edema and lymphocytes, plasma cells, and pigment on the posterior corneal surface, forming fine keratic precipitates, are secondary to chronic nongranulomatous uveitis.

Iris

I. The iris may undergo atrophy and necrosis with loss of dilator muscle, stroma, and even sphincter muscle and pigment epithelium.

II. Chronic anterior uveitis may induce peripheral anterior synechiae formation (see Fig. 3.5C).

III. Neovascularization of the anterior surface of the iris (rubeosis iridis or red iris, as seen clinically) may cause secondary anterior-chamber angle synechiae and secondary angle closure.

Shrinkage of the fibrovascular membrane on the anterior iris surface may evert the pupillary border of the iris, termed an *ectropion uveae* (Fig. 3.11; see Fig. 15.5).

IV. Inflammatory and fibrous iris membranes may attach the pupillary margin of the iris to an underlying lens, to a lens implant or lens capsule in pseudophakic eyes, or to the anterior surface of the vitreous in aphakic eyes, resulting in an immobile pupil, *seclusio pupillae* (Fig. 3.12).

The same membrane may grow over the pupil and cover or occlude the area completely, called *occlusio pupillae* (see Fig. 3.12).

The same membrane that binds the pupil down to surrounding structures usually grows across the pupil, so that seclusio pupillae and occlusio pupillae are often found together. Also, shrinkage of the membrane between iris and lens may cause the pupillary border to become inverted, termed *entropion uveae*.

V. Total (i.e., 360°) posterior synechiae cause a complete pupillary block, preventing aqueous flow into the anterior chamber.

A. The pressure builds up in the posterior chamber, bowing the iris forward (*iris bombé*; see Fig. 3.12).

B. An iris bombé forces the anterior peripheral iris to touch the peripheral posterior cornea, resulting in peripheral anterior synechiae and, if aqueous secretion is adequate, secondary closed-angle glaucoma.

Such eyes often have reduced aqueous flow and hypotony may result even in the face of a completely closed angle.

Lens

I. Intraocular inflammation frequently induces the lens epithelium to migrate posteriorly. The presence of the aberrant cells under the posterior lens capsule produces a posterior subcapsular cataract.

Although posterior subcapsular cataract can be induced by intraocular inflammation anywhere in the eye, it most likely is secondary to posterior inflammation (choroiditis).

II. An anterior subcapsular cataract frequently results from an anterior uveitis (e.g., iritis or iridocyclitis), especially when posterior synechiae are present.

Ciliary Body

I. With chronic intraocular inflammation, the ciliary processes or crests tend to become flattened and attenuated and their cores fibrosed (hyalinized).

II. The ciliary epithelium (nonpigmented, pigmented, or both) may proliferate, sometimes to a marked degree (i.e., massive proliferation of ciliary epithelium).

III. Intraocular inflammation may organize and fibrose behind the lens or lens implant (or behind the pupil in an aphakic eye) between portions of the pars plicata of the ciliary body. Such a fibrous membrane spanning the retrolental space and often incorporating proliferated ciliary epithelium and vitreous base is called a *cyclitic membrane* (see Fig. 3.12C; Fig. 3.13).

When a cyclitic membrane shrinks, the vitreous base, ciliary body pars plana, and peripheral neural retina are drawn inward to cause

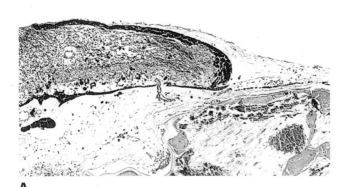
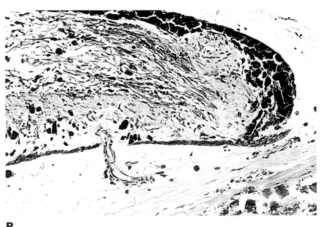

A **B**

Fig. 3.11 Ectropion uveae. **A,** The sphincter muscle and pigment epithelium (PE) of the iris are bowed forward, along with anterior proliferation of the PE. The iris is adherent to the underlying lens (posterior synechia), and neovascularization is arising from the posterior iris (shown with increased magnification in **B**).

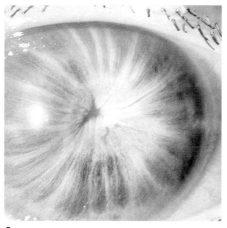

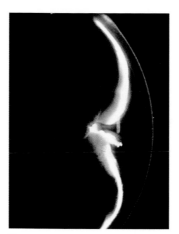

A   **B**

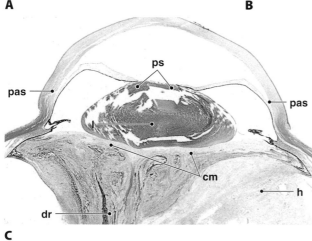

C

Fig. 3.12 Seclusion and occlusion of pupil. **A,** A membrane has grown across the pupil (occlusion of the pupil) and has adhered to the underlying lens, preventing the pupil from moving (seclusion of the pupil). **B,** Aqueous in the posterior chamber has bowed the iris forward (*iris bombé*), resulting in peripheral anterior synechiae. **C,** Histologic section of another case shows iris bombé, posterior synechiae (ps) of the iris to the anterior surface of the lens, a cyclitic membrane (cm), and a neural retinal detachment (dr). All are the result of long-standing chronic uveitis (pas, peripheral, anterior synechia; l, lens; h, hemorrhage under retina). (**A** and **B,** Courtesy of Dr. GOH Naumann.)

a total ciliary body and neural retinal detachment (see Fig. 3.13). Ciliary body degeneration diminishes aqueous production and leads to hypotony.

Vitreous Compartment

I. Newly formed blood vessels from the neural retina or optic disc, or both, may grow into the vitreous compartment of the eye.

    A. They usually grow between the vitreous and internal surface of the neural retina, along the posterior surface of a detached vitreous, or into Cloquet's canal.

    B. The newly formed blood vessels almost never grow into the formed vitreous.

II. The vitreous body may collapse (i.e., become detached posteriorly).

III. Inflammatory products in the vitreous body may induce organization of the vitreous. Fibrous membranes, including a cyclitic membrane and anterior vitreal organization, usually result.

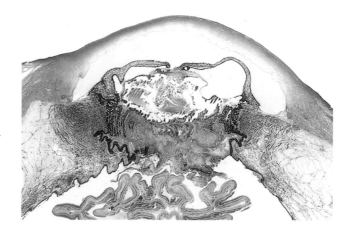

Fig. 3.13 Shrinkage of a cyclitic membrane, a fibrous membrane that spans the retrolental space and incorporates proliferated ciliary epithelium and vitreous base, has caused a neural retinal detachment. Massive ciliary body edema ("detachment"), posterior synechiae of iris to lens, and iris bombé are also present.

Choroid

I. As an aftermath of choroiditis, the choroid may show focal or diffuse areas of atrophy or scarring.
II. Retinochoroiditis or chorioretinitis may destroy Bruch's membrane and retinal pigment epithelium, the choroid and retina may become fused by fibrosis, and a chorioretinal scar or adhesion results.

Chorioretinal adhesions may result without choroidal involvement. This occurs when proliferated retinal pigment epithelium adheres overlying neural retina to the underlying choroid.

Retina

I. Inflammation anywhere in the eye, even in the cornea, frequently causes a neural retinal perivasculitis with lymphocytes surrounding the blood vessels. If extensive, the perivasculitis can be noted clinically as vascular sheathing.

Permanent vascular sheathing results from organization and cicatrization of a perivascular inflammatory infiltrate or from involution of the blood vessels and thickening of their walls.

II. Intraocular inflammation, especially involving the peripheral neural retina or ciliary body, may be accompanied by fluid in the macular retina (i.e., cystoid macular edema).
III. Retinochoroiditis or chorioretinitis may result in chorioretinal scarring.
IV. The neural retina may become detached secondary to subneural retinal exudation or hemorrhage or to organization and formation of vitreal fibrous membranes or a cyclitic membrane.
V. The retinal pigment epithelium is a very reactive tissue and may undergo massive hyperplasia after inflammation. It may also show alternating areas of mild hyperplasia and atrophy, or it may be associated with intraocular ossification.

Glaucoma

I. Glaucoma may result from inflammatory cells and debris clogging an open anterior-chamber angle; from peripheral anterior synechiae and secondary angle closure; from posterior synechiae, pupillary block, iris bombé, and secondary angle closure; or from trabecular damage (inflammation, i.e., trabeculitis and scarring).
II. The proper combination of factors must be present for glaucoma to develop; for example, peripheral anterior synechiae may be present, but if the inflammation damages the capacity for the ciliary body to secrete aqueous, glaucoma does not develop; in fact, hypotony may result.

When hypotony or a normal intraocular pressure is present in an eye with iris bombé and complete closure of the anterior-chamber angle, aqueous is not being secreted. Intraocular surgery in such an eye often hastens the development of phthisis bulbi.

END STAGE OF DIFFUSE OCULAR DISEASES

I. Atrophy without shrinkage
   A. This refers to atrophy of intraocular structures such as the retina and uvea in a normal-size or even enlarged eye (e.g., buphthalmos).
   B. The best example is the diffuse atrophy with longstanding glaucoma.
II. Atrophy with shrinkage (*atrophia bulbi*; Fig. 3.14)
   A. This refers to atrophy of intraocular structures, which remain recognizable, plus atrophy of the globe so that it is smaller than normal.
   B. The best example is chronic, long-standing uveitis (especially when it starts in childhood) that goes on to hypotony in the presence of an anterior-chamber angle closed by peripheral anterior synechiae.

Clinically, the eye is soft and partially collapsed. The pull of the horizontal and vertical rectus muscles causes the shrunken eye to appear cuboid ("squared-off") instead of spherical when viewed with the lids widely separated. A soft, squared-off atrophic eye when seen clinically is called a *phthisical eye* or a *phthisis bulbi*. Histologically, however, the eye does not usually show phthisis bulbi (see later), but rather atrophia bulbi.

III. Atrophy with shrinkage and disorganization (*phthisis bulbi*; see Fig. 3.14)
   A. This refers to a markedly thickened sclera and atrophy of intraocular structures sufficiently profound to make them unrecognizable.
   B. The best example is an unchecked purulent endophthalmitis that results in destruction of all the intraocular structures and widespread intraocular scarring and shrinkage.
IV. Intraocular ossification
   A. This is common in atrophia bulbi (see Fig. 3.14, and Fig. 18.11) and phthisis bulbi.
   B. The bone, which forms without cartilage, seems to require pigment epithelium for its formation, either as an inducer or from actual metaplasia.

A fatty marrow is often present in the bone. In younger patients (<20 years of age), the marrow usually possesses hematopoietic elements.

V. Calcium, often as calcium oxalate, may be deposited in a band keratopathy, a cataractous lens, intraocular bone, sclera, a gliotic neural retina, or optic nerve.

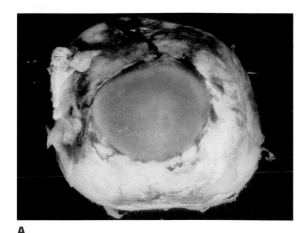

A

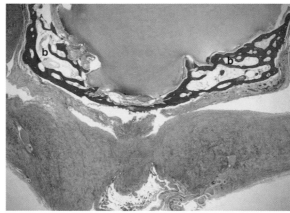

B

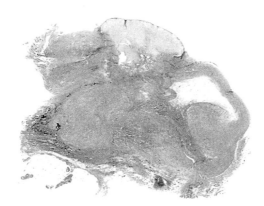

C

Fig. 3.14 End stage of diffuse ocular disease. **A,** The enucleated eye shows the characteristic squared-off appearance of hypotony. The pull of the horizontal and vertical rectus muscles causes the soft, often shrunken, eye to appear squared-off or cuboidal. Clinically, this type of eye is called a *phthisical eye* or *phthisis bulbi.* **B,** Histologic section through the posterior aspect of a small atrophic eye shows extensive bone (b) in the inner choroid. **C,** In this histologic section, the globe is so disorganized that the normal structures are unrecognizable. The condition is called *phthisis bulbi.* The eye has been completely scarred owing to purulent endophthalmitis.

BIBLIOGRAPHY

Suppurative Endophthalmitis and Panophthalmitis

Boyd SR, Young S, Lightman S: Immunopathology of the noninfectious posterior and intermediate uveitides. *Surv Ophthalmol* 46:209, 2001

Demirôglu H, Baralsta_ I, Dündar S: Risk factor assessment and prognosis of eye involvement in Behçet's disease in Turkey. *Ophthalmology* 104:701, 1997

Dominguez LN, Irvine AR: Fundus changes in Behçet's disease. *Trans Am Ophthalmol Soc* 95:367, 1997

Garcher C, Bielefeld P, Desvaux C et al.: Bilateral loss of vision and macular ischemia related to Behçet disease. *Am J Ophthalmol* 124:116, 1997

George RK, Chan C-C, Whitcup SM et al.: Ocular immunology of Behçet's disease. *Surv Ophthalmol* 42:157, 1997

Jackson TL, Eykyn SJ, Graham EM et al.: Endogenous bacterial endophthalmitis: a 17-year prospective series and review of 267 reported cases. *Surv Ophthalmol* 48:403, 2003

Inomota H, Yoshikawa H, Rao NA: Phacoanaphylaxis in Behçet's disease. A clinicopathologic and immunohistochemicsal study. *Ophthalmology* 110:1942, 2003

Kresloff MS, Castellarin AA, Zarbin MA: Endophthalmitis. *Surv Ophthalmol* 43:193, 1998

Margo CE, Mames RN, Guy JR: Endogenous *Klebsiella* endophthalmitis: Report of two cases and review of the literature. *Ophthalmology* 101:1298, 1994

Matsuo T, Notohara K, Shiraga F et al.: Endogenous amoebic endophthalmitis. *Arch Ophthalmol* 119:125, 2001

Mizuki N, Ota M, Yabuki K et al.: Localization of the pathogenic gene of Behçet's disease by microsatellite analysis of three different populations. *Invest Ophthalmol Vis Sci* 41:3702, 2000

Probst K, Fijnheer R, Rothova A: Endothelial cell activation and hypercoagulability in ocular Behçet's disease. *Am J Ophthalmol* 137:850, 2004

Shayegani A, MacFarlane D, Kazim M et al.: Streptococcal gangrene of the eyelids and orbit. *Am J Ophthalmol* 120:784, 1995

deSmet MD, Dayan M: Prospective determination of T-cell responses to S-antigen in Behçet's disease patients and controls. *Invest Ophthalmol Vis Sci* 41:3480, 2000

Tugal-Tutkun I, Onal S, Altan-Yaycioglu R et al.: Uveitis in Behçet disease: an analysis of 880 patients. *Am J Ophthalmol* 38:375, 2004

Verity DH, Vaughan RW, Madanat W et al.: Factor V Leiden mutation is associated with ocular involvement in Behçet's disease. *Am J Ophthalmol* 128:352, 1999

Zamir E, Bodaghi B, Tugal-Ttutkun I et al.: Conjunctival ulcers in Behçet's disease. *Ophthalmology* 110:1137. 2003

Nonsuppurative, Chronic Nongranulomatous Uveitis and Endophthalmitis

Barile GR, Flynn TE: Syphilis exposure in patients with uveitis. *Ophthalmology* 104:1605, 1997

Bechtel RT, Haught KA, Mets MB: Lymphocytic choriomeningitis virus: A new addition to the TORCH evaluation. *Arch Ophthalmol* 115:680, 1997

Berker N, Batman C, Guven A et al.: Optic atrophy and macular degeneration as initial presentations of subacute sclerosing encephalitis. *Am J Ophthalmol* 138:879, 2004

Bora NS, Bora PS, Kaplan HJ: Identification, quantitation, and purification of a 36 kDa circulating protein associated with active pars planitis. *Invest Ophthalmol Vis Sci* 37:1870, 1996

Bora NS, Bora PS, Kaplan HJ: Molecular cloning, sequencing, and expression of the 36 kDa protein present in pars planitis. *Invest Ophthalmol Vis Sci* 37:1877, 1996

Chodosh J, Gan Y-J, Sixbey JW: Detection of Epstein–Barr virus genome in ocular tissues. *Ophthalmology* 103:687, 1996

Chung E-V, Wilhelmus KR, Matoba AY, et al.: Herpes simplex keratitis in children. *Am J Ophthalmol* 138:474, 2004

Diaz-Valle D, del Castillo JMB, Aceñero MJF et al.: Bilateral lid margin ulcers as the initial manifestation of Crohn disease. *Am J Ophthalmol* 138:292, 2004

Ernst BB, Lowder CY, Meisler DM et al.: Posterior segment manifestations of inflammatory bowel disease. *Ophthalmology* 98:1272, 1991

Floegal I, Haas A, El-Shabrawi Y: Acute multifocal placoid pigment epitheliopathy-like lesion as an early sign of subacute sclerosing panencephalitis. *Am J Ophthalmol* 135:103, 2003

Foster CS, Barrett F: Cataract development and cataract surgery in patients with juvenile rheumatoid arthritis-associated iridocyclitis. *Ophthalmology* 100:809, 1993

Gardner BP, Margolis TP, Mondino BJ: Conjunctival lymphocytic nodule associated with the Epstein–Barr virus. *Am J Ophthalmol* 112:567, 1991

Goldstein DA, Edward DP, Tessler HH: Iris crystals in Fuchs heterochromic iridocyclitis. *Arch Ophthalmol* 116:1692, 1998

Grossniklaus HE, Aaberg TM, Purnell EW et al.: Retinal necrosis in X-linked lymphoproliferative disease. *Ophthalmology* 101:705, 1994

Kerkhoff FT, Lamberts QJ, van den Bieson PR et al.: Rhegmatogenous retinal detachment and uveitis. *Ophthalmology* 110:427, 2003

Kotaniemi K, Savolainen A, Karma A et al.: Recent advances in uveitis of juvenile idiopathic arthritis. *Surv Ophthalmol* 48:489, 2003

Liesegang TJ: Discussion of Wirostko E, Johnson LA, Wirostko BM et al.: *Mycoplasma*-like organisms and ophthalmic disease. *Trans Am Ophthalmol Soc* 91:95, 1993

Linssen A, Meenken C: Outcomes of HLA-B27-positive and HLA-B27-negative acute anterior uveitis. *Am J Ophthalmol* 120:351, 1995

Malinowski SM, Pulido JS, Folk JC: Long-term visual outcome and complications associated with pars planitis. *Ophthalmology* 100:818, 1993

Matoba AY: Ocular disease associated with Epstein–Barr virus infection. *Surv Ophthalmol* 35:145, 1990

Needham AD, Harding SP: Bilateral multifocal choroiditis in Reiter syndrome. *Arch Ophthalmol* 115:684, 1997

Nelson DA, Weiner A, Yanoff M et al.: Retinal lesions in subacute sclerosing panencephalitis. *Arch Ophthalmol* 84:613, 1970

O'Keefe JS, Sippy BD, Martin DF et al.: Anterior chamber infiltrates associated with systemic lymphoma. Report of two cases and review of the literature. *Ophthalmology* 109:253, 2002

Perry H, Yanoff M, Scheie HG: Fuchs's heterochromic iridocyclitis. *Arch Ophthalmol* 93:337, 1975

Quentin CD, Reiber H: Fuchs heterochromi cyclitis: rubella virus antibodies and genome in aqueous humor. *Am J Ophthalmol* 138:45, 2004

Rahhal FM, Siegel LM, Russak V et al.: Clinicopathologic correlations in acute retinal necrosis caused by herpes simplex virus type 2. *Arch Ophthalmol* 114:1416, 1996

Raja SC, Jabs DA, Dunn JP et al.: Pars planitis. Clinical features and class II HLA associations. *Ophthalmology* 106:594, 1999

Rieux-Laucat F, LeDeist F, Hivroz C et al.: Mutations in Fas associated with human lymphoproliferative syndrome. *Science* 268:1347, 1995

Rothova A, La Hey E, Baarsma GS et al.: Iris nodules in Fuchs' heterochromic uveitis. *Am J Ophthalmol* 118:338, 1994

Ruby AJ, Jampol LM: Crohn's disease and retinal vascular disease. *Am J Ophthalmol* 110:349, 1990

Schwab IR: The epidemiologic association of Fuchs' heterochromic iridocyclitis and ocular toxoplasmosis. *Am J Ophthalmol* 111:356, 1991

Soheilian M, Markomichelakis N, Foeter CS: Intermediate uveitis and retinal vasculitis as manifestations of cat scratch disease. *Am J Ophthalmol* 122:582, 1996

Tang WM, Pulido JS, Eckels DD et al.: The association of HLA-DR15 and intermediate uveitis. *Am J Ophthalmol* 123:70, 1997

Tay-Kearney M-L, Schwam BL, Lowder C et al.: Clinical features and associated systemic diseases of HLA-B27 uveitis. *Am J Ophthalmol* 121:47, 1996

Teyssot N, Cassoux N, Lehoang P et al.: Fuchs heterochromic cyclitis and ocular toxocariasis. *Am J Ophthalmol* 139:915, 2005

Tugal-Tutkun I, Havrlikova K, Power JP et al.: Changing patterns in uveitis of childhood. *Ophthalmology* 103:375, 1996

Wirostko E, Johnson LA, Wirostko BM et al.: *Mycoplasma*-like organisms and ophthalmic disease. *Trans Am Ophthalmol Soc* 91:86, 1993

Woda BA, Sullivan JL: Reactive histiocytic disorders. *Am J Clin Pathol* 99:459, 1993

Wolf CV II, Wolf JR, Parker JS: Kawasaki's syndrome in a man with the human immunodeficiency virus. *Am J Ophthalmol* 120:117, 1995

Yanoff M, Allman MI: Congenital herpes simplex virus, type 2, bilateral endophthalmitis. *Trans Am Ophthalmol Soc* 75:325, 1977

Yin Y, Manoury B, Fåhraeus R: Self-inhibition of synthesis and antigen presentation by Epstein–Barr virus-encoded EBNA1. *Science* 301:1371, 2003

Zamir E, Margalit E, Chowers I: Iris crystals in Fuchs' heterochromic iridocyclitis. *Arch Ophthalmol* 116:1394, 1998

Sequelae of Uveitis, Endophthalmitis, and Panophthalmitis

Chan C-C, Fujikawa LS, Rodrigues MM et al.: Immunohistochemistry and electron microscopy of cyclitic membrane. Report of a case. *Arch Ophthalmol* 104:1040, 1986

Kampik A, Patrinely JR, Green WR: Morphologic and clinical features of retrocorneal melanin pigmentation and pigmented pupillary membranes: review of 225 cases. *Surv Ophthalmol* 27:161, 1982

Winslow RL, Stevenson W III, Yanoff M: Spontaneous expulsive choroidal hemorrhage. *Arch Ophthalmol* 92:126, 1974

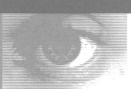

4

Granulomatous Inflammation

INTRODUCTION

Chronic granulomatous inflammation is a proliferative inflammation characterized by a cellular infiltrate of epithelioid cells [and sometimes inflammatory giant cells, lymphocytes, plasma cells, polymorphonuclear leukocytes (PMNs), and eosinophils; see p. 12 in Chapter 1].

POSTTRAUMATIC

Sympathetic Uveitis (Sympathetic Ophthalmia, Sympathetic Ophthalmitis)

I. Sympathetic uveitis (Figs 4.1 and 4.2) is a bilateral, diffuse, granulomatous, T-cell-mediated uveitis that occurs from 2 weeks to many years after penetrating or perforating ocular injury and is associated with traumatic uveal incarceration or prolapse.

   A. Although the uveitis may start as early as 5 days or as late as 50 years after injury, well over 90% of cases occur after 2 weeks but within 1 year. Most of these (80%) occur within 3 weeks to 3 months postinjury.

   B. Removal of the injured eye before sympathetic uveitis occurs usually completely protects against inflammation developing in the noninjured eye.* Once the inflammation starts, however, removal of the injured ("exciting") eye probably has little effect on the course of the disease, especially after 3 to 6 months.

Rarely, sympathetic uveitis has been reported to have developed in the sympathizing eye after the injured eye has been enucleated.

Evidence exists that early enucleation of the exciting eye can favorably affect visual prognosis, especially early enucleation, within the first 3 to 6 months. Sympathetic uveitis has been reported in nontraumatized eyes in a few isolated cases. However, unless the whole eye is serially sectioned and carefully examined for evidence of perforation, the clinician can never be sure that some long-forgotten penetrating ocular wound is not present. A diagnosis of sympathetic uveitis in the absence of an ocular injury should be viewed with marked skepticism.

II. Blurred vision and photophobia in the noninjured (sympathizing) eye are usually the first symptoms. Vision and photophobia worsen concurrently in the injured (exciting) eye, and a granulomatous uveitis develops, especially mutton-fat keratic precipitates (see Fig. 4.1A), which are collections of epithelioid cells plus lymphocytes, macrophages, inflammatory multinucleated giant cells, or pigment on the posterior surface of the cornea.

Glaucoma may develop owing to blockage of the angle by cellular debris or peripheral anterior synechiae, or hypotony may occur from decreased aqueous output by the inflamed ciliary body.

III. The cause appears to be a delayed-type hypersensitivity reaction of the uvea to antigens localized on the retinal pigment epithelium or on uveal melanocytes.

   A. The lymphocytic infiltrate consists almost exclusively of T lymphocytes.

   B. B cells found in some cases, usually of long duration, may represent the end stage of the disease.

Phacoanaphylactic endophthalmitis (PE) was found in approximately 25% of patients who had sympathetic uveitis in cases submitted to the Armed Forces Institute of Pathology before

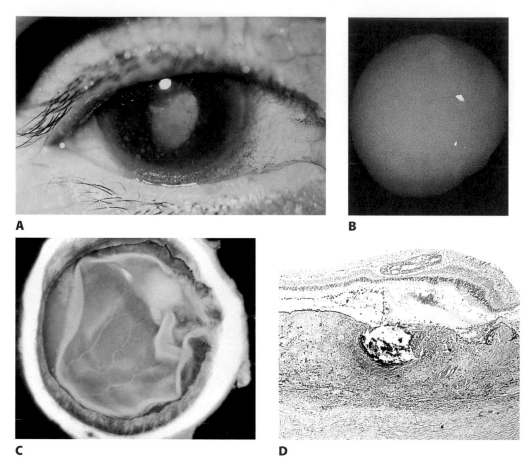

Fig. 4.1 Sympathetic uveitis. **A,** Large, "greasy," mutton-fat keratic precipitates (KPs: collections of epithelioid cells, lymphocytes, and plasma cells on posterior surface of cornea) seen in patient with sympathetic uveitis. **B,** Another patient had a perforating injury to his eye. The other (sympathizing) eye developed photophobia and mutton-fat KPs; the injured (exciting) eye was enucleated. Radiograph of enucleated eye shows two metallic foreign bodies in eye. **C,** Gross specimen shows massive, diffuse thickening of choroid. **D,** Granulomatous inflammation fills and thickens the choroid (see also Fig. 4.2A and B). The Perl stain is positive (blue) for iron in the large, dark foreign body in the choroid. (**B–D,** Courtesy of Dr. TH Chou.)

1950, whereas since 1950, only approximately 5% of cases of sympathetic uveitis have also had PE. The marked reduction in the association of the two diseases is probably attributable to advances in the management of penetrating wounds. It has been suggested that sympathetic uveitis represents a forme fruste of Vogt–Koyanagi–Harada (VKH) syndrome (see subsection on *Vogt–Koyanagi–Harada Syndrome* (*Uveomeningoencaphalitic Syndrome*), later). The relationship between the two entities is still uncertain.

C. Human leukocyte antigen (HLA)-DRB1*04, DQA1*03, and DQB1*04 are significantly associated with sympathetic uveitis.

Both the clinical manifestations and immunogenetic background of sympathetic uveitis and VKH syndrome (see later) are quite similar.

IV. Histologically, sympathetic uveitis has certain characteristics that are suggestive of the disorder but not diagnostic.

A. Sympathetic uveitis is a clinicopathologic diagnosis, never a histologic diagnosis alone.

The uveal inflammatory reaction tends to be more vigorous in black than in white patients.

B. The following four histologic findings are characteristic of both sympathizing and exciting eyes:
1. Diffuse granulomatous uveal inflammation composed predominantly of epithelioid cells and lymphocytes. Eosinophils may be plentiful. Plasma cells are few or moderate in number. Neutrophils are rare or absent
2. Sparing of the choriocapillaris
3. Epithelioid cells containing phagocytosed uveal pigment
4. Dalen–Fuchs nodules (i.e., collections of epithelioid cells lying between Bruch's membrane and the retinal pigment epithelium with no involvement of

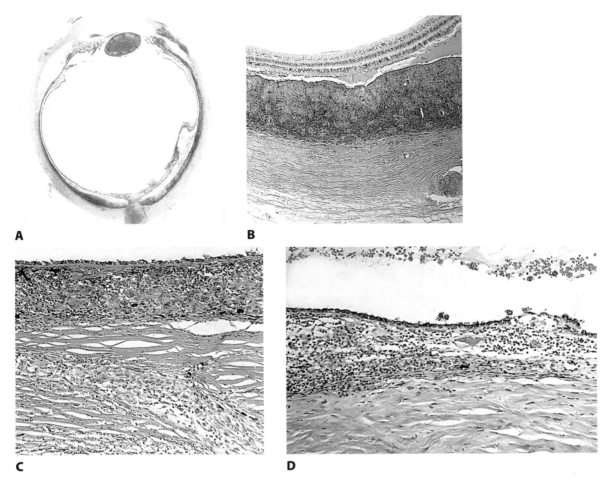

Fig. 4.2 Sympathetic uveitis. **A,** Enucleated eye from Figure 4.1B and C shows diffuse thickening of the choroid (shown with increased magnification in **B**) by granulomatous inflammation. The pale areas represent epithelioid cells and the dark areas consist mainly of lymphocytes. **C,** Sparing of the choriocapillaris and pigment phagocytosis by epithelioid cells is seen. Note granulomatous inflammation of scleral canal in lower right corner (reason why evisceration does not protect against sympathetic uveitis). **D,** Dalen–Fuchs nodule of epithelioid cells between retinal pigment epithelium and Bruch's membrane is seen. Underlying choriocapillaris is spared and overlying neural retina is free of inflammatory process. (Courtesy of Dr. TH Chou.)

the overlying neural retina and sparing of the underlying choriocapillaris*)

Because the signs of the trauma are usually in the anterior portion of the eye, the posterior choroid is the best place to look for the granulomatous inflammation. Typically the neural retina is not involved, except near the ora serrata. Localized neural retinal detachments may be seen, especially in areas where Dalen–Fuchs nodules coalesce.

C. Other findings:
1. Tissue damage caused by the trauma
2. Extension of the granulomatous inflammation into the scleral canals and optic disc

Because uveal tissue is normally found in the scleral canals and in the vicinity of the optic disc, evisceration, which

does not reach these areas, does *not* protect against sympathetic uveitis. If surgery is being done to prevent sympathetic uveitis, the procedure must be an enucleation, not an evisceration.

Phacoanaphylactic (Phacoimmune)

Endophthalmitis

I. PE (Fig. 4.3) is a rare, autoimmune, unilateral (sometimes bilateral if the lens capsule is ruptured in each eye), zonal, granulomatous inflammation centered around lens material. It depends on a ruptured lens capsule for its development.

Spontaneous rupture of the lens in Behçet's disease can cause PE.

II. The disease occurs under special conditions that involve an abrogation of tolerance to lens prottein.

*Some studies suggest that most of the epithelial cells occurring in the Dalen–Fuchs nodule are derived from monocytes and macrophages. Some cells may also come from transformation of retinal pigment epithelial cells.

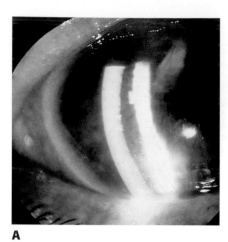
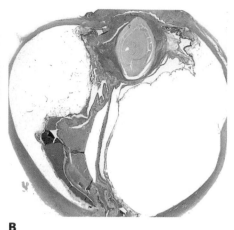
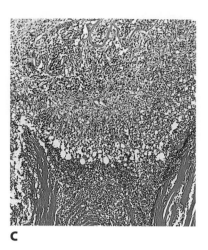

A B C

Fig. 4.3 Phacoanaphylactic endophthalmitis. **A,** The patient had an iridencleisis in 1971. The eye was injured by blunt trauma in an automobile accident in May 1973. In September 1973, signs of an anterior uveitis developed. Note the small mutton-fat keratic precipitates just to the right of the corneal slit-lamp section in the lower third of the picture. The eye was enucleated in May 1974. **B,** The enucleated globe shows iris in the subconjunctival tissue. The lens remnant, mainly nucleus, shows a zonal type of granulomatous reaction, consisting of surrounding epithelioid cells and giant cells, in turn surrounded by lymphocytes and plasma cells, in turn surrounded by granulation tissue. The lens capsule is ruptured posteriorly. **C,** Under increased magnification, the typical zonal pattern is seen around the remnant of the lens nucleus (periodic acid–Schiff stain).

Lens proteins are organ-specific but not species-specific. Lens proteins, if exposed to the systemic circulation, are normally recognized as "self." If they were not, PE would occur regularly, instead of rarely, after disruption of the lens capsule.

A. PE may result from the breakdown or reversal of central tolerance at the T-cell level. Small amounts of circulating lens protein normally maintain T-cell tolerance, but it may be altered as a result of trauma, possibly through the adjuvant effects of wound contamination or bacterial products, or both.

B. After the abrogation of tolerance to lens protein, antilens antibodies are produced. The antibodies reach the lens remnants in the eye and an antibody–antigen reaction takes place (PE).

Presumably the lens protein that leaks through an intact capsule (e.g., in a mature or hypermature lens) is denatured (unlike the nondenatured lens protein that escapes through a ruptured lens capsule). Thus, it is incapable of acting as an antigen and eliciting an antibody response. The denatured lens protein, however, may incite a mild foreign-body macrophagic response. The macrophages, swollen with engulfed denatured lens material, may block the anterior-chamber drainage angle and cause an acute secondary open-angle glaucoma called *phacolytic glaucoma* (see p. 384 in Chapter 10).

III. Histologically, in addition to the findings at the site of injury, a zonal granulomatous inflammation is found.
   A. Activated neutrophils surround and seem to dissolve or eat away lens material, probably releasing proteolytic enzymes, arachidonic acid metabolites, and oxygen-derived free radicals.
   B. Epithelioid cells and occasional (sometimes in abundance) multinucleated inflammatory giant cells are seen beyond the neutrophils.
   C. Lymphocytes, plasma cells, fibroblasts, and blood vessels (granulation tissue) surround the epithelioid cells.
   D. Usually the iris is encased in, and inseparable from, the inflammatory reaction.
   E. The uveal tract usually shows a reactive, chronic non-granulomatous inflammatory reaction.
      Sometimes, however, the same trauma that ruptures the lens and sets off the PE initiates a sympathetic uveitis and results in a diffuse, chronic, granulomatous inflammation.

Foreign-Body Granulomas

I. Foreign-body granulomas may develop around exogenous foreign bodies that are usually introduced into the eye at the time of a penetrating ocular wound, or they may develop around endogenous products such as cholesterol or blood in the vitreous.

An unusual cause of inflammatory granuloma of the conjunctiva is the synthetic fiber found in teddy bears, called a ("teddy-bear") granuloma.

Rarely, blood in the vitreous incites a marked foreign-body inflammatory response. When this occurs, the intravitreal hemorrhage almost is invariably traumatic in origin, rather than spontaneous.

II. Histologically, a zonal type of granulomatous inflammatory reaction surrounds the foreign body.

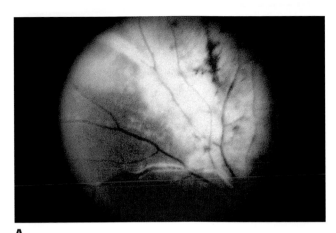

A

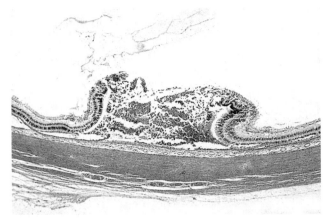

B

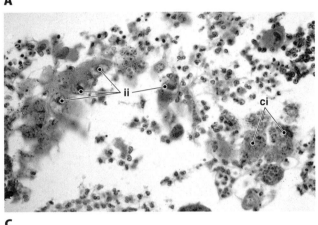

C

Fig. 4.4 Cytomegalic inclusion disease. **A,** The fundus picture shows the characteristic hemorrhagic exudation ("pizza-pie" appearance) along the retinal vessels. **B,** Histologic section shows the relatively normal neural retina sharply demarcated on each side from the central area of coagulative retinal necrosis, secondary to the infection. The choroid shows a secondary mild and diffuse granulomatous inflammation. **C,** Increased magnification shows typical eosinophilic intranuclear inclusion bodies (ii) and small, round basophilic and cytoplasmic inclusion bodies (ci). (**A,** Courtesy of Dr. SH Sinclair; **B** and **C,** presented by Dr. Daniel Toussaint at the meeting of the Verhoeff Society, 1976.)

NONTRAUMATIC INFECTIONS

Viral

I. Cytomegalic inclusion disease (salivary gland disease; Fig. 4.4)

  A. Cytomegalic inclusion disease is caused by systemic infection with the salivary gland virus, cytomegalovirus (CMV), an enveloped herpesvirus formed by an icosahedral capsid and a double-stranded DNA.

> CMV is huge, containing more than 200 genes (compared with its modest relative, herpes simplex virus, which contains only 84 genes). It is estimated that CMV infects 80% to 85% of people by 40 years of age. In otherwise healthy, immunocompetent people, CMV infection usually runs a benign, asymptomatic course (rarely, a heterophile-negative mononucleosis syndrome occurs). After primary exposure, CMV may establish a latent infection and the virus genome may persist in cells undetectable by conventional culture assays.

    1. Congenital: characterized by retinochoroiditis, prematurity, jaundice, thrombocytopenia, anemia, hepatosplenomegaly, neurologic involvement, and intracranial calcification

> Cytomegalic inclusion disease is the most common viral infection of the neonate, with an incidence of 5 to 20 per 1000 live births. Most of the infants are asymptomatic at birth. The differential diagnosis consists of the TORCH syndrome (toxoplasmosis, rubella, CMV, and herpes simplex; see p. 62 in Chapter 3).

    2. Acquired: mainly found in patients whose immune mechanisms have been modified [e.g., acquired immunodeficiency syndrome (AIDS), acute leukemia, malignant lymphomas, chemotherapy, and immunosuppressive therapy for renal transplantation]

> CMV retinitis occurs in approximately 30% of patients with AIDS (35% have bilateral CMV retinitis at time of presentation, and up to 75% will become bilateral). Patients who have AIDS and have a low CD4+ and CD8+ T-lymphocyte cell count are at a high risk for the development of CMV retinitis. CMV retinitis in patients with and without AIDS, treated with highly active antiretroviral therapy, has a similar course, except the incidence of retinal detachment is higher in the AIDS' patients.

  B. Clinically, a central retinochoroiditis seen in the congenital form is similar to that seen in toxoplasmosis.

1. The acquired form starts with scattered, yellow-white retinal dots or granular patches that may become confluent and are associated with sheathing of adjacent vessels and retinal hemorrhages (characteristic hemorrhagic exudation with "pizza-pie" or "cottage cheese with catsup" appearance).
2. Neural retinal detachments may develop in 15% of affected eyes.
3. Other ocular findings include iridocyclitis, punctate keratitis, and optic neuritis.

> A periphlebitis that mimics *acute frosted retinitis* may occur. Other conditions that may mimic CMV retinitis include other herpesviruses, measles, syphilis, fungal retinitis (*Cryptococcus neoformans* and *Candida albicans*), toxoplasmosis, and acute retinal necrosis.

4. Immune recovery uveitis, associated with the potent antiviral therapies, refers to a condition in which heightened intraocular inflammation occurs in some patients who have pre-existing CMV retinitis.

C. Histologically, a primary coagulative necrotizing retinitis and a secondary diffuse granulomatous choroiditis are seen.
1. The infected neural retinal cells show large eosinophilic intranuclear inclusions and small, multiple, basophilic intracytoplasmic inclusions.

2. In areas of healed retinitis, clinically seen focal yellow-white plaques contain calcium when examined histologically.

> The cytoplasmic inclusions consist of numerous virions closely associated with dense masses of matter (periodic acid–Schiff-positive on light microscopy) that are highly characteristic of CMV. An additional highly characteristic feature is the presence of the virions in a mass of viral subunit material that forms a lacy, centrally located pattern in the nucleus. The nucleolus is marginated and free of virions. Clumping of peripheral chromatin is lacking.

3. The location and character of the retinal vascular changes in AIDS indicate an ischemic pathogenesis, most profound in CMV retinitis.

II. Varicella/herpes zoster virus (VZV; Figs 4.5 and 4.6)
A. VZV causes varicella (chickenpox) and herpes zoster (shingles).
1. The virus, a member of the herpesvirus family, consists of a lipid envelope surrounding an icosahedral nucleocapsid with a central, double-stranded DNA core; only the enveloped virions are infectious.
2. Congenital infection is rare (differential diagnosis consists of the TORCH syndrome; see p. 62 in Chapter 3).
3. In immunocompetent individuals, VZV is a major cause of the acute retinal necrosis syndrome (see p. 417 in Chapter 11).

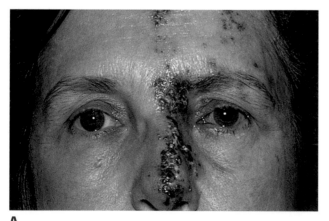

A

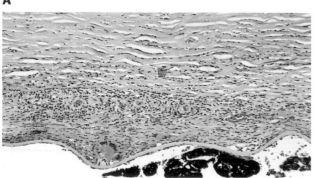

C

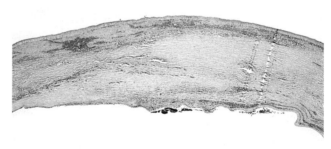

B

Fig. 4.5 Herpes zoster. **A,** Ophthalmic branch of trigeminal nerve involved, including tip of nose; the patient had iritis. **B,** Evisceration specimen from another patient who had herpes zoster ophthalmicus shows corneal thickening, scarring, and inflammation. **C,** Increased magnification shows granulomatous inflammation, with epithelioid cells and inflammatory giant cells, mainly centered around Descemet's membrane (granulomatous reaction to Descemet's membrane).

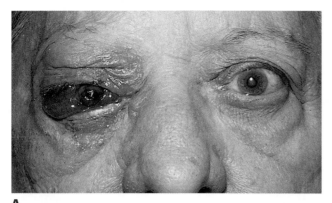

A

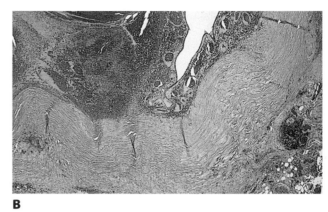

B

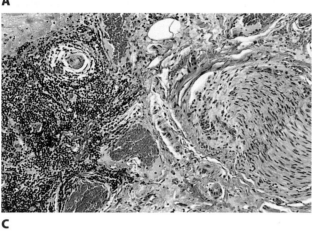

C

Fig. 4.6 Herpes zoster. **A,** Patient with herpes zoster ophthalmicus developed chronic herpes keratitis and then corneal perforation; the eye was enucleated. **B,** Nongranulomatous inflammatory infiltrates centered around ciliary nerves in posterior episclera (no granulomatous inflammation present), shown with increased magnification in **C.**

B. Ocular complications occur in approximately 50% of cases of herpes zoster ophthalmicus:

1. Cornea: dendritic ulcer (rare), ulceration, perforation, peripheral erosions, bullous keratopathy, epidermidalization (keratinization), band keratopathy, pannus formation, stromal vascularization, hypertrophy of corneal nerves, ring abscess, granulomatous reaction to Descemet's membrane, and endothelial degeneration
2. Anterior-chamber: iridocyclitis followed by peripheral anterior synechiae, exudate, and hyphema
3. Iris: patchy necrosis and postnecrotic atrophy (mimics iris after attack of acute angle closure glaucoma), chronic nongranulomatous inflammation, and anterior-surface fibrovascular membrane
4. Ciliary body: patchy necrosis of anterior portion, especially of circular and radial portions of ciliary muscle
5. Choroid: chronic nongranulomatous inflammation and, less commonly, granulomatous inflammation
6. Lens: cataract and posterior synechiae
7. Neural retina: perivasculitis and vasculitis
8. Vitreous: mild mononuclear inflammatory infiltrate
9. Sclera: acute or chronic episcleritis and scleritis
10. Optic nerve: perivasculitis and chronic leptomeningitis
11. Long posterior ciliary nerves and vessels: striking perineural and, less commonly, intraneural nongranulomatous and occasionally granulomatous inflammation and perivasculitis and vasculitis

C. Histologically, the most characteristic findings are lymphocytic (chronic nongranulomatous) infiltrations involving the posterior ciliary nerves and vessels, often in a segmental distribution, and a diffuse or patchy necrosis involving the iris and pars plicata of the ciliary body.

1. Granulomatous inflammatory lesions may also be seen.
2. Inclusion bodies have not been demonstrated in the chronic inflammatory lesions.

Bacterial

I. Tuberculosis (*Mycobacterium tuberculosis*; Figs 4.7 and 4.8)

A. Tuberculosis has re-emerged as a serious public health problem, mainly because of the human immunodeficiency virus (HIV) epidemic and newly developed resistance to standard antibiotic therapy.

It is estimated that about one-third of the world's population is infected by *Mycobacterium tuberculosis*. It may present in

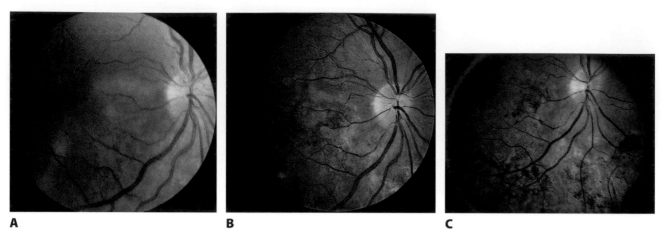

Fig. 4.7 Tuberculosis. **A,** Archeology college student presented with a granulomatous posterior choroiditis. Active pulmonary tuberculosis was documented; antituberculous therapy was instituted. Appearance of lesion 2 months (**B**) and 16 months (**C**) later. At time of last photograph (**C**), the tuberculosis was considered cured.

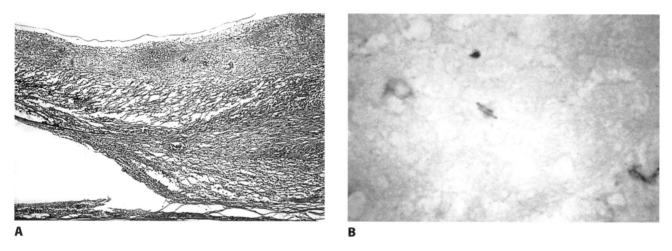

Fig. 4.8 Tuberculosis. **A,** Tuberculous zonal granuloma involves retina and choroid. Caseation necrosis is present. **B,** In the middle of the field, typical acid-fast organisms are shown by the Ziehl–Neelsen method. (Courtesy of Dr. AH Friedman.)

children initially as a preceptal cellulitis unresponsive to systemic antibiotic therapy.

B. Tubercle bacilli reach the eye through the blood stream, after lung infection.

Tubercle bacilli survive within macrophages because they secrete eukaryocyte-like serine/threonine protein kinase G within macrophage phagosomes, inhibiting phagosome–lysosome fusion and mediating intracellular survival of mycobacterium. Rarely, intraocular tuberculosis can occur without obvious systemic infection.

1. The most common form of ocular involvement is a cyclitis that rapidly becomes an iridocyclitis and may also spread posteriorly to cause a choroiditis.

Tuberculous choroiditis may mimic serpiginous choroiditis.

2. Clinically, mutton-fat keratic precipitates are seen on the posterior surface of the cornea and deep infiltrates in the choroid, often in the posterior pole.

Retinal tuberculosis usually spreads from an underlying choroiditis. The involvement may become massive to form a large tuberculoma involving all the coats of the eye (i.e., a panophthalmitis). Tuberculoprotein hypersensitivity may play a role in the pathogenesis of phlyctenules and Eales' disease.

C. Miliary tuberculosis usually causes a multifocal, discrete (sarcoidal, tuberculoidal) granulomatous choroiditis.
D. Histologically, the classic pattern of caseation necrosis consists of a zonal type of granulomatous reaction around the area of coagulative necrosis.
   1. A smooth, acid-fast bacillus can be demonstrated by acid-fast (Ziehl–Neelsen) or fluorescent acid-fast stains.

2. The polymerase chain reaction, prepared from formaldehyde-fixed and paraffin-embedded tissue, can be helpful in making the diagnosis.

II. Leprosy (Hansen's disease; *M. leprae*; Fig. 4.9)

Distinction in gene expression correlates with and accurately classifies the clinical forms of the disease

---

A. In *lepromatous leprosy*, the lepromin test (analogous to the tuberculin test) is negative, suggesting little or no immunity.

Genes belonging to the leukocyte immunoglobulin-like receptor (LIR) family are significantly upregulated in lesions of lepromatous patients suffering from the disseminated form of the infection.

---

1. The prognosis is poor.
2. Lepromas of the skin result in leonine facies and neurologic changes.
3. The eyeballs are involved, usually in their anterior portions.

4. Histologically, a diffuse type of granulomatous inflammatory reaction, known as a *leproma*, is present.
   a. The leproma shows large, pale-staining histiocytes that are called *lepra cells* when their cytoplasm is amorphous and *Virchow's cells* when vacuolated.
   b. The lepra cells and Virchow's cells teem with beaded bacilli (no immunity).
   c. The lepromas involve mainly cornea, anterior sclera, and iris.

The bacteria may grow better in the cooler, anterior portion of the eye, rather than in the warmer, posterior portion, just as they do in the cooler skin instead of in the warmer, deeper structures of the body.

B. In *tuberculoid leprosy*, the lepromin test is positive, suggesting immunity.
   1. The prognosis is good.
   2. A neural involvement predominates with hypopigmented (vitiliginous), hypoesthetic lesions and thickened nerves.

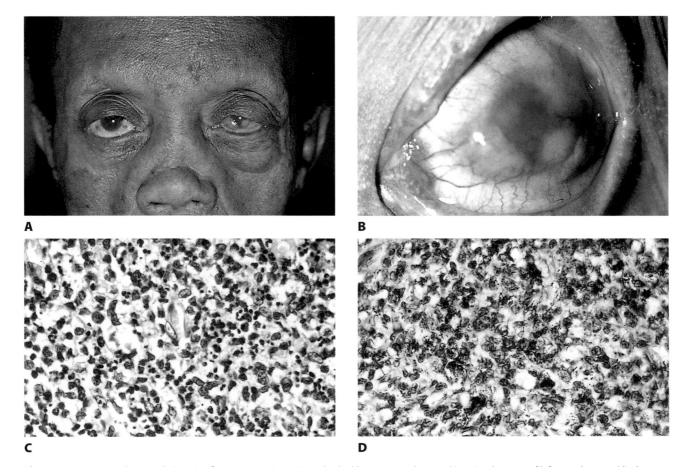

A

B

C

D

Fig. 4.9 Lepromatous leprosy. **A,** Leonine facies present in patient who had lepromatous leprosy. Note involvement of left eye, shown with closer view in **B. C,** Many "clear" cells are seen with hematoxylin and eosin-stained section. **D,** Same cells are teeming with acid-fast leprous organisms (red) as seen with the Ziehl–Neelsen method. (**A** and **B,** Courtesy of Dr. B Blaise; **C** and **D,** courtesy of Dr. P Henkind.)

The ulnar nerve is particularly vulnerable, leading to the characteristic claw hand.

3. The ocular adnexa and orbital structures are involved, especially the ciliary nerves, but not the eyeballs.
4. Histologically, a discrete (sarcoidal, tuberculoidal) type of granulomatous inflammatory reaction is seen, mainly centered around nerves.
   a. The individual nodules tend to be much more variably sized than those in sarcoidosis or miliary tuberculosis.
   b. Organisms are extremely hard to find (good immunity) and are usually located in an area of nerve degeneration.

III. Syphilis (*Treponema pallidum*; Fig. 4.10)
   A. Both the congenital and acquired forms of syphilis may produce a nongranulomatous interstitial keratitis (see p. 267 in Chapter 8) or anterior or posterior uveitis.

The two most commonly used nontreponemal tests (which detect antibody to cardiolipin–lecithin–cholesterol antigen) are the Venereal Disease Research Laboratory (VDRL) and the rapid plasma reagin. The treponemal tests (which detect antibody against treponemal antigens) include the fluorescent treponemal antibody absorption test (FTA-ABS), hemagglutination treponemal test for syphilis, *T. pallidum* hemagglutination assay, and the microhemagglutination test. Routine screening with VDRL and FTA-ABS is recommended in patients who have unexplained uveitis or other ocular inflammation.

Syphilis may occur in immunologically deficient patients (e.g., those with AIDS).

   B. Syphilis, a venereal disease, is divided into three chronologically overlapping stages.

The nonvenereal treponematoses caused by subspecies *T. p. pertenue* (yaws) and *T. p. endemicum* (bejel) are morphologically indistinguishable from *T. pallidum*, and display only subtle immunologic differences.

1. Primary stage: characterized by an ulcerative lesion, chancre, occurring at the site where *T. pallidum* penetrates the skin or mucous membrane. Primary lesions heal spontaneously in 2 to 8 weeks and rarely cause systemic symptoms.

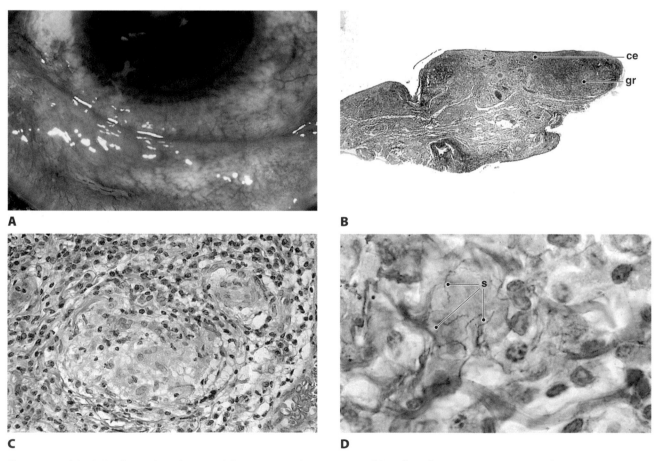

Fig. 4.10 Syphilis. **A,** Small, round translucent nodules are seen in the conjunctiva of the inferior fornix. **B,** Biopsy of nodules shows numerous granulomas under the conjunctival epithelium (ce, surface conjunctival epithelium; gr, granulomatous reaction in substantia propia). **C,** Increased magnification reveals epithelioid cells in the inflammatory nodules. **D,** A special stain, Dieteria, demonstrates spirochetes (s) in the inflammatory infiltrate. (Case reported in Spektor FE, *et al.: Ophthalmology* 88:863, 1981.)

2. Secondary stage: the period when the systemic treponemal concentration is greatest, usually 2 to 12 weeks after contact.
   a. This stage may be manifest by fever, malaise, lymphadenopathy, and mucocutaneous lesions.
   b. The secondary stage subsides in weeks to months but may recur within 1 to 4 years.
3. Tertiary stage: the late sequelae such as cardiovascular effects and neurosyphilis. Focal granulomatous vascular lesions (gummas) can affect any organ.

C. The common form of posterior uveitis is a smoldering, indolent, chronic, nongranulomatous inflammation.
   1. Disseminated, large, atrophic scars surrounded by hyperplastic retinal pigment epithelium (part of the differential diagnosis of "salt-and-pepper" fundus) characterize the lesions.
   2. A more virulent type of uveitis may occur with a granulomatous inflammation.

In the nongranulomatous and granulomatous forms, the overlying neural retina is often involved.

D. Histologic findings
   1. The chronic nongranulomatous disseminated form of posterior choroiditis:
      a. In the atrophic scar, the outer neural retinal layers, the retinal pigment epithelium, and the inner choroidal layers disappear.
      b. Dehiscences in Bruch's membrane may be present through which neural retinal elements may "invade" the choroid.
      c. Bruch's membrane may be folded into the atrophic, sclerosed choroid.
      d. Scattered lymphocytes and plasma cells may be present.
      e. The *Treponema* spirochete is a helical bacterium 5 to 15 μm in length and less than 0.18 μm in width, and can be demonstrated in the ocular tissue with special stains, often in areas devoid of inflammatory cells.

T. pallidum belongs to the same family (Spirochaetaceae) as *Borrelia* (see later) and *Leptospira*.

---

   2. The granulomatous form of posterior chorioretinitis:
      a. The inflammatory process usually involves the choroid and the overlying neural retina and is quite vascular.
      b. Epithelioid cells, lymphocytes, and plasma cells are seen.
      c. Spirochetes can be demonstrated in the inflammatory tissue.
   3. The preceding two types of reactions may also involve the anterior uvea.

Spirochetes may be obtained by aspiration of aqueous from the anterior chamber and identified by dark-field microscopy.

IV. Lyme disease (*Borrelia burgdorferi*; Fig. 4.11)
   A. Lyme disease is a worldwide, tickborne, multisystem disorder, heralded by a red rash and erythema migrans, which forms at the site of the tick bite, usually within 4 to 20 days.
      1. It enlarges with central clearing (forming a ring), and can last several weeks.
      2. It may return and become chronic (erythema chronicum migrans).
   B. The tick, an *Ixodes* species, transmits the infectious agent, *B. burgdorferi*, through its bite.
   The enzyme-linked immunosorbent assay (ELISA) and the indirect immunofluorescence antibody are the most commonly used tests to diagnose Lyme disease.
   C. Like syphilis, Lyme disease is divided into three chronologically overlapping stages. Not all patients exhibit each stage, and the signs and symptoms are variable within each stage.
      1. Stage 1 is characterized by the local erythema migrans, which may be accompanied by flulike symptoms, including headache, fever, malaise, and lymphadenopathy.

Ocular findings include follicular conjunctivitis and photophobia.

---

   2. Stage 2 occurs within days, weeks, or even months and reflects systemic dissemination of the spirochete.
      a. Multiple skin lesions may occur (e.g., the purple nodule, lymphocytoma, especially on the earlobe or breast).
      b. Other findings include cardiac problems, arthritis (rare in stage 2), and the neurologic triad of meningitis, cranial neuritis, and painful radiculitis.

Ocular findings include blepharitis, blepharospasm, iridocyclitis, uveitis, neuroretinitis, vitritis, pars planitis, macular edema, anterior ischemic optic neuropathy (ANION), optic neuritis, optic neuropathy, temporal arteritis, pseudotumor cerebri, optic disc edema, optic disc pallor, cranial ocular nerve palsies, Horner's syndrome, and Argyll–Robertson pupil.

---

   3. Stage 3 can follow a disease-free period and may last years.
      a. "Lyme arthritis" is the hallmark of stage 3, appearing in over 50% of untreated cases.
      b. Other findings include acrodermatitis chronica atrophicans and late neurologic sequelae, especially an encephalopathy.

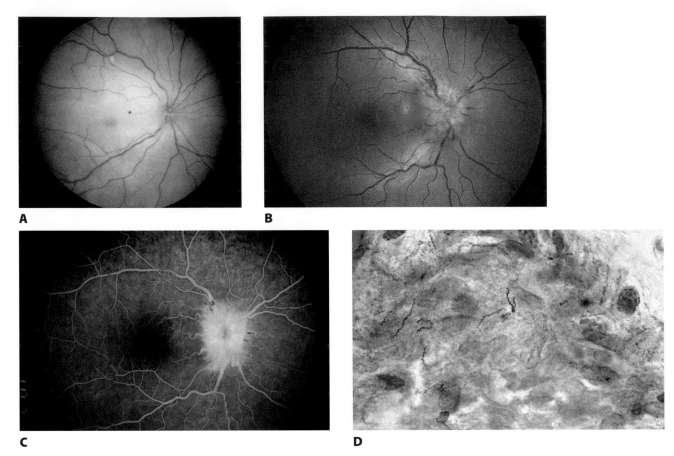

Fig. 4.11 Lyme disease. Lyme disease can cause a choroiditis (**A**) or an optic neuritis (**B** and **C**). Another patient had a chronic bilateral uveitis with a unilateral exudative retinal detachment and inflammatory pupillary membrane. Surgical iridectomy and membrane excision were performed. Spirochetes (*Borrelia burgdorferi*) were demonstrated by silver stain (**D**) and cultured in MKP medium (in the 16th subculture) from the excised tissue. (**A–C**, Courtesy of Prof. GOH Naumann; **D,** courtesy of Prof. HE Völcker and reported by Preac-Mursic V, *et al.: J Clin Neuroophthalmol* 13:155, 1993.)

Ocular findings include stromal keratitis, episcleritis, orbital myositis, and cortical blindness.

D. The pathologic mechanisms include direct invasion of tissues by the spirochete, vasculitis and small-vessel obliteration, perivascular plasma cell infiltration, and immunologic reactions.

V. Streptothrix (*Actinomyces*; Fig. 4.12)

A. The organism responsible for streptothrix infection of the lacrimal sac (see p. 210 in Chapter 6) and for a chronic form of conjunctivitis belongs to the class Schizomycetes, which contains the genera *Actinomyces* and *Nocardia*. The organism superficially resembles a fungus, but it is a bacterium.

The organism is best classified as an anaerobic and facultative capnophilic bacterium of the genus *Actinomyces*. The bacteria can be found in the normal microflora of the mouth of humans and animals.

B. Histologically, the organisms are seen in colonies as delicate, branching, intertwined filaments surrounded by necrotic tissue with little or no inflammatory component (e.g., the lacrimal cast from the nasolacrimal system). The organisms are weakly Gram-positive and acid-fast.

The colonies can be seen macroscopically as gray or yellow "sulfur" granules. Inflammatory giant cells are seen on occasion.

VI. Cat-scratch disease [CSD: *Bartonella* (previously called *Rochalimaea*) *henselae* cat-scratch bacillus]

A. CSD is a subacute regional lymphadenitis following a scratch by a kitten or cat (or perhaps a bite from the cat flea, *Ctenocephalides felis*), caused by the cat-scratch bacillus, *B. henselae*, a slow-growing, fastidious, Gram-negative, pleomorphic bacillus, which is a member of the α$_2$ subgroup of the class Probacteria, order Rickettsiales, family Rickettsiaceae.

Another possible cause is *Afipia felis*, a polymorphous bacillus that is a fastidious and facultative intercellular bacterium.

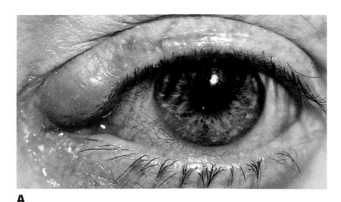

A

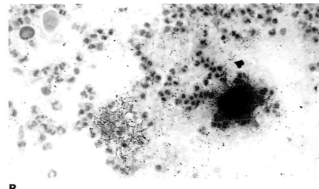

B

Fig. 4.12 Streptothrix (*Actinomyces*). **A,** Clinical appearance of acute canaliculitis. **B,** Smear of lacrimal cast stained with peridic acid–Schiff shows large colonies of organisms. (**A,** Courtesy of Dr. HG Scheie.)

1. Systemic manifestations in severe cases include splenohepatomegaly, splenic abscesses, mediastinal masses, encephalopathy, and osteolytic lesions.
2. Ocular findings include Parinaud's oculoglandular fever (see p. 232 in Chapter 7), neuroretinitis, branch retinal artery or vein occlusion, multifocal retinitis (retinal white-dot syndrome), focal choroiditis, optic disc edema associated with peripapillary serous retinal detachment, optic nerve head inflammation, and orbital infiltrates.
3. CSD antigen skin test is positive in infected patients.

CSD may occur in immunologically deficient patients (e.g., AIDS; see p. 21 in Chapter 1). Infection with *Bartonella* may also cause bacillary angiomatosis in immunologically deficient patients.

B. The contemporary infections caused by the *Bartonella* species include CSD, bacillary angiomatosis, relapsing bacteremia, endocarditis, and hepatic and splenic peliosis. CSD is the most common, affecting an estimated 22 000 people annually in the United States.
C. The domestic cat and its fleas are the major reservoir for *B. henselae*.
D. Histopathologically, the characteristics are discrete granulomas (which in time become suppurative) and follicular hyperplasia with general preservation of the lymph node architecture.
   1. Warthin–Starry silver stain demonstrates the cat-scratch bacillus in tissue sections.
   2. Electron microscopy shows extracellular rod-shaped bacteria.
VII. Tularemia (*Francisella tularensis*, also called *Pasteurella tularensis*; Fig. 4.13)
   A. The common ocular manifestation of tularemia is Parinaud's oculoglandular syndrome [i.e., conjunctivitis and regional (preauricular) lymphadenopathy, which may progress to suppuration].

B. Histologically, a granulomatous inflammation is found in the involved tissue. Organisms are extremely difficult to demonstrate histologically in the granulomatous tissue.
VIII. Other bacterial diseases
   A. Crohn's disease (see p. 67 in Chapter 3)
   B. Rhinoscleroma is a chronic, destructive granulomatous disease caused by *Klebsiella rhinoscleromatis*, a Gram-negative, encapsulated rod. The infection can spread from the nose, pharynx, and larynx to involve the nasolacrimal duct, lacrimal sac, and other orbital structures.

Fungal

I. Blastomycosis (*Blastomyces dermatitidis*, thermally dimorphic fungus)
   A. North American blastomycosis may involve the eyes in the form of an endophthalmitis as part of a secondary generalized blastomycosis that follows primary pulmonary blastomycosis, or it may involve the skin about the eyes in the form of single or multiple elevated red ulcers.
      1. Cutaneous blastomycosis does not usually become generalized.
      2. Involvement of the cornea, sclera, eyelid, and orbit, as well as choroiditis, endophthalmitis, and panophthalmitis, can occur.
   B. Histologically, the use of special stains demonstrates single budding cells in a granulomatous reaction.
II. Cryptococcosis (*Cryptococcus neoformans*)
   A. Cryptococcosis has also been called *torulosis*; another name for the causative agent is *Torula histolytica*. Cryptococcosis has increased in frequency because the causative agent is an opportunistic fungus that infects immunocompromised patients, especially those who are HIV-positive.
   B. The fungus tends to spread from its primary pulmonary involvement to central nervous system tissue, including the optic nerve and retina.

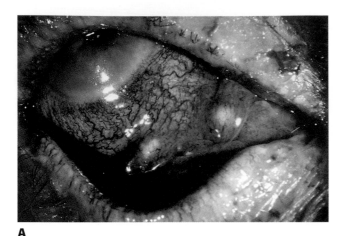

A

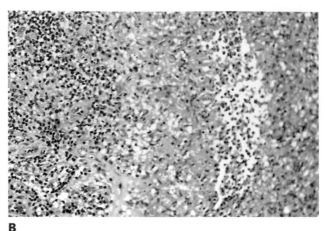

B

Fig. 4.13 Tularemia. **A,** Corneal ulcer and conjunctival granulomas developed in inflamed right eye. Palpable right preauricular node present. **B,** Central neutrophilic microabscess surrounded by granulomatous inflammation. *Francisella tularensis* cultured. (Presented by Dr. H Brown at 1996 combined meeting of Verhoeff and European Ophthalmic Pathology Societies and reported by Steinemann TL, *et al.: Arch Ophthalmol* 117:132, 1999.)

C. Histologically, special stains demonstrate the budding organism surrounded by a thick, gelatinous capsule, often in inflammatory giant cells in a granulomatous reaction.

III. Coccidioidomycosis (*Coccidioides immitis*)
    A. Coccidioidomycosis, endemic to the arid soils of the southern, central, southwestern, and western United States and Mexico, usually starts as a primary pulmonary infection that may spread to the eyes and cause an endophthalmitis.
    Rarely, it may present as an anterior-segment ocular coccidioidomycosis without any clinical evidence of systemic involvement.
    B. Histologically, spherules containing multiple spores (endospores) are noted in a granulomatous inflammatory reaction.

IV. Aspergillosis (*Aspergillus fumigatus*; Fig. 4.14B and C)
    A. Aspergillosis can cause a painful fungal keratitis, a very indolent chronic inflammation of the orbit, or an endophthalmitis; the latter condition is usually found in patients on immunosuppressive therapy.
    B. Histologically, septate, branching hyphae are frequently found in giant cells in a granulomatous reaction.

V. Rhinosporidiosis (*Rhinosporidium seeberi*)
    A. Rhinosporidiosis is caused by a fungus of uncertain classification.
    B. The main ocular manifestation of rhinosporidiosis is lid or conjunctival infection.
    C. Histologically, relatively large sacs or spherules (200 to 300 µm in diameter) filled with spores are seen. The organisms may be surrounded by a granulomatous reaction but are more likely to be surrounded by a nongranulomatous reaction of plasma cells and lymphocytes.

VI. Phycomycosis (mucormycosis, zygomycosis; see Fig. 14.7)
    A. The family Mucoraceae of the order Mucorales, in the class of fungi Phycomycetes, contains the genera *Mucor* and *Rhizopus*, which can cause human infections called *phycomycoses*, usually in patients who have severe acidosis [e.g., diabetes, burns, diarrhea, and immunosuppression (see p. 532 in Chapter 14)] or iron overload (e.g., in primary hemochromatosis).

The term *mucormycosis* should only refer to those infections caused by agents in the genus *Mucor*. Because the hyphae of species in the two genera, *Mucor* and *Rhizopus*, look identical histologically, and because *Mucor* may be difficult to culture, the term *phycomycosis* (or *zygomycosis*) is preferred to mucormycosis.

    B. The fungi can infect the orbit or eyeball, usually in patients with acidosis from any cause, but most commonly from diabetes mellitus.
    C. Histologically, the hyphae of *Mucor* and *Rhizo*pus are nonseptate, very broad (3 to 12 µm in diameter), and branch freely.
      1. Unlike most other fungi, the Mucoraceae readily take the hematoxylin stain and are easily identified in routine hematoxylin and eosin-stained sections.
      2. Typically, the hyphae infiltrate and cause thrombosis of blood vessels, leading to infarction.
      3. Inflammatory reactions vary from acute suppurative to chronic nongranulomatous to granulomatous.

VII. Candidiasis (*Candida albicans*; see Fig. 4.13A)
    A. *C. albicans* may cause a keratitis or an endophthalmitis.
    B. The endophthalmitis is most likely to occur in patients who have an underlying disease that has rendered them immunologically deficient.

The increased incidence of disseminated candidiasis correlates with the use of modern chemotherapy and the increase in immunologically deficient patients (e.g., those with AIDS).

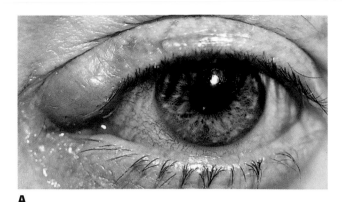

A

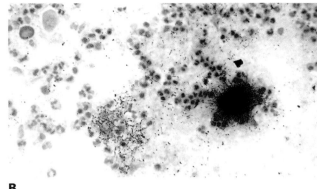

B

Fig. 4.12 Streptothrix (*Actinomyces*). **A,** Clinical appearance of acute canaliculitis. **B,** Smear of lacrimal cast stained with peridic acid–Schiff shows large colonies of organisms. (**A,** Courtesy of Dr. HG Scheie.)

1. Systemic manifestations in severe cases include splenohepatomegaly, splenic abscesses, mediastinal masses, encephalopathy, and osteolytic lesions.
2. Ocular findings include Parinaud's oculoglandular fever (see p. 232 in Chapter 7), neuroretinitis, branch retinal artery or vein occlusion, multifocal retinitis (retinal white-dot syndrome), focal choroiditis, optic disc edema associated with peripapillary serous retinal detachment, optic nerve head inflammation, and orbital infiltrates.
3. CSD antigen skin test is positive in infected patients.

> CSD may occur in immunologically deficient patients (e.g., AIDS; see p. 21 in Chapter 1). Infection with *Bartonella* may also cause bacillary angiomatosis in immunologically deficient patients.

B. The contemporary infections caused by the *Bartonella* species include CSD, bacillary angiomatosis, relapsing bacteremia, endocarditis, and hepatic and splenic peliosis. CSD is the most common, affecting an estimated 22 000 people annually in the United States.
C. The domestic cat and its fleas are the major reservoir for *B. henselae*.
D. Histopathologically, the characteristics are discrete granulomas (which in time become suppurative) and follicular hyperplasia with general preservation of the lymph node architecture.
   1. Warthin–Starry silver stain demonstrates the cat-scratch bacillus in tissue sections.
   2. Electron microscopy shows extracellular rod-shaped bacteria.
VII. Tularemia (*Francisella tularensis*, also called *Pasteurella tularensis*; Fig. 4.13)
   A. The common ocular manifestation of tularemia is Parinaud's oculoglandular syndrome [i.e., conjunctivitis and regional (preauricular) lymphadenopathy, which may progress to suppuration].

B. Histologically, a granulomatous inflammation is found in the involved tissue. Organisms are extremely difficult to demonstrate histologically in the granulomatous tissue.
VIII. Other bacterial diseases
   A. Crohn's disease (see p. 67 in Chapter 3)
   B. Rhinoscleroma is a chronic, destructive granulomatous disease caused by *Klebsiella rhinoscleromatis*, a Gram-negative, encapsulated rod. The infection can spread from the nose, pharynx, and larynx to involve the nasolacrimal duct, lacrimal sac, and other orbital structures.

Fungal

I. Blastomycosis (*Blastomyces dermatitidis*, thermally dimorphic fungus)
   A. North American blastomycosis may involve the eyes in the form of an endophthalmitis as part of a secondary generalized blastomycosis that follows primary pulmonary blastomycosis, or it may involve the skin about the eyes in the form of single or multiple elevated red ulcers.
      1. Cutaneous blastomycosis does not usually become generalized.
      2. Involvement of the cornea, sclera, eyelid, and orbit, as well as choroiditis, endophthalmitis, and panophthalmitis, can occur.
   B. Histologically, the use of special stains demonstrates single budding cells in a granulomatous reaction.
II. Cryptococcosis (*Cryptococcus neoformans*)
   A. Cryptococcosis has also been called *torulosis*; another name for the causative agent is *Torula histolytica*. Cryptococcosis has increased in frequency because the causative agent is an opportunistic fungus that infects immunocompromised patients, especially those who are HIV-positive.
   B. The fungus tends to spread from its primary pulmonary involvement to central nervous system tissue, including the optic nerve and retina.

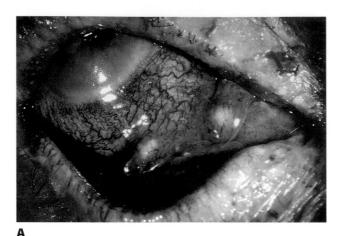

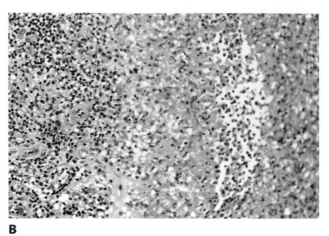

A

B

Fig. 4.13 Tularemia. **A,** Corneal ulcer and conjunctival granulomas developed in inflamed right eye. Palpable right preauricular node present. **B,** Central neutrophilic microabscess surrounded by granulomatous inflammation. *Francisella tularensis* cultured. (Presented by Dr. H Brown at 1996 combined meeting of Verhoeff and European Ophthalmic Pathology Societies and reported by Steinemann TL, *et al.: Arch Ophthalmol* 117:132, 1999.)

C. Histologically, special stains demonstrate the budding organism surrounded by a thick, gelatinous capsule, often in inflammatory giant cells in a granulomatous reaction.

III. Coccidioidomycosis (*Coccidioides immitis*)
  A. Coccidioidomycosis, endemic to the arid soils of the southern, central, southwestern, and western United States and Mexico, usually starts as a primary pulmonary infection that may spread to the eyes and cause an endophthalmitis.
  Rarely, it may present as an anterior-segment ocular coccidioidomycosis without any clinical evidence of systemic involvement.
  B. Histologically, spherules containing multiple spores (endospores) are noted in a granulomatous inflammatory reaction.

IV. Aspergillosis (*Aspergillus fumigatus*; Fig. 4.14B and C)
  A. Aspergillosis can cause a painful fungal keratitis, a very indolent chronic inflammation of the orbit, or an endophthalmitis; the latter condition is usually found in patients on immunosuppressive therapy.
  B. Histologically, septate, branching hyphae are frequently found in giant cells in a granulomatous reaction.

V. Rhinosporidiosis (*Rhinosporidium seeberi*)
  A. Rhinosporidiosis is caused by a fungus of uncertain classification.
  B. The main ocular manifestation of rhinosporidiosis is lid or conjunctival infection.
  C. Histologically, relatively large sacs or spherules (200 to 300 μm in diameter) filled with spores are seen. The organisms may be surrounded by a granulomatous reaction but are more likely to be surrounded by a nongranulomatous reaction of plasma cells and lymphocytes.

VI. Phycomycosis (mucormycosis, zygomycosis; see Fig. 14.7)
  A. The family Mucoraceae of the order Mucorales, in the class of fungi Phycomycetes, contains the genera *Mucor* and *Rhizopus*, which can cause human infections called

phycomycoses, usually in patients who have severe acidosis [e.g., diabetes, burns, diarrhea, and immunosuppression (see p. 532 in Chapter 14)] or iron overload (e.g., in primary hemochromatosis).

The term *mucormycosis* should only refer to those infections caused by agents in the genus *Mucor*. Because the hyphae of species in the two genera, *Mucor* and *Rhizopus*, look identical histologically, and because *Mucor* may be difficult to culture, the term *phycomycosis* (or *zygomycosis*) is preferred to mucormycosis.

  B. The fungi can infect the orbit or eyeball, usually in patients with acidosis from any cause, but most commonly from diabetes mellitus.
  C. Histologically, the hyphae of *Mucor* and *Rhizo*pus are nonseptate, very broad (3 to 12 μm in diameter), and branch freely.
    1. Unlike most other fungi, the Mucoraceae readily take the hematoxylin stain and are easily identified in routine hematoxylin and eosin-stained sections.
    2. Typically, the hyphae infiltrate and cause thrombosis of blood vessels, leading to infarction.
    3. Inflammatory reactions vary from acute suppurative to chronic nongranulomatous to granulomatous.

VII. Candidiasis (*Candida albicans*; see Fig. 4.13A)
  A. *C. albicans* may cause a keratitis or an endophthalmitis.
  B. The endophthalmitis is most likely to occur in patients who have an underlying disease that has rendered them immunologically deficient.

The increased incidence of disseminated candidiasis correlates with the use of modern chemotherapy and the increase in immunologically deficient patients (e.g., those with AIDS).

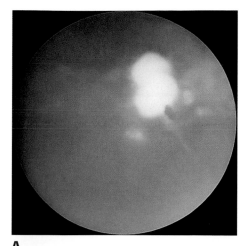

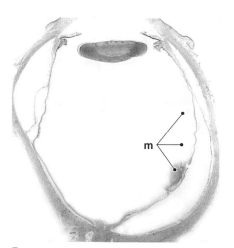

A   **B**

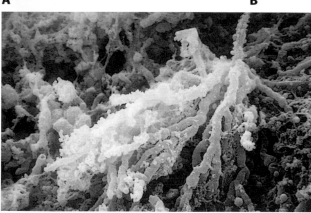

C

Fig. 4.14 Fungal endophthalmitis. **A,** Immunosuppressed patient developed endophthalmitis. Note "snowball" opacities in the vitreous (near the optic nerve head, just to right of opacities). *Candida albicans* was cultured from the blood. **B** and **C,** Another patient experienced decreased vision in his right eye, followed by renal failure 2 months after a kidney transplantation. He died 1 month later. The histologic section shows microabscesses (m) in the vitreous body characteristic of fungal infection (bacterial infection causes a diffuse vitreous abscess). **C,** Scanning electron microscopy demonstrates septate branching *Aspergillus* hyphae. (**C,** Courtesy of Dr. RC Eagle, Jr.)

C. Histologically, budding yeasts and pseudohyphal forms are seen surrounded by a chronic nongranulomatous inflammatory reaction, but sometimes by a granulomatous one.

VIII. Histoplasmosis (*Histoplasma capsulatum*)
Disseminated histoplasmosis with ocular involvement can be seen in immunologically deficient patients (e.g., in HIV-positive persons; see p. 433 in Chapter 11).

IX. Sporotrichosis (*Sporotrichum schenkii*)
A. Ocular involvement in sporotrichosis is usually the result of direct extension from primary cutaneous lesions of the lids and conjunctiva eroding into the eye and orbit.
   1. Lesions in adjacent bony structures may encroach on ophthalmic tissues.
   2. Less frequently, ocular and adnexal lesions may result from hematogenous dissemination of the fungus.
B. Histologically, the fungi are seen as round to cigar-shaped organisms, 3 to 6 μm in length, often surrounded by granulomatous inflammation.

X. *Pneumocystis carinii* (PC; Fig. 4.15)
A. PC pneumonia is the most common opportunistic infection in patients who have AIDS, occurring in more than 80% of such patients. The causative organism, PC, exists exclusively in the extracellular space.

Previously classified as a protozoan, molecular genetic evidence has shown that PC has more morphologic similarities to a fungus than to a protozoan. PC is now classified as a fungus.

B. Clinically, choroidal lesions are yellow to pale yellow, usually seen in the posterior pole.
   1. An association exists between PC and CMV in immunologically deficient patients so that PC choroiditis and CMV retinitis can exist concurrently in the same person.
   2. In addition, PC and *Mycobacterium avium-intracellulare*, two opportunistic organisms, have been reported in the same choroid at the same time in a patient with AIDS.
C. Histologically, choroidal lesions show "cysts," few or no inflammatory cells, and characteristic abundant, eosinophilic, frothy material, probably composed of dead and degenerating microorganisms.

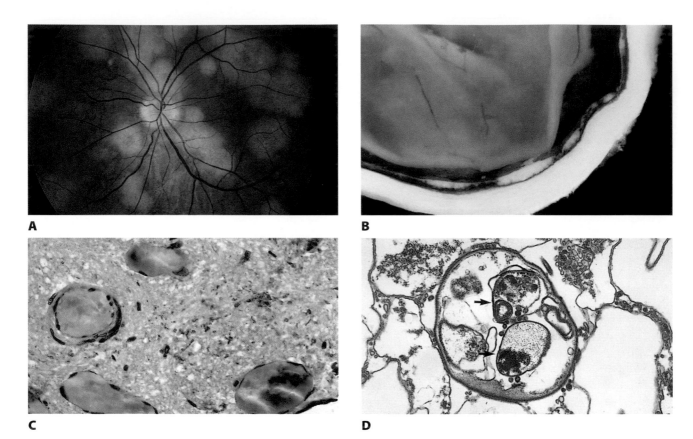

A

B

C

D

Fig. 4.15 *Pneumocystis carinii.* Scattered choroidal infiltrates can be seen in the fundus clinically (**A**) and in the gross specimen (**B**) in a patient who had acquired immunodeficiency syndrome (AIDS). **C,** The characteristic foamy, eosinophilic, and mostly acellular choroidal infiltrate is seen between dilated capillaries. **D,** An example of the electron microscopic appearance of *P. carinii* (*arrows*), previously thought to be a protozoan parasite of the Sporozoa subphylum, but now believed to be a fungus. (Case presented by Dr. NA Rao at the meeting of the Verhoeff Society, 1989.)

Parasitic

I. Protozoa
   A. Toxoplasmosis (*Toxoplasma gondii*; Figs 4.16 and 4.17)
     1. The definitive host of the intracellular protozoan *T. gondii* is the cat, but many intermediate hosts (e.g., humans, rodents, fowl) are known.
     2. The parasite primarily invades retinal cells directly.
     3. Clinically, the infestation starts as a focal area of retinitis, with an overlying vitritis.

Atypical, severe toxoplasmic retinochoroiditis in the elderly can mimic acute retinal necrosis.

---

     4. The lesions slowly clear centrally, destroying most of the retina and choroid, and become pigmented peripherally, so that "healed" lesions appear as atrophic white scars surrounded by a broad ring of pigment.
       Immunoglobulin G (IgG) is the major class involved in the humoral immune response to *T. gondii*, followed by IgA.
     5. Years later, reactivation can occur in the areas of the scars, or sometimes in new areas.

Even after the fifth decade, ocular toxoplasmosis remains an important cause of posterior uveitis. A subgroup of Fuchs' heterochromic iridocyclitis has an association, which may be causal, with toxoplasmic retinochoroiditis.

     6. Both congenital and acquired forms are recognized.
       a. The congenital form is associated with encephalomyelitis, visceral infestation (hepatosplenomegaly), and retinochoroiditis.

If a woman has dye-test antibodies when pregnancy is established, she will not transmit the disease to her fetus. If she is dye-negative at the onset of pregnancy, there is some risk of her transmitting toxoplasmosis to her infant if she acquires the disease during pregnancy. There is a 14% chance of the child showing severe manifestations of the disease. If the woman acquires toxoplasmosis during the first trimester, pregnancy may cause activation of ocular disease in the mother.

---

       b. The acquired form usually presents as a posterior uveitis and sometimes as an optic neuritis.

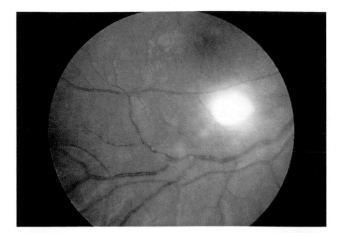

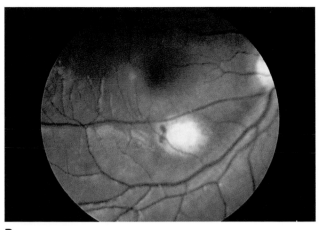

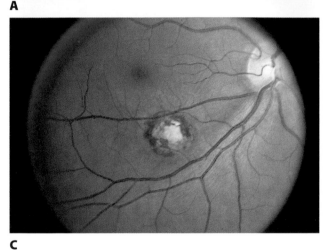

Fig. 4.16 Toxoplasmosis. **A,** Acute attack in right eye in 12-year-old girl (white spots on blood vessels represent granulomatous cellular reaction on surface of retina). **B,** Early pigmentation present 7 years later. **C,** Twelve years later, lesion looks like "typical" toxoplasmosis.

The acquired form, usually a retinitis, rarely a scleritis, may occur in persons who have immunologic abnormalities of many types, especially in AIDS.

7. Histologically, the protozoa are found in three forms: free, in pseudocysts, or in true cysts.
   a. Rarely, the protozoa may be found in a *free form* in the neural retina.
      1). The free parasite, called a *trophozoite*, resides in an intracellular vacuole that is completely unable to fuse with other endocytic or biosynthetic vacuoles.
      2). The protozoa are seen in an area of coagulative necrosis of the neural retina, sharply demarcated from the contiguous normal-appearing neural retina.
      3). They may also be seen in the optic nerve.
   b. Commonly, a protozoan enters a retinal cell (neural retina or retinal pigment epithelium) and multiplies in the confines of the cell membrane. All that is seen histologically, therefore, is a group of protozoa surrounded by the retinal cell membrane; the whole assemblage is called a *pseudocyst*.

   c. If the environment becomes inhospitable, an intracellular protozoan (trophozoite) may transform itself into a bradyzoite, surround itself with a self-made membrane, multiply, and then form a *true cyst* that extrudes from the cell and lies free in the tissue.
      1). It is found in the late stage of the disease, at the time of remission.
      2). The true cyst is resistant to the host's defenses and can remain in this latent form indefinitely.
   d. The underlying choroid, and sometimes sclera, contains a secondary diffuse granulomatous inflammation.
B. *Pneumocystis carinii* (see earlier, under *Fungal*)
C. Malaria (*Plasmodium*)
   1. Ocular complications occur in approximately 10% to 20% of malarial patients, and include conjunctival pigmentation; conjunctival, epibulbar, and retinal hemorrhages; keratitis; optic neuritis; peripapillary edema; and temporary loss of vision.
   2. Histologically, in a case of *Plasmodium falciparum* malaria, cytoadherence and rosetting of parasitized erythrocytes partially occluded small retinal and

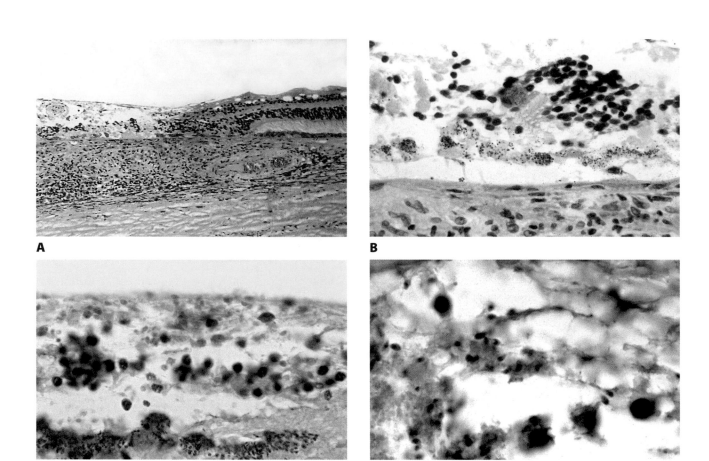

Fig. 4.17 Toxoplasmosis. **A,** Histologic section showing an acute coagulative retinal necrosis, whereas the choroid shows a secondary diffuse granulomatous inflammation. **B,** A toxoplasmic cyst is present in the neural retina; note the tiny nuclei in the cyst. **C,** In another section, free forms of the protozoa are present in the necrotic neural retina. The tiny nuclei are eccentrically placed and the opposite end of the cytoplasm tends to taper, shown with increased magnification in **D.**

uveal blood vessels; malarial pigment (hemozoin) can be demonstrated by polarized light.

D. Microsporidiosis (*Encephalitozoon, Enterocytozoon, Nosema,* and *Pleistophora*)

1. Diseases caused by microsporidia, which are obligate intracellular parasitic protozoa, have increased in prevalence because of the increase in the prevalence of AIDS.

2. Clinically, ocular findings include punctate epithelial keratopathy, keratitis, and keratoconjunctivitis.

3. Histologically, extracellular and intracellular spores are found in and around degenerating keratocytes. Electron microscopy shows encapsulated oval structures, approximately 3.5 to 4 μm in length and 1.5 μm in width.

E. *Acanthamoeba* species (*A. casttellani, A. polyphaga, A. culbertsoni*; see p. 273 in Chapter 8)

II. Nematodes

A. Toxocariasis (*Toxocara canis*; see Fig. 18.19)

1. Ocular toxocariasis is a manifestation of visceral larva migrans (i.e., larvae of the nematode *T. canis*).

Toxocara cati may also cause toxocariasis. *Nematodiasis* is not a correct term for the condition because nematodes other than *Toxocara* can also infest the eye (e.g., *Onchocercus*; see Fig. 8.11).

a. One eye tends to be involved, usually in children 6 to 11 years of age.

b. Rarely, bilateral ocular toxocariasis can be demonstrated by aqueous humor ELISA.

c. Often the child's history shows that the family possesses a puppy rather than an adult dog.

2. The condition may take at least three ocular forms:

a. Leukokoria with multiple retinal folds radiating out toward the peripheral retina, where the necrotic worm is present

b. A discrete lesion, usually in the posterior pole and seen through clear media

c. A painless endophthalmitis

3. In all three forms, the eye is not inflamed externally; the only complaint is loss of vision; and only one eye is involved.

Although the condition presumably follows widespread migration of larvae, only one eye is involved and only one worm can be found. No inflammatory reaction occurs until the worm dies. The eosinophil appears to be the major killer cell of *Toxocara*. Toxocaral fluorescent antibody tests may be helpful in making the diagnosis of toxocariasis.

4. Histologically, a granulomatous inflammatory infiltrate, usually with many eosinophils, surrounds the necrotic worm. The infiltrate is zonal, with the necrotic worm surrounded by an abscess containing eosinophils, neutrophils, and necrotic debris; granulomatous inflammation surrounds the abscess.

Splendore–Hoeppli phenomenon is a local eosinophilic, amorphous precipitate consisting of debris (mainly from eosinophils) and granular material (probably an antigen–antibody complex). It is presumed to be caused by a parasite, perhaps a nematode, but the exact cause is unclear.

B. Diffuse unilateral subacute neuroretinitis (DUSN; unilateral wipe-out syndrome)
 1. DUSN, which typically affects young, healthy people, is probably caused by more than one type of motile, subneural retinal, nematode roundworm.

Clinically, if the worm can be identified, it can be destroyed by focal photocoagulation.

 2. The early stage of the disease is characterized by unilateral vision loss, vitritis, mild optic disc edema, and successive crops of multiple, evanescent, gray-white, deep retinal lesions.
 3. Over a period of many months, widespread, diffuse, focal depigmentation of the retinal pigment epithelium develops, accompanied by retinal arterial narrowing, optic atrophy, severe vision loss, and electroretinographic abnormalities.
 4. Worms seen in the fundi of patients from the southern United States seem to be approximately one-half the size of those seen in patients from the northern and western United States, and the exact type of the small variant roundworm is not known. The large nematode variant is probably not caused by *Toxocara* but by the raccoon roundworm larva, *Baylisascaris procyonis*.

DUSN has been reported in Europe, probably caused by *T. canis*, but with banding distinct from the usual human toxocariasis.

C. Trichinosis (*Trichinella spiralis*; Fig. 4.18)
 1. The nematode *T. spiralis* is obtained by eating undercooked meat, classically pork that contains the trichina cysts.

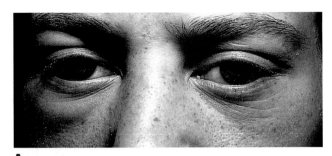

A

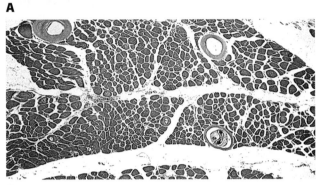

B

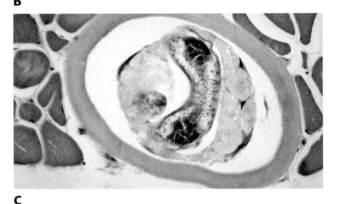

C

Fig. 4.18 Trichinosis. **A,** Acute trichinosis with orbital involvement. Note swelling of lids. **B,** Top two cysts are empty; bottom cyst shows larva of *Trichinella spiralis* (pork nematode); seen with increased magnification in **C.** (**A,** Courtesy of Dr. ME Smith.)

 2. Clinically, the lids and extraocular muscles may be involved as the larvae migrate systemically.
 3. Histologically, the larvae encapsulate or encyst in striated muscle and cause little or no inflammatory reaction. If the larvae die before they encapsulate, however, a zonal granulomatous inflammatory reaction around the necrotic worm results.
D. *Loa loa* (Fig. 4.19)
 1. The adult *L. loa* filarial worm wanders in the subcutaneous tissues. It may wander into the periorbital tissues and eyelids and often into the subconjunctival tissues, where its length makes it easily visible.
 2. Histologically, little inflammatory reaction occurs while the worm is alive.

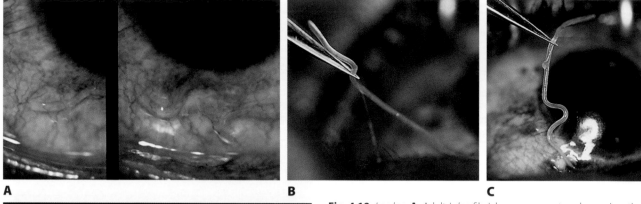

A   **B**   **C**

Fig. 4.19 *Loa loa.* **A,** Adult *L. loa* filarial worm present under conjunctiva. Note: position of end of worm changes (left to right—pictures taken a few minutes apart). **B,** Worm grasped by forceps during removal. **C,** Worm almost completely removed. **D,** Removed worm. (Courtesy of Dr. LA Karp.)

D

E. Dracunculiasis (*Dracunculus medinensis;* guinea worm; serpent worm)
   1. Dracunculiasis, caused by the obligate, nematode parasite, *D. medinensis,* affects the skin, subcutaneous tissues, and orbit.
   2. Histologically, the worm, when dead, is surrounded by an abscess.
III. Cestoidea (tapeworms)
   A. Cysticercosis (*Cysticercus cellulosae;* Fig. 4.20)
      1. *C. cellulosae* is the larval stage of the pork tapeworm *Taenia solium.* The larvae, or bladderworms, hatch in the intestine, and the resultant systemic infestation is called *cysticercosis.*

> Cysticercosis is the most common ocular tapeworm infestation and the most common parasitic infection of the central nervous system. The prognosis in untreated cases is uniformly poor. The best chance for cure is early surgical removal, although destruction of the parasite in situ by diathermy, light coagulation, or cryoapplication may prove successful.

   2. The bladderworm has a predilection for the central nervous system and eyes. It induces no inflammatory response when alive.
   3. Histologically, the necrotic bladderworm is surrounded by a zonal granulomatous inflammatory reaction that usually contains many eosinophils.
   B. Hydatid cyst (*Echinococcus granulosus*)
      1. The onchospheres of the dog tapeworm *E. granulosus* may enter humans and form a cyst called a

hydatid cyst that contains the larval form of the tapeworm.
   a. In this form, the tapeworms appear as multiple scolices provided with hooklets.
   b. Each scolex is the future head of an adult tapeworm.
   2. In humans, the tapeworm has a predilection for the orbit.
   3. Histologically, multiple scolices are seen adjacent to a thick, acellular, amorphous membrane that represents the wall of the cyst.
   C. Coenurus (*Multiceps multiceps*)
      1. Coenurus is a large, single bladderworm (larval cystic stage of *M. multiceps*), 5 cm or more in diameter. It contains several hundred scolices.
      2. The bladderworm may involve the subconjunctival or orbital regions, or occur in the eye.
      3. The adult tapeworm mainly has the domestic dog as its definitive host, but may also be found in other animals. The larval stage is usually found in sheep, but primates can be involved as incidental intermediate hosts.
      4. Histologically, multiple inverted scolices line up against an outer cuticular wall.
IV. Trematodes (flukes): Schistosomiasis (*Schistosoma haematobium, S. mansoni,* and *S. japonicum*)
   A. Trematodes of the genus *Schistosoma* can cause a chronic conjunctivitis or blepharitis in areas of the world where they are endemic.
   B. The eggs of schistosomes hatch in water into miracidia, which penetrate snails, undergo metamorphosis, and

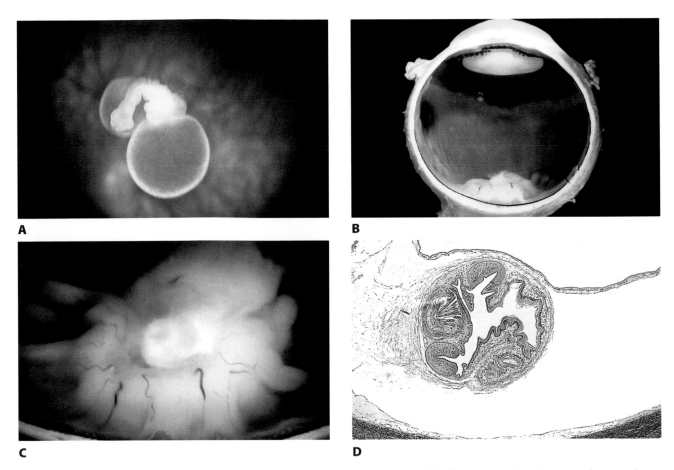

Fig. 4.20 Cysticercosis. **A,** Fundus picture shows bladderworm in vitreous. **B** and **C,** A 6-year-old girl had eye enucleated because of suspected retinoblastoma. Gross specimen shows bladderworm cyst over optic nerve head. **D,** Scolex area with hooks (birefringent to polarized light) and sucker is surrounded by a granulomatous reaction. (**A,** Courtesy of Dr. AH Friedman.)

form cercariae. The cercariae emerge from the snail and enter the skin of humans as metacercariae or adolescariae.

C. Histologically, the eggs and necrotic adult worms incite a marked zonal granulomatous inflammatory response.

Other trematodes that may infest the eye include *Paragonimus* and *Alaria* species.

V. Ophthalmomyiasis (fly larva)
  A. Myiasis is a rare condition in which fly larvae (maggots) invade and feed on dead tissue. Numerous different causative agents may be found, e.g., *Cochliomyia macellaria*, *Oestrus ovis*, *Gasterophilus* species, *Hypoderma bovis*, and *Cuterebera* species.
  B. Usually the larvae can be seen macroscopically, but exact identification relies on microscopic features.
VI. Retinal pigment epitheliopathy associated with the amyotrophic lateral sclerosis/parkinsonism–dementia complex of Guam—see p. 418 in Chapter 11.
VII. Many other parasites, including *Leishmania* (leishmaniasis), *Trypanosoma* (trypanosomiasis), *Ascaris* lumbricoides

(ascariasis), and *Dirofilaria* (dirofilariasis), can cause ocular infestations.

NONTRAUMATIC NONINFECTIOUS

Sarcoidosis (Figs 4.21 to 4.26)

I. Sarcoidosis is a systemic disease, affecting black people predominantly, and having an equal sex incidence.
II. Systemic findings include hypercalcemia, bilateral hilar adenopathy and lung parenchymal changes, peripheral lymphadenopathy, skin lesions varying from extensive erythematous infiltrates to nondescript plaques and papules, hepatosplenomegaly, occasional enlargement of lacrimal and salivary glands, and osteolytic lesions of distal phalanges. Central nervous system findings are seen in 5% of sarcoid patients, usually the result of basilar meningitis with infiltration or compression of adjacent structures.

The Kveim test appears to be based on an immunologic reaction associated with persistent lymphadenopathy of diverse causes and

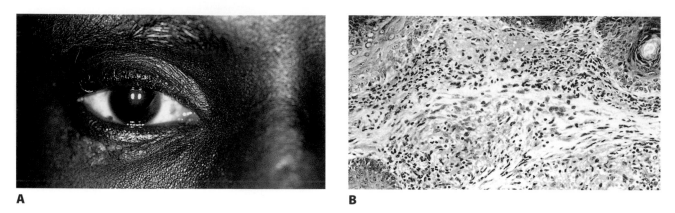

A **B**

Fig. 4.21 Sarcoidosis. **A,** Skin lesions in sarcoidosis. **B,** Biopsy shows granulomatous inflammation in the dermis.

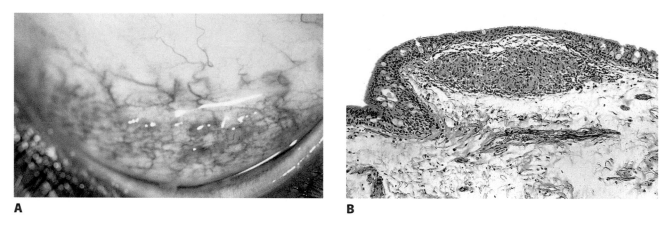

A **B**

Fig. 4.22 Sarcoidosis. **A,** The patient shows numerous, small, round, translucent cysts in the conjunctival fornix. **B,** A conjunctival biopsy reveals a discrete granuloma, composed of epithelioid cells and surrounded by a rim of lymphocytes and plasma cells. Such granulomas may be found histologically even if no conjunctival nodules are noted clinically.

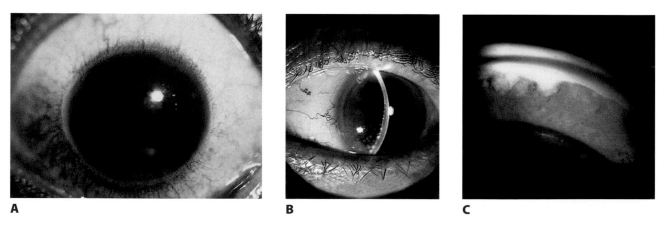

A **B** **C**

Fig. 4.23 Sarcoidosis. **A,** The iris is involved in the granulomatous process and shows numerous large granulomas. **B,** Slit-lamp section shows many mutton-fat keratic precipitates on the posterior corneal surface. **C,** Granulomas and peripheral anterior synechiae are noted in the angle of the anterior chamber.

is not specific for sarcoidosis. Elevated serum or tear angiotensin-converting enzyme levels and, to a lesser extent, serum collagenase levels may be helpful in assessing the activity of sarcoidosis. *Hamazaki–Wesenberg bodies* may be found in macrophages or free in peripheral portions of lymph nodes in sarcoid patients, isolated lymphoid tumors, or hyperplastic lymph nodes associated with carcinoma of the head and neck. The bodies are a form of ceroid and not, as previously thought, bacteria or other infectious agents. They are not, therefore, pathognomonic for sarcoidosis.

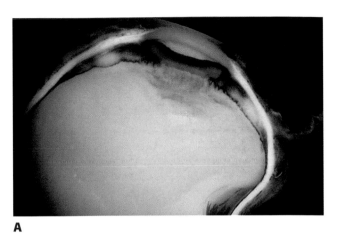

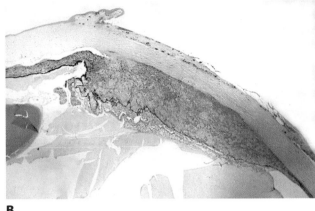

A   **B**

Fig. 4.24 Sarcoidosis. **A,** The enucleated globe shows an infiltrate in the ciliary body. **B,** The infiltrate consists of a discrete granulomatous inflammation.

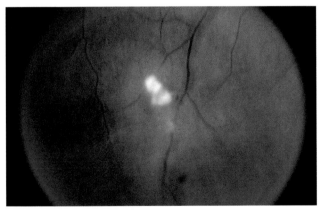

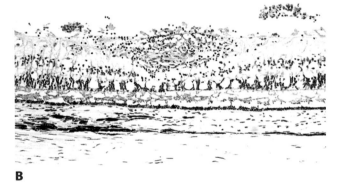

A   **B**

Fig. 4.25 Sarcoidosis. **A,** White cellular masses ("balls") are seen in the vitreous compartment on the surface of the inferior neural retina, along with early "candle-wax drippings." **B,** Candle-wax drippings are caused by perivascular, retinal, granulomatous infiltration. White balls are caused by accumulations of granulomatous inflammation in the vitreous. **C,** A large Dalen–Fuchs nodule is seen in this case of sarcoidosis. (**B** and **C,** Reported by Gass JDM, Olsen CL: *Arch Ophthalmol* 94:945, 1976.)

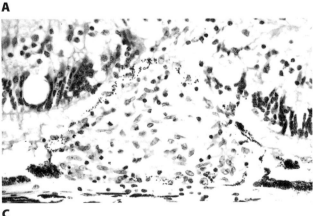

C

III. The most common ocular manifestation is an anterior granulomatous uveitis that occurs in approximately one-fifth of people who have sarcoidosis.

    A. Other findings include millet-shaped eyelid nodules; bilateral, white, focal discrete, conjunctival spots; nodular infiltrates in the bulbar conjunctiva; episcleral nodules; interstitial keratitis with a predilection for the lower half of the cornea; band keratopathy (especially with hypercalcemia); secondary closed-angle glaucoma; retinochoroidal granulomas; central or peripheral retinal neovascularization (sea fan); neovascularization of the optic nerve; retinal periphlebitis; "candle-wax drippings" (taches de bougie) on or near retinal vessels; retinal hemorrhages; whitish masses in dependent portion of vitreous; optic disc edema; optic neuritis; proptosis; and extraocular muscle palsies.

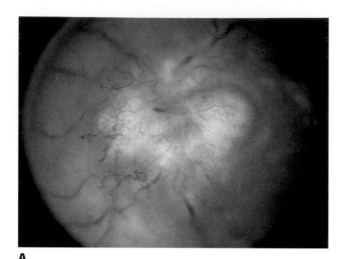

A

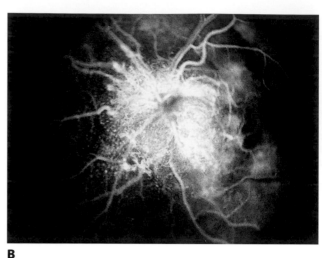

B

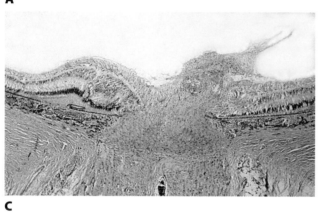

C

Fig. 4.26 Sarcoidosis. **A,** Patient with sarcoidosis presented with bilateral optic disc edema. **B,** Fluorescein angiogram. **C,** Granuloma involving edge of optic disc and adjacent retina. (**A** and **B,** Courtesy of Dr. AJ Brucker; case in **C,** reported by Gass JDM, Olsen CL: *Arch Ophthalmol* 94:945, 1976.)

The retinal form of sarcoidosis is rare and carries a grave prognosis for life because of its association with central nervous system sarcoidosis.

IV. Histologically, a noncaseating, granulomatous, inflammation of the discrete (sarcoidal, tuberculoidal) type, frequently with inflammatory foreign-body giant cells, is found.

A. Most of the granulomatous nodules are approximately the same size.

B. Slight central necrosis may be seen, but caseation is rare.

C. Star-shaped, acidophilic bodies (*asteroids*); small, macrophage-related, calcium oxalate, birefringent, ovoid bodies; and spherical or ovoid, basophilic, calcium oxalate, frequently laminated, birefringent bodies (*Schaumann bodies*) may be found in, or surrounded by, epithelioid or inflammatory foreign-body giant cells. These bodies may also be seen in conditions other than sarcoidosis.

D. Small granulomas may be present histologically in the submucosa of the conjunctiva even in the absence of visible clinical lesions.

1. The yield of positive lesions is higher, however, if a nodule is seen clinically.

2. A biopsy of conjunctiva from the lower cul de sac may help to establish the diagnosis of sarcoidosis even when no clinically visible lesions are seen.

A conjunctival biopsy is a safe and simple method for diagnosing sarcoidosis in a high percentage of suspected patients. It is important that the pathologist take sections from at least three levels and a "ribbon" of tissue (approximately six to eight sections) on each slide from the three levels. From the resultant 18 to 24 sections, granulomas may be found in only 1 or 2.

Granulomatous Scleritis

I. Granulomatous scleritis, anterior or posterior (see Fig. 8.59), is associated with rheumatoid arthritis (or other collagen disease) in approximately 15% of patients (see section on *Scleritis* in Chapter 8), and approximately 45% have a known systemic condition.

Up to 42% of patients who have scleritis have an associated uveitis. Acute scleritis may occur in Wegener's granulomatosis and porphyria cutanea tarda.

II. Histologically, a zonal type of granulomatous inflammatory infiltrate surrounds a nidus of necrotic scleral collagen.

A. Typically, the inflammation is in the sclera between the limbus and equator.

B. The lesions, which may be focal or diffuse, closely resemble subcutaneous rheumatoid nodules but have more plasma cells around the periphery.

> The sclera may become thickened or markedly thinned (see Fig. 8.58 in Chapter 8). An intense nongranulomatous anterior uveitis may accompany the scleritis. *Pseudorheumatoid nodule (granuloma annulare)* is a necrobiotic granuloma that usually occurs in subcutaneous tissue but can occur in the episclera and orbit. Immune complex vasculitis occurs.

Chalazion

See p. 174 in Chapter 6.

Xanthogranulomas (Juvenile Xanthogranuloma and Langerhans' Granulomatoses; Histiocytosis X)

See p. 343 in Chapter 9 and subsection on *Reticuloendothelial System* in Chapter 14.

Granulomatous Reaction to Descemet's Membrane

I. In approximately 10% of eyes with corneal ulcer or keratitis that are examined histologically, a granulomatous reaction to Descemet's membrane is found (see Fig. 4.5B and C). Most frequently, the corneas have a disciform keratitis with or without a history of herpes simplex or zoster keratitis.

II. The peculiar reaction to Descemet's membrane may be the result of altered antigenicity of the membrane and subsequent development of an autosensitivity reaction.

Chédiak–Higashi Syndrome

See p. 396 in Chapter 11.

Allergic Granulomatosis and Midline Lethal Granuloma Syndrome

See section on *Collagen Diseases* in Chapter 6.

Weber–Christian Disease (Relapsing Febrile Nodular Nonsuppurative Panniculitis)

See p. 188 in Chapter 6.

Vogt–Koyanagi–Harada Syndrome (Uveomeningoencephalitic Syndrome)

I. VKH syndrome (Fig. 4.27) is a multisystem disorder that reflects the integration of Vogt–Koyanagi syndrome with Harada's disease.

A. Although mainly a syndrome of adults, it rarely occurs in children, even those as young as 4 years of age.

B. VKH syndrome consists of a severe, acute, often bilateral, anterior uveitis associated with vitiligo (leukodermia), poliosis (whitened hair or canities), alopecia, and dysacusia.

1. Harada's disease consists primarily of a posterior granulomatous uveitis, usually bilateral and associ-

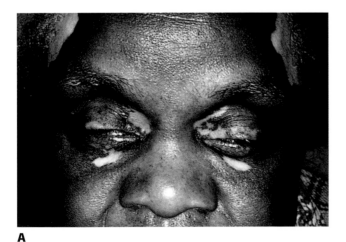

A

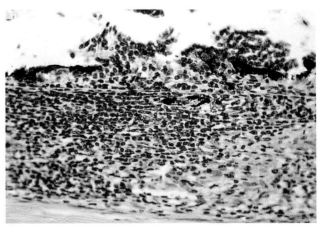

B

Fig. 4.27 Vogt–Koyanagi–Harada syndrome. **A,** Patient shows vitiligo, poliosis, and alopecia. **B,** Diffuse thickening of choroid by granulomatous inflammation resembles that seen in sympathetic uveitis. However, unlike in sympathetic uveitis, inflammation does not spare choriocapillaris and has broken through the retinal pigment epithelium into the subneural retinal area. (**A,** Case reported by Fine BS, Gilligan JH: *Am J Ophthalmol* 43:433, 1957; **B,** case presented at the 1980 Verhoeff Society Meeting by Dr. H Inomata and reported in Ikui H, Hiyama H: *Acta Soc Ophthalmol Jpn* 60:1687, 1956.)

ated with bilateral serous retinal detachments, accompanied by fluctuating meningeal symptoms, both central and peripheral.

2. Glaucoma, cataract, subretinal neovascularization, late subretinal fibrosis, and Sugiura's sign (perilimbal vitiligo) may occur.

C. The cerebrospinal fluid shows increased protein levels and pleocytosis.

> Melanin-laden macrophages may be found in the cerebrospinal fluid in the early stages (within 25 days) of the onset of VKH syndrome.

II. Autoaggressive cell-bound responses to uveal pigment may play a role in the histogenesis of VKH syndrome.
   A. VKH syndrome is associated with HLA-DR53, HLA-DR4, and HLA-DQ4 antigens (and HLA-DR1 in Hispanic patients).
   B. VKH may be a syndrome of combined allelic predisposition in which DQA1*0301 acts as the primary and HLA-DR4 acts as an additive factor, whereas DQB1*0604 may be protective, in the development of the prolonged form of the syndrome.

> It has been suggested that sympathetic uveitis represents a forme fruste of VKH syndrome. Rarely, VKH syndrome can occur after cutaneous injury such as laceration, burn, and contact dermatitis. Thus, both the clinical manifestations and immunogenetic background of sympathetic uveitis and VKH syndrome are quite similar.

   C. Also, T lymphocytes are decreased in the peripheral blood.

III. Histologically, a chronic, diffuse, granulomatous uveitis, closely resembling sympathetic uveitis, is seen.
   A. Multiple histologic sections, however, usually show one or more areas in the posterior segment where the inflammatory reaction does not spare the choriocapillaris and involves the overlying neural retina.
   B. An accompanying disciform degeneration of the macula is common. Immunocytology shows that the uveal infiltrates are composed of T lymphocytes and HLA-DR+ macrophages; nondendritic-appearing CD1 (Leu-6)-positive cells are localized to the choroid in close proximity to melanocytes. Scattered plasma cells and T lymphocytes occur in the retina.

Familial Chronic Granulomatous Disease of Childhood

I. Familial chronic granulomatous disease (FCGD) is characterized by chronic suppurative lymphadenitis, eczematoid dermatitis, osteomyelitis, hepatosplenomegaly, pulmonary infiltrates, abscesses of soft tissues caused by saprophytic organisms, pigmented lipid histiocytosis, and hypergammaglobulinemia.

> Approximately 60% have an X-linked, 40% an autosomal recessive, and less than 1% an autosomal dominant inheritance pattern.

II. FCGD is a heterogeneous group of disorders of phagocytic, oxidative metabolism.
   A. A lesion anywhere in the biochemical pathway that leads to hydrogen peroxide production has the potential to cause the disease.
   B. The patients have a common phenotype of recurrent bacterial infections with catalase-positive microbes (e.g., *Staphylococcus aureus* and *Serratia, Pseudomonas, Klebsiella, Chromobacterium, Escherichia, Nocardia,* and *Aspergillus* species).

   PMNs in patients with FCGD ingest bacteria but do not kill them because of a deficiency in leukocyte hydrogen peroxide metabolism. Furthermore, lysosomal hydrolytic enzymes (acid phosphatase and β-glucuronidase) are released in decreased amounts by PMNs during phagocytosis, resulting in abnormal (lessened) degranulation of the PMNs.
   C. Humoral immunity, cell-mediated immunity, and inflammatory responses are normal.

III. Ocular findings include lid dermatitis, keratoconjunctivitis, and chorioretinitis.

IV. Histologically, suppurative and granulomatous inflammatory lesions characteristically coexist.
   A. The suppurative component may be secondary to infection, whereas the granulomatous component is likely caused by inadequate breakdown of antigenic debris or inadequate feedback inhibition of inflammation by toxic oxygen products.
   B. The choroid and sclera show multiple foci of granulomatous inflammation.

BIBLIOGRAPHY

Sympathetic Uveitis

Boyd SR, Young S, Lightman S: Immunopathology of the noninfectious posterior and intermediate uveitides. *Surv Ophthalmol* 46:209, 2001

Chan C-C, Roberge FG, Whitcup SM *et al.*: 32 cases of sympathetic ophthalmia. *Arch Ophthalmol* 113:597, 1995

Davis JL, Mittal KK, Freidlin V *et al.*: HLA associations and ancestry in Vogt–Koyanagi–Harada disease and sympathetic ophthalmia. *Ophthalmology* 97:1137, 1990

Easom HA, Zimmerman LE: Sympathetic ophthalmia and bilateral phacoanaphylaxis: A clinicopathologic correlation of the sympathogenic and sympathizing eyes. *Arch Ophthalmol* 72:9, 1964

Fine BS, Gilligan JH: The Vogt–Koyanagi syndrome: A variant of sympathetic ophthalmia. Report of two cases. *Am J Ophthalmol* 43:433, 1957

Font RL, Fine BS, Messmer E *et al.*: Light and electron microscopic study of Dálen–Fuchs nodules in sympathetic ophthalmia. *Ophthalmology* 89:66, 1982

Gass JDM: Sympathetic ophthalmia following vitrectomy. *Am J Ophthalmol* 93:552, 1982

Green WR, Maumenee AE, Saunders TE *et al.*: Sympathetic uveitis following evisceration. *Trans Am Acad Ophthalmol Otolaryngol* 76:625, 1972

Kay ML, Yanoff M, Katowitz JA: Sympathetic uveitis: Development in spite of corticosteroid therapy. *Am J Ophthalmol* 78:90, 1974

Kinyoun JL, Bensinger RE, Chuang EL: Thirty-year history of sympathetic ophthalmia. *Ophthalmology* 90:59, 1983

Lubin JR, Albert DM: Early enucleation in sympathetic ophthalmia. *Ocul Inflamm Ther* 1:47, 1983

Marak GE Jr, Font RL, Zimmerman LE: Histologic variations related to race in sympathetic ophthalmia. *Am J Ophthalmol* 78:935, 1974

Shindo Y, Ohno S, Usi M et al.: Immunogenetic study of sympathetic ophthalmia. *Tissue Antigens* 49:111, 1997

Stafford WR: Sympathetic ophthalmia: Report of a case occurring ten and one half days after injury. *Arch Ophthalmol* 74:521, 1965

Yanoff M: Pseudo-sympathetic uveitis. *Trans Pa Acad Ophthalmol Otolaryngol* 30:118, 1977

Phacoanaphylactic Endophthalmitis

Apple DJ, Mamalis N, Steinmetz RL et al.: Phacoanaphylactic endophthalmitis associated with extracapsular cataract extraction and posterior chamber intraocular lens. *Arch Ophthalmol* 102:1528, 1984

Caudill JW, Streeten BW, Tso MOM: Phacoanaphylactoid reaction in persistent hyperplastic primary vitreous. *Ophthalmology* 92:1153, 1985

Chan C-C: Relationship between sympathetic ophthalmia, phacoanaphylactic endophthalmitis, and Vogt–Koyanagi–Harada disease. *Ophthalmology* 95:619, 1988

Chishti M, Henkind P: Spontaneous rupture of anterior lens capsule (phacoanaphylactic endophthalmitis). *Am J Ophthalmol* 69:264, 1970

Easom HA, Zimmerman LE: Sympathetic ophthalmia and bilateral phacoanaphylaxis: A clinicopathologic correlation of the sympathogenic and sympathizing eyes. *Arch Ophthalmol* 72:9, 1964

Inomota H, Yoshikawa H. Rao NA: Phacoanaphylaxis in Behçet's disease. A clinicopathologic and immunohistochemicsal study. *Ophthalmology* 110:1942, 2003

Marak GE: Phacoanaphylactic endophthalmitis. *Surv Ophthalmol* 36: 325, 1992

Yanoff M, Scheie HG: Cytology of human lens aspirate: Its relationship to phacolytic glaucoma and phacoanaphylactic endophthalmitis. *Arch Ophthalmol* 80:166, 1968

Foreign-Body Granulomas

Ferry AP: Synthetic fiber granuloma: "Teddy bear" granuloma of the conjunctiva. *Arch Ophthalmol* 112:1339, 1994

Naumann GOH, Völcker HE: Endophthalmitis haemogranulomatosa (eine spezielle Reaktionsform auf intraokulare Blutungen). *Klin Monatsbl Augenheilkd* 171:352, 1977

Riddle PJ, Font RL, Johnson FB et al.: Silica granuloma of eyelid and ocular adnexa. *Arch Ophthalmol* 99:683, 1981

Wilson MW, Grossniklaus HE, Heathcote JG: Focal choroidal granulomatous inflammation. *Am J Ophthalmol* 121:397, 1996

Viral

Anand R, Font RL, Fish RH et al.: Pathology of cytomegalovirus retinitis treated with sustained release intravitreal gancyclovir. *Ophthalmology* 100:1032, 1993

Bresnahan WA, Shenk T: A subset of viral transcripts packaged within human cytomegalovirus particles. *Science* 288:2373, 2000

deVenecia G, Rhein GMZ, Pratt M et al.: Cytomegalic inclusion retinitis in an adult: A clinical, histopathologic and ultrastructural study. *Arch Ophthalmol* 86:44, 1971

Foster DJ, Dugel PU, Frangieh GT et al.: Rapidly progressive outer retinal necrosis in the acquired immunodeficiency syndrome. *Am J Ophthalmol* 110:341, 1990

Friedman AH: The retinal lesions of the acquired immune deficiency syndrome. *Trans Am Ophthalmol Soc* 82:447, 1984

Glasgow BJ, Weisberger AK: A quantitative and cartographic study of retinal microvasculopathy in acquired immunodeficiency syndrome. *Am J Ophthalmol* 118:46, 1994

Gross JG, Bozzette SA, Mathews WC et al.: Longitudinal study of cytomegalovirus retinitis in acquired immune deficiency syndrome. *Ophthalmology* 97:681, 1990

Jabs DA, Martin BK, Forman MS et al.: Cytomegalovirus resistance to ganciclovir and clinical outcomes of patients with cytomegalovirus retinitis. *Am J Ophthalmol* 135:26, 2003

Karbassi M, Raizman MB, Schuman JS: Herpes zoster ophthalmicus . *Surv Ophthalmol* 36:395, 1992

Kempen JH, Jabs DA, Wilson LA et al.: Risk of vision loss in patients with cytomegalovirus and the acquired immunodeficiency syndrome. *Arch Ophthalmol* 121:466, 2003

Kuo IC, Kempen JH, Dunn JP et al.: Clinical characteristics and outcomes of cytomegalovirus retinitis in persons without human immunodeficiency virus infection. *Am J Ophthalmol* 138:338, 2004

Kupperman BD, Quienco JI, Wiley C et al.: Clinical and histopathologic study of varicella zoster virus retinitis in patients with the acquired immunodeficiency syndrome. *Am J Ophthalmol* 118:589, 1994

Lowder CY, Butler CP, Dodds EM et al.: CD8+ T lymphocytes and cytomegalovirus retinitis in patients with the acquired immunodeficiency syndrome. *Am J Ophthalmol* 120:283, 1995

Nguyen QD, Kempen JH, Bolton SG et al.: Immune recovery uveitis in patients with AIDS and cytomegalovirus retinitis following highly active retroviral therapy. *Am J Ophthalmol* 129:634, 2000

Rummelt V, Rummelt C, Jahn G et al.: Triple retinal infection with human immunodeficiency virus type 1, cytomegalovirus, and herpes simplex virus type 1: Light and electron microscopy, immunohistochemistry, and in situ hybridization. *Ophthalmology* 101:270, 1994

Walter KA, Coulter VL, Palay DA et al.: Corneal endothelial deposits in patients with cytomegalovirus retinitis. *Am J Ophthalmol* 121:391, 1996

Yoser SL, Forster DJ, Rao NA: Systemic viral infections and their retinal and choroidal manifestations. *Surv Ophthalmol* 37:313, 1993

Bacterial

Anderson B, Kelly C, Threlkel R et al.: Detection of *Rochalimaea henselae* in cat-scratch disease skin test antigens. *J Infect Dis* 168:1034, 1993

Babu RB, Sudharshan S, Kumaraasamy N et al.: Ocular tuberculosis in acquired immunodefiency syndrome. *Am J Ophthalmol* 142:413, 2006

Barile GR, Llynn TE: Syphilis exposure in patients with uveitis. *Ophthalmology* 104:1605, 1997

Becerra LI, Ksiazek SM, Savino PJ et al.: Syphilitic uveitis in human immunodeficiency virus-infected and noninfected patients. *Ophthalmology* 96:1727, 1989

Berinstein DM, Gentile RC, McCormick SA et al.: Primary choroidal tuberculoma. *Arch Ophthalmol* 115:430, 1997

Bleharski JR, Li H, Meinken C et al.: Use of genetic profiling in leprosy to discriminate clinical forms of the disease. *Science* 301:1527, 2003

Bowyer JD, Gormley PD, Seth R et al.: Choroidal tuberculosis diagnosed by polymerase chain reaction: A clinicopathologic case report. *Ophthalmology* 106:290, 1999

Bullington RH Jr, Lanier JD, Font RL: Nontuberculous mycobacterial keratitis: Report of two cases and review of the literature. *Arch Ophthalmol* 110:519, 1992

Cameron JA, Nasr AM, Chavis R: Epibulbar and ocular tuberculosis. *Arch Ophthalmol* 114:770, 1996

Chao JR, Khurana RN, Fawzi AA et al.: Syphilis: reemergence of an old adversary. *Ophthalmology* 113:2074, 2006

Cunningham ET Jr, Koehler JE: Ocular bartonellosis. *Am J Ophthalmol* 130:340, 2000

Cunningham ET Jr, McDonald HR, Schatz H *et al.*: Inflammatory mass of the optic nerve head associated with systemic *Bartonella hensela e* infection. *Arch Ophthalmol* 115:1596, 1997

Dana M-R, Hochman MA, Viana MAG *et al.*: Ocular manifestations of leprosy in a noninstitutionalized community in the United States. *Arch Ophthalmol* 112:626, 1994

Dondey JC, Sullivan TJ, Robson JMB *et al.*: Application of polymerase chain reaction assay in the diagnosis of orbital granuloma complicating atypical oculoglandular cat scratch disease. *Ophthalmology* 115:430, 1997

Flach AJ, Lavoie PE: Episcleritis, conjunctivitis, and keratitis as ocular manifestations of Lyme disease. *Ophthalmology* 97:973, 1990

Fraser CM, Norris SJ, Weinstock GM *et al.*: Complete genome sequence of *Treponema pallidum*, the syphilis spirochete. *Science* 281:375, 1998

Gass JDM, Braunstein RA, Chenoweth RG: Acute syphilitic posterior placoid chorioretinitis. *Ophthalmology* 97:1288, 1990

Gopal L, Rao SK, Biswas J *et al.*: Tuberculous granuloma managed by full thickness eye wall resection. *Am J Ophthalmol* 135:93, 2003

Gray AV, Wendel RT, Morse LS: *Bartonella henselae* infection associated with peripapillary angioma, branch retinal artery occlusion, and severe vision loss. *Am J Ophthalmol* 127:223, 1999

Gupta V, Gupta A, Arora S *et al.*: Presumed tubercular serpiginous choroiditis: clinical presentations and management. *Ophthalmology* 110:1744, 2003

Haas CJ, Zink A, Pàlfi G *et al.*: Detection of leprosy in ancient human skeletal remains by molecular identification of *Mycobacterium leprae*. *Am J Clin Pathol* 114:427, 2000

Helm CJ, Holland GN: Ocular tuberculosis. *Surv Ophthalmol* 38:229, 1993

Isogai E, Isogai H, Kotake S *et al.*: Detection of antibodies against *Borrelia burgdorferi* in patients with uveitis. *Am J Ophthalmol* 112:23, 1991

Karma A, Seppälä I, Mikkila H *et al.*: Diagnosis and clinical characteristics of ocular Lyme borreliosis. *Am J Ophthalmol* 119:127, 1995

Kestelyn P: Rhinoscleroma with bilateral orbital involvement. *Am J Ophthalmol* 101:381, 1986

Lee WR, Chawla JC, Reid R: Bacillary angiomatosis of the conjunctiva. *Am J Ophthalmol* 118:152, 1994

Margo CE, Hamed LM: Ocular syphilis. *Surv Ophthalmol* 37:203, 1992

Mikkilä HO, Seppälä IJT, Viljanen MK *et al.*: The expanding clinical spectrum of ocular Lyme borreliosis. *Ophthalmology* 107:581, 2000

Neneth GG, Fish RH, Itani KM *et al.*: Hansen's disease. *Arch Ophthalmol* 110:1482, 1992

Nepal BP, Shresha UD: Ocular findings in leprosy patients in Nepal in the era of multidrug therapy. *Am J Ophthalmol* 137:888, 2004

Ormerod LD, Skolnick KA, Menosky MM *et al.*: Retinal and choroidal manifestations of cat-scratch disease. *Ophthalmology* 105:1024, 1998

Preac-Mursic V, Pfister HW, Spiegel H *et al.*: First isolation of *Borrelia burgdorferi* from an iris biopsy. *J Clin Neuroophthalmol* 13:155, 1993

Rao NA, Hidayat AA: Endogenous mycotic endophthalmitis: variations in clinical and histologic changes in candidiasis compared with aspergillosis. *Am J Ophthalmol* 132:244, 2001

Raina UK, Jain S, Monga S *et al.*: Tubercular preseptal cellulites in children. A presenting sign of underlying systemic tuberculosis. *Ophthalmology* 111:291, 2004

Sarvananthan N, Wiselka M, Bibby K: Intraocular tuberculosis without detectable systemic infection. *Arch Ophthalmol* 116:1386, 1998

Scott IU, Silva-Lepe A, Siatkowski RM: Chiasmal optic neuritis in Lyme disease. *Am J Ophthalmol* 123:136, 1997

Shalaby IA, Dunn JP, Semba RD *et al.*: Syphilitic uveitis in human deficiency virus-infected patients. *Arch Ophthalmol* 115:469, 1997

Solley WA, Martin DF, Newman NJ *et al.*: Cat scratch disease: Posterior segment manifestations. *Ophthalmology* 106:1546, 1999

Spektor FE, Eagle RC, Nichols CW: Granulomatous conjunctivitis secondary to *Treponema pallidum*. *Ophthalmology* 88:863, 1981

Steinemann TL, Sheikholeslami MR, Brown HH *et al.*: Oculoglandular tularemia. *Arch Ophthalmol* 117:132, 1999

Tierno PM, Inglima K, Parisi MT: Detection of *Bartonella* (*Rochalimaea*) *henselae* bacteremia using BacT/Alert blood culture system. *Am J Clin Pathol* 104:530, 1995

Ulrich GG, Waecker NJ Jr, Meister SJ *et al.*: Cat scratch disease associated with neuroretinitis in a 6-year-old girl. *Ophthalmology* 99:246, 1992

Wade NK, Levi L, Jones MR *et al.*: Optic edema associated with peripapillary retinal detachment: an early sign of systemic *Bartonella henselae* infection. *Am J Ophthalmol* 130:327, 2000

Walburger A, Koul A, Ferrari G *et al.*: Protein kinase G from pathogenic mycobacteria promotes survival within macrophages. *Science* 304:1800, 2004

Whitcup SM, Fenton RM, Pluda JM *et al.*: *Pneumocystis carinii* and *Mycobacterium* infection of the choroid. *Retina* 12:331, 1992

Zacchei AC, Newman NJ, Sternberg P: Serous retinal detachment of the macula associated with cat scratch disease. *Am J Ophthalmol* 120:796, 1995

Zangwill KM, Hamilton DH, Perkins BA *et al.*: Cat scratch disease in Connecticut: Epidemiology, risk factors, and evaluation of a new diagnostic test. *N Engl J Med* 329:8, 1993

Fungal

Bartley GB: Blastomycosis of the eyelid. *Ophthalmology* 102:2020, 1995

Charles NC, Boxrud CA, Small EA: Cryptococcosis of the anterior chamber in acquired immune deficiency syndrome. *Ophthalmology* 99:813, 1992

Cohen DB, Glascow BJ: Bilateral optic nerve cryptococcosis in sudden blindness in patients with acquired immune deficiency syndrome. *Ophthalmology* 100:1689, 1993

Cohen J, Carvalho RC, Guimarães R *et al.*: Oculosporidiosis. *Arch Ophthalmol* 115:1340, 1997

Cunningham ET, Seiff SR, Berger TG *et al.*: Intraocular coccidioidomycosis diagnosed by skin biopsy. *Arch Ophthalmol* 116:674, 1998

Custis PH, Haller JA, de Juan E Jr: An unusual case of cryptococcal endophthalmitis. *Retina* 15:300, 1995

Donahue SP, Greven CM, Zuravleff JJ *et al.*: Intraocular candidiasis in patients with candidemia: Clinical implications derived from a prospective multicenter study. *Ophthalmology* 101:1302, 1994

Fairley C, Sullivan TJ, Bartley P *et al.*: Survival after rhino-orbital-cerebral mucormycosis in an immunocompetent. *Ophthalmology* 107:555, 2000

Font RL, Jakobiec FA: Granulomatous necrotizing retinochoroiditis caused by *Sporotrichum schenkii*. Report of a case including immunofluorescence and electron microscopical studies. *Arch Ophthalmol* 94:1513, 1976

Glasgow BJ, Brown HH, Foos RY: Miliary retinitis in coccidioidomycosis. *Am J Ophthalmol* 104:24, 1987

Gottlieb JL, McAllister IL, Guttman FA *et al.*: Choroidal blastomycosis: A report of two cases. *Retina* 15:248, 1995

Levin LA, Avery R, Shore JW *et al.*: The spectrum of orbital aspergillosis: A clinicopathological review. *Surv Ophthalmol* 41:142, 1996

Levy MG, Meuten DJ, Breitschwerdt EB: Cultivation of *Rhinosporidium seeberi* in vitro: Interaction with epithelial cells. *Science* 234:474, 1986

Li S, Perlman JI, Edward DP *et al.*: Unilateral *Blastomyces* dermatitidis endophthalmitis and orbital cellulitis: A case report and literature review. *Ophthalmology* 105:1467, 1998

Lin JC, Ward TP, Belyea DA *et al.*: Treatment of *Nocardia asteroides* keratitis with polyhexamethylene biguanide. *Ophthalmology* 104:1306, 7199

McNab AA, McKelvie P: Iron overload is a risk factor for zygomycosis. *Arch Ophthalmol* 115:919, 1997

Moorthy RS, Rao NA, Sidikaro Y *et al.*: Coccidioidomycosis iridocyclitis. *Ophthalmology* 101:1923, 1994

Safneck JR, Hogg GA, Napier LB: Endophthalmitis due to *Blastomyces dermatitidis*: Case report and review of the literature. *Ophthalmology* 97:212, 1990

Sheu S-J, Chen Y-C, Kuo N-W *et al.*: Endogenous cryptococcal endophthalmitis. *Ophthalmology* 105:377, 1998

Slade MP, McNab AA: Fatal mucormycosis therapy associated with deferoxamine (letter). *Am J Ophthalmol* 112:594, 1991

Specht CS, Mitchell KT, Bauman AE *et al.*: Ocular histoplasmosis with retinitis in a patient with acquired immune deficiency syndrome. *Ophthalmology* 98:1356, 1991

Sponsler TA, Sassani JW, Johnson LN *et al.*: Ocular invasion in mucormycosis. *Surv Ophthalmol* 36:345, 1992

Stone JL, Kalina RE: Ocular coccidioidomycosis. *Am J Ophthalmol* 116:249, 1993

Parasitic

Agrawal S, Agrawal J, Agrawal TP: Orbital cysticercosis-associated scleral indentation presenting with pseudo-retinal detachment. *Am J Ophthalmol* 137:1153, 2004

Bartlett MS, Smith JW: *Pneumocystis carinii*, an opportunist in immunocompromised patients. *Clin Microbiol Rev* 4:137, 1991

Benitez del Castillo JM, Herreros G, Guillen JL *et al.*: Bilateral ocular toxocariasis demonstrated by aqueous humor enzyme-linked immunosorbent assay. *Am J Ophthalmol* 119:514, 1995

Berger BB, Egwuagu CE, Freeman WR *et al.*: Miliary toxoplasmic retinitis in acquired immune deficiency syndrome. *Arch Ophthalmol* 111:373, 1993

Bernard EM, Sepkowitz KA, Telzak EE *et al.*: Pneumocystinosis. *Med Clin North Am* 76:107, 1992

Biswas J, Fogla R, Srinivasan P *et al.*: Ocular malaria. A clinical and histopathologic study. *Ophthalmology* 103:1471, 1996

Buettner H: Ophthalmomyiasis interna. *Arch Ophthalmol* 120:1582, 2002

Burnier M, Hidayat AA, Neafdiue R: Dracunculiasis of the orbit and eyelid: Light and electron microscopic observations of two cases. *Ophthalmology* 98:919, 1991

Campbell RJ, Steele JC, Cox TA *et al.*: Pathologic findings in the retinal pigment epitheliopathy associated with the amyotrophic lateral sclerosis/Parkinsonism-dementia complex (ALS/PDC) of Guam. *Ophthalmology* 100:37, 1993

Chan CML, Theng JTS, Li L, *et al.*: Microsporidial keratoconjunctivitis in healthy individuals: a case series. *Ophthalmology* 110:1420, 2003

Chang GY, Keane JR: Visual loss in cysticercosis. *Neurology* 57:545, 2001

Chuck RS, Olk RJ, Weil GJ *et al.*: Surgical removal of a subretinal proliferating cysticercus of *Taeniaeformis crassiceps*. *Arch Ophthalmol* 115:562, 1997

Fahnehjelm KT, Malm G, Ygge J *et al.*: Ophthalmological findings in children with congenital toxoplasmosis. Report from a Swedish prospective screening study of congenital toxoplasmosis with two years of follow-up. *Acta Ophthalmol Scand* 78:569, 2000

Font RL, Samaha AN, Keener MJ *et al.*: Corneal microsporidiosis: Report of a case, including electron microscopic observations. *Ophthalmology* 107:1769, 2000

Freeman WR, Gross JG, Labelle J *et al.*: *Pneumocystis carinii* choroidopathy: A new clinical entity. *Arch Ophthalmol* 107:863, 1989

Gendelman D, Blumberg R, Sadun A: Ocular *Loa loa* with cryoprobe extraction of subconjunctival worm. *Ophthalmology* 91:300, 1984

Glasgow BJ, Maggiano JM: Cuterebra ophthalmomyiasis. *Am J Ophthalmol* 119:512, 1995

Grevin CM, Teot LA: Cytologic identification of *Toxoplasma gondii* from vitreous fluid. *Arch Ophthalmol* 112:1086, 1994

Gupta NK, Sachdev MS, Bhardwaj Y *et al.*: Intraocular *Ascaris* larva. *Arch Ophthalmol* 106:880, 1988

Hidayat AA, Nalbandian RM, Sammons DW *et al.*: The diagnostic histopathologic features of ocular malaria. *Ophthalmology* 100:1183, 1993

Holland GN: Ocular toxoplasmosis: a global reassessment. Part I: epidemiology and course of the disease (LX Edward Jackson memorial lecture). *Am J Ophthalmol* 136:973, 2003

Holland GN: Ocular toxoplasmosis: a global reassessment. Part II: disease manifestations and management. (LX Edward Jackson memorial lecture). *Am J Ophthalmol* 137:1, 2004

Holland GN, MacArthur LJ, Foos RY: Choroidal pneumocystosis. *Arch Ophthalmol* 109:1454, 1991

Jackson HC, Colthurst D, Hancock V *et al.*: No detection of characteristic fungal protein elongation factor EF-3 in *Pneumocystis carinii*. *J Infect Dis* 163:675, 1991

Jakobiec FA, Gess L, Zimmerman LE: Granulomatous dacryoadenitis caused by *Schistosoma haematobium*. *Arch Ophthalmol* 95:278, 1977

Johnson MW, Greven CM, Jaffe GJ *et al.*: Atypical, severe toxoplasmic retinochoroiditis in elderly patients. *Ophthalmology* 104:48, 1997

Kırath H, Biliç S, Öztürkmen C *et al.*: Intramuscular hydatid cyst of the medial rectus. *Am J Ophthalmol* 135:98, 2003

Labalette P, Delhaes L, Margaron F *et al.*: Ocular toxoplasmosis after the fifth decade. *Am J Ophthalmol* 133:506, 2002

Lawson JMM, Dart JKG, McCartney ACE: Conjunctival nodules associated with the Splendore–Hoeppli phenomenon. *Arch Ophthalmol* 109:426, 1991

Mets MB, Holfels E, Boyer KM *et al.*: Eye manifestations of congenital toxoplasmosis. *Am J Ophthalmol* 123:1, 1997

Mohammad AE-NA, Ray CJ, Karcioglu ZA: *Echinococcus* cysts of the orbit and substernum. *Am J Ophthalmol* 118:676, 1994

Moorthy RS, Smith RE, Rao NA: Progressive toxoplasmosis in patients with the acquired immunodeficiency syndrome. *Am J Ophthalmol* 115:742, 1993

Morales LR, Cialdini AP, Avila MP *et al.*: Identifying live nematodes in diffuse unilateral subacute neuroretinitis by using the scanning laser ophthalmoscope. *Arch Ophthalmol* 120:135, 2002

Naumann GOH, Knorr HLJ: DUSN occurs in Europe (letter). *Ophthalmology* 101:971, 1994

Perry HD, Donnenfeld ED, Font RL: Intracorneal ophthalmomyasis. *Am J Ophthalmol* 109:741, 1990

Raithinam S, Fritsche TR, Srinivascan M *et al.*: An outbreak of trematode-induced granulomas of the conjunctiva. *Ophthalmology* 108:1223, 2001

Risco JM, Al-Dosari F, Millar L: Sheep nasal botfly (*Oestrus ovis*) larvae infestation of the conjunctiva. *Arch Ophthalmol* 113:529, 1995

Roberts F, Mets MB, Ferguson DJP *et al.*: Histopathological features of ocular toxoplasmosis in the fetus and infant. *Arch Ophthalmol* 119:51, 2001

Ronday MJ, Ongkosuwito JV, Rothova A *et al.*: Intraocular anti-*Toxoplasma gondii* IgA antibody production in patients with ocular toxoplasmosis. *Am J Ophthalmol* 127:294, 1999

Sakai R, Kawashima H, Shibui H *et al.*: *Toxocara cati*-induced ocular toxocariasis. *Arch Ophthalmol* 116:1686, 1998

Schwab IR: The epidemiologic association of Fuchs' heterochromic iridocyclitis and toxoplasmosis. *Am J Ophthalmol* 111:356, 1991

Schwartz DA, Visvesvara GS, Diesenhouse MC et al.: Pathologic features and immunofluorescent antibody demonstration of ocular microsporidiosis (*Encephalitozoon hellem*) in seven patients with acquired immunodeficiency syndrome. *Am J Ophthalmol* 115:285, 1993

Sekhar GC, Hanavar SG: Mycocysticercosis: Experience with imaging and therapy. *Ophthalmology* 106:2336, 1999

Sekhar GC, Lemke BN: Orbital cysticercosis. *Ophthalmology* 104:1599, 1997

Shami MJ, Freeman W, Friedberg D et al.: A multicenter study of *Pneumocystis* choroidopathy. *Am J Ophthalmol* 112:15, 1991

Sharma T, Sinha S, Shah N et al.: Intraocular cysticercosis: Clinical characteristics and visual outcome after vitrectomy surgery. *Ophthalmology* 110:1005, 2003

Werner JC, Ross RD, Green WR et al.: Pars plana vitrectomy and subretinal surgery for ocular toxocariasis. *Arch Ophthalmol* 117:332, 1999

Whitcup SM, Fenton RM, Pluda JM et al.: *Pneumocystis carinii* and *Mycobacterium* infection of the choroid. *Retina* 12:331, 1992

Wilder HC: Nematode endophthalmitis. *Trans Am Acad Ophthalmol Otolaryngol* 54:99, 1950

Wilder HC: *Toxoplasma* chorioretinitis in adults. *Arch Ophthalmol* 48:127, 1952

Sarcoidosis

Boyd SR, Young S, Lightman S: Immunopathology of the noninfectious posterior and intermediate uveitides. *Surv Ophthalmol* 46:209, 2001

Cornblath WT, Elner V, Rolfe M: Extraocular muscle involvement in sarcoidosis. *Ophthalmology* 100:501, 1993

Farr AK, Jabs DA, Green WR: Optic disc sarcoid granuloma. *Arch Ophthalmol* 118:728, 2000

Frohman L, Grigorian R, Slamovits T: Evolution of sarcoid granulomas of the retina. *Am J Ophthalmol* 131:661, 2001

Garcia GH, Harris GJ: Sarcoid inflammation and obstruction of the nasolacrimal system. *Arch Ophthalmol* 118:719, 2000

Gass JDM, Olson CL: Sarcoidosis with optic nerve and retinal involvement. *Arch Ophthalmol* 94:945, 1976

Hall JG, Cohen KL: Sarcoidosis of the eyelid and skin. *Am J Ophthalmol* 119:100, 1995

Khalatbari D, Stinnett S, McCallum RM et al.: Demographic-related variations in posterior segmet ocular sarcoidosis. *Ophthalmology* 111:357, 2004

Lower EE, Broderick JP, Brott TG et al.: Diagnosis and management of neurological sarcoidosis. *Arch Intern Med* 157:1864, 1997

Nichols CW, Eagle RC Jr, Yanoff M et al.: Conjunctival biopsy as an aid in the evaluation of the patient with suspected sarcoidosis. *Ophthalmology* 87:287, 1980

Nichols CW, Mishkin M, Yanoff M: Presumed orbital sarcoidosis: Report of a case followed by computerized axial tomography and conjunctival biopsy. *Trans Am Ophthalmol Soc* 76:67, 1978

Pelton RW, Lee AG, Orengo-Nania SD et al.: Bilateral optic disk edema caused by sarcoidosis mimicking pseudotumor cerebri. *Am J Ophthalmol* 127:229, 1999

Peterson EA, Hymas DC, Pratt DV et al.: Sarcoidosis with orbital tumor outside the lacrimal gland: Initial manifestation in 2 elderly white women. *Arch Ophthalmol* 116:804, 1998

Qazi A, Thorne JE, Jabs DA: Scleral nodule associated with sarcoidosis. *Am J Ophthalmol* 136, 2003

Reid JD, Andersen ME: Calcium oxalate in sarcoid granules: With particular reference to the small ovoid body and a note on the finding of dolomite. *Am J Clin Pathol* 90:545, 1988

Schaumann J: On nature of certain peculiar corpuscles present in tissue of lymphogranulomatosis benigna. *Acta Med Scand* 106:239, 1941

Sherman MD, Pince KJ, Farahmand SM: Sarcoidosis manifesting as uveitis and menometrorrhagia. *Am J Ophthalmol* 123:703, 1997

Westlake WH, Heath JD, Spalton DJ: Sarcoidosis involving the optic nerve and hypothalamus. *Arch Ophthalmol* 113:669, 1995

Granulomatous Scleritis

Brod RD, Saul RF: Nodular scleritis. *Arch Ophthalmol* 108:1170, 1990

Fong LP, de la Maza MS, Rice BA et al.: Immunopathology of scleritis. *Ophthalmology* 98:472, 1991

Hinzpeter EN, Naumann G, Gartelheimer HK: Ocular histopathology in Still's disease. *Ophthalmic Res* 2:16, 1971

Lebowitz MA, Jakobiec FA, Donnenfeld ED et al.: Bilateral epibulbar rheumatoid nodulosis: A new ocular entity. *Ophthalmology* 95:1256, 1988

de la Maza MS, Foster CS, Jabbur NS: Scleritis associated with rheumatoid arthritis and with other systemic immune-mediated diseases. *Ophthalmology* 101:1281, 1994

de la Maza MS, Foster CS, Jabbur NS: Scleritis associated with systemic vasculitic diseases. *Ophthalmology* 102:687, 1995

Sacks RD, Stock EL, Crawford SE et al.: Scleritis and Wegener's granulomatosis in children. *Am J Ophthalmol* 111:430, 1991

Salmon JF, Strauss PC, Todd G et al.: Acute scleritis in porphyria cutanea tarda. *Am J Ophthalmol* 109:400, 1990

Tuft SJ, Watson PG: Progression of scleral disease. *Ophthalmology* 98:467, 1991

Watson PG, Hayreh SS: Scleritis and episcleritis. *Br J Ophthalmol* 60:163, 1976

Granulomatous Reaction to Descemet's Membrane

Green WR, Zimmerman LE: Granulomatous reaction to Descemet's membrane. *Am J Ophthalmol* 64:555, 1967

Holbach LM, Font RL, Naumann GOH: Herpes simplex stromal and endothelial keratitis: Granulomatous cell reactions at the level of Descemet's membrane, the stroma, and Bowman's layer. *Ophthalmology* 97:722, 1990

Vogt–Koyanagi–Harada Syndrome

Boyd SR, Young S, Lightman S: Immunopathology of the noninfectious posterior and intermediate uveitides. *Surv Ophthalmol* 46:209, 2001

Cunningham ET, Demetrius R, Frieden IJ et al.: Vogt–Koya nagi–Harada syndrome in a 4-year-old child. *Am J Ophthalmol* 120:675, 1995

Davis JL, Mittal KK, Freidlin V et al.: HLA associations and ancestry in Vogt–Koyanagi–Harada disease and sympathetic ophthalmia. *Ophthalmology* 97:1137, 1990

Fine BS, Gilligan JH: The Vogt–Koyanagi syndrome: A variant of sympathetic ophthalmia: report of two cases. *Am J Ophthalmol* 43:433, 1957

Friedman AH, Deutsch-Sokol RH: Sugiura's sign. Perilimbal vitiligo in the Vogt–Koyanagi–Harada syndrome. *Ophthalmology* 88:1159, 1981

Gocho K, Kondo I, Yamaki K: Identification of autoreactive T cells in Vogt–Koyanagi–Harada disease. *Invest Ophthalmol Vis Sci* 42:2037, 2001

Goldberg AC, Yamamota JH, Chiarella JM et al.: DRB1*0405 is the predominant allele in Brazilian patients with Vogt–Koyanagi–Harada disease. *Hum Immunol* 59:183, 1998

Inomata H, Rao NA: Depigmented atrophic lesions in sunset glow fundi of Vogt–Koyanagi–Harada disease. *Am J Ophthalmol* 131:607, 2001

Keino H, Goto H, Mori H et al.: Association between severity of inflammation in CNS and development of sunset glow fundus in Vogh-Koyanagi-Herada disease. *Am J Ophthalmol* 141:1140, 2006

Kim M-H, Seong M-C, Kwak N-H *et al.*: Association of HLA with Vogt–Koyanagi–Harada syndrome in Koreans. *Am J Ophthalmol* 129:173, 2000

Kuo IC, Rechdouni A, Rao NA *et al.*: Subretinal fibrosis in patients with Vogt–Koyanagi–Harada disease. *Ophthalmology* 107:1721, 2000

Moorthy RS, Inomata H, Rao NA: Vogt–Koyanagi–Harada syndrome. *Surv Ophthalmol* 39:265, 1995

Najman-Vainer J, Levinson RD, Graves MC *et al.*: An association between Vogt–Koyanagi–Harada disease and Guillain Barré syndrome. *Am J Ophthalmol* 131:615, 2001

Nakamura S, Nakazawa M, Yoshioka M *et al.*: Melanin-laden macrophages in Vogt–Koyanagi–Harada syndrome. *Arch Ophthalmol* 114:1184, 1996

Pivetti-Pezzi P, Accorinti M, Colabelli-Gisoldi RAM *et al.*: Vogt–Koyanagi–Harada disease and HLA type in Italian patients. *Am J Ophthalmol* 122:889, 1996

Rathinam SR, Namperumalsamy P, Nozik RA *et al.*: Vogt–Koyanagi–Harada syndrome after cutaneous injury. *Ophthalmology* 106:635, 1999

Read RW, Holland GN, Rao NA *et al.*: Revised diagnostic criteria for Vogt–Koyanagi–Harada disease: Report of an international committee on nomenclature. *Am J Ophthalmol* 131:647, 2001

Read RW, Rechodouni A, Butani N *et al.*: Complications and prognostic factors in Vogt–Koyanagi–Harada disease. *Am J Ophthalmol* 131:599, 2001

Rutzen AR, Ortega-Larrocea G, Scwab IR *et al.*: Simultaneous onset of Vogt–Koyanagi–Harada syndrome in monozygotic twins. *Am J Ophthalmol* 119:239, 1995

Shindo Y, Inoko H, Yamamoto T *et al.*: HLA-DRB1 typing of Vogt–Koyanagi–Harada's disease by PCR-RFLP and the strong association with DRB1*0405 and DRB1*0410. *Br J Ophthalmol* 78:223, 1994

Shindo Y, Ohno S, Yamamoto T *et al.*: Complete association of the HLA-DRB*1 and -DQB1*04 alleles with Vogt–Koyanagi–Harada's disease. *Hum Immunol* 39:169, 1994

Taylor S, Lightman S: Recurrent anterior uveitis in patients with Vogt–Koyanagi–Harada syndrome. *Arch Ophthalmol* 122:922, 2004

Weisz JM, Holland GN, Roer LN *et al.*: Association between Vogt–Koyanagi–Harada syndrome and HLA-DR1 HLA-DR4 in Hispanic patients living in Southern California. *Ophthalmology* 102:1012, 1995

Familial Chronic Granulomatous Disease of Childhood

Gallin JI, Malech HL: Update on chronic granulomatous diseases of childhood. Immunotherapy and potential for gene therapy. *JAMA* 263:1533, 1990

Grossniklaus HE, Frank KE, Jacobs G: Chorioretinal lesions in chronic granulomatous disease of childhood: Clinicopathologic correlations. *Retina* 8:270, 1988

White CJ, Kwon-Chung KJ, Gallin JI: Chronic granulomatous disease of childhood: An unusual case of infection with *Aspergillus nidulans* var. *echinulatus*. *Am J Clin Pathol* 90:312, 1988

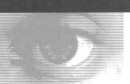

5

Surgical and Nonsurgical Trauma

CAUSES OF ENUCLEATION

I. Causes of enucleation are many and varied.
II. As can be seen in Figure 5.1, trauma (surgical and nonsurgical) is the number-one cause of enucleations, accounting for 35% of all enucleations.

COMPLICATIONS OF INTRAOCULAR SURGERY*

Immediate

Complications occurring from the time the decision is made to perform surgery until the patient leaves the operating room are considered immediate.

Cataract surgery of any type falls into the category of refractive surgery.

I. "Surgical confusion"
   A. Misdiagnosis: not all cataracts are primary, but they may be secondary to such things as trauma, inflammation, neoplasm (Fig. 5.2), or metabolic disease. When opaque media are caused by a cataract, ultrasonography, magnetic resonance imaging, or computed tomographic scanning can be helpful in establishing whether a neoplasm or a retinal detachment is present behind the cataract.

This section refers to a cataract or glaucoma incision that usually involves a wound to the limbal region so that conjunctiva, cornea, sclera, and iris can all be considered.

Many technical complications can be avoided by the use of topical and intracameral anesthesia, and a clear-cornea, temporal, no-stitch incision.

   B. Faulty technique may result in and/or from:
      1. Inadequate anesthesia
      2. Perforation of the globe, which may occur at the time of the retrobulbar or peribulbar anesthetic injection or when a bridle suture is inadvertently placed through the sclera

The risk of perforating the globe during retrobulbar anesthesia is approximately 1:1000 if the eye is less than 26 mm in axial length, and approximately 1:140 in longer eyes. The main risk factor for perforation is a posterior staphyloma.

         a. Localized, extreme scleral thinning can predispose to scleral rupture during strabismus surgery.
      3. Increased intraocular pressure because of a retrobulbar hemorrhage or poorly placed lid speculum
      4. Misalignment of the entering incision

If the corneal-entering incision into the anterior chamber is too far peripheral, iris prolapse may occur. If the incision is too far central, corneal striae and poor visibility may result. Ideally, the corneal-entering incision into the anterior chamber should be 1 to 2 mm into clear cornea.

      5. "Buttonhole" of the conjunctiva (not serious in cataract surgery but may lead to failure in filtering procedures)

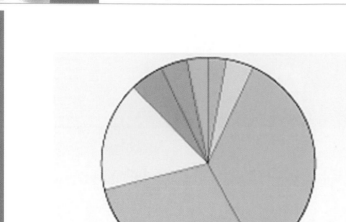

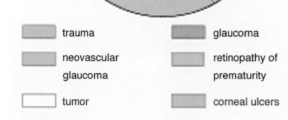

trauma   glaucoma

neovascular glaucoma   retinopathy of prematurity

tumor   corneal ulcers

endophthalmitis   other

Fig. 5.1 Reasons for enucleation. In this study of the incidence of enucleation in a defined population, trauma was the number-one cause. (Modified from Erie JC *et al.: Am J Ophthalmol* 113:138. Copyright Elsevier 1992.)

6. Splitting off (stripping) of Descemet's membrane from the posterior cornea (can lead to postoperative corneal edema; Fig. 5.3)

> Most commonly, the stripping may occur at the time of the introduction of the phacoemulsifier or the irrigation–aspiration tip, the placement of the lens implant into the eye, during the injection of a viscous agent into the eye. Many detachments resolve spontaneously and do not require surgical repair. Intracameral treatment of Descemet's membrane detachment with perfluoropropane gas has been successful.

7. Iridodialysis (although usually innocuous, may lead to anterior-chamber hemorrhage or problems with pupillary distortion)
8. Photic retinal toxicity (believed to occur from a too-strong surgical light, especially after a cataract is removed, the lens implant is in place, and the surgical light is focused on the macula)

> After the lens implant is in place, if further surgery is indicated, it is advisable to place an opaque or semiopaque cover over the cornea, or an air bubble in the anterior chamber to reduce the effect of light focused on the posterior pole.

II. Anterior-chamber bleeding
   A. This usually occurs from the scleral side of the cut edge of the wound, especially at the end of the incision.

B. It may also occur at the iridectomy site.
C. Bleeding invariably stops in a short time if patience and continuous saline irrigation are used.

III. Radial tear of the anterior capsulectomy (either capsulorhexis or "can-opener incision"), rupture of the posterior lens capsule, or a zonular dialysis
   A. This makes surgery more difficult and leads to an increased incidence of vitreous loss, posterior displacement of lens nucleus or nuclear fragments into the vitreous compartment, retained cortex, and complicated wound healing.
   B. It also predisposes to malposition of the lens implant and irregular pupil.

IV. Loss of vitreous, which occurs in approximately 3% to 9% of cataract cases, leads to an increased incidence of iris prolapse, bullous keratopathy, epithelial downgrowth, stromal ingrowth, wound infection, endophthalmitis, updrawn or misshapen pupil, vitreous bands, postoperative flat chamber, secondary glaucoma, poor wound healing, neural retinal detachment, cystoid macular and optic disc edema, vitreous opacities and hemorrhage, expulsive choroidal hemorrhage, and "chronic ocular irritability."
   A. Modern surgical techniques can reduce the incidence of vitreous loss associated with cataract surgery in patients with pseudoexfoliation to that in unaffected individuals.
   B. Lens fragments retained within the vitreous compartment at the time of cataract surgery are associated with an increased incidence of inflammation, increased intraocular pressure, and cystoid macular edema (CME). Vitrectomy to remove such fragments is associated with faster visual rehabilitation and better quality of vision.

V. Expulsive choroidal hemorrhage (Fig. 5.4; see also Figs 16.27 and 16.28).
   A. This is a rare (it occurs in approximately 0.13% with nuclear expression and 0.03% with phacoemulsification), catastrophic complication and may result in loss of the eye.

> Risk factors include glaucoma, increased axial length, elevated intraocular pressure, generalized atherosclerosis, and elevated systemic blood pressure

   B. The hemorrhage usually results from rupture of a sclerotic choroidal (ciliary) artery or arteriole as it makes a right-angle turn crossing the suprachoroidal space from its scleral canal. The sudden hypotony after penetration of the globe straightens the sclerotic vessel and causes the rupture.
   C. Although most hemorrhages are massive and immediate, occasionally they are delayed and may not occur for days to weeks.

> Spontaneous choroidal effusion may occur during intraocular surgery and mimic expulsive choroidal hemorrhage.

   D. Histologically, massive intraocular hemorrhage, a totally detached choroid and neural retina, and a gaping wound are seen. A ruptured ciliary artery may be found.

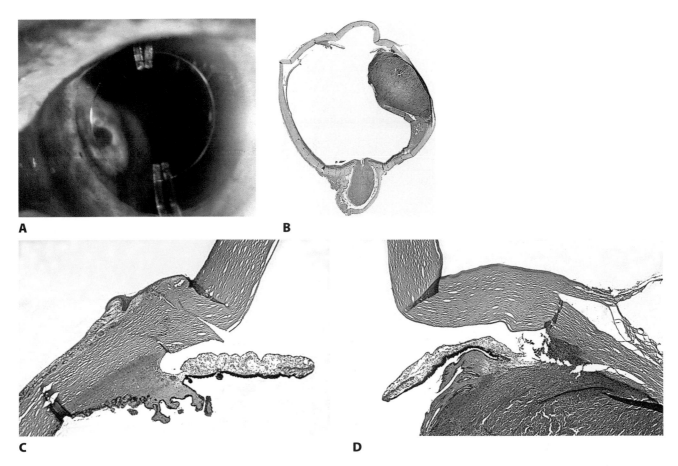

Fig. 5.2 Surgical confusion. **A,** Unsuspected mass noted in pupil after cataract extraction and anterior-chamber lens implantation; eye enucleated some time later. **B,** Large uveal melanoma extends from ciliary body to equator. **C,** Rounded anterior face of ciliary body shows where anterior-chamber lens footplate was. **D,** In this section, footplate had rested within the melanoma. Cataracts are not all primary but may be secondary to intraocular disease. (Presented by Dr. J Chess at the meeting of the Eastern Ophthalmic Pathology Society, 1983.)

VI. Foreign bodies may be introduced into the eye at the time of surgery.
   A. Cilia within the eye can have a variable response from endophthalmitis to prolonged periods of tolerance. Surgical removal of such foreign bodies is a clinical decision that must be individualized based on the patient response to the foreign material.
   B. Material placed within the anterior segment to facilitate cataract surgery, such as indocyanine green (ICG) dye, may prove toxic if it migrates posteriorly to involve the retina.
   C. Rarely, metallic foreign bodies may be introduced into the eye at the time of intraocular surgery and should be considered in the differential diagnosis of recalcitrant postoperative inflammation. Nevertheless, frequently there is no inflammatory response, and removal is not necessary.

Postoperative

Postoperative complications may arise from the time the patient leaves the operating room until approximately 2 or 3 months after surgery.

I. Atonic pupil
   A. Dilated, fixed pupil is rare, but when present, even with 20/20 acuity, can cause annoying, sometimes disabling, problems because of glare.

   An atonic pupil develops in less than 2% of eyes after cataract surgery and posterior-chamber lens implantation.
   B. The site of the lesion appears to be in the iris sphincter.
II. Flat anterior chamber*—most chambers refill within 4 to 8 hours after surgery.

Today, with phacoemulsification cataract surgery techniques and careful attention to wound construction and closure, including "no-stitch" closure, flat anterior chamber is quite rare. It is more commonly seen after filtration surgery than after cataract surgery.

A flat anterior chamber is one in which the iris comes up against the posterior cornea and completely obliterates the anterior chamber. This must be differentiated from a shallow chamber, in which some space is still present. If the chamber is flat for 5 days or more, peripheral anterior synechiae often develop on the posterior corneal surface (e.g., broad-based). With a shallow anterior chamber, synechiae take much longer to form.

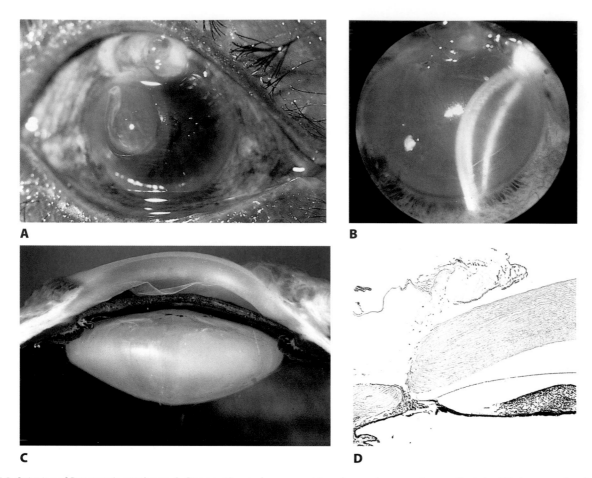

Fig. 5.3 Stripping of Descemet's membrane. **A,** Descemet's membrane was stripped over a large area temporally during filtering procedure (scleral cautery and peripheral iridectomy). **B,** Clinical appearance approximately 9 months later; eye enucleated. **C** and **D,** Gross and histologic appearance, respectively, of stripped Descemet's membrane. (Adapted from Kozart DM, Eagle RC Jr: Stripping of Descemet's membrane after glaucoma surgery. *Ophthalm Surg* 12:420–423, 1981. Adapted with permission from SLACK incorporated.)

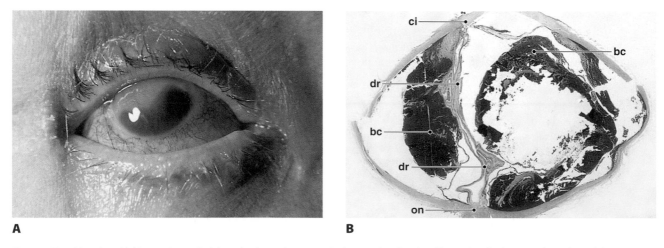

Fig. 5.4 Expulsive choroidal hemorrhage. **A,** A large hyphema is present in the anterior chamber. The patient had an expulsive choroidal hemorrhage during surgery. **B,** Histologic section shows hemorrhage in the choroid and subretinal space. The neural retina is in the corneoscleral wound (ci, cataract incision; dr, detached retina; bc, blood clot; on, optic nerve). (**A,** Courtesy of Dr. HG Scheie.)

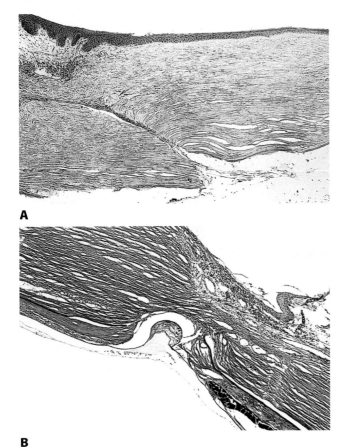

A

B

Fig. 5.5 Poor apposition of wound edges. **A,** Poor apposition of posterior edges of wound after cataract extraction. Vitreous is seen in wound. **B,** Vitreous incarcerated in wound just in front of anterior synechia (periodic acid–Schiff stain). Fibrous ingrowth formation present deep to cut edges of Descemet's membrane (see also Fig. 5.10B).

A. Secondary to hypotony

Most of the complications that cause hypotony are reduced or negated by clear-cornea, temporal, no-stitch phacoemulsification technique.

1. *Faulty wound closure* (Fig. 5.5): faulty apposition of the wound edges can lead to poor wound healing and a "leaky" wound. Hypotony and a flat anterior chamber result.
2. *Choroidal detachment* ("combined" choroidal detachment) is not a true detachment, but rather, an effusion or edema of the choroid (*hydrops*), and is always associated with a similar process in the ciliary body. This complication occurs much more commonly following glaucoma surgery than following cataract surgery.
    a. The choroidal detachment, instead of causing the flat chamber, is usually secondary to it; a leaky wound is the cause.

b. Once choroidal hydrops occurs, however, slowing of aqueous production by the edematous ciliary body and anterior displacement of the iris lens diaphragm by the increased volume within the vitreous compartment or by ciliary body "detachment" may further complicate the flat chamber and hypotonic eye.
    c. Histologically, the choroid and ciliary body, especially the outer layers, appear spread out like a fan, and the spaces are filled with an eosinophilic coagulum.
    Frequently, the edema fluid is "washed out" of tissue sections and the spaces appear empty.
3. *Iris incarceration* (Fig. 5.6; iris within the surgical wound) or iris prolapse (iris through the wound into the subconjunctival area) acts as a wick through which aqueous can escape, resulting in a flat chamber.

Other ocular structures such as ciliary body, lens remnants, vitreous, or even choroid and retina can become incarcerated in, or prolapsed through, the wound and lead to a flat chamber. All these structures are more likely to enter the wound after nonsurgical trauma than after surgical trauma. Rarely, a lens implant loop may prolapse through the surgical wound.

4. Histologically, iris (recognized by heavy pigmentation) may be seen in the limbal scar, in the limbal episclera, or in both areas.
5. *Fistulization* of the wound (Fig. 5.7) is usually of no clinical significance, but on occasion, it may be marked and lead to a large bleb, hypotony, flat chamber, corneal astigmatism, and epiphora.
6. *Vitreous wick syndrome* consists of microscopic-scale wound breakdown leading to subsequent vitreous prolapse, thus creating a tiny wick draining to the external surface of the eye.
    a. In some cases, severe intraocular inflammation develops and resembles a bacterial endophthalmitis.
    b. Infection can gain entrance into the eye through a vitreous wick.
7. Poor wound healing per se, without an identifiable cause, can lead to aqueous leakage, a filtering bleb, or a flat chamber.

B. Secondary to glaucoma
1. *Pseudophakic, pupillary block glaucoma* may occur from an intraocular lens. The prevalence varies with different types of intraocular lenses and from surgeon to surgeon.
    a. Most cases occur in eyes that have anterior-chamber intraocular lenses placed, but do not have a peripheral iridectomy performed (Fig. 5.8). However, most surgeons do not routinely perform a peripheral iridectomy when placing a posterior-chamber intraocular lens, and pseudophakic, pupillary block glaucoma is extremely rare in these cases.

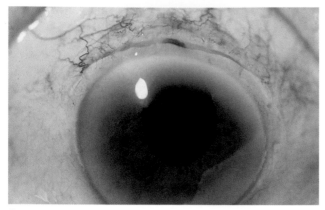

A

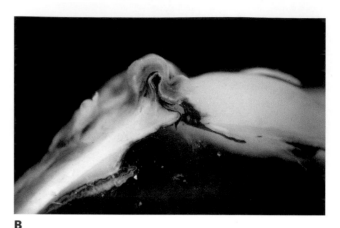

B

Fig. 5.6 Iris in the wound. **A,** Two weeks after surgery, the iris has prolapsed through the wound and presents subconjunctivally at the 12-o'clock position. **B,** Gross specimen of another case shows iris prolapsed through wound into subconjunctival space (as contrasted to iris incarceration, which is iris into, but not through, wound—see **C**). **C,** In this case, the iris has become incarcerated in the wound, causing the internal portion of the wound to gape.

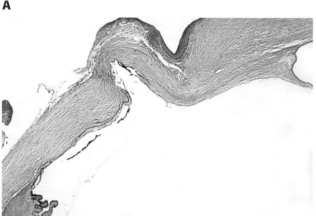

C

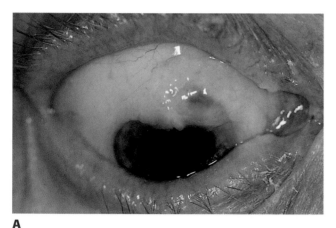

A

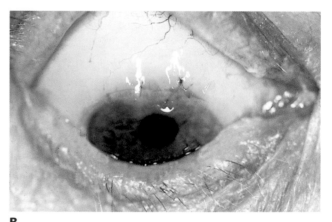

B

Fig. 5.7 Fistulization of wound. **A,** A filtering bleb appeared shortly after cataract surgery; the bleb enlarged and hypotony and irritability developed. The bleb was excised and the wound repaired. **B,** Eight months later. **C,** Histologic section of another excised bleb shows marked edema of the conjunctival substantia propria. Note the increased thickness of the epithelial basement membrane.

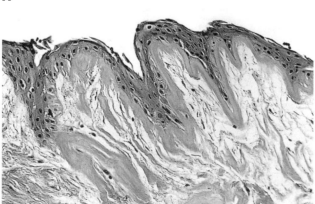

C

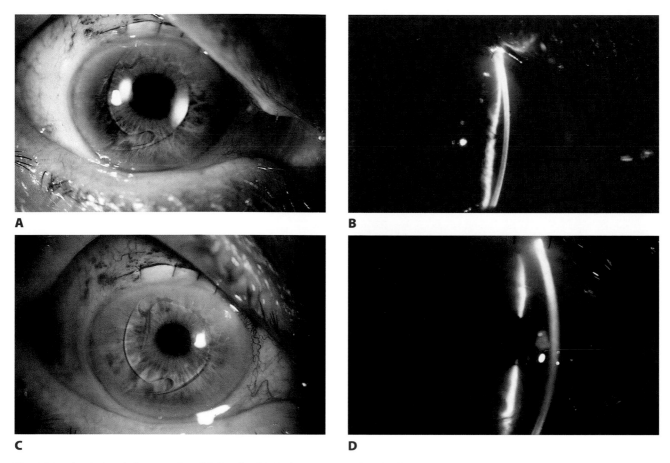

Fig. 5.8 Implant-induced glaucoma. **A** and **B,** Pupillary block glaucoma is noted on the first postoperative day in an eye with anterior-chamber lens implant. **C** and **D,** An yttrium aluminum garnet (YAG) laser iridectomy "cures" the glaucoma.

Aphakic glaucoma, or glaucoma in an aphakic eye, is almost never seen today because intracapsular cataract extraction is so rarely performed. The glaucoma in the postoperative period is usually caused by a pupillary block mechanism.

---

   b. Histologically, posterior synechiae form between the iris, lens capsule, and lens implant (or lens remnants, including cortex). In eyes that have had an intracapsular cataract extraction, synechiae form between the posterior pupillary portion of the iris and the anterior vitreous face.

2. A choroidal hemorrhage can occur slowly rather than abruptly and cause anterior vitreous displacement, resulting in an anterior displacement of the iris or iris lens implant diaphragm. The hemorrhage may remain confined to the uvea or may break through into the subretinal space, the vitreous, or even the anterior chamber.

An unusual hemorrhage is one in which blood collects in the narrow space between the posterior lens implant surface and posterior capsule (*endocapsular* hematoma) in an "in the bag" implant.

---

3. Sodium hyaluronate trapped within the vitreous compartment at the time of cataract surgery complicated by posterior capsule tear has resulted in intractable glaucoma.

III. Striate keratopathy ("keratitis")

   A. Damage to the corneal endothelium results in linear striae caused by posterior corneal edema and folding of Descemet's membrane.

   B. Vigorous bending or folding of the cornea during surgery was the usual cause in the days of intracapsular cataract surgery.

      Striate keratopathy occurs less commonly and is milder after phacoemulsification. In this setting it is most commonly secondary to endothelial injury resulting from aqueous turbulence, or from direct endothelial trauma by nuclear or instrument contact or from nuclear particles. Nevertheless, striate keratopathy is not uncommon after nuclear expression or intracapsular cataract extraction.

   C. Striate keratopathy is usually completely reversible and disappears within a week.

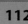

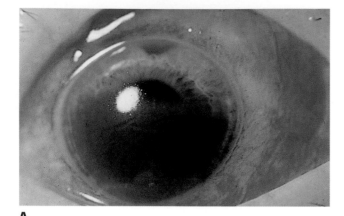

A

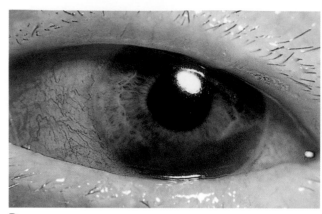

B

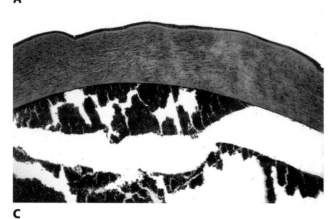

C

Fig. 5.9 Hyphema. **A,** Blood in anterior chamber (hyphema) the first day after cataract surgery. **B,** Two days later; in another 2 days, it was gone. **C,** In this case, the blood did not resolve and the eye ultimately had to be enucleated.

IV. Hyphema (Fig. 5.9)
  A. Most postoperative hyphemas occur within 24 to 72 hours after surgery.
  B. They tend not to be as serious as nonsurgical traumatic hyphemas, and usually clear with or without specific therapy.
V. Corneal edema
  A. Causes
    1. "Traumatic" extracapsular cataract extraction
      a. Pseudophakic or aphakic bullous keratopathy can develop after traumatic (complicated) extracapsular cataract extraction and anterior-chamber lens implantation, or no lens implantation, respectively.
      b. The bullous keratopathy may be associated with operative rupture of the posterior lens capsule and vitreous loss, followed by significant intraocular inflammation.
    2. Glaucoma, usually pupillary block glaucoma (pseudophakic glaucoma)
    3. Vitreous (Fig. 5.10) or iris adherent to the surgical wound or within it or adherent to the corneal endothelium
    4. Splitting of Descemet's membrane from the posterior cornea (Descemet's membrane detachment) (see Fig. 5.3)
    5. "Aggravation" of Fuchs' corneal dystrophy. The result is a combined endothelial dystrophy and epi-

thelial degeneration accompanied by guttata formation on Descemet's membrane.
    6. The scleral tunnel incision for cataract surgery is associated with less postoperative endothelial damage than clear corneal incisions, probably because of the more posterior location of the clear corneal incision.
    7. Idiopathic causes (i.e., unknown)
  B. Histologically (see Figs 8.45, 8.50, 16.26, and 16.27), the basal layer of epithelium is edematous early.
    1. In time, subepithelial collections of fluid (bullae or vesicles) may occur.
    2. Ultimately, a *degenerative pannus* may result from fibrous tissue growing between epithelium and Bowman's membrane.
VI. "Acute" band keratopathy
  This may develop when materials that contain excess phosphates, especially improperly buffered viscous substances, are placed in the eye during surgery. It has been postulated that the use of phosphate buffered irrigating fluid in the treatment of chemical eye injury may result in acute calcium phosphate deposition in some instances. Similarly, corneal calcification has occurred following intensified treatment with sodium hyaluronate artificial tears, which have a high concentration of phosphate.
VII. Subretinal hemorrhage
  It is usually secondary to extension of a choroidal hemorrhage.

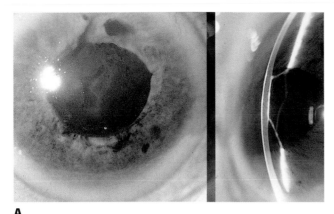

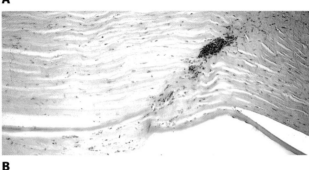

Fig. 5.10 Vitreous. **A,** Vitreous comes through pupil and touches posterior cornea, producing corneal edema (*left*). Slit-lamp view (*right*) shows thickening of cornea in area of vitreous touch. **B,** Histologic section of another case (see also Fig. 5.5B) shows vitreous in posterior aspect of corneal wound. (**A,** Courtesy of Dr. GOH Naumann.)

Hemorrhage is frequently found, however, in the vitreous inferiorly after intraocular surgery. The cause is unknown; however a careful search for retinal holes is mandatory in such cases.

VIII. Viscoelastic materials, and even air introduced into the anterior chamber, can cause a transient elevation of intraocular pressure that rarely lasts more than 24 to 48 hours. Although now only of historical interest, α-chymotrypsin used during intracapsular cataract surgery was associated with glaucoma in the early postoperative period.

IX. Inflammation

A. Endophthalmitis (see Fig. 3.1)

The incidence of postoperative endophthalmitis is about 0.128%.

---

1. In the first day or two after surgery, the disease is usually purulent, fulminating (i.e., rapid), and caused by bacteria frequently from contaminated solutions or intraocular lenses introduced during the surgical procedure (see also section on toxic anterior-segment syndrome (TASS), below, for a simulating condition).

A bacterial infection is also a possible cause in a delayed endophthalmitis, especially with less virulent bacteria such

---

as *Staphylococcus epidermidis* and *Propionibacterium acnes* (see later, p. 121). A delayed endophthalmitis, however, also suggests a fungal infection.

---

2. A form of aseptic endophthalmitis of unknown cause may be seen during the first few weeks after surgery.
3. An increased prevalence of endophthalmitis is seen in diabetic patients.

B. Uveitis

1. This may occur as an aggravation of a previous uveitis, a reaction to a noxious stimulus, or de novo, and may be chronic granulomatous or nongranulomatous.
2. Granulomatous reaction (mainly inflammatory giant cells) on the lens implant often is associated with a nongranulomatous anterior uveitis.

If acute iritis or anterior uveitis occurs in the first 5 days after cataract surgery, it is usually caused by (1) *bacterial endophthalmitis* or (2) *aseptic iritis* (see discussion of TASS later in this chapter). Bacterial endophthalmitis usually results in permanent vision impairment. Other causes of aseptic iritis include inert foreign materials and trauma. A common form of aseptic iritis caused by an inert foreign body was the *UGH* (uveitis, glaucoma, and hyphema) *syndrome*, most often associated with an anterior-chamber lens implant. The incidence of this syndrome has been greatly reduced by modern intraocular lens implant designs. Aseptic iritis may heal completely without any problems, may lead to complete blindness, or anything in between.

---

3. Nodular episcleritis, peripheral corneal ulceration, wound necrosis, and even wound dehiscence may be related to sutures that were used in cataract surgery, especially virgin silk sutures; however, modern synthetic monofilament sutures have made this complication very rare.
4. Uveitis secondary to non-Hodgkin lymphoma has presented after blunt trauma with the trauma possibly leading to the migration of atypical cells into the eye.

C. Toxic anterior segment syndrome (TASS) and toxic endothelial destruction syndrome (TEDS).

1. TASS is an acute, sterile, postoperative inflammation that manifests itself in the first 12 to 48 hours following surgery.
2. Possible causes that have been cited include intraocular solutions with inappropriate chemical composition, concentration, pH, or osmolality; preservatives; denatured ophthalmic viscosurgical devices; enzymatic detergents; bacterial endotoxin; oxidized metal deposits and residues; and factors related to intraocular lenses such as residues from polishing or sterilizing compounds.
3. In some cases of TASS, an oily substance has been noted in the anterior chamber of affected individuals and possessed the same gas chromatograph–

mass spectrometry characteristics as the ointment used postoperatively, thereby strongly suggesting intraocular migration ophthalmic ointment instilled at the end of the surgical procedure as a likely source for the inflammation. Poor wound construction and tight surgical dressings have been postulated to contribute to the entrance of the ointment into the anterior chamber.

4. Impurities in an autoclave steam mixture have also been cited as causing one outbreak of TASS.

5. An iris-supported phakic intraocular lens has been associated with TASS.

6. Some authors differentiate TASS from TEDS based on the less prominent corneal edema in TASS, and its more prominent inflammation in comparison to TEDS. Moreover, corneal edema, timing, impairment of iris sphincter function, and increased intraocular pressure to a level between 40 and 70 mm Hg also are said to help differentiate TASS from endophthalmitis.

X. Intraocular lens implantation

A. Lens implant subluxation and dislocation (Fig. 5.11)

1. The posterior-chamber lens implant may subluxate nasally, temporally, superiorly (sunrise syndrome), or inferiorly (sunset syndrome).

a. Bilateral spontaneous dislocation of intraocular lenses within the capsule bag has been related to the presence of retinitis pigmentosa, gyrate atrophy, and intermediate uveitis.

b. The lens implant may also dislocate into the anterior chamber partially (iris capture) or completely (rare), or into the vitreous compartment. Dislocation into the anterior chamber may be associated with pseudophakic bullous keratopathy.

c. Blunt trauma may result in the expulsion of an intraocular lens through a clear corneal wound.

d. The loops of the implant may prolapse through the corneoscleral wound or into the anterior-chamber angle.

e. Other forms of implantable devices, such as endocapsular tension rings, that are being utilized as adjuncts to cataract surgery, may also become dislocated into the vitreous compartment, or even into the anterior-chamber angle.

2. Anterior-chamber lens implants may dislocate posteriorly into the posterior chamber or vitreous compartment.

3. Dislocation of a posterior-chamber intraocular lens under the conjunctiva secondary to blunt trauma

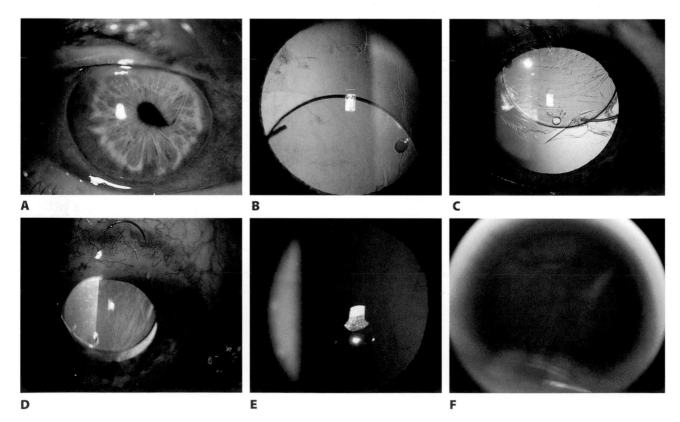

A	B	C
D	E	F

Fig. 5.11 Implant "movement." **A,** The implant's loop may migrate, as here, into the anterior chamber. The implant's optic may also migrate into the anterior chamber, causing iris capture or entrapment (see Fig. 5.19A). The implant may subluxate downward (sunset syndrome, **B**), upward (sunrise syndrome, **C**), out of the eye, as has the superior loop here (**D**), or it may dislocate, as here, into the vitreous (**E,** first postoperative day—no implant visible, **F,** implant is in the inferior anterior vitreous compartment).

and resulting in a pseudophacocele has been reported.

4. Intraocular lenses implanted for refractive correction in phakic individuals may exhibit zonular dehiscence, and even may dislocate into the vitreous cavity.

5. Fragments of a surgically removed intraocular lens may be retained in the anterior chamber and contribute to corneal endothelial decompensation.

6. The proper handling of an intraocular lens dislocated into the vitreous compartment has been a matter for discussion.

B. "Cocoon" formation may envelop an intraocular lens following implantation after a perforating injury.

C. Postcataract surgery intraocular lens opacification has occurred related to several types of intraocular lenses. Late opacification of hydrophilic acrylic intraocular lenses may be associated with calcific deposits on the lens surface, and/or ultrastructural changes within the lens material proper. Such opacification in association with aggravated uveitis in a patient with Behçet's disease has been reported.

XI. Surgical confusion

Misinterpretation of ocular signs by the clinician constitutes surgical confusion—for example, a postoperative choroidal detachment misdiagnosed as a uveal malignant melanoma with subsequent enucleation of the eye.

Delayed

Delayed complications are those that occur after the second or third month after surgery.

I. Corneal edema secondary to:

A. The seven entities listed under *Corneal edema* in the preceding subsection, *Postoperative*.

B. Intraocular lenses, especially iris-clip lenses (almost never used anymore), may cause delayed corneal edema (Fig. 5.12).

C. Peripheral corneal edema (Brown–McLean syndrome)

1. Onset of edema, often delayed 6 years after surgery, is bilateral when the surgery is bilateral, and mainly occurs in women.

2. It usually follows intracapsular cataract extraction and may be associated with peripheral iris atrophy.

3. The edema involves the stroma and epithelium and spares the superior and central cornea.

4. Discrete, orange, punctate pigmentation of unknown origin is frequently seen on the endothelial surface behind the edematous areas of the cornea.

5. Cornea guttata are often present.

6. The cause of the edema is unknown.

II. Cataract

A. Cataracts may be caused or accelerated by glaucoma surgery, even if the lens is in no way damaged physically by the surgery.

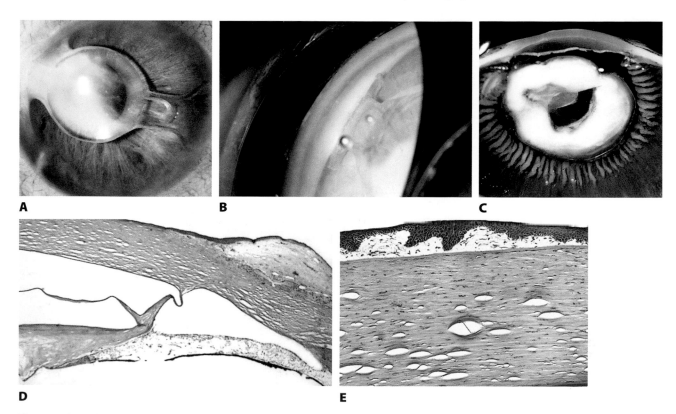

Fig. 5.12 Corneal edema. **A,** Corneal edema developed 30 years after successful anterior-chamber lens implantation of a rigid Schreck total *para-*methoxymethamphetamine (PMMA) lens. **B,** Footplate in anterior-chamber angle. **C,** Enucleated eye shows Soemmerring's ring cataract. **D,** Membrane in anterior chamber marks where footplate had been on opposite side from **B. E,** Cornea shows a degenerative pannus secondary to corneal edema. (Case reported by Rummelt V *et al.: Arch Ophthalmol* 108:401, 1990. © American Medical Association. All rights reserved.)

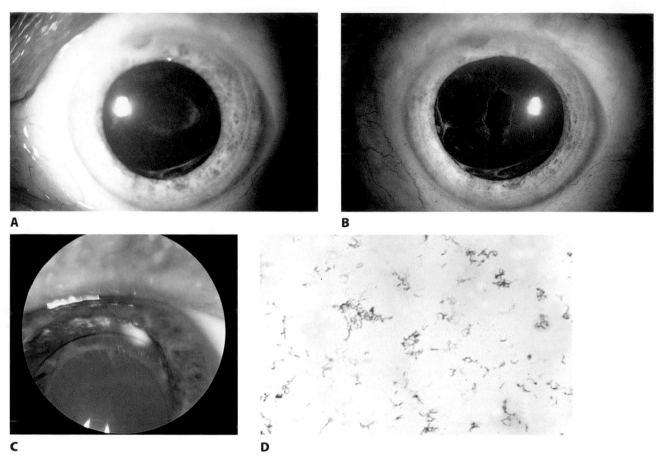

Fig. 5.13 Cicatrization of posterior lens capsule. A thickened, cicatrized posterior lens capsule (**A**) has caused a significant decrease in vision, necessitating a posterior yttrium aluminum garnet (YAG) laser capsulectomy (**B**). In another case, after capsulectomy a thick plaque was noted on the posterior surface of the cornea (**C**). Examination of the surgically removed plaque shows a mass of *Propionibacterium acnes* (**D**). (**C** and **D,** Courtesy of Dr. AH Friedman.)

The cataract may be a result of "shunting" of the aqueous through the iridectomy, so that the anterior and posterior surfaces of the lens are no longer properly nourished.

  B. Lens opacities may be the sequelae of posterior-chamber phakic intraocular lens implantation.

  C. Secondary ("after") cataract

    1. Posterior capsule opacification (Fig. 5.13)

      a. This results from proliferation of anterior lens epithelium on to the posterior capsule, and has been reported in 8% to 50% of cases (probable true prevalence approximately 25%) after extracapsular cataract extraction and lens implantation during the first 5 years after surgery.

The incidence of posterior capsular opacification is increased in patients who have large capsulorhexis (6 to 7 mm) and who have cataracts secondary to uveitis. Intraocular lenses made of polyacrylic seem to be associated with significantly less posterior capsular opacification than polymethylmethacrylate or silicone

---

lenses. Also, diabetic patients develop significantly greater posterior capsular opacifications than nondiabetic patients.

---

      b. In addition to Elschnig's pearl formation, vision is decreased in two ways: (1) multiple layers of proliferated lens epithelium produce a frank opacity; and (2) myofibroblastic and fibroblastic differentiation of the lens epithelium produce contraction, resulting in tiny wrinkles in the posterior capsule and vision distortion. The relationship between intraocular lens design and composition relative to postoperative anterior or posterior capsule opacification is a matter of discussion.

Proliferation of anterior lens epithelium on to the anterior capsule rarely causes problems because of the acapsular zone corresponding to the anterior capsulectomy. Rarely, a "pull-cord" effect pulls the capsulectomy edge centrad, reducing the clear opening, and results in visual symptoms (Fig. 5.14). Anterior capsular

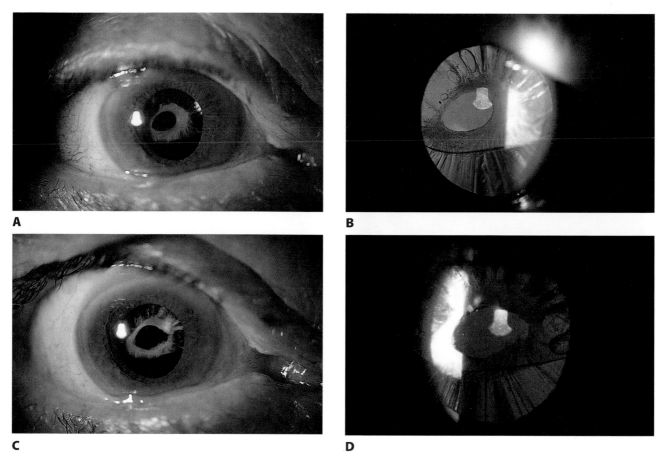

Fig. 5.14 Cicatrization of anterior lens capsule. **A** and **B,** Proliferation of anterior lens epithelium on to the anterior surface of a posterior-chamber lens implant has caused a "pull-cord" effect, resulting in visual symptoms. **C** and **D,** An anterior yttrium aluminum garnet (YAG) laser capsulectomy has alleviated the problem.

opacification appears to be most common with silicone intraocular lens implants.

---

c. Electron and immunoelectron microscopy show that the fibrous opacification consists of lens epithelial cells and extracellular matrix (ECM) composed of collagen types I and III and basement membrane-like material associated with collagen type IV.

2. *Elschnig's pearls* (Fig. 5.15) result from aberrant attempts by remaining lens cells attached to the capsule to form new lens "fibers."
Histologically, large, clear lens cells (bladder cells) are seen behind the iris, in the pupillary space, or in both areas.

3. *Soemmerring's ring* cataract (Detmar Wilhelm Soemmerring, 1793–1871; see Fig. 5.15) results from loss of anterior and posterior cortex, and nucleus but with retention of equatorial cortex.
   a. Apposition of the central portions of the anterior and posterior lens capsule causes a doughnut configuration.
   b. Frequently, the doughnut or ring is not complete, so that C- or J-shaped configurations

result. Previously, the most common cause was extracapsular cataract surgery; but is very uncommon following uncomplicated phacoemulsification procedures.

   c. Histologically, when the eye is sectioned vertical to the plane of the posterior lens capsule, two balls of degenerated and proliferated lens cells are seen encapsulated behind the peripheral iris leaf and connected by adherent anterior and posterior lens capsule in the form of a dumbbell.

4. Anterior-capsule contraction (phimosis syndrome) may lead to intraocular lens displacement and visual degradation following cataract surgery. Neodymium:yttrium aluminum garnet (YAG) laser anterior capsulotomy may be helpful in correcting this syndrome. Choroidal effusion and hypotony are reported complications of ciliary body traction from severe anterior-capsule contraction.

III. Neural retinal detachment (Fig. 5.16)
   A. The prevalence of retinal detachment in the general population is between 0.005% and 0.01%.
   B. Retinal detachment occurs in approximately 1.7% to 3% of aphakic patients (50% of these within 1 year after

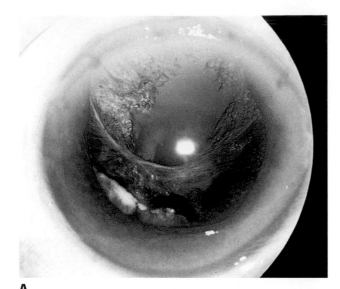

A

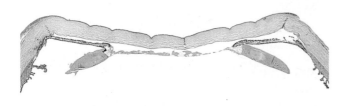

B

Fig. 5.15 Elschnig's pearls and Soemmerring's ring cataract.
A, Elschnig's pearls, noted as tiny, translucent spheres in superior pupillary space. Cortical remnants in the form of a Soemmerring's ring cataract are noted from 6 to 8 o'clock. **B,** Soemmerring's ring cataract is seen as cortical material trapped in equatorial portion of lens, giving a doughnut configuration (see Fig. 5.12C).

cataract surgery) or in as much as 25% of aphakic patients if a neural retinal detachment has previously occurred in either eye.

Retinal detachment can occur in up to 8% of very highly myopic eyes (~15 to −30 diopters).

C. The incidence of retinal detachment is decreased to 0.4% to 1.4% after nuclear expression extracapsular cataract surgery, to about .41% after phacoemulsification cataract extraction, and is lowest when the posterior capsule is intact.

1. If axial myopia (25.5 mm) exists, retinal detachment develops in approximately 1.3% of patients after extracapsular cataract extraction and posterior-chamber implant. Vitreous loss increases the incidence of postoperative detachments.

Anterior vitrectomy at the time of vitreous loss seems to have little or no effect on any of the expected complications that follow vitreous loss. The damage is probably done at the moment of loss (i.e., the vitreous pulls on the neural retina at the vitreous base or ora serrata). Subsequent vitrectomy, repair, and so forth cannot undo the initial trauma.

---

2. Following vitreous loss during cataract surgery, about 3% of eyes that receive posterior-chamber lenses and 2.4% of eyes that receive anterior-chamber lenses develop retinal detachment.

IV. Pseudophakic or aphakic glaucoma

A. In the delayed phase, this glaucoma is mainly caused by secondary chronic closed-angle glaucoma; a preexisting simple open-angle glaucoma, however, may be the cause.

B. *Peripheral anterior synechiae*, leading to secondary chronic closed-angle glaucoma, are usually secondary to persistent postoperative flat chamber (a rare event with modern phacoemulsification cataract surgery).

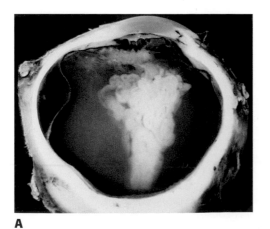

A

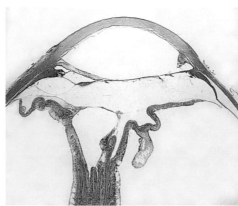

B

Fig. 5.16 Neural retinal detachment (RD). **A,** RD noted some time after cataract surgery. Total RD seen with a gelatinous material present in the subneural retinal space. **B,** Histologic section shows a total RD. Note that no lens is present (surgical aphakia). (**B,** Courtesy of Armed Forces Institute of Pathology acc. no. 1145406.)

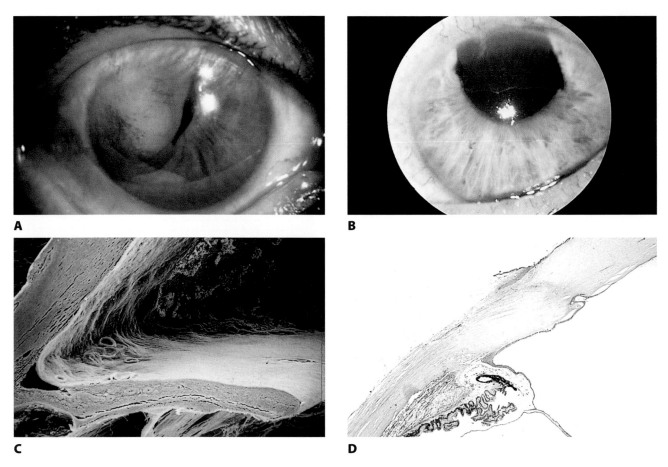

Fig. 5.17 Epithelial iris cyst and downgrowth. **A,** Implantation of epithelium on the iris at the time of surgery has resulted in the formation of a large epithelial cyst that obstructs most of the pupil. The milky material in the cyst consists of desquamated epithelial cells. **B,** In another case, the epithelium has grown into the eye through the cataract incision and is developing as a downgrowth on the back of the superior one-third of the cornea and on to the superior iris. The line of transition between epithelium and endothelium is clearly seen on the posterior cornea as a horizontal line. **C,** Scanning electron microscopy shows a sheet of epithelium covering trabecular meshwork, anterior face of ciliary body, anterior iris, and pupillary margin. **D,** Epithelium lines posterior cornea, anterior-chamber angle, and peripheral iris and extends on to vitreous posteriorly in surgically aphakic eye. (**B,** Case reported by Yanoff M: *Trans Am Ophthalmol Soc* 73:571, 1975.)

This type of secondary glaucoma seems to be easier to control medically than other types of secondary closed-angle glaucoma.

Histologically, the iris is adherent to posterior cornea, frequently central to Schwalbe's ring.

C. Posterior synechiae, usually the result of posterior-chamber inflammation (caused by iridocyclitis, endophthalmitis, hyphema, and so forth), result in iris bombé (see Figs 3.12 and 3.13) and secondary peripheral anterior synechiae.

Histologically, the posterior pupillary portion of the iris is adherent to the anterior face of the vitreous, to lens remnants, or to both. The anterior peripheral iris is adherent to the posterior cornea, frequently central to Schwalbe's ring.

D. *Epithelial downgrowth* (ingrowth; Fig. 5.17) is most likely to occur in eyes with problems in wound closure such as vitreous loss, wound incarceration of tissue,

delayed reformation of the anterior chamber, or frank rupture of the limbal incision; and when instruments are contaminated with surface epithelium before they are introduced into the eye.*

The clinical prevalence of epithelial downgrowth has been reported at 0.09% to 0.12%. In eyes enucleated after cataract extraction and examined histologically, the prevalence is as great as 16%. The prevalence is much lower with small-incision, sutureless cataract surgery. However, although extremely rare, epithelial downgrowth can occur after phacoemulsification through a clear corneal incision.

---

1. Epithelial downgrowth either causes secondary closed-angle glaucoma through peripheral anterior

Experimental evidence shows that healthy endothelium inhibits the growth of epithelium (i.e., contact inhibition). Epithelium, therefore, probably only grows into the eye if the endothelium is unhealthy, removed by trauma, or covered (e.g., by iris incarceration, vitreous, or lens remnants).

synechia formation or lines an open anterior-chamber angle, resulting in secondary open-angle glaucoma.

2. Histologically, the epithelium is seen to grow most luxuriously and in multiple layers on the iris, where a good blood supply exists, whereas it tends to grow sparsely and in a single layer on the posterior surface of the avascular cornea. The epithelium may extend behind the iris, over the ciliary body, and far into the interior of the eye through the pupil.

E. *Iris cyst* formation (see Fig. 5.17) is caused by implantation of surface epithelium on to the iris at the time of surgery.

1. The cyst usually grows slowly and is accompanied by peripheral anterior synechiae. If extensive, it may cause secondary chronic closed-angle glaucoma.

The cysts may be sonolucent or show variable internal reflectivity by ultrasound biomicroscopy.

---

2. Histologically, the cyst is lined by stratified squamous or columnar epithelium, sometimes containing mucous cells, and is filled with either keratin debris (white or pearl cysts) or mucous fluid (clear cysts).

Some pearl implantation cysts are thought to be derived from the epidermal layers at the root of an implanted cilium.

F. Endothelialization of anterior-chamber angle (see p. 642 in Chapter 16).

G. *Stromal ingrowth* is most apt to occur after vitreous loss or tissue incarceration into the surgical wound.

1. The stromal ingrowth (Fig. 5.18) may be localized, limited to the area of surgical perforation of Descemet's membrane, or may be quite extensive. It is frequently found on histopathologic examination of failed corneal transplants.

2. When the ingrowth is extensive, peripheral anterior synechiae and secondary closed-angle glaucoma result.

3. Histologically, fibrous tissue extends from corneal stroma through a large gap in Descemet's membrane.

After extracapsular surgery and penetrating keratoplasty, lens epithelium can rarely cover the posterior surface of the cornea along the surface of a retrocorneal fibrous membrane, a condition called *lensification* of the posterior corneal surface.

The fibrous tissue frequently covers the posterior cornea, fills part of the anterior chamber, and occludes the anterior-chamber angle.

V. Inflammation

A. Precipitates on implant

1. Both nonpigmented and pigmented precipitates (sometimes quite large) can appear on the anterior (most common) or posterior surfaces of the lens implant.

2. Histologically, the precipitates consist of histiocytes and multinucleated inflammatory giant cells (Fig. 5.19).

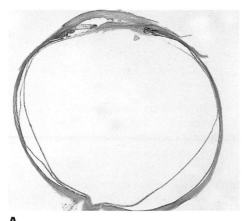

A

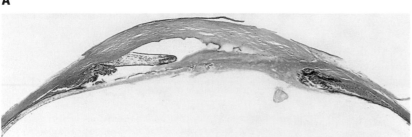

B

Fig. 5.18 Stromal overgrowth. **A,** Massive stromal overgrowth has occurred in region of cataract incision in surgically aphakic eye. **B,** Increased magnification shows fibrous tissue (stromal overgrowth) filling the anterior chamber in the area of the surgical iridectomy and extending behind the intact iris leaf into the posterior chamber.

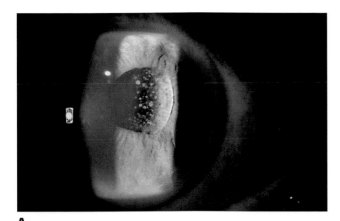

A

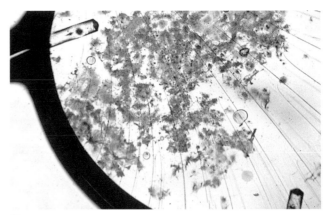

B

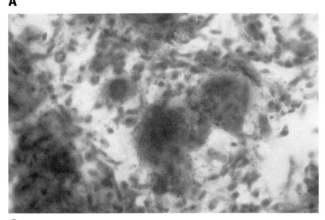

C

Fig. 5.19 Precipitates on implant. **A,** Large pigmented precipitates are present on the anterior and posterior surface of the lens implant. Entrapment of the posterior-chamber lens implant has taken place on the right-hand side of the pupil. **B,** This anterior-chamber lens was removed because of the uveitis, glaucoma, hyphema (UGH) syndrome. The lens is covered with precipitates. **C,** Increased magnification shows many histiocytes and multinucleated giant cells on the lens surface. (**B** and **C,** Courtesy of Dr. RC Eagle, Jr.)

B. Fungal infection (see p. 85 in Chapter 4) may take the form of a keratitis or an endophthalmitis (Fig. 5.20).
   1. Fungal endophthalmitis should be suspected when an endophthalmitis is seen in the delayed period.
   2. Clinically, the signs and symptoms are quite similar to the low-virulence, bacterial endophthalmitis seen in the delayed period (see later).
      Many saprophytic fungi can cause the infection, including *Aspergillus fumigatus,* *Candida albicans,* *Torulopsis candida* (*C. famata*), *Cephalosporium* species, *Sporotrichum schenckii,* *Histoplasma capsulatum,* and *Alternaria alternata.*
C. Bacterial endophthalmitis is unusual in the delayed period except when caused by bacteria of low virulence, such as *Staphylococcus epidermidis* and *P. acnes* (other causes include group G *Streptococcus,* *Nocardia asteroides,* and *Corynebacterium* species); filtering procedures can also provide bacteria access to the inside of the eye through the bleb.

Bacterial conjunctivitis in a patient with a filtering bleb must be considered a medical emergency. The earliest sign of an incipient endophthalmitis in a patient with a filtering bleb is opacification of the bleb. The thin blebs resulting from intra-operative or postoperative use of drugs such as 5-fluorouracil or mitomycin-C are much more susceptible to chronic bleb leaks and subsequent endophthalmitis, particularly if the bleb is placed inferiorly.

---

   1. Delayed bacterial endophthalmitis may present as a white intracapsular plaque, beaded fibrin strands in the anterior chamber, hypopyon, nongranulomatous or granulomatous uveitis, vitritis, and diffuse intraretinal hemorrhages.
   2. An unusual form of bacterial endophthalmitis results when *P. acnes,* trapped in the equatorial cortex after extracapsular cataract extraction, is liberated into the vitreous compartment at the time of a YAG laser capsulectomy (see Fig. 5.13).
D. Rubella endophthalmitis usually occurred after a two-stage needling and aspiration procedure of a congenital rubella cataract.
   1. When a "ripening" procedure performed by needling of a rubella cataract was followed after a delay of days to weeks by an aspiration procedure, an intractable endophthalmitis developed in a high percentage of patients. The advent of modern lensectomy procedures for these cases has eliminated the need for a two-stage procedure, and has greatly reduced the risk of such inflammatory events.

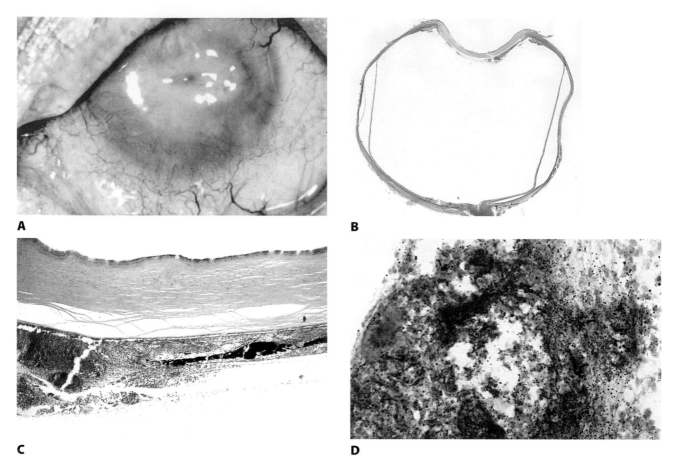

Fig. 5.20 Fungal endophthalmitis. **A,** Approximately 6 weeks after cataract extraction, the patient developed an intractable endophthalmitis. **B,** A number of microabscesses are present in the anterior and posterior chambers, shown with increased magnification in **C.** The anterior vitreous face and anterior vitreous are involved in the inflammatory process. **D,** Periodic acid–Schiff (PAS) stain shows PAS-positive fungi in the upper central field. (**A,** Courtesy of Dr. HG Scheie.)

Presumably, the virus is liberated into the eye and sets up a secondary viral endophthalmitis.

2. Histologically, fibrovascular organization centered about a chronic nongranulomatous inflammatory reaction contiguous with lens remnants results in cyclitic membrane formation and neural retinal detachment.

E. Multiple types of small foreign bodies, which may be inadvertently introduced at the time of surgery, can cause a delayed chronic nongranulomatous or granulomatous inflammatory reaction. For example, retained anterior-chamber cilia introduced into the anterior chamber at the time of phacoemulsification can result in endophthalmitis. Nevertheless, such cilia may be well tolerated so that the decision to remove one must be based on individual clinical examination.

F. Phacoanaphylactic endophthalmitis (see Fig. 4.3) rarely occurs with extracapsular cataract extraction.

G. Sympathetic uveitis (see Figs 4.1 and 4.2, and p. 73 in Chapter 4).

VI. Traumatic rupture of surgical wounds: blunt trauma to the eye may cause ocular rupture, often at the site of cataract or filtering surgery scars, or radial keratotomy incisions (see Fig. 5.29), which remain "weaker" than surrounding tissue.

A. A penetrating eye injury received in Iraq was the first such war-related injury resulting in sympathetic ophthalmia since World War II.

VII. Cystoid macular edema (CME) and optic disc edema (Irvine–Gass syndrome; Fig. 5.21)

A. CME can occur any time after cataract surgery (even up to 5 years after), but most cases occur within 2 months after surgery and are heralded by a sudden decrease in vision.

B. Most cases are self-limited, and the macular edema resolves completely with or without therapy within 6 months to a year.

Fluorescein angiography demonstrates CME in over 50% of eyes after cataract surgery, with or without lens implantation. Fortunately, only a small percentage of these patients will have clinical CME, approximately 75% of whom will obtain 20/30

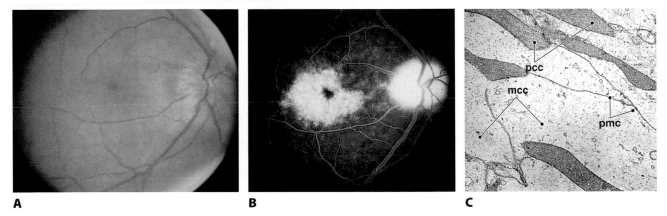

A **B** **C**

Fig. 5.21 Cystoid macular edema. After extracapsular cataract extraction and posterior-chamber lens implantation, the patient initially did well. Then, however, vision decreased. **A,** Examination of the fundus showed cystoid macular edema. **B,** The characteristic fluorescein appearance is present. The patient's vision decreased to 20/300. No treatment was given. Nine months later, the vision spontaneously returned to 20/20. **C,** Electron microscopy of another case shows accumulation of fluid in Müller cells. Initially, the fluid in cystoid macular edema appears to be intracellular and the condition is reversible. Further accumulation of fluid causes the cell membranes to break and fluid collects extracellularly; presumably, the condition is then irreversible (pmc, plasmalemma Müller cell; pcc, dense photoreceptor cell cytoplasm; mcc, lucent Müller cell cytoplasm). (**C,** Adapted from Yanoff M. Fine BS, Brucker AJ *et al., Pathology of human cystoid macular edema. Surv Ophthalmol* 28(suppl):505, 1984, with permission from Elsevier.)

vision or better after 6 months, leaving a prevalence of approximately 2% with clinical CME. The prevalence of clinical CME after extracapsular cataract surgery, when the posterior capsule is left intact, is much less, approximately 0.5% to 1%. In cases of persistent clinical CME, secondary permanent complications, such as lamellar macular hole formation, may occur. If clinically significant macular edema is present in diabetic eyes at the time of cataract surgery, it is unlikely to resolve spontaneously within a year; however, if it arises after surgery in diabetic eyes, especially if it is mild, it commonly resolves within a year. Optical coherence tomography (OCT) has greatly simplified the diagnosis and treatment of this disorder.

C. The condition can be precipitated or aggravated by topical prostaglandin analogue therapy for glaucoma.
D. The cause of the CME and optic disc edema is unknown, but may be related to prostaglandin secretion, vitreous traction (probably the minority), or a posterior vitritis.

Histologically, iritis, cyclitis, retinal phlebitis, and retinal periphlebitis have been noted. Whether these conditions cause the cystoid macular changes or whether they are simply incidental findings in enucleated eyes is not clear.

E. CME and degeneration have many causes (Table 5.1).
F. The macula shows multiple (usually four or five) intraretinal microcysts (clear bubbles) obscuring the normal foveal reflex. The cysts fill early during fluorescein angiography, and pooling causes a stellate geometric pattern that persists for 30 minutes or longer.
G. Sterile endophthalmitis may follow intravitreal injection of triamcinolone acetonide in the treatment of macular edema.
H. Histologically, an intracellular accumulation of fluid (water) produces cystoid areas and clouding of the neural retinal cells, probably Müller cells.

1. Intraretinal microvascular abnormalities resembling endothelial proliferation are seen with trypsin-digest preparations.
2. Whether the Müller-cell intracytoplasmic accumulation of fluid, as seen with electron microscopy, is a primary or secondary effect is not clear.
3. If excess fluid is present, it may break through cell membranes and accumulate intercellularly.

VIII. Failure of filtration following glaucoma surgery
A. Procedures to lower intraocular pressure function by transconjunctival filtration, absorption of aqueous into subconjunctival vessels, recanalization, reopening of drainage channels, passage through areas of perivascular degeneration, or any combination.
B. Filtration failure may be caused by incorrect placement of incision, hemorrhage, inflammation, prolapse of intraocular tissue into the filtration site, dense fibrosis, peripheral anterior synechiae and secondary chronic closed-angle glaucoma, endothelialization of the bleb, and unknown causes.
C. The histologic picture differs according to the cause.
IX. After surgery, atrophia bulbi (see Fig. 3.14) with or without disorganization may occur for no apparent clinical or histopathologic reason.

COMPLICATIONS OF NEURAL RETINAL DETACHMENT AND VITREOUS SURGERY

Immediate

I. Surgical confusion
A. Misdiagnosis

TABLE 5.1 Conditions that May Cause Cystoid Macular Edema (CME) or Pseudo-CME*

I. LEAKAGE OF PERIFOVEAL RETINAL CAPILLARIES
A. Postocular Surgery
1. Cataract extraction (Irvine–Gass syndrome)‡
2. Neural retinal reattachment†
3. Penetrating keratoplasty†
4. Filtering procedures†
5. Pars plana vitrectomy†
6. Cryotherapy, photocoagulation, or diathermy of neural retinal holes†

B. Retinal Vascular Disorders
1. Diabetic retinopathy†
2. Hypertensive retinopathy†
3. Branch retinal vein occlusion†
4. Central retinal vein occlusion†
5. Venous stasis retinopathy†
6. Retinal telangiectasia—Coats', macular, segmental†
7. Macroaneurysm†
8. Capillary hemangioma (von Hippel's disease)†
9. Retinal hamartoma†
10. Purtscher's retinopathy†
11. Systemic lupus erythematosus†
12. Hunter's syndrome‡
13. Internal limiting membrane contraction†

C. Intraocular Inflammation
1. Pars planitis, iridocyclitis, choroiditis†
2. Bird shot choroidopathy†
3. Vitritis†
4. Behçet's syndrome†
5. Sarcoidosis†
6. *Toxocara* endophthalmitis†
7. Peripheral (or posterior) retinitis (e.g., toxoplasmosis)†
8. Neurosyphilis†

D. Degeneration
1. Retinitis pigmentosa†
2. Surface wrinkling retinopathy†

E. Hypotony Following Surgery

F. Drugs
1. Hydrochlorothiazide†
2. Epinephrine†
3. Oral contraceptives†

G. Chronic Optic Disc Edema†

H. Electrical Injuries*

II. NO RETINAL VASCULAR LEAKAGE
A. Hereditary
1. Juvenile retinoschisis‡
2. Retinitis pigmentosa‡
3. Pit of the optic disc‡
4. Goldmann–Favre disease‡

B. Nicotinic Acid‡

C. Resolved (Leaking Neural Retinal or Subneural Retinal Cause with Permanent Structural Change)‡

D. Macular Hole Formation
1. Degenerative†
2. Traumatic‡
3. Myopic†

III. SUBNEURAL RETINAL LEAKAGE WITH CHRONIC SEROUS OR EXUDATIVE DETACHMENT OF NEURAL RETINA

A. Chronic Idiopathic Central Serous Choroidopathy†

B. Subneural Retinal (Choroidal) Neovascular Membrane (SRN)
1. Age-related macular degeneration (exudative, "wet" or involutional)†
2. Idiopathic, juvenile†
3. Angioid streaks†
4. Choroidal rupture†
5. Drusen of optic disc†
6. Ocular inflammation (e.g., histoplasmosis)†
7. Best's disease (vitelliform macular heredogeneration)†
8. Myopia†

C. After Severe Blunt Injury‡

D. Uveal Tumors
1. Nevi†
2. Malignant melanoma†
3. Hemangioma†
4. Metastasis†
5. Ciliary body cyst†

E. Serpiginous Choroiditis (When Causes SRN)†

CME has characteristic clinical and fluorescein appearance, whereas pseudo-CME has characteristic clinical appearance only.
†CME
‡Pseudo-CME.

Not all neural retinal detachments are rhegmatogenous (i.e., caused by a retinal hole). They may be secondary to intraocular inflammation (e.g., Harada's disease), neoplasm, or traction from membranes.
  B. Faulty technique
    1. Inadequate general anesthesia, a poor retrobulbar or facial block, or a retrobulbar hemorrhage may make the surgical procedure more difficult.

  2. Misplaced implant, explant, or scleral sutures can lead to an improper scleral buckle or to premature drainage of subneural retinal fluid.
  3. Diathermy, cryotherapy, or laser treatment that is misplaced, insufficient, or excessive can cause unsatisfactory results.
  4. Cut or obstructed vortex veins can cause choroidal detachment or hemorrhage.

5. The neural retina can be incarcerated.
II. Choroidal detachment or hemorrhage
    A. The most frequent cause of choroidal detachment is hypotony induced by surgical drainage of subneural retinal fluid.
    B. Choroidal hemorrhage may also result from hypotony induced by surgical drainage of subneural retinal fluid. Other causes may be cutting or obstructing vortex veins or incision of choroidal vessels at the time of surgical drainage of subneural retinal fluid.
    C. Histology [see p. 106 (subsection *Expulsive Choroidal Hemorrhage*) and p. 109 (subsection *Choroidal Detachment*) in this chapter].
III. Acute glaucoma
    A. The buckling procedure, especially if unaccompanied by drainage of subneural retinal fluid or by anterior-chamber paracentesis, may result in acute closed-angle glaucoma.

> The glaucoma should be recognized immediately during the surgical procedure and promptly treated. If unrecognized, it can cause central retinal artery occlusion, followed by subsequent blindness and optic atrophy.

    B. Depending on the characteristics of the gas utilized for intraocular gas tamponade during retinal reattachment surgery and the postoperative position of the patient's head, acute closed-angle glaucoma may result from the gas bubble floating against the iris lens diaphragm, and displacing it forward to close the angle. Similarly, expansion of the gas, particularly in a low ambient air pressure environment (airplane flight) may shift the iris lens diaphragm anteriorly to close the angle. Finally, overfill with gas at the time of surgery may also displace the iris lens diaphragm anteriorly to close the angle.
      1. The use of nitrous oxide during general anesthesia for retinal reattachment surgery in the presence of an existing intraocular gas bubble can result in a disastrous rise in intraocular pressure secondary to gas expansion.
    C. In phakic and even pseudophakic patients, silicone oil may cause pupillary block and secondary angle closure glaucoma, particularly in the presence of weak zonules, if an inferiorly placed iridotomy is not created at the time of retinal reattachment surgery.
    D. Histologically, the anterior-chamber angle is occluded by the peripheral iris.
IV. Toxic effects
    A. It has been suggested that some intraocular materials used during retinal reattachment surgery, such as perfluorohexyloctane (F_6H_8), may have a toxic effect on ocular tissues, leading to severe inflammatory-like reactions.

Postoperative

I. The original hole may still be open or a new one may develop.
II. Choroidal detachment or hemorrhage [see p. 106 (subsection *Expulsive Choroidal Hemorrhage*) and p. 109 (subsection *Choroidal Detachment*) in this chapter].

III. Inflammation
    A. Acute or subacute scleral necrosis may follow neural retinal detachment surgery in days or weeks, and is probably caused by ischemia rather than infection.
      1. In the acute form, the clinical picture starts a few days after surgery, and may resemble a true infectious scleritis, but without pain.
        a. There is a sudden onset of congestion, edema, and a dark red or purple appearance of the tissues over the implant (or explant). Discharge is not marked or is absent.
        b. The vitreous over the buckle usually becomes hazy.
        c. The cornea remains clear, but the involved area of sclera becomes completely necrotic.
      2. In the subacute form, pain starts after approximately 2 to 3 weeks.
        a. The globe may be congested, but no discharge occurs.
        b. The vitreous over the buckle may be hazy or clear.
        c. The sclera in the region of the buckle is necrotic.
    B. Infection in the form of scleral abscess, endophthalmitis, or keratitis may be secondary to bacteria (Fig. 5.22) or fungi (Fig. 5.23), and is characterized by redness of the globe, discharge, and pain.
    Histology (see section *Nontraumatic Infectious* in Chapter 4 and section *Suppurative Endophthalmitis and Panophthalmitis* in Chapter 3)
    C. Anterior-segment necrosis (ASN: anterior-segment ischemic syndrome; Fig. 5.24)
      1. ASN is thought to be secondary to interruption of the blood supply to the iris and ciliary body by temporary removal of one or more rectus muscles during surgery. The blood supply may also be compromised by encircling elements, lamellar dissection, implants, explants, cryotherapy, or diathermy.
      2. Clinically, keratopathy and intraocular inflammation develop, usually in the first postoperative week.
        a. Corneal changes consist of striate keratopathy and corneal edema.
        b. Intraocular inflammation is marked by chemosis, anterior-chamber flare and cells, large keratic precipitates, and white deposits on the lens capsule, findings often mistaken for infectious endophthalmitis.
        c. Later the pupil becomes dilated. Shrinkage of the iris toward the side of the greatest necrosis and hypoxia results in an irregular pupil.
        d. Cataract, hypotony, ectropion uveae, and, finally, phthisis bulbi develop.
      3. A high prevalence of the ASN syndrome is seen after scleral buckling procedures in patients who have hemoglobin sickle-cell (SC) disease.

> In hemoglobin SC disease, the increased frequency of ASN is most likely related to the increased blood viscosity and to the tendency toward erythrocyte packing that occurs

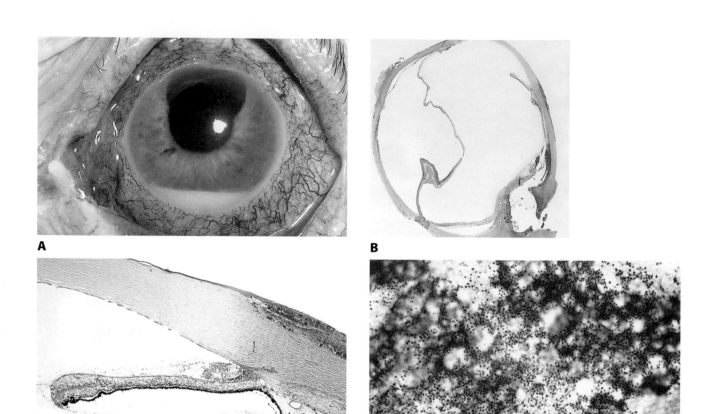

Fig. 5.22 Bacterial endophthalmitis. **A,** Patient had hypopyon and vitreous cells after neural retinal detachment repair; the eye was enucleated. **B,** Hypopyon present in anterior chamber (upper right of field—shown with increased magnification in **C**). Lower right field shows large intrascleral "empty space" where buckle had been. **D,** Special stain positive for Gram-positive cocci.

in these patients, especially with decreased oxygen tension.

4. Histologically, ischemic necrosis of the iris, ciliary body, and lens epithelial cells is present, often only on the side of the surgical procedure.

IV. Intraocular hemorrhage
   A. Choroidal hemorrhage may occur for the same reasons as described previously (see subsection *Immediate*, this chapter).
   B. Hemorrhage in the postoperative period may be caused by a delayed expulsive choroidal hemorrhage, most probably resulting from necrosis of a blood vessel induced by the original cryotherapy or from erosion of an implant or explant.

V. Glaucoma
   A. Acute secondary closed-angle glaucoma is usually seen after a neural retinal detachment procedure in which an encircling element or a very high buckle is created.

Acute secondary closed-angle glaucoma occurs in approximately 4% of scleral buckling procedures. Most commonly, the pathogenesis of the closed angle is pupillary block, and swelling of the ciliary body are among the mechanisms for this.

1. The buckle decreases the volume of the vitreous compartment, displacing vitreous and the lens iris diaphragm anteriorly.

Corneal edema on the first postoperative day, especially if accompanied by ocular pain, should be considered glaucomatous in origin until proved otherwise.

2. Histologically, anterior displacement of intraocular structures causes the iris to encroach on the anterior-chamber angle with resultant closed-angle glaucoma.
3. Chronic elevated intraocular pressure is associated with 11% of procedures in which pars plana vitrectomy with silicone oil injection is performed.
   a. The amount of emulsified silicone oil in the anterior chamber correlates with the incidence of a significant rise in intraocular pressure associated with retinal reattachment surgery.
   B. Primary open-angle glaucoma may become apparent when hypotony of a neural retinal detachment is alleviated by surgery.

VI. Miscellaneous
   A. Silicone oil (see also discussion relative to glaucoma).
      1. May be utilized as an adjunct to retinal reattachment surgery, and can form fixed preretinal oil

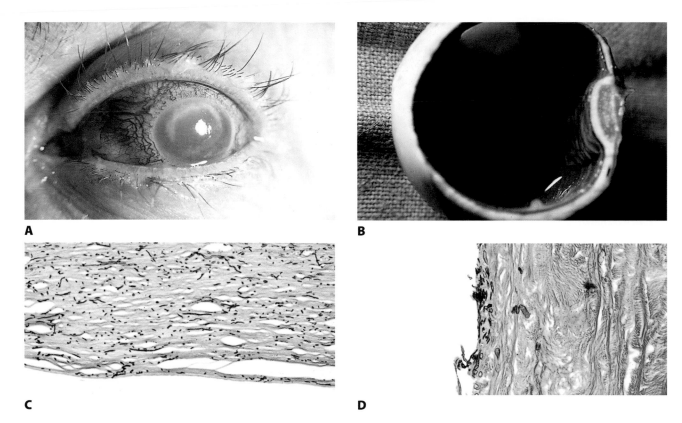

Fig. 5.23 Fungal endophthalmitis. **A,** Approximately 3 weeks after neural retinal detachment repair, a corneal ring abscess developed and extended into a central corneal ulcer; the eye was enucleated. **B,** The gross specimen shows the scleral buckle. Gomori's methenamine silver stain is positive for fungi throughout the cornea (**C**) and in the scleral wall of the buckle (**D**).

bubbles. The bubbles appear not to cause retinal damage.

2. Extrusion of silicone oil into periocular tissue can result in lipogranuloma formation and, even, blepharoptosis.

3. Silicone oil migration into the cerebral ventricles may be associated with poorly controlled high intraocular pressure and optic disc atrophy. It has also been postulated that infiltration of the subarachnoid space by silicone oil may contribute to its entry into the brain.

4. Intraocular silicone oil can lead to periretinal foreign-body granulomas, which may be associated with progressive proliferative vitreoretinopathy (PVR).

B. Myopia may be induced by elongation of the eye secondary to encircling element placement during retinal reattachment surgery.

C. Macular displacement secondary to retinal reattachment surgery can result in "retinal diplopia."

Delayed

I. Vitreous retraction
   A. This condition by itself is of little importance; however, when vitreous retraction is associated with fibrous, retinal pigment epithelium (RPE), or glial membranous proliferations on the internal or external surface of the neural retina, it can result in neural retinal detachment and new neural retinal holes.

   B. When the process is extensive and associated with a total neural retinal detachment, it is called *proliferative vitreoretinopathy* (see p. 494 in Chapter 12); the older terminology was *massive vitreous retraction* or *massive periretinal* proliferation.

   PVR may occur at any postoperative stage of neural retinal detachment surgery. Ominous preoperative signs of incipient PVR are star-shaped neural retinal folds; incarceration of neural retina into a drainage site from previous neural retinal surgery; fixed folds; fibrous, RPE, or glial vitreoretinal membranes; and "cellophane" neural retina.

   C. Histologically, glial, fibrous, or RPE membranes, or any combination, are seen on the internal, or external, or both surfaces of the neural retina. As the membranes shrink or contract, fixed folds of the neural retina develop.

   D. Interleukin-6 and interleukin-8 may be involved in the pathogenesis of PVR.

II. Migration of implant or explant (Fig. 5.25, p. 129)
   A. The explant or implant may migrate in its own plane from loosening of sutures. A misplaced buckle results.

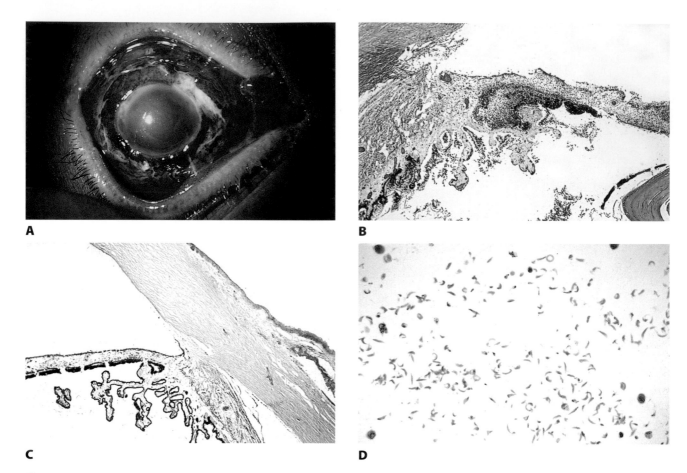

Fig. 5.24 Anterior-segment necrosis (ASN). **A,** ASN followed retinal detachment repair. **B,** Another case of ASN after retinal detachment repair in patient with hemoglobin sickle-cell disease. The ciliary body and iris show marked necrosis on side of scleral buckle. **C,** The side opposite the buckle is not involved in ASN. **D,** Sickled erythrocytes present in vitreous. (**B–D,** From Eagle RC *et al.: Am J Ophthalmol* 75:426. Copyright Elsevier 1973.)

B. Internal migration may result in intraocular penetration and hemorrhage, neural retinal detachment, or infection.

With internal migration of the scleral explant (or implant), conjunctival epithelium may gain access to the interior of the eye, complicating an already compromised eye.

C. External migration results in extrusion.
III. Heterophoria or heterotropia—these conditions may result when muscles have been removed during surgery.
Exotropia commonly occurs in adults when good visual acuity does not return after surgery.
IV. A new hole—a hole may develop de novo or secondary to an obvious vitreous pathologic process, to internal migration of implant or explant, or to improper use of cryotherapy or diathermy.
V. Disturbances of lid position and motility
VI. Secondary glaucoma
Glaucoma may be secondary to many causes [e.g., secondary closed-angle glaucoma, hemorrhage associated with

hemolytic (ghost cell) glaucoma, or inflammation with peripheral anterior or posterior synechiae].

Secondary chronic closed-angle glaucoma may result from iris neovascularization (neovascular glaucoma), which often occurs in diabetic patients after vitrectomy.

VII. Macular degeneration and puckering can occur after scleral buckling procedures or if cryotherapy or diathermy is used alone (see Irvine–Gass syndrome, p. 122 in this chapter).
VIII. Catgut granulomas result when catgut sutures, which were often used in removal and reattachment of rectus muscles, were retained instead of being reabsorbed. Such complications have been greatly reduced through the use of modern synthetic absorbable sutures.
A. Sequestered catgut acts as a foreign body.
B. Histologically, amorphous, eosinophilic, weakly birefringent material (catgut) is surrounded by a foreign-body giant cell granulomatous inflammatory reaction.

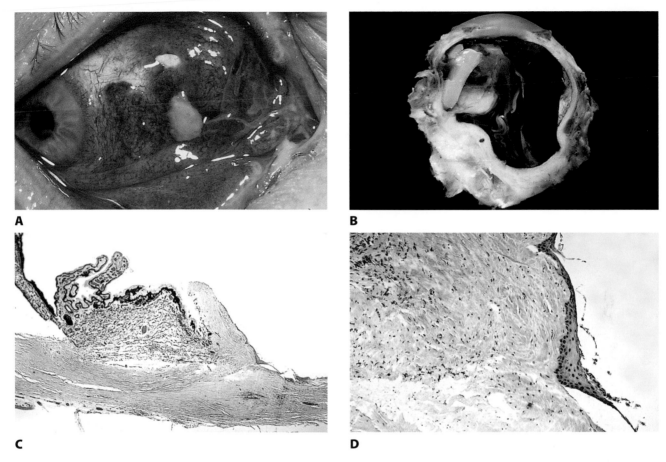

Fig. 5.25 Migration of explant. **A,** Explant has migrated externally so that a white-gray silicon explant is seen nasally. **B,** A gross specimen of another case shows internal migration of a silicon explant. **C,** Histologic section demonstrates an internal scleral flap lined by epithelium (epithelial ingrowth)—shown with increased magnification in **D.**

IX. Vitrectomy is a risk factor for progression of nuclear sclerosis; however, the risk is not related to the duration of the procedure.

X. Epithelial cysts
   A. Epithelial cysts may occur subconjunctivally, in the orbit, or, rarely, in the eye in association with an internally migrating implant (see Fig. 5.25).
   B. Histologically, epithelial-lined inclusion cysts are found.

XI. Phacoanaphylactic endophthalmitis (phacoantigenic uveitis) (Fig. 5.26 and p. 75 in Chapter 4) may occur if the lens is ruptured during surgery (e.g., during a vitrectomy).

XII. Sympathetic uveitis (see p. 73 in Chapter 4) may occur if uveal tissue becomes incarcerated or prolapsed during surgery.

XIII. MIRAgel scleral buckle material has been reported to enlarge greatly over a period of years, and may simulate an orbital tumor. Moreover, the material is said to be friable, and may lead to extensive postoperative inflammation following attempted removal.

COMPLICATIONS OF CORNEAL SURGERY

Corneal surgery of any type falls into the category of refractive surgery.

Penetrating Keratoplasty (Graft)

I. Immediate (see previous section *Complications of Intraocular Surgery*)
   A. Grafting into vascularized corneas often fails because of a markedly increased incidence of homograft reactions.

The major primary mechanism mediating rejection of corneal allografts appears to be delayed-type hypersensitivity directed against minor (as opposed to major) histocompatability antigens.

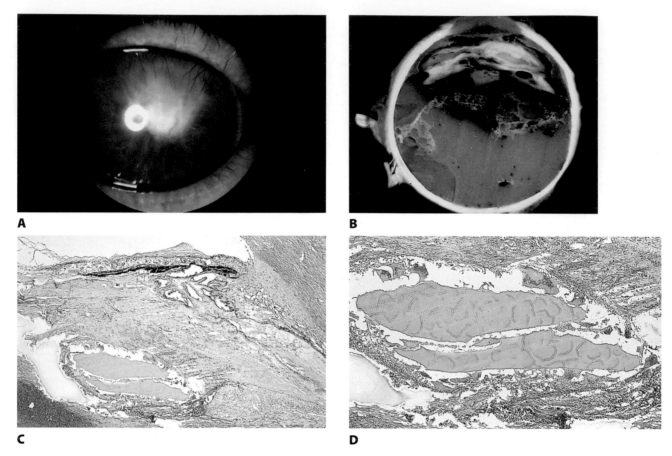

Fig. 5.26 Phacoanaphylactic endophthalmitis (phacoantigenic uveitis). **A,** After vitrectomy, intractable inflammation developed and the eye was enucleated. **B,** Gross specimen shows inflammation centered anteriorly around lens. **C,** Histologic section demonstrates a granulomatous reaction around lens remnants (lens was damaged during vitrectomy). **D,** Increased magnification shows epithelioid and giant cells comprising reaction. (Courtesy of Dr. KA Gitter.)

B. The donor cornea needs to be checked carefully to avoid using a diseased cornea (e.g., cornea guttata).

C. Poor technique can result in incomplete removal of part or even of the entire recipient's Descemet's membrane when the corneal button is removed.
   1. Conversely, poor technique can also result in failure to remove part or all of Descemet's membrane and endothelium when removing the donor's corneal button.
   2. Damage to the iris or lens can also result, as well as vitreous loss, especially in aphakic eyes.
   3. Rarely, inadvertent corneal button inversion may occur, leading to graft failure.

II. Postoperative (see previous section *Complications of Intraocular Surgery*)

Endophthalmitis occurs in about 0.2% of cases

A. Homograft reaction (immune reaction; Fig. 5.27)
   1. The reaction usually starts 2 or 3 weeks after surgery, and is characterized by iridocyclitis and fine keratic precipitates, ciliary flush, vascularization of the cornea starting peripherally and then extending into the stroma centrally, and epithelial edema followed by stromal edema.
   2. A classic late sign of rejection is the presence of a horizontal line of precipitates (Khodadoust's line) that progresses from the graft–host junction and moves across the posterior surface of the graft.
   3. Histologically, polymorphonuclear leukocytes and tissue necrosis are present in a sharply demarcated zone in the donor cornea.
      a. Central to the zone, the donor cornea undergoes necrosis.
      b. Peripheral to the zone, lymphocytes and plasma cells are seen.

B. Defective cicatrization of the stroma may result in marked gaping of the graft site and ultimate graft failure.

C. Corneal vascularization and cicatrization (Fig. 5.28)

III. Delayed (see previous section *Complications of Intraocular Surgery*)
   A. Retrocorneal fibrous membrane (stromal overgrowth, postgraft membrane)

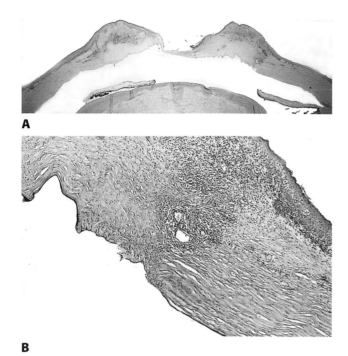

A

B

Fig. 5.27 Homograft reaction. **A,** An inflammatory reaction and tissue necrosis are present in a sharply demarcated zone in the region of the graft incision—shown with increased magnification in **B.**

1. Retrocorneal fibrous membrane is apt to follow graft rejection (immune reaction), faulty wound apposition, poor health of the recipient or donor endothelium, or from iris adhesions.

2. Retrocorneal fibrous membrane may result from a proliferation of corneal keratocytes, new mesenchymal tissue derived from mononuclear cells, endothelial cells that have undergone fibrous metaplasia,* fibroblast-like cells from the angle tissues, or any combination thereof.

After extracapsular surgery and penetrating keratoplasty, lens epithelium can rarely cover the posterior surface of the cornea along the surface of a retrocorneal fibrous membrane, a condition called *lensification* of the posterior corneal surface.

---

3. Histologically, a fibrous membrane covers part or all of the posterior surface of the donor and recipient cornea and may extend over the anterior-chamber angle and occlude it.

Retrocorneal fibrous membrane is found in approximately 50% of failed corneal grafts examined histologically.

The corneal endothelium, although derived from neuroectoderm, acts like a mesothelium and has the ability to act as connective tissue in various pathologic conditions. The corneal endothelium may undergo fibrous metaplasia given the appropriate stimulus (e.g., inflammation).

4. An unusual presentation of acute myeloid leukemia was as a corneal pseudomembrane that on histopathologic examination was comprised of myeloblasts admixed with an acute inflammatory response.

   A. Cornea guttata may be present in the donor cornea and lead to graft failure.

IV. Descemet's stripping with endothelial keratoplasty (DSEK) is an alternative to corneal transplantation for patients in whom the primary dysfunction is of the endothelium. Reported advantages over traditional keratoplasty for this procedure include minimal refractive change, more rapid visual recovery, and maintenance of the structural integrity of the recipient's cornea.

Other Refractive Keratoplasties

Types: radial and transverse keratotomies [e.g., phototherapeutic keratectomy (PTK)], keratomileusis [including laser-assisted in situ keratomileusis (LASIK)], epikeratophakia, keratophakia, photorefractive keratectomy (PRK), and thermal stromal coagulation.

I. All of the complications described previously under *Complications of Corneal Surgery* apply here.

   A. Late corneal perforation has occurred after PRK associated with topical diclofenac, and matrix metalloproteinases 9 and 3 may have been involved in delayed corneal wound closure and corneal melting.

II. Special problems

   A. Infection of the incision site (Fig. 5.29)

   B. Perforation during radial keratotomy procedures may lead to epithelial downgrowth or endophthalmitis. Radial keratotomy incisions also weaken the cornea, and may rupture after insignificant trauma.

   C. Keratophakia specimens may show viable epithelium in the recipient–donor lenticule interface, disruption of the normal collagen lamellar pattern in the lenticule, and absence of keratocytes.

   D. Keratomileusis and epikeratophakia lenticules may show variable keratocyte population, irregular epithelial maturation, and folds or breaks in Bowman's membrane.

   E. Scarring and corneal ulceration or melt (especially in patients who have collagen vascular disease or in whom diclofenac treatment is prolonged) may occur after PRK treatment.

   F. LASIK

      1. Dislocation of the LASIK flap even 7 years following surgery may occur as a late complication secondary to trauma. This complication is associated with diffuse lamellar keratitis and epithelial ingrowth.

         a. Epithelial ingrowth (growth of epithelium in the flap–corneal interface) may follow traumatic dislocation of the LASIK flap.

      2. Intraoperative epithelial defects after LASIK can be a severe complication that may result in diffuse lamellar keratitis, reduce final visual outcome,

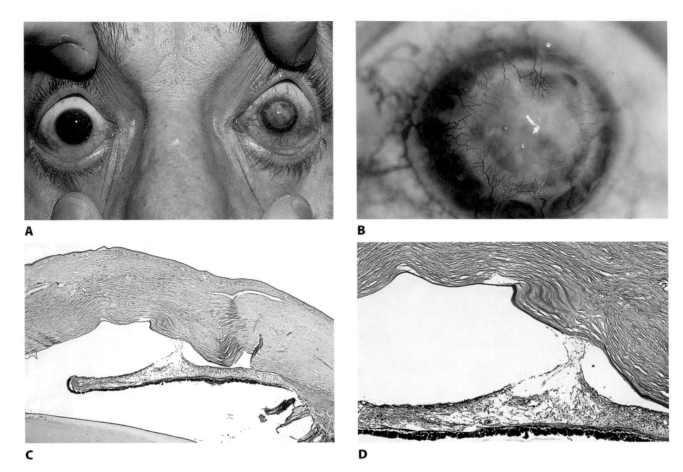

Fig. 5.28 Corneal vascularization and cicatrization. **A,** Penetrating graft in the left eye failed. **B,** Graft is vascularized and scarred; the eye was enucleated. **C,** Histologic section shows iris adherent to internal graft incision (adherent leukoma) between cut ends of Descemet's membrane—shown with increased magnification in **D.**

delay recovery of visual acuity, and induce undercorrection.

3. Tearing of the LASIK flap may occur during retreatment.

4. LASIK can be helpful in correcting high myopic astigmatism resulting from perforating ocular injury.

5. Anterior basement membrane dystrophy following LASIK is associated with visual complaints and/or recurrent erosion symptoms.

6. Corneal bed perforation by laser ablation may occur during LASIK.

7. Corneal ectasia had been reported following otherwise uncomplicated LASIK even in the absence of apparent preoperative risk factors. Factors associated with the development of ectasia after LASIK are high myopia, forme fruste keratoconus, and low residual stromal bed thickness. Ectasia may be transient and related to intraocular pressure elevation in such patients.

8. Salzmann's-like nodular corneal changes have followed LASIK.

9. Peripheral sterile corneal infiltrates may be sequelae to LASIK.

10. In general, LASIK after flap complications is usually associated with good visual outcome; however, there is a higher risk for intraoperative and postoperative complications after the second surgery.

11. Type I diabetes may increase the risk of epithelial downgrowth in LASIK.

12. Elevated intraocular pressure may be a cause of postoperative interlamellar keratitis following LASIK.

13. Epithelial ingrowth between the flap and underlying stroma may occur in between 1 and 20% of LASIK procedures.

G. Laser subepithelial keratomileusis (LASEK) may also be complicated by flap detachment.

H. Deep lamellar keratectomy is indicated in the treatment of patients with corneal stromal opacity without endothelial abnormalities.

1. Postoperative complications include loose sutures, ocular hypertension, Descemet's membrane detachment, and corneal melting.

I. Keratoprosthesis

1. Posterior-segment complications of keratoprosthesis implantation include membrane formation, retinal detachment, and vitreous opacities.

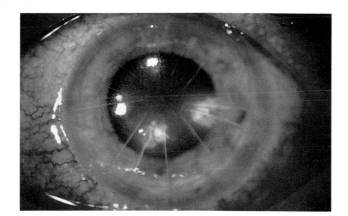

A

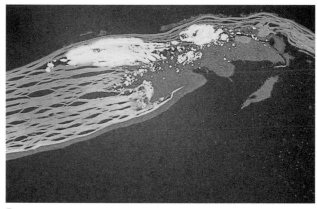

B

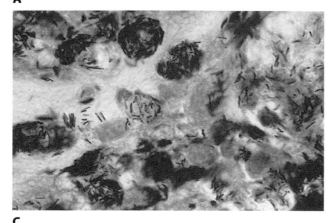

C

Fig. 5.29 Radial keratotomy infection. **A,** Corneal infiltrates present at 3:30 and 7 o'clock. **B,** Histologic section stained with acridine orange shows positive staining in area of clusters of mycobacteria. **C,** Ziehl–Neelsen-positive staining of many acid-fast atypical mycobacteria bacilli, both in clusters and individually. (Case presented by Dr. NA Rao at the combined Verhoeff and European Ophthalmic Pathology Society meeting, 1986, and reported in Robin JB *et al.: Am J Ophthalmol* 102:72. Copyright Elsevier 1986.)

2. Systemic risk factors for retroprosthetic membrane formation relative to the AlphaCor corneal prosthesis are race, hypertension, and diabetes mellitus.
3. Histopathology of these membranes reveals fibrovascular tissue resembling scarred corneal tissue.
   a. Corneal melting may occur following implantation of a keratoprosthesis, and is associated with the presence of immune related corneal surface disease.

COMPLICATIONS OF GLAUCOMA SURGERY

I. Cataract may follow glaucoma surgery even without direct lens contact during the procedure.
II. Subretinal suture misdirection may rarely occur during 360° suture trabeculotomy.
III. Bleb-related inflammation (blebitis) following trabeculectomy is associated with thin and/or chronically leaking filtering blebs secondary to the use of 5-fluorouracil or mitomycin-C.
A. It is usually infectious in origin, but rarely may result from retained material, such as sponge fragments, introduced at the time of surgery.
B. Mitomycin-C filtering blebs that have large, avascular areas or that are subjected to digital pressure are more likely to be associated with leaks.
   1. Limbal stem cell deficiency may follow mitomycin-C treatment for trabeculectomy.
   2. Peripheral anterior synechiae may progress following laser iridotomy for primary angle closure, particularly in those with a plateau iris configuration.
   3. In a national survey of first-time trabeculectomy for open-angle glaucoma in the United Kingdom, the complication rate for trabeculectomy was 46.6% (early) and 42.3% (late). The most common early complications in this report were hyphema (24.6%), shallow anterior chamber (23.9%), hypotony (24.3%), wound leak (17.8%), and choroidal detachment (14.1%). Late complications included cataract (20.2%), visual loss (18.8%), and encapsulated bleb (3.4%).

COMPLICATIONS OF NONSURGICAL TRAUMA

Contusion

Contusion is an injury to tissue caused by an external direct (e.g., a blow) or indirect (e.g., a shock wave) force that usually does not break (lacerate) the overlying tissue surface (e.g., cornea or sclera).

A contusion is the injury that results from a concussion (i.e., a violent jar or shake) caused by the external force.

I. Cornea
  A. Abrasion
    1. An abrasion results when some or all of the layers of epithelium are removed, but Bowman's membrane remains intact.

    Epidermal growth factor provides an important stimulus for initial human corneal epithelial cell migration.

    2. The wound heals by epithelial sliding and mitotic proliferation. If healing is uncomplicated, no scar occurs.
    3. After a wound, reorganization of the remaining epithelium occurs over several hours.
       a. The normal epithelium from the edge of the abraded area flattens and slides inward to cover the gap.
       b. The earliest sliding cells are wing cells.
       c. The basal cells then flatten and slide after releasing their lateral desmosomal attachments.

       Expression of genes, such as *c-fos*, happens within minutes of wounding, may be important for directing epithelial reorganization, and interacts with cell receptors and growth factor. If the entire corneal epithelium is lost, the gap is covered by sliding conjunctival epithelium in 48 to 72 hours. Over a period of weeks to a few months, the conjunctival epithelium takes on the complete morphologic characteristics of corneal epithelium.

    4. A subpopulation of normally slow-cycling, corneal epithelial basal cells resides in the limbal region. These stem cells are stimulated to proliferate in response to wounding of the central cornea. Impression cytology and immunocytochemistry for CK19- and CK3- combine to provide a simple and practical method to evaluate limbal stem cell deficiency. Treatment with autologous cultured limbal and conjunctival stem cells may be helpful to patients with ocular surface injuries, such as by acid burns.

Expression of α-enolase is elevated during corneal migration initiating from the stem cell population.

    5. Mitotic division by the basal cells (limbal stem cells) restores the normal epithelial layer thickness. Mitotic activity of the epithelium is first noted some distance from the wound, often not until 36 hours after injury, and seems to occur as a mitotic burst of activity.

    The proliferating epithelial cells can continue to slide along the original basement membrane for approximately 3 days. Basement membrane, if lost, may not be noted under the new epithelialized area until the third day. Polymorphonuclear leukocytes, derived from conjunctival blood vessels, arrive within the first hour and may persist up to 2 days or until complete healing has taken place.

    6. The corneal epithelium adheres to the underlying tissue through a series of linked structures termed, collectively, the *hemidesmosome* or the *adhesion complex*.

    Intermediate filaments (e.g., cytokeratin) play a part in the formation of hemidesmosomes.

    7. ECM proteins, mediated by integrins, play a role during wound healing.

    ECM proteins include components of basement membrane such as laminins, type IV collagen, nidogen, fibronectins, and tenascins. The functions of ECM appear to be mediated by heterodimeric transmembrane glycoproteins called *integrins*.

    8. Failure of successful reformation of the epithelial adhesion complex to Bowman's membrane following corneal epithelial abrasion can result in recurrent erosion in which the epithelial abrasion recurs spontaneously, resulting in the sudden onset of pain. Such episodes most frequently occur upon awakening in the morning when the epithelium is relatively hydrated and least strongly adherent to underlying structures.
       a. Defective collagen fibrils that anchor the corneal epithelial basement membrane to Bowman's layer have been documented to be related to recurrent erosions following trauma. Hemidesmosomes do not appear to be impaired.
    9. In vivo confocal microscopy may be helpful in the evaluation of corneal injuries.
  B. Blood staining (a secondary phenomenon)—see discussion of *Anterior Chamber and its Angle*, later, and p. 310 in Chapter 8.
  C. Traumatic corneal endothelial rings (traumatic annular keratopathy)
    1. Contusion to the eye may result in multiple, small, gray ring opacities of the corneal endothelium.

2. The lesions become visible immediately after injury, and become even more pronounced during the next few hours. The rings disappear within days, and result in no permanent loss of visual acuity.

3. Histologically, an annular area of endothelial cell disruption and a loss of cell-to-cell contact are seen along with swelling, irregular cell membranes, and sporadic absence of cells.

D. Ruptures of Descemet's membrane (see Fig. 16.6 in Chapter 16) most commonly occur as a result of birth trauma.

1. They tend to be unilateral, most often in the left eye (most common fetal presentation is left occiput anterior), and usually run in a diagonal direction across the central cornea.

2. Histologically, whether the rupture is caused by birth trauma, congenital glaucoma, or trauma after birth, a gap is seen in Descemet's membrane (see Fig. 16.6).

   a. Endothelium may cover the gap and form a new Descemet's membrane.

   b. In attempting to cover the gap, endothelium may grow over the free, rolled end of the ruptured Descemet's membrane and form a scroll-like structure.

c. Combinations of the preceding two possibilities may occur.

E. Keloid of the cornea occasionally follows ocular injury.

1. Most keloids appear as glistening white masses that extend outward from the eye in the region of the cornea (i.e., protuberant white corneal masses).

2. Histologically, corneal perforation is often present. Haphazardly arranged fibroblasts, collagen, and blood vessels form a hypertrophic corneal scar.

II. Conjunctiva may show edema, hemorrhage, or laceration (Fig. 5.30).

After a blow to the eye, the conjunctiva should always be carefully explored for lacerations, which may be a clue to a missile entry wound into the globe.

III. Anterior chamber and its angle

A. Hyphema or blood in the anterior-chamber angle may lead to a number of secondary complications.

1. Blood staining of a cornea that has healthy endothelium (Fig. 5.31) may result if intraocular pressure is uninterruptedly elevated for approximately 48 hours.

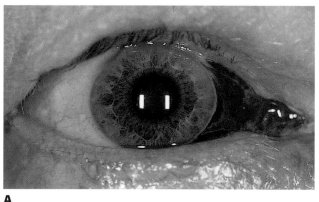

A

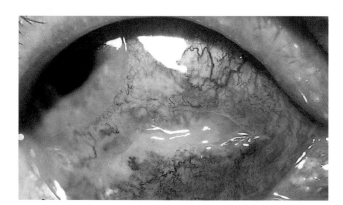

B

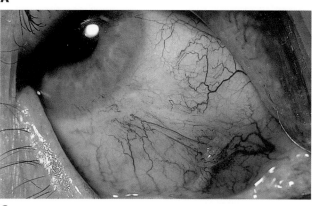

C

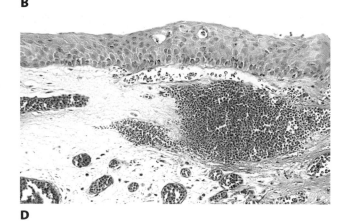

D

Fig. 5.30 Conjunctival hemorrhage and laceration. **A,** Trauma resulted in a large hemorrhage in the nasal conjunctiva. **B,** Conjunctival laceration present in another patient. **C,** The laceration healed without treatment. **D,** Histologic section of another case of conjunctival hemorrhage shows blood in the substantia propria of the conjunctiva.

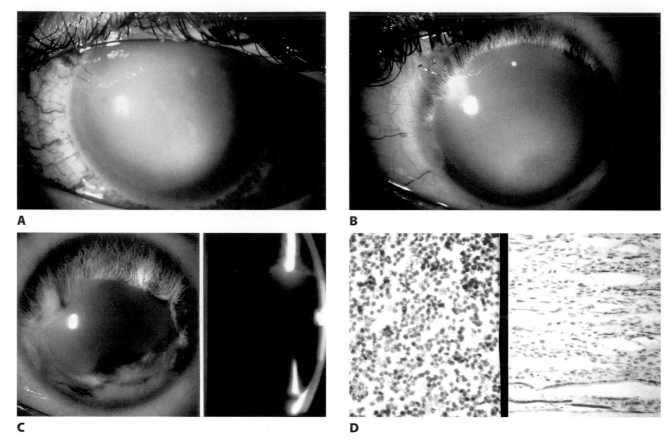

Fig. 5.31 Hyphema. **A,** The patient sustained a blunt trauma that resulted in a total hyphema. One month later, blood staining has occurred. **B,** Three months after the initial injury, the hyphema has started to clear peripherally. **C,** One year after the trauma, most of the cornea has cleared. **D,** Histologic sections from a case of corneal blood staining show intact red blood cells in the anterior chamber on the left side. The right side, taken at the same magnification, shows the cornea; both sides are stained for iron. The red blood cells in the cornea have broken up into hemoglobin particles and do not stain for iron. The only positive staining for iron is within the cytoplasm of corneal keratocytes (**D,** *left* and *right*, Perls' stain).

> Excessively high intraocular pressure causes blood staining of the cornea more rapidly than minimal or intermittently elevated intraocular pressure. If the endothelium is unhealthy, blood staining can occur without a rise in intraocular pressure.

2. The blood may mechanically occlude the anterior-chamber angle and lead to a secondary open-angle glaucoma.
3. Organization of the blood may result in peripheral anterior synechiae and secondary closed-angle glaucoma.
4. The blood may extend posteriorly, especially in an aphakic eye, and result in *hemophthalmos* (i.e., an eye completely filled with blood).
5. Iron may be deposited in the tissue (hemosiderosis bulbi), cause heterochromia (the darker iris is the affected iris), and a toxic effect on the retina and trabecular meshwork.
6. Cholesterolosis of anterior chamber (see p. 142 in this chapter)

B. Angle recession (postcontusion deformity of anterior-chamber angle; Figs 5.32 and 5.33) consists of a posterior displacement of the iris root and inner pars plicata (including ciliary processes or crests, circular ciliary muscles, and some or all of the oblique ciliary muscles, but *not* the meridional ciliary muscle).
   1. The posterior displacement is caused by a laceration into the anterior face of the ciliary body.
      Glaucoma may develop in approximately 7% to 9% of eyes with angle recession, most often when the recession is 240° or greater.
   2. An injury severe enough to cause a hyphema causes an angle recession in more than 70% of eyes and, if the hyphema fills three-fourths of the volume of the anterior chamber, a traumatic cataract and vitreous hemorrhage occur in approximately 50% of eyes.
   3. The acute angle recession probably has little or nothing to do directly with the development of glaucoma, but rather is a sign that indicates a concussive force sufficient in magnitude to damage to the drainage angle.

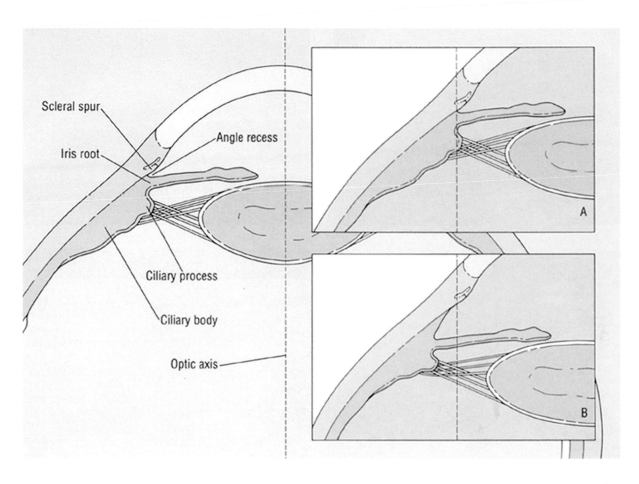

Fig. 5.32 Angle recession. Normal anterior segment. **Inset A,** Line drawn parallel to the optic axis in a normal eye passes through the scleral spur, the angle recess, the iris root, and the most anterior portion of the ciliary processes. The ciliary body has a wedge shape (i.e., is pointed at its posterior portion but straight-sided anteriorly). **Inset B,** In an eye that has an angle recession (also called *postcontusion deformity of the anterior-chamber angle*), the line parallel to the optic axis that passes through the scleral spur will pass anterior to the angle recess, the iris root, and the most anterior portion of the ciliary body. The ciliary body is fusiform (i.e., pointed posteriorly and anteriorly). (In a fetal or neonatal eye, the line parallel to the optic axis that passes through the scleral spur will pass posterior to the angle recess, the iris root, and the most anterior portion of the ciliary body; the ciliary body has a normal wedge shape.)

4. The glaucoma, if it develops, may result from a number of factors:
   a. The initial injury may stimulate corneal endothelium to grow over the trabecular meshwork and form a new Descemet's membrane.
      A secondary open-angle glaucoma results from mechanical obstruction of aqueous outflow (either by the new membrane or by endothelium acting as a reverse pump in turning the aqueous inward).
   b. The initial injury may stimulate fibroblastic activity in the drainage angle and lead to sclerosis and a secondary open-angle glaucoma.
   c. The initial injury may cause hemorrhage or inflammation with subsequent organization, and lead to peripheral anterior synechiae and a secondary closed-angle glaucoma.
   d. Approximately one-third of the patients who develop glaucoma in the injured eye will develop primary open-angle glaucoma in the noninjured eye. The angle recession glaucoma, therefore, may develop in susceptible eyes, already at risk for primary open-angle glaucoma.
   e. The initial injury may lead to cataract and phacolytic glaucoma. Approximately 25% of enucleated eyes that show phacolytic glaucoma also show angle recession.
5. Histologically, the inner part of the pars plicata and the iris root are displaced posteriorly.

Complicating factors such as overgrowth of Descemet's membrane (Fig. 5.34), trabecular meshwork sclerosis, and peripheral anterior synechiae may be seen in a deeply recessed anterior-chamber angle. If a secondary peripheral anterior synechia occurs, a new anterior-chamber angle, commonly called a *pseudoangle*, forms between the posterior cornea and the anterior surface of the pupillary end of the iris synechia. It is common for endothelial cell proliferation to occur over the pseudoangle in the setting of ocular trauma.

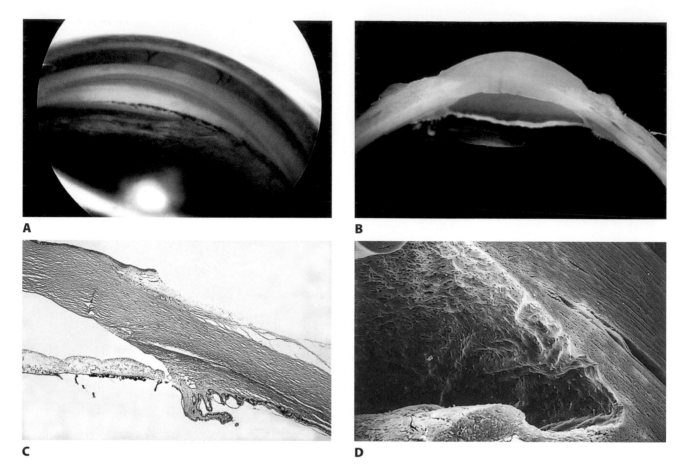

Fig. 5.33 Angle recession. **A,** The angle of the anterior chamber in the eye of a patient who had sustained a blunt trauma is of normal depth over the right side of the figure, except for peripheral anterior synechiae, but is markedly deepened and recessed over the left side. **B,** A gross specimen from another case shows the deepened anterior chamber and recessed angle. The fusiform (pointed at both ends) shape of the ciliary body (most clearly seen on the right) is characteristic of angle recession. **C,** The ciliary body inserts into the scleral spur normally. The oblique and circular muscles of the ciliary body have atrophied after a laceration into the anterior face of the ciliary body, and the resulting scar tissue has contracted, pulling the angle recess, iris root, and ciliary process posteriorly. The anterior wedge shape of the ciliary body has been lost. The entire process results in a fusiform shape of the ciliary body. A number of mechanisms, such as trabecular damage and late scarring, peripheral anterior synechiae, and endothelialization of an open angle, can lead to secondary glaucoma that would result in optic nerve damage. **D,** Scanning electron microscopy shows the pointed anterior ciliary body (instead of the normal wedge shape) and the angle recession. (**D,** Courtesy of Dr. RC Eagle, Jr.)

a. Frequently, a scar extends into the anterior face of the ciliary body.

C. Cyclodialysis (Fig. 5.35) differs from an angle recession in that the entire pars plicata of the ciliary body, *including* the meridional muscles, is stripped completely free from the sclera at the scleral spur.

D. An iridodialysis (Fig. 5.36) or a tear in the iris at its thinnest part (the iris root) often leads to a hyphema.

Other traumatic tears in the iris such as sphincter tears and iridoschisis may occur, but are not usually serious.

E. The trabecular meshwork not only may develop scarring, but may be torn and disrupted by the initial injury.

F. Traumatic iridocyclitis is quite common, frequently severe, and, if untreated, may lead to posterior syn-

echiae, then peripheral anterior synechiae, and finally to secondary closed-angle glaucoma.

IV. Lens

A. Cataract can result immediately, in weeks, months, or even years later.

Posttraumatic cataracts may collect different kinds of material (e.g., calcium and cholesterol). A condition called *calcific phacolysis* exists when intraocular dispersal of calcified lens particles occurs after disruption of the lens capsule in long-standing posttraumatic cataracts (a similar process can cause anterior-chamber cholesterolosis when cholesterol-containing lenses rupture).

B. Anterior and posterior subcapsular cataracts (see p. 373)

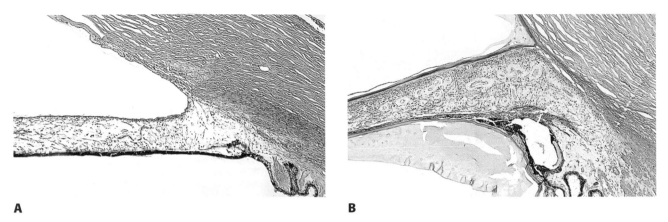

A **B**

Fig. 5.34 Angle recession. **A,** Following angle recession, a peripheral anterior synechia developed. Corneal endothelium has grown over the pseudoangle and on to the anterior surface of the iris and has laid down a new Descemet's membrane. **B,** Another case shows endothelialization of the pseudoangle and a thick, periodic acid–Schiff-positive Descemet's membrane.

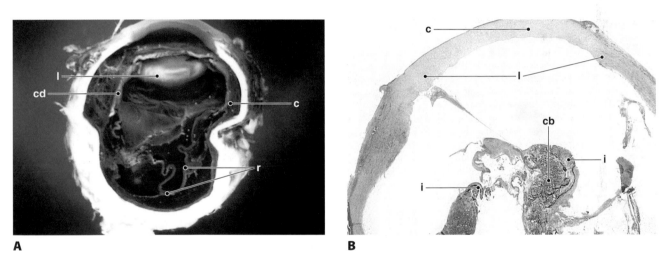

A **B**

Fig. 5.35 Cyclodialysis. **A,** The gross eye shows the ciliary body attached to the scleral spur on the right side. The entire ciliary body on the left side, however, is avulsed from the scleral spur, resulting in a cyclodialysis (cd) (c, choroid; r, retina; l, lens). **B,** Histologic section from another case shows the ciliary body (cb) and iris (i) in the center of the eye, avulsed from the scleral spur 360° (c, cornea; l, limbus).

A special type of anterior or posterior cataract is frequently seen after trauma. The lens opacities take the form of petals (Fig. 5.37), usually 10, in the anterior or posterior cortex, or both, and are called *rosette* or *flower-like cataracts*.

C. Rupture of the lens capsule, if small, may be sealed by overlying iris or healed by proliferation of lens epithelium (see Fig. 10.7A).
   1. A small rupture is noted clinically as a tiny white opacity.
      Histologically, it is seen as a break in the lens capsule associated with contiguous lens epithelial and superficial cortical cell degeneration.
   2. A large rupture usually results in the rapid development of a cataract with considerable lens material in the anterior chamber (see Fig. 10.7B). This con-

dition may progress to phacolytic glaucoma if the inflammatory response primarily is to lens cortex, or phacoantigenic uveitis if the inflammation is allowed to involve the lens nucleus.
   a. Histologically, lens cortex, admixed with macrophages, is seen.
   b. *Elschnig's pearls* or a *Soemmerring's ring* cataract (see Fig. 5.15) may result.
   3. Phacoanaphylactic (phacogenic) endophthalmitis (see p. 75 in Chapter 4)
D. Phacolytic glaucoma (see p. 384 in Chapter 10)
E. *Vossius' ring,* a pigmented ring on the anterior surface of the lens just behind the pupil, may occur immediately after trauma.
   1. It represents iris pigment epithelium from the posterior iris near the pupil that has deposited as a ring (i.e., iris fingerprints).

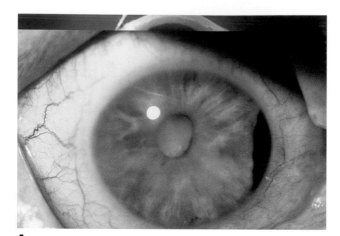

A

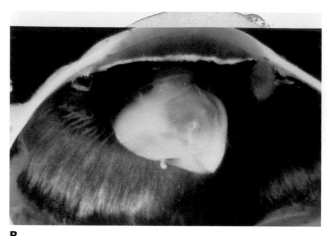

B

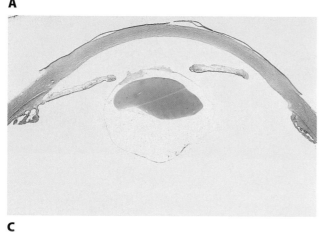

C

Fig. 5.36 Iridodialysis. **A,** The patient sustained blunt trauma that resulted in an iridodialysis. Over the next few months, a mature cataract developed. The no-light-perception eye was enucleated. **B,** Gross appearance of eye in **A**. **C,** Histologic section shows that the liquefied cortex has completely leaked out from the lens during tissue processing; all that remains is the nucleus, surrounded by a clear area where the cortex had been, encircled in turn by the lens capsule. Note the anterior subcapsular cataract. The iridodialysis is seen on the right. In addition, the fusiform shape of the ciliary body, best seen on the left, indicates that an angle recession is present. (**C,** periodic acid–Schiff stain.)

2. If delayed, it may represent initial damage to the lens with subsequent deposition of pigment from the aqueous.

3. An annular pigmented band corresponding to the adherence of the hyaloideocapsulare ligament to the posterior capsule has been reported following blunt ocular trauma.

F. *Dislocation (luxation)* and *subluxation* of the lens may occur after trauma (Fig. 5.38).

1. Dislocation is caused by total zonular rupture with the lens completely out of the posterior chamber (into the anterior chamber or vitreous compartment).

2. Subluxation is caused by incomplete zonular rupture with the lens still in the posterior chamber but not in its normal position.

3. Dislocation of the crystalline lens into the subretinal space has been reported.

4. Transient myopia resulting from blunt trauma is caused by anatomic changes in the ciliary body and lens, particularly anterior shift of the iris lens diaphragm caused by ciliochoroidal effusion and ciliary body edema, and thickening of the lens.

The trauma that altered the position of the lens may also cause a cataract. A subluxated lens is frequently suspected because the anterior chamber is obviously deepened by recession of the unsupported iris diaphragm, which tends to undulate with eye movement (*iridodonesis* or "shimmering iris"). A small bead or herniation of vitreous may also be observed in the anterior chamber. Glaucoma may frequently be associated with a posteriorly dislocated lens. The glaucoma is usually a direct result of the initial blunt trauma to the tissues of the drainage angle. Glaucoma may be caused indirectly by the lens when the lens material itself participates (e.g., phacolytic glaucoma). Zonular weakening or loss may permit the lens to move forward, resulting in pupillary-block angle-closure glaucoma. Dislocation of the lens into the anterior chamber may result in an unusual pupillary-block mechanism in which the pupil is occluded as the iris moves anteriorly against the posterior surface of the dislocated lens. An unusual hybrid form of pupillary-block angle-closure glaucoma can result from traumatic vitreous prolapse in the presence of a posterior-chamber intraocular lens implant.

V. Vitreous

A. Blood and inflammatory cells may be seen early in the vitreous; fibrous membranes are noted late.

B. The vitreous may become detached, commonly posteriorly, but its base may also become detached.

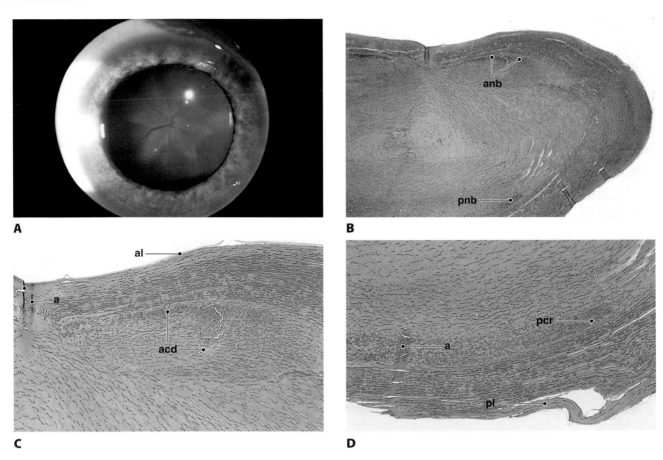

Fig. 5.37 Traumatic cataract. **A,** The patient had blunt trauma several years earlier. A typical petal-shaped cataract has developed. This may develop in the cortex, under the anterior capsule, or under the posterior capsule. In this case, the cataract is present in both the anterior and posterior cortex. **B,** Histologic section of another petal-shaped traumatic cataract shows anterior and posterior cortical degeneration in the form of narrow bands (anb, anterior narrow band; pnb, posterior narrow band)—seen under increased magnification in **C** and **D.** (**C:** a, artifactitious folds; acd, band of anterior cortical degeneration; al, anterior lens. **D:** a, artifact; pl, posterior lens; pcr, band of posterior cortical degeneration). The bands are responsible for the "petals" seen clinically.

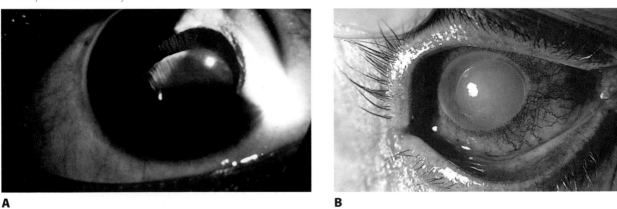

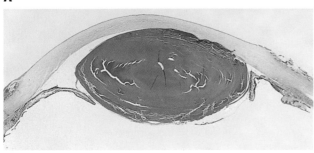

Fig. 5.38 Lens subluxation and dislocation. **A,** The lens is subluxated inferiorly so that the zonular fibers are easily noted in the superior pupil. When a lens is subluxated, it is still in the posterior chamber, but not in its normal position. **B,** The lens is dislocated into the anterior chamber. Pupillary block has resulted in peripheral anterior synechiae and closed-angle glaucoma (a similar case is shown histologically in **C**).

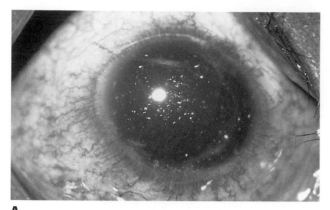

A

B

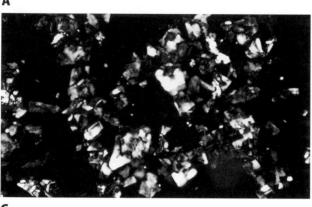

C

Fig. 5.39 Cholesterolosis. **A,** Traumatic hyphema has been absorbed, but cholesterol remains in the anterior chamber. **B,** An anterior-chamber aspirate of another case shows cholesterol crystals. **C,** The cholesterol crystals are birefringent to polarized light. (**B,** unstained; **C,** unstained and polarized.)

Detachment of the vitreous base is almost always caused by severe trauma (see Fig. 11.23B).

C. Cholesterolosis (synchysis scintillans; Figs 5.39 and 5.40) most often results after a vitreous hemorrhage.
1. Cholesterolosis in the vitreous compartment is mainly found in men in their fourth or fifth decade and is usually unilateral. The cholesterolosis appears as glistening, brilliant yellow crystals that tend to settle inferiorly when the eye is stationary, but that fill the vitreous compartment on movement of the eye.
2. In aphakic eyes, the cholesterol-containing vitreous may pass forward through the pupil, presenting as anterior-chamber cholesterolosis.

Cholesterolosis of the anterior chamber may also occur in phakic eyes and result from a hyphema without vitreous hemorrhage, from rupture of the lens capsule in cholesterol-containing cataracts, or with Coats' disease. The glistening, brilliant crystals of cholesterol in the anterior chamber can temporarily be dissolved by applying heat (e.g., from a hair dryer). Cholesterol may also be found under the neural retina in eyes that have long-standing subneural retinal exudation or hemorrhage.

---

3. Histologically, the cholesterol may be free in the vitreous, may incite a foreign-body granulomatous

inflammatory reaction, may be phagocytosed by macrophages, or may be surrounded by dense fibrous tissue without any inflammatory reaction.
   a. The cholesterol crystals are birefringent to polarized light and stain with fat stains in freshly fixed, frozen-sectioned tissue, but are dissolved out by alcohol and xylene in the normal processing of tissue for embedding in paraffin.
   b. In processed tissue, cholesterol appears as empty spaces, often described as *cholesterol clefts.*
D. In aphakic eyes or eyes that have subluxated or dislocated lenses, the vitreous may herniate into the pupil or anterior chamber and may result in pupillary block and iris bombé.
VI. Ciliary body and choroid
   A. Ciliary body and choroidal hemorrhage and detachment may result from trauma.

Hemorrhage and inflammation in the posterior chamber may result in the formation of a cyclitic membrane (Fig. 5.41).

   B. Indirect (posterior) choroidal ruptures (Fig. 5.42) are usually crescent-shaped and concentric to the optic disc between the fovea and optic disc. Direct or anterior choroidal ruptures at the site of impact may also occur.
   1. The indirect or posterior type is more common than the direct or anterior type.

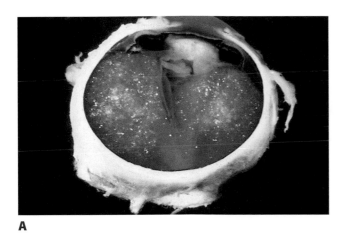

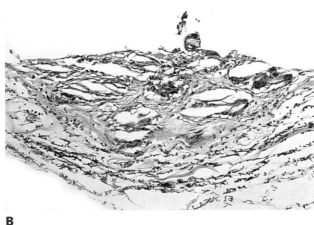

A **B**

Fig. 5.40 Cholesterolosis. **A,** The subneural retinal space is filled with an exudate containing many cholesterol crystals. Cholesterol often settles out after vitreous or subneural retinal hemorrhages. The cholesterol may be seen free, as in **A** and in Fig. 5.39, or the clefts may appear as empty spaces surrounded by foreign-body giant cells (**B**). The cholesterol itself is dissolved out by processing of the tissue, and only the space remains where the cleft had been.

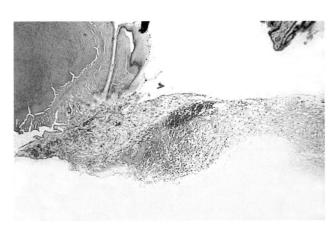

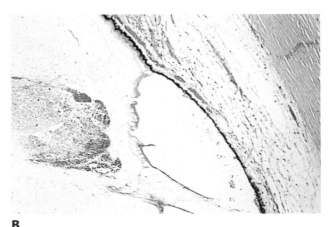

A **B**

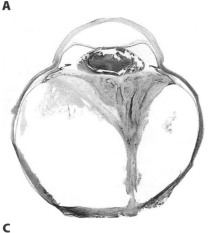

C

Fig. 5.41 Cyclitic membrane. **A** and **B,** A perforating wound of the cornea and penetrating wound of globe produced hemorrhage and inflammation in the posterior chamber. Organization of the hemorrhage (**A**) results in early cyclitic membrane formation. Note the inward traction of the peripheral retina and nonpigmented ciliary epithelium (**B**). **C,** Another case shows shrinkage of cyclitic membrane, resulting in total neural retinal detachment.

2. Most often, the overlying neural retina is intact, but rarely, it too is ruptured.

Subneural retinal neovascularization and chorioretinal vascular anastomoses may be seen after blunt trauma to the eye, and are best detected by fluorescein angiography.

3. Histologically, either Bruch's membrane and choriocapillaris, or the full thickness of the choroid is ruptured. The overlying RPE and neural retina may be normal, atrophic, or, rarely, ruptured.

C. The late appearance of traumatic chorioretinopathy can resemble retinitis pigmentosa clinically and histologically.

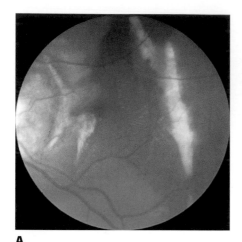

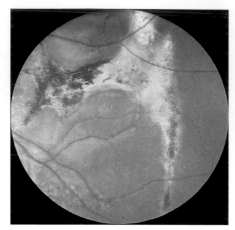

A

B

Fig. 5.42 Choroidal rupture. **A,** The patient sustained a blunt trauma that resulted in choroidal ruptures in the posterior pole and in subneural retinal hemorrhages. The optic nerve head is on the left in this eye. **B,** One year later, considerable scarring has taken place. These patients must be watched closely for the occurrence of subneural retinal neovascularization that may occur at the edge of the healed rupture. **C,** Histologic section of another case shows rupture of the choroid after blunt trauma. (**C,** Courtesy of Dr. WR Green, reported in Aguilar JP, Green WR: *Retina* 4:269, 1984.)

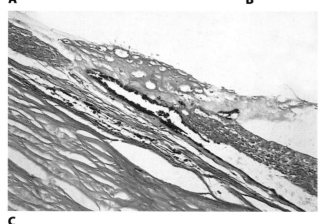

C

D. Delayed, spontaneous, suprachoroidal hemorrhage can be a complication of blunt trauma in individuals with coagulopathy such as factor VIII deficiency.

Retinitis sclopetaria is a specific type of traumatic chorioreti-nopathy that results indirectly from blunt injury produced by a missile entering the orbit to ricochet off the sclera.

E. Sympathetic uveitis (see p. 73 in Chapter 4).

VII. Retina

A. Commotio retinae (Fig. 5.43; Berlin's edema) occurs as a result of contrecoup injury and is usually visible within 24 hours of blunt injury to the globe (see Table 5.2, p. 153).

1. Experimental evidence, histologic evidence in a human eye, and clinical observation all suggest that changes at the level of the photoreceptor outer segment–RPE junction in the foveal and macular areas cause the neural retina to appear pale and white, an appearance that mimics that seen in central retinal artery occlusion and the cherry-red spot of some storage diseases (e.g., Tay–Sachs disease).

Similar patches of pallor, which tend to heal by pigmenta-tion, may be seen in the peripheral neural retina.

2. No fluid leak or edema is evident by fluorescein angiography. Mild blocking of the choroidal fluo-rescence pattern is sometimes seen.

3. The process may resolve completely without sequelae, or damage to photoreceptors may cause vision loss.

4. Cystoid macular degeneration, with cyst and hole formation, may occur months or years later.

The origin of the cysts is obscure. Presumably, loss of tissue from the initial damage may result, in some cases, in microcystoid degeneration of the foveal region. Alter-nately, perhaps after the acute injury, the region becomes edematous and leads to microcystoid degeneration. Once microcystoid degeneration occurs, the septa between the microcysts may break down, resulting in posterior polar retinoschisis (macular cyst). A hole may develop in the inner layer of the cyst (*lamellar hole*); rarely, a hole may develop in both inner and outer layers, causing a true neural retinal hole (see Fig. 5.43B).

5. Histologically, photoreceptor outer-segment dis-ruption and damage to the RPE are noted in the foveal and macular areas.

a. RPE then phagocytizes outer-segment ma-terials.

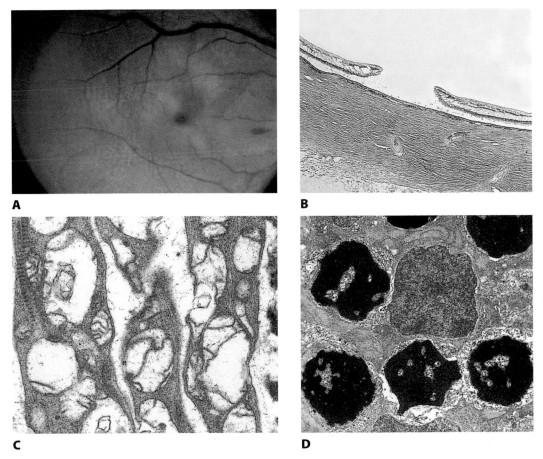

Fig. 5.43 Commotio retinae (Berlin's edema). **A,** The posterior pole is milky and opaque because of damage in the form of vacuolization and degeneration of the inner portion of the photoreceptor and outer nuclear layers. **B,** After commotio retinae, some cases heal with pigmentation. In other cases, fluid enters the macular retinal region and causes microcystoid degeneration. Hole formation may ultimately result, as shown here. **C,** Marked disruption of mitochondria of photoreceptor inner segments 21 hours after trauma. **D,** Nuclei in outer nuclear layer are pyknotic 48 hours after trauma. (**C** and **D,** Reproduced from Owl monkeys; from Sipperley JO *et al.: Arch Ophthalmol* 96:2267, 1978. © American Medical Association. All rights reserved.)

b. RPE next undergoes hyperplasia and may migrate into the neural retina.
c. Late effects may include microcystoid degeneration of the fovea, macrocyst formation, lamellar hole formation, and through-and-through neural retinal hole formation.

B. Neural retinal hemorrhages
1. Flame-shaped retinal hemorrhage (see pp. 406 and 407 in Chapter 11 and p. 610 in Chapter 15)
2. Dot-and-blot neural retinal hemorrhages (see pp. 406 and 407 in Chapter 11 and p. 610 in Chapter 15)
3. Globular, confluent, and massive neural retinal hemorrhages (see p. 610 in Chapter 15)
4. Intraneural retinal submembranous hemorrhage (see Fig. 12.11D in Chapter 12)
5. Terson's syndrome (see p. 439 in Chapter 12)

C. Neural retinal tears (see section *Neural Retinal Detachment* in Chapter 11)

VIII. Optic nerve
A. Partial or complete rupture or avulsion (Fig. 5.44) may occur.

B. Hemorrhage may occur into the nerve parenchyma or into the sheaths (meninges) of the optic nerve.
C. Optic disc edema may result from trauma.

IX. Sclera (see subsection *Penetrating and Perforating Injuries*, next)

Penetrating and Perforating Injuries

I. Penetrating injury
In this type of injury, a structure is partially cut or torn (Fig. 5.45).
A. Ocular injuries from Hymenoptera insect stings may result in corneal edema or decompensation, anterior-chamber inflammation, and cataract requiring surgery. The injuries tend to be more severe in wasp stings and less severe in bee stings.
B. In rural areas, most ocular penetrating injuries are related to: repair and maintenance work (35.7%), wood chopping (25%), machine use (17.8%), simple instrument use (10.7%), falls (7.1%), and cow horn injuries (3.6%), and result in blindness in 64% of cases.

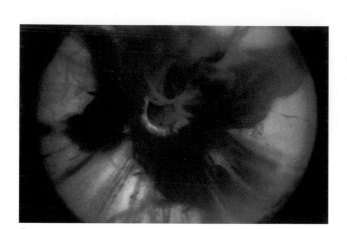
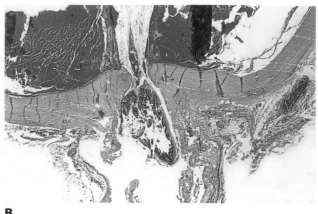

A   **B**

Fig. 5.44 Avulsion of the optic nerve. **A,** After trauma, the optic nerve has been avulsed. Note the hole opening into the orbit, where the optic nerve had been. **B,** The scleral optic nerve canal is not filled with optic nerve but contains retina. (**A,** Courtesy of Dr. ME Smith.)

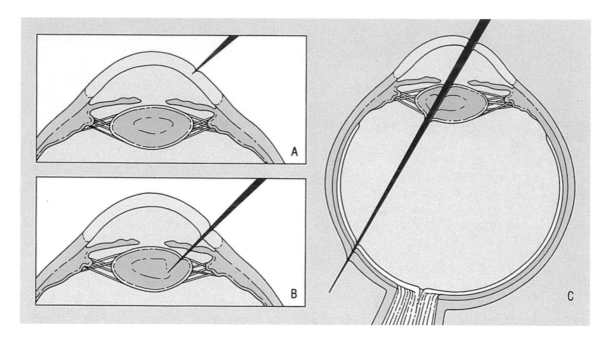

Fig. 5.45 Penetration and perforation of the globe. **A,** The arrow shows a penetrating wound of the cornea. **B,** The arrow shows a perforating wound of the cornea and iris and a penetrating wound of the lens and globe. **C,** The arrow shows a perforating wound of the cornea, lens, retina, choroid, sclera, and globe.

II. Perforating injury

In this type of injury, a structure is cut or torn through completely (see Fig. 5.45).

A. If a missile goes through the cornea and into the globe but not through it, a perforating injury of the cornea and a penetrating injury of the globe result.

B. If a missile goes through the cornea, into the eye, and then through the sclera into the orbit, a perforating injury of the cornea, sclera, and globe results.

III. Corneal and scleral rupture caused by contusion (Figs. 5.46 to 5.48; see Fig. 5.45)

A. Direct rupture of the globe occurs at the site of impact, most commonly the limbus or cornea, but the sclera is also frequently involved, either alone or by extension of the cornea or limbal rupture.

B. Indirect rupture of the globe results from force vectors set up at the point of impact on the essentially incompressible globe.

The globe tends to rupture at its thinnest parts (i.e., limbus and sclera just posterior to the insertion of the rectus muscles, or just adjacent to the optic nerve) in a plane in the direction of the force (contrecoup), or in a plane perpendicular to the direction of the force.

Because most blows strike the unprotected inferior temporal aspect of the eye, the resultant forces frequently cause a supe-

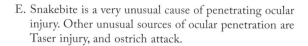

rior nasal limbal rupture. The limbus region is relatively thin (0.8 mm) and is weakened by the internal scleral sulcus, Schlemm's canal, and collecting aqueous channels. Another frequent site of rupture is the superior sclera just behind the insertion of the superior rectus muscle. Both are ruptured by forces set in motion perpendicular to the original line of contusion force. A posterior scleral rupture may result from a contrecoup, usually just temporal to the optic nerve, in the same directional line as the contusion force.

C. Complications (see sections *Complications of Intraocular Surgery* and *Complications of Nonsurgical Trauma*, in this chapter)

D. Corneal perforation may occur even with minor trauma in predisposed eyes, such as in Ehlers–Danlos syndrome.

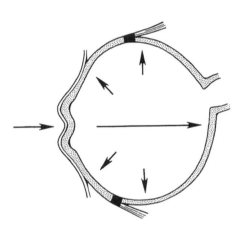

Fig. 5.46 Blunt injury to eye. Diagram shows intraocular pressure effects and regions vulnerable to tear on blunt injury to eye. Arrow in front (to left) of eye shows direction of blunt force to eye. Horizontal arrow within eye shows propagation of force vector in same direction toward macular region (contrecoup). Other arrows represent force vectors set in motion in planes perpendicular to direction of main force.

E. Snakebite is a very unusual cause of penetrating ocular injury. Other unusual sources of ocular penetration are Taser injury, and ostrich attack.

Intraocular Foreign Bodies

I. The amount of damage done by an intraocular foreign body depends on the size, number, location, composition, path through eye, and time retained. For nonmetallic and nonmagnetic intraocular foreign bodies, the final visual outcome may be independent of size and type of foreign body. Moreover, pars plana extraction may be associated with a higher rate of retinal break formation and subsequent retinal detachment in these cases, particularly if the foreign body is glass.

Even if a missile is "clean" and inert, it may carry fungi, bacteria, vegetable matter, cilia, or bone into the eye. Any hemorrhagic area in the conjunctiva should be suspected as a possible site of entrance of a foreign body. After ocular trauma, hypotony, an intravitreal hemorrhage, or a deeper or shallower anterior chamber than in the nontraumatized eye should be considered evidence of a perforated globe until proved otherwise.

II. Inorganic

A. Gold, silver (see Fig. 7.10), platinum, aluminum, and glass are almost inert and cause little or no reaction.

The materials, however, can cause intraocular damage both by their path through the eye and their final position. Glass, for example, may lie in the anterior-chamber angle inferiorly and cause a recalcitrant localized corneal edema months to years after injury. Unexplainable localized corneal edema, therefore, especially inferiorly, should arouse suspicion of glass in the anterior-chamber angle.

B. Lead and zinc, although capable of causing an inflammatory reaction, which is usually chronic nongranulo-

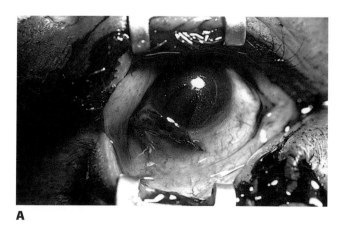

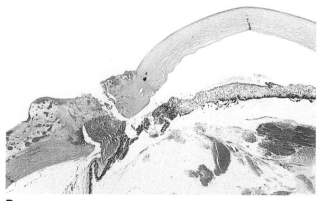

A   **B**

Fig. 5.47 Penetration of globe. **A,** Explosion caused corneoscleral laceration with iris prolapse. Patient later developed sympathetic uveitis. **B,** Another patient had blunt trauma to the eye that caused rupture of the limbal region at the site of previous filtering surgery. The ciliary body herniated into the wound. Spongy subconjunctival tissue represents a filtering bleb. A second scar, a corneal scar, is the site of previous cataract surgery. (**A,** Case reported by Kay ML *et al.: Am J Ophthalmol* 78:90. Copyright Elsevier 1974.)

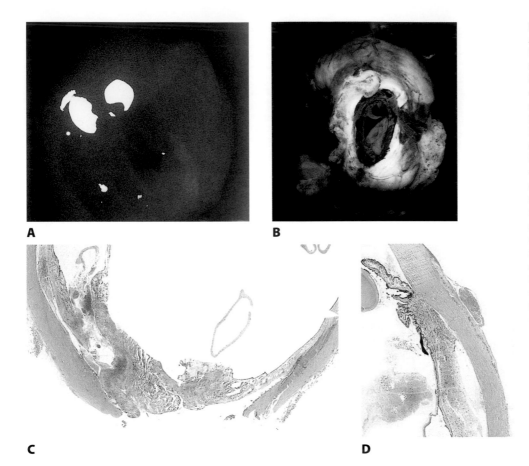

A

B

C

D

Fig. 5.48 Perforation of globe. **A,** The patient had a gunshot injury to the eye. Radiograph shows multiple metallic foreign bodies in the globe. Both cornea and scleral entrance, and scleral exit wounds are present. **B,** Gross specimen shows a large "button-hole" in the back of the eye. In enucleating the hypotonic globe, the surgeon cut across the sclera, leaving the optic nerve head with its surrounding sclera, choroid, and retina in the orbit, creating a situation where the patient is a candidate for sympathetic uveitis. **C,** Histologic section shows the large posterior button-hole. The neural retina is detached and disorganized. **D,** An opaque foreign body (black object) is present on the internal surface of the ciliary body.

matous, are usually tolerated by the eye with few adverse effects except those caused by the initial injury.

C. Iron can ionize and diffuse throughout the eye, and then be deposited, mainly as ferritin and sometimes as cytoplasmic siderosomes, in many of its structures—a condition called *siderosis bulbi*.

1. Bivalent iron (ferrous) is more toxic to ocular tissues than trivalent iron (ferric).

2. The iron ionizes and spreads to all ocular tissues (siderosis bulbi; Fig. 5.49), but is mainly concentrated in epithelial cells (corneal; iris pigmented; ciliary, pigmented and nonpigmented; lens; and RPE), iris dilator and sphincter muscles, trabecular meshwork, and neural retina.

3. Toxicity resulting from interference by excess intracellular free iron with some essential enzyme processes leads to neural retinal degeneration and gliosis, anterior subcapsular cataract (*siderosis lentis*; see Fig. 5.49), trabecular meshwork scarring, and secondary chronic open-angle glaucoma.

> Structures such as the iris, lens, and neural retina can appear "rusty" clinically and macroscopically. The lens is frequently yellow-brown with clumping of rusty material in the anterior subcapsular area. The iris is stained dark so that heterochromia results (darker iris in siderotic eye). The iron may be seen in the anterior-chamber angle as irregu-
> lar, scattered black blotches that may resemble a malignant melanoma.

4. Histologically, Prussian blue or Perls' stain colors the iron blue, and shows it to be present in all ocular epithelial structures, iris dilator and sphincter muscles, neural retina, and trabecular meshwork.

> Intraocular hemorrhage can produce the same clinical and histopathologic changes as are found with an intraocular foreign body. Iron deposition in tissues from an intraocular hemorrhage is called *hemosiderosis bulbi* (Fig. 5.50). In long-standing cases, trabecular meshwork scarring and degeneration, and gliosis of the neural retina are seen.

D. Copper can ionize in the eye and deposit in many ocular structures—a condition called *chalcosis*.

1. Rather than causing the slowly evolving chalcosis, pure copper tends to cause a violent purulent reaction, often leading to panophthalmitis and loss of the eye.

2. Alloy metals with high concentrations of copper tend to cause chalcosis.

3. The copper has an affinity for basement membranes (e.g., internal limiting membrane of retina). It may also be deposited in Descemet's membrane and lens capsule.

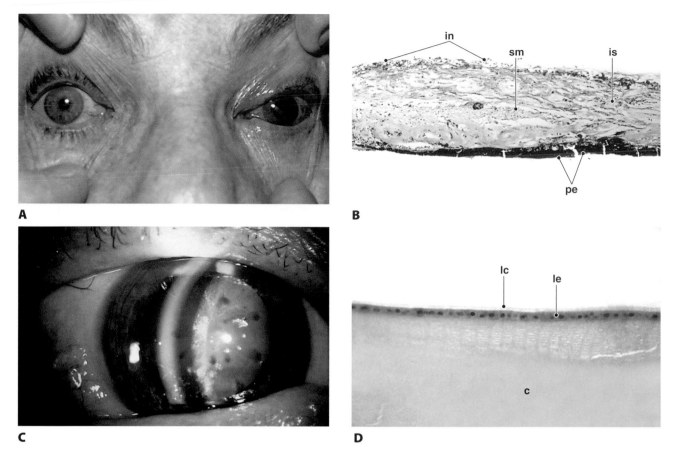

Fig. 5.49 Siderosis bulbi (see also Fig. 10.26). **A,** The patient has an iron foreign body in his left eye. Pigmentation has caused the left iris to become dark. **B,** Perls' stain shows blue in the presence of iron and indicates iron diffusely in the stroma (is) of the iris. Iron was also present in the anterior layer of the iris pigment epithelium (pe). Note the presence of iris neovascularization (in) (sm, sphincter muscle). **C,** The patient had a long-standing hemorrhage in the eye. Iron deposition in the lens had caused hemosiderosis lentis. Hemosiderosis and siderosis are indistinguishable histologically. **D,** Iron, as indicated by the blue color (Perls' stain), is deposited in the lens epithelium (le) and not in the lens capsule (lc) or cortex (c).

4. Clinically, the copper can be seen in the cornea as a *Kayser–Fleischer ring* (see p. 310 in Chapter 8) and in the anterior and posterior central lens capsule as a green-gray, almost metallic, disciform opacity, often with serrated edges and lateral radiations [i.e., a *sunflower* cataract (*chalcosis lentis*)].

5. Histologically, no adequate stain specific for copper exists; however, the copper itself functions as a vital stain and can be seen as tiny opaque (black) dots in unstained sections.

E. Barium sulfate and zinc disulfide
1. These materials are contained under enormous pressure in the core of golf balls. If cut into, the contents of the core travel at great speed and can penetrate deeply into the tissues of the lids and conjunctiva.
2. Histologically, an amorphous mass without inflammation is present in the tissue. The mass is birefringent to polarized light.

III. Organic material (Fig. 5.51)
A. Materials such as cilia, vegetable matter, and bone may be carried into the eye and tend to cause a marked granulomatous reaction.

B. Fungi accompanying the organic material may infect the eye secondarily.
C. Rarely, autologous bone from an orbital fracture may penetrate the globe, resulting in an intraocular foreign body.

Chemical Injuries

I. Acid burns
A. Tear film can buffer acids unless the amount is excessive or the pH is low—less than 3.0.

Explosions of car batteries can cause eye injuries, especially acid-induced corneal abrasions, conjunctivitis, and iridocyclitis.

B. Acid causes an instantaneous coagulation necrosis and precipitation of protein, mainly at the epithelial level, which helps to neutralize the acid, and acts to limit the penetrating ability of the acid, so that the damage tends to be superficial.

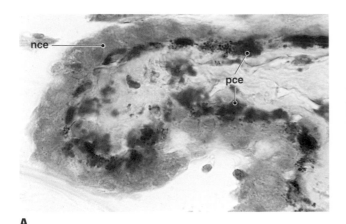

A

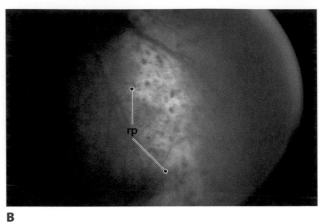

B

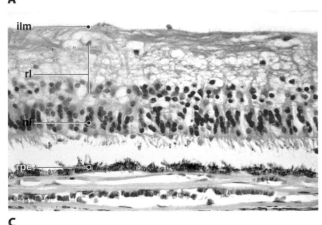

C

Fig. 5.50 Siderosis and hemosiderosis bulbi. **A,** In both conditions, iron may be deposited in neuroepithelial structures such as iris pigment epithelium, lens epithelium, and ciliary epithelium, and in pigment epithelium of the retina. Iron may also be deposited in the iris stroma, the neural retina, and the trabecular meshwork. The toxic effect of iron may cause neural retinal damage and scarring in the trabecular meshwork, as well as a secondary chronic open-angle glaucoma (nce, nonpigmented ciliary epithelium; pce, pigmented ciliary epithelium). **B,** Distinctive changes in the pigment epithelium are caused by an intraocular iron foreign body (rp, retinal pigment epithelial changes). **C,** In another case, iron is deposited in the neural retina and in the retinal pigment epithelium (ilm, inner limiting membrane; rl, degeneration of inner retinal layers; nl, outer nuclear layer; rpe, retinal pigment epithelium). (**A** and **C,** Perls' stains; **B,** courtesy of Dr. AJ Brucker.)

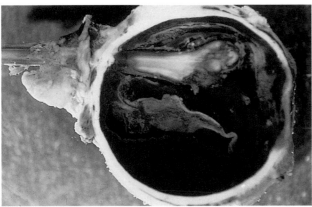

A

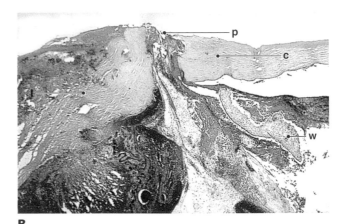

B

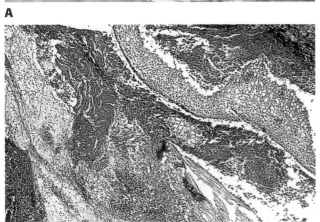

C

Fig. 5.51 Intraocular foreign body. **A,** The gross specimen shows a large splinter of wood in the eye. **B,** Histology shows a perforation through the limbal cornea. The ciliary body, lower left, is filled with blood. Wood (shown under increased magnification in **C**) is present in the anterior chamber and in the wound (p, penetration; c, cornea; w, wood; l, limbus). (Case courtesy of Dr. WR Green.)

If the corneal epithelium is defective or the amount of acid is excessive so that the epithelium can no longer act as a protective barrier, the acid can penetrate into the eye and cause extensive damage.

   C. Histologically, the main finding is a coagulation necrosis of corneal and conjunctival epithelium.

II. Alkali burns (Fig. 5.52)

   A. The eye is unable to deal with alkali nearly as effectively as it does with acids.

   B. Alkali produces an immediate swelling of the epithelium followed by desquamation (rather than precipitation of protein, as does acid).

     Thus, the alkali is allowed direct access to the corneal stroma, through which it can penetrate rapidly.

   C. Alkali coagulates conjunctival blood vessels.

     If it gains access to the interior of the eye, it kills the corneal keratocytes and endothelium, and the lens epithelial cells, and causes a severe nongranulomatous iridocyclitis.

Clinically, the conjunctiva has a porcelain-white appearance caused by coagulation of the blood vessels. Alkali on the conjunctiva and lids frequently leads to symblepharon, entropion, and so forth, as late sequelae.

   D. During the first few weeks of the healing phase, enzymes, mainly collagenase, are derived from corneal epithelium and, to a lesser extent, from neutrophils and keratocytes.

     1. The enzymes can lead to keratomalacia.

Collagenase is a zinc-dependent endoproteinase and is a member of the matrix metalloproteinase family of enzymes.

---

     2. Neutrophils are drawn to the region by chemotactic tripeptides, probably derived from corneal collagen. The early arrival of neutrophils and their elaboration of collagenase compound the problem in alkali burns.

   E. Histologically, widespread necrosis of conjunctiva and cornea is seen, accompanied by a loss of conjunctival blood vessels.

     1. If the alkali has gained access to the inner eye, corneal keratocytes and endothelial cells, and lens nuclei disappear.

       a. Corneal edema and cortical degeneration take place.

     2. A chronic nongranulomatous iridocyclitis is found, and peripheral anterior synechiae frequently result.

III. Tear gas (chloroacetophenone) causes an epithelial exfoliation that heals without sequelae.

IV. Mustard gas (dichlorodiethyl sulfide) causes an immediate and sometimes a delayed reaction.

   A. The immediate reaction consists of a conjunctivitis that is usually self-limiting and heals without damage.

   B. The delayed reaction occurs some decades after the initial injury, and its onset is heralded by an attack of conjunctivitis that becomes chronic, followed by corneal clouding (in the area of the interpalpebral fissure) caused by interstitial keratitis.

     1. The entire cornea may be involved, and areas of stromal calcification and vascularization may develop.

     2. The epithelium overlying the calcified areas characteristically breaks down.

     3. Limbal or perilimbal avascular and calcific patches develop on the conjunctiva, producing a marbling effect.

     4. Aneurysmal dilatations and tortuosity of conjunctiva vessels complete the picture.

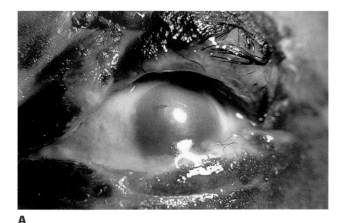
A

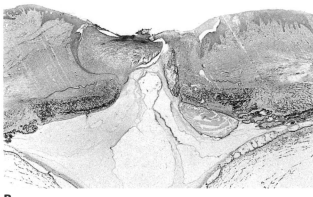
B

Fig. 5.52 Alkali burn. **A,** Considerable lye has caused a massive burn to the conjunctiva and cornea in the patient's left eye. The "whiteness" of the eye is a measure of the avascularity of the conjunctiva and is always a bad sign in a lye burn. Ultimately, the cornea became necrotic and perforation occurred. **B,** Histologic section of another case shows corneal perforation. Lens remnants, including the capsule, are within the corneal wound. Note the thickened cornea and proliferation of corneal epithelium into the stroma. The proliferating epithelium, along with keratocytes and polymorphonuclear leukocytes, secretes collagenase that causes a "melting" of the corneal stroma. The eye shows hypotony, as evidenced by the massive choroidal detachment. (**B,** Periodic acid–Schiff stain.)

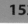

5. Histologically, degenerative changes in all layers of the cornea consist of thinning and atrophy along with areas of thickening of the epithelium; amorphous granular masses beneath the epithelium and sometimes beneath Bowman's membrane; disorganization of the stroma with deposition of hyalin, calcium, and crystals; and vascularization.

Burns

I. Thermal
   A. The blink reflex protects the eyes from most burn injuries.
   B. The eyes, especially the cornea and conjunctiva, may suffer extensive secondary exposure effects when the lids and face are burned severely.
   C. True exfoliation of lens (see p. 368 in Chapter 10)
   D. Holmium laser (2006 nm; Fig. 5.53)
      1. Holmium laser, used in the refractive surgical treatment of hyperopia and hyperopic astigmatism, causes an iatrogenic corneal thermal coagulation.
      2. Histologically, a triangular area (the base in the region of Bowman's membrane and the apex pointing posteriorly almost to Descemet's membrane) of collagen densification and shrinkage is seen.

II. Electric
   A. Electrical injuries, especially if in the area of the head, can cause lens opacities.
      1. Industrial accidents mainly affect the anterior superficial lens cortex.
      2. Lightning affects both the anterior and posterior subcapsular areas.
   B. The earliest changes are subcapsular vacuoles in the anterior mid-periphery.
      1. The changes can be missed if the pupil is not widely dilated.
      2. The vacuoles form a ring, then enlarge and coalesce, and gradually alter into sunflower-like anterior subcapsular opacities that extend into the visual axis.
      3. The last change may be delayed several months to over a year.
      4. Posterior subcapsular cataract may also occur.

> If the electric energy is close to the eye and intense, an anterior uveitis or even anterior-tissue necrosis may result.

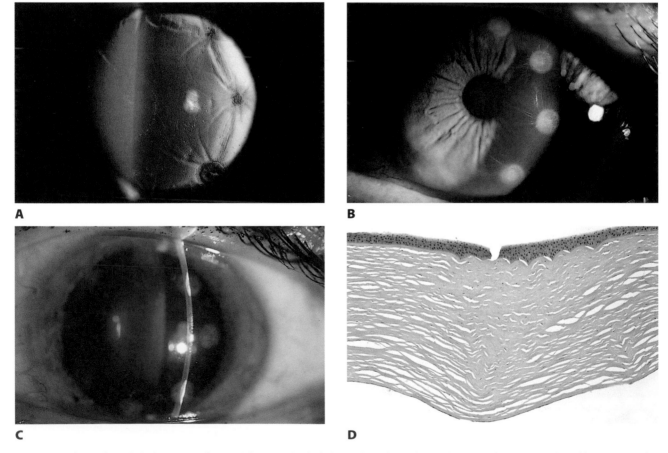

A **B** **C** **D**

Fig. 5.53 Holmium laser. **A,** Patient 1 year after an eight-spot, circular holmium laser thermokeratoplasty (LTK) for the correction of hyperopia. Each spot has radiating lines 360°, some of which connect with the next spot, causing a "belt" effect that bulges the central cornea. **B,** This patient, 1 day post-LTK, demonstrates the belt effect. **C,** Another patient, 2 years post-LTK, shows the typical wedge-shaped spot. **D,** The cornea in a human 6 weeks post-LTK shows a wedge-shaped area (apex toward endothelium) of a relatively homogeneous corneal stroma and acellularity.

C. Histologically, anterior lens opacities are caused by proliferation and abnormal differentiation of lens epithelial cells, whereas posterior lens opacities are caused by faulty formation of lens fibers.

Ocular Effects of Injuries to Other Parts of the Body

I. Purtscher's retinopathy (Table 5.2).
   A. Purtscher's retinopathy usually follows chest compression and is characterized by superficial white exudates in the neural retina, often accompanied by neural retinal hemorrhages.
   B. Fluorescein angiography shows staining of retinal arteriolar walls and profuse leakage from posterior retinal capillaries.

A clinical appearance of the fundus identical to Purtscher's retinopathy may be seen after acute pancreatitis. The retinopathy is probably caused by retinal vascular occlusion secondary to fat embolism or to thrombosis. The syndromes of posttraumatic fat embolism, compression cyanosis, and ophthalmologic hydrostatic pressure also all manifest with a similar retinopathy, as can maternal postchildbirth retinopathy. Other conditions, unrelated to trauma, in which a Purtscher's-like retinopathy can be seen, include lupus erythematosus, dermatomyositis, scleroderma, amniotic fluid embolism, and thrombotic thrombocytopenic purpura.

   C. The clinical picture is probably caused by damage to retinal vessels secondary to sudden changes in intraluminal pressure that are related directly or indirectly to the compression of the chest; microemboli, however, cannot be ruled out.

D. Histologically, the neural retinal changes are probably cotton-wool spots and hemorrhages.
E. Without treatment, most patients recover some visual function. Although systemic steroids may benefit some patients, there is not enough evidence to support their routine use.

II. Traumatic asphyxia (compression cyanosis; see Table 5.2)
   A. The condition usually follows chest compression, which is accompanied by cyanosis and characterized by retinal hemorrhages.
   B. Histologically, hemorrhages are seen in the middle neural retinal layers.

III. Neural retinal fat emboli (see Table 5.2; Fig. 5.54)
   A. Neural retinal fat embolization usually follows fractures, frequently of chest bones or long bones of extremities, and after a delay of a day or two is characterized by neural retinal exudates, edema, and hemorrhage.
   B. Histologically, fat globules are seen in many retinal and ciliary vessels.

IV. Talc and cornstarch emboli
   A. Talc and cornstarch emboli may occur in drug addicts after intravenous injections, such as with crushed methylphenidate hydrochloride tablets.
   B. Clinically, tiny glistening crystals are found in small vessels around the macula.
   C. Histologically, talc and cornstarch particles are found in the neural retina and choroid.

V. Caisson disease (barometric decompression sickness)
   A. Caisson disease (the bends) results from a too-sudden decompression, so that nitrogen "bubbles out" of solution in the blood.
   B. The nitrogen bubbles can embolize to retinal arterioles and lead to ischemic retinal effects.

TABLE 5.2 Comparison of Findings in Four Types of Traumatic Retinopathies

	Purtscher's Retinopathy	**Traumatic Asphyxia**	**Commotio Retinae**	**Neural Retinal Fat Embolism**
TRAUMA	Chest compression	Chest compression	Local to eye	Fractures
VISION				
Initially	Variable	Variable	~20/200	Rarely reduced
Duration of loss	Several weeks	Several weeks	Days	Several weeks
Ultimate	Normal	Variable	Normal*	Normal
SYSTEMIC SIGNS				
Picture	None	Cyanosis	None	Cerebral and cutaneous
Onset	None	Immediate	None	After 48 hours
CONJUNCTIVA	Normal	Subconjunctival hemorrhages	Variable	None or petechiae
FUNDUS				
Picture	Exudates and hemorrhages	Normal or hemorrhages	Neural retinal whitening	Exudates, hemorrhages, and edema
Onset	1–2 days	Immediate to a few hours	Few hours	1–2 days

*Unless a cystic macula results.
(Modified from Kelley JS: Am J Ophthalmol 74:278, 1972. Copyright Elsevier 1972.)

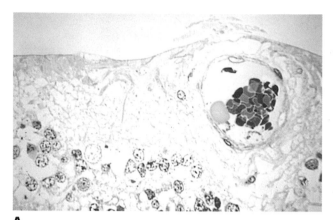

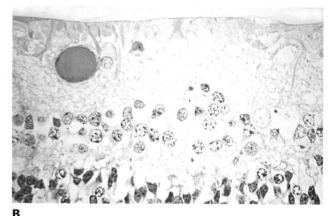

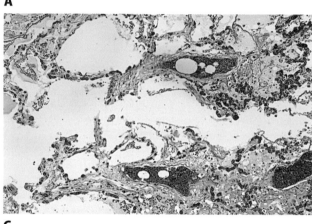

Fig. 5.54 Retinal fat emboli. **A,** Gray-blue, homogeneous fat embolus present in lower left side of the retinal arteriole (erythrocytes stain dark blue) in this thin section prepared for electron microscopy. **B,** In another thin section, the fat embolus completely occludes a small retinal vessel (*upper left*). **C,** Many fat emboli (clear, round bodies of different sizes) present in lung from the same patient. Patient had closed-chest cardiac massage. Multiple rib fractures resulted.

VI. Child abuse (nonaccidental trauma, battered-baby, shaken-baby) syndrome
  A. The ocular findings include neural retinal (most common finding), vitreous, and subdural optic nerve hemorrhages; direct trauma to the eyes and adnexa; and neural retinal tears, detachments, schisis, and folds.
    1. The retinal hemorrhage may extend into the vitreous through a break in the internal limiting membrane.
    2. The distribution of retinal hemorrhages accompanying head injury is said to correlate with acute and evolving regional cerebral parenchymal injury patterns.
    3. Intraocular hemorrhage accompanying subdural hematoma is strongly suggestive of nonaccidental trauma.
    4. In general, the severity of retinal and intracranial injury is correlated in children with nonaccidental trauma.
    5. Epiretinal membrane formation may be a late manifestation of nonaccidental trauma.
  B. Systemic findings include subdural hematoma, fractures, evidence of sexual molestation, cigarette burns, and human bites.
VII. Neural retinal hemorrhages in the newborn
  A. Splinter and flame-shaped neural retinal hemorrhages are most commonly found; lake or geographic and dense, round "blob" hemorrhages may also be seen.
  B. Neural retinal hemorrhages are present in 20% to 30% of newborns.
  C. The neural retinal hemorrhages are probably caused by a mechanical rise in pressure inside the skull during labor; increased blood viscosity and obstetric instrumentation during delivery may also play a role.
VIII. Carotid–cavernous fistula
  A. Traumatic carotid–cavernous fistula causes exophthalmos, often pulsating, marked chemosis, conjunctival vascular engorgement, frequently glaucoma, and in half the patients, abnormal neuro-ophthalmologic signs.
  B. It may close off spontaneously, but usually needs surgical correction.
IX. Acceleration injuries
  A. Positive G from rapid acceleration may force blood downward from the head and result in arterial pressure reduced below the intraocular pressure. Retinal arterioles collapse and retinal ischemia result.
  B. Negative G (redout), such as occurs in tumbling rotations, forces blood away from the center of rotation toward the head so that arterial and venous pressures may approach each other, causing cessation of retinal circulation.
  C. Transverse G due to rapid deceleration may slam blood from back to front of the head and produce subconjunctival and neural retinal hemorrhages.

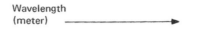

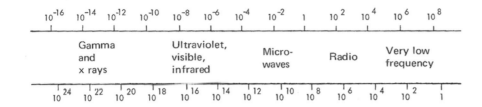

Fig. 5.55 Electromagnetic spectrum. Top numbers show wavelength (meters), bottom numbers show frequency (hertz).

Radiation Injuries (Electromagnetic)

I. Types of radiation (Fig. 5.55)

  A. *Long waves* (3000 to 30 m) are found in radio and diathermy.

  B. *Microwaves* (1 mm to 1 m) are found in radar and rapid-cooking ovens.

  C. *Infrared waves* (12 000 to 770 nm*) are found in furnaces (e.g., glass works). The holmium laser is in the infrared range at 2060 nm (see earlier subsection *Thermal*).

  D. *Visible light waves* (770 to 390 nm) are found in sunlight, electric light, and nuclear fission.

  E. *Ultraviolet (UV) waves* (390 to 180 nm) are found in sunlight and welding arc.

   1. Chronic exposure to UV light during arc welding may be related to the development of corneal spheroidal degeneration.

   2. UV-A (long-wave, near UV, blacklight; 400 to 320 nm)
      Levels 800 to 100 times higher than UV-B are required to cause erythema because a substantial amount is absorbed in the ozone, but more UV-A than UV-B is present in the solar spectrum.

   3. UV-B (middle UV, "sunburn" radiation; 320 to 290 nm)
      Virtually none is absorbed in ozone. UV-B, especially the shorter wavelengths (340 to 320 nm), is most efficient in causing erythema and sunburn.

   4. UV-C (short-wave, far UV, germicidal radiation; below 290 nm)
      Virtually all is absorbed in ozone, and therefore it plays no role in photobiology of natural sunlight.

The *excimer laser*, used in refractive surgery mainly to correct myopia, is in the UV-C at 190 nm.

F. *Laser* (light amplification by stimulated emission of radiation) *radiations* are coherent, monochromatic, directional, and powerful and currently are produced in the UV, visible, and infrared parts of the spectrum.

   1. Cyclodiode laser therapy results in damage to the ciliary body pars plicata; however, some ciliary processes are frequently spared within the treatment zone. Ciliary epithelial proliferation is associated with longer time after treatment. Regeneration of ciliary processes with fibrovascular cores is not seen.

G. *Ionizing radiation* is the term applied to those very short waves of the electromagnetic spectrum that disturb the electrical neutrality of the atoms that constitute matter (e.g., X-rays and γ-rays).

II. Types of injuries

  A. Microwaves can cause cataracts in the experimental animal.

Although cataracts (posterior cortical) can be produced under severe experimental conditions in animals, microwave-induced cataracts from cumulative exposure have yet to be adequately demonstrated in humans.

  B. Infrared waves can cause true exfoliation of the lens (see p. 368 in Chapter 10).

  C. If visible light waves are sufficiently intense and viewed directly, they can cause chorioretinal burns (photic maculopathy).

Prior to the availability of true lasers, for clinical use, visible light waves from sources such as the xenon arc photocoagulator (i.e., focused, incoherent white light) or even focused sunlight were used clinically in producing desirable chorioretinal adhesions.

Indirectly, over time, visible light waves probably play a role in the development of cataract, and may play a role in age-related macular degeneration.

The old symbol μm (millimicron) has been replaced by nm (nanometer).

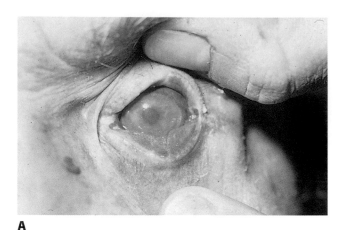

A

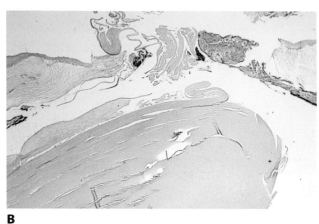

B

Fig. 5.56 Radiation injury. **A,** The patient had radiation therapy for sebaceous carcinoma of the eyelid. Note the scarring of the cornea and ciliary injection. **B,** Another patient who received radiation therapy for basal cell carcinoma of the eyelid shows corneal perforation. Note the vascularized cornea. Lens remnants and iris are present in the corneal perforation.

D. UV waves, especially UV-B light (320 to 290 nm), are absorbed by the conjunctiva and cornea and can cause conjunctivitis and keratitis, and are thought to be causative or contributory in pterygia, conjunctival dysplasia and squamous cell carcinoma, elastotic (climatic, Labrador, spheroidal) degeneration keratopathy, cortical cataract, and perhaps age-related macular degeneration.

Superficial punctate keratitis often follows overzealous use of sunlamps. Although painful, it is self-limited and heals without treatment within 24 hours. A similar picture can be caused by reflected sunlight (e.g., snow blindness). Use of topical anesthetic drops as an inappropriate treatment can cause topical anesthetic-abuse keratopathy.

If the waves are of sufficient power (e.g., from an UV laser), they can reach the lens.

E. Laser (e.g., ruby, argon, krypton, and neodymium) radiations can cause chorioretinal injuries. Lasers of longer wavelengths (e.g., CO_2, YAG, excimer, and erbium) can cause burns of the cornea and conjunctiva.

F. Ionizing radiations (Fig. 5.56) can produce conjunctival telangiectasis; corneal vascularization and keratinization; cataract; and neural retinal atrophy, telangiectasis, hemorrhage, and exudation; all occur mainly as late effects.

1. Acute radiation sickness may result from large doses of radiation.

2. Neural retinal and vitreous hemorrhages may develop in these patients.

3. Histologically, bacterial colonies can be found in the choroid and neural retina.

G. Lightning strike may result in maculopathy. Iridocyclitis and ocular hypertension may also be associated with lightning injuries.

BIBLIOGRAPHY

Causes of Enucleation

Erie JC, Nevitt MP, Hodge D *et al.*: Incidence of enucleation in a defined population. *Am J Ophthalmol* 113:138, 1992

Wong TY, Klein BEK, Klein R: The prevalence and 5-year incidence of ocular trauma: The Beaver Dam Study. *Ophthalmology* 107:2196, 2000

Complications of Intraocular Surgery

Allen RC, Russell SR, Schluter ML *et al.*: Retained posterior segment indocyanine green dye after phacoemulsification. *J Cataract Refract Surg* 32:357, 2006

Apple DJ, Mamalis N, Loftfield K *et al.*: Complications of intraocular lenses: A historical and histopathological review. *Surv Ophthalmol* 29:1, 1984

Apple D, Solomon KD, Tetz MR *et al.*: Posterior capsule opacification. *Surv Ophthalmol* 37:73, 1992

Assia E, Apple D, Tsai J *et al.*: Mechanism of radial tear formation and extension after anterior capsulectomy. *Ophthalmology* 98:432, 1991

Auffarth GU, Brezin A, Caporossi A *et al.*: Comparison of Nd : YAG capsulotomy rates following phacoemulsification with implantation of PMMA, silicone, or acrylic intra-ocular lenses in four European countries. *Ophthalmic Epidemiol* 11:319, 2004

Ayaki M, Ohara K, Ibaraki N *et al.*: The outgrowth of lens epithelial cells onto the anterior capsule after intraocular lens implantation (letter). *Am J Ophthalmol* 115:668, 1993

Aydin E, Bayramlar H, Totan Y *et al.*: Dislocation of a scleral-fixated posterior chamber intraocular lens into the anterior chamber associated with pseudophakic bullous keratopathy. *Ophthalmic Surg Lasers Imaging* 35:67, 2004

Bandyopadhyay R, Banerjee A, Bhaduri G *et al.*: Traumatic pseudophacocele. *J Indian Med Assoc* 102:731, 2004

Beltrame G, Salvetat ML, Driussi G *et al.*: Effect of incision size and site on corneal endothelial changes in cataract surgery. *J Cataract Refract Surg* 28:118, 2002

Bergsma DR Jr, McCaa CS: Extensive detachment of Descemet membrane after holmium laser sclerostomy. *Ophthalmology* 103:678, 1996

Bernauer W, Thiel MA, Kurrer M et al.: Corneal calcification following intensified treatment with sodium hyaluronate artificial tears. *Br J Ophthalmol* 90:285, 2006

Binder PS, Deg JK, Kohl FS: Calcific band keratopathy after intraocular chondroitin sulfate. *Arch Ophthalmol* 105:1243, 1987

Blomquist PH: Expulsion of an intraocular lens through a clear corneal wound. *J Cataract Refract Surg* 29:592, 2003

Bobergg-Ans G, Villumsen J, Henning V: Retinal detachment after phacoemusification cataract extraction. *J Cataract Refract Surg* 29:1333, 2003

Boniuk V, Nockowitz R: Perforation of the globe during retrobulbar injection: Medicolegal aspects of four cases. *Surv Ophthalmol* 39:141, 1994

Bourne WM, Nelson LR, Hodge DO: Continued endothelial cell loss ten years after lens implantation. *Ophthalmology* 101:1014, 1994

Breebaart A, Nuyts R, Pels E et al.: Toxic endothelial cell destruction of the cornea after routine extracapsular cataract surgery. *Arch Ophthalmol* 108:1121, 1990

Brilakis HS, Lustbader JM: Bilateral dislocation of in-the-bag posterior chamber intraocular lenses in a patient with intermediate uveitis. *J Cataract Refract Surg* 29:2013, 2003

Bullock JD, Warwar RE, Green WR: Ocular explosion from periocular anesthetic injections: A clinical, histopathologic, experimental, and biophysical study. *Ophthalmology* 106:2341, 1999

Busbee BG, Recchia FM, Kaiser R et al.: Bleb-associated endophthalmitis: clinical characteristics and visual outcomes. *Ophthalmology* 111:1495, 2004

Caballero A, Garcia-Elskamp C, Losada M et al.: Natural evolution of Elschnig pearl posterior capsule opacification after posterior capsulotomy. *J Cataract Refract Surg* 27:1979, 2001

Champion R, McDonnell PJ, Green WR: Intraocular lenses: Histopathologic characteristics of a large series of autopsy eye. *Surv Ophthalmol* 30:1, 1985

Chien A, Raber I, Fischer D et al.: *Propionibacterium acnes* endophthalmitis after intracapsular cataract extraction. *Ophthalmology* 99:487, 1992

Daly M, Tuft SJ, Munro PM: Acute corneal calcification following chemical injury. *Cornea* 24:761, 2005

Dana MR, Chatzistefanou K, Schaumberg DA et al.: Posterior capsule opacification after cataract surgery in patients with uveitis. *Ophthalmology* 104:1387, 1997

Deka S, Deka A, Bhattacharjee H: Management of posteriorly dislocated endocapsular tension ring and intraocular lens complex. *J Cataract Refract Surg* 32:887, 2006

Deokule SP, Mukherjee SS, Chew CK: Neodymium:YAG laser anterior capsulotomy for capsular contraction syndrome. *Ophthalmic Surg Lasers Imaging* 37:99, 2006

Dowler JGF, Sehmi KS, Hykin PG et al.: The natural history of macular edema after cataract surgery in diabetes. *Ophthalmology* 106:663, 1999

Edge R, Navon S: Scleral perforation during retrobulbar and peribulbar anesthesia: Risk factors and outcome in 50 000 cases. *J Cataract Refract Surg* 25:1237, 1999

Eleftheriadis H, Amoros S, Bilbao R et al.: Spontaneous dislocation of a phakic refractive lens into the vitreous cavity. *J Cataract Refract Surg* 30:2013, 2004

Eriksson A, Koranyi G, Seregard S et al.: Risk of acute suprachoroidal hemorrhage with phacoemulsification. *J Cataract Refract Surg* 24:793, 1998

Fine BS, Brucker AJ: Macular edema and cystoid macular edema. *Am J Ophthalmol* 92:466, 1981

Finger PT, McCormick SA, Lombardo J et al.: Epithelial inclusion cyst. *Arch Ophthalmol* 113:777, 1995

Flach A, Jampol L, Weinberg D et al.: Improvement in visual acuity in chronic aphakic and pseudophakic cystoid macular edema after treatment with topical 0.5% ketorolac tromethamine. *Am J Ophthalmol* 112:514, 1991

Fox G, Joondeph B, Flynn HW et al.: Delayed-onset pseudophakic endophthalmitis. *Am J Ophthalmol* 111:163, 1991

Freidlin J, Pak J, Tessler HH et al.: Sympathetic ophthalmia after injury in the Iraq war. *Ophthalm Plast Reconstr Surg* 22:133, 2006

Friberg T, Kuzma P: *Propionibacterium acnes* endophthalmitis two years after extracapsular cataract extraction. *Am J Ophthalmol* 109:609, 1990

Friedberg M, Pilkerton AR: A new technique for repositioning and fixating a dislocated intraocular lens. *Arch Ophthalmol* 110:413, 1992

Galloway GD, Ang GS, Shenoy R et al.: Retained anterior chamber cilium causing endophthalmitis after phacoemulsification. *J Cataract Refract Surg* 30:521, 2004

Gass JDM, Norton EWD: Cystoid macular edema and papilledema following cataract extraction. *Arch Ophthalmol* 76:646, 1966

Gothard TW, Hardten DR, Lane SS et al.: Clinical findings in Brown–McLean syndrome. *Am J Ophthalmol* 115:729, 1993

Hagan J, Gaasterland DE: Endocapsular hematoma. *Arch Ophthalmol* 109:514, 1991

Halpern BL, Pavilack MA, Gallagher SP: The incidence of atonic pupil following cataract surgery. *Arch Ophthalmol* 113:448, 1995

Haugen OH, Kjeka O: Localized, extreme scleral thinning causing globe rupture during strabismus surgery. *J AAPOS* 9:595, 2005

Hay A, Flynn H, Hoffman J et al.: Needle penetration of the globe during retrobulbar and peribulbar injections. *Ophthalmology* 98:1017, 1991

Hayashi K, Hayashi H, Nakao F et al.: Posterior capsule opacification after cataract surgery in patients with diabetes mellitus. *Am J Ophthalmol* 134:10, 2002

Hellinger WC, Hasan SA, Bacalis LP et al.: Outbreak of toxic anterior segment syndrome following cataract surgery associated with impurities in autoclave steam moisture. *Infect Control Hosp Epidemiol* 27:294, 2006

Hoffman RS, Fine IH, Packer M: Retained IOL fragment and corneal decompensation after pseudophakic IOL exchange. *J Cataract Refract Surg* 30:1362, 2004

Hollick EJ, Spalton DJ, Meacock WER: The effect of capsulorhexis size on posterior capsular opacification: One-year results of a randomized prospective trial. *Am J Ophthalmol* 128:271, 1999

Hollick EJ, Spalton DJ, Ursell PJ et al.: The effect of polymethylmethacrylate, silicone, and polyacrylic lenses on posterior capsular opacification 3 years after cataract surgery. *Ophthalmology* 106:54, 1999

Holliday J, Buller C, Bourne W: Specular microscopy and fluorophotometry in the diagnosis of epithelial downgrowth after a sutureless cataract operation. *Am J Ophthalmol* 116:238, 1993

Hoover DL, Giangiacomo J, Benson RL: Descemet's membrane detachment by sodium hyaluronate. *Arch Ophthalmol* 103:805, 1985

Hoyos JE, Cigales M, Hoyos-Chacon J: Zonular dehiscence two years after phakic refractive lens (PRL) implantation. *J Refract Surg* 21:13, 2005

Irvine SR: A newly defined vitreous syndrome following cataract extraction. *Am J Ophthalmol* 36:599, 1953

Ishibashi T, Hatae T, Inomata H: Collagen types in human posterior opacification. *J Cataract Refract Surg* 20:643, 1994

Islam N, Dabbagh A: Inert intraocular eyelash foreign body following phacoemulsification cataract surgery. *Acta Ophthalmol Scand* 84:432, 2006

Izak AM, Apple DJ, Werner L et al.: Bipseudophakia: clinicopathological correlation of a dropped lens. *J Cataract Refract Surg* 28:874, 2002

Jamal S, Solomon L: Risk factors for posterior capsular pearling after uncomplicated extracapsular cataract extraction and plano-convex posterior chamber lens implantation. *J Cataract Refract Surg* 19:333, 1993

Kappelhof JP, Vrensen GFJM, deJong PTVM *et al.*: An ultrastructural study of Elschnig's pearls in the pseudophakic eye. *Am J Ophthalmol* 101:58, 1986

Karabatsas CH, Hoh HB, Easty DL: Epithelial downgrowth following penetrating keratoplasty with a running adjustable suture. *J Cataract Refract Surg* 22:1242, 1996

Kargi SH, Oz O, Erdinc E *et al.*: Tolerated cilium in the anterior chamber. *Ocul Immunol Inflamm* 11:73, 2003

Karp LA, Scheie HG: Results of 1000 consecutive intracapsular cataract extractions. *Ann Ophthalmol* 13:1201, 1981

Katsimpris JM, Koliakou K, Petropoulos IK *et al.*: Opacification of hydrophilic acrylic intraocular lenses: a clinical and ultrastructural analysis of three explanted lenses. *Klin Monatsbl Augenheilkd* 220:165, 2003

Kattan H, Flynn HW, Pflugfelder S *et al.*: Nosocomial endophthalmitis. *Surv Ophthalmol* 98:227, 1991

Kim CY, Kang SJ, Lee SJ *et al.*: Opacification of a hydrophilic acrylic intraocular lens with exacerbation of Behçet's uveitis. *J Cataract Refract Surg* 28:1276, 2002

Knauf HP, Rowsey JJ, Margo CE: Cystic epithelial downgrowth following clear-cornea cataract extraction. *Arch Ophthalmol* 115:668, 1997

Kohnen T, Koch DD, Font RL: Lensification of the posterior corneal surface: An unusual proliferation of lens epithelial cells. *Ophthalmology* 104:1343, 1997

Kozart DM, Eagle RC Jr: Stripping of Descemet's membrane after glaucoma surgery. *Ophthalmic Surg* 12:420, 1981

Lahav M: The decreased incidence of retinal detachment after cataract surgery. *Trans Am Ophthalmol Soc* 86:321, 1988

Lanzl IM, Mertz M, Kopp C: Choroidal effusions and hypotony caused by severe anterior lens capsule contraction after cataract surgery. *Am J Ophthalmol* 133:165, 2002

Lee BL, Gaton DD, Weinreb RN: Epithelial downgrowth following phacoemulsification through a clear cornea. *Arch Ophthalmol* 117:283, 1999

Lee BL, Manche EE, Glascow BJ: Rupture of radial and arcuate keratotomy scars by blunt trauma 91 months after incisional keratotomy. *Am J Ophthalmol* 120:108, 1995

Lee HJ, Min SH, Kim TY: Bilateral spontaneous dislocation of intraocular lenses within the capsular bag in a retinitis pigmentosa patient. *Korean J Ophthalmol* 18:52, 2004

Little BC, Richardson T, Morris S: Removal of a capsular tension ring from the anterior chamber angle. *J Cataract Refract Surg* 30:1832, 2004

Mader T, Stulting R: Penetrating keratoplasty in ectodermal dysplasia. *Am J Ophthalmol* 110:319, 1990

Mamalis N, Edelhauser HF, Dawson DG *et al.*: Toxic anterior segment syndrome. *J Cataract Refract Surg* 32:324, 2006

Marcon AS, Rapuano CJ, Jones MR *et al.*: Descemet's membrane detachment after cataract surgery: management and outcome. *Ophthalmology* 109:2325, 2002

Marcon AS, Rapuano CJ, Jones MR *et al.*: Descemet's membrane detachment after cataract surgery: management and outcome. *Ophthalmology* 109:2325, 2002

Marigo FA, Finger PT, McCormick SA *et al.*: Anterior segment implantation cysts: Ultrasound biomicroscopy with histopathologic correlation. *Arch Ophthalmol* 116:1569, 1998

McCombe M, Heriot W: Penetrating ocular injury following local anaesthesia. *Aust N Z J Ophthalmol* 23:33, 1995

McDonald PR: Evolution of cataract surgery since the de Schweinitz era. *Ophthalmic Surg* 10:44, 1979

McDonnell PJ, Patel A, Green WR: Comparison of intracapsular and extracapsular cataract surgery: Histopathologic study of eyes obtained postmortem. *Ophthalmology* 92:1208, 1985

Melamed S, Cahane M, Gutman I *et al.*: Postoperative complications after Molteno implant surgery. *Am J Ophthalmol* 111:319, 1991

Michael JC, de Venecia G: Retinal trypsin digest study of cystoid macular edema associated with choroidal melanoma. *Am J Ophthalmol* 119:152, 1995

Miller K, Glasgow B: Bacterial endophthalmitis following sutureless cataract surgery. *Arch Ophthalmol* 111:377, 1993

Moshirfar M, Whitehead G, Beutler BC *et al.*: Toxic anterior segment syndrome after Verisyse iris-supported phakic intraocular lens implantation. *J Cataract Refract Surg* 32:1233, 2006

Musa F, Aralikatti AK, Prasad S: Choroidal effusion and hypotony caused by severe anterior lens capsule contraction following cataract surgery. *Eur J Ophthalmol* 14:153, 2004

Nagashima RJ: Decreased incidence of capsule complications and vitreous loss during phacoemulsification in eyes with pseudoexfoliation syndrome. *J Cataract Refract Surg* 30:127, 2004

Naumann G, Rummelt V: Block excision of cystic and diffuse epithelial ingrowth of the anterior chamber. *Arch Ophthalmol* 110:223, 1992

Neuhann IM, Kleinmann G, Apple DJ *et al.*: Cocooning of an iris-fixated intraocular lens in a 3-year-old child after perforating injury: clinicopathologic correlation. *J Cataract Refract Surg* 31:1826, 2005

Nevyas AS, Raber IM, Eagle RC *et al.*: Acute band keratopathy following intracameral Viscoat. *Arch Ophthalmol* 105:958, 1987

Nissen KR, Fuchs J, Goldschmidt E *et al.*: Retinal detachment after cataract extraction in myopic eyes. *J Cataract Refract Surg* 24:772, 1998

Parikh CH, Edelhauser HF: Ocular surgical pharmacology: corneal endothelial safety and toxicity. *Curr Opin Ophthalmol* 14:178, 2003

Pearson P, Owen D, Van Meter W *et al.*: Vitreous loss rates in extracapsular cataract surgery by residents. *Ophthalmology* 96:1225, 1989

Peng Q, Henning A, Vasavada AR *et al.*: Posterior capsular plaque: A common feature of cataract surgery in the developing world. *Am J Ophthalmol* 125:621, 1998

Peterson WC, Yanoff M: Why retrobulbar anesthesia? *Trans Am Ophthalmol Soc* 88:136, 1990

Pohjalainen T, Vesti E, Uusitalo RJ *et al.*: Posterior capsular opacification in pseudophakic eyes with a silicone or acrylic intraocular lens. *Eur J Ophthalmol* 12:212, 2002

Pokroy R, Pollack A, Bukelman A: Retinal detachment in eyes with vitreous loss and an anterior chamber or posterior chamber intraocular lens. *J Cataract Refract Surg* 28:1997, 2000

Pulido J, Folberg R, Carter KO *et al.*: *Histoplasma capsulatum* endophthalmitis after cataract extraction. *Ophthalmology* 97:217, 1990

Putnam D, Wilson DJ, Morrison JC: Epithelial ingrowth and apparent filtering bleb encapsulation. *Am J Ophthalmol* 118:113, 1994

Rao GN, Aquavella JV, Goldberg SH *et al.*: Pseudophakic bullous keratopathy: Relationship to preoperative corneal endothelial status. *Ophthalmology* 91:1135, 1984

Riandelli G, Scassa C, Parisi V *et al.*: Cataract surgery as a risk factor for retinal detachment in very highly myopic eyes. *Ophthalmology* 110:2355, 2003

Rinkoff J, Doft B, Lobes L: Management of ocular penetration from injection of local anesthesia preceding cataract surgery. *Arch Ophthalmol* 109, 1991

Rossetti A, Doro D: Retained intravitreal lens fragments after phacoemulsification: complications and visual outcome in vitrectomized and nonvitrectomized eyes. *J Cataract Refract Surg* 28:310, 2002

Roy PN, Mehra KS, Deshpande PJ: Cataract surgery performed before 800 BC. *Br J Ophthalmol* 59:171, 1975

Rummelt V, Lang G, Yanoff M *et al.*: A 32-year follow-up of the rigid Schreck anterior chamber lens. *Arch Ophthalmol* 108:401, 1990

Rummelt V, Ruprecht KW, Boltze HJ *et al.*: Chronic *Alternaria alternata* endophthalmitis following intraocular lens implantation. *Arch Ophthalmol* 109:178, 1991

Sanchez-Galeana CA, Smith RJ, Sanders DR *et al.*: Lens opacities after posterior chamber phakic intraocular lens implantation. *Ophthalmology* 110:781, 2003

Sandhu R, Hunter P: Late spontaneous prolapse of a posterior chamber intraocular lens. *J Cataract Refract Surg* 31:2425, 2005

Sandvig KU, Dannevig L: Postoperative endophthalmitis: establishment and results of a national registry. *J Cataract Refract Surg* 29:1273, 2003

Schaumberg DA, Dana MR, Christen WG *et al.*: A systematic overview of the incidence of posterior capsule opacification. *Ophthalmology* 105:1213, 1998

Scott IU, Flynn HW Jr, Feuer W: Endophthalmitis after secondary intraocular lens implantation: A case-control study. *Ophthalmology* 102:1925, 1995

Seitzman GD: Cataract surgery in Fuchs' dystrophy. *Curr Opin Ophthalmol* 16:241, 2005

Shah M, Bathia J, Kothari K: Repair of late Descemet's membrane detachment with perfluoropropane gas. *J Cataract Refract Surg* 29:1242, 2003

Shirai K, Saika S, Okada Y *et al.*: Histology and immunochemistry of fibrous posterior capsule opacification in an infant. *J Cataract Refract Surg* 30:523, 2004

Sidoti PA, Minckler DS, Baerveldt G *et al.*: Epithelial ingrowth and glaucoma drainage implants. *Ophthalmology* 101:872, 1994

Sihota R, Saxena R, Agarwal HC: Intravitreal sodium hyaluronate and secondary glaucoma after complicated phacoemulsification. *J Cataract Refract Surg* 29:1226, 2003

Smith PW, Stark WJ, Maumenee AE *et al.*: Retinal detachment after extracapsular cataract extraction with posterior chamber intraocular lens. *Ophthalmology* 94:495, 1987

Smith RS, Boyle E, Rudt LA: Cyclocryotherapy: A light and electron microscopic study. *Arch Ophthalmol* 95:284, 1977

Sonada Y, Sano Y, Ksander B *et al.*: Characterization of cell-mediated immune responses elicited by orthotopic corneal allografts in mice. *Invest Ophthalmol Vis Sci* 36:427, 1995

Song A, Scott IU, Flynn HW Jr *et al.*: Delayed-onset bleb-associated endophthalmitis: clinical features and visual outcomes. *Ophthalmology* 109:985, 2002

Soylu M, Ozcan AA, Okay O *et al.*: Non-Hodgkin lymphoma presenting with uveitis occurring after blunt trauma. *Pediatr Hematol Oncol* 22:53, 2005

Speaker M, Guerrriero P, Met J *et al.*: A case-control study of risk factors for intraoperative suprachoroidal expulsive hemorrhage. *Ophthalmology* 98:202, 1991

Stangos AN, Pournaras CJ, Petropoulos IK: Occult anterior-chamber metallic fragment post-phacoemulsification masquerading as chronic recalcitrant postoperative inflammation. *Am J Ophthalmol* 139:541, 2005

Steinert R, Puliafito C, Kumar S *et al.*: Cystoid macular edema, retinal detachment, and glaucoma after Nd:YAG laser posterior capsulotomy. *Am J Ophthalmol* 112:373, 1991

Stonecipher K, Parmley V, Jensen H *et al.*: Infectious endophthalmitis following sutureless cataract surgery. *Arch Ophthalmol* 109:1562, 1991

Su WW, Chang SH: Spontaneous, late, in-the-bag intraocular lens subluxation in a patient with a previous acute angle-closure glaucoma attack. *J Cataract Refract Surg* 30:1805, 2004

Taban M, Behrens A, Newcomb RL *et al.*: Acute endophthalmitis following cataract surgery. A systematic review of the literature. *Arch Ophthalmol* 123:613, 2005

Tetz MR, Nimsgern C: Posterior capsule opacification: Part 2. Clinical findings. *J Cataract Refract Surg* 25:1662, 1999

Trivedi RH, Werner L, Apple DJ *et al.*: Post cataract-intraocular lens (IOL) surgery opacification. *Eye* 16:217, 2002

Tsilou E, Rubin BI, Abraham FA *et al.*: Bilateral late posterior chamber intraocular lens dislocation with the capsular bag in a patient with gyrate atrophy. *J Cataract Refract Surg* 30:1593, 2004

Vargas LG, Vroman DT, Solomon KD *et al.*: Epithelial downgrowth after clear cornea phacoemusification: report of two cases and review of literature. *Ophthalmology* 109:2331, 2002

Vinger PF, Mieler WF, Oestreicher JH *et al.*: Ruptured globes following radial and hexagonal keratotomy surgery. *Arch Ophthalmol* 114:129, 1996

Walker J, Dangel ME, Makley TA *et al.*: Postoperative *Propionibacterium granulosum* endophthalmitis. *Arch Ophthalmol* 108, 1990

Wang LC, Yang CM: Sterile endophthalmitis following intravitreal injection of triamcinolone acetonide. *Ocul Immunol Inflamm* 13:295, 2005

Wasserman D, Apple D, Castaneda V *et al.*: Anterior capsular tears and loop fixation of posterior chamber intraocular lenses. *Ophthalmology* 98:425, 1991

Werner L, Pandey SK, Escobar-Gomez M *et al.*: Anterior capsule opacification: A histopathological study comparing different IOL styles. *Ophthalmology* 107:463, 2000

Werner L, Pandey SK, Apple DJ *et al.*: Anterior capsule opacification: correlation of pathologic findings with clinical sequelae. *Ophthalmology* 108:1675, 2001

Werner L, Sher JH, Taylor JR *et al.*: Toxic anterior segment syndrome and possible association with ointment in the anterior chamber following cataract surgery. *J Cataract Refract Surg* 32:227, 2006

Whitcup SM, Belfort R Jr, de Smet MD *et al.*: Immunohistochemistry of the inflammatory response in *Propionibacterium acnes* endophthalmitis. *Arch Ophthalmol* 109:978, 1991

Wirostko WJ, Han DP, Mieler WF *et al.*: Suprachoroidal hemorrhage: outcome of surgical management according to hemorrhagic severity. *Ophthalmology* 105:2276, 1998

Wolner B, Liebmann JM, Sassani JW *et al.*: Late bleb-related endophthalmitis after trabeculectomy with adjunctive 5-fluorouracil. *Ophthalmology* 98:1053, 1991

Yanoff M, Redovan E: Anterior eyewall perforation during subconjunctival cataract block (abstract). *Ophthalmic Surg* 21:362, 1990

Yanoff M, Fine BS, Brucker AJ *et al.*: Pathology of human cystoid macular edema. *Surv Ophthalmol* 28(Suppl):505, 1984

Yanoff M, Scheie HG, Allman MI: Endothelialization of filtering bleb in iris nevus syndrome. *Arch Ophthalmol* 94:1933, 1976

Zimmerman P, Mamalis N, Alder J *et al.*: Chronic *Nocardia asteroides* endophthalmitis after extracapsular cataract extraction. *Arch Ophthalmol* 111:837, 1993

Complications of Retinal Detachment and Vitreous Surgery

Al-Jazzaf AM, Netland PA, Charles S: Incidence and management of elevated intraocular pressure after silicone oil injection. *J Glaucoma* 14:40, 2005

Avitabile T, Bonfiglio V, Cicero A *et al.*: Correlation between quantity of silicone oil emulsified in the anterior chamber and high pressure in vitrectomized eyes. *Retina* 22:443, 2002

Barr C: The histopathology of successful retinal reattachment. *Retina* 120:189, 1990

Barton JJ: "Retinal diplopia" associated with macular wrinkling. *Neurology* 63:925, 2004

Betis F, Leguay JM, Gastaud P *et al.*: Multinucleated giant cells in periretinal silicone granulomas are associated with progressive proliferative vitreoretinopathy. *Eur J Ophthalmol* 13:634, 2003

Canataroglu H, Varinli I, Ozcan AA *et al.*: Interleukin (IL)-6, interleukin (IL)-8 levels and cellular composition of the vitreous humor in proliferative diabetic retinopathy, proliferative vitreoretinopathy, and traumatic proliferative vitreoretinopathy. *Ocul Immunol Inflamm* 13:375, 2005

Chang C-J, Lai WW, Edward DP *et al.*: Apoptotic photoreceptor cell death after traumatic retinal detachment in humans. *Arch Ophthalmol* 113:880, 1995

Cheng L, Azen SP, El-Bradey MH *et al.*: Duration of vitrectomy and postoperative cataract in the vitrectomy for macular hole study. *Am J Ophthalmol* 132:881, 2001

Colosi NJ, Yanoff M: Intrusion of scleral implant associated with conjunctival epithelial ingrowth. *Am J Ophthalmol* 83:504, 1977

Cox MS, Schepens CL, Freeman HM: Retinal detachment due to ocular contusion. *Arch Ophthalmol* 76:678, 1966

Donker DL, Paridaens D, Mooy CM *et al.*: Blepharoptosis and upper eyelid swelling due to lipogranulomatous inflammation caused by silicone oil. *Am J Ophthalmol* 140:934, 2005

Eagle RC, Yanoff M, Morse PH: Anterior segment necrosis following scleral buckling in hemoglobin SC disease. *Am J Ophthalmol* 75:426, 1973

Fangtian D, Rongping D, Lin Z *et al.*: Migration of intraocular silicone into the cerebral ventricles. *Am J Ophthalmol* 140:156, 2005

Fasternberg D, Perry H, Donnenfeld E: Expulsive suprachoroidal hemorrhage with scleral buckling surgery. *Arch Ophthal*mol 109, 1991

Ferry AP: Histopathologic observations on human eyes following cyclocryotherapy for glaucoma. *Trans Am Acad Ophthalmol Otolaryngol* 83:90, 1977

Fu AD, McDonald HR, Eliott D *et al.*: Complications of general anesthesia using nitrous oxide in eyes with preexisting gas bubbles. *Retina* 22:569, 2002

Gedde SJ: Management of glaucoma after retinal detachment surgery. *Curr Opin Ophthalmol* 13:103, 2002

Jackson TL, Thiagarajan M, Murthy R *et al.*: Pupil block glaucoma in phakic and pseudophakic patients after vitrectomy with silicone oil injection. *Am J Ophthalmol* 132:414, 2001

Johnson D, Bartley G, Garrity J *et al.*: Massive epithelium-lined inclusion cysts after scleral buckling. *Am J Ophthalmol* 113:439, 1992

Kushner B: Subconjunctival cysts as a complication of strabismus surgery. *Arch Ophthalmol* 110:1243, 1992

Lobes LA Jr, Grand MG: Incidence of cystoid macular edema following scleral buckling procedure. *Arch Ophthalmol* 98:1230, 1980

Lois N, Wong D: Pseudophakic retinal detachment. *Surv Ophthalmol* 48:467, 2003

Meredith TA, Reeser FH, Topping TM *et al.*: Cystoid macular edema after retinal detachment surgery. *Ophthalmology* 87:1090, 1980

Mertens S, Bednarz J, Engelmann K: Evidence of toxic side effects of perfluorohexyloctane after vitreoretinal surgery as well as in previously established in vitro models with ocular cell types. *Graefes Arch Clin Exp Ophthalmol* 240:989, 2002

van Meurs JC: Slit-lamp visualization of aqueous flow through an inferior iridectomy. *Am J Ophthalmol* 136:364, 2003

Papp A, Toth J, Kerenyi T *et al.*: Silicone oil in the subarachnoidal space—a possible route to the brain? *Pathol Res Pract* 200:247, 2004

Perez RN, Phelps CD, Burton TC: Angle-closure glaucoma following scleral buckling operations. *Trans Am Acad Ophthal*mol *Otolaryngol* 81:247, 1976

Pulhorn G, Teichmann KD, Teichmann I: Intraocular fibrous proliferation as an incisional complication in pars plana vitrectomy. *Am J Ophthalmol* 83:810, 1977

Shields CL, Demirci H, Marr BP *et al.*: Expanding MIRAgel scleral buckle simulating an orbital tumor in four cases. *Ophthalm Plast Reconstr Surg* 21:32, 2005

Vukojevic N, Sikic J, Curkovic T *et al.*: Axial eye length after retinal detachment surgery. *Coll Antropol* 29(Suppl. 1):25:25, 2005

Wang LC, Wang TJ, Yang CM: Entrapped preretinal oil bubble: report of two cases. *Jpn J Ophthalmol* 50:277, 2006

Complications of Corneal Surgery

Asano-Kato N, Toda I, Hori-Komai Y *et al.*: Epithelial ingrowth after laser in situ keratomileusis: clinical features and possible mechanisms. *Am J Ophthalmol* 134:801, 2002

Bechera S, Grossniklaus HE, Waring GO: Subepithelial fibrosis after myopic epikeratoplasty: Report of a case. *Arch Ophthal*mol 110:228, 1992

Belin MW, Hannush SB, Yau CW *et al.*: Elevated intraocular pressure-induced interlamellar stromal keratitis. *Ophthalmology* 109:1929, 2002

Binder PS, Baumgartner SD, Fogle JA: Histopathology of a case of epikeratophakia (aphakic epikeratoplasty). *Arch Ophthalmol* 103:1357, 1985

Braunstein RE, Airiani S, Chang S: Epithelial ingrowth under a laser in situ keraomileusis flap after phacoemulsification. *J Cataract Refract Surg* 29:2239, 2003

Campos M, Hertzog L, Garbus J *et al.*: Photorefractive keratectomy for severe postkeratoplasty astigmatism. *Am J Ophthalmol* 114:429, 1992

Cheng AC, Rao SK, Leung GY *et al.*: Late traumatic flap dislocations after LASIK. *J Refract Surg* 22:500, 2006

Cockerham GC, Bijwaard K, Sheng Z-M: Primary graft failure: A clinicopathologic and molecular analysis. *Ophthalmology* 107:2083, 2000

Davidson RS, Brandt JD, Mannis MJ: Intraocular pressure-induced interlamellar keratitis after LASIK surgery. *J Glaucoma* 12:23, 2003

Donnenfeld ED, O'Brien TP, Solomon R *et al.*: Infectious keratitis after photorefractive keratectomy. *Ophthalmology* 110:743, 2003

Dudenhoefer EJ, Nouri M, Gipson IK *et al.*: Histopathology of explanted collar button keratoprostheses: a clinicopathologic correlation. *Cornea* 22:424, 2003

Esquenazi S, Bui V: Long-term refractive results of myopic LASIK complicated with intraoperative epithelial defects. *J Refract Surg* 22:54, 2006

Ferry AP, Madge GE, Mayer W: Epithelialization of the anterior chamber as a complication of penetrating keratoplasty. *Ann Ophthalmol* 17:414, 1985

Freitas D, Alvarenga L, Sampaio J *et al.*: An outbreak of *Mycobacterium chelonae* after Lasik. *Ophthalmology* 110:276, 2003

Fulton JC, Cohen EJ, Rapuano CJ: Bacterial ulcer 3 days after excimer laser keratectomy. *Arch Ophthalmol* 114:626, 1996

Gabison EE, Chastang P, Menashi S *et al.*: Late corneal perforation after photorefractive keratectomy associated with topical diclofenac: involvement of matrix metalloproteinases. *Ophthalmology* 110:1626, 2003

Garg P, Bansal AK, Sharma S *et al.*: Bilateral infectious keratitis after laser in situ keratomileusis: A case report and review of the literature. *Ophthalmology* 108:121, 2001

Glasgow B, Brown H, Aizuss D *et al.*: Traumatic dehiscence of incisions seven years after radial keratotomy. *Am J Ophthalmol* 106:703, 1988

Grimmett MR, Holland EJ, Krachmer JH: Therapeutic keratoplasty after radial keratotomy. *Am J Ophthalmol* 118:108, 1994

Gussler JR, Miller D, Jaffe M *et al.*: Infection after radial keratotomy. *Am J Ophthalmol* 119:798, 1995

Heidemann DG, Dunn SP, Watts JC: *Aspergillus* keratitis after radial keratotomy. *Am J Ophthalmol* 120:254, 1995

Hicks CR, Crawford GJ: Melting after keratoprosthesis implantation: the effects of medroxyprogesterone. *Cornea* 22:497, 2003

Hicks CR, Hamilton S: Retroprosthetic membranes in AlphaCor patients: risk factors and prevention. *Cornea* 24:692, 2005

Hill VE, Brownstein S, Jackson WB *et al.*: Infectious keratopathy complicating photorefractive keratectomy. *Arch Ophthalmol* 116:1383, 1998

Imamura A, Amano S, Oshika T: Corneal bed perforation by laser ablation during laser in situ keratomileusis. *J Cataract Refract Surg* 29:1638, 2003

Jabbur NS, Chicani CF, Kuo IC *et al.*: Risk factors in interface epithelialization after laser in situ keratomileusis. *J Refract Surg* 20:343, 2004

Joo C-K, Pepose JS, Stuart PM: T-cell mediated responses in a murine model of orthotopic corneal transplantation. *Invest* Ophthalmol Vis Sci 36:1530, 1995

Kahle G, Stradter H, Seiler T *et al.*: Gas chromatographic and mass spectroscopic analysis of excimer and erbium: yttrium aluminum garnet laser-ablated human cornea. *Invest Ophthalmol Vis Sci* 33:2180, 1992

Karp CL, Tuli SS, Yoo SH *et al.*: Infectious keratitis after LASIK. *Ophthalmology* 110:503, 2003

Khoury JM, Haddad WF, Noureddin B: LASIK for high myopic astigmatism resulting from perforating ocular injury. *J Refract Surg* 21:756, 2005

Klein SR, Epstein RJ, Randleman JB *et al.*: Corneal ectasia after laser in situ keratomileusis in patients without apparent preoperative risk factors. *Cornea* 25:388, 2006

Kohnen T, Koch DD, Font RL: Lensification of the posterior corneal surface: An unusual proliferation of lens epithelial cells. *Ophthalmology* 104:1343, 1997

Kremer I, Rapuano C, Cohen E *et al.*: Retrocorneal fibrous membranes in failed corneal grafts. *Am J Ophthalmol* 115:478, 1993

Kurup SK, Coleman H, Chan CC: Corneal pseudomembrane from acute inflammatory response and fibrin formation to acute myeloid leukemic infiltrate. *Am J Ophthalmol* 139:921, 2005

Lang GK, Green WR, Maumenee AE: Clinicopathologic studies of keratoplasty eyes obtained post mortem. *Am J Ophthalmol* 101:28, 1986

Lee BL, Manche EE, Glascow BJ: Rupture of radial and arcuate keratotomy scars by blunt trauma 91 months after incisional keratotomy. *Am J Ophthalmol* 120:108, 1995

Leger F, Mortemousque B, Morel D *et al.*: Penetrating corneal transplant with inadvertent corneal button inversion. *Am J Ophthalmol* 135:91, 2003

Levartovsky S, Rosenwaser GOD, Goodman DF: Bacterial keratitis after laser in situ keratomileusis. *Ophthalmology* 108:321, 2001

Lifshitz T, Levy J, Mahler O *et al.*: Peripheral sterile corneal infiltrates after refractive surgery. *J Cataract Refract Surg* 31:1392, 2005

Maldonado MJ, Juberias JR, Pinero DP *et al.*: Flap tearing during lift-flap laser in situ keratomileusis retreatment. *J Cataract Refract Surg* 31:2016, 2005

McDonald M, Liu J, Byrd T *et al.*: Central photorefractive keratectomy for myopia. *Ophthalmology* 98:1327, 1991

McLeod SD, Flowers CW, Lopez PF *et al.*: Endophthalmitis and orbital cellulitis after radial keratotomy. *Ophthalmology* 102:1902, 1995

Meyer JC, Stulting RD, Thompson KP *et al.*: Late onset of corneal scar after laser photorefractive keratectomy. *Am J Ophthalmol* 121:529, 1996

Moshirfar M, Marx DP, Barsam CA *et al.*: Salzmann's-like nodular degeneration following laser in situ keratomileusis. *J Cataract Refract Surg* 31:2021, 2005

Mulhern MG, Naor J, Rootman DS: The role of epithelial defects in intralamellar inflammation after laser in situ keratomileusis. *Can J Ophthalmol* 37:409, 2002

Naoumidi I, Papadaki T, Zacharopoulos I *et al.*: Epithelial ingrowth after laser in situ keratomileussi: a histopathologic study in human corneas. *Arch Ophthalmol* 121:950, 2003

Nirankari VS, Karesh JW: Cystoid macular edema following penetrating keratoplasty: incidence and prognosis. *Ophthalmic Surg* 17:404, 1986

Ozler S, Liaw L, Neev J *et al.*: Acute ultrastructural changes of cornea after excimer laser ablation. *Invest Ophthalmol Vis Sci* 33:540, 1992

Panda A, Das GK, Vanathi M *et al.*: Corneal infection after radial keratotomy. *J Cataract Refract Surg* 24:331, 1998

Pande M, Hillman J: Optical zone centration in keratorefractive surgery. *Ophthalmology* 100:1230, 1993

Perez VL, Colby KA, Azar DT: Epithelial ingrowth in the flap-graf interface after microkeratome-assisted posterior penetrating keratoplasty. *J Cataract Refract Surg* 29:2225, 2003

Perry H, Donnenfeld E: Cryptococcal keratitis after keratoplasty. *Am J Ophthalmol* 110:320, 1990

Price FW Jr, Price MO: Descemet's stripping with endothelial keratoplasty in 50 eyes: a refractive neutral corneal transplant. *J Refract Surg* 21:339, 2005

Randleman JB, Thompson KP, Staver PR: Wavefront aberrations from corneal ectasia after laser in situ keratomileusis demonstrated by Inter-Wave aberrometry. *J Refract Surg* 20:170, 2004

Ray S, Khan BF, Dohlman CH *et al.*: Management of vitreoretinal complications in eyes with permanent keratoprosthesis. *Arch Ophthalmol* 120:559, 2002

Read RW, Chuck RSH, Rao NA *et al.*: Traumatic *Acremonium atrogriseum* keratitis following laser-assisted in situ keratomileusis. *Arch Ophthalmol* 118:418, 2000

Rezende RA, Uchoa UC, Cohen EJ *et al.*: Complications associated with anterior basement membrane dystrophy after laser in situ keratomileusis. *J Cataract Refract Surg* 30:2328, 2004

Sano-Kato N, Toda I, Fukumoto T *et al.*: Detection of neutrophils in late-onset interface inflammation associated with flap injury after laser in situ keratomileusis. *Cornea* 23:306, 2004

Seiler T, Wollensak J: Myopic photorefractive keratectomy with the excimer laser. *Ophthalmology* 98:1156, 1991

Seiler T, Derse M, Pham T: Repeated excimer laser treatment after photorefractive keratectomy. *Arch Ophthalmol* 110:1230, 1992

Sharma N, Ghate D, Agarwal T *et al.*: Refractive outcomes of laser in situ keratomileusis after flap complications. *J Cataract Refract Surg* 31:1334, 2005

Sinbawy A, McDonnell P, Moreira H: Surface ultrastructure after excimer laser ablation. *Arch Ophthalmol* 109:1531, 1991

Solomon R, Donnenfeld ED, Azar DT *et al.*: Infectious keratitis after laser in situ keratmileusis: results of an ASCRS survey. *J Refract Surg* 29:2003, 2001

Sonavane MS, Sharma S, Gangopadhyaca N *et al.*: Clinico-microbiologoical correlation of suture-related graft infection following penetrating keratoplasty. *Am J Ophthalmol* 135:89, 2003

Sridhar MS, Garg P, Bansal MS *et al.*: *Aspergillus flavus* keratitis after laser in situ keratomileusis. *Am J Ophthalmol* 129:802, 2000

Sternberg P, Meredith T, Stewart M *et al.*: Retinal detachment in penetrating keratoplasty patients. *Am J Ophthalmol* 109:148, 1990

Swartz M: Histology of macular photocoagulation. *Ophthalmology* 93:959, 1986

Taban M, Behrens A, Newcomb RL *et al.*: Incidence of acute endophthalmitis following penetrating keratoplasty. A systematic review. *Arch Ophthalmol* 123:605, 2005

Toshino A, Uno T, Ohashi Y *et al.*: Transient keratectasia caused by intraocular pressure elevation after laser in situ keratomileusis. *J Cataract Refract Surg* 31:202, 2005

Tsuji K, Yamamoto T, Hori-Komai Y *et al.*: Traumatic epithelial flap detachment after laser subepithelial keratomileusis. *J Refract Surg* 22:305, 2006

Vinger PF, Mieler WF, Oestreicher JH *et al.*: Ruptured globes following radial and hexagonal keratotomy surgery. *Arch Ophthalmol* 114:129, 1996

Wang MY, Maloney RK: Epithelial ingrowth after laser in situ keratomileusis. *Am J Ophthalmol* 129:746, 2000

Waring GO: Making sense of keratospeak IV. *Arch Ophthalmol* 110:1385, 1992

Wilson DJ, Green WR: Histopathologic study of the effect of retinal detachment surgery on 49 eyes obtained post mortem. *Am J Ophthalmol* 103:167, 1987

Wu W, Stark W, Green WR: Corneal wound healing after 193-nm excimer laser keratectomy. *Arch Ophthalmol* 109:1426, 1991

Wylegala E, Tarnawska D, Dobrowolski D: Deep lamellar keratoplasty for various corneal lesions. *Eur J Ophthalmol* 14:467, 2004

Yeh DL, Bushley DM, Kim T: Treatment of traumatic LASIK flap dislocation and epithelial ingrowth with fibrin glue. *Am J Ophthalmol* 141:960, 2006

Complications of Glaucoma Surgery

Al-Shahwan S, Edward DP: Foreign body granulomas secondary to retained sponge fragment following mitomycin C trabeculectomy. *Graefes Arch Clin Exp Ophthalmol* 243:178, 2005

Choi JS, Kim YY: Progression of peripheral anterior synechiae after laser iridotomy. *Am J Ophthalmol* 140:1125, 2005

Edmunds B, Thompson JR, Salmon JF et al.: The National Survey of Trabeculectomy. III. Early and late complications. *Eye* 16:297, 2002

Hu CY, Matsuo H, Tomita G et al.: Clinical characteristics and leakage of functioning blebs after trabeculectomy with mitomycin-C in primary glaucoma patients. *Ophthalmology* 110:345, 2003

Sauder G, Jonas JB: Limbal stem cell deficiency after subconjunctival mitomycin C injection for trabeculectomy. *Am J Ophthalmol* 141:1129, 2006

Verner-Cole EA, Ortiz S, Bell NP et al.: Subretinal suture misdirection during 360 degrees suture trabeculotomy. *Am J Ophthalmol* 141:391, 2006

Complications of Nonsurgical Trauma

Agrawal A, McKibbin MA: Purtscher's and Purtscher-like retinopathies: a review. *Surv Ophthalmol* 51:129, 2006

Aguilar JP, Green WR: Choroidal rupture: A histopathologic study of 47 cases. *Retina* 4:269, 1984

Al-Towerki AE: Corneal honeybee sting. *Cornea* 22:672, 2003

Anand A, Harrison RJ: Annular pigment band on the posterior capsule following blunt ocular trauma: a case report. *BMC Ophthalmol* 20:13, 2005

Arcieri ES, Franca ET, de Oliveria HB et al.: Ocular lesions arising after stings by hymenopteran insects. *Cornea* 21:328, 2002

Blodi FC: Mustard gas keratopathy. *Int Ophthalmol Clin* 11:1, 1971

Blodi B, Johnson M, Gass D et al.: Purtscher's-like retinopathy after childbirth. *Ophthalmology* 97:1654, 1990

Chang C-J, Lai WW, Edward DP et al.: Apoptotic photoreceptor cell death after traumatic retinal detachment in humans. *Arch Ophthalmol* 113:880, 1995

Charles NC, Rabin S: Calcific phacolysis. *Arch Ophthalmol* 113:786, 1995

Chaudhry IA, Al-Sharif AM, Hamdi M: Severe ocular and periocular injuries caused by an ostrich. *Ophthalm Plast Reconstr Surg* 19:246, 2003

Chaudhuri Z, Pandey PK, Bhatia A: Electrical cataract: a case study. *Ophthalmic Surg Lasers* 33:166, 2002

Chen CC, Yang CM, Hu FC et al.: Penetrating ocular injury caused by venomous snakebite. *Am J Ophthalmol* 140:544, 2005

Chen YT, Huang CW, Huang FC et al.: The cleavage plane of corneal epithelial adhesion complex in traumatic recurrent corneal erosion. *Mol Vis* 12:196, 2006

Chorich LJ III, Davidorf FH, Chambers RB et al.: Bungee cord-associated ocular injuries. *Am J Ophthalmol* 125:270, 1998

Cogan DG: Pseudoretinitis pigmentosa. *Arch Ophthalmol* 81:45, 1969

Colosi NJ, Yanoff M: Reactive corneal endothelialization. *Am J Ophthalmol* 83:219, 1977

Cosar CB, Ceyhan N, Sevim S et al.: Corneal perforation with minor trauma: Ehlers–Danlos syndrome type VI. *Ophthalmic Surg Lasers Imaging* 36:350, 2005

Donisi PM, Rama P, Fasolo A et al.: Analysis of limbal stem cell deficiency by corneal impression cytology. *Cornea* 22:533, 2003

Dubovy SR, Guyton DL, Green WR: Clinicopathologic correlation of chorioretinitis sclopetaria. *Retina* 17:510, 1997

Eagle RC, Yanoff M: Cholesterolosis of the anterior chamber. *Graefes Arch Ophthalmol* 193:121, 1975

Eagle R, Yanoff M: Anterior chamber cholesterolosis. *Arch Ophthalmol* 108, 1990

Eagle RC Jr, Shields JA, Canny CLB et al.: Intraocular wooden foreign body clinically resembling a pearl cyst. *Arch Ophthalmol* 95:835, 1977

Ells AL, Kherani A, Lee D: Epiretinal membrane formation is a late manifestation of shaken baby syndrome. *J AAPOS* 7:223, 2003

Elner S, Elner V, Arnall M et al.: Ocular and associated systemic findings in suspected child abuse. *Arch Ophthalmol* 108:1094, 1990

Emerson GG: Extension of retinal hemorrhage into the vitreous of a shaken baby through a break in the internal limiting membrane. *Arch Ophthalmol* 122:792, 2004

Fenton RH, Zimmerman LE: Hemolytic glaucoma: An unusual cause of acute open-angle secondary glaucoma. *Arch Ophthalmol* 70:236, 1963

Finkelstein M, Legmann A, Rubin PAD: Projectile metallic foreign bodies in the orbit: A retrospective study of epidemiologic factors, management, and outcomes. *Ophthalmology* 104:96, 1997

Foster BS, March GA, Lucarelli MJ et al.: Optic nerve avulsion. *Arch Ophthalmol* 115:623, 1997

Frangieh GT, Green WR, Engel HM: A histopathologic study of macular cysts and holes. *Retina* 1:311, 1981

Fraunfelder FT, Hanna C: Electric cataracts: I. Sequential changes, unusual and prognostic findings. *Arch Ophthalmol* 87:179, 1972

Garg SJ, Benson W, Fineman M et al.: Bone from an orbital floor fracture causing an intraocular foreign body. *Am J Ophthalmol* 139:543, 2005

Gilles EE, McGregor ML, Levy-Clarke G: Retinal hemorrhage asymmetry in inflicted head injury: a clue to pathogenesis? *J Pediatr* 143:494, 2003

Giovinazzo VJ, Yannuzzi LA, Sorenson JA et al.: The ocular complications of boxing. *Ophthalmology* 94:587, 1987

Goldberg MF: Chorioretinal vascular anastomoses after perforating trauma to the eye. *Am J Ophthalmol* 85:171, 1978

Green WR, Robertson D: Pathologic findings of photic retinopathy in the human eye. *Am J Ophthalmol* 112:520, 1991

Hanna C, Fraunfelder FT: Electric cataracts: II. Ultrastructural lens changes. *Arch Ophthalmol* 87:184, 1972

Humayun M, de la Cruz Z, Maguire A et al.: Intraocular cilia. *Arch Ophthalmol* 111:1396, 1993

Ikeda N, Ikeda T, Nagata M et al.: Pathogenesis of transient high myopia after blunt eye trauma. *Ophthalmology* 109:501, 2002

Inkeles DM, Walsh JB, Matz R: Purtscher's retinopathy in acute pancreatitis. *Am J Med Sci* 272:335, 1976

Johnson RN, McDonald HR, Lewis H et al.: Traumatic macular hole: observations, pathogenesis, and results of vitrectomy surgery. *Ophthalmology* 108:853, 2001

Jonas JB, Knorr HLJ, Buddle WM: Prognostic factors in ocular injuries caused by intraocular or retrobulbar foreign bodies. *Ophthalmology* 107:823, 2000

Kay ML, Yanoff M, Katowitz JA: Development of sympathetic uveitis in spite of corticosteroid therapy. *Am J Ophthalmol* 78:90, 1974

Kobayashi A, Maeda A, Sugiyama K: In vivo confocal microscopy in the acute phase of corneal inflammation. *Ophthalmic Surg Lasers Imaging* 34:433, 2003

Kozart DM, Yanoff M, Katowitz JA: Tolerated eyelash embedded in the retina. *Arch Ophthalmol* 91:235, 1974

Liem ATA, Keunen JEE, van Norren D: Reversible cone photoreceptor injury in commotio retinae of the macula. *Retina* 15:58, 1995

Lovejoy B, Cleasby A, Hassell AM et al.: Structure of the catalytic domain of fibroblast collagenase complexed with an inhibitor. *Science* 263:375, 1994

Lucas DR, Dunham AC, Lee WR et al.: Ocular injuries from liquid golf ball cores. *Br J Ophthalmol* 60:740, 1976

Mackiewicz J, Howicz-Matejko E, Salaga-Pylak M et al.: Work-related, penetrating eye injuries in rural environments. *Ann Agric Environ Med* 12:27, 2005

Magovern M, Wright JD Jr, Mohammed A: Spheroidal degeneration of the cornea: a clinicopathologic case report. *Cornea* 23:84, 2004

Maguluri S, Bueno CL, Fuller IB et al.: Delayed suprachoroidal hemorrhage and factor VIII deficiency. *Am J Ophthalmol* 139:195, 2005

Mansour A, Green WR, Hogge C: Histopathology of commotio retinae. *Retina* 12:24, 1992

McDonnell PJ, Green WR, Stevens RE et al.: Blood staining of the cornea: Light microscopic and ultrastructural features. *Ophthalmology* 92:1668, 1985

McKelvie PA, Walland MJ: Pathology of cyclodiode laser: a series of nine enucleated eyes. *Br J Ophthalmol* 86:381, 2002

Meyer RF, Hood CI: Fungus implantation with wooden intraocular foreign bodies. *Ann Ophthalmol* 9:271, 1977

Minatoya HK: Eye injuries from exploding car batteries. *Arch Ophthalmol* 96:477, 1978

Moon SJ, Kim JE, Han DP: Lightning-induced maculopathy. *Retina* 25:380, 2005

Morad Y, Kim YM, Armstrong DC et al.: Correlation between retinal abnormalities and intracranial abnormalities in the shaken baby syndrome. *Am J Ophthalmol* 134:354, 2002

Ng W, Chehade M: Taser penetrating ocular injury. *Am J Ophthalmol* 139:713, 2005

Orlin S, Farber M, Brucker A et al.: The unexpected guest: Problem of iris reposition. *Surv Ophthalmol* 35:59, 1990

Perry HD, Rahn EK: Chorioretinitis sclopetaria. *Arch Ophthalmol* 95:328, 1977

Pfister RR, Haddox JL, Sommers CI et al.: Identification and synthesis of chemotactic tripeptides from alkali-degraded corneas. *Invest Ophthalmol Vis Sci* 36:1306, 1995

Pierre-Kahn V, Roche O, Dureau P et al.: Ophthalmologic findings in suspected child abuse victims with subdural hematomas. *Ophthalmology* 110:1718, 2003

Pilger IS, Khwarg SG: Angle recession glaucoma: Review and two case reports. *Ann Ophthalmol* 17:197, 1985

Portellos M, Orlin SE, Kozart DM: Electric cataracts. *Arch Ophthalmol* 114:1022, 1996

Potts AM, Distler JA: Shape factor in the penetration of intraocular foreign bodies. *Am J Ophthalmol* 100:183, 1985

Power MH, Regillo CD, Custis, PH: Thrombotic thrombocytopenic purpura associated with Purtscher's retinopathy. *Arch Ophthalmol* 115:128, 1997

Rani A, Pal N, Vohra R et al.: Subretinal dislocation of the crystalline lens: unusual complication of phacoemulsification. *J Cataract Refract Surg* 31:1843, 2005

Riffenburgh R, Sathyavagiswaran L: Ocular findings at autopsy of child abuse victims. *Ophthalmology* 98:1519, 1991

Risco J, Millar L: Ultrastructural alterations in the endothelium in a patient with topical anesthetic abuse keratopathy. *Ophthalmology* 99:628, 1992

Rosenthal AR, Marmor MF, Leuenberger P et al.: Chalcosis: A study of natural history. *Ophthalmology* 86:1956, 1979

Sangwan VS, Vemuganti GK, Iftekhar G et al.: Use of autologous cultured limbal and conjunctival epithelium in a patient with severe bilateral ocular surface disease induced by acid injury: a case report of unique application. *Cornea* 22:478, 2003

Schatz H, Drake M: Self-injected retinal emboli. *Ophthalmology* 86:468, 1979

Scroggs M, Proia A, Charles NC et al.: Calcific phacolysis. *Ophthalmology* 100:377, 1993

Shields JA, Fammartino J, Shields CL: Coats' disease as a cause of anterior chamber cholesterolosis. *Arch Ophthalmol* 113:975, 1995

Sloan SH: Champagne cork injury to the eye. *Trans Am Acad Ophthalmol Otolaryngol* 79:889, 1975

Snady-McCoy L, Morse PH: Retinopathy associated with acute pancreatitis. *Am J Ophthalmol* 100:246, 1985

Soheilian M, Feghi M, Yazdani S et al.: Surgical management of non-metallic and non-magnetic metallic intraocular foreign bodies. *Ophthalmic Surg Lasers Imaging* 36:189, 2005

Sommer LK, Lund-Andersen H: Skin burn, bilateral iridocyclitis and amnesia following a lightning injury. *Acta Ophthalmol Scand* 82:596, 2004

Sowka JW: Pupil block glaucoma from traumatic vitreous prolapse in a patient with posterior chamber lens implantation. *Optometry* 73:685, 2002

Stern JD, Goldfarb IW, Slater H: Ophthalmological complications as a manifestation of burn injury. *Burns* 22:135, 1996

Stulting RD, Rodrigues MM, Nay RE: Ultrastructure of traumatic corneal endothelial rings. *Am J Ophthalmol* 101:156, 1986

Talamo JH, Topping TM, Maumenee AE et al.: Ultrastructural studies of cornea, iris and lens in a case of siderosis bulbi. *Ophthalmology* 92:1675, 1985

Tawara A: Transformation and cytotoxicity of iron in siderosis bulbi. *Invest Ophthalmol Vis Sci* 27:226, 1986

Tesluk GC, Spaeth GL: The occurrence of primary open-angle glaucoma in the fellow eye of patients with unilateral angle-cleavage glaucoma. *Ophthalmology* 92:904, 1985

Thomas MA, Parrish RK II, Feuer WJ: Rebleeding after traumatic hyphema. *Arch Ophthalmol* 104:206, 1986

Weingeist TA, Goldman EJ, Folk JC et al.: Terson's syndrome: Clinicopathologic correlations. *Ophthalmology* 93:1435, 1986

Wolff SM, Zimmerman LE: Chronic secondary glaucoma associated with retrodisplacement of iris root and deepening of the anterior chamber angle secondary to contusion. *Am J Ophthalmol* 54:547, 1962

Wong TY, Seet B, Ang C-L: Eye injuries in twentieth century warfare: a historical perspective. *Surv Ophthalmol* 22:135, 1997

Wright PL, Wilkinson CP, Balyeat HD et al.: Angiographic cystoid macular edema after posterior chamber lens implantation. *Arch Ophthalmol* 106:740, 1988

Yanoff M: Incidence of bone-marrow embolism due to closed-chest cardiac massage. *N Engl J Med* 269:837, 1963

Yanoff M, Kurata F, Lamensdorf M: Inexpensive device to reduce surgical light exposure. *Ophthalmology* 90(Suppl):137, 1983

Zion VM, Burton TC: Retinal dialysis. *Arch Ophthalmol* 98:1971, 1980

6

Skin and Lacrimal Drainage System

NORMAL ANATOMY (Figs 6.1 and 6.2)

Epidermis

Lid skin is quite thin.
- I. The epidermis is composed of only a few layers of squamous cells (keratinocytes) and a basal layer; the typical large rete ridge or peg (digitated) pattern is absent.
- II. Admixed with the epithelial cells are dendritic melanocytes and Langerhans' cells (dendritic-appearing cells expressing class II antigen).
  - A. Multiple coloboma-like defects of the eyelids have been noted in association with eyelid involvement in Langerhans' cell histiocytosis, which is a proliferation of histiocytes of the mononuclear phagocyte system.

Dermis

The dermis is sparse, composed of delicate collagen fibrils, and contains the epidermal appendages (i.e., sebaceous glands, apocrine and eccrine sweat glands, and hair complex) and vasculature.

Subcutaneous Tissue

The subcutaneous layer is mostly composed of adipose tissue.

TERMINOLOGY

Orthokeratosis and Parakeratosis

- I. The stratum corneum (keratin layer) is thickened.

> *Hyperkeratosis* means "increased scale" and includes both orthokeratosis and parakeratosis. In orthokeratosis, a thick granular layer is usually found because the epidermal cells slowly migrate upward; when the migration upward is rapid, no granular cells are seen and parakeratosis results. *Orthokeratosis* is hyperkeratosis composed of cells that have complete keratinization and no nuclear remnants, whereas *parakeratosis* is hyperkeratosis that shows incomplete keratinization in which nuclei are retained in the cells of the stratum corneum. Orthokeratosis and parakeratosis often exist in the same lesion (Fig. 6.3A).

- II. Orthokeratosis commonly is seen in verruca and the scaly lesions such as actinic and seborrheic keratoses.
- III. Parakeratosis is characteristic of psoriasis and other inflammatory conditions (e.g., seborrheic keratosis).

Acanthosis

- I. The stratum spinosum (squamous or prickle-cell layer) of the epidermis shows increased thickness (see Fig. 6.3B).
- II. It is commonly seen in many proliferative epithelial lesions (e.g., papilloma, actinic keratosis, squamous cell carcinomas, and pseudoepitheliomatous hyperplasia).

Dyskeratosis

- I. Dyskeratosis is keratinization of individual cells within the stratum spinosum, where the cells are not normally

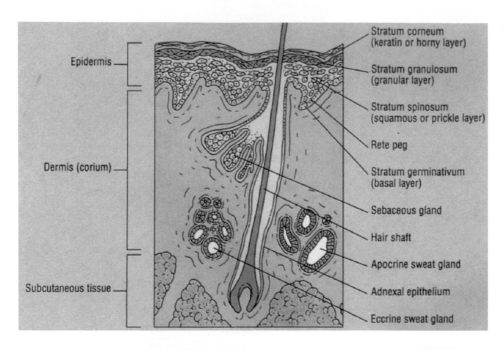

Epidermis

Dermis (corium)

Subcutaneous tissue

Stratum corneum
(keratin or horny layer)

Stratum granulosum
(granular layer)

Stratum spinosum
(squamous or prickle layer)

Rete peg

Stratum germinativum
(basal layer)

Sebaceous gland

Hair shaft

Apocrine sweat gland

Adnexal epithelium

Eccrine sweat gland

Fig. 6.1 Normal layers of skin.

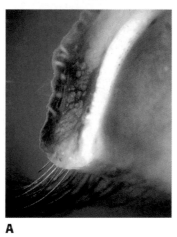

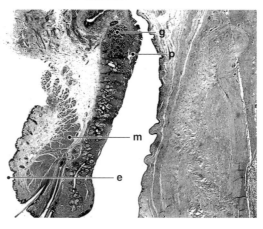

A   **B**

Fig. 6.2 Normal anatomy. **A,** Cross-section of the eyelid shows the inner white tarsal plate, the middle layers of muscle fibers, and the surface epithelium. Note the cilia coming out of the lid margin inferiorly. **B,** Histologic section shows the inner tarsal plate (p) containing the meibomian glands, the middle muscular bundles (m), and the surface epithelium (e). The cilia exit from the middle portion of the lid margin inferiorly. Apocrine sweat glands, eccrine sweat glands, sebaceous glands of Zeis, and hair follicles of the surface lanugo hairs are also seen in the lids (see also Figs 1.26C and 7.1) (g, accessory lacrimal glands). (**A,** Courtesy of Dr. RC Eagle, Jr.)

keratinized (Fig. 6.4A; see Fig. 7.17). The keratinizing cells show abundant pink (eosinophilic) cytoplasm and small, normal-appearing nuclei.

In contrast, necrotic keratinocytes have homogeneous pink cytoplasm and nuclear karyolysis and pyknosis.

II. Dyskeratosis is characteristic of benign familial intraepithelial dyskeratosis, Darier's disease, and Bowen's disease, and is sometimes seen in actinic keratosis, in squamous cell carcinoma, and after sunburn.

Acantholysis

I. Acantholysis is a separation of epidermal cells that results from a variety of pathologic processes, and causes a dissolution or degeneration of the intercellular connections (see Figs 6.5 and 6.27).

II. Acantholysis is commonly seen in viral vesicles (e.g., herpes simplex), inverted follicular keratosis (IFK), pemphigus, and Darier's disease.

Bulla

I. A bulla is a fluid-filled space in the epidermis or beneath it (see Fig. 6.5).

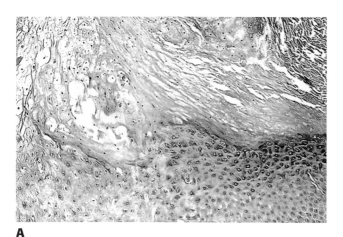

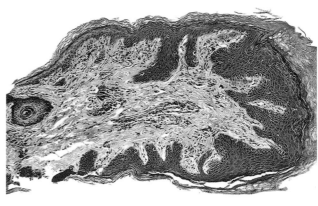

A   **B**

Fig. 6.3 Orthokeratosis, parakeratosis, and acanthosis. **A,** In this actinic keratosis, orthokeratosis (hyperkeratosis) is present (right half of picture) where the granular cell layer is prominent. Parakeratosis is present (left half of picture) where nuclei are retained in cells of keratin layer; granular cell layer is not prominent. **B,** In this squamous papilloma, acanthosis is present, especially on right side, evidenced by thickening of prickle-cell (squamous) layer. The granular cell layer is also thickened and orthokeratosis is present.

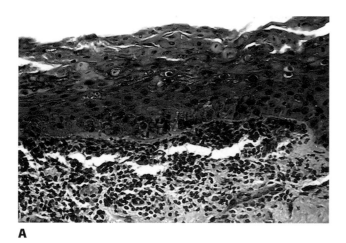

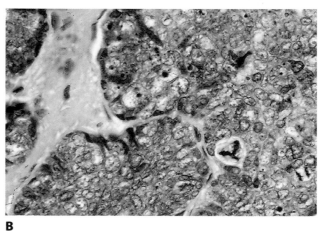

A   **B**

Fig. 6.4 Dyskeratosis and atypical cells. **A,** In this case of hereditary benign intraepithelial dyskeratosis, keratinization of individual cells is present in the stratum spinosum (squamous or prickle-cell layer)—see also Fig. 7.17B. **B,** In this sebaceous gland carcinoma, many atypical cells are seen, including a tripolar mitotic figure.

Spongiosis is fluid accumulation between keratinocytes (intercellular edema), which may lead to cleft or vesicle formation. It is commonly seen in inflammatory conditions, especially the spectrum of dermatitides. *Ballooning* is intracellular edema characteristic of virally infected cells.

II. A small bulla is arbitrarily called a *vesicle*.

Vesicles and bullae may arise from primary cell damage or acantholysis. They may be located under the keratin layer (subcorneal), between the epithelium and dermis (junctional), or in the middle layers of epithelium.

Atrophy

I. Atrophy (see subsection *Atrophy* later, under *Aging*, and Fig. 6.8) is: (1) thinning of the epidermis; (2) smoothing or diminution (effacement) of rete ridges ("pegs"); (3) disorder of epidermal architecture; (4) diminution or loss of epidermal appendages such as hair; and (5) alterations of the collagen and elastic dermal fibers.

II. Atrophy is commonly seen in aging.

It may also be seen in the epidermis overlying a slow-growing tumor in the corium.

Atypical Cell

I. An atypical cell (see Fig. 6.4B) is one in which the normal nucleus-to-cytoplasm ratio is altered in favor of the nucleus, which stains darker than normal (*hyperchromasia*), may show an abnormal configuration (giant form or multinucleated form), may have an abnormal nuclear configuration (e.g., indented, cerebriform, multinucleated), or may

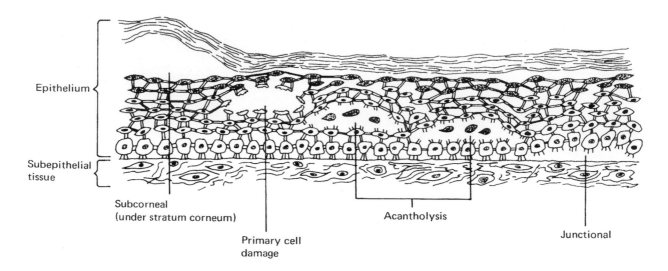

Epithelium

Subepithelial tissue

Subcorneal (under stratum corneum)

Primary cell damage

Acantholysis

Junctional

Fig. 6.5 Varieties of bullae encountered in skin.

contain an abnormal mitotic figure (e.g., tripolar metaphase).

If sufficiently atypical, according to generally accepted criteria, the cell may be classified as cancerous.

> It is the overall pattern of the tissue rather than any one individual cell that aids in the diagnosis of cancer; one dyskeratotic or atypical cell does not necessarily mean the tissue is cancerous.

II. Isolated atypical cells may be found in benign conditions such as actinic keratosis and pseudoepitheliomatous hyperplasia.

Atypical cells may be abundant in malignant conditions such as carcinoma in situ and squamous cell carcinoma.

Leukoplakia

I. Leukoplakia (white plaque) is a clinical term (*not* a histopathologic term) that is usually applied to mucous membrane lesions. The clinical appearance is caused by the orthokeratosis (hyperkeratosis).
II. Clinically, any mucous membrane (conjunctival) lesion that contains orthokeratosis appears as a white plaque (leukoplakia; e.g., orthokeratosis induced by an underlying pinguecula, pterygium, papilloma, or carcinoma in situ).

Polarity

I. Tissue polarity refers to the arrangement of epithelial cells in the epithelium [i.e., in normal polarity an orderly transition exists from basal cells to prickle (acanthocytes), to squamous cells, and so forth].
II. Complete loss of polarity (see Fig. 7.21) has occurred when the cells at the surface are indistinguishable from the cells at the base because of loss of the normal sequence of cell maturation (e.g., in squamous cell carcinoma).

A. Spatial relationships between cells are also disturbed.
B. Disorganized epithelial architecture is often a better means of diagnosing epithelial malignancy than is individual cell morphology.

CONGENITAL ABNORMALITIES

Dermoid and Epidermoid Cysts

See p. 540 in Chapter 14.

Phakomatous Choristoma

I. Phakomatous choristoma (Fig. 6.6) is a rare, congenital, choristomatous tumor (i.e., a tumor of tissue not normally found in the area) of lenticular anlage, usually involving the inner aspect of the lower lid.
II. Histologically, cells resembling lens epithelial cells and lens "bladder" cells along with patches of a thick, irregular periodic acid–Schiff (PAS)-positive membrane closely simulating lens capsule are seen growing irregularly in a dense fibrous tissue matrix.

Positive staining for vimentin, S-100 protein, and numerous antibodies against lens-specific proteins strongly support the lenticular anlage origin.

> An unusual complex choristoma of the lateral canthus has been reported to contain elements of hair follicle nevus, bulbar dermoid, epibulbar osseous choristoma, and accessory tragus. It is proposed that the lesion is the result of faulty migration of pluripotential cells during embryogenesis.

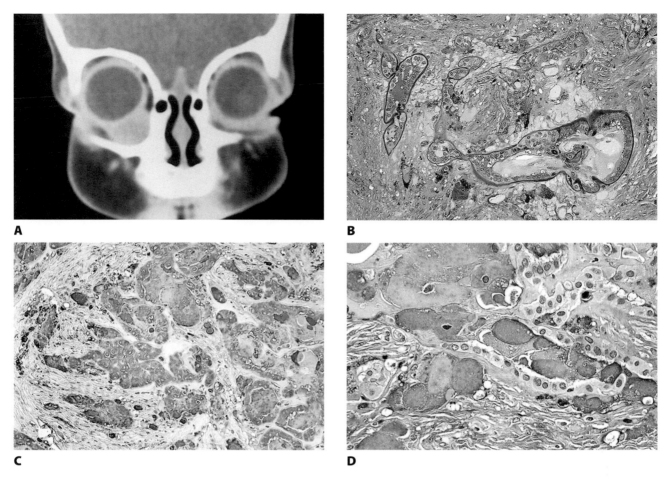

Fig. 6.6 Phakomatous choristoma. **A,** Mass, present since birth, seen in lower lid of 10-week-old infant. **B,** Nests of benign cells resembling lens epithelial cells present in abnormal (choristomatous) location in dermis of lower lid. Periodic acid–Schiff-positive membrane mimics lens capsule. Anti-α lens protein (**C**) and anti-β crystallin (**D**) immunohistochemical stains are both positive. (Case presented by Dr. RC Eagle, Jr. to the meeting of the Verhoeff Society in 1992 and reported in Ellis FJ *et al.: Ophthalmology* 100:955, 1993.)

Miscellaneous Choristomas and Hamartomas

I. Nevus lipomatosus (pedunculated nevus) has been reported on the eyelid of an 11-year-old boy having an eyelid papule that had been present since birth and was gradually enlarging. Histologically, the lesion was polypoid in shape and consisted of mature adipocytes within the dermis and subconjunctival mucosa consistent with nevus lipomatosus.

II. Juvenile hyaline fibromatosis is characterized by multiple facial nodules, gingival fibromatosis, and osteolytic lesions in the proximal metaphysis of the tibia and humerus symmetrically. It has presented as an eyelid tumor scalloping the superior orbital osseous rim and resulting in blepharoptosis.

III. Neurocutaneous pattern syndromes are a group of disorders characterized by congenital abnormalities involving both the skin and the nervous system for which no identifiable cause has been isolated. Examples are encephalocraniocutaneous lipomatosis, oculocerebrocutaneous syndrome, and linear nevus sebaceous syndrome.

A. Encephalocraniocutaneous lipomatosis is rare and characterized by congenital cutaneous, ocular, and neurologic abnormalities, particularly involving the head and neck. It has been reported in a boy with lipomatous brown pigmented plaques of the top of the skull with accompanying alopecia, ptosis, bulbar conjunctival lipodermoid, microcalcifications, and atrophy of the cerebral parenchyma, and widening of the frontal subarachnoid space and the fissure of Sylvius. There were accompanying intraoral lesions, maxillary compound odontoma, and juvenile extranasopharyngeal angiofibroma of the gingiva.

B. Congenital lipoblastoma of the scalp involving the eyelid has been reported. Histopathologic examination revealed lobular adipose tissue separated by fibrous septa.

Cryptophthalmos (Ablepharon)

I. Cryptophthalmos is a rare condition in which the embryonic lid folds fail to develop.

II. Conjunctiva, cornea, and lid folds are replaced by skin that passes smoothly over the orbital margins. Palpebral structures and eyebrows cannot be identified.

Because the cornea is not formed or is rudimentary, an incision through the skin covering the anterior orbit may enter directly into the inside of the eye.

Microblepharon

Microblepharon is a rare condition in which the lids are usually normally formed but shortened; the shortening results in incomplete lid closure.

Coloboma

I. A coloboma of the lid is a defect that ranges from simple notching at the lid margin to complete absence of a segment of lid.
II. Other ocular and systemic anomalies may be found (see discussion of Goldenhar's syndrome, p. 265 in Chapter 8).
   A. Eyelid colobomas may be seen in the amniotic deformity, adhesion, and mutilation (ADAM) sequence in which a broad spectrum of anomalies having intrinsic causes (germ plasm defect, vascular disruption, and disturbance of threshold boundaries of morphogens during early gastrulation) alternate with extrinsic causes (amniotic band rupture) to explain the condition. In addition to mutilation (reduction) and deformity (ring constriction) of distal extremities there can be acrania, cephalocele, typical or atypical facial clefts, and celosomia in addition to skin evidence of a constriction band.

Epicanthus

I. Epicanthus consists of a rounded, downward-directed fold of skin covering the caruncular area of the eye. It is usually bilateral and is often inherited as an autosomal-dominant trait.

Epicanthus inversus is an upward-directed, rounded fold of skin.

II. Ptosis may be associated with epicanthus.

Ectopic Caruncle

A clinically and histologically normal caruncle may be present in the tarsal area of the lower lid.

Lid Margin Anomalies

I. Congenital entropion—this anomaly may result from an absence of the tarsal plate, or from hypertrophy of the tarsal plate or the marginal (ciliary) portion of the orbicularis muscle.
II. Primary congenital ectropion
   A. This is a rare disorder.
   B. Most cases are secondary to conditions such as microphthalmos, buphthalmos, or an orbitopalpebral cyst.
   C. Congenital entropion and atrichosis of the lower eyelids may be associated with tarsal hypoplasia. It may be an

isolated occurrence or inherited as an autosomal-dominant trait.
   D. Kabuki (make-up) syndrome includes characteristic facies with long palpebral fissures, everted lower lateral eyelids, and arched eyebrows. Systemic findings include mild to moderate mental retardation, fetal pads, and cleft palate. Additionally, postnatal growth retardation, skeletal and visceral anomalies are present in a large percentage of patients.
   E. Oculoauriculofrontonasal syndrome can have features of oculoauriculovertebral spectrum and frontonasal dysplasia sequence. Findings have included preauricular skin tag, hypoplastic pinna lacking an ear canal, everted and hypoplastic eyelid, cleft lip and palate, bifid nasal tip, ocular hypertelorism, micrognathia, hypoplastic mandible, extra cervical rib, hemivertebrae, agenesis of the posterior corpus callosum with midline lipoma, and an extrarenal pelvis.
III. Ankyloblepharon—this defect consists of partial fusion of the lid margins, most commonly the temporal aspects.

Eyelash Anomalies

I. Hypotrichosis (madarosis)
   A. Primary hypotrichosis (underdevelopment of the lashes) is rare.

Schopf–Schulz–Passarage syndrome is a rare ectodermal dysplasia characterized by hypodontia, hypotrichosis, nail dystrophy, palmoplantar keratoderma, and periocular and eyelid margin hidrocystomas. Multiple palmoplantar eccrine syringofibroadenomas have also been associated with the syndrome.

   B. Most cases are secondary to chronic blepharitis or any condition that causes lid margin scarring or lid neoplasms.
   C. Secondary eyelash loss may be associated with hyperthyroidism.
II. Hypertrichosis is an increase in length or number of lashes.
   A. *Trichomegaly* is an increase in the length of the lashes.

Increased eyelash length is associated with allergic diseases.

   B. *Polytrichia* is an increase in the number of lashes.
      1. Distichiasis—two rows of cilia
      2. Tristichiasis—three rows of cilia
      3. Tetrastichiasis—four rows of cilia

Distichiasis is the term used for the congenital presence of an extra row of lashes, whereas *trichiasis* is the term used for the acquired condition, which is usually secondary to lid scarring. Distichiasis may be associated with late-onset hereditary lymphedema (see section on *Congenital Conjunctival Lymphedema* in Chapter 7). The syndrome is characterized by lymphedema of the limbs, with variable age of onset, and extra aberrant growth of eyelashes from the meibomian glands. Mutation of the *FOXC2* gene (a member of the forkhead/winged family of transcription factors) has been associated with the lymphedema–distichiasis syndrome. It has been postulated that hereditary distichiasis and lymphedema–distichiasis may not be separate genetic disorders but different phenotypic expressions of the same underlying disorder.

A form of congenital hypertrichosis in the periorbital region, associated with cutaneous hyperpigmentation, may overlie a neurofibroma.

III. Ectopic cilia
  A. Ectopic cilia is a rare choristomatous anomaly in which a cluster of lashes grows in a location (lid or conjunctiva) remote from the eyelid margin.
  B. A case of complex eyelid choristoma containing ectopic cilia and a functioning lacrimal gland has been reported.

Ptosis

I. Ptosis is a condition in which lid elevation is partially or completely impaired.

II. It may be congenital, associated with other anomalies, or caused by trauma, third cranial nerve damage, or many other causes.
III. Histologically, the levator muscle may show atrophy or may appear normal.

Ichthyosis Congenita

I. Ichthyosis (Fig. 6.7) can be divided into four types:
  A. Autosomal-dominant ichthyosis vulgaris (onset usually in first year of life)
  B. Autosomal-dominant ichthyosis congenita (ichthyosiform erythroderma, onset at birth), with a generalized bullous form and a localized nonbullous form (ichthyosis hystrix)
  C. X-linked recessive ichthyosis vulgaris [the rarest type (Xp22.32), onset at 1 to 3 weeks]
  D. Autosomal-recessive ichthyosis congenita with a severe harlequin type and a less severe lamellar type (onset at birth)

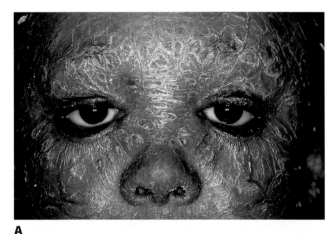

A

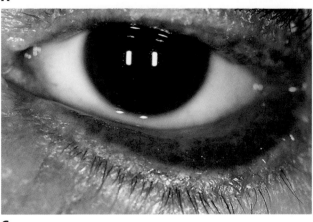

C

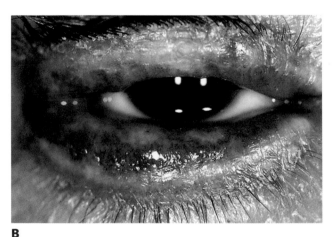

B

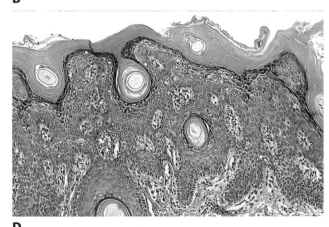

D

Fig. 6.7 Ichthyosis congenita. **A,** Child has severe ichthyosis congenita. **B** and **C,** Right and left eyes show thickened, scaly skin and keratinization (white-gray plaques) of palpebral conjunctiva. **D,** Thickened epidermis and very prominent granular cell and keratin layers are seen (conjunctiva also showed papillary reaction with keratinization). (**D,** Modified from Katowitz JA *et al.: Arch Ophthalmol* 91:208, 1974, with permission. © American Medical Association. All rights reserved.)

1. Keratinocyte transglutaminase (TGK) activity mediates the cross-linkage during the formation of the normal cornified cell membrane.
2. Intact cross-linkage of cornified cell envelopes is required for epidermal tissue homeostasis.
3. In lamellar ichthyosis, TGK levels are drastically reduced, causing the keratinocytic defect in the disease.

II. All types have in common dryness of the skin with variable amounts of profuse scaling.

Only in the autosomal-recessive type do ectropion of the lids and conjunctival changes develop.

III. Cicatricial ectropion is a common finding in recessive ichthyosis congenita.
   A. Corneal changes such as gray stromal opacities (dystrophica punctiformis profunda) occur in ichthyosis vulgaris and autosomal-recessive ichthyosis congenita.

In X-linked ichthyosis, corneal changes may occur that electron microscopically resemble the changes in lecithin cholesterol acyltransferase disease.

   B. Superficial corneal changes (punctate epithelial erosions, gray elevated nodules, and band-shaped keratopathy) also occur.

IV. The differential diagnosis includes ectodermal dysplasia, poikiloderma congenitale (Rothmund–Thomson syndrome), adult progeria (Werner's syndrome), keratosis palmaris et plantaris, keratosis follicularis spinulosa decalvans (Siemens' disease), epidermolysis bullosa, and the syndrome of ichthyosis follicularis, atrichia, and photophobia (IFAP syndrome, a rare neuroichthyosis that is probably X-linked recessive).

Keratitis–ichthyosis–deafness (KID) syndrome is a rare congenital ectodermal dysplasia characterized by the presence of hyperkeratotic skin lesions, moderate to profound sensorineural hearing loss, and vascularizing keratitis. Genetic mutations in the *GJB2* gene coding for connexin 26, which is a component of gap junctions in epithelial cells, have been detected in the disorder. Specific associated ocular and adnexal findings are lid abnormalities, corneal surface instability, limbal stem cell deficiency with resulting corneal complications, and dry eye.

V. Histologically, the epidermis is thickened and covered by a thick, dense, orthokeratotic scale.

In the autosomal-recessive type, the conjunctiva may show a papillary reaction with hyperkeratosis and parakeratosis of the epithelium.

Xeroderma Pigmentosum

I. Xeroderma pigmentosum is one of the inherited DNA repair disorders, which also include Cockayne syndrome, trichothiodystrophy, Bloom syndrome, Rothmund–Thomson syndrome, and Werner syndrome. It is inherited as an autosomal-recessive disorder, is characterized by a hypersensitivity of the skin to ultraviolet radiation, a deficiency in the repair of damaged DNA, and a resultant high incidence of skin cancers.

Squamous and basal cell carcinomas, fibrosarcoma, and malignant melanoma may all develop on areas of skin exposed to sun. Multiple malignancies of different types may develop in an individual even in children.

II. Skin lesions show three stages: mild, diffuse erythema associated with scaling and tiny, hyperpigmented macules; atrophy of the skin, mottled pigmentation, and telangiectasis—the picture resembles radiation dermatitis; and development of skin malignancies.

III. Histology
   A. Early, the epidermis shows orthokeratotic and atrophic foci associated with epidermal cells and macrophages showing pigment phagocytosis. Subepidermal perivascular infiltrates of lymphocytes and plasma cells are found.
   B. Later, the orthokeratosis and pigment deposition become more marked. An associated acanthosis of the epidermis and basophilic degeneration of the collagen are found in the corium.
   C. The histopathologic appearance of the malignancies is identical to that in patients who do not have xeroderma pigmentosum.

AGING

Atrophy

See subsection *Atrophy*, earlier, under *Terminology*.
   I. "Aging" skin appears dry, rough, wrinkled, lax, and unevenly pigmented.
   II. Because the collagen of the corium is altered, it stains basophilic instead of eosinophilic with hematoxylin and eosin. The collagen stains positively for elastin; the positivity is not changed if the tissue is pretreated with elastase.

It is the altered staining characteristic of the corium that has led to the use of terms such as *basophilic degeneration*, *actinic changes*, and *senile elastosis*.

   III. The elastic tissue is also altered and tremendously increased; it, along with the changed collagen, helps to explain the characteristic wrinkling of senile skin.

Senile Ectropion and Entropion

I. An accentuation of the aging changes may result in an ectropion (turning-out) or an entropion (turning-in) of the lower lid.
II. Histologically, both ectropion and entropion show chronic nongranulomatous inflammation and cicatrization of the skin and conjunctiva.

A. Ectropion exhibits increased orbicularis and Riolan's muscle ischemia, fragmentation of elastic and collagenous tissues in the orbital septum and tarsus, and hypertrophy of the tarsus. Actinic damage of the anterior eyelid lamella of the lower eyelid has been cited as a contributing factor in patients with involutional eyelid changes, and is most marked in those with ectropion.

B. Entropion shows increased atrophy of the orbital septum and tarsus.

Dermatochalasis

I. Dermatochalasis (Fig. 6.8) is an aging change characterized by lax, redundant skin of the lids. The folds may cover the palpebral fissure, even impairing vision.

Dermatochalasis should not be confused with *blepharochalasis*, an uncommon condition characterized by permanent changes in the eyelids after recurrent and unpredictable attacks of edema, usually in people younger than 20 years of age. Elastin mRNA expression in cultured fibroblasts from blepharochalasis is not decreased, suggesting that environmental factors or other matrix components of elastic fibers may be involved in the loss of elastic fibers found in the disorder. Also, the *Melkersson–Rosenthal syndrome* (triad of recurrent labial edema, relapsing facial paralysis, and fissured tongue) can present with eyelid edema of "unknown cause."

II. Histologically, the epidermis appears thin and smooth with decreased or absent rete ridges.
In the corium, some loss of elastic and collagen tissue occurs along with an increase in capillary vascularity, an often basophilic degeneration of the collagen (actinic elastosis), and a mild lymphocytic inflammatory reaction.

Herniation of Orbital Fat

I. Defects or dehiscences in the orbital septum produced by aging changes, often associated with dermatochalasis, may result in herniated orbital fat, simulating an orbital lipoma.

II. Histologically, mature fat is found that looks similar to that in a lipoma.

Frequently, the distinction between a primary orbital lipoma and herniated orbital fat is made more readily clinically than histologically.

Floppy-Eyelid Syndrome

A. Upregulation of elastolytic enzymes, probably related to repeated mechanical stress, has been postulated to participate in elastic fiber degradation and subsequent tarsal laxity with eyelash ptosis in floppy-eyelid syndrome.

INFLAMMATION

Terminology

I. Dermatitis (synonymous with *eczema*, *eczematous dermatitis*)

A. Dermatitis is a diffuse inflammation of the skin caused by a variety of cutaneous disorders, some quite specific and others nonspecific.

B. It may be acute (erythema and edema progressing to vesiculation and oozing, then to crusting and scaling), subacute (intermediate between acute and chronic), or chronic (papules, plaques with indistinct borders, less intense erythema, increased skin markings—lichenification—containing fine scales and firm or indurated to palpation).

Dermatitis of the lids is called *blepharitis*.

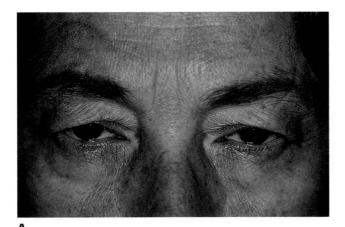

A

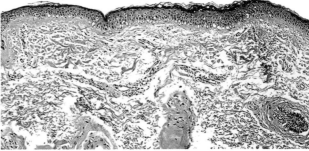

B

Fig. 6.8 Dermatochalasis. **A,** Lax, redundant lid skin is hanging in folds and partially occludes pupils. A blepharoplasty was performed. **B,** Histologic section shows an atrophic, thin, smooth epidermis with a decrease in the number and size of the rete pegs. The corium shows some loss of elastic and collagen tissue, as well as basophilic degeneration of the collagen, along with an increase in capillary vascularity and a mild lymphocytic inflammatory reaction.

II. Blepharitis
  A. Blepharitis is a simple diffuse inflammation of the lids.

  A granulomatous blepharitis, which is part of *Melkersson–Rosenthal syndrome* (triad of recurrent labial edema, relapsing facial paralysis, and fissured tongue), may present along with lid edema.

  B. Seborrheic blepharitis refers to a specific type of chronic blepharitis primarily involving the lid margins and often associated with dandruff and greasy scaling of the scalp, eyebrows, central face, chest, and pubic areas.
    1. Red, inflamed lid margins and yellow, greasy scales on the lashes are characteristic.
    2. Histologically, the epidermis shows spongiosis, a mild, superficial perivascular, predominantly lymphohistiocytic, mononuclear cell infiltrate in the superficial dermis, and even acanthosis, orthokeratosis, or parakeratosis, alone or in combination.
  C. Blepharoconjunctivitis refers to a specific type of chronic blepharitis involving the lid margins primarily and the conjunctiva secondarily.
    1. Sensitivity to *Staphylococcus* is the likely cause.
    2. The chronic inflammation may result in loss (madarosis) or abnormalities (e.g., trichiasis) of the eyelashes along with secondary phenomena such as hordeolum and chalazion. The lid margins may be thickened and ulcerated with gray, tenacious scales at the base of the remaining lashes.
    3. Histologically, a vascularized, chronic, nongranulomatous inflammation, often containing neutrophils, is associated with acanthosis, orthokeratosis, or parakeratosis of the epidermis.
  D. Cellulitis refers to a specific type of acute, infectious blepharitis primarily involving the subepithelial tissues.
    1. Histologically, polymorphonuclear leukocytes, vascular congestion, and edema predominate.
    2. Bacteria, especially *Streptococcus*, are the usual cause.

  Erysipelas is a specific type of acute cellulitis caused by group A hemolytic streptococci that is characterized by a sharply demarcated, red, warm, dermal and subcutaneous facial plaque.

III. Hordeolum (Fig. 6.9)
  A. An *external hordeolum* (*stye*) results from an acute purulent inflammation of the superficial glands (sweat and sebaceous) and hair follicles of the eyelids.
    1. It presents clinically as a discrete, superficial, elevated, erythematous, warm, tender papule or pustule, usually on or near the lid margin.
    2. Histologically, polymorphonuclear leukocytes, edema, and vascular congestion are centered primarily around hair follicles and adjacent structures.

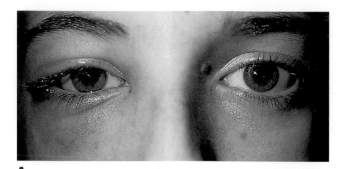

A

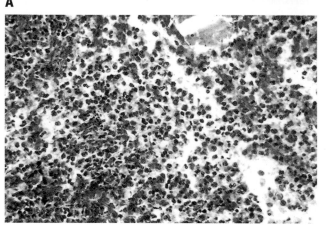

B

Fig. 6.9 Hordeolum. **A,** The patient complained of swelling, redness, and pain in the right lower lid over a few days. The inflammation is mainly located in the outer layers of the lid and is called an *external hordeolum*. Similar inflammation in the inner layers is called an *internal hordeolum*. **B,** Histologic section of another case shows a purulent exudate consisting of polymorphonuclear leukocytes and cellular debris.

  B. An *internal hordeolum* results from an acute purulent inflammation of the meibomian glands in the tarsal plate of the eyelids.
    It presents clinically as a diffuse, deep, tender, warm erythematous area involving most of the lid.

  Hordeolum can be considered simply as an inflammatory papule or pustule (pimple) of the lid. An external hordeolum is located superficially; an internal hordeolum is deep and points internally.

IV. Chalazion (Fig. 6.10)

  A chalazion may result from an internal hordeolum or may start de novo.

  A. Chronic inflammation of the meibomian glands (deep chalazion) or Zeis sebaceous glands (superficial chalazion) results in a hard, painless nodule in the eyelid called a *chalazion* or *lipogranuloma of* the lid.

  A lipogranuloma is composed of an extracellular accumulation of fat, as apposed to a xanthoma, which consists of an intracellular accumulation of fat. Lipogranulomatous eyelid inflamma-

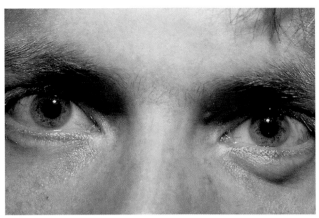

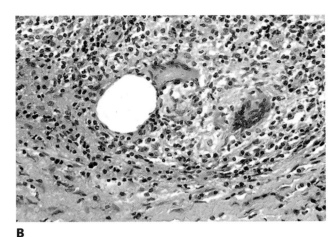

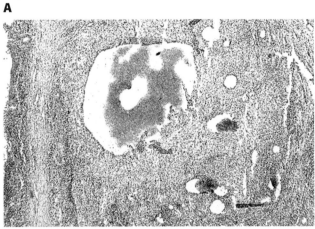

Fig. 6.10 Chalazion. **A,** The hard, painless lump was present in the left lower lid for at least a few weeks. **B,** Histologic section shows a clear circular area surrounded by epithelioid cells and multinucleated giant cells. In processing the tissue, fat is dissolved out, and the area where the fat had been appears clear. **C,** Fresh frozen tissue that has not been processed through solvents stains positively for fat in the circular areas. (**C,** oil red-O stain.)

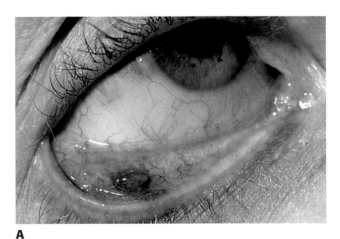

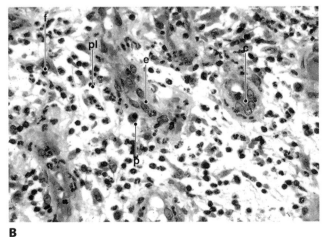

Fig. 6.11 Granuloma pyogenicum. **A,** The patient who had a hard, painless lump in the right lower lid for over a month presented complaining of a red, fleshy area inside the lid. **B,** Histologic section shows a vascularized tissue (granulation tissue) that consists of inflammatory cells (polymorphonuclear lymphocytes (pl), fibroblasts (f), and the endothelial cells (e) of budding capillaries (c) (p, plasma cell).

tion has resulted from leakage into the eyelid of silicone oil used in vitreoretinal surgery.

B. If the chalazion ruptures through the tarsal conjunctiva, granulation tissue growth (fibroblasts, young capillaries, lymphocytes, and plasma cells) may result in a rapidly enlarging, painless, polypoid mass (*granuloma pyogenicum*; Fig. 6.11).

C. Histologically, a zonal lipogranulomatous inflammation is centered around clear spaces previously filled with lipid but dissolved out during tissue processing.

1. Polymorphonuclear leukocytes, plasma cells, and lymphocytes may also be found in abundance.
2. Not infrequently, multinucleated giant cells (resembling foreign-body giant cells or Langhans' giant cells) and even asteroid and Schaumann's bodies—all nonspecific findings—may be seen.

Recurrent giant chalazia may be found in the hyperimmunoglobulin E (Job) syndrome. The syndrome is a rare immunodeficiency and multisystem disorder characterized by recurrent skin and pulmonary abscesses, connective tissue abnormalities, and elevated levels of serum immunoglobulin E (IgE).

V. Acne rosacea
   A. Acne rosacea affects mainly the skin of the middle face, nose, cheeks, forehead, and chin, and presents in three types, which may occur separately or together: (1) an erythematous telangiectatic type with erythema, telangiectasis, follicular pustules, and occasional abscesses; (2) a glandular hyperplastic type with enlargement of the nose (rhinophyma); and (3) a papular type with numerous, moderately firm, slightly raised papules 1 to 2 mm in diameter and associated with diffuse erythema.

Many dermatologists believe that some cases of acne rosacea are caused by large numbers of *Demodex* (see subsection *Demodicosis*, later).

   B. Ocular involvement is commonly found and consists of blepharitis, chalazion, conjunctival and lid granulomas, episcleritis, hyperemic conjunctivitis, internal hordeolum, keratitis, lid margin telangiectasis, meibomianitis, squamous metaplasia of the meibomian duct, and superficial punctate keratopathy.
   C. Histology
      1. Type 1 shows dilated blood vessels and a nonspecific, dermal, chronic nongranulomatous inflammatory infiltrate often associated with pustules (i.e., intrafollicular accumulations of neutrophils).
      2. Type 2 shows hyperplasia of sebaceous glands along with the findings seen in type 1.
      3. Type 3 shows papules composed of either a chronic nongranulomatous inflammatory infiltrate or, frequently, a granulomatous inflammatory infiltrate simulating tuberculosis (formerly called *rosacea-like*, *tuberculid*, or *lupoid rosacea*).
VI. Relapsing febrile nodular nonsuppurative panniculitis (Weber–Christian disease)—see p. 188 in this chapter.

Viral Diseases

I. Molluscum contagiosum (Fig. 6.12)
   A. Clinically, a dome-shaped, small (1 to 3 mm), discrete, waxy papule, often multiple, is seen with a characteristic umbilicated center (central dell).

Blepharoconjunctivitis associated with molluscum contagiosum may occur in the *Wiskott–Aldrich syndrome* (WAS), which is characterized by atopic dermatitis, thrombocytopenic purpura, normal-appearing megakaryocytes but small, defective platelets, and increased susceptibility to infections. The syndrome represents an immunologically deficient state (decreased levels of serum IgM and increased levels of IgA and IgE) and is transmitted as an X-linked recessive trait (abnormal gene on Xp11–11.3 chromosome). WASp, the protein made by the gene that is defective in WAS, is impaired. Another condition, *acquired immunodeficiency syndrome* (AIDS; see p. 21 in Chapter 1), may show multiple eyelid lesions of molluscum or present initially with molluscum eyelid lesions. In addition, multiple epibulbar molluscum lesions have been reported in association with atopic dermatitis.

   B. The large pox virus replicates in the cytoplasm and is seen histologically as large, homogeneous, purple, intracytoplasmic inclusion bodies (molluscum bodies) in a markedly acanthotic epidermis.
      1. In the deeper layers of the epidermis, near the basal layer, viruses are present as tiny, eosinophilic, intracytoplasmic inclusions. As the bodies extend toward the surface, they grow so enormous that they exceed the size of the invaded cells.
      2. At the level of the epidermal granular layer, the large bodies change from eosinophilic to basophilic.
II. Verruca (wart; Fig. 6.13)
   A. Verruca vulgaris (anywhere on the skin), verruca plana (mainly on face and dorsa of hands), verruca plantaris (soles of feet), and condyloma acuminatum (glans penis, mucosa of female genitalia, and around anus) are all caused by a variety of the papillomaviruses.
   B. Verruca vulgaris appears as a small papule containing a digitated surface or an elongated, filiform wart around the eyelids, usually at or near the lid margin.
   C. Histologically, massive papillomatosis, marked by acanthosis, parakeratosis, and orthokeratosis, and containing collections of serum in the stratum corneum at the tips of the digitations, is seen.
      1. Characteristically, in early lesions, cells in the upper part of the squamous layer and in the granular layer are vacuolated.
      2. In the vacuolated keratocytes, condensation and clumping of dark-staining keratohyaline granules and occasional intranuclear eosinophilic inclusion bodies, which represent virus inclusions, are noted.
III. Viral vesicular lesions
   A. Infections with the viruses of variola (smallpox), vaccinia (cowpox), varicella (chickenpox), herpes zoster (shingles), and primary and recurrent herpes simplex all produce similar erythematous–vesicular–pustular and crusted papular eruptions.
   B. Histologically, an intraepidermal vesicle characterizes all five diseases (see Fig. 6.5).
      1. Marked interepidermal spongiosis involves the deep epidermis and results in swollen epidermal cells that lose their intercellular bridges, causing acantholysis and intraepidermal vesicle formation.

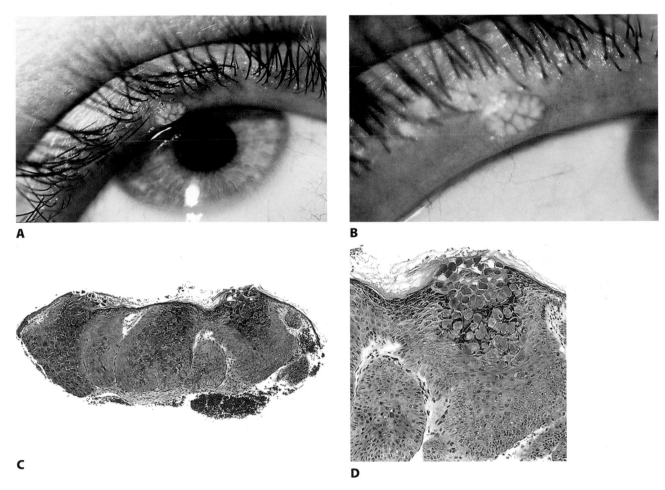

Fig. 6.12 Molluscum contagiosum. **A,** Lesion of molluscum contagiosum on upper-lid margin had caused follicular conjunctival reaction in inferior bulbar conjunctiva. **B,** Increased magnification shows an umbilicated lesion that contains whitish packets of material. **C,** Typical molluscum bodies present in epithelium. **D,** Intracytoplasmic, small, eosinophilic molluscum bodies occur in the deep layers of epidermis. The bodies become enormous and basophilic near the surface. The bodies may be shed into the tear film where they cause a secondary, irritative follicular conjunctivitis. (**A** and **B,** Courtesy of Dr. WC Frayer.)

2. Reticular degeneration and necrosis and massive ballooning degeneration involve the superficial and peripheral epidermis and result in enormous swelling of the squamous cells (intracellular edema), causing them to burst so that only the resistant parts of cell walls remain as septa forming a multilocular vesicle.

Ballooning degeneration is specific for viral vesicles, whereas reticular degeneration is seen in acute dermatitis (e.g., poison ivy).

---

3. Multinucleated epithelial giant cells, often with steel-gray nuclei showing peripheral margination of clumped chromatin, may be seen with herpes simplex and herpes zoster.
4. A dense, superficial, dermal, perivascular lymphohistiocytic inflammation, often with neutrophils infiltrating the epidermis, is seen.

5. Eosinophilic inclusion bodies are found in all five diseases, mainly in the cytoplasm in variola and in vaccinia (Guarnieri bodies). They are occasionally found in the nucleus in variola, but exclusively in the nucleus (usually surrounded by a halo or clear zone) in varicella, herpes zoster, and herpes simplex.

IV. Trachoma and lymphogranuloma venereum (see pp. 231 and 232 in Chapter 7).

Bacterial Diseases

I. Impetigo
   A. Impetigo may be caused by staphylococci or streptococci (less common), both of which cause a bullous eruption.
   B. Histologically, a superficial bulla directly under the keratin layer is filled with polymorphonuclear leukocytes; cocci are found in neutrophils or free in the bulla.

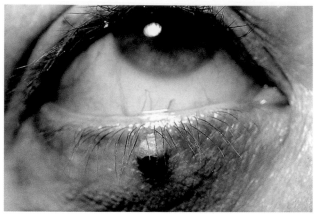

A

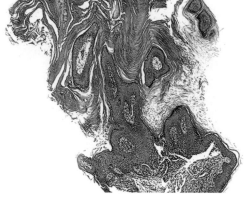

B

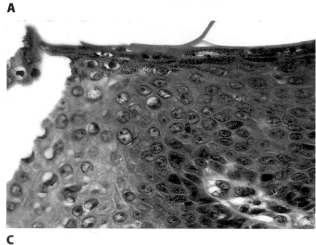

C

Fig. 6.13 Verruca vulgaris. **A,** Clinical appearance of a typical "warty" lesion near the lid margin. **B,** Histologic section demonstrates papillomatous lesion with marked orthokeratosis (hyperkeratosis) and elongated rete ridges characteristically bent inward (i.e., radiating toward central focus). **C,** High magnification shows acanthosis, orthokeratosis (hyperkeratosis), intracellular dark-staining keratohyaline granules, and occasional intranuclear eosinophilic inclusion bodies, which represent virus inclusions. Most vacuolated cells contain smaller eosinophilic particles, probably representing degenerative products.

    II. *Staphylococcus*—see under *Impetigo* (previous entry) and *Blepharoconjunctivitis* (p. 174 in this chapter).

    III. Parinaud's oculoglandular syndrome (see p. 232 in Chapter 7).

Fungal and Parasitic Diseases

See subsections on fungal and parasitic nontraumatic infections, pp. 85–93 in Chapter 4.

    I. Demodicosis (Fig. 6.14)

      A. The parasitic mite, *Demodex folliculorum*, lives in the hair follicles in humans and certain other mammals, especially around the nose and eyelashes. *D. brevis* lives in eyelash and small hair sebaceous glands, and in lobules of meibomian glands.

      B. Although present in almost all middle-aged and elderly people, and in a significant percentage of younger people, the mites seem relatively innocuous and only rarely produce any symptoms.

> Many dermatologists believe that some cases of acne rosacea and folliculitis are caused by large numbers of *Demodex*, especially in immunosuppressed patients.

      C. Histologically, the mite is often seen as an incidental finding in a hair follicle in skin sections.

      D. No inflammatory reaction is associated with the mite.

    II. *Phthirus pubis* (Fig. 6.15)

      A. Infestation of the eyelashes and brow by *P. pubis*, the crab louse, is called *phthiriasis palpebrarum.*

      B. Transmission from the primary site of infestation, the pubic hair, is usually by hand.

        1. The louse, or several lice, grips the bottom of the lash with its claw.

        2. The ova (nits) are often present in considerable numbers, adhering to the lashes.

        3. A secondary blepharoconjunctivitis may be present.

LID MANIFESTATIONS OF SYSTEMIC DERMATOSES OR DISEASE

Ichthyosis Congenita

See section *Congenital Abnormalities* earlier in this chapter.

Xeroderma Pigmentosum

See section *Congenital Abnormalities* earlier in this chapter.

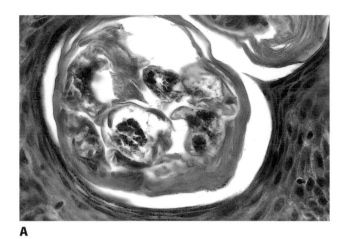

A

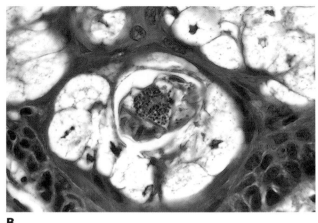

B

Fig. 6.14 *Demodex folliculorum. Demodex* seen in hair follicle (**A**) and in sebaceous gland of hair follicle (**B**). Tiny dots represent nuclei of mite. **C,** Photomicrograph of mite. (**C,** Courtesy of Dr. HJ Nevyas.)

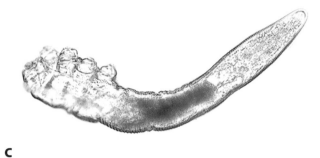

C

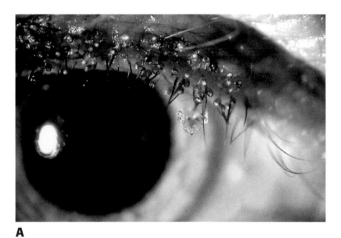

A

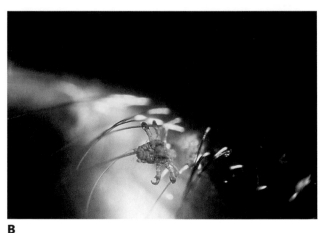

B

Fig. 6.15 *Phthirus pubis.* **A,** One crab louse and many nits (ova) are present amongst the lashes toward the lid margin. **B,** Different view of the crab louse.

Pemphigus

See p. 229 in Chapter 7.

Ocular involvement in pemphigus vulgaris occurs rarely, and is usually limited to the conjunctiva and/or the eyelids. In contrast, pemphigus foliaceus involves the skin of the eyelid and not the conjunctiva.

Ehlers–Danlos Syndrome ("India-Rubber Man")

I. Ehlers–Danlos (ED) syndrome consists of a rare, heterogeneous group of disorders characterized by loose-jointed-ness, hyperextensibility, fragile and bruisable skin with "cigarette paper" scarring, generalized friability of tissues, vascular abnormalities with rupture of great vessels, hernias, gastrointestinal diverticula, and friability of the bowel and lungs.

Most cases are inherited as autosomal-dominant traits, and the others show an X-linked recessive or autosomal-recessive pattern (including one probably distinct "ocular" form, i.e. type VI).

The skin in ED syndrome is hyperextensible but not lax. When it is pulled, it stretches; when let go, it quickly springs to the original position. The skin in cutis laxa (see subsection *Cutis Laxa*, later), on the other hand, tends to return slowly after it is pulled.

II. The basic problem appears to be an abnormal organization of collagen bundles into an intermeshing network; a defect in the collagen interferes with cross-linking.

> Most patients with ED syndrome type VI (ocular type) lack lysyl hydroxylase, an enzyme that catalyzes the hydroxylation of lysine to hydroxylysine. In hydroxylysine deficiency, the structural integrity of collagen is thought to be diminished because hydroxylysine is an important source of cross-links in collagen. A few cases of ED syndrome type VI, however, show normal activity of the enzyme lysyl hydroxylase. Therefore, two variants of ED syndrome type VI may exist.

III. Ocular findings include epicanthus (the most common finding), hypertelorism, poliosis, strabismus, blue sclera, microcornea, megalocornea, myopia, keratoconus, ectopia lentis, intraocular hemorrhage, neural retinal abnormalities, and angioid streaks.

IV. Histologically, conjunctival biopsies studied by light and electron microscopy showed no abnormalities.

The pathologic lesions in ED syndrome are controversial.

Cutis Laxa

I. In cutis laxa (Fig. 6.16), the extensible skin hangs in loose folds over all parts of the body, especially in those areas where it is normally loose (e.g., around the eyes).
   A. The lungs may be involved with emphysema.
   B. Cor pulmonale may result in early death.
   C. Both autosomal-dominant and recessive forms have been reported.
   D. It may also be an acquired condition.
      1. Rarely, it is found to involve only the face without a preceding inflammatory condition or systemic involvement.

II. The basic defect seems to be in the elastic fibers, which are reduced in number, shortened, and show granular degeneration.

III. Ocular findings include hypertelorism, blepharochalasis, ectropion, and corneal opacities.

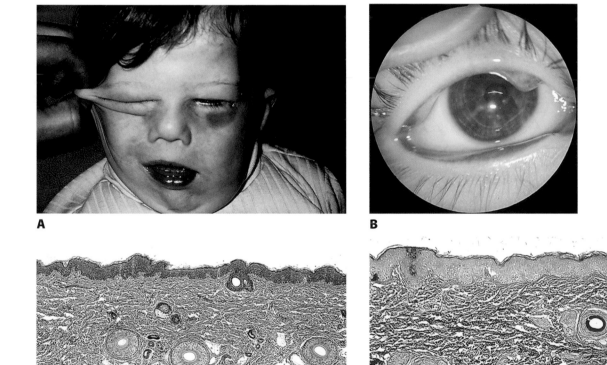

Fig. 6.16 Cutis laxa. **A,** Pulling easily extends loose skin of face. **B,** Corneal opacities occur in all layers of stroma. **C,** Skin appears relatively normal at low magnification. **D,** Verhoeff's elastica stain shows fragmentation and granular degeneration of dermal elastic tissue. (**A** and **B,** Courtesy of Dr. JA Katowitz.)

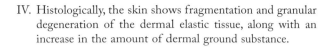

IV. Histologically, the skin shows fragmentation and granular degeneration of the dermal elastic tissue, along with an increase in the amount of dermal ground substance.

Pseudoxanthoma Elasticum

I. Pseudoxanthoma elasticum is mostly inherited in an autosomal-recessive manner, but also in an autosomal-dominant pattern, and mainly involves the skin, the eyes, and the cardiovascular system.

Linkage analysis and mutation detection techniques have shown mutations in the *ABCC6* gene.

  A. The skin of the face, neck, axillary folds, cubital areas, inguinal folds, and periumbilical area (often with an umbilical hernia) becomes thickened and grooved, with the areas between the grooves diamond-shaped, rectangular, polygonal, elevated, and yellowish (resembling chicken skin).
     1. The skin in the involved areas becomes lax, redundant, and relatively inelastic.
     2. The skin changes are often not noted until the second decade of life or later.
  B. The eyes show angioid streaks (see Fig. 11.38), often with subretinal neovascularization.
     1. Examination of the fundus may show a background pattern, called *peau d'orange*, in the posterior aspect of the eyes, caused by multiple breaks in Bruch's membrane.
     2. The optic nerve may contain drusen.

Drusen of the optic nerve occurs 20 to 50 times more often in pseudoxanthoma elasticum than in the general, healthy population.

  C. The cardiovascular system manifestations include weak or absent peripheral pulses, intermittent claudication, angina pectoris, and internal hemorrhages.
II. The basic defect seems to be related to a dystrophy of elastic fibers, but some think collagen fibers are at fault.
III. Histologically, the skin shows elastin abnormalities only in the midepidermis, with elastin band swelling, granular degeneration, and fragmentation. Angioid streaks consist of breaks in Bruch's membrane.

Erythema Multiforme

I. Erythema multiforme, an acute, self-limited dermatosis, is a common-pathway, cutaneous reaction to drugs, viral or bacterial infections, or unknown causes.
II. Erythema multiforme shows multiform lesions of macules, papules (most common lesion), vesicles, and bullae.

Characteristic "target" lesions are noted as round to oval erythematous plaques that contain central darkening and marginal erythema.

III. A severe form of erythema multiforme, starting suddenly with high fever and prostration and showing predominantly a bullous eruption of the skin and mucous membranes, including conjunctiva, is *Stevens–Johnson* syndrome. The systemic syndrome may lead to death.
IV. Another severe variant of erythema multiforme is *toxic epidermal necrolysis* (see later).
V. Histologic findings
  A. In the skin of Stevens–Johnson syndrome, a dense lymphohistiocytic inflammation obscures the dermoepidermal junction and is associated with progressive necrosis of keratinocytes from the basilar to the uppermost portions of the epidermis.
  B. In the conjunctiva, epithelial goblet cells and openings of the accessory lacrimal glands may be destroyed, leading to marked drying of the conjunctiva and epidermidalization.
     Both intraepidermal and subepidermal vesiculation may lead to severe scarring, including symblepharon and entropion.
  C. The cellular infiltrate consists largely of lymphocytes, mainly T4+ (helper) cells in the dermis and T8+ (cytotoxic) cells in the epidermis.

Toxic Epidermal Necrolysis

I. Toxic epidermal necrolysis (Lyell's disease; epidermolysis necroticans combustiformis; acute epidermal necrolysis; scalded-skin syndrome) really consists of two different diseases, *Lyell's disease* (subepidermal type or true toxic epidermal necrolysis—probably a variant of severe erythema multiforme), and *Ritter's disease* (subcorneal type or staphylococcal scalded-skin syndrome—not related to toxic epidermal necrolysis).
  A. Toxic epidermal necrolysis (Lyell's disease) is probably a variant of severe erythema multiforme, frequently occurs as a drug allergy, often overlaps with Stevens–Johnson syndrome, and histologically resembles the epidermal type of erythema multiforme.
  B. Staphylococcal scalded-skin syndrome (Ritter's disease) is not related to erythema multiforme, occurs largely in the newborn and in children younger than 5 years, and occurs as an acute disease.
     1. Its onset begins abruptly with diffuse erythema accompanied by severe malaise and high fever.
     2. Large areas of epidermis form clear fluid-filled, flaccid bullae, which exfoliate almost immediately, so that the denuded areas resemble scalded skin.

Phage group II staphylococci are absent from the bullae but are present at a distant site (e.g., purulent conjunctivitis, rhinitis, or pharyngitis). The bullae are caused by a staphylococcal toxin called *exfoliatin*.

---

     3. The disease runs an acute course and is fatal in fewer than 4% of cases.

It rarely occurs in adults, but when it does, it may have a mortality rate of over 50%.

II. Histologically, most cases of toxic epidermal necrolysis show a severe degeneration and necrosis of epidermal cells resulting in detachment of the entire epidermis (flaccid bullae).

Epidermolysis Bullosa

I. Epidermolysis bullosa hereditaria (mechanobullous diseases) includes a group of rare, inherited, noninflammatory, nonimmunologic diseases characterized by the susceptibility of the skin to blister after even mild trauma.

An unrelated acquired form is thought to be an autoimmune disease.

II. Ocular complications (especially in recessive epidermolysis bullosa) include loss of eyelashes, obstruction of the lacrimal ducts, and epiphora. Late complications include cicatricial ectropion, exposure keratitis, recurrent corneal erosions and ulcers, and even corneal perforation.

III. Histologically, according to the different types, blisters can form in the epidermis, at the lamina lucida, or below the lamina lucida.

Underlying the plasma membrane of the basal epithelial cells is a comparatively electron-lucent zone, the *lamina lucida*, which separates the trilaminar plasma membrane (approximately 8 nm wide) from the medium-dense basement membrane (lamina densa).

Contact Dermatitis

I. An allergenic or irritating substance applied to the skin may result in contact dermatitis, which is a type IV immunologic reaction requiring a primary exposure, sensitization, and re-exposure to an allergen, and then an immunologic delay before clinical expression of the dermatitis.
   A. Contact dermatitis is one of the most common abnormal conditions affecting the lids.
   B. Agents such as cosmetics and locally applied atropine and epinephrine may produce a contact dermatitis.
   C. Contact dermatitis may be present in three forms:
      1. An acute form with diffuse erythema, edema, oozing, vesicles, bullae, and crusting
      2. A chronic form with erythema, scaling, and thick, hard, leathery skin (*lichenification*)
      3. A subacute form showing characteristics of acute and chronic forms

Anterior subcapsular cataracts (usual form) and posterior subcapsular cataracts (rare form) seem to occur with increased frequency in patients who have a history of atopia.

II. Histology
   A. In the acute stage, epidermal (intraepidermal vesicles) and dermal edema predominate along with a lympho-cytic infiltrate.

Spongiosis or intercellular edema between squamous cells contributes to the formation of vesicles (unilocular bullae). Intracellular edema, however, results in reticular degeneration and the formation of multilocular bullae.

   B. In the chronic stage, there is acanthosis, orthokeratosis, and some parakeratosis together with elongation of rete pegs.
      1. Mild spongiosis is present, but vesicle formation does not occur.
      2. In the dermis, perivascular lymphocytes, eosinophils, histiocytes, and fibroblasts are found.

Histologically, a distinction cannot be made between a primary allergic contact dermatitis and an irritant-induced or toxic dermatitis, except possibly in the early stage. *Atopic dermatitis*, which is a chronic, severely pruritic dermatitis associated with a personal or family history of atopy (asthma, allergic rhinitis, atopic dermatitis), does not show vesicles, although it does show lichenified and scaling erythematous areas, which when active may show oozing and crusting, but no vesicles.

Collagen Diseases

I. Dermatomyositis (see p. 540 in Chapter 14).
II. Periarteritis (polyarteritis) nodosa
   A. Periarteritis nodosa is a disease of unknown cause characterized by a panarteritis of small- and medium-sized, muscular-type arteries of kidney, muscle, heart, gastrointestinal tract, and pancreas, but not of the central nervous system or lungs, and rarely of the skin.

A benign cutaneous form of periarteritis nodosa exists as a chronic disease limited to the skin and subcutaneous tissue.

   B. Histologically, four stages may be seen:
      1. The degenerative or necrotic stage: foci of necrosis (fibrinoid necrosis) involve the coats of the artery and may result in localized dehiscences or aneurysms.
      2. The inflammatory stage: inflammatory cells, predominantly neutrophils but also eosinophils and lymphocytes, infiltrate the necrotic areas.
      3. The granulation stage: healing occurs with the formation of granulation tissue, which may occlude the vascular lumens.
      4. The fibrotic stage: healing ends with scar formation.
III. Lupus erythematosus can be subdivided into three types:
      1. Chronic discoid, which is limited to the skin
         a. Discoid lupus erythematosus involving the eyelids is rare. It may present as madarosis.
         b. Periorbital edema and erythema are rare cutaneous manifestations of discoid lupus erythematosus.
      2. Intermediate or subacute, which has systemic symptoms in addition to skin lesions

3. Systemic, which is dominated by visceral lesions

Transition from the chronic discoid type to the systemic type occurs infrequently.

A. Histology shows five main characteristics (when they involve the skin, the three types of lupus erythematosus differ only in degree of involvement; the systemic form is the most severe).
B. All five histologic characteristics are not necessarily present in each case.
1. Orthokeratosis with keratotic plugging found mainly in the follicular openings but also found elsewhere
2. Atrophy of the squamous layer of epidermis and of rete pegs
3. Liquefaction degeneration of basal cells (i.e., vacuolation and dissolution of basal cells—most significant finding)
4. Focal lymphocytic dermal infiltrates mainly around dermal appendages
5. Edema, vasodilatation, and extravasation of erythrocytes in the upper dermis
IV. Scleroderma (Fig. 6.17) exists in two forms: (1) a benign circumscribed (morphea) form, which almost never pro-

gresses or transforms to the systemic form; and (2) a systemic form (progressive systemic sclerosis), which may prove fatal.
A. The characteristic lesion is a sclerotic plaque with an ivory-colored center and appearing bound-down when palpated.
B. Ocular findings include pseudoptosis secondary to swollen lids, hyposecretion of tears with trophic changes in the cornea and conjunctiva (Sjögren's syndrome), ocular muscle palsies, temporal arteritis, unilateral glaucoma, exophthalmos, neural retinal cotton-wool patches, signs of hypertensive retinopathy, defects of the retinal pigment epithelium near the macula, central serous choroidopathy, and fluorescein leaks of thickened retinal capillaries.
C. Histologically, the morphea and the systemic forms are similar, if not identical.
1. Early, the dermal collagen bundles appear swollen and homogeneous and are separated by edema. Round inflammatory cells, mainly lymphocytes, are found around edematous blood vessel walls and between collagen bundles (panniculitis).
2. In the intermediate stages, the subcutaneous tissue is infiltrated by round inflammatory cells, dermal collagen becomes further thickened, and dermal adnexa are involved in the process.

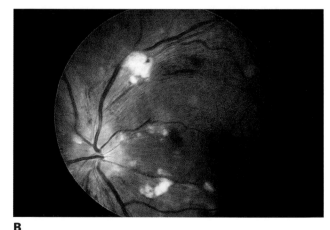

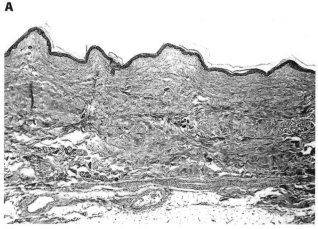

A

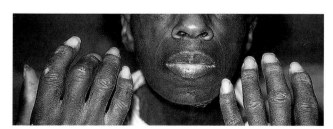

B

C

Fig. 6.17 Scleroderma. **A,** Typical changes in face and hands of patient who has scleroderma. **B,** Cotton-wool spots seen in fundus of person with advanced scleroderma. **C,** Dermis thickened and subcutaneous tissue mostly replaced by collagen. Atrophic sweat glands appear trapped in midst of collagen bundles.

Blood vessel walls show edema with intimal prolif-eration and narrowing of their lumina.

3. In the late stages, the dermis is thickened by the addition of new collagen at the expense of subcutaneous tissue.

   a. The subcutaneous fat is replaced by collagen and blood vessels are fibrotic.

   b. The thickened dermis contains hyalinized, hypertrophic, closely packed collagen bundles, atrophic sweat glands trapped in the midst of collagen bundles, decreased fibrocytes, and few or no sebaceous glands or hair structures.

   c. Inflammation is minor or absent.

4. The overlying epidermal structure, including rete ridges, is rather well preserved except in the late stages of the systemic form, when atrophy occurs.

5. The underlying muscle, especially in the systemic form, may be involved and shows early degeneration, swelling, and inflammation, followed by late fibrosis.

Granulomatous Vasculitis

I. Wegener's granulomatosis

  A. The classic form of Wegener's granulomatosis is characterized by generalized small-vessel vasculitis, necrotizing granulomas, focal necrotizing glomerulonephritis, and vasculitis of the upper and lower respiratory tract.

    1. Typical presentation is a persistent inflammatory nasal and sinus disease associated with systemic symptoms of fever, malaise, and migratory arthritis.

    2. Serum antineutrophilic cytoplasmic antibodies (ANCAs) are a sensitive and rather specific marker for Wegener's granulomatosis.

    3. A limited form of Wegener's granulomatosis lacks renal involvement (see Fig. 8.59).

    4. In both the classic and limited forms, most of the ocular findings can occur.

    5. Ocular involvement, most commonly orbital, occurs in up to 50%, and neurologic involvement in up to 54% of cases.

  B. Ocular findings include dry eyes, nasolacrimal obstruction, blepharitis, conjunctivitis, scleritis or episcleritis, corneoscleral ulceration, uveitis, retinal vein occlusion, retinal pigmentary changes, acute retinal necrosis, choroidal folds, optic neuritis, and exophthalmos secondary to orbital involvement. It has presented as cicatricial conjunctival inflammation with trichiasis.

  C. Histologically, the classic triad of necrotizing vasculitis (granulomatous and disseminated small-vessel), tissue necrosis, and granulomatous inflammation are characteristic.

  The vasculitis can be seen in three forms:

    1. Microvasculitis or capillaritis—infiltration and destruction of capillaries, venules, and arterioles by neutrophils

    2. Granulomatous vasculitis (most characteristic)—granulomatous vasculitis involving small or medium-sized arteries and veins

    3. Necrotizing vasculitis involving small or medium-sized arteries and veins but not associated with granulomatous inflammation

II. Allergic granulomatosis (allergic vasculitis, Churg–Strauss syndrome) involves the same-size arteries as periarteritis but differs in having respiratory symptoms, pulmonary infiltrates, systemic and local eosinophilia, intravascular and extravascular granulomatous lesions, and often cutaneous and subcutaneous nodules and petechial lesions.

III. Temporal arteritis (see p. 507 in Chapter 13)

Vasculitis-Like Disorders and Leukemia/Lymphoma

I. Natural killer (NK) T-cell lymphoma (polymorphic reticulosis or angiocentric T-cell lymphoma)

  A. NK cells are a distinct non-T, non-B lineage of lymphocytes that mediate major histocompatibility complex-unrestricted cytotoxicity.

  B. NK/T-cell malignancies are uncommon and were previously known as polymorphic reticulosis or angiocentric T-cell lymphomas. The World Health Organization further divides these lesions into NK/T-cell lymphoma (nasal and extranasal) type and aggressive NK-cell leukemia.

    1. Its lymphoma cells are CD2$^+$, CD56$^+$, and CD3epsilon$^+$.

  C. Relatively common in Asia, Mexico, and South America, but extremely rare in most western countries.

  D. Lethal midline granuloma form of NK/T-cell lymphoma.

    1. Rare entity that usually arises in the nasal cavity.

    2. It has a male preponderance, and a wide age range.

    3. It is extremely aggressive, and has approximately a 20% 5-year survival.

  E. Apoptosis, necrosis, and angioinvasion are typical features of the lymphoma.

  F. Invasion and blockage of blood vessels by lymphoma cells result in marked ischemic necrosis of normal and neoplastic tissues.

  G. The leukemic form tends to affect younger patients, who often present with advanced disease and multiple organ involvement.

    1. Survival is particularly brief.

  H. Gamma-delta T-cell receptor clonality is the most common T-cell receptor rearrangement in several T-cell lymphomas, including NK/T-cell lymphoma.

  I. Characteristic patterns of genomic alteration typify aggressive NK-cell leukemia and extranodal NK/T-cell lymphoma, nasal type.

  J. Epstein–Barr virus (EBV) can encode multiple genes that drive cell proliferation and confer resistance to cell death, including two viral proteins that mimic the effects of activated cellular signaling proteins.

    1. Infection with the virus is associated with a variety of lymphomas and lymphoproliferative disorders, including Burkitt's lymphoma; NK/T-cell lymphoma, lymphoma and lymphoproliferative dis-

eases in immunocompromised individuals, and Hodgkin's lymphoma.

2. The presence of EBV-infected cells in the aqueous humor originating from nasal NK/T-cell lymphoma has been reported.

K. The majority of ocular adnexal lymphomas are marginal zone B-cell (mucosal-associated lymphoid tissue: MALT) lymphomas.

L. In one Korean study, only 2/68 cases were NK/T cell lesions.

M. NK/T-cell lymphoma has occasionally involved the eye.

N. Extranodal nasal type NK/T-cell lymphoma has involved the posterior orbit, lungs, uterus, adrenal gland, pericardium, and meninges in a 41-year-old woman with a rapidly fatal clinical course.

O. Lethal midline granuloma in NK/T-cell lymphoma has presented as conjunctival swelling of the left upper eyelid. The tumor was exceptional because this patient was Caucasian and was not immunosuppressed.

P. Other rare T-cell lymphomas involving the eyelids have been reported.

II. Symmetrical leukemia cutis of the eyelids accompanied by B-cell chronic lymphocytic leukemia has been reported. The differential diagnosis for a cause of such eyelid swelling includes other tumors, hyperthyroidism, nephrotic syndrome, and hypoalbuminemia. Additionally, metastasis from the histiocytoid form of breast carcinoma may produce eyelid swelling.

III. Primary diffuse large B-cell lymphoma has presented as an ulcerating lesion of the eyelid tarsal surface. Positivity of monoclonal antibodies for CD20 and CD79a, and polyclonal antibodies for lambda chains, confirmed the diagnosis.

IV. Mycosis fungoides, which is a cutaneous T-cell lymphoma, has presented as a severe, progressive, full-thickness, lower-eyelid ulceration in a 72-year-old man.

Xanthelasma

I. Xanthelasma (Fig. 6.18) most commonly occurs in middle-aged or elderly people who usually, but not always, have normal serum cholesterol levels.

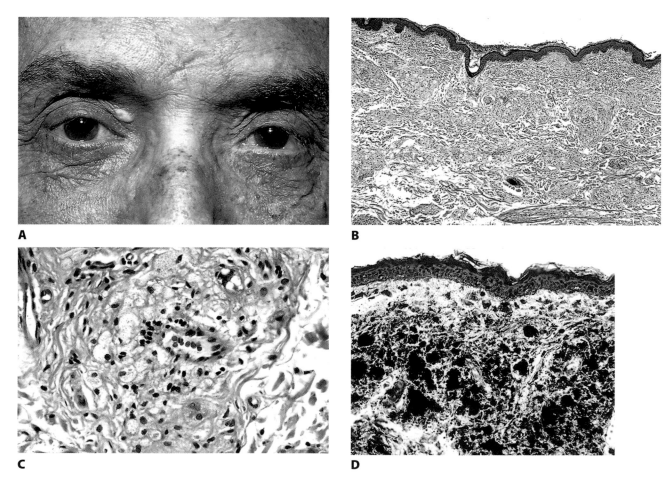

Fig. 6.18 Xanthelasma. **A,** Characteristic clinical appearance of xanthelasmas which involve inner aspect of each upper lid. **B,** Lipid-laden foam cells are present in dermis and tend to cluster around blood vessels. **C,** High magnification of foam cells clustered around blood vessels. **D,** Oil red-O stain for fat demonstrates dermal lipid positivity (red globules).

A. Xanthelasma is a form of xanthoma [i.e., a tumor containing fat mainly within cells (intracellular)], whereas a lipogranuloma (e.g., a chalazion) is a tumor containing fat mainly outside cells (extracellular).
B. It may occur in primary hypercholesterolemia or with nonfamilial serum cholesterol elevation.

Evidence suggests that xanthelasma may be associated with qualitative and quantitative abnormalities of lipid metabolism (increased levels of serum cholesterol, low-density lipoprotein cholesterol, and apolipoprotein B; and decreased levels of high-density lipoprotein subfraction 2 cholesterol) that may favor lipid deposition in the skin and arterial wall, that xanthelasma is a marker of dyslipidemia, and that patients who have xanthelasma should undergo a full lipid profile to identify those who are at an increased risk for cardiovascular disease.

C. Xanthelasma is associated with other xanthomas or with hyperlipemia syndromes in approximately 5% of patients.
II. After initial surgical excision, the recurrence rate is slightly less than half.
III. Recurrence is more likely if all four lids are involved, if an underlying hyperlipemia syndrome is present, or if there have been previous recurrences.

Lid lesions resembling xanthelasma occur in *Erdheim–Chester disease*, which is an idiopathic, widespread, multifocal, granulomatous disorder characterized by cholesterol-containing foam cells infiltrating viscera and bones, including the orbit, and sometimes bilateral xanthelasmas. When the orbit is involved, there tends to be bilateral involvement. Histologically, the lesions show broad sheets of lipid-filled xanthoma cells and scattered foci of chronic inflammatory cells, mainly lymphocytes and plasma cells, along with significant fibrosis. Touton giant cells may be found. A localized, adult-onset, periocular xanthogranuloma with severe asthma may be a distinct entity (pseudo Erdheim–Chester disease), or may be a variant of Erdheim–Chester disease or of necrobiotic xanthogranuloma, and needs to be differentiated from other histiocytic proliferations.

IV. Xanthelasmas appear as multiple, soft, yellowish plaques most commonly at the inner aspects of the upper and lower lids.
V. Histologically, lipid-containing foam cells are found in the superficial dermis. The cells cluster around blood vessels and may even involve their walls.

Necrobiotic Xanthogranuloma

I. Necrobiotic xanthogranuloma, an entity of unknown cause, affects both sexes equally.
A. Cutaneous involvement is universal, with the periorbital region a site of predilection.
B. The typical lesion is an indurated papule, nodule, or plaque that is violaceous to red-orange, often with a central ulceration or atrophy.
II. The most characteristic abnormal laboratory finding is a paraproteinemia.

A. Monoclonal gammopathy associated with IgG is most common, but gammopathy may also be associated with IgA and others.
B. Bone marrow biopsy may show different abnormalities, the most serious of which is multiple myeloma.
III. Systemic findings include hepatomegaly, splenomegaly, lymphadenopathy, arthralgia or arthritis, pulmonary disease, and hypertension.
IV. Histologically, granulomatous masses are separated by broad bands of hyaline necrobiosis. Giant cells are of the foreign-body type and often the Touton type.

The lesions most closely resemble necrobiosis lipoidica diabeticorum, but they may also be confused with juvenile xanthogranuloma, granuloma annulare, erythema induratum, atypical sarcoidosis, Erdheim–Chester disease, Rothman–Makai panniculitis, foreign-body granulomas, various xanthomas, nodular tenosynovitis, and the extra-articular lesions of proliferative synovitis.

Juvenile Xanthogranuloma

Juvenile xanthogranuloma of the eyelid is uncommon; however, it has presented as a large, solitary, pedunculated lesion involving the eyelid in a 31-month-old Japanese girl. Systemic evaluation was unremarkable.

See also p. 343 in Chapter 9.

Amyloidosis

Rarely, nodular cutaneous amyloid tumors of the eyelid may occur in the absence of systemic amyloidosis.

See also p. 238 in Chapter 7.

Malignant Atrophic Papulosis (Degos' Disease)

I. The syndrome is a rare cutaneovisceral syndrome of unknown cause characterized by the diffuse eruption of asymptomatic, porcelain-white skin lesions. Death usually occurs within a few months.
II. Ocular lesions include porcelain-white lid lesions; a characteristic white, avascular thickened plaque of the conjunctiva; telangiectasis of conjunctival blood vessels and microaneurysms; strabismus; posterior subcapsular cataract, choroidal lesions such as peripheral choroiditis, small plaques of atrophic choroiditis, gray avascular areas, and discrete loss of choroidal pigment and peripheral retinal pigment epithelium; visual field changes; and intermittent diplopia and papilledema associated with progressive central nervous system involvement.
III. Histologically, capillaries are occluded by endothelial proliferation and swelling; the endarterioles show endothelial proliferation, swelling, and fibrinoid necrosis involving only the intima; arterial involvement is greater than venous; thrombosis may occur secondary to endothelial changes; and no significant inflammatory cellular response is noted.

Calcinosis Cutis

I. Calcinosis cutis has three forms
  A. *Metastatic calcinosis cutis*, or calcium deposition secondary to either hypercalcemia (e.g., with parathyroid neoplasm, hypervitaminosis D, excessive intake of milk and alkali, and extensive destruction of bone by osteomyelitis or metastatic carcinoma) or hyperphosphatemia (e.g., with chronic renal disease and secondary hyperparathyroidism)
  B. *Dystrophic calcinosis cutis* (i.e., deposition in previously damaged tissue)
  C. *Subepidermal calcified nodule* [i.e., a single (rarely two), small, raised, hard nodule, occasionally present at birth]
II. Histologically, forms A and B show large deposits of calcium in the subcutaneous tissue and small, granular deposits in the dermis, whereas form C shows deposits of irregular granules and globules in the upper dermis. The calcium appears as deep blue or purple granules.

Lipoid Proteinosis

I. Lipoid proteinosis (Fig. 6.19) is a rare condition of the lids and mucous membranes that has an autosomal-recessive inheritance pattern. It has been reported to involve siblings. The disorder maps to 1q21, and is caused by mutations in the extracellular matrix protein 1 gene.
II. Multiple, waxy, pearly nodules, 2 to 3 mm in diameter, cover the lid margins linearly along the roots of the cilia. The lesions are said to be pathognomonic for the disorder.
III. Whitish plaques are found on mucous membranes.
IV. Histologically, a papillomatosis of the epidermis occurs along with large dermal collections of an amorphous, eosinophilic, PAS-positive material without inflammation.
  Electron microscopy shows large masses of an extracellular, finely granular, amorphous material without a fibrillar structure.

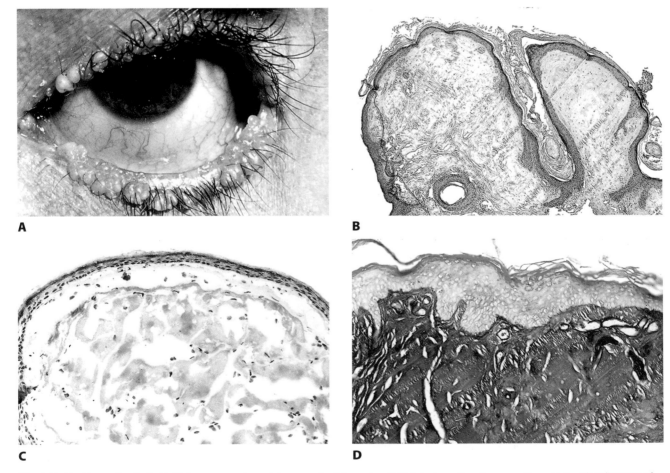

Fig. 6.19 Lipoid proteinosis. **A,** Multiple, waxy, pearly nodules cover the lid margins. **B,** Histologic section shows papillomatosis with collections of amorphous material in dermis. Material is positive for lipid (**C,** Sudan IV stain) and is also periodic acid–Schiff-positive (**D**). (Case presented by Dr. J Duke at the Eastern Ophthalmic Pathology Society meeting, 1966.)

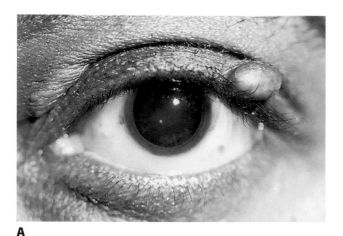

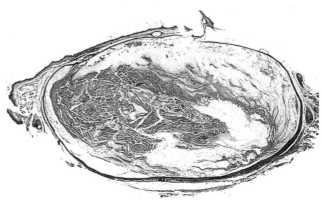

A

B

Fig. 6.20 Epidermoid cyst. **A,** Large epidermoid cyst present on outer third of left upper lid. Note xanthelasma in corner of left upper lid. **B,** The cyst has no dermal appendages in its wall and is lined by stratified squamous epithelium that desquamates keratin into its lumen. Histologically, an epidermoid cyst is identical to an epithelial inclusion cyst, but differs from a dermoid cyst in that the latter has epidermal appendages in its wall.

Idiopathic Hemochromatosis

I. Brown pigmentation of the lid margin, conjunctiva, cornea, and around the disc margin has been described (see p. 24 in Chapter 1).

II. Histologically, the brown pigmentation of the lid margin and conjunctiva is caused by an increased melanin content of the epidermis, especially the basal layer.

    A. The peripapillary pigmentation may result from small amounts of iron in the peripapillary retinal pigment epithelium.

    B. Intraocular deposition of iron is most prominent in the nonpigmented ciliary epithelium but may also be found in the sclera, corneal epithelium, and peripapillary retinal pigment epithelium.

Relapsing Febrile Nodular Nonsuppurative Panniculitis (Weber–Christian Disease)

I. The condition, which is of unknown cause, occurs most often in middle-aged and elderly women. It is characterized by malaise and fever and by the appearance of crops of tender nodules and papules in the subcutaneous fat, usually on the trunk and extremities.

II. Ocular findings include necrotic eyelid and subconjunctival nodules and, rarely, ocular proptosis, anterior uveitis, and macular hemorrhage.

III. Histologically, three stages can be seen.

    A. An early, rapid phase shows fat necrosis and an acute inflammatory infiltrate of neutrophils, lymphocytes, and histiocytes.

    B. A second stage shows a granulomatous inflammation with lipid-filled macrophages, epithelioid cells, and foreign-body giant cells.

    C. A third stage of fibrosis may result clinically in depression of the overlying skin.

Pigmentation

I. Argyrosis

    A. Periocular and eyelid skin can be involved in argyrosis, resulting in the typical grayish discoloration.

      1. Chronic use of eyelash tint has been an unusual cause for the disorder.

II. Bimatoprost treatment for glaucoma may result in increased melanin pigmentation of the periocular skin without melanocyte proliferation. The keratinocytes in these patients have abundant mature melanosomes compared to controls.

CYSTS, PSEUDONEOPLASMS, AND NEOPLASMS

Benign Cystic Lesions

I. Epidermoid (Fig. 6.20) and dermoid (see Figs 14.12 and 14.13) cysts* are congenital lesions that tend to occur at the outer upper portion of the upper lid.

II. Epidermal inclusion cysts* (see Fig. 6.20) appear identical histologically to congenital epidermoid cysts; the former, however, instead of occurring congenitally, are caused by traumatic dermal implantation of epidermis or are follicular cysts of the hair follicle infundibulum that result from occlusion of its orifice, sometimes the result of trauma.

Milia are identical histologically to epidermal inclusion cysts; they differ only in size, milia being the smaller. They may represent retention cysts, caused by the occlusion of a pilosebaceous follicle

---

Rupture of any of these cysts results in a marked granulomatous, foreign-body inflammatory reaction in the adjacent tissue (see Fig. 14.13).

or of sweat pores, may represent benign keratinizing tumors, or they may have a dual origin. Multiple epidermal inclusion cysts, especially of the face and scalp, may occur in Gardner's syndrome.

Histologically, the cyst is lined by epithelial cells essentially identical to surface epithelium. The cavity contains loose, laminated keratin.

III. Sebaceous (pilar, trichilemmal) cysts* (see footnote on p. 188) are caused by obstruction of the glands of Zeis, of the meibomian glands, or of the isthmus portion of the hair follicle, from which keratinization analogous to the outer root sheath of the hair or trichilemma arises.

Histologically, the cyst is lined by epithelial cells that possess no clearly visible intercellular bridges.

   A. The peripheral layer of cells shows a palisade arrangement, and the cells closest to the cavity are swollen without distinct cell borders.
   B. The cyst cavity contains an amorphous eosinophilic material.

The epithelial cells lining the sebaceous cyst are different from the typical cells lining an epidermal inclusion cyst, in which the cells are stratified squamous epithelium. The cystic contents of the sebaceous cyst are different from the horny (keratinous) material filling the epidermal inclusion cyst. "Old" sebaceous cysts, however, may show stratified squamous epithelial metaplasia of the lining, resulting in keratinous material filling the cyst and producing a picture identical to an epidermal inclusion cyst, unless a microscopic section accidentally passes through the occluded pore of the sebaceous cyst.

IV. Comedo (blackhead, primary lesion of acne vulgaris) presents clinically as follicular papules and pustules.
   A. The comedo occludes the sebaceous glands of the pilosebaceous follicle, which may undergo atrophy.
   B. Histologically, the comedo results from intrafollicular orthokeratosis that leads to a cystic collection of sebum and keratin.
   C. With rupture of the cyst wall, sebum and keratin are released, causing a foreign-body giant cell granulomatous reaction.
      Bacteria, especially *Propionibacterium acnes*, may be found.
   D. Eventually, epithelium grows downward and encapsulates the inflammatory infiltrate.
   E. The lesion heals by fibrosis.
V. Steatocystoma
   A. Steatocystoma may occur as a solitary cyst (simplex) or as multiple cysts (multiplex), the latter often inherited as an autosomal-dominant trait.
   B. The small, firm cysts, which exude an oily or creamy fluid when punctured, are derived from cystic dilatation of the sebaceous duct that empties into the hair follicle.
   C. Histologically, a thick, eosinophilic cuticle covers the several layers of epithelial cells lining the cyst wall. Sebaceous lobules are present either within or close to the cyst wall.

VI. Calcifying epithelioma of Malherbe (pilomatricoma; Fig. 6.21)
   A. Calcifying epithelioma of Malherbe is a cyst derived from the hair matrix that forms the hair.
   B. It can occur at any age, but most appear in the first two decades of life; it presents as a solitary tumor, firm, deep-seated, and covered by normal skin. Nevertheless, it is frequently misdiagnosed when occurring in young adults.
      1. If superficial, it produces a blue-red discoloration.
   C. Histologically, the tumor is sharply demarcated and composed of basophilic and shadow cells.
      1. Basophilic cells closely resemble the basaloid cells of a basal cell carcinoma (dark basophilic nucleus surrounded by scant basophilic cytoplasm).
      2. Shadow cells stain faintly eosinophilic, have distinct cell borders, and instead of nuclei show central, unstained regions where the nuclei should be.
         a. In older tumors, basophilic cells may have disappeared completely so that only shadow cells remain.
      3. The stroma may show areas of keratinization, fibrosis, calcification, foreign-body granuloma, and ossification.
      4. Follicular hybrid cyst of the tarsus, which had features of pilomatricoma and steatocystoma, has been reported to perforate the palpebral surface of the conjunctiva.
   D. *Pilomatrix carcinoma* may develop from malignant transformation of a benign pilomatricoma or may arise de novo.
VII. Hidrocystoma (Figs 6.22 and 6.23)
   A. Cysts resulting from occlusion of the eccrine or apocrine duct are referred to as *hidrocystomas*.
      1. Apocrine hidrocystomas usually occur in adults as solitary (sometimes multiple) lesions, often with a blue tint, and are usually located in the skin near the eyes.
      2. Eccrine hidrocystomas may be solitary or multiple, and clinically are indistinguishable from apocrine hidrocystomas.
   B. Histologically, the apocrine hidrocystoma, which is derived from the apocrine sweat glands of Moll, is an irregularly shaped cyst, and has an outer myoepithelium layer and an inner (luminal) layer of columnar epithelium, showing apical decapitation secretion.
      The eccrine hidrocystoma, which is derived from the eccrine sweat glands, is more rounded and shows a flattened wall that contains one or two layers of cuboidal epithelium and sometimes contains papillary projections into the lumen of the cysts. Mean age at diagnosis is 59 years; 71% of lesions are single; and 87% are located near but not on the eyelid margin.

The apocrine hidrocystoma is more likely to be proliferative than the eccrine hidrocystoma.

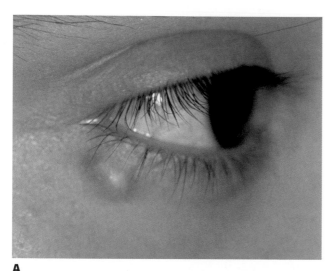

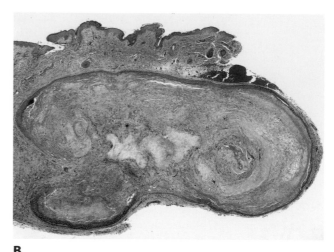

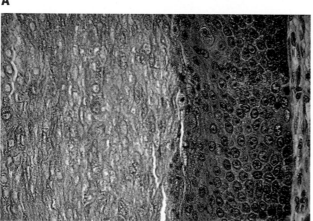

Fig. 6.21 Calcifying epithelioma of Malherbe (pilomatricoma). **A,** Clinical photo of lesion involving the lateral aspect of the right lower eyelid. **B,** Low-magnification photomicrograph demonstration position of lesion relative to the skin surface and light areas of necrosis containing shadow cells and dark basophilic cells. **C,** High magnification of pale shadow cells on left and dark basophilic cells on right. (**A** and **B,** Courtesy of Dr. Morton Smith; **C,** courtesy of Armed Forces Institute of Pathology, Washington, DC, accession number 984935.)

Benign Tumors of the Surface Epithelium

I. Papilloma (Figs 6.24 and 6.25)

   A. Papilloma is an upward proliferation of skin resulting in an elevated irregular lesion with an undulating surface.

   B. Six conditions show this type of proliferation as a predominant feature: (1) nonspecific papilloma (most common); (2) nevus verrucosus (epidermal cell nevus; Jadassohn); (3) acanthosis nigricans; (4) verruca vulgaris (see earlier under subsection *Viral Diseases*); (5) seborrheic keratosis; and (6) actinic keratosis (see later under section *Precancerous Tumors of the Surface Epithelium*).

   C. Histologically, a papilloma is characterized by finger-like projections or fronds of papillary dermis covered by epidermis showing a normal polarity but some degree of acanthosis and hyperkeratosis, along with variable parakeratosis and elongation of rete pegs.

      1. The dermal component may have a prominent vascular element.

      2. Usually, histologic examination of a papillomatous lesion indicates which of the different papillomatous conditions is involved.

   D. Nonspecific papilloma (see Fig. 6.25)

      1. Nonspecific papilloma, a polyp of the skin, is usually further subdivided into a broad-based and a narrow-based type.

         a. The broad-based type is called a *sessile papilloma*.

         b. The narrow-based type is called a *pedunculated papilloma*, a *fibroepithelial papilloma*, *acrochordon*, or simply a *skin tag*.

      2. Histologically, finger-like projections of papillary dermis are covered by normal-thickness epithelium showing elongation of rete ridges and orthokeratosis.

   E. Nevus verrucosus (epidermal cell nevus; Jadassohn)

      1. Nevus verrucosus consists of a single lesion present at birth or appearing early in life.

      2. Histologically, the lesion consists of closely set, papillomatous, orthokeratotic papules, marked acanthosis, and elongation of rete pegs.

   F. Acanthosis nigricans

      1. Acanthosis nigricans exists in five types, all showing papillomatous and verrucous brownish patches predominantly in the axillae, on the dorsum of fingers, on the neck, or in the genital and submammary regions.

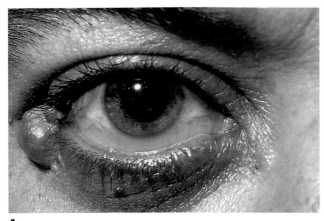

A

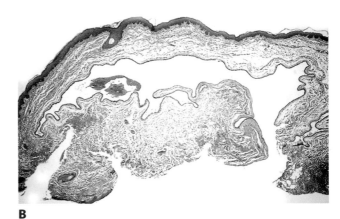

B

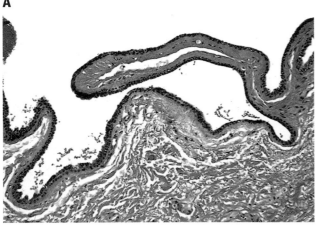

C

Fig. 6.22 Ductal cyst, probably apocrine, caused by clogged sweat duct, may take many forms. **A,** Ductal cyst noted near the outer margin of the right lower lid. **B,** Multiloculated large ductal cyst appears empty. **C,** The cyst is lined by a double layer of epithelium.

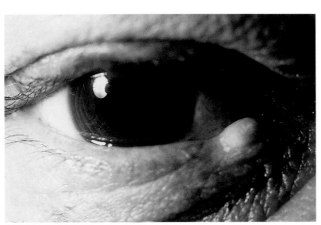

A

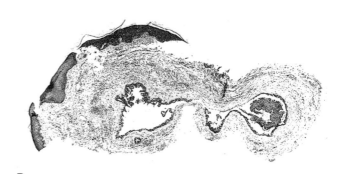

B

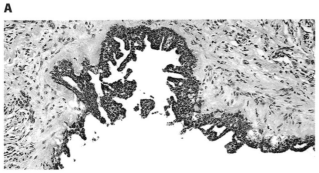

C

Fig. 6.23 Eccrine hidrocystoma. **A,** Clinical appearance of lesion. **B,** Histologic section shows a flattened wall lined by one or two layers of cuboidal epithelium and containing papillary projections into the lumen of the cysts. **C,** Increased magnification of papillary projections.

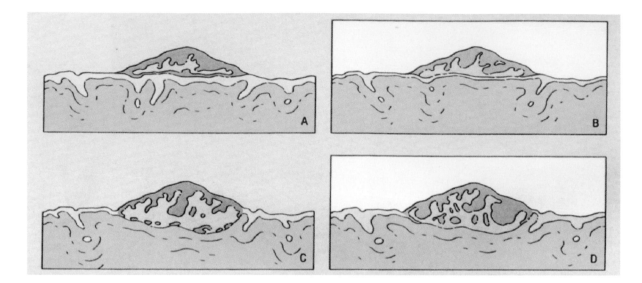

Fig. 6.24 Differences between benign and malignant skin lesions. **A,** An elevated skin lesion sitting as a "button" on the skin surface. This is characteristic of benign papillomatous lesions. When such lesions appear red histologically under low magnification, they show acanthosis, as in actinic keratosis. **B,** Lesions structurally similar to **A** but that appear blue under low magnification are caused by proliferation of basal cells, as in seborrheic keratosis. **C,** An elevated lesion that invades the underlying skin is characteristic of a malignancy. Invasive lesions that appear red under low magnification are caused by proliferation of the squamous layer (acanthosis), as in squamous cell carcinoma. **D,** A lesion structurally similar to **C** but that appears blue under low magnification represents proliferation of basal cells, as seen in basal cell carcinoma.

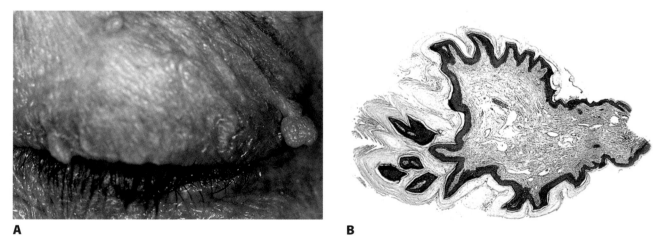

A

B

Fig. 6.25 Fibroepithelial papilloma. **A,** Clinical appearance of two skin tags (fibroepithelial papillomas) of left upper lid. **B,** Fibroepithelial papilloma consists of a narrow-based (to the right) papilloma whose fibrovascular core and finger-like projections are covered by acanthotic, orthokeratotic (hyperkeratotic) epithelium.

a. Hereditary (benign) type: not associated with an internal adenocarcinoma, other syndromes, or endocrinopathy

b. Benign type: associated with insulin resistance, endocrine disorders, and other disorders such as Crouzon's disease

c. Pseudoacanthosis nigricans: a reversible condition related to obesity

d. Drug-induced type

e. Adult (malignant) type: associated with an internal adenocarcinoma, most commonly of the stomach

f. Histologically, the first four are identical and show marked orthokeratosis and papillomatosis and mild acanthosis and hyperpigmentation. The fifth has additional malignant cytologic changes.

G. Seborrheic keratosis results from an intraepidermal proliferation of benign basal cells (basal cell acanthoma; see Fig 6.24; Fig. 6.26).

1. Seborrheic keratosis increases in size and number with increasing age and is most common in the elderly.

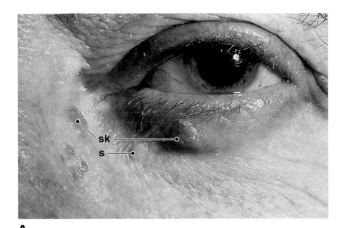

A

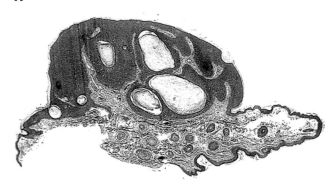

B

Fig. 6.26 Seborrheic keratosis. **A,** The "greasy" elevated lesion is present in the middle nasal portion of the left lower lid. Biopsy showed this to be a seborrheic keratosis (sk). The smaller lesion just inferior and nasal to the seborrheic keratosis proved to be a syringoma (s; see Fig. 6.38). Another seborrheic keratosis is present on the side of the nose. **B,** Histologic section shows a papillomatous lesion that lies above the skin surface and is blue. The lesion contains proliferated basaloid cells and keratin-filled cysts.

2. The lesions tend to be sharply defined, brownish, softly lobulated papules or plaques with a rough, almost warty surface.
3. Histologically, the lesion has a papillomatous configuration and an upward acanthosis so that it sits as a "button" on the surface of the skin and contains a proliferation of cells closely resembling normal basal cells, called *basaloid cells.*

The histologic appearance of a seborrheic keratosis is variable. The lesion frequently contains cystic accumulations of horny (keratinous) material. Six subtypes are recognized: acanthotic, hyperkeratotic, reticulated (adenoid), clonal, irritated (IFK; see later), and melanoacanthoma. All show acanthosis, orthokeratosis, and papillomatosis. Some may show an epithelial thickening (acanthotic) or a peculiar adenoid pattern in which the epithelium proliferates in the dermis in narrow, interconnecting cords or tracts (reticulated). It may be deeply pigmented (melanoacan-

---

thoma) and even confused clinically with a malignant melanoma.

---

4. IFK (irritated seborrheic keratosis, basosquamous cell epidermal tumor, basosquamous cell acanthoma; Fig. 6.27) resembles a seborrheic keratosis but has an additional squamous element.
   a. IFK is a benign epithelial skin lesion found most frequently on the face.
      1). Middle-aged or older people are usually affected.
      2). The lesion typically presents as an asymptomatic, pink to flesh-colored, small papule, rarely pigmented.

Rarely, IFK may recur rapidly after excision. Re-excision cures the lesion.

---

   b. It usually shows a papillomatous configuration, exists as a solitary lesion, and may exhibit rapid growth.
   c. Most IFKs are identical to irritated seborrheic keratoses, whereas others may be forms of verruca vulgaris or a reactive phenomenon related to pseudoepitheliomatous hyperplasia (see later).
   d. Histologically, IFK is similar to a seborrheic keratosis or verruca vulgaris but with the addition of basaloid cells around whorls of squamous epithelium forming squamous eddies.

II. Pseudoepitheliomatous hyperplasia (invasive acanthosis, invasive acanthoma, carcinomatoid hyperplasia; Fig. 6.28) consists of a benign proliferation of the epidermis simulating an epithelial neoplasm.
   A. It is seen frequently at the edge of burns or ulcers, near neoplasms such as basal cell carcinoma, malignant melanoma, or granular cell tumor, around areas of chronic inflammation such as blastomycosis, scrofuloderma, and gumma, or in lesions such as keratoacanthoma and perhaps IFK.
   B. Histologically, the usual type of pseudoepitheliomatous hyperplasia, no matter what the associated lesion, if any, has the following characteristics:
      1. Irregular invasion of the dermis by squamous cells that may show mitotic figures but do not show dyskeratosis or atypia
      2. Frequent infiltration of the squamous proliferations by leukocytes, mainly neutrophils

---

Although an inflammatory infiltrate is frequently seen under or around a squamous cell carcinoma, the inflammatory cells almost never infiltrate the neoplastic cells directly. If inflammatory cells admixed with squamous cells are seen, especially if the inflammatory cells are neutrophils, a reactive lesion such as pseudoepitheliomatous hyperplasia should be considered.

III. Keratoacanthoma (Fig. 6.29)
   A. Keratoacanthoma may be a type of pseudoepitheliomatous hyperplasia, although most dermatopathologists

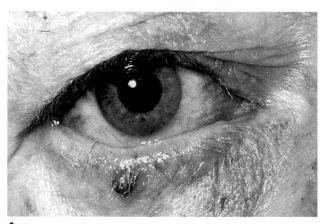

A

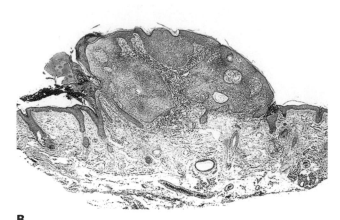

B

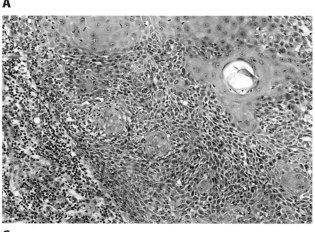

C

Fig. 6.27 Inverted follicular keratosis. **A,** Clinical appearance of lesion in the middle of the right lower lid. **B,** Histologic section shows a papillomatous lesion above the skin surface composed mainly of acanthotic epithelium. **C,** Increased magnification shows separation or acantholysis of individual squamous cells that surround the characteristic squamous eddies.

now believe it is a type of low-grade squamous cell carcinoma.

B. It consists of a solitary lesion (occasionally grouped lesions) that develops on exposed (usually hairy) areas of skin in middle-aged or elderly people, grows rapidly for 2 to 6 weeks, shows a raised, smooth edge and an umbilicated, crusted center, and then involutes in a few months to a year, leaving a depressed scar.

> Rarely, keratoacanthoma can occur on the conjunctiva.

C. Histologically, keratoacanthoma is characterized by its dome- or cup-shaped configuration with elevated wall and central keratin mass seen under low magnification, and by acanthosis with normal polarity seen under high magnification.

The deep edges of the tumor appear wide and blunt, rather than infiltrative.

> In the past, the tumor has been confused with "aggressive" squamous cell carcinoma. The typical noninvasive, elevated cup shape with a large central keratin core, as seen under low-power light microscopy, along with the benign cytology and wide and blunt deep edges seen under high-power light microscopy, should lead to the proper diagnosis of keratoacanthoma with no difficulty. If, however, only a small piece of

tissue (e.g., a partial biopsy) is available for histopathologic examination, it may be difficult or impossible to differentiate a keratoacanthoma from squamous cell carcinoma, and indeed, some keratoacanthomas show areas of undisputed squamous cell carcinoma differentiation. The superficially invasive variant of keratoacanthoma, called *invasive keratoacanthoma*, may not involute spontaneously and probably represents a form of squamous cell carcinoma.

IV. Warty dyskeratoma

A. It presents primarily on the scalp, face, or neck as an umbilicated, keratotic papule, resembling a keratoacanthoma.

B. Histologically, a cup-shaped invagination is filled with keratin and acantholytic, dyskeratotic cells. Villi of dermal papillae lined by a single layer of basal cells project into the base of the crater.

> Corps ronds (i.e., dyskeratotic cells containing pyknotic nuclei, surrounded by a clear halo, present in the granular layer at the entrance to the invagination) are reminiscent of Darier's disease.

V. Large cell acanthoma

A. Large cell acanthoma appears as a slightly keratotic, solitary lesion, usually smaller than 1 cm, and has a

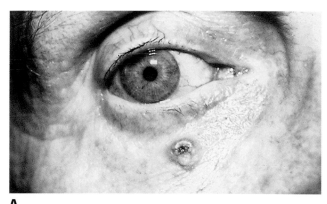

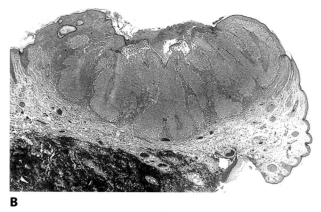

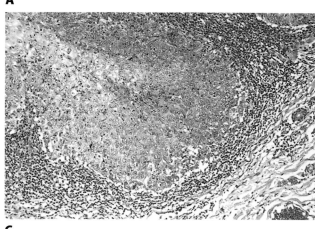

Fig. 6.28 Pseudoepitheliomatous hyperplasia. **A,** Clinical appearance. **B,** Histologic section shows marked acanthosis, mild orthokeratosis, and inflammation characteristically present in dermis and epidermis. **C,** High magnification shows polymorphonuclear leukocytes in dermis and epidermis.

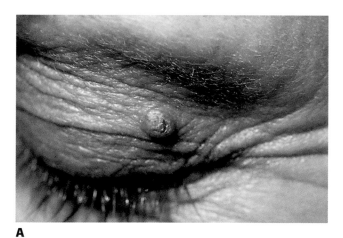

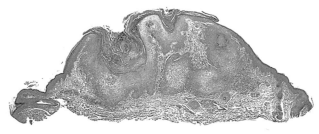

Fig. 6.29 Keratoacanthoma. **A,** This patient had a 6-week history of a rapidly enlarging lesion. Note the umbilicated central area. **B,** Histologic section shows that the lesion is above the surface epithelium, and has a cup-shaped configuration, and a central keratin core. The base of the acanthotic epithelium is blunted (rather than invasive) at the junction of the dermis.

predilection for the face and neck, followed by the upper extremities.

B. Histologically, it is a benign epidermal lesion showing a moderately acanthotic epidermis that contains sharply circumscribed, uniformly hyperplastic keratinocytes, a wavy, orthokeratotic, and parakeratotic granular cell layer, and sometimes a papillomatosis.

Dysplastic enlarged keratinocytes and an increased number of *Civatte bodies* (necrotic keratinocytes) may be found.

VI. Benign keratosis consists of a benign proliferation of epidermal cells, usually acanthotic in form, which does not fit into any known classification.

Precancerous Tumors of the Surface Epithelium

I. Leukoplakia—this is a clinical term that describes a white plaque but gives no information about the underlying cause or prognosis; the term should not be used in histopathology.

II. Xeroderma pigmentosum—see section *Congenital Abnormalities* earlier in this chapter.

III. Radiation dermatosis
   A. The chronic effects include atrophy of epidermis, dermal appendages, and noncapillary blood vessels; dilatation or telangiectasis of capillaries; and frequently hyperpigmentation.
   B. Squamous cell carcinoma (most common), basal cell carcinoma, or mesenchymal sarcomas such as fibrosarcoma may develop years after skin irradiations (e.g., after radiation for retinoblastoma).

IV. Actinic keratosis (senile keratosis; solar keratosis) occurs as multiple lesions on areas of skin exposed to sun (Fig. 6.30; see Fig. 6.24).

A. Fair-skinned people are prone to development of multiple neoplasms, including solar keratosis and basal and squamous cell carcinomas.

B. The lesions tend to be minimally elevated, slightly scaly, and flesh-colored to pink, but present as a papilloma or as a projecting cutaneous horn.

A *cutaneous horn* (*cornu cutaneum*) is a descriptive clinical term. The lesion has many causes. Actinic keratosis frequently presents clinically as a cutaneous horn, but so may verruca vulgaris, seborrheic keratosis, IFK, squamous cell carcinoma (uncommonly), and even sebaceous gland carcinoma (rarely). Approximately 77% are associated with benign lesions at the base, 15% are premalignant, and 8% are associated with malignant lesions. The most common histopathologic benign diagnosis is seborrheic keratosis; premalignant, actinic keratosis; and malignant, squamous cell carcinoma.

C. Histologically, actinic keratosis is characterized by focal to confluent parakeratosis overlying an epidermis of variable thickness.
   1. Both cellular atypia and mitotic figures appear in the deeper epidermal layers, which may form buds extending into the superficial dermis.

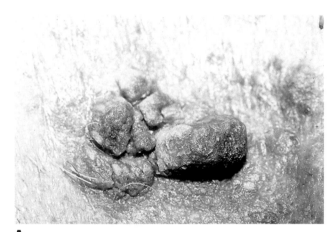

A

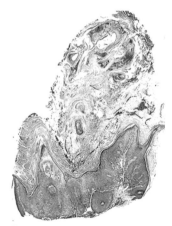

B

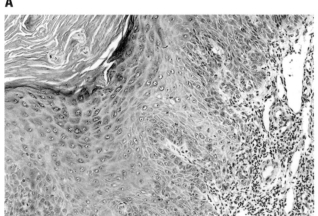

C

Fig. 6.30 Actinic keratosis. **A,** The clinical appearance of a lesion involving the left upper lid. **B,** Histologic section shows a papillomatous lesion that is above the skin surface, appears red, and has marked hyperkeratosis and acanthosis. **C,** Although the squamous layer of the skin is increased in thickness (acanthosis) and the basal layer shows atypical cells, the normal polarity of the epidermis is preserved.

Actinic keratosis may become quite pigmented and then mimic, both clinically and histopathologically, a primary melanocytic tumor.

2. The underlying dermis usually shows actinic elastosis and an inflammatory reaction mainly of lymphocytes and some plasma cells.

Actinic keratosis may resemble squamous cell carcinoma or Bowen's disease. It differs from the former in not being invasive and from the latter in not showing total replacement (loss of polarity) of the epidermis by atypical cells.

Squamous cell carcinoma infrequently and basal cell carcinoma rarely may arise from actinic keratosis.

Cancerous Tumors of the Surface Epithelium

In general, the strongest evidence from published reports regarding the treatment of malignant eyelid tumors supports complete surgical removal using histologic controls for verifying tumor-free surgical margins.

I. Basal cell carcinoma (Figs 6.31 and 6.32; see Fig. 6.24)
    A. Over 500 000 new cases of skin cancer occur each year in the United States; at least 75% are basal cell carci-

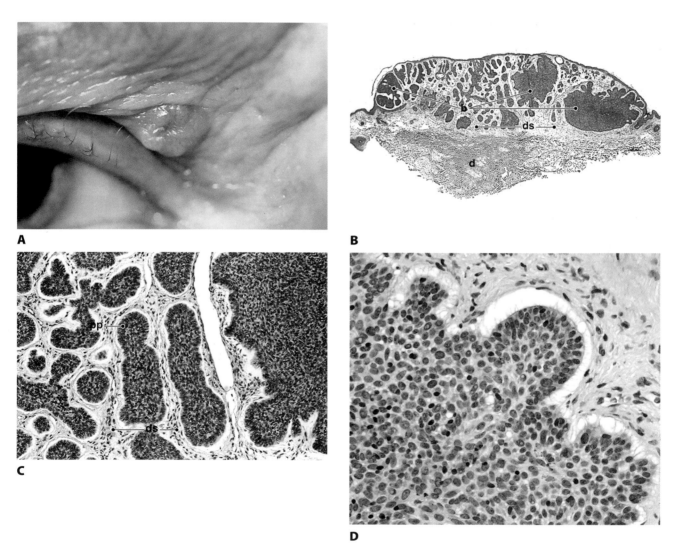

A

B

C

D

Fig. 6.31 Basal cell carcinoma. **A,** This firm, indurated painless lesion had been present and growing for approximately 8 months. **B,** Excisional biopsy shows epithelial proliferation arising from the basal layer of the epidermis (b, basal cell carcinoma). The proliferated cells appear blue and are present in nests of different sizes. Note the sharp demarcation of the pale-pink area of stroma supporting the neoplastic cells from the underlying (normal) dark-pink dermis (d, relatively normal dermis). This stromal change, called *desmoplasia* (ds, desmoplastic stroma), is characteristic of neoplastic lesions. Compare with the benign lesions in Figs 6.24 to 6.27, where the dermis does not show such a change. **C,** The nests are composed of atypical basal cells and show peripheral palisading (pp). Mitotic figures are present. Again, note the pseudosarcomatous change (desmoplasia) (ds, desmoplastic stroma) of the surrounding supporting stroma, which is light-pink and contains proliferating fibroblasts. (**A,** Courtesy of Dr. HG Scheie.) **D,** Higher magnification illustrates characteristic features of basal cell carcinoma, including atypical cells and separation artifact between nests of cells and desmoplastic surrounding connective tissue. (A, Courtesy of Dr. Hc Scheie; Courtesy of Dr. Morton Smith.)

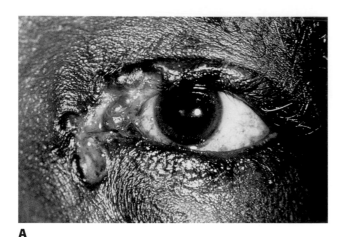

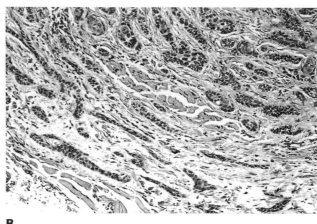

A

B

Fig. 6.32 Basal cell carcinoma. **A,** The inner aspect of the eyelids is ulcerated by the infiltrating tumor. **B,** Histologic section shows the morphea-like or fibrosing type, where the basal cells grow in thin strands or cords, often only one cell layer thick, closely resembling metastatic scirrhous carcinoma of the breast ("Indian file" pattern). This uncommon type of basal cell carcinoma has a much worse prognosis than the more common types [i.e., nodular (Fig. 6.31), ulcerative, and multicentric].

noma. Approximately 16% are located on the eyelids, most commonly on the lower eyelids.

B. Basal cell carcinoma is by far the most common malignant tumor of the eyelids, occurring most frequently on the lower eyelid, followed by the inner canthus, the upper eyelid, and then the lateral canthus. It occurs most commonly in fair-skinned people on skin areas exposed to ultraviolet radiation (i.e., sun-exposed areas).

C. The neoplasm has no sex predilection, is found most often in whites, mainly in the seventh decade of life, and tends to be only locally invasive, almost never metastasizing.

> The overproduction of sonic hedgehog, the ligand for PTC (tumor suppressor gene *PATCHED*) mimics loss of *ptc* function and induces basal cell carcinomas in mice; it may play a role in human tumorigenesis.

D. The clinical appearance varies greatly, but most present as a painless, shiny, waxy, indurated, firm, pearly nodule with a rolled border and fine telangiectases.
    1. Ulceration and pigmentation may occur.
    2. Rarely, metastases may occur.

E. Histologically and clinically, the tumor has considerable variation, but it can be grouped into three types: nodular, superficial, and morpheaform.
    1. Nodular (garden-variety) type occurs most commonly (96%):
        a. Small, moderate-sized, or large groups or nests of cells resembling basal cells show peripheral palisading.
            1). Cells in the nests contain large, oval, or elongated nuclei and little cytoplasm, may be pleomorphic and atypical but tend to be fairly uniform, and may contain mitotic figures.

2). The abnormal cells show continuity with the basal layer of surface epithelium.
        b. The neoplasm may show surface ulceration, large areas of necrosis resulting in a cystic structure, areas of glandular formation, and squamous or sebaceous differentiation (nodular basal cell carcinoma variants include keratotic, adenoidal, and pigmented).

> Basal cell carcinomas with areas of squamous differentiation, even if quite large, behave clinically as a basal cell carcinoma, not as a squamous cell carcinoma. Thus, classifying them separately and calling them *basal–squamous* (*basalosquamous*) *cell carcinomas* serves no clinically useful purpose. Similarly, in lesions with mature sebaceous differentiation, there is no useful reason to call them *sebaceous epitheliomas*. Some basal cell carcinomas may be heavily pigmented from melanin deposition and clinically simulate malignant melanomas.

c. The surrounding and intervening invaded dermis undergoes a characteristic pseudosarcomatous (resembling a sarcoma) change called *desmoplasia* (i.e., the fibroblasts become large, numerous, and often bizarre, and the mesenchymal tissue becomes mucinous, loose, and "juicy" in appearance).

> The stromal desmoplastic reaction is typical of the basal cell neoplasm and helps differentiate the tumor from the similarly appearing adenoid cystic carcinoma (see Fig. 14.37), which frequently has an amorphous, relatively acellular surrounding stroma.

d. Ductal and glandular differentiation may occur in basal cell carcinoma. Such tumors are more common on the eyelid, face, and scalp, and display the presence of ducts of varying size and glandular structures occasionally suggesting apocrine secretion.

  e. There is a significantly increased prevalence and density of demodicosis in patents with eyelid basal cell carcinoma compared to control individuals, and may act as a triggering factor for carcinogenesis in individuals predisposed by trauma, irritation, or chronic inflammation.

  f. Eyelid location is a predictive factor for extensive subclinical spread of basal cell carcinoma.

2. Superficial basal cell carcinoma shows irregular buds of basaloid cells arising from a unicentric focus or multicentric foci of the epidermal undersurface.

The superficial location makes this type the easiest to cure.

---

3. Morpheaform (fibrosing) type
  a. Rather than growing in nests of cells with peripheral palisading, the neoplastic basaloid cells grow in thin, elongated strands or cords, often only one cell layer thick, closely resembling metastatic scirrhous carcinoma of the breast ("Indian file" pattern).
  b. The stroma, rather than being juicy and loose (desmoplastic), shows considerable proliferation of connective tissue into a dense fibrous stroma, reminiscent of scleroderma or morphea.

    The tumor strands tend to shrink in processing, leaving surrounding retraction spaces.
  c. In the morpheaform variant, it is difficult clinically to determine the limits of the lesion. The tumor tends to be much more aggressive, to invade much deeper into underlying tissue, and to recur more often than the nodular or superficial type.

4. Linear basal cell carcinoma has been proposed as a distinct clinical entity found along relaxing skin tension lines of the lower eyelid and cheek, characterized by increased subclinical extension and an aggressive tumor behavior.

The *basal cell nevus syndrome* (*Gorlin's syndrome*), inherited in an autosomal-dominant fashion, consists of multiple basal cell carcinomas of the skin associated with defects in other tissues such as odontogenic cysts of the jaw, bifid rib, abnormalities of the vertebrae, and keratinizing pits on the palms and soles. Histologically, the skin tumors are indistinguishable from the noninherited form of basal cell carcinoma. The defective gene is in the tumor suppressor gene *PATCHED*, a gene on chromosome 9q.

II. Squamous cell skin carcinoma (Fig. 6.33; see Fig. 6.24)
  A. Squamous cell carcinoma rarely involves the eyelid and is seen at least 40 times less frequently than eyelid basal cell carcinoma.

1. The most frequent sites of periocular involvement are the lower eyelid (49%), medial canthus (36%), and the upper eyelid (23%).

The opposite situation exists in the conjunctiva (see p. 245–247 in Chapter 7), where squamous cell carcinoma is the most common epithelial malignancy and basal cell carcinoma is the rarest.

  B. From the 1960s to the 1980s, the incidence of squamous cell skin carcinoma increased 2.6 times in men and 3.1 times in women, attributed to presumed voluntary exposure to sunlight (ultraviolet radiation).
  C. Intraepidermal squamous cell carcinoma (squamous cell carcinoma in situ)
    1. When epidermal atypia becomes full-thickness, intraepidermal squamous cell carcinoma (carcinoma in situ) is present. It may arise de novo or from precancerous keratoses (e.g., actinic keratosis).
    2. Clinically, the area is indurated and plaquelike.
    3. Histologically, the lesion resembles the precancerous keratoses except for more advanced changes.
      a. Carcinoma in situ is characterized by replacement of the epidermis by an atypical proliferation of keratinocytes showing loss of polarity, nuclear hyperchromatism and pleomorphism, cellular atypia, and mitotic figures. Better differentiation may be accompanied by the presence of "squamous pearls or dyskeratotic pearls" formed by clusters of abnormal gradually keratinizing atypical squamous cells. These structures must be differentiated from "horn cysts" that are common in benign squamous lesions and consist of keratin-filled cysts that do not display the gradual keratinization commonly found in dyskeratotic pearls, or with the "squamous eddy" typical of IFK.
      b. The overlying stratum corneum is parakeratotic.
  D. Invasive squamous cell carcinoma
    1. Carcinoma in situ may remain fairly stationary or enlarge slowly and invade the dermis (i.e., invasive squamous cell carcinoma).
    2. Histologically, if the intraepidermal squamous cell carcinoma penetrates through the epidermal basement membrane and invades the dermis, the lesion is classified as invasive squamous cell carcinoma.

      The supporting dermal stroma then undergoes a proliferative, desmoplastic, pseudosarcomatous reaction.

Human papillomavirus (HPV) type 16 viral DNA has been found in a recurrent squamous cell carcinoma of the lid.

---

    3. Squamous cell skin carcinomas less than 2 mm thick (approximately 50% of total) almost never metastasize ("no-risk carcinomas"); of those

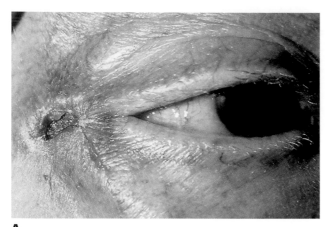

A

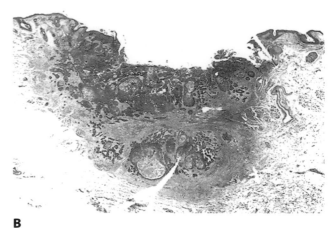

B

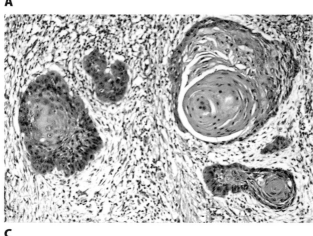

C

Fig. 6.33 Squamous cell carcinoma. **A,** The patient had an ulcerated lesion of the lateral aspect of the eyelids that increased in size over many months. **B,** Histologic section of the excisional biopsy shows epithelial cells with an overall pink color that infiltrate the dermis deeply. The overlying region is ulcerated. **C,** Increased magnification shows the invasive squamous neoplastic cells making keratin (pearls) in an abnormal location (dyskeratosis). Numerous mitotic figures are present. Note the pseudosarcomatous (dysplastic) change in the surrounding stroma.

between 2 and 6 mm thick (moderate differentiation and invasion not extending beyond the subcutis), approximately 4.5% metastasize ("low-risk carcinomas"); and of those over 6 mm thick, especially with infiltration of the musculature, perichondrium, or periosteum, approximately 15% metastasize ("high-risk carcinomas").

  a. The rate of regional lymph node metastasis in patients with eyelid or periocular squamous cell carcinoma may be as high as 24%. Sentinel lymph node biopsy may be helpful in the evaluation of conjunctival and eyelid malignancies. Preoperative lymphoscintigraphy facilitates identifying sentinel lymph nodes.

  b. Overexpression of cluster of differentiation 44 variant 6 is correlated with the progress and metastasis of ocular squamous cell carcinoma and is associated with proliferating cell nuclear antigen labeling index.

  c. Perineural invasion is an adverse prognostic finding. Cutaneous squamous cell carcinoma may show perineural spread of the neoplasm through the orbit. They may also metastasize to regional lymph nodes in about 24% of patients.

4. Squamous cell carcinoma needs to be differentiated from pseudocarcinomatous (pseudoepithelioma-tous) hyperplasia, which shows minimal or absent individual cell keratinization and nuclear atypia (see Fig. 6.28).

E. Bowen's disease (intraepidermal squamous cell carcinoma, Bowen type)

  1. Bowen's disease is a clinicopathologic entity that consists of an indolent, solitary (or multiple), erythematous, sharply demarcated, scaly patch. It grows slowly in a superficial, centrifugal manner, forming irregular, serpiginous borders.

The lesions may remain relatively stationary for up to 30 years.

---

  2. Bowen's disease is associated with other skin tumors, both malignant and premalignant, in up to 50% of patients, and with an internal cancer in up to 80% of patients.

Arsenic concentration in Bowen's disease lesions is high and may even cause them. Recently, the relationship of Bowen's disease to internal cancer has been questioned; the final word has yet to be written.

---

  3. Rarely, Bowen's disease may invade the underlying dermis, and then it behaves like an invasive squamous cell carcinoma.

4. Histologically, the lesion is characterized by a loss of polarity of the epidermis so that the normal epidermal cells are replaced by atypical, sometimes vacuolated or multinucleated, haphazardly arranged cells not infrequently showing dyskeratosis and mitotic figures that are often bizarre.

The basal cell layer is intact, and the underlying dermis is not invaded.

Histologically, the clinicopathologic entity of Bowen's disease and intraepidermal squamous cell carcinoma unrelated to Bowen's disease (see earlier) cannot be distinguished. Bowen's disease is *not* a histopathologic diagnosis but rather a clinicopathologic one.

F. Adenoacanthoma, a rare tumor, may represent a pseudoglandular (tubular and alveolar formations in the tumor) form of squamous cell carcinoma, or it may be an independent neoplasm.

The prognosis is somewhat more favorable than for the usual squamous cell carcinoma.

Clear cell acanthoma (Degos' acanthoma) is a benign, solitary, well-circumscribed, noninvasive neoplasm. Histologically, there is a proliferation of glycogen-rich, clear, large epidermal cells.

Tumors of the Epidermal Appendages (Adnexal Skin Structures)

Benign adnexal tumors include apocrine or eccrine hydrocystoma (80%), pilomatrixoma (5%), syringoma (5%), trichilemmoma (5%), syringocystadenoma papilliferum (2%), trichoepithelioma 1%, and trichofolliculoma (1%).

I. Tumors of, or resembling, sebaceous glands

A. Congenital sebaceous gland hyperplasia (organoid nevus syndrome, nevus sebaceus of Jadassohn, congenital sebaceous gland hamartoma)

1. Congenital sebaceous gland hyperplasia consists of a single, hairless patch, usually on the face or scalp, that usually reaches its full size at puberty.

2. The tumor seems to be a developmental error, resulting in a localized hyperplasia of sebaceous glands frequently associated with numerous imperfectly developed hair follicles and occasionally apocrine glands.

The tumor can be considered hamartomatous.

Epibulbar choristoma and conjunctival choristomas, choroidal colobomas, macro optic discs, and focal yellow discoloration in the fundus may occur in the nevus sebaceus of Jadassohn. *Linear nevus sebaceus syndrome* consists of nevus sebaceus of Jadassohn, seizures, and mental retardation.

---

3. Histologically, a group or groups of mature sebaceous gland lobules, with or without hair follicles, and frequently with underlying apocrine glands, are present just under the epidermis, along with overlying papillomatosis.

Basal cell carcinoma may develop in up to 20% of the lesions, and more rarely other tumors may develop (e.g., syringocystadenoma papilliferum and sebaceous carcinoma). Moreover, syringocystadenoma papilliferum may mimic basal cell carcinoma clinically.

B. Acquired sebaceous gland hyperplasia (senile sebaceous gland hyperplasia, senile sebaceous nevi, adenomatoid sebaceous gland hyperplasia)

1. Acquired sebaceous gland hyperplasia consists of one or more small, elevated, soft, yellowish, slightly umbilicated nodules occurring on the face (especially the forehead) in the elderly.

2. Histologically, a greatly enlarged sebaceous gland is composed of numerous lobules grouped around a central large sebaceous duct.

Sebaceous gland hyperplasia may follow chronic dermatitis, especially acne rosacea and rhinophyma.

C. Adenoma sebaceum of Pringle (angiofibromas of face; Fig. 6.34)

1. The small, reddish, smooth papules seen on the nasolabial folds, on the cheeks, and on the chin in people with *tuberous sclerosis* (see p. 34 in Chapter 2) have been called adenoma sebaceum (Pringle) but are truly angiofibromas.

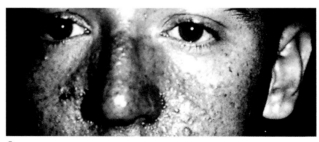

A

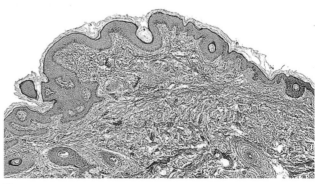

B

Fig. 6.34 Adenoma sebaceum of Pringle in tuberous sclerosis. **A,** Clinical appearance. **B,** Dermal capillary dilatation and fibrosis are typical components of the lesion (i.e., angiofibroma).

2. Histologically, the sebaceous glands are usually atrophic.

   Dilated capillaries and fibrosis are seen in the smaller lesions, whereas capillary dilatation is minimal or absent in the larger lesions, where markedly sclerotic collagen is arranged in thick concentric layers around atrophic hair follicles.

D. Sebaceous adenoma

   1. Although rare, it has a predilection for the eyebrow and eyelid and appears as a single, firm, yellowish nodule.

   The presence of a solitary sebaceous gland lesion (mainly adenoma) may be associated with a visceral malignancy, primarily of the gastrointestinal tract (*Muir–Torre syndrome*). Both clear-cut benign sebaceous and transitional squamosebaceous neoplasms should be considered as possible manifestations of the syndrome. Multiple sebaceous adenomas and extraocular sebaceous carcinoma have been reported in a patient with multiple sclerosis.

   ---

   2. Histologically, the irregularly shaped lobules are composed of three types of cells.
      a. Generative or undifferentiated cells

      These are identical in appearance to the cells present at the periphery of normal sebaceous glands. Their presence allows the diagnosis to be made.

      ---

      b. Mature sebaceous cells
      c. Transitional cells between the preceding two types

E. Sebaceous gland carcinoma (Fig. 6.35; see Fig. 6.4B)

   1. Sebaceous gland carcinoma is more common in middle-aged women, has a predilection for the eyelids, and arises mainly from the meibomian glands but also from the glands of Zeis.
      a. It is the most common eyelid malignancy after basal cell carcinoma
      b. In descending order of frequency, it affects the upper lid (two to three times more often than the lower), the lower lid, the caruncle, then the brow.

   2. Clinically, a sebaceous gland carcinoma is often mistaken for a chalazion. The lesion, however, may mimic many conditions, and is called the *great masquerader*.

   Any recurrent chalazion should be considered for histologic study, and any chronic, recalcitrant, atypical blepharitis or atypical unilateral papillary conjunctivitis should be considered for biopsy.

   ---

   3. The mortality rate is approximately 22%.

   Treatment by Mohs micrographic surgery may significantly reduce the mortality.

   ---

4. Histologically, irregular lobular masses of cells resemble sebaceous adenoma but tend to be more bizarre and to show distinct invasiveness.

   Mutational inactivation of p53 may be involved in the progression of sebaceous carcinoma.

   ---

   a. Focally, cells show abundant cytoplasm signifying sebaceous differentiation.
   b. Fat stains of frozen sections of fixed tissue show that many of the cells are lipid-positive.
   c. The malignant epithelial cells may invade the epidermis, producing an overlying change resembling Paget's disease called *pagetoid change*.

   Intraepithelial sebaceous carcinoma (pagetoid change) can spread to the conjunctiva and cornea. Resultant diffuse loss of lashes may simulate a blepharitis. Rarely, intraepithelial sebaceous carcinoma may be the only evidence of the lesion with no underlying invasion present. The intraepithelial invasion may involve the lids and conjunctiva together, or only the conjunctiva and cornea.

II. Tumors of or resembling hair follicles

   A. Trichoepithelioma (epithelioma adenoides cysticum, benign cystic epithelioma)

   Trichoepithelioma is probably a special variety of trichoblastoma, characterized by its almost universal facial location, its dermal rather than subcutaneous location, its mainly cribriform pattern, and its compartmentalized clefts between fibroepithelial units. Trichoblastoma, a benign tumor of hair germ cells (follicular germinative cells), includes the entities panfolliculoma, trichoblastoma with advanced follicular differentiation, immature trichoepithelioma, and trichoepithelioma.

   ---

   1. The tumor may occur as a single nodule (Fig. 6.36), as a few isolated nodules, or as multiple symmetric nodules with onset at puberty. It occurs predominantly on the face and is inherited as an autosomal-dominant trait (Brooke's tumor).
   2. The nodule is small and rosy yellow or glistening flesh-colored, and tends to grow to several millimeters or even to 1 cm.
   3. Histologically, multiple squamous cell cysts (i.e., *horn cysts*, consisting of a keratinized center surrounded by basaloid cells) are the characteristic finding and represent immature hair structures.
      a. Basaloid cells, indistinguishable from the cells that constitute basal cell carcinoma, are present around the horn cysts and in the surrounding tissue as a lacework or as solid islands.
      b. Occasionally the cysts have openings to the skin surface and resemble abortive hair follicles.
      c. The cysts may rupture, inducing granulomatous inflammation, or they may become calcified.

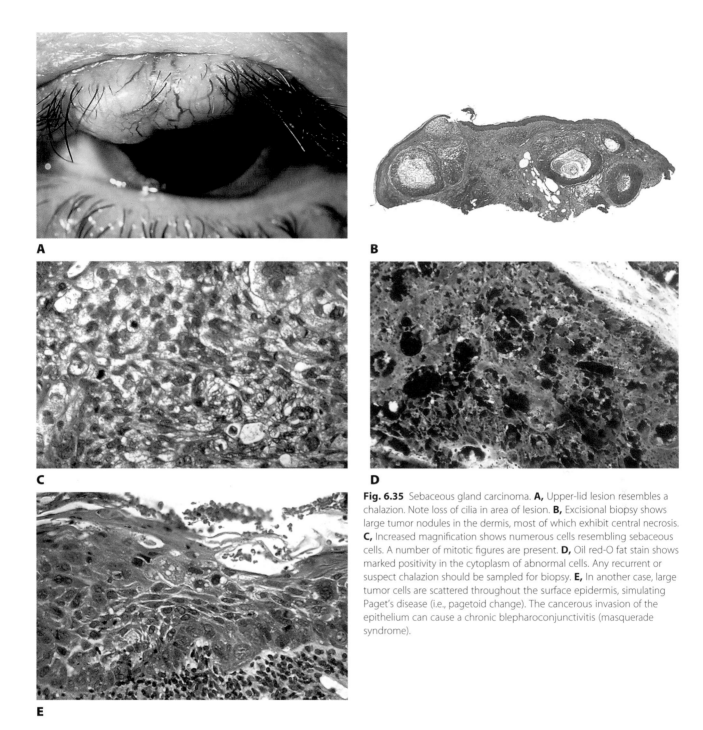

Fig. 6.35 Sebaceous gland carcinoma. **A,** Upper-lid lesion resembles a chalazion. Note loss of cilia in area of lesion. **B,** Excisional biopsy shows large tumor nodules in the dermis, most of which exhibit central necrosis. **C,** Increased magnification shows numerous cells resembling sebaceous cells. A number of mitotic figures are present. **D,** Oil red-O fat stain shows marked positivity in the cytoplasm of abnormal cells. Any recurrent or suspect chalazion should be sampled for biopsy. **E,** In another case, large tumor cells are scattered throughout the surface epidermis, simulating Paget's disease (i.e., pagetoid change). The cancerous invasion of the epithelium can cause a chronic blepharoconjunctivitis (masquerade syndrome).

The horn cyst shows complete and abrupt keratinization, thereby distinguishing it from the *horn* pearl of squamous cell carcinoma, which shows incomplete and gradual keratinization.

Trichoadenoma, a rare benign cutaneous tumor, resembles trichofolliculoma, but the cells appear less mature; conversely, the cells appear more mature than the cells in trichoepithelioma.

B. Trichofolliculoma
1. Trichofolliculoma is found in adults and consists of a small, solitary lesion frequently with a central pore.

2. Histologically, a large dermal cystic space lined by squamous epithelium and containing keratin and hair shaft fragments is surrounded by smaller, well-differentiated, secondary hair follicles.

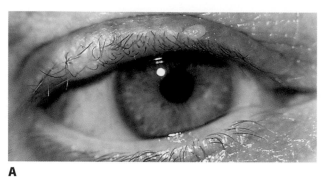

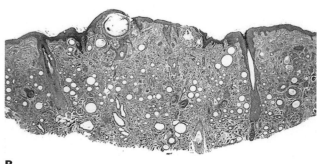

A

B

Fig. 6.36 Trichoepithelioma. **A,** Clinical appearance of a lesion in the middle of the right upper lid near the margin. **B,** Histologic section shows the tumor diffusely present throughout the dermis. The tumor is composed of multiple squamous cell horn cysts that represent immature hair structures.

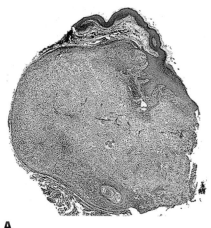

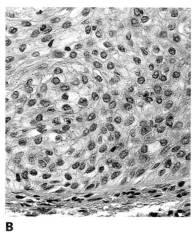

A

B

Fig. 6.37 Trichilemmoma. **A,** Histologic section shows lobular acanthosis of clear cells (shown with increased magnification in **B**) oriented around hair follicles. **C,** The clear cells are strongly periodic acid–Schiff-positive.

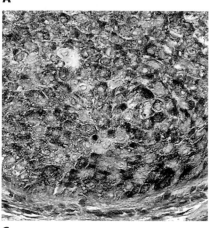

C

C. Trichilemmoma (Fig. 6.37)
1. It tends to be a solitary, asymptomatic lesion located on the face and mainly found in middle-aged people. The lesion has no sex predilection.
2. Characteristically, trichilemmoma often shows a central pore that contains a tuft of wool-like hair.

Patients who have multiple (not solitary) facial trichilemmomas may have *Cowden's disease* (*multiple hamartoma syndrome*), an autosomal-dominant disease characterized by multiple trichilemmomas, acral keratoses, occasional Merkel cell carcinoma, oral papillomas, goiter, hypothyroidism, ovarian cysts, uterine leiomyomas, oral and gastrointestinal polyps, and breast disease.

3. Histologically, a central cystic space represents an enlarged hair follicle.
   a. A lobular acanthosis of glycogen-rich cells is oriented about hair follicles.
   b. The edge of the lesion usually shows a palisade of columnar cells that resemble the outer root sheath of a hair follicle and rest on a well-formed basement membrane.

4. Desmoplastic trichilemmoma may simulate a verruca, follicular keratosis, or a basal cell carcinoma. It is characterized by the presence of central desmoplasia, outer root sheath differentiation of the tumor cells, and CD34 positivity. These features help differentiate it from basal cell carcinoma.

D. Trichilemmal carcinoma

1. Trichilemmal carcinoma is a rare tumor that arises from the hair sheath, mainly on the face or ears of the elderly. Actinic damage, long-term low-dose irradiation, and transformation from benign trichilemmoma have been postulated as possible pathogenetic mechanisms.

2. Histologically, it is composed of follicular-oriented, lobular sheets of atypical, clear, glycogen-containing cells resembling the outer root sheath of a hair follicle.

3. Malignant proliferating trichilemmal tumor of the eyelid has ben reported. It was characterized by proliferation of outer hair sheath epithelium with multiple central areas of trichilemmal keratinization.

E. Calcifying epithelioma of Malherbe (pilomatricoma; see earlier section *Benign Cystic Lesions*)

F. Adnexal carcinoma—the term *adnexal carcinoma* should be restricted to those tumors that are histologically identical to basal cell carcinoma but in which the site of origin (e.g., epidermis, hair follicle, sweat gland, sebaceous gland) cannot be determined.

III. Tumors of or resembling sweat glands: Apocrine sweat glands are represented in the eyelids by Moll's glands; eccrine sweat glands are present in the lids both at the lid margin and in the dermis over the surface of the eyelid.

A. Syringoma (Fig. 6.38)

1. Syringoma is a common, benign, adenomatous tumor of the eccrine sweat structure occurring mainly in young women and consisting of small, soft papules, usually only 1 or 2 mm in size, found predominantly on the lower eyelids. It probably arises from intraepidermal eccrine ducts.

Rarely, malignant syringoma (well-differentiated eccrine carcinoma) may occur on the eyelid.

---

2. Histologically, dermal epithelial strands of small basophilic cells are characteristic, as are cystic ducts lined by a double layer of flattened epithelial cells and containing a colloidal material. The ducts often have comma-like tails that give them the appearance of tadpoles.

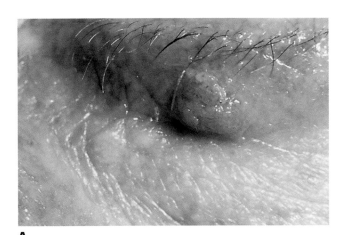

A

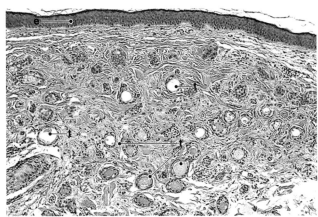

B

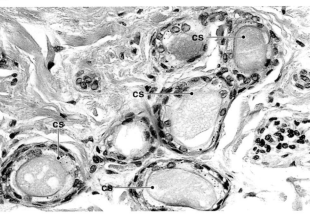

C

Fig. 6.38 Syringoma. **A,** Clinical appearance of lesions just below and nasal to seborrheic keratosis of left lower lid (same patient as in Fig. 6.26). **B,** Histologic section shows that the dermis contains proliferated eccrine sweat gland structures that form epithelial strands and cystic spaces (e, surface epithelium; t, tumor "ducts" and epithelial strands). **C,** Increased magnification demonstrates epithelial strands and cystic spaces lined by a double-layered epithelium (cs).

A variant of syringoma is the chondroid syringoma (mixed tumor of the skin—see later). Fewer than 30 cases have been reported to involve the periorbital area. The lesions are classified into an apocrine type having tubular cystic branching lumens lined by two layers of epithelial cells, and the eccrine type having small tubular lumens lined by a single layer of epithelial cells. Each of these types may have benign, atypical, and malignant variants. There is also a myxoid, adipocytic, chondroid, and/or fibrous stroma. Complete excision and regular follow-up of even cytologically benign lesions are recommended because they may recur with malignant transformation.

B. Syringomatous carcinoma
1. Many names have been given to the entity of syringomatous carcinoma: syringoid eccrine carcinoma, eccrine epithelioma, basal cell epithelioma with eccrine differentiation, eccrine carcinoma with syringomatous features, sclerosing sweat duct carcinoma, many examples of microcystic adnexal carcinoma, malignant syringoma, sclerosing sweat duct syringomatous carcinoma, sweat gland carcinoma with syringomatous features, basal cell carcinoma with eccrine differentiation, and eccrine basaloma.
   a. Eighty-one percent of cases of microcystic adnexal carcinoma that have histopathology checked in the initial assessment are misdiagnosed.
2. The tumor usually occurs as a single nodule and can be classified as well, moderately, or poorly differentiated syringomatous carcinoma.
   a. Well-differentiated syringomatous carcinoma is characterized by many discrete tubules, lack of nuclear atypia, some mitotic figures, often aggregations of cells showing a solid basaloid or cribriform, adenoid cyst-like pattern, and usually desmoplastic or sclerotic stroma.
   b. Moderately differentiated syringomatous carcinoma consists of easily recognized, well-formed tubules, nuclear atypia, few or no mitotic figures, and usually desmoplastic or sclerotic stroma.
   c. Poorly differentiated syringomatous carcinoma consists of focal subtle tubular differentiation, striking nuclear atypia, numerous mitotic figures, strands of neoplastic cells between collagen bundles, and usually desmoplastic or sclerotic stroma.
3. Infiltration of the underlying subcutaneous tissue, perineural spaces, and muscle, often with focal inflammation, is common.
4. In addition to PAS positivity in some lumina and lining cells, immunohistochemical staining is positive for S-100 protein, high-molecular-weight cytokeratins (AE1/AE3), and epithelial membrane antigen (negative for K-10 and the low-molecular-weight cytokeratin CAM 5.2).
C. Syringocystadenoma papilliferum (papillary syringadenoma)

1. Syringocystadenoma papilliferum represents an adenoma of apocrine sweat structures that differentiates toward apocrine ducts.
2. The lesion is usually solitary and occurs in the scalp as a hairless, smooth plaque until puberty, after which it becomes raised, nodular, and verrucous. In 75% of cases, the lesion arises in a pre-existent nevus sebaceous (see p. 201 in this chapter); the other 25% occur as an isolated finding.
3. Histologically, the epidermis is papillomatous.
   a. One or more cystic invaginations (frequently forming villus-like projections), lined by a double layer of cells composed of luminal high columnar cells and outer myoepithelial cells, extend into the dermis.
   b. The cystic spaces open from the surface epithelium rather than representing closed spaces entirely within the dermis.

In most cases, a heavy plasma cell inflammatory infiltrate is present. Congenital abnormalities of sebaceous glands and hair follicles are often also present.

D. Eccrine spiradenoma (nodular hidradenoma, clear cell hidradenoma, clear cell carcinoma, clear cell myoepithelioma, myoepithelioma)
1. Eccrine spiradenomas usually occur in adults as deep, solitary, characteristically painful dermal nodules that arise from eccrine structures.
2. Histologically, the tumor is composed of one or more basophilic dermal islands arranged in intertwining bands, as well as tubules containing two types of cells and surrounded by a connective tissue capsule.
   a. Small, dark cells with dark nuclei and scant cytoplasm are present toward the periphery of the bands and tubules.

Previously, these undifferentiated basal cells were incorrectly thought to be myoepithelial cells.

   b. Cells with large, pale nuclei and scant cytoplasm are present in the center of the bands and tubules, and line the few small lumina usually present.

A possible variant of the eccrine spiradenoma is a tumor composed primarily of cells containing clear cytoplasm called a *clear cell hidradenoma* (*eccrine acrospiroma*, clear cell myoepithelioma, solid cystic hidradenoma, clear cell papillary carcinoma, porosyringoma, nodular hidradenoma). An intradermal nodule that may ulcerate or enlarge rapidly secondary to internal hemorrhage, the clear cell hidradenoma shows two cell types: a polyhedral to fusiform cell with slightly basophilic or eosinophilic cytoplasm, and a clear (glycogen-containing) cell. The epithelial cells stain positively for cytokeratins AE1 and AE3 (high-molecular-weight cytokeratins), epithelial membrane and carcinoembryonic antigens, and muscle-specific actin. Although the clear cell hidradenoma is thought to be of eccrine origin, it may be of apocrine gland origin. A further variant of the clear cell hydradenoma is the *apocrine mixed tumor*. The histologic appearance is the same as that of the lacrimal gland mixed tumor. A more probable variant of eccrine spiradenoma is the *eccrine hidrocystoma* (see earlier subsection *Benign Cystic Lesions*).

E. Eccrine mixed tumor (chondroid syringoma; see earlier)
 1. Eccrine mixed tumor is rarer than the apocrine mixed tumor, but is histologically similar.
 2. Histologically, it has tubular lumina lined by a single layer of flat epithelial cells.

Conversely, the epithelial lining of apocrine mixed tumors is larger, more irregularly shaped, and consists of at least a double layer of epithelial cells.

 a. The epithelial lining stains positively for cytokeratin, carcinoembryonic antigen, and epithelial membrane antigen.
 b. The outer layers prove positive for vimentin, S-100 protein, neuron-specific enolase, and sometimes glial acidic protein.
 c. The stroma stains immunohistochemically like the outer cell layers.
F. Cylindroma (turban tumor)
 1. Cylindroma is probably of apocrine origin, is benign, often has an autosomal-dominant inheritance pattern, has a predilection for the scalp, and appears in early adulthood.

Cylindromas and trichoepitheliomas are frequently associated and may occur in such numbers as to cover the whole scalp like a turban, hence the name *turban tumor*.

 2. Histologically, islands of cells fit together like pieces of a jigsaw puzzle and consist of two types of cells, irregular in size and shape, separated from each other by an amorphous, hyaline-like stroma.
 a. Cells with small, dark nuclei and scant cytoplasm are found in the periphery of the islands.
 b. Cells with large, pale nuclei and scant cytoplasm are present in the center of the islands.
 c. Tubular lumina are usually present and are lined by cells demonstrating decapitation secretion, like cells seen in apocrine glands.
G. Eccrine poroma
 1. Eccrine poroma usually occurs on the soles of the feet as firm, dome-shaped, slightly pedunculated, pinkish-red tumors, but it may occur elsewhere. It arises from the eccrine duct as it courses through the epidermis.
 2. Histologically, it consists of intraepidermal masses of cells that thicken the epidermis and extend down into the dermal area.

 a. The cells are connected by intercellular bridges.
 b. The cells resemble squamous cells but are more cuboidal and smaller, and have a basophilic nucleus.
 c. Small ductal lumina are usually present and are lined by a PAS-positive, diastase-resistant cuticle.

Eccrine porocarcinoma is a rare form of eccrine adenocarcinoma. Most commonly it arises on the lower extremity and has a variable prognosis. Rarely it has been reported to occur on the eyelid.

H. Oncocytoma
 1. Oncocytoma may occur on the caruncle (see Fig. 7.19), lacrimal gland, lacrimal sac, and much more rarely on the lids. It arises from apocrine glands.
 2. Histologically, the tumor usually shows cystic and papillary components.
 3. Electron microscopy shows malformed mitochondria in the tumor cells.
I. Sweat gland carcinomas are rare.
 1. Eccrine sweat gland carcinomas

Two groups occur: one arises from benign eccrine tumors (or de novo) as a malignant counterpart. These include eccrine porocarcinoma, malignant eccrine spiradenoma, malignant hidradenoma, and malignant chondroid syringoma. The second group comprises primary eccrine carcinomas and includes classic eccrine adenocarcinoma (ductal eccrine carcinoma), syringomatous carcinoma (see earlier), microcystic adnexal carcinoma (see later), mucinous (adenocystic) carcinoma, and aggressive digital papillary adenocarcinoma. Mucinous eccrine adenocarcinoma is a rare ocular adnexal tumor that can involve the eyelid and periocular skin, can be locally invasive, and has a high risk of local recurrence even after Mohs surgery. Nevertheless, the prognosis following excision with confirmed tumor-free margins is good.

 a. They have a tubular, or rarely, an adenomatous (adenocarcinoma) structure.

A rare histiocytoid variant may be seen.

 b. Histologically, it is difficult to differentiate eccrine carcinoma from metastatic carcinoma; the diagnosis of metastatic carcinoma should therefore always be considered before making a final diagnosis of eccrine carcinoma.

Signet-ring carcinoma of eccrine or apocrine gland origin has been described.

 c. Microcystic adnexal carcinoma
 1). Usually solitary and occurs as a nodule or indurated, deep-seated plaque

Many tumors previously diagnosed as microcystic adnexal carcinomas are really syringomatous carcinoma. Also, signet-ring cell carcinoma of the eccrine sweat glands of the eyelid should not be confused with syringomatous carcinoma.

2). In the superficial part of the tumor, small keratocytes are often seen, whereas deeper in the tumor, microtubules and thin trabeculae predominate.

3). Infiltration of the underlying subcutaneous tissue, perineural spaces, and muscle, often with focal inflammation, is common.

4). The histogenesis is unknown—theories include eccrine and pilar origin.

2. Apocrine sweat gland carcinomas (from Moll's glands in the eyelid) are adenocarcinomas and occur in two varieties: a ductopapillary tumor located exclusively in the dermis, and an intraepidermal proliferation (i.e., extramammary Paget's disease) that rarely invades the dermis. Apocrine carcinoma

of the eyelids may demonstrate an aggressive behavior, including distant metastasis.

a. Histiocytoid variant of eccrine sweat gland carcinoma of the eyelid may present as an insidious tumor and diffusely invade the orbit. Histopathologically, the tumor consists of cells with a histiocytoid to signet-ring appearance, which are positive for low- and high-molecular-weight cytokeratins, carcinoembryonic antigen, and epithelial membrane antigen.

Merkel Cell Carcinoma (Neuroendocrine Carcinoma, Trabecular Carcinoma) (Fig. 6.39)

I. The Merkel cell, first described by Friedrich Merkel in 1875, is a distinctive, nondendritic, nonkeratinocytic epithelial clear cell believed to migrate from the neural crest to the epidermis and dermis.

Merkel cells, specialized epithelial cells that probably act as touch receptors, are sporadically present at the undersurface of the epi-

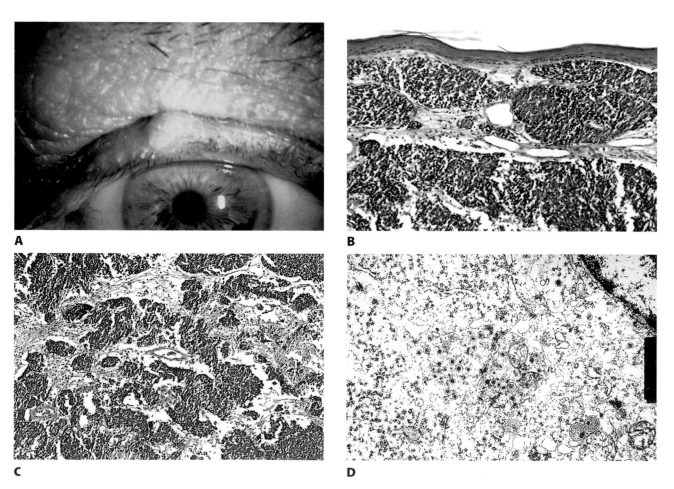

Fig. 6.39 Merkel cell tumor. **A,** Patient has lesions on the middle portion of upper lid. **B,** Excisional biopsy shows nests of dark, poorly differentiated cells in the dermis. **C,** Increased magnification demonstrates round cells that resemble large lymphoma cells. Numerous mitotic figures are seen. **D,** Electron micrograph shows the nucleus in the upper right corner. Many cytoplasmic, small, dense-core, neurosecretory granules are seen. (Case presented by Dr. DA Morris at the meeting of the Eastern Ophthalmic Pathology Section, 1985; **D,** Courtesy of Dr. A di Sant'Agnese and Ms. KWJ de Mesy Jensen.)

dermis. Other specialized cells present in the epidermis include the three types of dendritic cell (i.e., Langerhans' cells, melanocytes, and the intermediate dendritic cells).

A. Tumors arising from Merkel cells occur on the head and neck area, the trunk, arms, and legs, mainly (75%) in patients 65 years of age or older.

Merkel cell carcinoma, like other neuroectodermal tumors (e.g., neuroblastoma, malignant melanoma, and pheochromocytoma), may show a distal deletion involving chromosome 1p35–36. Also, Merkel cell carcinoma may occur in Cowden's disease (see earlier discussion of trichilemmoma).

B. Clinically, the most common appearance is that of a nonulcerated, reddish-purple nodule.
C. The tumor is aggressive, has variable clinical manifestations, tends to spread early to regional lymph nodes, and should probably be treated with radical surgical therapy.
II. Histologically, they resemble a primary cutaneous lymphoma or cutaneous metastasis of lymphoma or carcinoma.
A. The tumor is composed of solid arrangements of neoplastic cells, simulating large cell malignant lymphoma cells, separated from the epidermis by a clear space.
B. Immunohistochemical staining is strongly positive for neuron-specific enolase, chromogranin, and cytokeratins 8, 18, and 19 (low–molecular-weight type); it is weakly positive for synaptophysin, but negative for leukocytic markers.
C. Electron microscopy shows characteristic membrane-bound, dense-core neurosecretory granules; paranuclear aggregates of intermediate filaments; and cytoplasmic actin filaments.

After excision, a high frequency of recurrence exists, and metastases can occur.

Malacoplakia

I. Malacoplakia is a rare disorder in which tumors occur subjacent to an epithelial surface.
A. Malacoplakia often arises in immunodeficient or immunosuppressed patients.
B. It is characterized by persistent bacterial infection, most often with *Escherichia coli*.
II. Histologically, aggregates of histiocytes (von Hansemann histiocytes) contain characteristic inclusions (Michaelis–Gutmann bodies).

Pigmented Tumors

See Chapter 17.

Mesenchymal Tumors

The same mesenchymal tumors that may occur in the orbit may also occur in the eyelid and are histopathologically identical (see subsection *Mesenchymal Tumors* in Chapter 14).

Metastatic Tumors

I. Metastasis to the eyelids is uncommon and usually a late manifestation of the disease.
A. The most frequent primary tumor is breast carcinoma, followed by lung carcinoma and cutaneous melanoma.
B. More rare primary tumors include stomach, colon, thyroid, parotid, and trachea carcinomas.
C. Although metastatic cancer is usually unilateral, the presence of lesions involving eyelids of both eyes does not exclude the possibility of metastatic disease.
II. The histologic appearance depends on the nature of the primary tumor.

LACRIMAL DRAINAGE SYSTEM

NORMAL ANATOMY (Fig. 6.40)

The excretory portion of the lacrimal system consists of the canaliculi (upper and lower), common canaliculus, lacrimal sac, and nasolacrimal duct. The nasolacrimal apparatus develops during the sixth week of prenatal life as a line of epithelium formed by the overlapping of lateral nasal processes by the maxillary processes.
I. Tears pool toward the medial canthus at the lacus lacrimalis and then enter the lacrimal puncta that lie near the nasal end of each eyelid.
A. The lower punctum lies slightly lateral to the upper.
B. Normally, both are turned inward to receive tears, and therefore are not visible to direct inspection.
C. The puncta vary from 0.5 to 1.5 mm in diameter.
II. The canaliculi are lined by stratified, nonkeratinized squamous epithelium.
III. The lacrimal sac is also lined with nonkeratinized squamous epithelium but, unlike the canaliculi, it contains

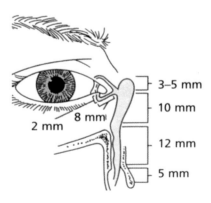

Fig. 6.40 Schematic functional anatomy of the lacrimal excretory system. (From de Toledo AR *et al.*: In Podos SM, Yanoff M, eds: *Textbook of Ophthalmology*, vol. 8. Copyright Elsevier 1994.)

many goblet cells and foci of columnar ciliated (respiratory-type) epithelium. The vascular plexus (cavernous body) that surrounds the lacrimal sac and nasolacrimal duct is subject to autonomic control and plays an important role in regulating the rate of tear outflow.

IV. The nasolacrimal duct occupies roughly 75% of the 3- to 4-mm-wide bony nasolacrimal canal.

Many so-called valves have been described in the duct, but these represent folds of the mucosa rather than true valves, although presumably they may retard flow in some individuals.

V. Tear duct-associated lymphoid tissue is commonly found in individuals with symptomatically normal nasolacrimal ducts, and appears to be most associated with the scarring of symptomatic dacryostenosis.

CONGENITAL ABNORMALITIES

Atresia of the Nasolacrimal Duct

I. The nasolacrimal duct usually becomes completely canalized and opens into the nose by the eighth month of fetal life.

II. The duct may fail to canalize (usually at its lower end) or epithelial debris may clog it.

III. Most ducts not open at birth open spontaneously during the first 6 months postpartum.

IV. Congenital dacryocystocele is a rare anomaly accompanied by swelling of the lacrimal sac that is present at birth and resulting from obstruction of the lacrimal system either above or below the lacrimal sac.

Atresia of the Punctum

I. Atresia of the punctum may occur alone or be associated with atresia of the nasolacrimal duct.

II. An acquired form may result secondary to scarring from any cause.

Lacrimal outflow dysgenesis may involve multiple components of the system, including absent or hypoplastic punctum, canaliculus, lacrimal sac, and/or nasolacrimal duct. The dysgenesis is proximal in 89%, distal in 33%, and both in 22%. Systemic syndrome or dysmorphism is present in 40% of cases and positive family history is noted in 36%.

III. Punctal stenosis may be an acquired condition having a variety of causes, including: chronic blepharitis, 45%; unknown etiology, 27%; ectropion, 23%; and drug-related 5%. Punctal stenosis may be accompanied by obstruction of the lacrimal drainage system at other levels.

Congenital Fistula of Lacrimal Sac (Minimal Facial Fissure)

I. An opening of the lacrimal sac directly into the nose (internal fistula) or out on to the cheek (external fistula—

the more common of the two) is a not uncommon finding.

II. The opening, which may be unilateral or bilateral, is quite narrow and may be overlooked.

There are many other anomalies of the lacrimal puncta, canaliculus, sac, and nasolacrimal duct, but these are beyond the scope of this book.

INFLAMMATION—DACRYOCYSTITIS (Fig. 6.41)

Blockage of Tear Flow into the Nose

I. Most inflammations and infections of the lacrimal sac are secondary to a blockage of tear flow at the level of the sac opening into the nasolacrimal duct or distal to that point.

II. A cast of the lacrimal sac (see Fig. 4.12) may be formed by *Streptothrix* (*Actinomyces*), which also can cause a secondary conjunctivitis.

III. Treatment for dry-eye syndromes utilizing punctal plugs or of canalicular injury with stents may occasionally result in pyogenic granuloma formation. Such lesions may eventuate in extrusion of the punctal plug in 4.2% of such plugs. Other complications have been reported.

IV. Lacrimal sac biopsies represent approximately 1.8% of the specimens sent to a busy ophthalmic pathology laboratory.

The most common diagnoses were: nongranulomatous inflammation, 85.1%; granulomatous inflammation consistent with sarcoidosis, 2.1%; lymphoma, 1.9%; papilloma, 1.11%; lymphoplasmacytic infiltrate, 1.1%; transitional cell carcinoma, 0.5%; and single cases of adenocarcinoma, undifferentiated carcinoma, granular cell tumor, plasmacytoma, and leukemic infiltrate. Another study of the histopathology of the lacrimal drainage system found the following diagnoses: dacryocystitis, 79%; dacryolithiasis, 7.9%; tumor, 4.5%; trauma, 3.0%; congenital malformation, 1.4%; canaliculitis, 1.2%; and granulomatous inflammation, 1.2%. B-cell lymphoma was the most common malignant tumor detected. There is some disagreement regarding the relative involvement of the lacrimal drainage system by leukemia/lymphoma, and leukemia may be the more common lesion. Nevertheless, even NK/T-cell lymphoma has occurred in the lacrimal sac.

A. One study reported that an unsuspected malignant tumor was found on lacrimal sac biopsy in 0.6% of cases with a clinical diagnosis of dacryocystitis/lithiasis. Another study found unsuspected tumors in 2.1%. Some have questioned the value of routine biopsy of the lacrimal sac during dacryocystorhinostomy surgery; however, most ophthalmic pathologists would probably maintain the utility of histopathologic examination of such biopsy specimens.

1. Wegener's granulomatosis may rarely involve the wall of the lacrimal sac and present as a mass lesion.

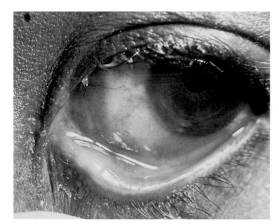

A

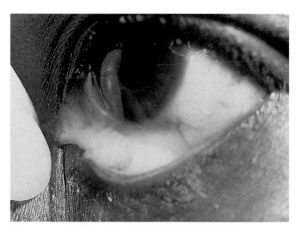

B

Fig. 6.41 Dacryocystitis. **A** and **B,** The patient had a history of tearing and a lump in the region of the lacrimal sac. Pressure over the lacrimal sac shows increasing amounts of pus coming through the punctum. **C,** Another patient had an acute canaliculitis. A smear of the lacrimal cast obtained at biopsy shows large colonies of delicate, branching, intertwined filaments characteristics of *Streptothrix* (*Actinomyces*).

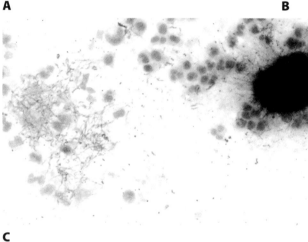

C

2. Canaliculitis and dacryolith formation are uncommon in children but may occur as a cause of chronic or recurrent nasolacrimal obstruction in them.
3. Hematoma of the lacrimal sac may mimic a tumor.
4. Adenocarcinoma of the lacrimal sac may arise from pleomorphic adenoma. Another rare tumor that has arisen in this region is mucoepidermoid carcinoma.

V. Treatment with docetaxel may result in lacrimal drainage obstruction by inducing stromal fibrosis in the mucosal lining of the lacrimal drainage apparatus.

VI. Ascending inflammation from the nose or descending inflammation from the eye may precipitate and maintain a cascade of changes that contribute to acquired malfunction of the lacrimal drainage system.

TUMORS

Epithelial

Malignant tumors constitute 70% of lacrimal sac neoplasms and squamous cell carcinoma accounts for most of these lesions.

I. From lacrimal sac lining epithelium
   A. The epithelial lining of the lacrimal sac is the same as the rest of the upper respiratory tract (i.e., pseudostratified columnar epithelium).

   Tumors, therefore, are similar to those found elsewhere in the upper respiratory system, namely, papillomas, squamous cell carcinomas, transitional cell carcinomas, and adenocarcinomas.

   HPV appear to be involved in the genesis of both benign (HPV 11) and malignant (HPV 18) neoplasms of the epithelium of the lacrimal sac.
   B. Tumors of the lacrimal sac, however, are relatively rare. They usually cause early symptoms of epiphora.
   C. Histology
      1. The papillomas may be squamous (see p. 242 in Chapter 7), transitional, or adenomatous.

      Rarely, a lacrimal sac papilloma may undergo oncocytic metaplasia (i.e., an eosinophilic cystadenoma or oncocytoma).

      ---

      2. Squamous cell carcinomas (Fig. 6.42) are identical to those found elsewhere (see pp. 245–247 in Chapter 7) and are the most common.

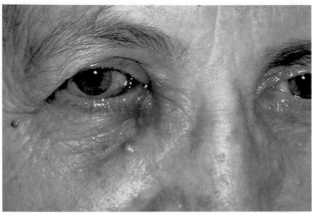

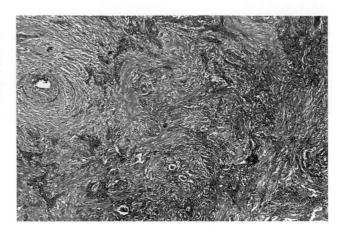

A   B

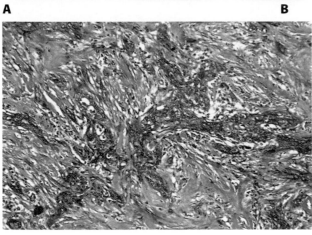

C

Fig. 6.42 Squamous cell carcinoma of the lacrimal sac. **A,** Clinical appearance of tumor in region of right lacrimal sac. **B,** Strands and cords of cells are infiltrating the tissues surrounding the lacrimal sac. **C,** Increased magnification shows the cells to be undifferentiated malignant squamous cells. (Case presented by Dr. AC Spalding to the meeting of the Verhoeff Society, 1982.)

3. Transitional cell carcinomas are composed of transitional cell epithelium showing greater or lesser degrees of differentiation.
4. Inverted papilloma is an uncommon neoplasm that has a tendency to recur; is associated with malignancy; and may invade adjacent structures. It has been reported to invade the orbit through the nasolacrimal duct.
5. Primary lymphoma of the lacrimal drainage system is extremely rare, and is usually a B-cell lesion when it does occur. Female sex may be an unfavorable prognostic factor for these lesions. Primary non-Hodgkin's lymphoma has rarely been reported to involve the lacrimal sac in children.

II. From lacrimal sac glandular elements
   A. Benign
      1. Oncocytoma (eosinophilic cystadenoma)
      2. Benign mixed tumor (pleomorphic adenoma)
      3. Adenoacanthoma
   B. Malignant
      1. Oncocytic adenocarcinoma
      2. Adenoid cystic carcinoma
      3. Adenocarcinoma

Melanotic

Melanotic tumors arising from the lacrimal sac (i.e., malignant melanomas) are quite rare and are similar histologically to those found in the lid (see section *Melanotic Tumors of Eyelids* in Chapter 17).

Mesenchymal

The same mesenchymal tumors that may involve the lids and orbit may involve the lacrimal sac (see subsection *Mesenchymal Tumors* in Chapter 14).

Miscellaneous

Localized amyloidosis may rarely involve the lacrimal sac and nasolacrimal duct, resulting in tearing.

BIBLIOGRAPHY

Skin

Normal Anatomy

Jakobiec FA, Iwamoto T: The ocular adnexa: Lids, conjunctiva, and orbit. In Fine BS, Yanoff M, eds: *Ocular Histology: A Text and Atlas*, 2nd edn. Hagerstown, MD, Harper & Row, 1979:289, 294

Kuwabara T, Cogan DG, Johnson CC: Structure of the muscles of the upper eyelid. *Arch Ophthalmol* 93:1189, 1975

Lever WF, Schaumburg-Lever G: *Histopathology of the Skin*, 7th edn. Philadelphia, JB Lippincott, 1990

Wat CS, Yuen HK, Tse KK et al.: Multiple eyelid defects in cutaneous Langerhans cell histiocytosis. *Ophthalm Plast Reconstr Surg* 22:216, 2006

Yanoff M, Fine BS: *Ocular Pathology: A Color Atlas*, 2nd edn. New York, Gower Medical Publishing, 1992:6.1

Congenital Abnormalities

Amacher AG III, Mazzoli RA, Gilbert BN et al.: Dominant familial congenital entropion with tarsal hypoplasia and atrichosis. *Ophthalm Plast Reconstr Surg* 18:381, 2002

Andreadis DA, Rizos CB, Belazi M et al.: Encephalocraniocutaneous lipomatosis accompanied by maxillary compound odontoma and juvenile angiofibroma: report of a case. *Birth Defects Res A Clin Mol Teratol* 70:889, 2004

Brooks BP, Dagenais SL, Nelson CC et al.: Mutation of the FOXC2 gene in familial distichiasis. *J AAPOS* 7:354, 2003

Brown KE, Goldstein SM, Douglas RS et al.: Encephalocraniocutaneous lipomatosis: a neurocutaneous syndrome. *J AAPOS* 7:148, 2003

Casady DR, Carlson JA, Meyer DR: Unusual complex choristoma of the lateral canthus. *Ophthalm Plast Reconstr Surg* 21:161, 2005

Chu G, Chang E: Xeroderma pigmentosum group E cells lack a nuclear factor that binds to damaged DNA. *Science* 242:564, 1988

Cockerham KP, Hidayat AA, Cockerham GC et al.: Melkersson–Rosenthal syndrome: New clinicopathologic findings in 4 cases. *Arch Ophthalmol* 118:227, 2000

Cruz AAV, Menezes FAH, Chaves R et al.: Eyelid abnormalities in lamellar ichthyoses. *Ophthalmology* 107:1895, 2000

Cursiefen C, Schlötzer-Schrehardt U, Holbach LM et al.: Ocular findings in ichthyosis follicularis, atrichia, and photophobia syndrome. *Arch Ophthalmol* 117:681, 1999

De WJ, Evens F, De MA: Eyelid tumour and juvenile hyaline fibromatosis. *Br J Plast Surg* 58:106, 2005

Dollfus H, Porto F, Caussade P et al.: Ocular manifestations in the inherited DNA repair disorders. *Surv Ophthalmol* 48:107, 2003

El-Hayek M, Lestringant GG, Frossard PM: Xeroderma pigmentosum in four siblings with three different types of malignancies simultaneously in one. *J Pediatr Hematol Oncol* 26:473, 2004

Ellis FJ, Eagle RC, Shields JA et al.: Phakomatous choristoma (Zimmerman's tumor). *Ophthalmology* 100:955, 1993

Erickson RP, Dagenais SL, Caulder MS et al.: Clinical heterogeneity in lymphoedema-distichiasis with FOXC2 truncating mutations. *J Med Genet* 38:761, 2001

Ettl A, Marinkovic M, Koorneef L: Localized hypertrichosis associated with periorbital neurofibroma: Clinical findings and differential diagnosis. *Ophthalmology* 103:942, 1996

Gordon AJ, Patrinely JR, Knupp JA et al.: Complex choristoma of the eyelid containing ectopic cilia and lacrimal gland. *Ophthalmology* 98:1547, 1991

Hampton PJ, Angus B, Carmichael AJ: A case of Schopf–Schulz–Passarge syndrome. *Clin Exp Dermatol* 30:528, 2005

Higuchi T, Satoh T, Yokozeki H et al.: Palpebral edema as a cutaneous manifestation of hyperthyroidism. *J Am Acad Dermatol* 48:617, 2003

Hu X, Plomp AS, van Soest S et al.: Pseudoxanthoma elasticum: a clinical, histopathological, and molecular update. *Surv Ophthalmol* 48:4243, 2003

Huber M, Rettler I, Bernasconi K et al.: Mutations of keratinocyte transglutaminase in lamellar ichthyosis. *Science* 267:525, 1995

Ishmael HA, Begleiter ML, Regier EJ et al.: Oculoauriculofrontonasal syndrome (OAFNS) in a nine-month-old male. *Am J Med Genet* 107:169, 2002

Jordan DR, Ahuja N, Khouri L: Eyelash loss associated with hyperthyroidism. *Ophthalm Plast Reconstr Surg* 18:219, 2002

Kaneoya K, Momota Y, Hatamochi A et al.: Elastin gene expression in blepharochalasis. *J Dermatol* 32:26, 2005

Katowitz JA, Yolles EA, Yanoff M: Ichthyosis congenita. *Arch Ophthalmol* 91:208, 1974

Kaw P, Carlson A, Meyer DR: Nevus lipomatosus (pedunculated lipofibroma) of the eyelid. *Ophthalm Plast Reconstr Surg* 21:74, 2005

Kempster RC, Hirst LW, de la Cruz Z et al.: Clinicopathologic study of the cornea in X-linked ichthyosis. *Arch Ophthalmol* 115:409, 1997

Kraemer KH, Lee MM, Scotto J: Xeroderma pigmentosum. *Arch Dermatol* 123:241, 1987

Kriederman BM, Myloyde TL, Witte MH et al.: FOXC2 haploinsufficient mice are a model for human autosomal dominant lymphedema–distichiasis syndrome. *Hum Mol Genet* 12:1179, 2003

Levy Y, Segal N, Ben-Amitai D et al.: Eyelash length in children and adolescents with allergic diseases. *Pediatr Dermatol* 21:534, 2004

Marshall JA, Valenzuela AA, Strutton GM et al.: Anterior lamella actinic changes as a factor in involutional eyelid malposition. *Ophthalm Plast Reconstr Surg* 22:192, 2006

Messmer EM, Kenyon KR, Rittinger O et al.: Ocular manifestations of keratitis-ichthyosis-deafness (KID) syndrome. *Ophthalmology* 112:e1, 2005

Oestreicher JH, Nelson CC: Lamellar ichthyosis and congenital ectropion. *Arch Ophthalmol* 108:1772, 1990

Orioli IM, Ribeiro MG, Castilla EE: Clinical and epidemiological studies of amniotic deformity, adhesion, and mutilation (ADAM) sequence in a South American (ECLAMC) population. *Am J Med Genet A* 118:135, 2003

Pe'er J, BenEzra D: Heterotopic smooth muscle in the choroid of two patients with cryptophthalmos. *Arch Ophthalmol* 104:1665, 1986

Rosenbaum PS, Kress Y, Slamovits T et al.: Phakomatous choristoma of the eyelid. *Ophthalmology* 99:1779, 1992

Schlotzer-Schrehardt U, Stojkovic M, Hofmann-Rummelt C et al.: The pathogenesis of floppy eyelid syndrome: involvement of matrix metalloproteinases in elastic fiber degradation. *Ophthalmology* 112:694, 2005

Singh V, Raju R, Singh M et al.: Congenital lipoblastoma of the scalp. *Am J Perinatol* 21:377, 2004

Traboulsi EI, Al-Khayer K, Matsumota M et al.: Lymphedema–distichiasis syndrome and FOXC2 gene mutation. *Am J Ophthalmol* 134:592, 2002

Traboulsi EI, Al-Khayer K, Matsumoto M et al.: Lymphedema–distichiasis syndrome and FOXC2 gene mutation. *Am J Ophthalmol* 134:592, 2002

Wessels MW, Brooks AS, Hoogeboom J et al.: Kabuki syndrome: a review study of three hundred patients. *Clin Dysmorphol* 11:95, 2002

Yeatts RP, White WL: Granulomatous blepharitis as a sign of Melkersson–Rosenthal syndrome. *Ophthalmology* 104:1185, 1997

Zimmerman LE: Phakomatous choristoma of the eyelid: a tumor of lenticular anlage. *Am J Ophthalmol* 71:169, 1971

Inflammation

Ashton N, Cook C: Allergic granulomatous nodules of the eyelid and conjunctiva. *Ophthalmology* 86:8, 1979

Bonnar E, Eustace P, Powell FC: The *Demodex* mite population in rosacea. *Am Acad Dermatol* 28:443, 1993

Cameron JA, Mahmood MA: Pyogenic granuloma of the cornea. *Ophthalmology* 102:1681, 1995

Crama N, Toolens AM, van der Meer JW *et al.*: Giant chalazia in the hyperimmunoglobulinemia E (hyper-IgE) syndrome. *Eur J Ophthalmol* 14:258, 2004

Donker DL, Paridaens D, Mooy CM *et al.*: Blepharoptosis and upper eyelid swelling due to lipogranulomatous inflammation caused by silicone oil. *Am J Ophthalmol* 140:934, 2005

English FP, Cohn D, Groeneveld ER: Demodectic mites and chalazion. *Am J Ophthalmol* 100:482, 1985

Ferry AP: Pyogenic granulomas of the eye and ocular adnexa: A study of 100 cases. *Trans Am Ophthalmol Soc* 87:327, 1989

Ficker L, Ramakrishnan M, Seal D *et al.*: Role of cell-mediated immunity to staphylococci in blepharitis. *Am J Ophthalmol* 111:473, 1991

Hoang-Xuan T, Rodriguez A, Zaltas MM *et al.*: Ocular rosacea. *Ophthalmology* 97:1468, 1990

Ingraham HJ, Schoenleber DB: Epibulbar molluscum contagiosum. *Am J Ophthalmol* 125:394, 1998

Kroft SH, Finn WG, Singleton TP *et al.*: Follicular lymphoma with immunoblastic features in a child with Wiscott–Aldrich syndrome: An unusual immunodeficiency-related neoplasm not associated with Epstein–Barr virus. *Am J Clin Pathol* 110:95, 1998

Lambert SR, Taylor D, Kriss A *et al.*: Ocular manifestations of the congenital varicella syndrome. *Arch Ophthalmol* 107:52, 1989

Leahey AB, Shane JJ, Listhaus A *et al.*: Molluscum contagiosum eyelid lesions as the initial manifestation of acquired immunodeficiency syndrome. *Am J Ophthalmol* 124:240, 1997

McCulley JP, Dougherty JM, Deneau DG: Classification of chronic blepharitis. *Ophthalmology* 89:1173, 1982

Patrinely JR, Font RL, Anderson RL: Granulomatous acne rosacea of the eyelids. *Arch Ophthalmol* 108:561, 1990

Raithinam S, Fritsche TR, Srinivascan M *et al*: An outbreak of trematode-induced granulomas of the conjunctiva. *Ophthalmology* 108:1223, 2001

To KW, Hoffman RJ, Jakobiec FA: Extensive squamous hyperplasia of the meibomian duct in acne rosacea. *Arch Ophthalmol* 112:160, 1994

Wear DJ, Malaty RH, Zimmerman LE: Cat scratch disease bacilli in the conjunctiva of patients with Parinaud's oculoglandular syndrome. *Ophthalmology* 92:1282, 1985

Yeatts RP, White WL: Granulomatous blepharitis as a sign of Melkersson–Rosenthal syndrome. *Ophthalmology* 104:1185, 1997

Lid Manifestations of Systemic Dermatoses or Disease

Akova YA, Jabbur NS, Foster CS: Ocular presentation of polyarteritis nodosa: Clinical course and management with steroid and cytotoxic therapy. *Ophthalmology* 100:1775, 1993

Ambinder RF: Epstein–Barr virus-associated lymphoproliferative disorders. *Rev Clin Exp Hematol* 7:362, 2003

Baba FE, Frangieh GT, Iliff WJ *et al.*: Morphea of the eyelids. *Ophthalmology* 89:1285, 1982

Braun RP, French LE, Massouye I *et al.*: Periorbital oedema and erythema as a manifestation of discoid lupus erythematosus. *Dermatology* 205:194, 2002

Bullock JD, Bartley RJ, Campbell RJ *et al.*: Necrobiotic xanthogranuloma with paraproteinemia: Case report and a pathogenetic theory. *Ophthalmology* 93:1233, 1986

Byard RW, Keeley FW, Smith CR: Type IV Ehlers–Danlos syndrome presenting as sudden infant death. *Am J Clin Pathol* 93:579, 1990

Chan JK, Sin VC, Wong KF *et al.*: Nonnasal lymphoma expressing the natural killer cell marker CD56: a clinicopathologic study of 49 cases of an uncommon aggressive neoplasm. *Blood* 89:4501, 1997

Cheung MM, Chan JK, Wong KF: Natural killer cell neoplasms: a distinctive group of highly aggressive lymphomas/leukemias. *Semin Hematol* 40:221, 2003

Cho EY, Han JJ, Ree HJ *et al.*: Clinicopathologic analysis of ocular adnexal lymphomas: extranodal marginal zone b-cell lymphoma constitutes the vast majority of ocular lymphomas among Koreans and affects younger patients. *Am J Hematol* 73:87, 2003

Chu FC, Rodrigues MM, Cogan DG *et al.*: The pathology of idiopathic midline destructive disease (IMDD) in the eyelid. *Ophthalmology* 90:1385, 1983

Cook JN, Kikkawa DO: Proptosis as the manifesting sign of Weber–Christian disease. *Am J Ophthalmol* 124:125, 1997

Daoud YJ, Cervantes R, Foster CS *et al.*: Ocular pemphigus. *J Am Acad Dermatol* 53:585, 2005

Daoud YJ, Foster CS, Ahmed R: Eyelid skin involvement in pemphigus foliaceus. *Ocul Immunol Inflamm* 13:389, 2005

Depot MJ, Jakobiec FA, Dodick JM *et al.*: Bilateral and extensive xanthelasma palpebrarum in a young man. *Ophthalmology* 91:522, 1984

Donzis PB, Insler MS, Buntin DM *et al.*: Discoid lupus erythematosus involving the eyelids. *Am J Ophthalmol* 98:32, 1984

Egan R, Lessell S: Posterior subcapsular cataract in Degos disease. *Am J Ophthalmol* 129:806, 2000

Evens AM, Gartenhaus RB: Molecular etiology of mature T-cell non-Hodgkin's lymphomas. *Front Biosci* 8: d156, 2003

Ferry AP: Subepidermal calcified nodules of the eyelid. *Am J Ophthalmol* 109:85, 1990

Finan MC, Winkelmann RK: Histopathology of necrobiotic xanthogranuloma with paraproteinemia. *J Cut Pathol* 15:18, 1987

Flach AJ, Smith RE, Fraunfelder FT: Stevens–Johnson syndrome associated with methazolamide treatment reported in Japanese-American women. *Ophthalmology* 102:1677, 1995

Font RL, Rosebaum PS, Smith JL: Lymphomatoid granulomatosis of eyelid and brow with progression to lymphoma. *J Am Acad Dermatol* 23:334, 1990

Gallardo MJ, Randleman JB, Price KM *et al.*: Ocular argyrosis after long-term self-application of eyelash tint. *Am J Ophthalmol* 141:198, 2006

Game JA, Davies R: Mycosis fungoides causing severe lower eyelid ulceration. *Clin Exp Ophthalmol* 30:369, 2002

Graham EM, Spalton DJ, Barnard RO *et al.*: Cerebral and retinal vascular changes in systemic lupus erythematosus. *Ophthalmology* 92:444, 1985

Hamada T, McLean WH, Ramsay M *et al.*: Lipoid proteinosis maps to 1q21 and is caused by mutations in the extracellular matrix protein 1 gene (ECM1). *Hum Mol Genet* 11:833, 2002

Hayashi N, Komatsu T, Komatsu T *et al.*: Juvenile xanthogranuloma presenting with unilateral prominent nodule of the eyelid: report of a case and clinicopathological findings. *Jpn J Ophthalmol* 48:435, 2004

Huerva V, Canto LM, Marti M: Primary diffuse large B-cell lymphoma of the lower eyelid. *Ophthalm Plast Reconstr Surg* 19:160, 2003

Ikeda T, Sakurane M, Uede K *et al.*: A case of symmetrical leukemia cutis on the eyelids complicated by B-cell chronic lymphocytic lymphoma. *J Dermatol* 31:560, 2004

Ing E, Hsieh E, Macdonald D: Cutaneous T-cell lymphoma with bilateral full-thickness eyelid ulceration. *Can J Ophthalmol* 40:467, 2005

Iwamoto M, Haik BG, Iwamoto T *et al.*: The ultrastructural defect in conjunctiva from a case of recessive dystrophic epidermolysis bullosa. *Arch Ophthalmol* 109:1382, 1991

Jakobiec FA, Mills MD, Hidayat AA *et al.*: Periocular xanthogranulomas associated with severe adult-onset asthma. *Trans Am Soc Ophthalmol* 91:99, 1993

Jensen AD, Khodadoust AA, Emery JM: Lipoid proteinosis. *Arch Ophthalmol* 88:273, 1972

Jordan DR, Addison DJ: Wegener's granulomatosis: Eyelid and conjunctival manifestations as the presenting feature in two individuals. *Ophthalmology* 101:602, 1994

Jordan DR, Zafar A, Brownstein S et al.: Cicatricial conjunctival inflammation with trichiasis as the presenting feature of Wegener granulomatosis. *Ophthalm Plast Reconstr Surg* 22:69, 2006

Kalina PH, Lie JT, Campbell J et al.: Diagnostic value and limitations of orbital biopsy in Wegener's granulomatosis. *Ophthalmology* 99:120, 1992

Kapur R, Osmanovic S, Toyran S et al.: Bimatoprost-induced periocular skin hyperpigmentation: histopathological study. *Arch Ophthalmol* 123:1541, 2005

Kase S, Namba K, Kitaichi N et al.: Epstein–Barr virus infected cells in the aqueous humour originated from nasal NK/T cell lymphoma. *Br J Ophthalmol* 90:244, 2006

Knoch DW, Lucarelli MJ, Dortzbach RK et al.: Limited Wegener granulomatosis with 40 years of follow-up. *Arch Ophthalmol* 121:1640, 2003

Koga M, Kubota Y, Kiryu H et al.: A case of discoid lupus erythematosus of the eyelid. *J Dermatol* 33:368, 2006

Kubota T, Hirose H: Ocular changes in a limited form of Wegener's granulomatosis: patient with cutaneous ulcer of upper eyelid. *Jpn J Ophthalmol* 47:398, 2003

Kwong YL: Natural killer-cell malignancies: diagnosis and treatment. *Leukemia* 19:2186, 2005

Lazzaro DR, Lin K, Stevens JA: Corneal findings in hemochromatosis. *Arch Ophthalmol* 116:1531, 1998

Lee DA, Su WPD, Liesegang TJ: Ophthalmic changes of Degos' disease (malignant atrophic papulosis). *Ophthalmology* 91:295, 1984

Liang R: Diagnosis and management of primary nasal lymphoma of T-cell or NK-cell origin. *Clin Lymphoma* 1:33, 2000

Lin AN, Murphy F, Brodie SE et al.: Review of ophthalmic findings in 204 patients with epidermolysis bullosa. *Am J Ophthalmol* 118:384, 1994

Loo H, Forman WB, Levine MR et al.: Periorbital ecchymoses as the initial sign in multiple myeloma. *Ann Ophthalmol* 14:1066, 1982

Lopez LR, Santos ME, Espinoza LR et al.: Clinical significance of immunoglobulin A versus immunoglobulins G and M anticardiolipin antibodies in patients with systemic lupus erythematosus. *Am J Clin Pathol* 98:449, 1992

Mendenhall WM, Olivier KR, Lynch JW Jr et al.: Lethal midline granuloma-nasal natural killer/T-cell lymphoma. *Am J Clin Oncol* 29:202, 2006

Michael CW, Flint A: The cytologic features of Wegener's granulomatosis. *Am J Clin Pathol* 110:17, 1998

Nakashima Y, Tagawa H, Suzuki R et al.: Genome-wide array-based comparative genomic hybridization of natural killer cell lymphoma/leukemia: different genomic alteration patterns of aggressive NK-cell leukemia and extranodal Nk/T-cell lymphoma, nasal type. *Genes Chromosomes Cancer* 44:247, 2005

Newman NJ, Slamovits TL, Friedland S et al.: Neuro-ophthalmic manifestations of meningocerebral inflammation from the limited form of Wegener's granulomatosis. *Am J Ophthalmol* 120:613, 1995

Onesti MG, Mazzocchi M, De LA et al.: T-cell lymphoma presenting as a rapidly enlarging tumor on the lower eyelid. *Acta Chir Plast* 47:65, 2005

Oshimi K: Leukemia and lymphoma of natural killer lineage cells. *Int J Hematol* 78:18, 2003

Papalkar D, Sharma S, Francis IC et al.: A rapidly fatal case of T-cell lymphoma presenting as idiopathic orbital inflammation. *Orbit* 24:131, 2005

Pelton RW, Desmond BP, Mamalis N et al.: Nodular cutaneous amyloid tumors of the eyelids in the absence of systemic amyloidosis. *Ophthalmic Surg Lasers* 32:422, 2001

Perry SR, Rootman J, White VA: The clinical and pathologic constellation of Wegener granulomatosis of the orbit. *Ophthalmology* 104:683, 1997

Pollack JS, Custer PL, Hart WH et al.: Ocular complications in Ehlers–Danlos syndrome type IV. *Arch Ophthalmol* 115:416, 1997

Power WJ, Ghoraishi M, Merayo-Lloves J et al.: Analysis of the acute ophthalmic manifestations of the erythema multiforme/Stevens–Johnson syndrome/toxic epidermal necrolysis disease spectrum. *Ophthalmology* 102:1669, 1995

Power WJ, Rodriguez A, Neves RA et al.: Disease relapse in patients with ocular manifestations of Wegener granulomatosis. *Ophthalmology* 102:154, 1995

Rao JK, Weinberger M, Oddone EZ et al.: The role of antineutrophil cytoplasmic antibody (c-ANCA) testing in the diagnosis of Wegener granulomatosis. *Ann Intern Med* 123:925, 1995

Rao NA, Font RL: Pseudorheumatoid nodules of the ocular adnexa. *Am J Ophthalmol* 79:471, 1975

Ribera M, Pintó X, Argimon JM et al.: Lipid metabolism and apolipoprotein E phenotypes in patients with xanthelasma. *Am J Med* 99:485, 1995

Riveros CJ, Gavilan MF, Franca LF et al.: Acquired localized cutis laxa confined to the face: case report and review of the literature. *Int J Dermatol* 43:931, 2004

Robertson DM, Winkelmann RK: Ophthalmic features of necrobiotic xanthogranuloma with paraproteinemia. *Am J Ophthalmol* 97:173, 1984

Robinson MR, Lee SS, Sneller MC et al.: Tarsal-conjunctival disease associated with Wegener's granulomatosis. *Ophthalmology* 110:1770, 2003

Selva D, Chen CS, James CL et al.: Discoid lupus erythematosus presenting as madarosis. *Am J Ophthalmol* 136:545, 2003

Sethuraman G, Tejasvi T, Khaitan BK et al.: Lipoid proteinosis in two siblings: a report from India. *J Dermatol* 30:562, 2003

Sharma V, Kashyap S, Betharia SM et al.: Lipoid proteinosis: a rare disorder with pathognomonic lid lesions. *Clin Exp Ophthalmol* 32:110, 2004

Shields CL, Shields JA, Rozanski TI: Conjunctival involvement in Churg–Strauss syndrome. *Am J Ophthalmol* 102:601, 1986

Shields JA, Karcioglu ZA, Shields CL et al.: Orbital and eyelid involvement with Erdheim–Chester disease: A report of two cases. *Arch Ophthalmol* 109:850, 1991

Shivaswamy KN, Thappa DM, Laxmisha C et al.: Lipoid proteinosis in two siblings: a report from south India. *Dermatol Online J* 9:12, 2003

Sneller MC: Wegener's granulomatosis. *JAMA* 273:1288, 1995

Soukiasian SH, Foster CS, Niles JL et al.: Diagnostic value of antineutrophil cytoplasmic antibodies in scleritis associated with Wegener's granulomatosis. *Ophthalmology* 99:125, 1992

Stavrou P, Deutsch J, Rene C et al.: Ocular manifestations of classical and limited Wegener's granulomatosis. *QJM* 86:719, 1993

Takanashu T, Uchida S, Arita M et al.: Orbital inflammatory pseudotumor and ischemic vasculitis in Churg–Strauss syndrome: report of two cases and review of the literature. *Ophthalmology* 108:1129, 2001

Tomasini C, Soro E, Pippione M: Eyelid swelling: think of metastasis of histiocytoid breast carcinoma. *Dermatology* 205:63, 2002

Trocme SD, Bartley GB, Campbell RJ et al.: Eosinophil and neutrophil degranulation in ophthalmic lesions of Wegener's granulomatosis. *Arch Ophthalmol* 109:1585, 1991

Tsokos M, Fauci AS, Costa J: Idiopathic midline destructive disease (IMDD): A subgroup of patients with the "midline granuloma" syndrome. *Am J Clin Pathol* 77:162, 1982

Valmaggia C, Neuweiler J, Fretz C et al.: A case of Erdheim–Chester disease with orbital involvement. *Arch Ophthalmol* 115:1467, 1997

Vedamurthy M: Lipoid proteinosis in siblings. *Dermatol Online J* 9:13, 2003

West RH, Barnett AJ: Ocular involvement in scleroderma. *Br J Ophthalmol* 63:845, 1979

Widmer S, Tinguely M, Egli F et al.: Lethal Epstein–Barr virus associated NK/T-cell lymphoma with primary manifestation in the conjunctiva. *Klin Monatsbl Augenheilkd* 222:255, 2005

Yanoff M: In discussion of Diddie KR, Aronson AJ, Ernest JT: Chorioretinopathy in a case of systemic lupus erythematosus. *Trans Am Ophthalmol Soc* 75:130, 1977

Cysts, Pseudoneoplasms, and Neoplasms

Abenoza P, Ackerman AB: Neoplasms with eccrine differentiation. In Ackerman AB, de Viragh PA, Chongchitnant N, eds: *Neoplasms with Follicular Differentiation.* Philadelphia, Lea & Febiger, 1990:181–218

Ackerman AB, de Viragh PA, Chongchitnant N, eds: *Neoplasms With Follicular Differentiation.* Philadelphia: Lea & Febiger, 1993:Table 7–1

Addison DJ: Malakoplakia of the eyelid. *Ophthalmology* 93:1064, 1986

Addison DJ: Merkel cell carcinoma of the eyelid. Presented at the meeting of the Eastern Ophthalmic Pathology Society, Bermuda, 1993

Akhtar S, Oza KK, Roulier RG: Multiple sebaceous adenomas and extraocular sebaceous carcinoma in a patient with multiple sclerosis: case report and review of literature. *J Cutan Med Surg* 5:490, 2001

Allaire GS, Corriveau C, Laflamme P et al.: Sebaceous carcinoma and hyperplasia of the caruncle: A clinicopathological report. *Can J Ophthalmol* 29:288, 1994

Amato M, Esmaeli B, Ahmadi MA et al.: Feasibility of preoperative lymphoscintigraphy for identification of sentinel lymph nodes in patients with conjunctival and periocular skin malignancies. *Ophthalm Plast Reconstr Surg* 19:102, 2003

Ansai S, Hashimoto H, Aoki T et al.: A histochemical and immunohistochemical study of extra-ocular sebaceous carcinoma. *Histopathology* 22:127, 1993

Argenyi ZB, Balogh K, Goeken JA: Immunohistochemical characterization of chondroid syringomas. *Am J Clin Pathol* 90:662, 1988

Askar S, Kilinc N, Aytekin S: Syringocystadenoma papilliferum mimicking basal cell carcinoma on the lower eyelid: a case report. *Acta Chir Plast* 44:117, 2002

Batra RS, Kelley LC: A risk scale for predicting extensive subclinical spread of nonmelanoma skin cancer. *Dermatol Surg* 28:107, 2002

Bindra M, Keegan DJ, Guenther T et al.: Primary cutaneous mucinous carcinoma of the eyelid in a young male. *Orbit* 24:211, 2005

Boynton JR, Markowitch W Jr: Mucinous eccrine carcinoma of the eyelid. *Arch Ophthalmol* 116:1130, 1998

Boynton JR, Markowitch W Jr: Porocarcinoma of the eyelid. *Ophthalmology* 104:1626, 1997

Braverman IM: Bowen's disease and internal cancer. *JAMA* 266:842, 1991

Breuninger H, Black B, Rassner G: Microstaging of squamous cell carcinomas. *Am J Clin Pathol* 94:624, 1990

Brownstein MH, Fernando S, Shapiro L: Clear cell adenoma: Clinicopathologic analysis of 37 new cases. *Am J Clin Pathol* 59:306, 1973

Burgdorf W, Pitha J, Falmy A: Muir–Torre syndrome: Histologic spectrum of sebaceous proliferations. *Am J Dermatopathol* 8:202, 1986

Cahill MT, Moriarty PM, Mooney DJ et al.: Pilomatrix carcinoma of the eyelid. *Am J Ophthalmol* 127:463, 1999

Chao AN, Shields CL, Krema H et al.: Outcome of patients with periocular sebaceous gland carcinoma with and without conjunctival intraepithelial invasion. *Ophthalmology* 108:1877, 2001

Chevez P, Patrinely JR, Font RL: Large-cell acanthoma of the eyelid. *Arch Ophthalmol* 109:1433, 1991

Chute CG, Chuang TY, Bergstralh EJ et al.: The subsequent risk of internal cancer with Bowen's disease. *JAMA* 266:816, 1991

Clement CI, Genge J, O'Donnell BA et al.: Orbital and periorbital microcystic adnexal carcinoma. *Ophthalm Plast Reconstr Surg* 21:97, 2005

Cook BE Jr, Bartley GB: Epidemiologic characteristics and clinical course of patients with malignant eyelid tumors in an incidence cohort in Olmsted County, Minnesota. *Ophthalmology* 106:746, 1999

Cook BE Jr, Bartley GB: Treatment options and future prospects for the management of eyelid malignancies: an evidence-based update. *Ophthalmology* 108:2088, 2001

Dailey JR, Helm KF, Goldberg SH: Tricholemmal carcinoma of the eyelid. *Am J Ophthalmol* 115:118, 1993

D'Ambrosia RA, Ward H, Parry E: Eccrine porocarcinoma of the eyelid treated with Mohs micrographic surgery. *Dermatol Surg* 30:570, 2004

Davies R, Briggs JH, Levine MR et al.: Metastatic basal cell carcinoma of the eyelid: Report of a case. *Arch Ophthalmol* 113:634, 1995

De Azevedo ML, Milani JAA, de Souza EC et al.: Pilomatrixoma: An unusual case with secondary corneal ulcer. *Arch Ophthalmol* 103:553, 1985

Diven DG, Solomon AR, McNeely MC et al.: Nevus sebaceus associated with major ophthalmologic abnormalities. *Arch Dermatol* 123:383, 1987

Donaldson MJ, Sullivan TJ, Whitehead KJ et al.: Squamous cell carcinoma of the eyelids. *Br J Ophthalmol* 86:1161, 2002

Donaldson MJ, Sullivan TJ, Whitehead KJ et al.: Periocular keratoacanthoma: clinical features, pathology, and management. *Ophthalmology* 110:1403, 2003

Douglas RS, Goldstein SM, Einhorn E et al.: Metastatic breast cancer to 4 eyelids: a clinicopathologic report. *Cutis* 70:291, 2002

Dudley TH, Moinuddin S: Cytologic and immunohistochemical diagnosis of neuroendocrine (Merkel cell) carcinoma in cerebrospinal fluid. *Am J Clin Pathol* 91:714, 1989

Duffy MT, Harrison W, Sassoon J et al.: Sclerosing sweat duct carcinoma of the eyelid margin: Unusual presentation of a rare tumor. *Ophthalmology* 106:751, 1999

Duncan JL, Golabi M, Fredrick DR et al.: Complex limbal choristomas in linear nevus sebaceous syndrome. *Ophthalmology* 105:1459, 1998

Durairaj VD, Hink EM, Kahook MY et al.: Mucinous eccrine adenocarcinoma of the periocular region. *Ophthalm Plast Reconstr Surg* 22:30, 2006

Erbagci Z, Erbagci I, Erkilic S: High incidence of demodicidosis in eyelid basal cell carcinomas. *Int J Dermatol* 42:567, 2003

Esmaeli B, Naderi A, Hidaji L et al.: Merkel cell carcinoma of the eyelid with a positive sentinel node. *Arch Ophthalmol* 120:646, 2002

Faustina M, Diba R, Ahmadi MA et al.: Patterns of regional and distant metastasis in patients with eyelid and periocular squamous cell carcinoma. *Ophthalmology* 111:1930, 2004

Font RL, Rishi K: Sebaceous gland adenoma of the tarsal conjunctiva in a patient with Muir–Torre syndrome. *Ophthalmology* 110:1833, 2003

Font RL, Stone MS, Schanzer MC et al.: Apocrine hidrocystomas of the lids, hypodontia, palmar-plantar hyperkeratosis, and onychodystrophy: A new variant of ectodermal dysplasia. *Arch Ophthalmol* 104:1811, 1986

Frucht-Pery J, Sugar J, Baum J et al.: Mitomycin C treatment for conjunctival-corneal intraepithelial neoplasia: A multicenter study. *Ophthalmology* 104:2085, 1997

Gardner TW, O'Grady RB: Mucinous adenocarcinoma of the eyelid: A case report. *Arch Ophthalmol* 102:912, 1984

Glass AG, Hoover RN: The emerging epidemic of melanoma and squamous cell skin cancer. *JAMA* 262:2097, 1989

Glatt HJ, Proia AD, Tsoy EA et al.: Malignant syringoma of the eyelid. *Ophthalmology* 91:987, 1984

Gloor P, Ansari I, Sinard J: Sebaceous carcinoma presenting as a unilateral papillary conjunctivitis. *Am J Ophthalmol* 127:458, 1999

Gonzalez-Fernandez F, Kaltreider SA, Patnaik BD *et al.*: Sebaceous carcinoma: Tumor progression through mutational inactivation of P53. *Ophthalmology* 105:497, 1998

Groos EB, Mannis MJ, Brumley TB *et al.*: Eyelid involvement in acanthosis nigricans. *Am J Ophthalmol* 115:42, 1993

Grossniklaus HE, Knight SH: Eccrine acrospiroma (clear cell hidradenoma) of the eyelid. *Ophthalmology* 98:347, 1991

Grossniklaus HE, Green WR, Luckenbach M *et al.*: Conjunctival lesions in adults: A clinical and histopathologic review. *Cornea* 6:78, 1987

Grossniklaus HE, Wojno TH, Yanoff M *et al.*: Invasive keratoacanthoma of the eyelid and ocular adnexa. *Ophthalmology* 103:937, 1996

Gunduz K, Demirel S, Heper AO *et al.*: A rare case of atypical chondroid syringoma of the lower eyelid and review of the literature. *Surv Ophthalmol* 51:280, 2006

Haibach H, Burns TW, Carlson HE *et al.*: Multiple hamartoma syndrome (Cowden's disease) associated with renal cell carcinoma and primary neuroendocrine carcinoma of the skin (Merkel cell carcinoma). *Am J Clin Pathol* 97:705, 1992

Herman DC, Chan CC, Bartley GB *et al.*: Immunohistochemical staining of sebaceous cell carcinoma of the eyelid. *Am J Ophthalmol* 107:127, 1989

Hess RJ, Scharfenberg JC, Ratz JL *et al.*: Eyelid microcystic adnexal carcinoma. *Arch Ophthalmol* 113:494, 1995

Hidayat A, Font RL: Trichilemmoma of eyelid and eyebrow: A clinicopathologic study of 31 cases. *Arch Ophthalmol* 98:844, 1980

Honavar SG, Shields CL, Maus M *et al.*: Primary intraepithelial sebaceous gland carcinoma of the palpebral conjunctiva. *Arch Ophthalmol* 119:764, 2001

Hood CI, Font RL, Zimmerman LE: Metastatic mammary carcinoma in the eyelid with histiocytoid appearance. *Cancer* 31:793, 1973

Hunts JH, Patel BCK, Langer PD *et al.*: Microcystic adnexal carcinoma of the eyebrow and eyelid. *Arch Ophthalmol* 113:1332, 1995

Jakobiec FA, Austin P, Iwamoto T *et al.*: Primary infiltrating signet ring carcinoma of the eyelids. *Ophthalmology* 90:291, 1983

Jakobiec FA, Zimmerman LE, La Piana F *et al.*: Unusual eyelid tumors with sebaceous differentiation in the Muir–Torre syndrome. *Ophthalmology* 95:1543, 1988

Kass LG, Hornblass A: Sebaceous carcinoma of the ocular adnexa. *Surv Ophthalmol* 33:477, 1989

Katz B, Wiley CA, Lee VW: Optic nerve hypoplasia and the nevus sebaceous of Jadassohn: A new association. *Ophthalmology* 94:1570, 1987

Keskinbora KH, Buyukbabani N, Terzi N: Desmoplastic trichilemmoma: a rare tumor of the eyelid. *Eur J Ophthalmol* 14:562, 2004

Kifuku K, Yoshikawa H, Sonoda K-H *et al.*: Conjunctival keratoacanthoma in an Asian. *Arch Ophthalmol* 121:118, 2003

Kim Y, Scolyer RA, Chia EM *et al.*: Eccrine porocarcinoma of the upper eyelid. *Australas J Dermatol* 46:278, 2005

Kivela T, Tarkkanen A: The Merkel cell and associated neoplasms in the eyelids and periocular region. *Surv Ophthalmol* 35:171, 1990

Klintworth GK: Chronic actinic keratopathy: A condition associated with conjunctival elastosis (pingueculae) and typified by characteristic extracellular concretions. *Am J Pathol* 67:327, 1972

Kramer TR, Grossniklaus HE, McLean IW *et al.*: Histiocytoid variant of eccrine sweat gland carcinoma of the eyelid and orbit. *Ophthalmology* 109:553, 2002

Krause FE, Rohrschneider K, Burk RO *et al.*: Nevus sebaceous of Jadassohn associated with macro optic discs and conjunctival choristomas. *Arch Ophthalmol* 116:1379, 1998

Krishnakumar S, Mohan ER, Babu K *et al.*: Eccrine duct carcinoma of the eyelid mimicking meibomian carcinoma: clinicopathological study of a case. *Surv Ophthalmol* 48:439, 2003

Lai TF, Huilgol SC, James CL *et al.*: Trichilemmal carcinoma of the upper eyelid. *Acta Ophthalmol Scand* 81:536, 2003

Lee SJ, Choi KH, Han JH *et al.*: Malignant proliferating trichilemmal tumor of the lower eyelid. *Ophthalm Plast Reconstr Surg* 21:349, 2005

Leshin B, Yeatts P, Anscher M *et al.*: Management of periocular basal cell carcinoma: Mohs' micrographic surgery versus radiotherapy. *Surv Ophthalmol* 38:193, 1993

Lisman RD, Jakobiec FA, Small P: Sebaceous carcinoma of the eyelids. *Ophthalmology* 96:1021, 1989

Lund HZ: The nosologic position of inverted follicular keratosis is still unsettled. *Am J Dermatopathol* 5:443, 1983

Mahoney MC, Burnett WS, Majerovics A *et al.*: The epidemiology of ophthalmic malignancies in New York State. *Ophthalmology* 97:1143, 1990

Mandeville JT, Roh JH, Woog JJ *et al.*: Cutaneous benign mixed tumor (chondroid syringoma) of the eyelid: clinical presentation and management. *Ophthalm Plast Reconstr Surg* 20:110, 2004

Mansour AM, Hidayat AA: Metastatic eyelid disease. *Ophthalmology* 94:667, 1987

Margo CE, Grossniklaus HE: Intraepithelial sebaceous neoplasm without underlying invasive carcinoma. *Surv Ophthalmol* 39:293, 1995

Margo CE, Mulla ZD: Malignant tumors of the eyelid: A population-based study of non-basal cell and non-squamous cell malignant neoplasms. *Arch Ophthalmol* 116:195, 1998

Margo CE, Waltz K: Basal cell carcinoma of the eyelid and periocular skin. *Surv Ophthalmol* 38:169, 1993

Mavrikakis I, Malhotra R, Barlow R *et al.*: Linear basal cell carcinoma: a distinct clinical entity in the periocular region. *Ophthalmology* 113:338, 2006

McDonnell JM, McDonnell PJ, Stout WC *et al.*: Human papillomavirus DNA in a recurrent squamous carcinoma of the eyelid. *Arch Ophthalmol* 107:1631, 1989

McNab AA, Francis IC, Benger R *et al.*: Perineural spread of cutaneous squamous cell carcinoma via the orbit. *Ophthalmology* 104:1457, 1997

Mencia-Gutierrez E, Gutierrez-Diaz E, Garcia-Suarez E *et al.*: Eyelid pilomatricomas in young adults: a report of 8 cases. *Cutis* 69:23, 2002

Mencia-Gutierrez E, Gutierrez-Diaz E, Redondo-Marcos I *et al.*: Cutaneous horns of the eyelid: a clinicopathological study of 48 cases. *J Cutan Pathol* 31:539, 2004

Misago N, Satoh T, Narisawa Y: Basal cell carcinoma with ductal and glandular differentiation: a clinicopathological and immunohistochemical study of 10 cases. *Eur J Dermatol* 14:383, 2004

Monshizadeh R, Cohen L, Rubin PA: Perforating follicular hybrid cyst of the tarsus. *J Am Acad Dermatol* 48:S33, 2003

Morand B, Bettega G, Bland V *et al.*: Oncocytoma of the eyelid: An aggressive benign tumor. *Ophthalmology* 105:2220, 1998

Morris DA: An eye-catching basal cell carcinoma. Presented at the meeting of the Eastern Ophthalmic Pathology Society, 1989

Munro S, Brownstein S, Liddy B: Conjunctival keratoacanthoma. *Am J Ophthalmol* 116:654, 1993

Nerad JA, Folberg R: Multiple cylindromas. The "turban tumor." *Arch Ophthalmol* 105:1137, 1987

Nerad JA, Whitaker DC: Periocular basal cell carcinoma in adults 35 years of age and younger. *Am J Ophthalmol* 106:723, 1988

Nijhawan N, Ross MI, Diba R *et al.*: Experience with sentinel lymph node biopsy for eyelid and conjunctival malignancies at a cancer center. *Ophthalm Plast Reconstr Surg* 20:291, 2004

Niu Y, Liu F, Zhou Z *et al.*: Expression of CD44V6 and PCNA in squamous cell carcinomas. *Chin Med J (Engl)* 115:1564, 2002

Olver JM, Muhtaseb M, Chauhan D *et al.*: Well-differentiated squamous cell carcinoma of the eyelid arising during a 20-year period. *Arch Ophthalmol* 118:422, 2000

Ozdal PC, Callejo SA, Codere F et al.: Benign ocular adnexal tumours of apocrine, eccrine or hair follicle origin. *Can J Ophthalmol* 38:357, 2003

Pe'er J, Ilsar M: Epibulbar complex choristoma associated with nevus sebaceus. *Arch Ophthalmol* 113:1301, 1995

Perlman JI, Urban RC, Edward DP et al.: Syringocystadenoma papilliferum of the eyelid. *Am J Ophthalmol* 117:647, 1994

Randall MB, Geisinger KR, Kute TE et al.: DNA content and proliferative index in cutaneous squamous cell carcinoma and keratoacanthoma. *Am J Clin Pathol* 93:259, 1990

Reifler DM, Ballitch HA II, Kessler DL et al.: Tricholemmoma of the eyelid. *Ophthalmology* 94:1272, 1987

Rodgers IR, Jakobiec FA, Krebs W et al.: Papillary oncocytoma of the eyelid. *Ophthalmology* 95:1071, 1988

Rumelt S, Hogan NR, Rubin PAD et al.: Four-eyelid sebaceous cell carcinoma following irradiation. *Arch Ophthalmol* 116:1670, 1998

Salama SD, Margo CE: Large pigmented actinic keratosis of the eyelid. *Arch Ophthalmol* 113:977, 1995

Salomon J, Bieniek A, Baran E et al.: Basal cell carcinoma on the eyelids: own experience. *Dermatol Surg* 30:257, 2004

Sassani JW, Yanoff M: Inverted follicular keratosis. *Am J Ophthalmol* 87:810, 1979

Scheie HG, Yanoff M, Frayer WC: Carcinoma of sebaceous glands of the eyelid. *Arch Ophthalmol* 72:800, 1964

Scheie HG, Yanoff M, Sassani JW: Inverted follicular keratosis clinically mimicking malignant melanoma. *Ann Ophthalmol* 9:949, 1977

Schuster SAD, Ferguson EC III, Marshall RB: Alveolar rhabdomyosarcoma of the eyelid. *Arch Ophthalmol* 87:646, 1972

Schweitzer JG, Yanoff M: Inverted follicular keratosis: A report of two recurrent cases. *Ophthalmology* 94:1465, 1987

Seregard S: Apocrine adenocarcinoma arising in moll gland cystadenoma. *Ophthalmology* 100:1716, 1993

Shields JA, Demirci H, Marr BP et al.: Sebaceous gland carcinoma of the eyelids. Personal experience with 60 cases. *Ophthalmology* 111:2151, 2004

Shields JA, Eagle RC, Shields CL et al.: Apocrine hidrocystoma of the eyelid. *Arch Ophthalmol* 3:866, 1993

Shields JA, Shields CL, Eagle RC Jr et al.: Ocular manifestations of the organoid nevus syndrome. *Ophthalmology* 104:549, 1997

Shields JA, Shields CL, Eagle RC Jr et al.: Ophthalmic features of the organoid nevus syndrome. *Trans Am Ophthalmol Soc* 94:66, 1997

Shields JA, Shields CL, Eagle RC Jr: Trichoadenoma of the eyelid. *Am J Ophthalmol* 126:846, 1998

Shields JA, Shields CL, Gundus K et al.: Intraocular invasion of conjunctival squamous cell carcinoma in five patients: The 1998 Pan American lecture. *Ophthalmol Plast Reconstr Surg* 15:153, 1999

Shintaku M, Tsuta K, Yoshida H et al.: Apocrine adenocarcinoma of the eyelid with aggressive biological behavior: report of a case. *Pathol Int* 52:169, 2002

Sinard JH: Immunohistochemical distinction of ocular sebaceous carcinoma from basal cell and squamous cell carcinoma. *Arch Ophthalmol* 117:776, 1999

Singh AD, McCloskey L, Parsons MA et al.: Eccrine hidrocystoma of the eyelid. *Eye* 19:77, 2005

Snow SN, Larson PO, Lucaelli MJ et al.: Sebaceous gland carcinoma of the eyelids treated by Mohs micrographic surgery: report of nine cases with review of the literature. *Dermatol Surg* 28:623, 2002

Soltau JB, Smith ME, Custer PL: Merkel cell carcinoma of the eyelid. *Am J Ophthalmol* 121:331, 1996

Staibano S, Lo Muzia L, Pannone G et al.: DNA ploidy and cyclin D1 expression in basal cell carcinoma of the head and neck. *Am J Clin Pathol* 115:805, 2001

Stern RS, Boudreaux KC, Arndt KA: Diagnostic accuracy and appropriateness of care for seborrheic keratoses. *JAMA* 265:74, 1991

Tay E, Schofield JB, Rowell NP et al.: Ophthalmic presentation of the Muir Torre syndrome. *Ophthalm Plast Reconstr Surg* 19:402, 2003

Tillawi I, Katz R, Pellettiere EV: Solitary tumors of meibomian gland origin and Torre's syndrome. *Am J Ophthalmol* 104:179, 1987

Vortmeyer AO, Merino MJ, Böni R et al.: Genetic changes associated with primary Merkel cell carcinoma. *Am J Pathol* 109:565, 1998

Wedge CC, Rootman DS, Hunter W et al.: Malignant acanthosis nigricans. *Ophthalmology* 100:1590, 1993

Wilson MW, Fleming JC, Fleming RM et al.: Sentinel node biopsy for orbital and ocular adnexal tumors. *Ophthalm Plast Reconstr Surg* 17:338, 2001

Yanoff M: Most inverted follicular keratoses are probably verruca vulgaris. *Am J Dermatopathol* 5:475, 1983

Zajdela A, Vielh P, Schlienger P et al.: Fine-needle cytology of 292 palpable orbital and eyelid tumors. *Am J Clin Pathol* 93:100, 1990

Züurcher M, Hintschich CR, Garner A et al.: Sebaceous carcinoma of the eyelids: A clinicopathological study. *Br J Ophthalmol* 82:1049, 1998

Lacrimal Drainage System

Normal Anatomy

Ayub M, Thale AB, Hedderich J et al.: The cavernous body of the human efferent tear ducts contributes to regulation of tear outflow. *Invest Ophthalmol Vis Sci* 44:4900, 2003

Chronister CL, Lee A, Kaiser H: Rarely reported cases of congenital atresia of nasolacrimal puncta. *Optometry* 73:237, 2002

Paulsen FP, Schaudig U, Maune S et al.: Loss of tear duct-associated lymphoid tissue in association with the scarring of symptomatic dacryostenosis. *Ophthalmology* 110:85, 2003

de Toledo AR, Chandler JW, Buffman FV: Lacrimal system: Dry-eye states and other conditions. In Podos SM, Yanoff M, eds: *Textbook of Ophthalmology*, vol. 8. London, Mosby, 1994:14.5–14.6

Congenital Abnormalities

Duke-Elder S: *System of Ophthalmology*, vol III, *Normal and Abnormal Development*. Part 2: Congenital Deformities. St. Louis, CV Mosby, 1963:911

Grossman T, Putz R: Anatomy, consequences and treatment of congenital stenosis of lacrimal passage in newborn infants. *Klin Monatsbl Augenheilkd* 160:563, 1972

Kashkouli MB, Beigi B, Murthy R et al.: Acquired external punctal stenosis: etiology and associated findings. *Am J Ophthalmol* 136:1079, 2003

Teixeira CC, Dias RJ, Falcao-Reis FM et al.: Congenital dacryocystocele with intranasal extension. *Eur J Ophthalmol* 15:126, 2005

Yuen SJ, Oley C, Sullivan TJ: Lacrimal outflow dysgenesis. *Ophthalmology* 111:1782, 2004

Inflammation

Anderson NG, Wojno TH, Grossniklaus HE: Clinicopathologic findings from lacrimal sac biopsy specimens obtained during dacryocystorhinostomy. *Ophthalm Plast Reconstr Surg* 19:173, 2003

Baredes S, Ludwin DB, Troublefield YL et al.: Adenocarcinoma expleomorphic adenoma of the lacrimal sac and nasolacrimal duct: a case report. *Laryngoscope* 113:940, 2003

Bernardini FP, Moin M, Kersten RC et al.: Routine histopathologic evaluation of the lacrimal sac during dacryocystorhinostomy: how useful is it? *Ophthalmology* 109:1214, 2002

Brook I, Frazier EH: Aerobic and anaerobic microbiology of dacryocystitis. *Am J Ophthalmol* 125:552, 1998

Esmaeli B, Burnstine MA, Ahmadi MA *et al.*: Docetaxel-induced histologic changes in the lacrimal sac and the nasal mucosa. *Ophthalm Plast Reconstr Surg* 19:305, 2003

Ghanem RC, Chang N, Aoki L *et al.*: Vasculitis of the lacrimal sac wall in Wegener granulomatosis. *Ophthalm Plast Reconstr Surg* 20:254, 2004

Hornblass A, Gross ND: Lacrimal sac cyst. *Ophthalmology* 94:706, 1987

Hsu HC, Lin SA, Lin HF: Pyogenic granuloma as a rare complication of silicone stent after canalicular injury. *J Trauma* 51:1197, 2001

Karesh JW, Perman KI, Rodrigues MM: Dacryocystitis associated with malignant lymphoma of the lacrimal sac. *Ophthalmology* 100:669, 1993

Kim BM, Osmanovic SS, Edward DP: Pyogenic granulomas after silicone punctal plugs: a clinical and histopathologic study. *Am J Ophthalmol* 139:678, 2005

Lee J, Flanagan JC: Complications associated with silicone intracanalicular plugs. *Ophthalm Plast Reconstr Surg* 17:465, 2001

Lee-Wing MW, Ashenhurst ME: Clinicopathologic analysis of 166 patients with primary acquired nasolacrimal duct obstruction. *Ophthalmology* 108:2038, 2001

Marthin JK, Lindegaard J, Prause JU *et al.*: Lesions of the lacrimal drainage system: a clinicopathological study of 643 biopsy specimens of the lacrimal drainage system in Denmark 1910–1999. *Acta Ophthalmol Scand* 83:94, 2005

Merkonidis C, Brewis C, Yung M *et al.*: Is routine biopsy of the lacrimal sac wall indicated at dacryocystorhinostomy? A prospective study and literature review. *Br J Ophthalmol* 89:1589, 2005

Mori T, Tokuhira M, Mori S *et al.*: Primary natural killer cell lymphoma of the lacrimal sac. *Ann Hematol* 80:607, 2001

Park A, Morgenstern KE, Kahwash SB *et al.*: Pediatric canaliculitis and stone formation. *Ophthalm Plast Reconstr Surg* 20:243, 2004

Paulsen FP, Thale AB, Maune S *et al.*: New insights into the pathophysiology of primary acquired dacryostenosis. *Ophthalmology* 108:2329, 2001

Pe'er JJ, Stefanysczyn M, Hidayat AA: Nonepithelial tumors of the lacrimal sac. *Am J Ophthalmol* 118:650, 1994

Sacks E, Jakobiec FA, Dodick J: Canaliculops. *Ophthalmology* 94:78, 1987

Smith S, Rootman J: Lacrimal ductal cysts. Presentation and management (review). *Surv Ophthalmol* 30:245, 1986

Williams JD, Agrawal A, Wakely PE Jr: Mucoepidermoid carcinoma of the lacrimal sac. *Ann Diagn Pathol* 7:31, 2003

Yen MT, Hipps WM: Nasolacrimal sac hematoma masquerading as an orbital mass. *Ophthalm Plast Reconstr Surg* 20:170, 2004

Yip CC, Bartley GB, Habermann TM *et al.*: Involvement of the lacrimal drainage system by leukemia or lymphoma. *Ophthalm Plast Reconstr Surg* 18:242, 2002

Yuen KS, Cheng AC, Chan WM: Pyogenic granulomas after silicone punctal plugs: a clinical and histopathologic study. *Am J Ophthalmol* 140:963, 2005

Tumors

Akhtar S, Oza KK, Roulier RG: Multiple sebaceous adenomas and extraocular sebaceous carcinoma in a patient with multiple sclerosis: case report and review of literature. *J Cutan Med Surg* 5:490, 2001

Amacher AG, III, Mazzoli RA, Gilbert BN *et al.*: Dominant familial congenital entropion with tarsal hypoplasia and atrichosis. *Ophthalm Plast Reconstr Surg* 18:381, 2002

Amato M, Esmaeli B, Ahmadi MA *et al.*: Feasibility of preoperative lymphoscintigraphy for identification of sentinel lymph nodes in patients with conjunctival and periocular skin malignancies. *Ophthalm Plast Reconstr Surg* 19:102, 2003

Ambinder RF: Epstein–Barr virus-associated lymphoproliferative disorders. *Rev Clin Exp Hematol* 7:362, 2003

Anderson KK, Lessner AM, Hood I *et al.*: Invasive transitional cell carcinoma of the lacrimal sac arising in an inverted papilloma. *Arch Ophthalmol* 112:306, 1994

Anderson NG, Wojno TH, Grossniklaus HE: Clinicopathologic findings from lacrimal sac biopsy specimens obtained during dacryocystorhinostomy. *Ophthalm Plast Reconstr Surg* 19:173, 2003

Andreadis DA, Rizos CB, Belazi M *et al.*: Encephalocraniocutaneous lipomatosis accompanied by maxillary compound odontoma and juvenile angiofibroma: report of a case. *Birth Defects Res A Clin Mol Teratol* 70:889, 2004

Askar S, Kilinc N, Aytekin S: Syringocystadenoma papilliferum mimicking basal cell carcinoma on the lower eyelid: a case report. *Acta Chir Plast* 44:117, 2002

Ayub M, Thale AB, Hedderich J *et al.*: The cavernous body of the human efferent tear ducts contributes to regulation of tear outflow. *Invest Ophthalmol Vis Sci* 44:4900, 2003

Bambirra EA, Miranda D, Rayes A: Mucoepidermoid tumor of the lacrimal sac. *Arch Ophthalmol* 99:2149, 1981

Baredes S, Ludwin DB, Troublefield YL *et al.*: Adenocarcinoma expleomorphic adenoma of the lacrimal sac and nasolacrimal duct: a case report. *Laryngoscope* 113:940, 2003

Batra RS, Kelley LC: A risk scale for predicting extensive subclinical spread of nonmelanoma skin cancer. *Dermatol Surg* 28:107, 2002

Bernardini FP, Moin M, Kersten RC *et al.*: Routine histopathologic evaluation of the lacrimal sac during dacryocystorhinostomy: how useful is it? *Ophthalmology* 109:1214, 2002

Bindra M, Keegan DJ, Guenther T, Lee V: Primary cutaneous mucinous carcinoma of the eyelid in a young male. *Orbit* 24:211, 2005

Bonder D, Fischer MJ, Levine MR: Squamous cell carcinoma of the lacrimal sac. *Ophthalmology* 90:1133, 1983

Braun RP, French LE, Massouye I *et al.*: Periorbital oedema and erythema as a manifestation of discoid lupus erythematosus. *Dermatology* 205:194, 2002

Brooks BP, Dagenais SL, Nelson CC *et al.*: Mutation of the FOXC2 gene in familial distichiasis. *J AAPOS* 7:354, 2003

Brown KE, Goldstein SM, Douglas RS *et al.*: Encephalocraniocutaneous lipomatosis: a neurocutaneous syndrome. *J AAPOS* 7:148, 2003

Casady DR, Carlson JA, Meyer DR: Unusual complex choristoma of the lateral canthus. *Ophthalm Plast Reconstr Surg* 21:161, 2005

Chan JK, Sin VC, Wong KF *et al.*: Nonnasal lymphoma expressing the natural killer cell marker CD56: a clinicopathologic study of 49 cases of an uncommon aggressive neoplasm. *Blood* 89:4501, 1997

Charles NC, Palu RN, Jagirdar JS: Hemangiopericytoma of the lacrimal sac. *Arch Ophthalmol* 116:1677, 1998

Chaudhry IA, Taiba K, Al-Sadhan Y *et al.*: Inverted papilloma invading the orbit through the nasolacrimal duct: a case report. *Orbit* 24:135, 2005

Cheung MM, Chan JK, Wong KF: Natural killer cell neoplasms: a distinctive group of highly aggressive lymphomas/leukemias. *Semin Hematol* 40:221, 2003

Cho EY, Han JJ, Ree HJ *et al.*: Clinicopathologic analysis of ocular adnexal lymphomas: extranodal marginal zone b-cell lymphoma constitutes the vast majority of ocular lymphomas among Koreans and affects younger patients. *Am J Hematol* 73:87, 2003

Chronister CL, Lee A, Kaiser H: Rarely reported cases of congenital atresia of nasolacrimal puncta. *Optometry* 73:237, 2002

Clement CI, Genge J, O'Donnell BA *et al.*: Orbital and periorbital microcystic adnexal carcinoma. *Ophthalm Plast Reconstr Surg* 21:97, 2005

Cook BE Jr, Bartley GB: Treatment options and future prospects for the management of eyelid malignancies: an evidence-based update. *Ophthalmology* 108:2088, 2001

Crama N, Toolens AM, van der Meer JW *et al.*: Giant chalazia in the hyperimmunoglobulinemia E (hyper-IgE) syndrome. *Eur J Ophthalmol* 14:258, 2004

D'Ambrosia RA, Ward H, Parry E: Eccrine porocarcinoma of the eyelid treated with Mohs micrographic surgery. *Dermatol Surg* 30:570, 2004

Daoud YJ, Cervantes R, Foster CS *et al.*: Ocular pemphigus. *J Am Acad Dermatol* 53:585, 2005

Daoud YJ, Foster CS, Ahmed R: Eyelid skin involvement in pemphigus foliaceus. *Ocul Immunol Inflamm* 13:389, 2005

De WJ, Evens F, De MA: Eyelid tumour and juvenile hyaline fibromatosis. *Br J Plast Surg* 58:106, 2005

Dollfus H, Porto F, Caussade P *et al.*: Ocular manifestations in the inherited DNA repair disorders. *Surv Ophthalmol* 48:107, 2003

Donaldson MJ, Sullivan TJ, Whitehead KJ *et al.*: Squamous cell carcinoma of the eyelids. *Br J Ophthalmol* 86:1161, 2002

Donker DL, Paridaens D, Mooy CM *et al.*: Blepharoptosis and upper eyelid swelling due to lipogranulomatous inflammation caused by silicone oil. *Am J Ophthalmol* 140:934, 2005

Douglas RS, Goldstein SM, Einhorn E *et al.*: Metastatic breast cancer to 4 eyelids: a clinicopathologic report. *Cutis* 70:291, 2002

Durairaj VD, Hink EM, Kahook MY *et al.*: Mucinous eccrine adenocarcinoma of the periocular region. *Ophthalm Plast Reconstr Surg* 22:30, 2006

El-Hayek M, Lestringant GG, Frossard PM: Xeroderma pigmentosum in four siblings with three different types of malignancies simultaneously in one. *J Pediatr Hematol Oncol* 26:473, 2004

Erbagci Z, Erbagci I, Erkilic S: High incidence of demodicidosis in eyelid basal cell carcinomas. *Int J Dermatol* 42:567, 2003

Erickson RP, Dagenais SL, Caulder MS *et al.*: Clinical heterogeneity in lymphoedema-distichiasis with FOXC2 truncating mutations. *J Med Genet* 38:761, 2001

Esmaeli B, Burnstine MA, Ahmadi MA *et al.*: Docetaxel-induced histologic changes in the lacrimal sac and the nasal mucosa. *Ophthalm Plast Reconstr Surg* 19:305, 2003

Evens AM, Gartenhaus RB: Molecular etiology of mature T-cell non-Hodgkin's lymphomas. *Front Biosci* 8:d156, 2003

Faustina M, Diba R, Ahmadi MA *et al.*: Patterns of regional and distant metastasis in patients with eyelid and periocular squamous cell carcinoma. *Ophthalmology* 111:1930, 2004

Ferry AP, Kaltreider SA: Cavernous hemangioma of the lacrimal sac. *Am J Ophthalmol* 110:316, 1990

Gallardo MJ, Randleman JB, Price KM *et al.*: Ocular argyrosis after long-term self-application of eyelash tint. *Am J Ophthalmol* 141:198, 2006

Game JA, Davies R: Mycosis fungoides causing severe lower eyelid ulceration. *Clin Exp Ophthalmol* 30:369, 2002

Gao HW, Lee HS, Lin YS *et al.*: Primary lymphoma of nasolacrimal drainage system: a case report and literature review. *Am J Otolaryngol* 26:356, 2005

Ghanem RC, Chang N, Aoki L *et al.*: Vasculitis of the lacrimal sac wall in Wegener granulomatosis. *Ophthalm Plast Reconstr Surg* 20:254, 2004

Gunduz K, Demirel S, Heper AO *et al.*: A rare case of atypical chondroid syringoma of the lower eyelid and review of the literature. *Surv Ophthalmol* 51:280, 2006

Hamada T, McLean WH, Ramsay M *et al.*: Lipoid proteinosis maps to 1q21 and is caused by mutations in the extracellular matrix protein 1 gene (ECM1). *Hum Mol Genet* 11:833, 2002

Hampton PJ, Angus B, Carmichael AJ: A case of Schopf–Schulz–Passarge syndrome. *Clin Exp Dermatol* 30:528, 2005

Hayashi N, Komatsu T, Komatsu T *et al.*: Juvenile xanthogranuloma presenting with unilateral prominent nodule of the eyelid: report of a case and clinicopathological findings. *Jpn J Ophthalmol* 48:435, 2004

Higuchi T, Satoh T, Yokozeki H *et al.*: Palpebral edema as a cutaneous manifestation of hyperthyroidism. *J Am Acad Dermatol* 48:617, 2003

Hsu HC, Lin SA, Lin HF: Pyogenic granuloma as a rare complication of silicone stent after canalicular injury. *J Trauma* 51:1197, 2001

Huerva V, Canto LM, Marti M: Primary diffuse large B-cell lymphoma of the lower eyelid. *Ophthalm Plast Reconstr Surg* 19:160, 2003

Ikeda T, Sakurane M, Uede K *et al.*: A case of symmetrical leukemia cutis on the eyelids complicated by B-cell chronic lymphocytic lymphoma. *J Dermatol* 31:560, 2004

Ing E, Hsieh E, Macdonald D: Cutaneous T-cell lymphoma with bilateral full-thickness eyelid ulceration. *Can J Ophthalmol* 40:467, 2005

Ishmael HA, Begleiter ML, Regier EJ *et al.*: Oculoauriculofrontonasal syndrome (OAFNS) in a nine-month-old male. *Am J Med Genet* 107:169, 2002

Jordan DR, Ahuja N, Khouri L: Eyelash loss associated with hyperthyroidism. *Ophthalm Plast Reconstr Surg* 18:219, 2002

Jordan DR, Zafar A, Brownstein S *et al.*: Cicatricial conjunctival inflammation with trichiasis as the presenting feature of Wegener granulomatosis. *Ophthalm Plast Reconstr Surg* 22:69, 2006

Kaneoya K, Momota Y, Hatamochi A *et al.*: Elastin gene expression in blepharochalasis. *J Dermatol* 32:26, 2005

Kapur R, Osmanovic S, Toyran S *et al.*: Bimatoprost-induced periocular skin hyperpigmentation: histopathological study. *Arch Ophthalmol* 123:1541, 2005

Kase S, Namba K, Kitaichi N *et al.*: Epstein–Barr virus infected cells in the aqueous humour originated from nasal NK/T cell lymphoma. *Br J Ophthalmol* 90:244, 2006

Kashkouli MB, Beigi B, Murthy R *et al.*: Acquired external punctal stenosis: etiology and associated findings. *Am J Ophthalmol* 136:1079, 2003

Kaw P, Carlson A, Meyer DR: Nevus lipomatosus (pedunculated lipofibroma) of the eyelid. *Ophthalm Plast Reconstr Surg* 21:74, 2005

Keskinbora KH, Buyukbabani N, Terzi N: Desmoplastic trichilemmoma: a rare tumor of the eyelid. *Eur J Ophthalmol* 14:562, 2004

Kim BM, Osmanovic SS, Edward DP: Pyogenic granulomas after silicone punctal plugs: a clinical and histopathologic study. *Am J Ophthalmol* 139:678, 2005

Kim Y, Scolyer RA, Chia EM *et al.*: Eccrine porocarcinoma of the upper eyelid. *Australas J Dermatol* 46:278, 2005

Koga M, Kubota Y, Kiryu H *et al.*: A case of discoid lupus erythematosus of the eyelid. *J Dermatol* 33:368, 2006

Koksal Y, Kiratli H, Varan A *et al.*: Primary lacrimal sac non-Hodgkin's lymphoma in a child. *Int J Pediatr Otorhinolaryngol* 69:1551, 2005

Kramer TR, Grossniklaus HE, McLean IW *et al.*: Histiocytoid variant of eccrine sweat gland carcinoma of the eyelid and orbit: report of five cases. *Ophthalmology* 109:553, 2002

Kriederman BM, Myloyde TL, Witte MH *et al.*: FOXC2 haploinsufficient mice are a model for human autosomal dominant lymphedema–distichiasis syndrome. *Hum Mol Genet* 12:1179, 2003

Kubota T, Hirose H: Ocular changes in a limited form of Wegener's granulomatosis: patient with cutaneous ulcer of upper eyelid. *Jpn J Ophthalmol* 47:398, 2003

Kwong YL: Natural killer-cell malignancies: diagnosis and treatment. *Leukemia* 19:2186, 2005

Lai TF, Huilgol SC, James CL *et al.*: Trichilemmal carcinoma of the upper eyelid. *Acta Ophthalmol Scand* 81:536, 2003

Lee J, Flanagan JC: Complications associated with silicone intracanalicular plugs. *Ophthalm Plast Reconstr Surg* 17:465, 2001

Lee SJ, Choi KH, Han JH *et al.*: Malignant proliferating trichilemmal tumor of the lower eyelid. *Ophthalm Plast Reconstr Surg* 21:349, 2005

Lee-Wing MW, Ashenhurst ME: Clinicopathologic analysis of 166 patients with primary acquired nasolacrimal duct obstruction. *Ophthalmology* 108:2038, 2001

Levy Y, Segal N, Ben-Amitai D *et al.*: Eyelash length in children and adolescents with allergic diseases. *Pediatr Dermatol* 21:534, 2004

Liang R: Diagnosis and management of primary nasal lymphoma of T-cell or NK-cell origin. *Clin Lymphoma* 1:33, 2000

Madreperla SA, Green WR, Daniel R *et al.*: Human papillomavirus in primary epithelial tumors of the lacrimal sac. *Ophthalmology* 100:569, 1993

Mandeville JT, Roh JH, Woog JJ *et al.*: Cutaneous benign mixed tumor (chondroid syringoma) of the eyelid: clinical presentation and management. *Ophthalm Plast Reconstr Surg* 20:110, 2004

Marback RL, Kincaid MC, Green WR *et al.*: Fibrous histiocytoma of the lacrimal sac. *Am J Ophthalmol* 93:511, 1982

Marcet MM, Roh JH, Mandeville JT *et al.*: Localized orbital amyloidosis involving the lacrimal sac and nasolacrimal duct. *Ophthalmology* 113:153, 2006

Marshall JA, Valenzuela AA, Strutton GM *et al.*: Anterior lamella actinic changes as a factor in involutional eyelid malposition. *Ophthalm Plast Reconstr Surg* 22:192, 2006

Marthin JK, Lindegaard J, Prause JU *et al.*: Lesions of the lacrimal drainage system: a clinicopathological study of 643 biopsy specimens of the lacrimal drainage system in Denmark 1910–1999. *Acta Ophthalmol Scand* 83:94, 2005

Mavrikakis I, Malhotra R, Barlow R *et al.*: Linear basal cell carcinoma: a distinct clinical entity in the periocular region. *Ophthalmology* 113:338, 2006

Mencia-Gutierrez E, Gutierrez-Diaz E, Garcia-Suarez E *et al.*: Eyelid pilomatricomas in young adults: a report of 8 cases. *Cutis* 69:23, 2002

Mencia-Gutierrez E, Gutierrez-Diaz E, Redondo-Marcos I *et al.*: Cutaneous horns of the eyelid: a clinicopathological study of 48 cases. *J Cutan Pathol* 31:539, 2004

Mendenhall WM, Olivier KR, Lynch JW Jr *et al.*: Lethal midline granuloma-nasal natural killer/T-cell lymphoma. *Am J Clin Oncol* 29:202, 2006

Merkonidis C, Brewis C, Yung M *et al.*: Is routine biopsy of the lacrimal sac wall indicated at dacryocystorhinostomy? A prospective study and literature review. *Br J Ophthalmol* 89:1589, 2005

Messmer EM, Kenyon KR, Rittinger O *et al.*: Ocular manifestations of keratitis-ichthyosis-deafness (KID) syndrome. *Ophthalmology* 112:e1, 2005

Misago N, Satoh T, Narisawa Y: Basal cell carcinoma with ductal and glandular differentiation: a clinicopathological and immunohistochemical study of 10 cases. *Eur J Dermatol* 14:383, 2004

Monshizadeh R, Cohen L, Rubin PA: Perforating follicular hybrid cyst of the tarsus. *J Am Acad Dermatol* 48:S33, 2003

Mori T, Tokuhira M, Mori S *et al.*: Primary natural killer cell lymphoma of the lacrimal sac. *Ann Hematol* 80:607, 2001

Nakashima Y, Tagawa H, Suzuki R *et al.*: Genome-wide array-based comparative genomic hybridization of natural killer cell lymphoma/leukemia: different genomic alteration patterns of aggressive NK-cell leukemia and extranodal Nk/T-cell lymphoma, nasal type. *Genes Chromosomes Cancer* 44:247, 2005

Nijhawan N, Ross MI, Diba R *et al.*: Experience with sentinel lymph node biopsy for eyelid and conjunctival malignancies at a cancer center. *Ophthalm Plast Reconstr Surg* 20:291, 2004

Niu Y, Liu F, Zhou Z *et al.*: Expression of CD44V6 and PCNA in squamous cell carcinomas. *Chin Med J (Engl)* 115:1564, 2002

Onesti MG, Mazzocchi M, De LA *et al.*: T-cell lymphoma presenting as a rapidly enlarging tumor on the lower eyelid. *Acta Chir Plast* 47:65, 2005

Orioli IM, Ribeiro MG, Castilla EE: Clinical and epidemiological studies of amniotic deformity, adhesion, and mutilation (ADAM) sequence in a South American (ECLAMC) population. *Am J Med Genet A* 118:135, 2003

Oshimi K: Leukemia and lymphoma of natural killer lineage cells. *Int J Hematol* 78:18, 2003

Ozdal PC, Callejo SA, Codere F *et al.*: Benign ocular adnexal tumours of apocrine, eccrine or hair follicle origin. *Can J Ophthalmol* 38:357, 2003

Papalkar D, Sharma S, Francis IC *et al.*: A rapidly fatal case of T-cell lymphoma presenting as idiopathic orbital inflammation. *Orbit* 24:131, 2005

Park A, Morgenstern KE, Kahwash SB *et al.*: Pediatric canaliculitis and stone formation. *Ophthalm Plast Reconstr Surg* 20:243, 2004

Paulsen FP, Schaudig U, Maune S *et al.*: Loss of tear duct-associated lymphoid tissue in association with the scarring of symptomatic dacryostenosis. *Ophthalmology* 110:85, 2003

Paulsen FP, Thale AB, Maune S *et al.*: New insights into the pathophysiology of primary acquired dacryostenosis. *Ophthalmology* 108:2329, 2001

Pe'er J, Hidayat AA, Ilsar M *et al.*: Glandular tumors of the lacrimal sac: Their histopathologic patterns and possible origin. *Ophthalmology* 103:1601, 1996

Pelton RW, Desmond BP, Mamalis N *et al.*: Nodular cutaneous amyloid tumors of the eyelids in the absence of systemic amyloidosis. *Ophthalmic Surg Lasers* 32:422, 2001

Peretz WL, Ettinghausen SE, Gray GF: Oncocytic adenocarcinoma of the lacrimal sac. *Arch Ophthalmol* 96:303, 1978

Preechawai P, la Roccad RC, Della RD *et al.*: Transitional cell carcinoma of the lacrimal sac. *J Med Assoc Thai* 88(Suppl. 9):S138, 2005

Riveros CJ, Gavilan MF, Franca LF *et al.*: Acquired localized cutis laxa confined to the face: case report and review of the literature. *Int J Dermatol* 43:931, 2004

Ryan SJ, Font RL: Primary epithelial neoplasms of the lacrimal sac. *Am J Ophthalmol* 76:73, 1973

Salomon J, Bieniek A, Baran E *et al.*: Basal cell carcinoma on the eyelids: own experience. *Dermatol Surg* 30:257, 2004

Schlotzer-Schrehardt U, Stojkovic M, Hofmann-Rummelt C *et al.*: The pathogenesis of floppy eyelid syndrome: involvement of matrix metalloproteinases in elastic fiber degradation. *Ophthalmology* 112:694, 2005

Selva D, Chen CS, James CL *et al.*: Discoid lupus erythematosus presenting as madarosis. *Am J Ophthalmol* 136:545, 2003

Sethuraman G, Tejasvi T, Khaitan BK *et al.*: Lipoid proteinosis in two siblings: a report from India. *J Dermatol* 30:562, 2003

Sharma V, Kashyap S, Betharia SM *et al.*: Lipoid proteinosis: a rare disorder with pathognomonic lid lesions. *Clin Exp Ophthalmol* 32:110, 2004

Shintaku M, Tsuta K, Yoshida H *et al.*: Apocrine adenocarcinoma of the eyelid with aggressive biological behavior: report of a case. *Pathol Int* 52:169, 2002

Shivaswamy KN, Thappa DM, Laxmisha C *et al.*: Lipoid proteinosis in two siblings: a report from south India. *Dermatol Online J* 9:12, 2003

Singh AD, McCloskey L, Parsons MA *et al.*: Eccrine hidrocystoma of the eyelid. *Eye* 19:77, 2005

Singh K, Mersol VF, Mastny VJ *et al.*: Adenoacanthoma of lacrimal sac. *Ann Ophthalmol* 9:1027, 1977

Singh V, Raju R, Singh M *et al.*: Congenital lipoblastoma of the scalp. *Am J Perinatol* 21:377, 2004

Tay E, Schofield JB, Rowell NP *et al.*: Ophthalmic presentation of the Muir Torre syndrome. *Ophthalm Plast Reconstr Surg* 19:402, 2003

Teixeira CC, Dias RJ, Falcao-Reis FM *et al.*: Congenital dacryocystocele with intranasal extension. *Eur J Ophthalmol* 15:126, 2005

Tomasini C, Soro E, Pippione M: Eyelid swelling: think of metastasis of histiocytoid breast carcinoma. *Dermatology* 205:63, 2002

Traboulsi EI, Al-Khayer K, Matsumoto M *et al.*: Lymphedema–distichiasis syndrome and FOXC2 gene mutation. *Am J Ophthalmol* 134:592, 2002

Vedamurthy M: Lipoid proteinosis in siblings. *Dermatol Online J* 9:13, 2003

Wat CS, Yuen HK, Tse KK *et al.*: Multiple eyelid defects in cutaneous Langerhans cell histiocytosis. *Ophthalm Plast Reconstr Surg* 22:216, 2006

Wessels MW, Brooks AS, Hoogeboom J *et al.*: Kabuki syndrome: a review study of three hundred patients. *Clin Dysmorphol* 11:95, 2002

Widmer S, Tinguely M, Egli F *et al.*: Lethal Epstein–Barr virus associated NK/T-cell lymphoma with primary manifestation in the conjunctiva. *Klin Monatsbl Augenheilkd* 222:255, 2005

Williams JD, Agrawal A, Wakely PE Jr: Mucoepidermoid carcinoma of the lacrimal sac. *Ann Diagn Pathol* 7:31, 2003

Wilson MW, Fleming JC, Fleming RM *et al.*: Sentinel node biopsy for orbital and ocular adnexal tumors. *Ophthalm Plast Reconstr Surg* 17:338, 2001

Yen MT, Hipps WM: Nasolacrimal sac hematoma masquerading as an orbital mass. *Ophthalm Plast Reconstr Surg* 20:170, 2004

Yip CC, Bartley GB, Habermann TM *et al.*: Involvement of the lacrimal drainage system by leukemia or lymphoma. *Ophthalm Plast Reconstr Surg* 18:242, 2002

Yuen KS, Cheng AC, Chan WM: Pyogenic granulomas after silicone punctal plugs: a clinical and histopathologic study. *Am J Ophthalmol* 140:963, 2005

Yuen SJ, Oley C, Sullivan TJ: Lacrimal outflow dysgenesis. *Ophthalmology* 111:1782, 2004

7

Conjunctiva

NORMAL ANATOMY

I. The conjunctiva (Fig. 7.1) is a mucous membrane, similar to mucous membranes elsewhere in the body, whose surface is composed of nonkeratinizing squamous epithelium, intermixed with goblet (mucus) cells, Langerhans' cells (dendritic-appearing cells expressing class II antigen), and occasional dendritic melanocytes. Stem cells for the epithelium are located near the limbus and their loss can result in exhaustion of the conjunctival epithelial population. Such stem cell loss may have many causes, including the use of mitomycin C in glaucoma filtration surgery, which may be exhibited as a late complication.

   A. *Idiopathic stem cell deficiency* is rare, most commonly found in women, and may be familial in some cases. Patients exhibit severe photophobia and, on clinical examination, have corneal vascularization accompanied by loss of the limbal palisades of Vogt, hazy peripheral corneal epithelium, and the presence of conjunctival goblet cells by impression cytology.

   A conjunctivalized pannus may develop on the cornea of those with total limbal stem cell deficiency. Characterization of this tissue demonstrates that it is not corneal, as evidenced by failure to stain for cornea-specific K12 mRNA and protein, but rather, it is conjunctival, as evidenced by the presence of goblet cells, the weak expression of K3, and the strong expression of K19.

   B. The homeostasis of the conjunctiva is dependent, in part, on the maintenance of a normal tear film, which is comprised of lipid, aqueous, and mucoid layers. Multiple disorders are associated with abnormal tear quantity and/or quality, and secondary ocular surface changes.

1. Cigarette smoking has a deteriorating effect on the tear film in general, and on its lipid layer in particular. It results in decreased quantity and quality of the tear film, decreased corneal sensitivity and squamous metaplasia, and this deterioration is related to the amount of smoking.

2. Tear film abnormalities have been documented in association with pseudoexfoliation syndrome and pseudoexfoliation glaucoma, and are reflected in abnormal conjunctival impression cytology and altered goblet cell morphology.

3. Although ocular surface glycocalyx is normally present in conjunctival epithelium, it is generally absent in patients with Sjögren's syndrome who have accompanying ultrastructural abnormalities of the apical conjunctival epithelium. Conjunctival biopsy specimens from patients with Sjögren's syndrome and non-Sjögren's keratoconjunctivitis sicca demonstrate lymphocytic infiltration and increased immunoreactivity for markers of immune activation.

4. The pattern of human leukocyte antigen (HLA)-DR expression in mild and moderate dry eyes appears to reflect disease progression, and suggests that inflammation may be a primary cause of ocular surface damage.

5. Abnormal tear film stability and meibomian gland dysfunction are associated with aniridia, and correlate with the severity of the disease. Impression cytology has confirmed varying degrees of limbal stem cell deficiency in these patients.

6. Squamous metaplasia of the ocular surface epithelium and ocular tear function abnormalities have been associated with interferon and ribavirin treatment for hepatitis C.

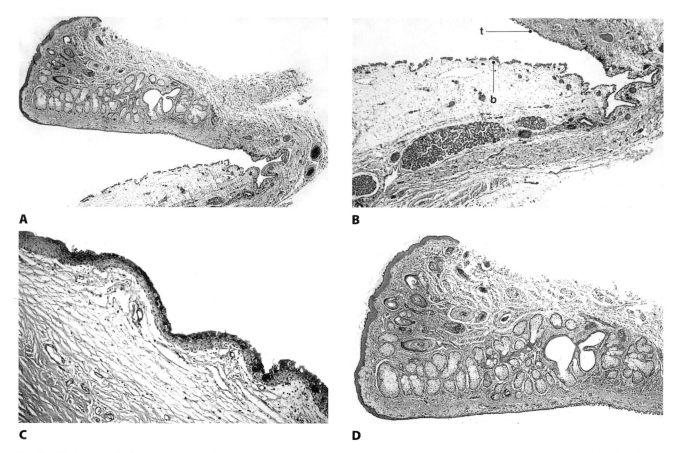

Fig. 7.1 Conjunctiva. **A,** The normal conjunctiva, a mucous membrane composed of nonkeratinizing squamous epithelium intermixed with goblet cells, sits on a connective tissue substantia propria. It is divided into three zones: tarsal, fornical–orbital, and bulbar. **B,** Increased magnification shows the tight adherence of the substantia propria of the tarsal (palpebral) conjunctival epithelium (t) to the underlying tarsal connective tissue and the loose adherence of the substantia propria of the bulbar conjunctival epithelium (b) to the underlying tissue. **C,** The goblet cells of the bulbar conjunctiva are seen easily with this periodic acid–Schiff stain. **D,** The tarsal conjunctiva becomes keratinized as it becomes continuous with the keratinized squamous epithelium of the skin on the intermarginal surface of the lid near its posterior border.

7. Conjunctiva in beta-thalassemia exhibits goblet cell loss and conjunctival squamous metaplasia.

8. There is increased expression of conjunctival epithelial beta-defensin-2 in patients with moderately dry eye, suggesting that the disorder may be mediated by proinflammatory cytokine activity.

9. Complete androgen-insensitivity syndrome may promote meibomian gland dysfunction and increase the signs and symptoms of dry eye.

10. The ocular surface disease in keratoconus is characterized by abnormal tear quality, squamous metaplasia, and goblet cell loss, all of which appear to relate to the extent of keratoconus progression.

11. In patients with dry eyes, the degree of conjunctival metaplasia, characterized by increased stratification, epithelial cellular size, and a general loss of goblet cells, correlates with the clinical severity of their disorder.

12. Marx's line represents a narrow line of epithelial cells posterior to the tarsal gland orifices along the lid marginal zone, averaging 0.10 mm in width, and is stained with lissamine green dye. It is believed to be the natural site of frictional contact between the eyelid margin and the surfaces of the bulbar conjunctiva and cornea, rather than the edge of the tear meniscus or location of the edge of the lacrimal river.

II. The conjunctival epithelium rests on a connective tissue, the substantia propria.

III. The conjunctiva is divided into three zones: tarsal, fornical–orbital, and bulbar.

A. The substantia propria of the tarsal conjunctiva adheres tightly to the underlying tarsal connective tissue, whereas the substantia propria of the bulbar conjunctiva (and even more so the fornical–orbital conjunctival substantia propria) adheres loosely to the underlying tissue (the fornical–orbital conjunctiva being thrown into folds).

The bulbar conjunctiva inserts anterior to Tenon's capsule toward the limbus. Small ectopic lacrimal *glands of Krause* are found in both the upper and lower fornices, with very few on the nasal side; *glands of Wolfring* are found around the upper border of the tarsus in the nasal half of the upper lid, and in lesser numbers, in the lower lid near the lower tarsal border; and *glands of Popoff* reside in the plica semilunaris and caruncle.

B. The periodic acid–Schiff (PAS) stain-positive goblet cells are most numerous in the fornices, the semilunar fold, and the caruncle. The latter is composed of modified conjunctiva containing hairs, sebaceous glands, acini of lacrimal glandlike cells, globules of fat, on occasion smooth-muscle fibers, and rarely cartilage.

C. The tarsal conjunctiva meets the keratinized squamous epithelium of the skin on the intermarginal surface of the lid near its posterior border.

CONGENITAL ANOMALIES

Cryptophthalmos (Ablepharon)

See p. 169 in Chapter 6.

Epitarsus

I. Epitarsus consists of a fold of conjunctiva attached to the palpebral surface of the lid or lids of one or both eyes. The fold has a free edge, and both surfaces (front and back) are covered by conjunctival epithelium.

II. Histologically, the folded conjunctival tissue looks like normal conjunctiva except for the occasional presence of islands of cartilage.

Hereditary Hemorrhagic Telangiectasia (Rendu–Osler–Weber Disease)

I. It is a generalized vascular dysplasia characterized by multiple telangiectases in the skin, mucous membranes, and viscera, with recurrent bleeding and an autosomal-dominant inheritance pattern.

No evidence of abnormalities in platelet aggregation or of qualitative abnormalities of factor VIII complex is found. Conjunctival hemorrhagic telangiectasia can give rise to "bloody tears." Occasionally, telangiectases are observed in the retina and may mimic hypertensive or diabetic retinopathy.

II. Dilated conjunctival blood vessels, frequently in a star or sunflower shape, may appear at birth but are not usually fully developed until late adolescence or early adult life.

III. Histologically, abnormal, dilated blood vessels are seen in the conjunctival substantia propria.

Ataxia–Telangiectasia (Louis–Bar Syndrome)

See p. 36 in Chapter 2.

Congenital Conjunctival Lymphedema (Milroy's Disease, Nonne–Milroy–Meige Disease)

I. This condition of hypoplastic lymphatics is characterized by massive edema, mainly of the lower extremities and rarely of the conjunctiva, and has an X-linked recessive inheritance pattern.

A. Mutations in the kinase domain of the vascular endothelial growth facor receptor-3 (VEGFR3) gene cause Milroy disease

B. Late-onset hereditary lymphedema may be associated with distichiasis *(lymphedema–distichiasis syndrome)* and has an autosomal-dominant inheritance pattern.

Lymphedema–distichiasis syndrome has been mapped to 16q23 and to mutations in the *FOXC2* gene.

II. The disease is thought to be due to a congenital dysplasia of the lymphatics, resulting in chronic lymphedema.

III. Histologically, dilated lymphatic channels and edematous tissue are seen.

Dermoids, Epidermoids, and Dermolipomas

See p. 240 in this chapter and p. 540 in Chapter 14.

Laryngo-Onycho-Cutaneous (LOC or Shabbir) Syndrome

I. LOC is an autosomal-recessive epithelial disorder characterized by cutaneous erosions, nail dystrophy, and exuberant vascular granulation in certain epithelia, especially the conjunctiva and larynx.

II. It is confined to the Punjabi Muslim population, and is caused by an unusual N-terminal deletion of the laminin alpha3a isoform, thereby demonstrating that the laminin alpha3a N-terminal domain is a key regulator of the granulation tissue response. The protein product is secreted by basal keratinocytes of stratified epithelia, and it has been postulated that LOC results from a dysfunction of keratinocyte–mesenchymal communication.

VASCULAR DISORDERS

Sickle-Cell Anemia

See p. 412 in Chapter 11.

I. In homozygous sickle-cell disease, conjunctival capillaries may show widespread sludging of blood, and the venules may show saccular dilatations.

II. The characteristic findings (marked in SS disease and mild in SC disease), however, are multiple, short, comma-shaped or curlicued conjunctival capillary segments, mostly near the limbus, often seemingly isolated from the vascular network *(Paton's sign)*.

Similar conjunctival capillary abnormalities may occasionally be seen in the nasal and temporal conjunctiva in patients without sickle-cell disease. Abnormalities in the inferior conjunctiva, however, are found almost exclusively in patients with sickle-cell disease. The vascular abnormalities seem positively related to the presence of sickled erythrocytes and may be useful in gauging the severity of the systemic disease. The comma-shaped capillaries are most easily seen after local application of phenylephrine.

III. Histologically, the capillary lumen is irregular and filled with sickled erythrocytes.

Conjunctival Hemorrhage (Subconjunctival Hemorrhage)

I. Intraconjunctival hemorrhage (see Fig. 5.30) into the substantia propria, or hemorrhage between conjunctiva and episclera, most often occurs as an isolated finding without any obvious cause.
II. The condition may occasionally result from trauma; severe conjunctival infection (e.g., leptospirosis and typhus); local vascular anomalies; sudden increase in venous pressure (e.g., after a paroxysm of coughing or sneezing); local manifestation of such systemic diseases as arteriolosclerosis, nephritis, diabetes mellitus, and chronic hepatic disease; blood dyscrasias, especially when anemia and thrombocytopenia coexist; acute febrile systemic infection (e.g., subacute bacterial endocarditis); spontaneously during menstruation; and trichinosis.
III. Histologically, blood is seen in the substantia propria of the conjunctiva.

Lymphangiectasia

I. Abnormal diffuse enlargement of lymphatics appears clinically as chemosis. Localized, dilated lymphatics appear clinically as a cyst or a series of cysts, the latter commonly in the area of the interpalpebral fissure.
II. When involvement is diffuse, the cause is not usually known.
An old scar, a pinguecula, or some other conjunctival lesion usually obstructs localized, dilated lymphatics secondarily.
III. Histologically, the lymphatic vessels are abnormally dilated.

Lymphangiectasia Hemorrhagica

Conjunctivae

I. The condition is characterized by a connection between a blood vessel and a lymphatic so that the latter is permanently or intermittently filled with blood.
II. The cause is not known.

Ataxia–Telangiectasia

See p. 36 in Chapter 2.

Diabetes Mellitus

See section *Conjunctiva and Cornea* in Chapter 15.

Hemangioma and Lymphangioma

See pp. 544 and 545 in Chapter 14.

INFLAMMATION

Basic Histologic Changes

I. Acute conjunctivitis (Fig. 7.2)
A. Edema (chemosis), hyperemia, and cellular exudates are characteristic of acute conjunctivitis.
B. Inflammatory membranes (Fig. 7.3)

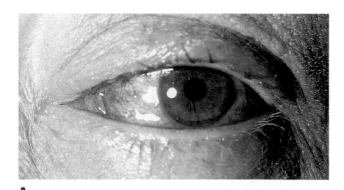

A

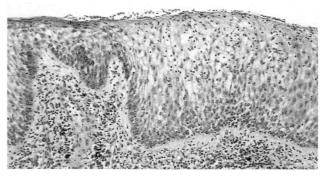

B

Fig. 7.2 Acute conjunctivitis. **A,** Clinical appearance of a mucopurulent conjunctivitis of the left eye. The pupil reacted normally. The conjunctival infection was least at the limbus and increased peripherally. **B,** The major inflammatory cell of acute bacterial conjunctivitis is the polymorphonuclear leukocyte, which here infiltrates the swollen edematous epithelium and the substantia propria.

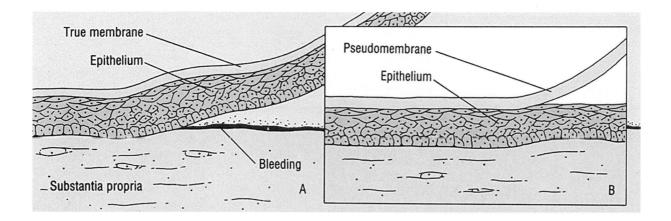

Fig. 7.3 Inflammatory membranes. **A,** In a true membrane, when the membrane is stripped off, the epithelium is also removed and a bleeding surface remains. **B,** In a pseudomembrane, when the membrane is stripped off, it separates from the epithelium, leaving it intact and causing no surface bleeding.

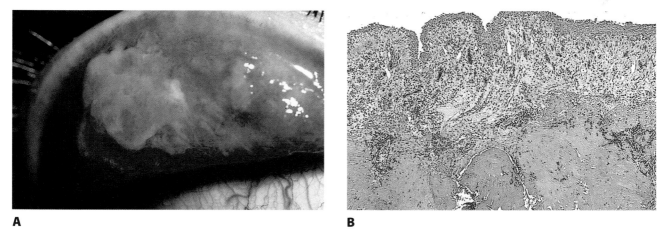

Fig. 7.4 Ligneous conjunctivitis. **A,** A thick membrane covers the upper palpebral conjunctiva. Ligneous conjunctivitis is a chronic, bilateral, recurrent, membranous or pseudomembranous conjunctivitis of childhood of unknown cause. **B,** Biopsy shows a thick, amorphous material contiguous with an inflammatory membrane composed mostly of mononuclear inflammatory cells, mainly plasma cells, and some lymphocytes. (Case presented by Dr. JS McGavic at the meeting of the Verhoeff Society, 1986).

1. A *true membrane* consists of an exudate of fibrin–cellular debris firmly attached to the underlying epithelium by fibrin.
   a. Characteristically, when the true membrane is removed, the epithelium is also stripped off, leaving a raw, bleeding surface.
   b. The condition may be seen in epidemic keratoconjunctivitis, Stevens–Johnson syndrome, and infections caused by *Pneumococcus, Staphylococcus aureus,* and *Corynebacterium diphtheriae.*
2. A *pseudomembrane* consists of a loose fibrin–cellular debris exudate not adherent to the underlying epithelium, from which it is easily stripped.
   a. This finding can be associated with epidemic keratoconjunctivitis, Stevens–Johnson syndrome, pharyngoconjunctival fever, vernal conjunctivitis, ligneous conjunctivitis, chemical burns (especially alkali), and infections caused by *C. diphtheriae* and *Streptococcus pyogenes.*
3. *Ligneous conjunctivitis* (Fig. 7.4) is an unusual type of bilateral, chronic, recurrent, membranous or pseudomembranous conjunctivitis of childhood, most commonly in girls, of unknown cause.
   a. The condition persists for months to years and may become massive.
   b. The conjunctivitis is characterized by wood-like induration of the palpebral conjunctiva, chronicity, and rapid recurrence after medical or surgical treatment.
   c. Severe corneal complications may occur.
   d. Similar lesions may also occur in the larynx, vocal cords, trachea, nose, vagina, cervix, and gingiva.

e. Rarely, the middle ear may exhibit a similar histopathologic process.

f. Histologically, the conjunctival epithelium is thickened and may be dyskeratotic.

The subepithelial tissue consists of an enormously thick membrane composed primarily of fibrin, albumin, immunoglobulin G (IgG), and an amorphous eosinophilic material containing a sprinkling of T and B lymphocytes and plasma cells.

C. *Ulceration*, or loss of epithelium with or without loss of subepithelial tissue associated with an inflammatory cellular infiltrate, may occur with acute conjunctivitis.

D. A *phlyctenule* usually starts as a localized, acute inflammatory reaction, followed by central necrosis and infiltration by lymphocytes and plasma cells.

II. Chronic conjunctivitis (Fig. 7.5)

A. The epithelium and its goblet cells increase in number (i.e., become hyperplastic).

> Infoldings of the proliferated epithelium and goblet cells may resemble glandular structures in tissue section and are called *pseudoglands* (Henle). Commonly, the surface openings of the pseudoglands, especially in the inferior palpebral conjunctiva, may become clogged by debris. They form clear or yellow cysts called *pseudoretention cysts*, containing mucinous secretions admixed with degenerative products of the epithelial cells.

B. The conjunctiva may undergo *papillary hypertrophy* (Fig. 7.6), which is caused by the conjunctiva being thrown into folds.

1. The folds or projections are covered by hyperplastic epithelium and contain a core of vessels surrounded

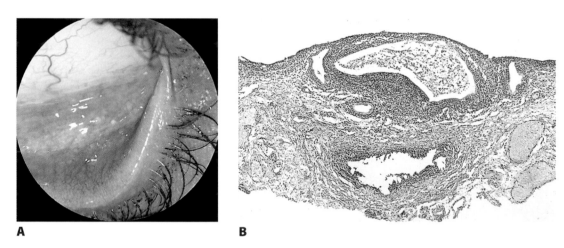

A   **B**

Fig. 7.5 Chronic conjunctivitis. **A,** The conjunctiva is thickened and contains tiny yellow cysts. **B,** Histologic section of the conjunctiva demonstrates the cyst lined by an epithelium that resembles ductal epithelium and that contains a pink granular material. A chronic nongranulomatous inflammation of lymphocytes and plasma cells surrounds the cyst, along with a proliferation of the epithelium of the palpebral conjunctiva, forming structures that resemble glands and are called *pseudoglands* (Henle).

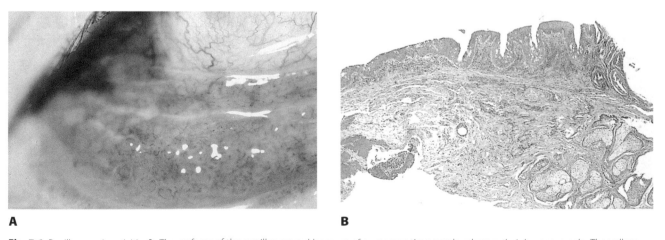

A   **B**

Fig. 7.6 Papillary conjunctivitis. **A,** The surfaces of the papillae are red because of numerous tiny vessels, whereas their bases are pale. The yellow staining is caused by fluorescein. **B,** Histologic section of the conjunctiva demonstrates an inflammatory infiltrate in the substantia propria and numerous small vessels coursing through the papillae. The inflammatory cells are lymphocytes and plasma cells.

by edematous subepithelial tissue infiltrated with chronic inflammatory cells (lymphocytes and plasma cells predominate).

2. Papillary hypertrophy is primarily a vascular response.

3. The lymphocyte (even lymphoid follicles) and plasma cell infiltrations are secondary.

> Clinically, the small (0.1 to 0.2 mm), hyperemic projections are fairly regular, are most marked in the upper palpebral conjunctiva, and contain a central tuft of vessels. The valleys between the projections are pale and relatively vessel-free. Papillae characterize the subacute stage of many inflammations (e.g., *vernal catarrh* and the *floppy-eyelid syndrome*; decreased tarsal elastin may contribute to the laxity of the tarsus in the floppy-eyelid syndrome).

C. The conjunctiva may undergo follicle formation. *Follicular hypertrophy* (Fig. 7.7) consists of lymphoid hyperplasia and secondary visualization.

> Lymphoid tissue is not present in the conjunctiva at birth but normally develops within the first few months. In *inclusion blennorrhea* of the newborn, therefore, a papillary reaction develops, whereas the same infection in adults may cause a follicular reaction. Lymphoid hyperplasia develops in such diverse conditions as drug toxicities (e.g., atropine, pilocarpine, eserine), allergic conditions, and infections (e.g., trachoma). It has been reported, presumably, as secondary to extremely thin sclera in high myopia. Clinically, lymphoid follicles are smaller and paler than papillae and lack the central vascular tuft.

D. Vitamin A deficiency or drying of the conjunctiva (e.g., chronic exposure with lid ectropion) may cause keratinization.

E. Chronic inflammation during healing may cause an overexuberant amount of granulation tissue to be formed (i.e., granuloma pyogenicum; see Fig. 6.11).

F. The conjunctiva may be the site of granulomatous inflammation (e.g., sarcoid; see p. 93 in Chapter 4).

G. Conjunctival epithelium of patients on chronic topical medical treatment, such as individuals with glaucoma, demonstrates increased expression of immunoinflammatory markers such as HLA-DR, and interleukins IL-6, IL-8, and IL-10 in impression cytology specimens.

H. Clinical and/or histopathologic demonstration of tarsal conjunctival disease may be evidenced by: (1) conjunctival hyperemia and granuloma formation, areas of necrosis, or active fibrovascular changes in the tarsus or conjunctiva; or (2) an inactive fibrovascular scar associated with subglottic stenosis and nasolacrimal duct obstruction in patients with Wegener's granulomatosis (WG).

III. Ligneous conjunctivitis (see earlier, this chapter).

IV. Scarring of conjunctiva

A. *Ocular cicatricial pemphigoid* (benign mucous membrane pemphigoid, pemphigus conjunctivae, chronic cicatrizing conjunctivitis, essential shrinkage of conjunctiva)

1. Ocular cicatricial pemphigoid is a rare, T-cell immune-mediated, bilateral (one eye may be involved first), blistering, chronic conjunctival disease. It may involve the conjunctiva alone or, more commonly, other mucous membranes and skin in elderly people.

> The conjunctiva is the only site of involvement in most cases. Drugs such as echothiophate iodide, pilocarpine, idoxuridine, and epinephrine may induce a pseudopemphigoid conjunctival reaction.

2. The disease results in shrinkage of the conjunctiva (secondary to scarring), trichiasis, xerosis, and finally reduced vision from secondary corneal scarring.

> At the onset of the condition, an acute or subacute papillary conjunctivitis and diffuse hyperemia are common. One or two small conjunctival ulcers covered by a gray membrane are often noted. Keratinization of the caruncu-

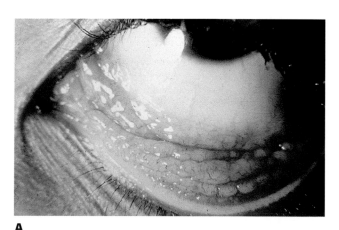

A

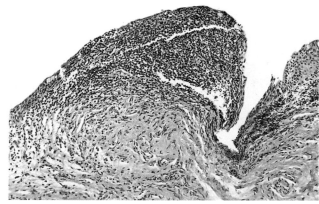

B

Fig. 7.7 Follicular conjunctivitis. **A,** The surfaces of the follicles are pale, whereas their bases are red. **B,** Histologic section of the conjunctiva shows a lymphoid follicle in the substantia propria.

lar region (i.e., medial canthal keratinization) is a reliable early sign of ocular cicatricial pemphigoid, especially if entities such as Stevens–Johnson are excluded. The ulcers heal by cicatrization, as new ulcers form. The condition occurs more frequently in women.

3. About 22% of patients who have systemic, nonocular, mucous membrane pemphigoid develop ocular disease.

4. Histology
   a. Subepithelial conjunctival bullae rupture and are replaced by fibrovascular tissue containing lymphocytes (especially T cells), dendritic (Langerhans') cells, and plasma cells.
      1). The epithelium has an immunoreactive deposition (immunoglobulin or complement) along its basement membrane zone. The presence of circulating antibodies to the epithelial basement membrane zone can also be helpful in making the diagnosis. Such immunohistochemical confirmation is important because the clinical characteristics of ocular mucous membrane pemphigoid and pseudopemphigoid are similar, which may lead to a clinical misdiagnosis.
         a). Increased conjunctival expression of IL-4 may play an important role in the regulation of local accumulation of macrophages by inducing macrophage colony-stimulating factor, and of matrix accumulation by inducing heat shock protein-47 during conjunctival scarring in patients with ocular cicatricial pemphigoid, thereby contributing to conjunctival inflammatory and subsequent fibrotic responses associated with the disorder. Moreover, increased expression of collagen-binding heat shock protein-47 and transforming growth factor beta1 by conjunctival fibroblasts in ocular cicatricial pemphigoid may regulate increased synthesis, assembly, and production of collagens, thereby further contributing to conjunctival scaring in pemphigoid.
         b). Increased expression of connective tissue growth factor has been demonstrated in the conjunctiva of patients with ocular cicatricial pemphigoid, and it is probably one of the factors involved in the pathogenesis of the typical conjunctival fibrosis in the disorder.
         c). Macrophage colony-stimulating factor has increased expression in conjunctiva in ocular cicatricial pemphigoid, and there is a positive correlation between its expression and the accumulation of macrophages in conjunctival biopsies in patients with pemphigoid.

2). The use of the immunoperoxidase technique in biopsy material may increase the diagnostic yield in clinically suspected cases.

Ocular cicatricial pemphigoid, *bullous pemphigoid*, and *benign mucous membrane pemphigoid*, all immune-mediated blistering diseases, resemble each other clinically, histopathologically, and immunologically. Ocular cicatricial pemphigoid, however, appears to be a unique entity separated from the others by antigenic specificity of autoantibodies. Another systemic blistering condition, *epidermolysis bullosa acquisita*, can cause symblepharon and small, subepithelial corneal vesicles.

---

         a). The vascular and inflammatory components lessen with chronicity, resulting in contracture of the fibrous tissue with subsequent shrinkage, scarring, symblepharon, ankyloblepharon, and so forth.
         3). Expression of macrophage migration inhibitory factor is increased in cicatricial pemphigoid and may help regulate the inflammatory events in this disorder.
         4). Elevated numbers of conjunctival mast cells are not only associated with atopic keratoconjunctivitis, but are also present in ocular cicatricial pemphigoid and Stevens–Johnson syndrome.

Pemphigus, a group of diseases that have circulating antibodies against intercellular substances or keratinocyte surface antigens, unlike pemphigoid, is characterized histologically by acantholysis, resulting in intraepidermal vesicles and bullae rather than subepithelial vesicles and bullae. The bullae of pemphigus, unlike those of pemphigoid, tend to heal without scarring. In pemphigus, the conjunctiva is rarely involved, and even then scarring is not a prominent feature. Unilateral refractory (erosive) conjunctivitis may be an unusual manifestation of pemphigus vulgaris.

B. Secondary scarring occurs in many conditions. Some examples are chemical burns, erythema multiforme (Stevens–Johnson syndrome), old membranous conjunctivitis (diphtheria, β-hemolytic *Streptococcus*, adenovirus, primary herpes simplex), trachoma, trauma (surgical or nonsurgical), paraneoplastic pemphigus, and pemphigus vulgaris. Deliberate chronic use of high-dose topical hydrogen peroxide has resulted in severe corneal and conjunctival changes that can mimic ocular cicatricial pemphigoid. Cicatricial conjunctivitis may be a manifestation of porphyria cutanea tarda.

C. Conjunctival involvement in toxic epidermal necrolysis has been reported in association with autoimmune polyglandular syndrome type I, which is defined as the presence of two of the following diseases: Addison's disease, hypoparathyroidism, and chronic mucocutaneous candidiasis.

Specific Inflammations

Infectious

 I. Virus—see subsection *Chronic Nongranulomatous Inflammation* in Chapter 1.
 II. Bacteria—see sections *Phases of Inflammation* in Chapter 1 and *Suppurative Endophthalmitis and Panophthalmitis* in Chapter 3.
 III. Chlamydiae cause trachoma, lymphogranuloma venereum, and ornithosis (psittacosis).
   A. Previously classified as "large" viruses, they have been shown to be Gram-negative, basophilic, coccoid or spheroid *bacteria*. Because of certain similarities to rickettsiae, they may be classified in that group.
   B. The chlamydiae are identified taxonomically into order Chlamydiales, family Chlamydiaceae, genus *Chlamydia*, and species *trachomatis* and *psittaci*.

The agents that cause trachoma and inclusion conjunctivitis, both classified as *Chlamydia trachomatis*, are almost indistinguishable from each other, and the term *TRIC* agent encompasses both. Reproduction of chlamydiae starts with the attachment and penetration of the *elementary body*, an infectious small particle 200 to 350 nm in diameter with an electron-dense nucleoid, into the host cell cytoplasm. The phagocytosed agent surrounded by the invaginated host cell membrane forms a cytoplasmic inclusion body. The elementary body then enlarges to approximately 700 to 1000 nm in diameter to form a nonmotile obligate intracellular (cytoplasmic) parasite (called an *energy parasite* because of its dependence on the host cell for energy) known as an *initial body* that does not contain electron-dense material. Initial bodies then divide by binary fission into numerous, small, highly infectious elementary bodies. The host cell ruptures, the elementary bodies are released, and a new infectious cycle begins.

   C. Trachoma (Fig. 7.8)
    1. Trachoma, caused by the bacterial agent *C. trachomatis* and one of the world's leading causes of blindness, primarily affects the conjunctival and corneal epithelium.
    2. Healing is marked by scarring or cicatrization.
    3. Histology of MacCallan's four stages:
      a. Stage I: early formation of conjunctival follicles, subepithelial conjunctival infiltrates, diffuse punctate keratitis, and early pannus
       1). The conjunctival epithelium undergoes a marked hyperplasia, and its cytoplasm contains clearly defined, glycogen-containing

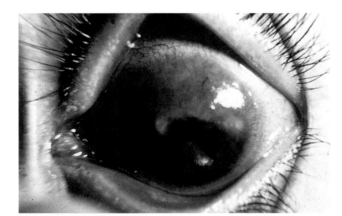

A

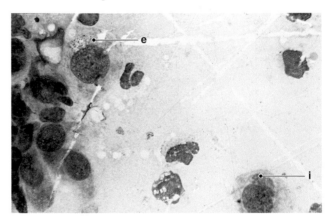

B

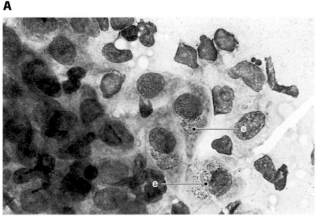

C

Fig. 7.8 Trachoma. **A,** The patient has a trachomatous pannus growing over the superior conjunctiva. With healing, the follicles disappear from the peripheral cornea, leaving areas filled with a thickened transparent epithelium called *Herbert's pits*. The palpebral conjunctiva scars by the formation of a linear, white, horizontal line or scar near the upper border of the tarsus, called *von Arlt's line*. **B,** A conjunctival smear from another case of trachoma shows a large cytoplasmic basophilic initial body (i). Small cytoplasmic elementary bodies (e) are seen in some of the other cells. **C,** Small cytoplasmic elementary bodies (e) are seen in numerous cells. (**A,** Courtesy of Dr. AP Ferry.)

intracellular microcolonies of minute elementary bodies and large basophilic initial bodies.

2). The bodies form the conjunctival and corneal epithelial cytoplasmic *inclusion bodies* of Halberstaedter and Prowazek.

3). The subepithelial tissue is edematous and infiltrated by round inflammatory cells.

4). Fibrovascular tissue from the substantia propria proliferates and starts to grow into the cornea under the epithelium, destroying Bowman's membrane; the tissue is then called an *inflammatory pannus*.

b. Stage II: florid inflammation, mainly of the upper tarsal conjunctiva with the early formation of follicles appearing like sago grains, and then like papillae

1). The corneal pannus increases and large macrophages with phagocytosed debris (Leber cells) appear in the conjunctival substantia propria.

2). The follicles cannot be differentiated histologically from lymphoid follicles secondary to other causes (e.g., allergic).

c. Stage III: scarring (cicatrization)

In the peripheral cornea, follicles disappear and the area is filled with thickened, transparent epithelium (*Herbert's pits*); as the palpebral conjunctiva heals, a white linear horizontal line or scar forms near the upper border of the tarsus (*von Arlt's line*). Cicatricial entropion and trichiasis may result.

1). Ocular rosacea can produce chronic cicatrizing conjunctivitis of the upper eyelids, which was previously thought to be unique to trachoma. Conjunctival impression cytology in ocular rosacea demonstrates significant ocular surface epithelial degeneration involving both the upper bulbar and inferonasal interpalpebral bulbar epithelium compared to normal individuals.

The inflammatory infiltrate of the tarsoconjunctiva is predominantly composed of T cells (CD4+ and CD8+), and suggests that T cells may be involved in the genesis of both tarsal thickening and conjunctival scarring in the late stages of trachoma.

---

d. Stage IV: arrest of the disease

D. Inclusion conjunctivitis (inclusion blennorrhea)

1. Inclusion conjunctivitis is caused by the bacterial agent *C. trachomatis* (*oculogenitale*).

2. It is an acute contagious disease of newborns quite similar clinically and histologically to trachoma, except the latter has a predilection for the upper rather than the lower palpebral conjunctiva and fornix.

Inclusion conjunctivitis can also occur in adults, commonly showing corneal involvement (mainly superficial epithelial keratitis, but also subepithelial nummular keratitis, marginal keratitis, and superior limbal swelling and pannus formation).

---

3. Histologically, a follicular reaction is present with epithelial cytoplasmic inclusion bodies indistinguishable from those of trachoma.

E. Lymphogranuloma venereum (inguinale)

1. Lymphogranuloma venereum, also caused by the bacterial agent *C. trachomatis*, is characterized by a follicular conjunctivitis or a nonulcerating conjunctival granuloma, usually near the limbus and associated with a nonsuppurative regional lymphadenopathy.

The clinical picture is that of *Parinaud's oculoglandular syndrome* (see later).

Keratitis may occur, usually with infiltrates in the upper corneal periphery, associated with stromal vascularization and thickened corneal nerves. An associated anterior uveitis may also occur.

---

2. Histologically, a granulomatous conjunctivitis and lymphadenitis occur, the latter containing stellate abscesses.

Elementary bodies and inclusion bodies cannot be identified in histologic sections.

IV. Fungal—see the subsection *Fungal*, section *Nontraumatic Infections* in Chapter 4.

V. Parasitic—see the subsection *Parasitic*, section *Nontraumatic Infections* in Chapter 4 and pp. 88, and 273 in Chapter 8.

VI. Rickettsial—because of certain similarities to rickettsias, chlamydiae may be classified in this group.

VII. *Parinaud's oculoglandular syndrome* (granulomatous conjunctivitis and ipsilateral enlargement of the preauricular lymph nodes) consists of a granulomatous inflammation and may be caused most commonly by cat-scratch disease, but also by Epstein–Barr virus infection, tuberculosis, sarcoidosis, syphilis, tularemia, Leptothrix infection, soft chancre (chancroid—*Haemophilus ducreyi*), glanders, lymphogranuloma venereum, Crohn's disease, and fungi.

Noninfectious

I. Physical—see subsections *Burns* and *Radiation Injuries* (*Electromagnetic*) in Chapter 5.

II. Chemical—see subsection *Chemical Injuries* in Chapter 5.

III. Allergic

A. Allergic conjunctivitis is usually associated with a type 1 hypersensitivity reaction. It can be further subdivided into acute disorders (seasonal allergic conjunctivitis and perennial allergic conjunctivitis), and chronic diseases (vernal conjunctivitis, atopic keratoconjunctivitis, giant papillary conjunctivitis). Mast cells play a central role in the pathogenesis of ocular allergy. Their numbers are increased in all forms of allergic conjunctivitis, and may participate in the process through their activation, resulting in the release of preformed and newly formed mediators. Chronic conjunctivitis may be accompanied by remodeling of the ocular surface tissues.

B. Vernal keratoconjunctivitis (vernal catarrh, spring catarrh; Fig. 7.9)

1. Vernal keratoconjunctivitis tends to be a bilateral, recurrent, self-limited conjunctival disease occurring mainly in warm weather and affecting young people (mainly boys).

   a. It is of unknown cause, but is presumed to be an immediate hypersensitivity reaction to exogenous antigens.

   b. The disease is associated with increased serum levels of total IgE, eosinophil-derived products, and nerve growth factor.

   > Nerve growth factor may play a role in vernal keratoconjunctivitis by modulating conjunctival mast cell proliferation, differentiation, and activation. Also, the enzymatic degradation of histamine in both tears and plasma appears to be significantly decreased in patients who have vernal keratoconjunctivitis.

   c. It has been postulated that vernal conjunctivitis is a Th2 lymphocyte-mediated disease in which mast cells, eosinophils, and their mediators play major roles in the clinical manifestations. This process, therefore, involves the Th2-derived cytokines, IL-4, IL-5, and IL-13, as well as other chemokines, growth factors, and enzymes, which are overexpressed in the disorder. Eventually, structural cells, such as epithelial cells and fibroblasts, are involved both in the inflammatory process and in tissue remodeling, eventuating in the characteristic giant papillae.

   d. Chronic conjunctival inflammation in vernal keratoconjunctivitis is associated with staining of alpha3, and alpha6 integrin subunits, epidermal growth factor (EGF) receptor, vascular endothelial growth factor, transforming growth factor-beta, basic fibroblast growth factor, and platelet-derived growth factor that might mediate conjunctival remodeling.

   e. The CXC chemokine Mig is selectively and highly expressed in vernal keratoconjunctivitis, and it has been suggested that this finding indicates a pathogenic role for the chemokine receptor CXCR3 and the ligand Mig in the recruitment of activated T lymphocytes.

   f. Unique intercellular communication between corneal epithelium and conjunctival cellular elements through the tear film, and mediated

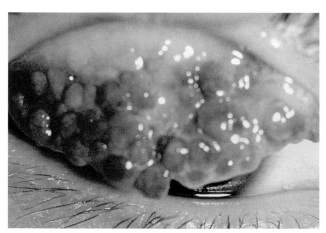

A

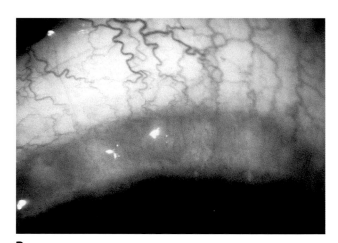

B

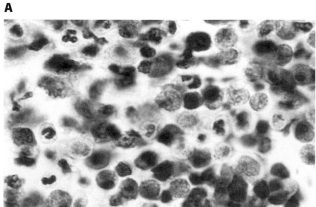

C

Fig. 7.9 Vernal catarrh. **A,** Clinical appearance of the papillary reaction of the palpebral conjunctiva. **B,** Clinical appearance of the less commonly seen limbal reaction. **C,** Histologic examination of a conjunctival smear shows the presence of many eosinophils. (**B** and **C,** Courtesy of Dr. IM Raber.)

by proinflammatory and T-helper 2 cytokines, chemokines such as eotaxin and thymus and activation-regulated chemokine (TARC), and adhesion molecules such as intercellular adhesion molecule 1 (ICAM-1) and vascular cell adhesion molecule 1 (VCAM-1), may contribute to the pathogenesis of vernal keratoconjunctivitis.

g. Cultured fibroblasts and conjunctival papillae from patients with vernal keratoconjunctivitis demonstrate that trypase increases conjunctival fibroblast proliferation, and this response appears to be mediated by protease-activated receptor (PAR)-2. Mast cells have been postulated to be the most likely source for the trypase.

A condition called *giant papillary conjunctivitis* resembles vernal conjunctivitis. It occurs in contact lens wearers as a syndrome consisting of excess mucus and itching, diminished or destroyed contact lens tolerance, and giant papillae in the upper tarsal conjunctiva.

---

2. Vernal conjunctivitis may be associated with, or accompanied by, keratoconus (or, more rarely, pellucid marginal corneal degeneration, keratoglobus, or superior corneal thinning).

3. Involvement may be limited to the tarsal conjunctiva (palpebral form), the bulbar conjunctiva (limbal form), or the cornea (vernal superficial punctate keratitis form), or combinations of all three. It is mediated, at least in part, by IgE antibodies produced in the conjunctiva.

4. Histology

   a. The tarsal conjunctiva may undergo hyperplasia of its epithelium and proliferation of fibrovascular connective tissue along with an infiltration of round inflammatory cells, especially eosinophils and basophils.

Papillae that form as a result can become quite large, clinically resembling cobblestones.

---

   b. The epithelium and subepithelial fibrovascular connective tissue of the limbal conjunctival region may undergo hyperplasia and round-cell inflammatory infiltration, with production of limbal nodules.

   c. In the larger yellow or gray vascularized nodules, concretions, containing eosinophils, appear clinically as white spots (*Horner–Trantas spots*).

   d. Degeneration and death of corneal epithelium result in punctate epithelial erosions that are especially prone to occur in the upper part of the cornea.

Eosinophilic granule major basic protein (the core of the eosinophilic granule) may play a role in the devel-

opment of corneal ulcers associated with vernal keratoconjunctivitis.

C. Inflammatory cells (eosinophils and neutrophils) in brush cytology specimens from the tarsus correlate with corneal damage in *atopic keratoconjunctivitis*. In atopic blepharoconjunctivitis, the tear content of group IIA phospholipase A_2 is decreased without any dependence on the quantity of different conjunctival cells.

Mast cell densities are increased in the bulbar and tarsal substantia propria in seasonal atopic keratoconjunctivitis and atopic blepharoconjunctivitis, but only in the bulbar substantia propria in atopic conjunctivitis. Ocular surface inflammation, tear film instability, and decreased conjunctival MUC5AC mRNA expression are thought to be important in the pathogenesis of noninfectious corneal shield ulcers in atopic ocular disease. Reactive oxygen species generated by NAD(P)H oxidases in pollen grains may intensify immediate allergic reactions and recruitment of inflammatory cells in the conjunctiva.

D. Hayfever conjunctivitis

E. Contact blepharoconjunctivitis

F. Phlyctenular keratoconjunctivitis

IV. Immunologic

A. Graft-versus-host disease (GvHD) conjunctivitis

1. A significant percentage (perhaps 10%) of patients who have had an allogeneic (an HLA-identical donor, e.g., a sibling) bone marrow transplantation develop a distinct type of conjunctivitis, representing GvHD of the conjunctiva.

2. It presents with pseudomembrane formation secondary to loss of the conjunctival epithelium.

3. In approximately 20% of these cases, the corneal epithelium also sloughs.

4. Conjunctival ICAM-1 expression is increased in GvHD patients, and the severity of the disease is associated with abnormal tear parameters, goblet cell decrease, and inflammatory markers such as ICAM-1.

5. After autologous bone marrow transplant there appears to be a subclinical cell-mediated immune reaction; moreover, T cells and macrophages are major contributors to the conjunctivitis of chronic GvHD.

Another ocular manifestation mediated by GvHD is *keratoconjunctivitis sicca*.

B. Wegerer's granulomatosis (WG) should be considered when conjunctival inflammation is recurrent and not typical of other conjunctival inflammatory conditions. Based on assessment of the presence of major basic protein and eosinophil cationic protein, it has been suggested that activated eosinophils in the sclera or conjunctiva of patients with ocular limited WG may predict the progression to complete WG.

C. Isolated congenital histiocytosis has involved the palpebral conjunctival in a newborn infant. Histopathologic examination revealed a cellular infiltrate composed of eosinophils and histiocytes without skin or systemic involvement. Immunohistochemistry was positive for S-100 and CD1 antigenic determinant.

D. Inflammatory pseudotumor, characterized by the presence of aggregates of chronic inflammatory cells (lymphocytes, plasma cells, neutrophils, and fibroblasts) without noncaseating epithelioid granuloma formation, has been reported to occur simultaneously in the conjunctiva and lung.

E. Rarely, conjunctival ulceration may be a manifestation of Behçet's disease, and is characterized on histopathologic examination by disrupted epithelium, infiltration by both acute and chronic inflammatory cells, and high endothelial venules. Immunohistologic studies of the inflammatory infiltrate reveal primarily T-cell populations admixed with several B cells and CD68-positive histiocytes.

V. Neoplastic processes (e.g., sebaceous gland carcinoma) can cause a chronic nongranulomatous blepharoconjunctivitis with cancerous invasion of the epithelium and subepithelial tissues.

A. Sebaceous carcinoma may involve the conjunctival epithelium in 47% of cases, of which the superior tarsal and forniceal conjunctiva are involved in 100%; inferior tarsal conjunctiva, 68%; inferior forniceal conjunctiva, 64%; superior bulbar conjunctiva, 68%; and inferior bulbar conjunctiva, 57%. The caruncle is involved in 54% and the cornea in 39%. Metastasis occur in 11%.

B. Impression cytology may be useful in the detection of conjunctival intraepithelial invasion by sebaceous gland carcinoma; however, full-thickness biopsies are necessary to confirm the diagnosis.

INJURIES

See Chapter 5.

CONJUNCTIVAL MANIFESTATIONS OF SYSTEMIC DISEASE

Deposition of Metabolic Products

I. Cystinosis (Lignac's disease)—see Fig. 8.41.
II. Ochronosis—see p. 314 in Chapter 8.
III. Hypercalcemia—see p. 279 in Chapter 8.
IV. Addison's disease: melanin is deposited in the basal layer of the epithelium.
V. Mucopolysaccharidoses—see p. 298 in Chapter 8.
VI. Lipidosis—see pp. 450–453 in Chapter 11.
VII. Dysproteinemias

VIII. Porphyria
IX. Jaundice
A. Bilirubin salts are deposited diffusely in the conjunctiva and episclera, but not usually in the sclera unless the jaundice is chronic and excessive; even in the latter case, the bulk of the bilirubin is in the conjunctiva (*scleral icterus*, therefore, is a misnomer).
B. Rarely, the icterus can extend into the cornea.
X. Malignant atrophic papulosis (Degos' syndrome)—see p. 186 in Chapter 6.
XI. The characteristic anterior-segment finding in Fabry disease is corneal verticillata, which is secondary to glycosphingolipid deposition in the cornea. *In vivo* confocal microscopy of the conjunctiva demonstrates abnormalities throughout the ocular surface, including bright roundish intracellular inclusions, which are more pronounced in tarsal than in bulbar conjunctiva.
XII. Consistent, qualitative abnormalities in conjunctival fibrillin-1 staining pattern can be seen in the conjunctiva of patients with Marfan syndrome with ectopia lentis.
XIII. Squamous metaplasia of the conjunctival epithelium and corneoconjunctival calcification frequently accompany chronic renal failure requiring hemodialysis. Abnormal tear function is associated with squamous metaplasia, but not with corneoconjunctival calcification. Similarly, although impression cytology demonstrates more frequent and extensive deposits of calcium deposits in the conjunctiva of chronic failure patients on regular hemodialysis compared to control patients, the severity of conjunctival squamous metaplasia associated with chronic renal failure appears not to be related to calcium deposition, but rather, to acute conjunctival inflammation.

Deposition of Drug Derivatives

I. Argyrosis (Fig. 7.10)
A. Long-term use of silver-containing medications may result in a slate-gray discoloration of the mucous membranes, including the conjunctiva, and of the skin, including the lids. The discoloration may also involve the nasolacrimal apparatus.
B. Histologically, silver is deposited in reticulin (i.e., loose collagenous) fibrils of subepithelial tissue and in basement membranes of epithelium, endothelium (e.g., Descemet's membrane), and blood vessels.
II. Chlorpromazine—see p. 313 in Chapter 8.
III. Atabrine
IV. Epinephrine
A. Conjunctival or corneal deposition can follow long-term use of epinephrine.
B. Epinephrine may deposit under an epithelial bleb, where it becomes oxidized to a compound similar to melanin.
1. Occasionally, the black corneal deposit (*black cornea*) has been mistaken for malignant melanoma of the cornea.
C. Histologically, an amorphous pink material that bleaches and reduces silver salts is found between

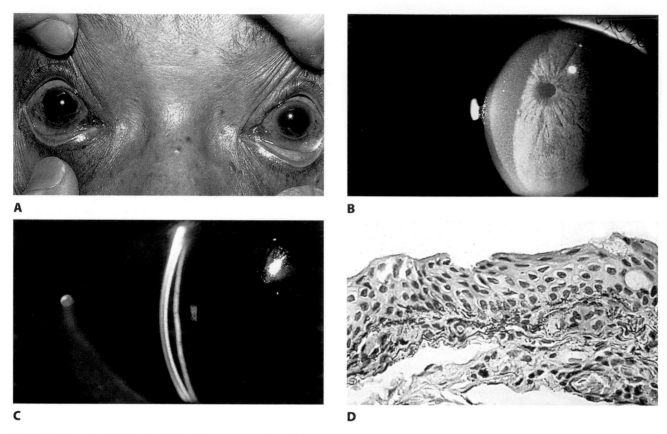

Fig. 7.10 Argyrosis. **A,** Patient had taken silver-containing drops for many years. Note the slate-gray appearance of conjunctiva. **B,** The cornea shows a diffuse granular appearance. **C,** The granular corneal appearance is caused by silver deposition in Descemet's membrane. **D,** Histologic section of another case shows silver deposited in the epithelium and in the mucosal basement membrane of the lacrimal sac. (**D,** Adapted from Yanoff M, Scheie HG: *Arch Ophthalmol* 72:57, 1964. © American Medical Association. All rights reserved.)

corneal epithelium and Bowman's membrane or in conjunctival cysts.

V. Mercury

VI. Arsenicals

VII. Minocycline hydrochloride, which is a semisynthetic derivative of tetracycline, may cause pigmentation of the sclera and conjunctiva, and other tissues, including skin, thyroid, nails, teeth, oral cavity, and bone.

Vitamin A Deficiency: Bitot's Spot

See p. 276 in Chapter 8.

Sjögren's Syndrome

See p. 274 in Chapter 8 and p. 533 in Chapter 14.

Skin Diseases

I. Erythema multiforme (Stevens–Johnson syndrome)—see p. 181 in Chapter 6.

II. Atopic dermatitis

III. Rosacea—see p. 176 in Chapter 6.

IV. Xeroderma pigmentosum—see p. 172 in Chapter 6.

V. Ichthyosis congenita—see p. 171 in Chapter 6.

VI. Molluscum contagiosum—see p. 176 in Chapter 6.

VII. Dermatitis herpetiformis, epidermolysis bullosa, erythema nodosum, and many others may show conjunctival manifestations.

DEGENERATIONS

Xerosis

I. Xerosis (dry eyes; Fig. 7.11) owing to conjunctival disease may result from keratoconjunctivitis sicca (Sjögren's syndrome), ocular pemphigoid, trachoma, measles, vitamin A deficiency, proptosis with exposure, familial dysautonomia, chemical burns, and erythema multiforme (Stevens–Johnson syndrome).

II. Histologically, the epithelium undergoes epidermidalization with keratin formation, and the underlying subepithelial tissue frequently shows cicatrization.

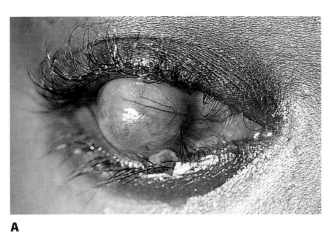

A

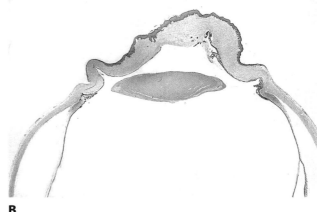

B

Fig. 7.11 Xerosis. **A,** After rubeola infection, the cornea and conjunctiva have become dry and appear skin-like. **B,** The corneal and limbal conjunctival epithelium show marked epidermidalization. The corneal stroma is thickened and scarred. (**A,** Courtesy of Dr. RE Shannon.)

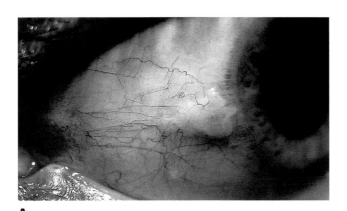

A

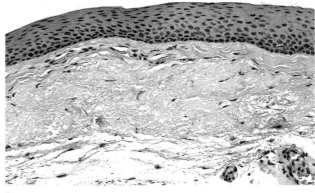

B

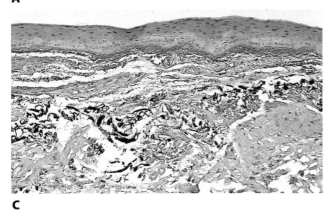

C

Fig. 7.12 Pinguecula. **A,** A pinguecula characteristically involves the limbal conjunctiva, most frequently nasally, and appears as a yellowish-white mound of tissue. **B,** Histologic section shows basophilic (actinic) degeneration of the conjunctival substantia propria. **C,** Another case shows even more marked basophilic degeneration that stains heavily black when the Verhoeff elastica stain is used.

Pterygium

See p. 277 in Chapter 8.

Pinguecula

I. Pinguecula (Fig. 7.12) is a localized, elevated, yellowish-white area near the limbus, usually found nasally and bilaterally, and seen predominantly in middle and late life.

Pigmented, triangular, brown pingueculae may appear during the second decade of *Gaucher's disease*. Lesions sampled for biopsy contain Gaucher cells. Patients with Gaucher's disease may also show congenital oculomotor apraxia (50%) and white retinal infiltrates (38%). Corneal opacities in the posterior two-thirds of the stroma may also occur in Gaucher's disease. The genetic defect in Gaucher's disease resides on chromosome 1q21.

II. Histologically, it appears identical to a pterygium except for lack of corneal involvement.

A. The subepithelial tissue shows senile elastosis (basophilic degeneration) and irregular, dense subepithelial concretions. The elastotic material stains positively for elastin but is not sensitive to elastase (*elastotic degeneration*).

B. The elastotic material is positive for elastin, microfibrillar protein, and amyloid P, components that never normally co-localize.

The control of elastogenesis is seriously defective so that the elastic fibers are not immature, but are abnormal in their biochemical organization. A marked reduction of elastic microfibrils, rather than an overproduction, appears to prevent normal assembly of elastic fibers. *p53* mutations in limbal epithelial cells, probably caused by ultraviolet irradiation, may be an early event in the development of pingueculae, pterygia, and some limbal tumors.

The subepithelial dense concretions stain positively for lysozyme.

Lipid Deposits

I. Biomicroscopic examination of peripheral bulbar conjunctiva and episcleral tissue, especially in the region of the palpebral fissure, often reveals lipid globules.
   A. The globules, which increase with age, vary from 30 to 80 nm in diameter, but tend to be fairly uniform in size in each patient.
   B. The deposits assume two basic patterns: most often, multiple globules lying adjacent to blood vessels; and sometimes globules occurring in isolated foci unrelated to blood vessels.
   C. Subconjunctival and episcleral lipid deposits are asymptomatic (except for rare granulomatous response to the lipids) and occur in approximately 30% of patients.
II. Histologically, lipid material may be present free within extracellular spaces in the subepithelial conjunctival and episcleral loose connective tissue or, rarely, a granulomatous inflammatory process may surround it.

Amyloidosis

I. Primary
   Primary conjunctival amyloidosis should be considered in any patient with recurrent hyposphagma (conjunctival hemorrhage) of unknown cause.
   A. Systemic (primary familial amyloidosis; see Fig. 12.10, p. 296 in Chapter 8, and p. 488 in Chapter 12)
      1. Primary amyloidosis, now designated *AL amy*loidosis (AL amyloid is the same type of amyloid found in myeloma-associated amyloid), is regarded as part of the spectrum of plasma cell dyscrasias with an associated derangement in the synthesis of immunoglobulin.
         a. Portions of immunoglobulin light chains, most often fragments of the variable region of the N-terminal end of the lambda light chain, are the major constituents of the amyloid filamentous substance (i.e., the deposited amyloid filaments found in tissues are portions of immunoglobulin light chains).
         b. Lambda light chains contain six variable-region subgroups.
         c. Survival in patients who have AL amyloidosis is shortened; congestive heart failure and hepatomegaly are poor prognostic signs.
      2. Vitreous opacities are the most important ocular finding, but ecchymosis of lids, proptosis, ocular palsies, internal ophthalmoplegia, neuroparalytic keratitis, and glaucoma may result from amyloid deposition in tissues (see p. 488 in Chapter 12).
      3. Amyloid deposition is found around and in walls of ocular blood vessels, especially retinal and uveal. Skin and conjunctiva may be involved, but this is not as important as involvement of other ocular structures.

Rarely, amyloidosis of the lid can be so severe as to cause ptosis. Numerous variants of primary systemic amyloidosis have been described. Some have peripheral neuropathy, which may or may not be associated with vitreous opacities.

   B. Familial amyloidotic polyneuropathy (see p. 488 in Chapter 12)
   C. Localized (localized nodular amyloidosis; see also p. 296 in Chapter 8)
      1. Small and large, brownish-red nodules may be found in the conjunctiva and lids.
      2. The intraocular structures are not involved.
      3. Based on autopsy analysis, the most frequently involved ocular tissues are: conjunctiva, 89%; iris, 44%; trabecular meshwork, 11%; and vitreous body, 11%.

Lattice corneal dystrophy, one of the inherited corneal dystrophies, is considered by some to be a primary, localized form of amyloidosis of the cornea (see p. 283 in Chapter 8). Rarely, a localized amyloidosis of the cornea unrelated to lattice corneal dystrophy may occur idiopathically (e.g., in climatic droplet keratopathy). Conversely, lattice corneal dystrophy occurs rarely in primary systemic amyloidosis.

II. Secondary
   A. Systemic (secondary amyloidosis)
      1. Unlike primary amyloidosis, the amyloid filaments in secondary amyloidosis, termed *AA amyloidosis*, are related to a nonimmunoglobulin serum protein.
      2. Systemic secondary amyloidosis may result from chronic inflammatory diseases such as leprosy, osteomyelitis, or rheumatoid arthritis, or it may be part of multiple myeloma (AL amyloid is found in myeloma-associated amyloid) or Waldenström's macroglobulinemia. The ocular structures are usually spared.

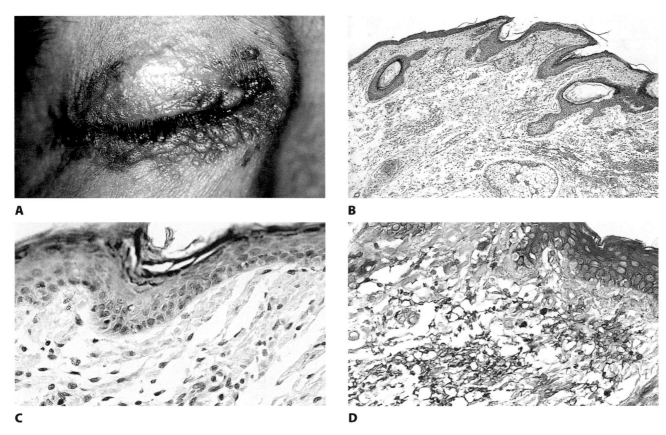

Fig. 7.13 Secondary systemic amyloidosis. **A,** Patient had bruises involving eyelids for 10 months and spontaneous bleeding for 4 months. **B,** Hematoxylin and eosin-stained section of lid biopsy shows increased superficial dermal vascularization and ribbons of an amorphic pink material, best seen in the middle dermis on the right. The material is Congo red-positive (**C**) and metachromatic with crystal violet (**D**). Approximately 1 year later, multiple myeloma was diagnosed.

The eyelids may show characteristic multiple purpuric lesions in secondary systemic amyloidosis, especially in multiple myeloma (Fig. 7.13).

---

3. Secondary localized amyloidosis (Fig. 7.14) may result from such chronic local inflammations of the conjunctiva and lids as trachoma and chronic nongranulomatous, idiopathic conjunctivitis, and blepharitis.

   The condition is not as common as primary local amyloidosis.

III. Histology

A. Amyloid appears as amorphous, eosinophilic, pale hyaline deposits free in the connective tissue, or around or in blood vessel walls.

   A nongranulomatous inflammatory reaction or, rarely, a foreign-body giant cell reaction or no inflammatory reaction may be present.

Amyloid may have a natural green positive birefringence in unstained sections, and in hematoxylin and eosin-stained sections. The green birefringence is enhanced by Congo red staining.

B. The material demonstrates metachromasia (polycationic dyes such as crystal violet change color from blue to purple), positive staining with Congo red, dichroism (change in color that varies with the plane of polarized light, usually from green to orange with rotation of polarizer), birefringence (double refraction with polarized light) of Congo red-stained material, and fluorescence with thioflavine-T.

Birefringence is the change in refractive indices with respect to light polarized in different directions through a substance. Dichroism is the property of a substance absorbing light polarized in a certain direction. When light is polarized at right angles to this direction, it is transmitted to a greater extent. In contrast to birefringence, dichroism can be specific for a particular substance. Dichroism can be observed in a microscope with the use of either a polarizer or an analyzer, but not both, because the dichroic substance itself (e.g., amyloid) serves as polarizer or analyzer, depending on the optical arrangement. Amyloid is only dichroic to green light.

C. Electron microscopically, amyloid is composed of ordered or disordered, or both, filaments that have a diameter of approximately 7.5 nm.

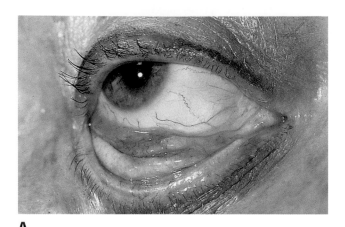

A

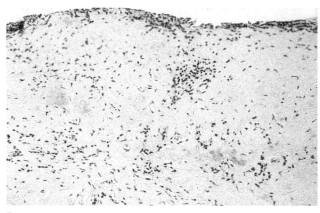

B

Fig. 7.14 Localized amyloidosis. **A,** The patient has a smooth "fish-flesh" redundant mass in the inferior conjunctiva of both eyes, present for many years. The underlying cause was unknown, and the patient had no systemic involvement. Clinically, this could be lymphoid hyperplasia, lymphoma, leukemia, or amyloidosis. The lesion was biopsied. **B,** Histologic section shows an amorphous pale hyaline deposit in the substantia propria of the conjunctiva that stains positively with Congo red stain. The scant inflammatory cellular infiltrate consists mainly of lymphocytes, and plasma and mast cells. (**B,** Congo red; reported in Glass R *et al.*; *Ann Ophthalmol* 3:823, 1971. Reproduced with kind permission of Springer Science and Business Media.)

D. Amyloid proteins
1. Amyloid fibril proteins derived from immunoglobulin light chains are designated AL (see p. 488 in Chapter 12) and are found in primary familial amyloidosis and secondary amyloidosis associated with multiple myeloma and Waldenström's macroglobulinemia (monoclonal gammopathies).
2. Other secondary amyloidoses show a tissue amyloid derived from a serum precursor (designated amyloid AA) or an amyloid that is a variant of prealbumin.
3. Another protein, protein AP, is found in all of the amyloidoses and may be bound to amyloid fibrils.

Conjunctivochalasis

I. Conjunctivochalasis is usually found in older individuals and consists of an elevation of the bulbar conjunctiva along the lateral or central lower-lid margin. It may also involve the upper bulbar conjunctiva. It is a cause for tearing, and may worsen dry-eye symptoms. A possible mechanism for its development is as a result of mechanical forces between the lower eyelid and conjunctiva interfering with lymphatic flow which, when chronic, may result in lymphatic dilatation and, eventually, conjunctivochalasis.
II. The most common histopathologic findings are elastosis or chronic nongranulomatous inflammation. Additionally, microscopic lymphangiectasia is typically present.

CYSTS, PSEUDONEOPLASMS, AND NEOPLASMS

Choristomas

I. Epidermoid cyst—see p. 540 in Chapter 14.
II. Dermoid cyst—see p. 540 in Chapter 14.
   Most limbal dermoids are solid and contain epidermal, dermal, and fatty tissue.

> Rarely, they may be cystic and may contain bone, cartilage, lacrimal gland, teeth, smooth muscle, brain, or respiratory epithelium.

III. Dermolipoma (Fig. 7.15)
   A. Dermolipoma usually presents as bilateral, large, yellowish-white soft tumors near the temporal canthus and extending backward and upward.
   B. It is a form of solid dermoid composed primarily of fatty tissue.

> Frequently, serial sections of the tumor must be made to find nonfatty elements such as stratified squamous epithelium and dermal appendages.

IV. Nevus lipomatosus (pedunculated nevus) has been reported on the eyelid of an 11-year-old boy having an eyelid papule that had been present since birth and was gradually enlarging. Histologically, the lesion was polypoid in shape and consisted of mature adipocytes within the dermis and subconjunctival mucosa consistent with nevus lipomatosus.
V. Epibulbar (episcleral) osseous choristoma (bone-containing choristoma of the conjunctiva) is usually located in the supratemporal quadrant (Fig. 8.60) and may contain

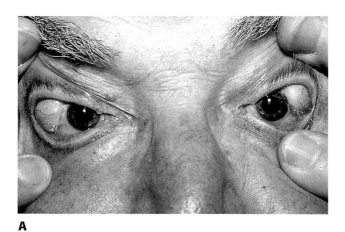

A

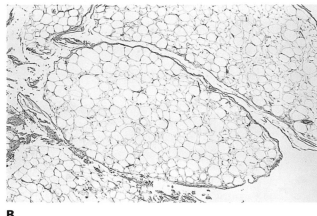

B

Fig. 7.15 Dermolipoma. **A,** The patient shows the typical clinical appearance of bilateral temporal dermolipomas. **B,** The histologic specimen shows that the dermolipoma is almost entirely composed of fatty tissue. Rarely, dermolipomas may also show structures such as epidermal appendages and fibrous tissue.

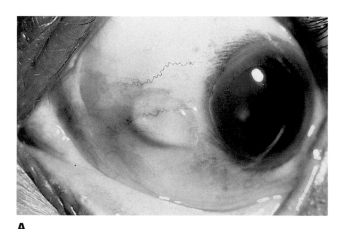

A

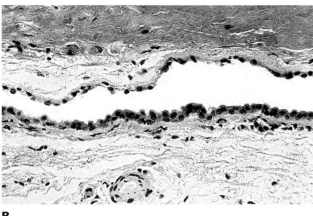

B

Fig. 7.16 Conjunctival cyst. **A,** A clear cyst is present just nasal to the limbus. **B,** Histologic section of another clear conjunctival cyst shows that it is lined by a double layer of epithelium, suggesting a ductal origin.

other choristomatous tissue as frequently as 10% of the time. The lesion may be attached to the underlying muscle or sclera.

Hamartomas

   I. Lymphangioma—see p. 545 in Chapter 14.
  II. Hemangioma—see p. 544 in Chapter 14.
 III. Phakomatoses—see p. 29 in Chapter 2.

Cysts

   I. Cysts of the conjunctiva (Fig. 7.16) may be congenital or acquired, with the latter predominating.
  II. Acquired conjunctival cysts are mainly implantation cysts of surface epithelium, resulting in an *epithelial inclusion cyst*. Other cysts may be ductal (e.g., from accessory lacrimal glands) or inflammatory.

 III. Histologically, the structure depends on the type of cyst.
    A. Epidermoid and dermoid cyst—see p. 540 in Chapter 14.
    B. Epithelial inclusion cysts, lined by conjunctival epithelium, contain a clear fluid.
    C. Ductal cysts (e.g., Wolfring dacryops) are lined by a double layer of epithelium and contain a PAS-positive material.
    D. Inflammatory cysts contain polymorphonuclear leukocytes and cellular debris.

Pseudocancerous Lesions

   I. Hereditary benign intraepithelial dyskeratosis (HBID; Fig. 7.17; see Fig. 6.4A)
    A. HBID is a bilateral dyskeratosis of the conjunctival epithelium associated with comparable lesions of the

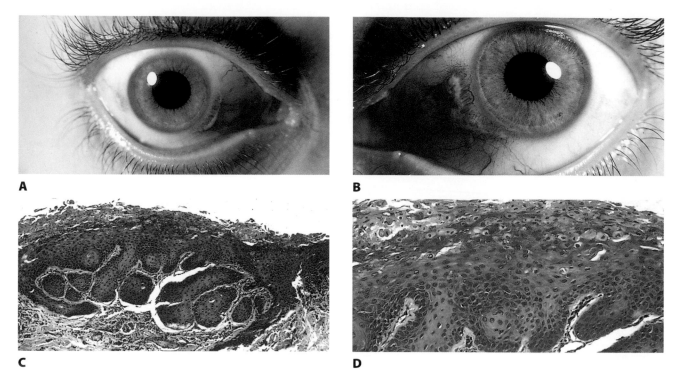

A **B** **C** **D**

Fig. 7.17 Hereditary benign intraepithelial dyskeratosis (HBID). The patient has limbal, nasal, vascularized pearly lesions in her right (**A**) and left (**B**) eyes. The patient also had bilateral temporal lesions, but they are difficult to see because of light reflection. The patient's mother had similar bilimbal, bilateral lesions. **C,** Histologic section shows an acanthotic epithelium that contains dyskeratotic cells, shown with increased magnification in **D**. HBID is indigenous to family members of a large triracial (Native American, black, and white) isolate from Halifax County, North Carolina. (Modified from Yanoff M: *Arch Ophthalmol* 79:291, 1968, with permission. © American Medical Association. All rights reserved.)

oral mucosa and inherited as an autosomal-dominant trait.

The disease is indigenous to family members of a large triracial (Native American, black, and white) isolate in Halifax County, North Carolina. Members of the family now live in other parts of the United States, so the lesion may be encountered outside North Carolina.

B. Clinically, irregularly raised, horseshoe-shaped plaques are present at the nasal and temporal limbus in each eye.
   1. They are granular-appearing, richly vascularized, and gray.
   2. A whitish placoid lesion of the mucous membrane of the mouth (tongue or buccal mucosa) is also present.

Corneal abnormalities may be found, especially stromal vascularization and dyskeratotic plaques of the corneal epithelium. The corneal plaques, like the conjunctival limbal plaques, invariably recur if excised.

C. Histologically, considerable acanthosis of the epithelium is present along with a chronic nongranulomatous inflammatory reaction and increased vascularization of the subepithelial tissue. A characteristic dyskera-

tosis, especially prominent in the superficial layers, is seen.

II. Pseudoepitheliomatous hyperplasia (PEH; see p. 193 in Chapter 6)
   A. PEH may mimic a neoplasm clinically and microscopically.
   B. Epithelial hyperplasia and a chronic nongranulomatous inflammatory reaction of the subepithelial tissue, along with neutrophilic infiltration of the hyperplastic epithelium, are characteristic of PEH.
      1. PEH may occur within a pinguecula or pterygium and cause sudden growth that simulates a neoplasm.
   C. Keratoacanthoma (see p. 193 in Chapter 6) may be a specific variant of PEH, perhaps caused by a virus, or more likely a low-grade type of squamous cell carcinoma.

III. Papilloma (squamous papilloma; Fig. 7.18)
   A. Conjunctival papillomas tend to be pedunculated when they arise at the lid margin or caruncle, but sessile with a broad base at the limbus.
      1. Papillomas are rare in locations other than the lid margin, interpalpebral conjunctiva, or caruncle.
      2. Approximately one-fourth of all the lesions of the caruncle are papillomas.

Although inverted papillomas (*schneiderian* or *mucoepidermoid papillomas*) typically involve mucous membranes

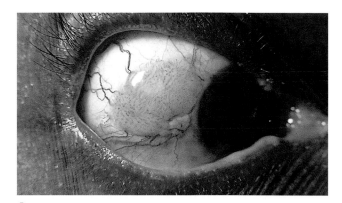

A

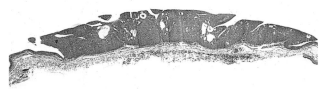

B

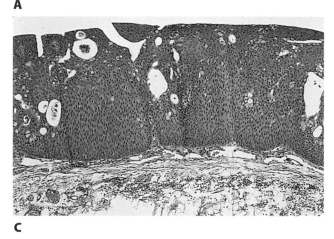

C

Fig. 7.18 Papilloma. **A,** A large sessile papilloma of the limbal conjunctiva is present. **B,** Histologic section shows a papillary lesion composed of acanthotic epithelium with many blood vessels going into the individual fronds, seen as red dots in the clinical picture in **A.** The base of the lesion is quite broad. **C,** Increased magnification shows the blood vessels and the acanthotic epithelium. Although the epithelium is thickened, the polarity from basal cell to surface cell is normal and shows an appropriate maturation. (**A,** Courtesy of Dr. DM Kozart.)

of the nose, paranasal sinuses, and lacrimal sac, they only occasionally involve the conjunctiva.

B. Human papillomavirus (HPV) types 6, 11, 16, 18, and 33 have been identified in conjunctival papillomas. Moreover, in subtropical Tanzania, where dysplastic lesions and neoplasms of the conjunctiva account for 2% of all malignant lesions, HPV 6/11, HPV-16, and HPV-18 characterize precancerous and squamous cell lesions of the conjunctiva. Co-infections are frequently observed. Higher signal intensity is observed in dysplasia grades 1 and 2, and in better-differentiated areas of the invasive component of conjunctival carcinoma compared to less-differentiated areas.

1. Focal epithelial hyperplasia is rare and caused by HPV-13 or -32. Although thought to infect the oral mucosa exclusively, HPV-13 has been reported to cause multiple conjunctival papillomas in an otherwise healthy patient.

p53 mutations in limbal epithelial cells, probably caused by ultraviolet irradiation, may be an early event in the development of some limbal tumors, including those associated with HPV.

C. Histologically, the fronds or finger-like projections are covered by acanthotic epithelium, tending toward slight

or moderate keratinization. The fronds have a core of fibrovascular tissue.

Goblet cells are common in the papillomas, except those arising at the limbus. Although most papillomas are infectious or irritative in origin and have little or no malignant potential, occasionally one may develop into a squamous cell carcinoma.

IV. Oncocytoma (eosinophilic cystadenoma, oxyphilic cell adenoma, apocrine cystadenoma; Fig. 7.19)

A. Oncocytoma is a rare tumor of the caruncle.

1. Most commonly, the tumor presents as a small, yellowish-tan or reddish mass arising not from surface epithelium but from accessory lacrimal glands in the caruncle, especially in elderly women. It can also arise from the conjunctival accessory lacrimal glands, lacrimal sac, or eyelid.

2. Rarely, the tumor may undergo carcinomatous transformation.

B. Histologically, one or more cystic cavities are lined by proliferating epithelium, resembling apocrine epithelium (hence, *apocrine cystadenoma*).

1. High-frequency ultrasound of the lesion reveals low internal reflectivity and a cystic component. Multiple hypoechogenic tumor stroma components correlate with multiple cystic glandular structures on histopathologic examination.

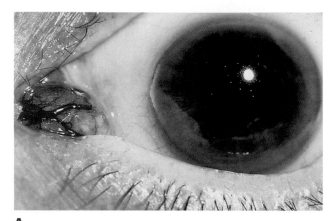

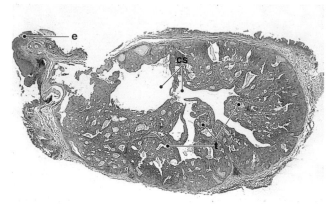

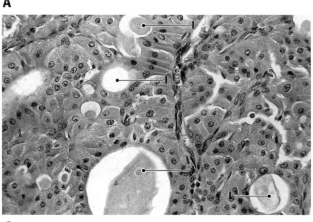

Fig. 7.19 Oncocytoma (eosinophilic cystadenoma, oxyphilic cell adenoma). **A,** A fleshy, vascularized lesion is present at the caruncle. **B,** Histologic section shows proliferating epithelium around a cystic cavity (e, surface epithelium; cs, cystic spaces; t, tumor). **C,** Increased magnification shows large eosinophilic cells that resemble apocrine cells and are forming glandlike spaces (l, lumina surrounded by epithelial cells). **A,** Courtesy of Dr. HG Scheie.)

V. Myxoma

    A. Myxomas are rare benign tumors that resemble primitive mesenchyme, and are often mistaken for cysts.

        1. They have a smooth, fleshy, gelatinous appearance and are slow-growing.

        2. Myxomas may be found in *Carney's syndrome,* an autosomal-dominantly inherited syndrome consisting of myxomas (especially cardiac but also eyelid), spotty mucocutaneous (including conjunctiva) pigmentation (see p. 668 in Chapter 17), and endocrine overactivity (especially Cushing's syndrome).

    B. Histologically, the tumor is hypocellular and composed of stellate and spindle-shaped cells, some of which have small intracytoplasmic and intranuclear vacuoles.

    The stroma contains abundant mucoid material, sparse reticulin, and delicate collagen fibers.

VI. Dacryoadenoma

    A. Dacryoadenoma is a rare benign conjunctival tumor arising from metaplasia of the surface epithelium.

    B. Histologically, an area of metaplastic surface epithelium with cuboidal to columnar cells invaginates into the underlying connective tissue, forming tubular and glandlike structures.

    C. Electron microscopy shows cells containing zymogen-type lacrimal secretory granules.

VII. Rarely, inverted follicular keratosis may arise on the conjunctiva.

Potentially Precancerous Epithelial Lesions

    I. Xeroderma pigmentosum—see p. 172 in Chapter 6.

    II. Other actinic keratoses—see p. 194–196 in Chapter 6.

Cancerous Epithelial Lesions

All such tumors may appear clinically as leukoplakia.* Reported cases of neoplasms involving orbits containing ocular prostheses highlight the importance of a periodic thorough examination of such sockets.

    I. From the 1960s to the 1980s, the incidence of cutaneous squamous cell carcinoma rose 2.6-fold in men and 3.1-fold in women.

        A. The rising incidence is probably attributable to increased voluntary exposure to sun and the depletion of the ozone layer.

        B. An emerging epidemic of squamous cell carcinoma seems to be occurring.

        C. Ki-67 labeling index, which is strictly associated with cell proliferation, is 46% in sebaceous gland carcinoma;

*Leukoplakia *is a clinical, descriptive term, not a clinical or a microscopic diagnosis. Histologieally lesions that present as leukoplakia may range from pinguecula to frank squamous cell carcinoma. The leukoplakic or white, shiny appearance is caused by keratinization of the normally nonkeratinized conjunctival epithelium.*

28% in squamous cell carcinoma; 20% in conjunctival intraepithelial neoplasia; 9% in pterygium,; and 7% in normal conjunctiva. These findings suggest that Ki-67 labeling index may be useful for malignant tumor grading of ocular surface tumors.

D. Cell proliferation and apoptosis markers are altered in the development of conjunctival squamous cell papillomas and squamous cell carcinomas. In papillomas, *p53* expression is observed in approximately 67%; Ki-67 in 31%; proliferating cell nuclear antigen in 98%, Bcl-2 in 53%; Bak in 62%; Bax in 69%; and Bcl-xl in 100%. In squamous cell carcinomas *p53* expression is observed in approximately 73%; Ki-67 in 18%; proliferating cell nuclear antigen in 73%, Bcl-2 in 45%; Bak in 91%; Bax in 91%; and Bcl-xl in 100%. Alterations in these cellular proliferation and apoptosis markers appear to be important events in cancer development.

II. Carcinoma derived from the squamous cells of conjunctival epithelium
A. Conjunctival intraepithelial neoplasm (CIN; dysplasia, carcinoma in situ, intraepithelial carcinoma, intraepithelial epithelioma, Bowen's disease, intraepithelioma; Figs 7.20 and 7.21)
1. Clinically it may appear as leukoplakia or a fleshy mass, usually located at or near the limbus. Occasionally, conjunctival squamous cell carcinoma may be pigmented, thereby clinically suggesting malignant melanoma. The papillomatous arrangement of blood vessels in such tumors may be helpful in clinically differentiating them from melanomas, even in the absence of leukoplakia.
2. Solar elastosis is found much more frequently in conjunctival squamous cell neoplasia patients than in control individuals.
3. Atopic eczema may be a risk factor for squamous cell carcinoma of the conjunctiva, and its development may be related to T-cell immunologic dysfunction.
4. High-frequency ultrasonography can be used to evaluate the tumor thickness, shape, internal reflectivity, and extent of conjunctival intraepithelial neoplasia and squamous cell carcinoma.

Human immunodeficiency virus (HIV) infection should be considered in any patient younger than 50 years of age who has a conjunctival intraepithelial neoplasia.

5. Histology
a. The lesions range from mild dysplasia with nuclear atypia, altered cytoplasmic-to-nuclear ratios, and abnormal cell maturation confined to the basal third of the epithelium, to full-thick-

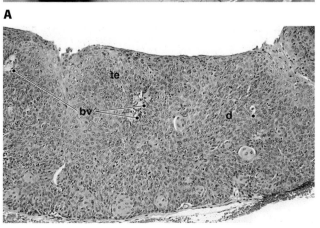

A

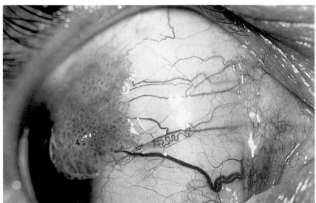

C

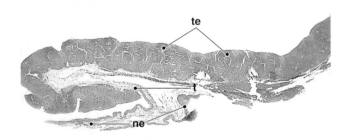

B

Fig. 7.20 Papilloma: with dysplasia. **A,** Clinical appearance of a typical limbal sessile conjunctival papilloma. **B,** Histologic section shows a sudden and abrupt transition (t) from the normal conjunctival epithelium (ne) to a markedly thickened epithelium (te). The lesion is broad-based and shows numerous blood vessels penetrating into the thickened epithelium. **C,** Increased magnification shows a tissue with normal polarity but which contains atypical cells and individual cells making keratin (dyskeratosis). Because the polarity is normal, a diagnosis of dysplasia was made. Approximately 8% of conjunctival dysplasias or squamous cell carcinomas contain human papillomavirus (te, thickened epithelium; bv, blood vessels; d, dyskeratotic cell).

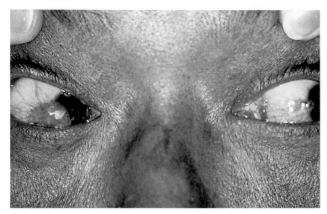

A

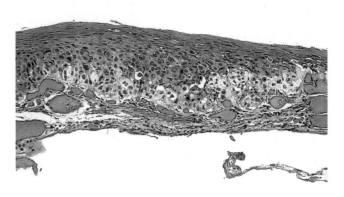

B

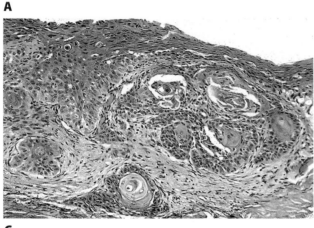

C

Fig. 7.21 Squamous cell carcinoma. **A,** The patient had a vascularized, elevated pearly lesion at the temporal limbus in the right eye. In addition, he had a pterygium nasally in the left eye. Excisional biopsy of the lesion in the right eye was diagnosed as carcinoma in situ. **B,** Histologic section of another case shows full-thickness atypia and loss of polarity. A diagnosis of carcinoma in situ would be made here. **C,** Other regions of this case show malignant epithelial cells in the substantia propria of the conjunctiva, forming keratin pearls in some areas representing invasive squamous cell carcinoma.

ness replacement of the epithelium by atypical, often bizarre and pleomorphic epithelial cells.

b. Dyskeratotic epithelial cells may be seen.

Rarely, mucoepidermoid differentiation can be seen in the neoplasm.

---

c. The involved epithelial area is thickened and sharply demarcated from the contiguous, normal-appearing conjunctival epithelium.

The thickening usually ranges from approximately two to five times normal thickness, but may be greater in malignant transformation of papillomas.

---

d. Polarity of the epithelium is lost.
e. Mitotic figures are commonly found.
f. The basement membrane of the epithelium is intact, and no invasion of the subepithelial tissue occurs.
g. Conjunctival squamous cell carcinoma intensely expresses immunoreactivity for the tyrosine kinase EGF receptor. Studies involving the induction of apoptosis in serum-deprived cultured conjunctival epithelial cell have demon-

strated that EGF and retinoic acid play key roles in the maintenance of the ocular surface.

h. Conjunctival intraepithelial neoplasia and squamous cell carcinoma are associated with preferential expression of *p63* in the immature dysplastic epithelial cells. The staining for *p63*, which is a homologue of the tumor suppressor gene *p53*, is not correlated with MIB-1 expression and, therefore, appears not to be linked to cell proliferation.

Never clinically, but occasionally histologically, CIN may resemble superficially the intraepithelial carcinoma of the skin described by Bowen (Bowen's disease) or the intraepithelial carcinoma of the glans penis described by Queyrat (erythroplasia of Queyrat). Both entities are specific clinicopathologic entities and their terms should be restricted to their proper use, which never includes carcinoma in situ of the conjunctiva or any conjunctival neoplasm.

B. Squamous cell carcinoma with superficial invasion (see Fig. 7.21)

In addition to the epithelial changes of CIN, invasion by the malignant, pleomorphic, atypical squamous epithelial cells occurs through the epithelial basement membrane into the superficial subepithelial tissue.

Rarely, squamous cell carcinoma with superficial (micro)stromal invasion can arise primarily in the cornea (squamous cell carcinoma of the cornea) without extension to the corneoscleral limbus.

C. Squamous cell carcinoma with deep invasion (see Fig. 7.21)

In addition to the epithelial changes of CIN, there is invasion by the malignant squamous epithelial cells through the epithelial basement membrane deep into the subepithelial tissue or even into adjacent structures.

Spindle-cell carcinoma is a rare variant of squamous cell carcinoma, and may arise from the conjunctiva. Positive staining with cytokeratin and epithelial membrane antigen markers is helpful in differentiating the variant from other spindle-cell tumors such as amelanotic melanoma, malignant schwannoma, fibrosarcoma, leiomyosarcoma, and malignant fibrous histiocytoma. Malignant fibrous histiocytoma rarely arises in the conjunctiva.

D. Squamous cell carcinoma with metastasis

All the features of squamous cell carcinoma with deep invasion are involved, plus evidence of metastasis. Metastatic squamous cell carcinoma may be an atypical presentation of HIV infection.

III. Carcinoma derived from the basal cells of conjunctival epithelium

Basal cell carcinoma rarely arises from the conjunctiva or caruncle.

The lid differs from the conjunctiva in being a site of preference for basal cell carcinoma.

IV. Carcinoma derived from the mucus-secreting cells and squamous cells of conjunctival epithelium

Mucoepidermoid carcinoma (Fig. 7.22) is a rare conjunctival tumor characteristically composed of mucus-secreting cells intermixed with epidermoid (squamous) cells.

Mucoepidermoid carcinoma can also arise from the caruncle. A third type of cell, called *intermediate* or *basal cell*, may also be found.

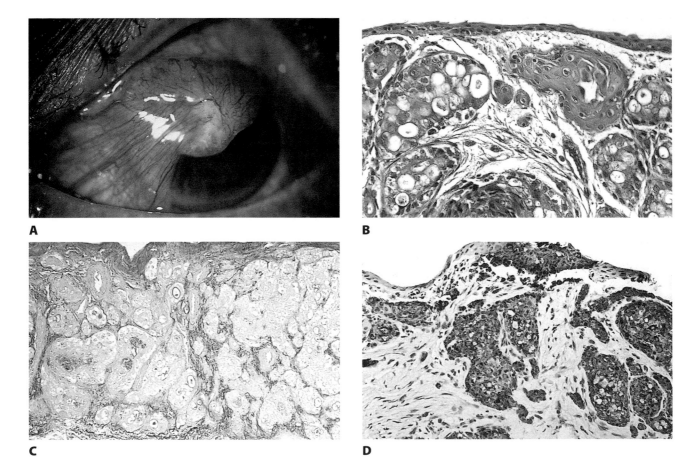

Fig. 7.22 Mucoepidermoid carcinoma. **A,** A pterygium-like growth present on the left eye was excised. **B,** Histologic section shows a malignant epithelial lesion containing both epidermoid and mucinous components. **C,** The blue color in the colloidal iron stain for acid mucopolysaccharides demonstrates the mucinous elements. **D,** The cytokeratin stain is positive (red-brown color) in the epidermoid elements. (Case presented by Dr. WC Frayer at the meeting of the Verhoeff Society, 1994.)

A. Some tumors show a predominance of epidermoid cells, whereas others have mainly mucus-secreting cells.

B. The tumors appear to be aggressive locally and tend to recur rapidly after excision; a wide local excision is therefore recommended.

C. Histologically, lobules of tumor cells show a variable admixture of epidermoid and mucus-secreting cells. Histochemical stains for mucin are most helpful in confirming the diagnosis.

Pigmented Lesions of the Conjunctiva

See section *Melanotic Tumors of Conjunctiva* in Chapter 17.

Laugier–Hunziker syndrome is a rare acquired hyperpigmentation of the oral mucosa and lips, which is often associated with longitudinal melanonychia (black pigmentation of the nails). It may also be associated with conjunctival and penile pigmentation. Histopathologic examination demonstrates basal epithelial melanosis, moderate acanthosis, and superficial pigmentary incontinence. Electron microscopic examination reveals increased number of normal-appearing melanosomes inside basal keratinocytes and dermal melanophages.

Stromal Neoplasms

I. Angiomatous—see discussions of hamartomas and vascular mesenchymal tumors on pp 543–548 in Chapter 14.

II. Pseudotumors, lymphoid hyperplasia, lymphomas, and leukemias (Fig. 7.23)—see discussions of tumors of the reticuloendothelial system, lymphatic system, and myeloid system on p. 568 in Chapter 14.

A. Extranodal marginal-zone B-cell lymphoma of mucosa-associated lymphoid tissue (MALT) constitutes about 88% of all lymphoma involving the ocular adnexa. It tends to appear in patients with a history of autoimmune disease or chronic inflammatory disorders. It has been reported in a child. Rarely, it may arise in Tenon's

capsule. These lesions respond well to conventional treatment; however, there is a high rate of recurrence.

At least three different site-specific chromosomal translocations involving the nuclear factor-kappaB have been implicated in the development and progression of MALT lymphoma. The most common such translocation is t(11;18) (q21;q21), resulting in the fusion of the cIAP2 region on chromosome 11q21 with the MALT1 gene on chromosome 18q21, and is said to be involved in more than one-third of cases. In gastric MALT lymphoma, t(11;18) (q21;q21) is significantly associated with infection by CagA-positive strains of *Helicobacter pylori*, and eradication of the organism is standard therapy for all *H. pylori*-positive gastric MALT lymphomas. Oxidative damage may play a role in the development of this translocation. Translocation t(14;18) (q32;q21) is also commonly found in this disorder, and the specific translocation varies considerably with the primary location of the disease. MALT lymphoma has also been found in a patient with adult inclusion conjunctivitis.

---

1. CD43-positive ocular lymphomas are associated with a higher rate of subsequent distant recurrence and rate of lymphoma-related death.

2. Uncommonly, conjunctival B-cell lymphoma may present as an ulcerating tarsal conjunctival mass.

The spontaneous regression of a large B-cell lymphoma involving the conjunctiva and orbit has been reported. Mantle cell lymphoma has presented as a marked follicular conjunctivitis in both eyes with a nodal mass in the right upper eyelid, and nuchal lymphadenopathy. The diagnosis was made on conjunctival biopsy.

B. Although rarely found in the conjunctiva, T-cell lymphoma must be considered in the differential diagnosis of gelatinous lesions of the conjunciva. It is characterized by positive staining with CD-45 RO (T-cell

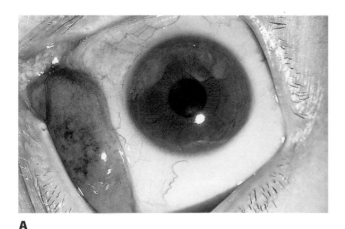

A

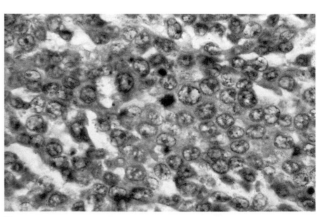

B

Fig. 7.23 Leukemia. **A,** The patient has a smooth "fish-flesh" lesion that had appeared a few weeks previously. The lesion resembles that seen in lymphoid hyperplasia, lymphoma, or amyloidosis. A diagnosis of acute leukemia had recently been made. **B,** Histologic section shows sheets of immature blastic leukemic cells, many of which exhibit mitotic figures.

marker) and negativity with CD-20 (B-cell marker). Additionally, positivity for T-cell receptor gene rearrangement with clonality confirms the diagnosis.

   C. Lethal midline granuloma associated with natural killer (NK)/T-cell lymphoma and Epstein–Barr virus infection has presented involving the conjunctiva. This lethal midline granuloma, which is a very rare, angiocentric NK/T-cell lymphoma associated with Epstein–Barr virus infection, demonstrated features of a highly malignant, CD3 and BCL2-positive T-cell lymphoma with features of an NK/T-cell origin (CD56⁺, T-cell intraceullar antigen (TIA⁺), T-cell receptor rearrangement: germline). All lymphoma cells were said to be positive for Epstein-Barr virus RNA. At presentation the patient was otherwise a healthy, immunocompetent, Caucasian.

   D. Benign lymphoid hyperplasia of the conjunctiva is particularly uncommon in children, but has been reported. Polymerase chain reaction for Epstein–Barr virus was negative, and immunohistochemistry and flow cytometry were consistent with the diagnosis.

   E. T-cell prolymphocytic leukemia, a rare and very aggressive hematological neoplasm, has presented with bilateral perilimbal conjunctival infiltrates, in which the diagnosis was confirmed on histopathologic examination. Conjunctival involvement has accompanied uveal (including anterior uveitis), palpebral, and orbital invasion by adult T-cell leukemia.

III. Juvenile xanthogranulomas—see p. 343 in Chapter 9.

IV. Neural tumors—see discussion of neural mesenchymal tumors on p. 558 in Chapter 14.

V. Fibrous tumors—see discussion of fibrous–histiocytic mesenchymal tumors on p. 551 in Chapter 14.

VI. Leiomyosarcoma and rhabdomyosarcoma—see discussion of muscle mesenchymal tumors on p. 554 in Chapter 14.

   A. Rarely, rhabdomyosarcoma may present as a conjunctival lesion without orbital extension.

VII. Metastatic

BIBLIOGRAPHY

Normal Anatomy

Altinors DD, Akca S, Akova YA *et al.*: Smoking associated with damage to the lipid layer of the ocular surface. *Am J Ophthalmol* 141:1016, 2006

Cermak JM, Krenzer KL, Sullivan RM *et al.*: Is complete androgen insensitivity syndrome associated with alterations in the meibomian gland and ocular surface? *Cornea* 22:516, 2003

Dogru M, Karakaya H, Ozcetin H *et al.*: Tear function and ocular surface changes in keratoconus. *Ophthalmology* 110:1110, 2003

Donald C, Hamilton L, Doughty MJ. A quantitative assessment of the location and width of Marx's line along the marginal zone of the human eyelid. *Optom Vis Sci* 80:564, 2003

Erdogan H, Arici DS, Toker MI *et al.*: Conjunctival impression cytology in pseudoexfoliative glaucoma and pseudoexfoliation syndrome. *Clin Exp Ophthalmol* 34:108, 2006

Espana EM, Di Pascuale MA, He H *et al.*: Characterization of corneal pannus removed from patients with total limbal stem cell deficiency. *Invest Ophthalmol Vis Sci* 45:2961, 2004

Espana EM, Grueterich M, Romano AC *et al.*: Idiopathic limbal stem cell deficiency. *Ophthalmology* 109:2004, 2002

Gartaganis SP, Georgakopoulos CD, Exarchou A *et al.*: Alterations in conjunctival cytology and tear film dysfunction in patients with beta-thalassemia. *Cornea* 22:591, 2003

Hayashi Y, Kao WW, Kohno N *et al.*: Expression patterns of sialylated epitope recognized by KL-6 monoclonal antibody in ocular surface epithelium of normals and dry eye patients. *Invest Ophthalmol Vis Sci* 45:2212, 2004

Huang FC, Shih MH, Tseng SH *et al.*: Tear function changes during interferon and ribavirin treatment in patients with chronic hepatitis C. *Cornea* 24:561, 2005

Jakobiec FA, Iwamoto T: The ocular adnexa: Lids, conjunctiva, and orbit. In Fine BS, Yanoff M, eds: *Ocular Histology: A Text and Atlas*, 2nd edn. Hagerstown, Harper & Row, 1979:308–310

Jastaneiah S, Al-Rajhi AA. Association of aniridia and dry eyes. *Ophthalmology* 112:1535, 2005

Koufakis DI, Karabatsas CH, Sakkas LI *et al.*: Conjunctival surface changes in patients with Sjögren's syndrome: a transmission electron microscopy study. *Invest Ophthalmol Vis Sci* 47:541, 2006

Kozobolis VP, Christodoulakis EV, Naoumidi II *et al.*: Study of conjunctival goblet cell morphology and tear film stability in pseudoexfoliation syndrome. *Graefes Arch Clin Exp Ophthalmol* 242:478, 2004

McCallum RM, Cobo LM, Haynes BF: Analysis of corneal and conjunctival microenvironments using monoclonal antibodies. *Invest Ophthalmol Vis Sci* 34:1793, 1993

Murube J, Rivas L. Biopsy of the conjunctiva in dry eye patients establishes a correlation between squamous metaplasia and dry eye clinical severity. *Eur J Ophthalmol* 13:246, 2003

Narayanan S, Miller WL, McDermott AM. Expression of human beta-defensins in conjunctival epithelium: relevance to dry eye disease. *Invest Ophthalmol Vis Sci* 44:3795, 2003

Rolando M, Barabino S, Mingari C *et al.*: Distribution of conjunctival HLA-DR expression and the pathogenesis of damage in early dry eyes. *Cornea* 24:951, 2005

Satici A, Bitiren M, Ozardali I *et al.*: The effects of chronic smoking on the ocular surface and tear characteristics: a clinical, histological and biochemical study. *Acta Ophthalmol Scand* 81:583, 2003

Sauder G, Jonas JB. Limbal stem cell deficiency after subconjunctival mitomycin C injection for trabeculectomy. *Am J Ophthalmol* 141:1129, 2006

Stern ME, Gao J, Schwalb TA *et al.*: Conjunctival T-cell subpopulations in Sjögren's and non-Sjögren's patients with dry eye. *Invest Ophthalmol Vis Sci* 43:2609, 2002

Yanoff M, Fine BS: *Ocular Pathology: A Color Atlas*, 2nd edn. New York, Gower Medical Publishing, 1992:7.1–7.2

Yoon KC, Song BY, Seo MS. Effects of smoking on tear film and ocular surface. *Korean J Ophthalmol* 19:18, 2005

Congenital Anomalies

Brant AM, Schachat AP, White RI: Ocular manifestations in hereditary hemorrhagic telangiectasia (Rendu–Osler–Weber disease). *Am J Ophthalmol* 107:642, 1989

Duke-Elder S: *System of Ophthalmology*, vol III, *Normal and Abnormal Development*, Part 2, *Congenital Deformities*. St. Louis, CV Mosby, 1963:908

Kolin T, Johns KJ, Wadlington WB *et al.*: Hereditary lymphedema and distichiasis. *Arch Ophthalmol* 109:980, 1991

McLean WH, Irvine AD, Hamill KJ *et al.*: An unusual N-terminal deletion of the laminin alpha3a isoform leads to the chronic granulation tissue disorder laryngo-onycho-cutaneous syndrome. *Hum Mol Genet* 12:2395, 2003

Steel D, Bovill EG, Golden E et al.: Hereditary hemorrhagic telangiectasia. *Am J Clin Pathol* 90:274, 1988

Traboulsi EI, Al-Khayer K, Matsumota M et al.: Lymphedema–distichiasis syndrome and FOXC2 gene mutation. *Am J Ophthalmol* 134:592, 2002

Zierhut H, Thiel HJ, Weidle EG et al.: Ocular involvement in epidermolysis bullosa acquisita. *Arch Ophthalmol* 107:398, 1989

Vascular Disorders

Jampol LM, Nagpal KC: Hemorrhagic lymphangiectasia of the conjunctiva. *Am J Ophthalmol* 85:419, 1978

Nagpal KC, Asdourian GK, Goldbaum MH et al.: The conjunctival sickling sign, hemoglobin S, and irreversibly sickled erythrocytes. *Arch Ophthalmol* 95:808, 1977

Inflammation

Aronni S, Cortes M, Sacchetti M et al.: Upregulation of ICAM-1 expression in the conjunctiva of patients with chronic graft-versus-host disease. *Eur J Ophthalmol* 16:17, 2006

Ashton N, Cook C: Allergic granulomatous nodules of the eyelid and conjunctiva. *Am J Ophthalmol* 87:1, 1978

Bacsi A, Dharajiya N, Choudhury BK et al.: Effect of pollen-mediated oxidative stress on immediate hypersensitivity reactions and late-phase inflammation in allergic conjunctivitis. *J Allergy Clin Immunol* 116:836, 2005

Baddeley SM, Bacon AS, McGill JI et al.: Mast cell distribution and neutral protease expression in chronic allergic conjunctivitis. *Clin Exp Allergy* 25:41, 1995

Baudouin C, Hamard P, Liang H et al.: Conjunctival epithelial cell expression of interleukins and inflammatory markers in glaucoma patients treated over the long term. *Ophthalmology* 111:2186, 2004

Bernauer W, Wright P, Dart JK et al.: The conjunctiva in acute and chronic mucous membrane pemphigoid. *Ophthalmology* 100:339, 1993

Bobo L, Munoz B, Viscidi R et al.: Diagnosis of *Chlamydia trachomatis* eye infection in Tanzania by polymerase chain reaction/enzyme immunoassay. *Lancet* 338:847, 1991

Bowman RJC, Jatta B, Cham B et al.: Natural history of trachomatous scarring in The Gambia: results of a 12-year longitudinal follow-up. *Ophthalmology* 108:2219, 2001

bu El-Asrar AM, Al-Mansouri S, Tabbara KF et al.: Immunopathogenesis of conjunctival remodelling in vernal keratoconjunctivitis. *Eye* 20:71, 2006

bu El-Asrar AM, Struyf S, Al-Kharashi SA et al.: The T-lymphocyte chemoattractant Mig is highly expressed in vernal keratoconjunctivitis. *Am J Ophthalmol* 136:853, 2003

Cameron JA, Al-Rajhi AA, Badr IA: Corneal ectasia in vernal keratoconjunctivitis. *Ophthalmology* 96:1615, 1989

Chan LS, Yancey KB, Hammerberg C et al.: Immune-mediated subepithelial blistering diseases of mucous membranes: Pure ocular cicatricial pemphigoid is a unique clinical and immunopathological entity distinct from bullous pemphigoid and other subsets identified by antigenic specificity of autoantibodies. *Arch Dermatol* 129:448, 1993

Chang SW, Hou PK, Chen MS: Conjunctival concretions. *Arch Ophthalmol* 108:405, 1990

Choopong P, Khan N, Sangwan VS et al.: Eosinophil activation in Wegener's granulomatosis: a harbinger of disease progression? *Ocul Immunol Inflamm* 13:439, 2005

de Cock R, Ficker LA, Dart JD et al.: Topical heparin in the treatment of ligneous conjunctivitis. *Ophthalmology* 102:1654, 1995

Dogru M, sano-Kato N, Tanaka M et al.: Ocular surface and MUC5AC alterations in atopic patients with corneal shield ulcers. *Curr Eye Res* 30:897, 2005

Ferry AP: Pyogenic granulomas of the eye and ocular adnexa: A study of 100 cases. *Trans Am Ophthalmol Soc* 87:327, 1989

Foster CS, Allansmith MR: Chronic unilateral blepharoconjunctivitis caused by sebaceous carcinoma. *Am J Ophthalmol* 86:218, 1978

Francs IC, McCluskey PJ, Wakefield D et al.: Medial canthal keratinization (MCK): A diagnostic sign of ocular cicatricial pemphigoid. *Aust N Z J Ophthalmol* 2:350, 1992

Friedlaender MH: Immunologic aspects of diseases of the eye. *JAMA* 268:2869, 1992

Goto Y, Ohaki Y, Ibaraki N. A clinicopathologic case report of inflammatory pseudotumors involving the conjunctiva and lung. *Jpn J Ophthalmol* 48:573, 2004

Greiner JV, Covington HI, Allansmith MR: Surface morphology of giant papillary conjunctivitis in contact lens wearers. *Am J Ophthalmol* 85:242, 1978

Hanna C, Lyford JH: Tularemia infection of the eye. *Ann Ophthalmol* 3:1321, 1971

Hidayat AA, Riddle PJ: Ligneous conjunctivitis: A clinicopathologic study of 17 cases. *Ophthalmology* 94:949, 1987

Hoang-Xuan T, Robin H, Demers PE et al.: Pure ocular pemphigoid: A distinct immunopathologic subset of cicatricial pemphigoid. *Ophthalmology* 106:355, 1999

Hyden D, Latkovic S, Brunk U et al.: Ear involvement in ligneous conjunctivitis: a rarity or an under-diagnosed condition? *J Laryngol Otol* 116:482, 2002

Jabs DA, Wingard J, Green WR et al.: The eye in bone marrow transplantation. *Arch Ophthalmol* 107:1343, 1989

Jordan DR, Zafar A, Brownstein S et al.: Cicatricial conjunctival inflammation with trichiasis as the presenting feature of Wegener granulomatosis. *Ophthalm Plast Reconstr Surg* 22:69, 2006

Kocak-Altintas AG, Kocak-Midillioglu I, Gul U et al.: Impression cytology and ocular characteristics in ocular rosacea. *Eur J Ophthalmol* 13:351, 2003

Kumagai N, Fukuda K, Fujitsu Y et al.: Role of structural cells of the cornea and conjunctiva in the pathogenesis of vernal keratoconjunctivitis. *Prog Retin Eye Res* 25:165, 2006

Laibson PR, Dhiri S, Oconer J et al.: Corneal infiltrates in epidemic keratoconjunctivitis. *Arch Ophthalmol* 84:36, 1970

Lam S, Stone MS, Goeken JA et al.: Paraneoplastic pemphigus, cicatricial conjunctivitis, and acanthosis nigricans with pachydermatoglyphy in a patient with bronchogenic squamous cell carcinoma. *Ophthalmology* 99:108, 1992

Lambiase A, Bonini S, Bonini S et al.: Increased plasma levels of nerve growth factor in vernal keratoconjunctivitis and relationship to conjunctival mast cells. *Invest Ophthalmol Vis Sci* 36:2127, 1995

Lee GA, Williams G, Hirst LW et al.: Risk factors in the development of ocular surface epithelial dysplasia. *Ophthalmology* 101:360, 1994

Leonardi A. The central role of conjunctival mast cells in the pathogenesis of ocular allergy. *Curr Allergy Asthma Rep* 2:325, 2002

Leonardi A. Vernal keratoconjunctivitis: pathogenesis and treatment. *Prog Retin Eye Res* 21:319, 2002

MacCallan AF: The epidemiology of trachoma. *Br J Ophthalmol* 15:369, 1931

Matoba AY: Ocular disease associated with Epstein–Barr virus infection (review). *Surv Ophthalmol* 35:145, 1990

Memarzadeh F, Shamie N, Gaster RN et al.: Corneal and conjunctival toxicity from hydrogen peroxide: a patient with chronic self-induced injury. *Ophthalmology* 111:1546, 2004

Mondino BJ: Inflammatory diseases of the peripheral cornea. *Ophthalmology* 95:463, 1988

Monos T, Levy J, Lifshitz T et al.: Isolated congenital histiocytosis in the palpebral conjunctiva in a newborn. *Am J Ophthalmol* 139:728, 2005

Naumann GO, Lang GK, Rummelt V et al.: Autologous nasal mucosa transplantation in severe bilateral conjunctival mucus deficiency syndrome. *Ophthalmology* 97:1011, 1990

Netland PA, Sugrue SP, Albert DM et al.: Histopathologic features of the floppy eyelid syndrome. *Ophthalmology* 101:174, 1994

Ono SJ, Abelson MB. Allergic conjunctivitis: update on pathophysiology and prospects for future treatment. *J Allergy Clin Immunol* 115:118, 2005

Park AJ, Webster GF, Penne RB et al.: Porphyria cutanea tarda presenting as cicatricial conjunctivitis. *Am J Ophthalmol* 134:619, 2002

Peuravuori H, Kari O, Peltonen S et al.: Group IIA phospholipase A2 content of tears in patients with atopic blepharoconjunctivitis. *Graefes Arch Clin Exp Ophthalmol* 242:986, 2004

Porzionato A, Zancaner S, Betterle C et al.: Fatal toxic epidermal necrolysis in autoimmune polyglandular syndrome type I. *J Endocrinol Invest* 27:475, 2004

Power WJ, Neves RA, Rodriguez A et al.: Increasing the diagnostic yield of conjunctival biopsy in patients with suspected ocular cicatricial pemphigoid. *Ophthalmology* 102:1158, 1995

Ravage ZB, Beck AP, Macsai MS et al.: Ocular rosacea can mimic trachoma: a case of cicatrizing conjunctivitis. *Cornea* 23:630, 2004

Razzaque MS, Ahmed BS, Foster CS et al.: Effects of IL-4 on conjunctival fibroblasts: possible role in ocular cicatricial pemphigoid. *Invest Ophthalmol Vis Sci* 44:3417, 2003

Razzaque MS, Foster CS, Ahmed AR. Role of collagen-binding heat shock protein 47 and transforming growth factor-beta1 in conjunctival scarring in ocular cicatricial pemphigoid. *Invest Ophthalmol Vis Sci* 44:1616, 2003

Razzaque MS, Foster CS, Ahmed AR: Role of enhanced expression of m-CSF in conjunctiva affected by cicatricial pemphigoid. *Invest Ophthalmol Vis Sci* 43:2977, 2002

Razzaque MS, Foster CS, Ahmed AR: Role of connective tissue growth factor in the pathogenesis of conjunctival scarring in ocular cicatricial pemphigoid. *Invest Ophthalmol Vis Sci* 44:1998, 2003

Razzaque MS, Foster CS, Ahmed AR: Role of macrophage migration inhibitory factor in conjunctival pathology in ocular cicatricial pemphigoid. *Invest Ophthalmol Vis Sci* 45:1174, 2004

Razzaque MS, Foster CS, Ahmed AR: Role of macrophage inhibitory factor in conjunctival pathology in ocular cicatricial pemphigoid. *Invest Ophthalmol Vis Sci* 45:1174, 2004

Reacher MH, Pe'er J, Rapoza PA et al.: T cells and trachoma. *Ophthalmology* 98:334, 1991

Robinson MR, Lee SS, Sneller MC et al.: Tarsal-conjunctival disease associated with Wegener's granulomatosis. *Ophthalmology* 110:1770, 2003

Rofail M, Lee LR, Whitehead K. Conjunctival benign reactive lymphoid hyperplasia associated with myopic scleral thinning. *Clin Exp Ophthalmol* 33:73, 2005

Rojas B, Cuhna R, Zafirakis P et al.: Cell populations and adhesion molecules expression in conjunctiva before and after bone marrow transplantation. *Exp Eye Res* 81:313, 2005

Sandstrom I, Kallings I, Melen B: Neonatal chlamydial conjunctivitis. *Acta Paediatr Scand* 77:207, 1988

sano-Kato N, Fukagawa K, Okada N et al.: Tryptase increases proliferative activity of human conjunctival fibroblasts through protease-activated receptor-2. *Invest Ophthalmol Vis Sci* 46:4622, 2005

Sawada Y, Fischer JL, Verm AM et al.: Detection by impression cytologic analysis of conjunctival intraepithelial invasion from eyelid sebaceous cell carcinoma. *Ophthalmology* 110:2045, 2003

Scheie HG, Crandall AS, Henle W: Keratitis associated with lymphogranuloma venereum. *JAMA* 135:333, 1947

Scheie HG, Yanoff M, Frayer WC: Carcinoma of the sebaceous glands of the eyelid. *Arch Ophthalmol* 72:800, 1964

Schuster V, Seregard S: Ligneous conjunctivitis. *Surv Ophthalmol* 48:369, 2003

Sehgal VN, Sharma S, Sardana K. Unilateral refractory (erosive) conjunctivitis: a peculiar manifestation of pemphigus vulgaris. *Skinmed* 4:250, 2005

Shields JA, Demirci H, Marr BP et al.: Conjunctival epithelial involvement by eyelid sebaceous carcinoma. The 2003 J. Howard Stokes lecture. *Ophthalm Plast Reconstr Surg* 21:92, 2005

Takano Y, Fukagawa K, Dogru M et al.: Inflammatory cells in brush cytology samples correlate with the severity of corneal lesions in atopic keratoconjunctivitis. *Br J Ophthalmol* 88:1504, 2004

Taylor HR, Rapoza PA, West S et al.: The epidemiology of infection in trachoma. *Invest Ophthalmol Vis Sci* 30:1823, 1989

Thorne JE, Anhalt GJ, Jabs DA: Mucous membrane pemphigoid and pseudopemphigoid. *Ophthalmology* 111:45, 2004

Thorne JF, Anhalt GJ, Jabs DA: Mucous membrane pemphigoid and pseudopemphigoid. *Ophthalmology* 111:45, 2004

Thygeson P: Historical review of oculogenital disease. *Am J Ophthalmol* 71:975, 1971

Trocme SD, Kephart GM, Bourne WM et al.: Eosinophil granule major basic protein deposition in corneal ulcers associated with vernal keratoconjunctivitis. *Am J Ophthalmol* 115:640, 1993

Yao L, Baltatzis S, Zafirakis P et al.: Human mast cell subtypes in conjunctiva of patients with atopic keratoconjunctivitis, ocular cicatricial pemphigoid and Stevens–Johnson syndrome. *Ocul Immunol Inflamm* 11:211, 2003

Zamir E, Bodaghi B, Tugal-Tutkun I et al.: Conjunctival ulcers in Behcet's disease. *Ophthalmology* 110:1137, 2003

Conjunctival Manifestations of Systemic Disease

Ashton N, Cook C: Allergic granulomatous nodules of the eyelid and conjunctiva. *Am J Ophthalmol* 87:1, 1978

Bakaris S, Ozdemir M, Isik IO et al.: Impression cytology changes and corneoconjunctival calcification in patients with chronic renal failure. *Acta Cytol* 49:1, 2005

Brothers DM, Hidayat AA: Conjunctival pigmentation associated with tetracycline medication. *Ophthalmology* 88:1212, 1981

Ferry AP, Safir A, Melikian HE: Ocular abnormalities in patients with gout. *Ann Ophthalmol* 71:632, 1985

Foster CS, Fong LP, Azar D et al.: Episodic conjunctival inflammation after Stevens–Johnson syndrome. *Ophthalmology* 95:453, 1988

Frazier PD, Wong VG: Cystinosis: Histologic and crystallographic examination of crystals in eye tissues. *Arch Ophthalmol* 80:87, 1968

Gallardo MJ, Randleman JB, Price KM et al.: Ocular argyrosis after long-term self-application of eyelash tint. *Am J Ophthalmol* 141:198, 2006

Ganesh A, Smith C, Chan W et al.: Immunohistochemical evaluation of conjunctival fibrillin-1 in Marfan syndrome. *Arch Ophthalmol* 124:205, 2006

Hanna C, Fraunfelder FT, Sanchez J: Ultrastructural study of argyrosis of the cornea and conjunctiva. *Arch Ophthalmol* 92:18, 1974

Katowitz JA, Yolles EA, Yanoff M: Ichthyosis congenita. *Arch Ophthalmol* 91:208, 1974

Mastropasqua L, Nubile M, Lanzini M et al.: Corneal and conjunctival manifestations in Fabry disease: in vivo confocal microscopy study. *Am J Ophthalmol* 141:709, 2006

Ozdemir M, Bakaris S, Ozdemir G et al.: Ocular surface disorders and tear function changes in patients with chronic renal failure. *Can J Ophthalmol* 39:526, 2004

Phinney RB, Mondino BJ, Abrahim A: Corneal icterus resulting from stromal bilirubin deposition. *Ophthalmology* 96:1212, 1989

Sanchez AR, Rogers RS, III, Sheridan PJ. Tetracycline and other tetracycline-derivative staining of the teeth and oral cavity. *Int J Dermatol* 43:709, 2004

Sevel D, Burger D: Ocular involvement in cutaneous porphyria: A clinical and histologic report. *Arch Ophthalmol* 85:580, 1971

Yanoff M, Scheie HG: Argyrosis of the conjunctiva and lacrimal sac. *Arch Ophthalmol* 72:57, 1964

Degenerations

Benjamin I, Taylor H, Spindler J: Orbital and conjunctival involvement in multiple myeloma. *Am J Clin Pathol* 63:811, 1975

Bordin GM: Natural green birefringence of amyloid (letter). *Am J Clin Pathol* 65:417, 1976

Brownstein S, Rodrigues MM, Fine BS *et al.*: The elastotic nature of hyaline corneal deposits: A histochemical, fluorescent and electron microscopic examination. *Am J Ophthalmol* 75:799, 1973

Brozou CG, Baglivo E, de GP *et al.*: Chronic hyposphagma revealing primary ocular amyloidosis. *Klin Monatsbl Augenheilkd* 220:196, 2003

Ciulla TA, Tolentino F, Morrow JF *et al.*: Vitreous amyloidosis in familial amyloidotic polyneuropathy: Report of a case with the ValsoMet transthyretin mutation. *Surv Ophthalmol* 40:197, 1995

Di Pascuale MA, Espana EM, Kawakita T *et al.*: Clinical characteristics of conjunctivochalasis with or without aqueous tear deficiency. *Br J Ophthalmol* 88:388, 2004

Dushku N, Hatcher SLS, Albert DM *et al.*: p53 expression and relation to human papillomavirus infection in pingueculae, pterygia, and limbal tumors. *Arch Ophthalmol* 1117:1593, 1999

Fine BS, Yanoff M, eds: *Ocular Histology: A Text and Atlas*, 2nd edn. Hagerstown, Harper & Row, 1979:41

Fong DS, Frederick AR, Krichter CU *et al.*: Adrenochrome deposit. *Arch Ophthalmol* 3:1142, 1993

Francis IC, Chan DG, Kim P *et al.*: Case-controlled clinical and histopathological study of conjunctivochalasis. *Br J Ophthalmol* 89:302, 2005

Fraunfelder FT, Garner A, Barras TC: Subconjunctival and episcleral lipid deposits. *Br J Ophthalmol* 60:532, 1976

Gertz MA, Kyle RA: Primary systemic amyloidosis: A diagnostic primer. *Mayo Clin Proc* 64:1505, 1989

Glass R, Scheie HG, Yanoff M: Conjunctival amyloidosis arising from a plasmacytoma. *Ann Ophthalmol* 3:823, 1971

Gorevic PD, Rodrigues MM: Ocular amyloidosis (perspective). *Am J Ophthalmol* 117:529, 1994

Guemes A, Kosmorsky GS, Moodie DS *et al.*: Corneal opacities in Gaucher's disease. *Am J Ophthalmol* 126:833, 1998

Haraoka K, Ando Y, Ando E *et al.*: Amyloid deposition in ocular tissues of patients with familial amyloidotic polyneuropathy (FAP). *Amyloid* 9:183, 2002

Hida T, Proia AD, Kigasawa K *et al.*: Histopathologic and immunochemical features of lattice corneal dystrophy type III. *Am J Ophthalmol* 104:249, 1987

Hill VE, Brownstein S, Jordan DR: Ptosis secondary to amyloidosis of the tarsal conjunctiva and tarsus. *Am J Ophthalmol* 123:852, 1997

Kaiser PK, Pineda R, Albert DM *et al.*: Black cornea after long-term epinephrine use. *Arch Ophthalmol* 110:1273, 1992

Levine RA, Rabb MF: Bitot's spot overlying a pinguecula. *Arch Ophthalmol* 86:525, 1971

Li ZY, Wallace RN, Streeten BW *et al.*: Elastic fiber components and protease inhibitors in pinguecula. *Invest Ophthalmol Vis Sci* 32:1573, 1991

Loo H, Forman WB, Levine MR *et al.*: Periorbital ecchymoses as the initial sign in multiple myeloma. *Ann Ophthalmol* 14:1066, 1982

Marsh WM, Streeten BW, Hoepner JA *et al.*: Localized conjunctival amyloidosis associated with extranodal lymphoma. *Ophthalmology* 94:61, 1987

Sandgren O: Ocular amyloidosis with special reference to the hereditary forms with vitreous involvement. *Surv Ophthalmol* 40:1173, 1995

Tso MOM, Bettman JW Jr: Occlusion of choriocapillaris in primary nonfamilial amyloidosis. *Arch Ophthalmol* 86:281, 1971

Watanabe A, Yokoi N, Kinoshita S *et al.*: Clinicopathologic study of conjunctivochalasis. *Cornea* 23:294, 2004

Wu SS-H, Brady K, Anderson JJ *et al.*: The predictive value of bone marrow morphologic characteristics and immunostaining in primary (AL) amyloidosis. *Am J Clin Pathol* 96:95, 1991

Yanoff M: Discussion of Maumenee AE: Keratinization of the conjunctiva. *Trans Am Ophthalmol Soc* 77:142, 1979

Cysts, Pseudoneoplasms, and Neoplasms

Al-Muammar A, Hodge WG, Farmer J: Conjunctival T-cell lymphoma: a clinicopathologic case report. *Ophthalmology* 113:459, 2006

Amstutz CA, Michel S, Thiel MA: Follicular conjunctivitis caused by a mantle cell lymphoma. *Klin Monatsbl Augenheilkd* 221:398, 2004

Arora R, Monga S, Mehta DK *et al.*: Malignant fibrous histiocytoma of the conjunctiva. *Clin Exp Ophthalmol* 34:275, 2006

Ayoub N, Barete S, Bouaziz JD *et al.*: Additional conjunctival and penile pigmentation in Laugier–Hunziker syndrome: a report of two cases. *Int J Dermatol* 43:571, 2004

Benjamin SN, Allen HF: Classification for limbal dermoid choristomas and branchial arch anomalies. Presentation of an unusual case. *Arch Ophthalmol* 87:305, 1972

Bertoni F, Zucca E: Delving deeper into MALT lymphoma biology. *J Clin Invest* 116:22, 2006

Brichard B, De PP, Godfraind C, *et al.*: Embryonal rhabdomyosarcoma presenting as conjunctival tumor. *J Pediatr Hematol Oncol* 25:651, 2003

Buggage RR, Smith JA, Shen D *et al.*: Conjunctival papillomas caused by papioomavirus type 33. *Arch Ophthalmol* 120:202, 2002

Buuns DR, Tse DT, Folberg R: Microscopically controlled excision of conjunctival squamous cell carcinoma. *Am J Ophthalmol* 117:97, 1994

Cakmak SS, Unlu MK, Bilek B *et al.*: Conjunctival inverted follicular keratosis: a case report. *Jpn J Ophthalmol* 48:497, 2004

Cameron JA, Hidayat AA: Squamous cell carcinoma of the cornea. *Am J Ophthalmol* 111:571, 1991

Chang YC, Chang CH, Liu YT *et al.*: Spontaneous regression of a large-cell lymphoma in the conjunctiva and orbit. *Ophthalm Plast Reconstr Surg* 20:461, 2004

Clarke B, Legodi E, Chrystal V *et al.*: Systemic anaplastic large cell lymphoma presenting with conjunctival involvement. *Arch Ophthalmol* 121:569, 2003

De Silva DJ, Tumuluri K, Joshi N: Conjunctival squamous cell carcinoma: atypical presentation of HIV. *Clin Exp Ophthalmol* 33:419, 2005

Dushku N, Hatcher SLS, Albert DM *et al.*: p53 expression and relation to human papillomavirus infection in pingueculae, pterygia, and limbal tumors. *Arch Ophthalmol* 1117:1593, 1999

Eagle RC Jr: Carney's syndrome. Presented at the meeting of the Verhoeff Society, 1990

Eng H-L, Lin T-M, Chen S-Y *et al.*: Failure to detect human papillomavirus DNA in malignant epithelial neoplasms of conjunctiva by polymerase chain reaction. *Am J Clin Pathol* 117:429, 2002

Erie JC, Campbell RJ, Liesegang TJ: Conjunctival and corneal intraepithelial and invasive neoplasia. *Ophthalmology* 93:176, 1986

Evides dos Santos PJ, Borborema dos Santos CM, Rufino MR *et al.*: Human papillomavirus type 13 infecting the conjunctiva. *Diagn Microbiol Infect Dis* 53:71, 2005

Finger PT, Tran HV, Turbin RE *et al.*: High-frequency ultrasonographic evaluation of conjunctival intraepithelial neoplasia and squamous cell carcinoma. *Arch Ophthalmol* 121:168, 2003

Gayre GS, Proia AD, Dutton JJ: Epibulbar osseous choristoma: case report and review of the literature. *Ophthalmic Surg Lasers* 33:410, 2002

Glass AG, Hoover RN: The emerging epidemic of melanoma and squamous cell skin cancer. *JAMA* 262:2097, 1989

Glasson WJ, Hirst LW, Axelsen RA *et al.*: Invasive squamous cell carcinoma of the conjunctiva. *Arch Ophthalmol* 112:1342, 1994

Gonnering RS, Sonneland PR: Oncocytic carcinoma of the plica semilunaris with orbital extension. *Ophthalmic Surg* 18:604, 1987

Heinz C, Fanihagh F, Steuhl KP: Squamous cell carcinoma of the conjunctiva in patients with atopic eczema. *Cornea* 22:135, 2003

Higuchi A, Shimmura S, Takeuchi T *et al.*: Elucidation of apoptosis induced by serum deprivation in cultured conjunctival epithelial cells. *Br J Ophthalmol* 90:760, 2006

Holland MJ, Hayes LJ, Whittle HC *et al.*: Conjunctival scarring in trachoma is associated with depressed cell-mediated immune responses to chlamydial antigens. *J Infect Dis* 168:1528, 1993

Huerva V, Canto LM, Marti M: Primary diffuse large B-cell lymphoma of the lower eyelid. *Ophthalm Plast Reconstr Surg* 19:160, 2003

Huntington AC, Langloss JM, Hidayat AA: Spindle cell carcinoma of the conjunctiva. *Ophthalmology* 97:711, 1990

Husain SE, Patrinely JR, Zimmerman LE *et al.*: Primary basal cell carcinoma of the limbal conjunctiva. *Ophthalmology* 100:1720, 1993

Hwang IP, Jordan DR, Brownstein S *et al.*: Mucoepidermoid carcinoma of the conjunctiva: A series of three cases. *Ophthalmology* 107:801, 2000

Jakobiec FA, Buckman G, Zimmerman LE *et al.*: Metastatic melanoma within and to the conjunctiva. *Ophthalmology* 96:999, 1989

Jakobiec FA, Harrison W, Aronian D: Inverted mucoepidermoid papillomas of the epibulbar conjunctiva. *Ophthalmology* 94:283, 1987

Jakobiec FA, Perry HD, Harrison W *et al.*: Dacryoadenoma. *Ophthalmology* 96:1014, 1989

Jakobiec FA, Sacks E, Lisman RL *et al.*: Epibulbar fibroma of the conjunctival substantia propria. *Arch Ophthalmol* 106:661, 1988

Karp CL, Scott IU, Chang TS *et al.*: Conjunctival intraepithelial neoplasm: A possible marker for human immunodeficiency virus infection? *Arch Ophthalmol* 114:257, 1996

Kaw P, Carlson A, Meyer DR: Nevus lipomatosus (pedunculated lipofibroma) of the eyelid. *Ophthalm Plast Reconstr Surg* 21:74, 2005

Kennedy RH, Flanagan JC, Eagle RC Jr *et al.*: The Carney complex with ocular signs suggestive of cardiac myxoma. *Am J Ophthalmol* 111:699, 1991

Kennedy RH, Waller RR, Carney JA: Ocular pigmented spots and eyelid myxomas. *Am J Ophthalmol* 104:533, 1987

Kifuku K, Yoshikawa H, Sonoda K-H *et al.*: Conjunctival keratoacanthoma in an Asian. *Arch Ophthalmol* 121:118, 2003

Kim P, Macken PL, Palfreeman S *et al.*: Bilateral benign lymphoid hyperplasia of the conjunctiva in a paediatric patient. *Clin Exp Ophthalmol* 33:285, 2005

Kurli M, Finger PT, Garcia JP Jr *et al.*: Peribulbar oncocytoma: high-frequency ultrasound with histopathologic correlation. *Ophthalmic Surg Lasers Imaging* 37:154, 2006

Lauer SA, Malter JS, Meier JR: Human papillomavirus type 18 in conjunctival intraepithelial neoplasia. *Am J Ophthalmol* 110:23, 1990

Lee GA, Hirst LW: Ocular surface squamous neoplasia. *Surv Ophthalmol* 39:429, 1995

Lee SS, Robinson MR, Morris JC *et al.*: Conjunctival involvement with T-cell prolymphocytic leukemia: report of a case and review of the literature. *Surv Ophthalmol* 49:525, 2004

Lewallen S, Shroyer KR, Keyser RB *et al.*: Aggressive conjunctival squamous cell carcinoma in three young Africans. *Arch Ophthalmol* 114:215, 1996

Mahmood MA, Al-Rajhi A, Riley F *et al.*: Sklerokeratitis. An unusual presentation of squamous cell carcinoma of the conjunctiva. *Ophthalmology* 108:553, 2001

Malek SN, Hatfield AJ, Flinn IW: MALT Lymphomas. *Curr Treat Options Oncol* 4:269, 2003

Margo CE, Grossniklaus HE: Pseudoepitheliomatous hyperplasia of the conjunctiva. *Ophthalmology* 108:135, 2001

Margo CE, Mack W, Guffey JM: Squamous cell carcinoma and human immunodeficiency virus infection. *Arch Ophthalmol* 114:257, 1996

McDonnell JM, McDonnell PJ, Sun YY: Human papillomavirus DNA in tissues and ocular surface swabs of patients with conjunctival epithelial neoplasia. *Invest Ophthalmol Vis Sci* 33:184, 1992

Meier P, Sterker I, Meier T: Primary basal cell carcinoma of the caruncle. *Arch Ophthalmol* 116:1373, 1998

Morand B, Bettega G, Bland V *et al.*: Oncocytoma of the eyelid: An aggressive benign tumor. *Ophthalmology* 105:2220, 1998

Mori A, Deguchi HE, Mishima K *et al.*: A case of uveal, palpebral, and orbital invasions in adult T-cell leukemia. *Jpn J Ophthalmol* 47:599, 2003

Moubayed P, Mwakyoma H, Schneider DT: High frequency of human papillomavirus 6/11, 16, and 18 infections in precancerous lesions and squamous cell carcinoma of the conjunctiva in subtropical Tanzania. *Am J Clin Pathol* 122:938, 2004

Munro S, Brownstein S, Liddy B: Conjunctival keratoacanthoma. *Am J Ophthalmol* 116:654, 1993

Murga Penas EM, Hinz K, Roser K *et al.*: Translocations t(11;18)(q21;q21) and t(14;18)(q32;q21) are the main chromosomal abnormalities involving MLT/MALT1 in MALT lymphomas. *Leukemia* 17:2225, 2003

Nola M, Lukenda A, Bollmann M *et al.*: Outcome and prognostic factors in ocular adnexal lymphoma. *Croat Med J* 45:328, 2004

Obata H, Mori K, Tsuru T: Subconjunctival mucosa-associated lymphoid tissue (MALT) lymphoma arising in Tenon's capsule. *Graefes Arch Clin Exp Ophthalmol* 244:118, 2006

Odrich MG, Jakobiec FA, Lancaster WD *et al.*: A spectrum of bilateral squamous conjunctival tumors associated with human papillomavirus type 16. *Ophthalmology* 98:628, 1991

Ohara M, Sotozono C, Tsuchihashi Y *et al.*: Ki-67 labeling index as a marker of malignancy in ocular surface neoplasms. *Jpn J Ophthalmol* 48:524, 2004

Pe'er J, Neufeld M, Ilsar M: Peripunctal eyelid oncocytoma. *Am J Ophthalmol* 116:385, 1993

Poon A, Sloan B, McKelvie P *et al.*: Primary basal cell carcinoma of the caruncle. *Arch Ophthalmol* 115:1585, 1997

Quillen DA, Goldberg SH, Rosenwasser GO *et al.*: Basal cell carcinoma of the conjunctiva. *Am J Ophthalmol* 116:244, 1993

Reszec J, Sulkowska M, Koda M *et al.*: Expression of cell proliferation and apoptosis markers in papillomas and cancers of conjunctiva and eyelid. *Ann N Y Acad Sci* 1030:419–26.:419, 2004

Rodman RC, Frueh BR, Elner VM: Mucoepidermoid carcinoma of the caruncle. *Am J Ophthalmol* 123:564, 1997

Roth AM: Solitary keratoacanthoma of the conjunctiva. *Am J Ophthalmol* 85:647, 1978

Santos A, Gómez-Leal A: Lesions of the lacrimal caruncle: Clinico-pathologic features. *Ophthalmology* 101:943, 1994

Scholzen T, Gerdes J: The Ki-67 protein: from the known and the unknown. *J Cell Physiol* 182:311, 2000

Scott IU, Karp CL, Nuovo GJ: Human papillomavirus 16 and 18 expression in conjunctival intraepithelial neoplasia. *Ophthalmology* 109:542, 2002

Seitz B, Fischer M, Hollbach LM *et al.*: Differentialdiagnose und Prognose bei 112 exzidierten epibulbären Tumoren [Differential diagnosis and prognosis of 112 excised epibulbar epithelial neoplasias]. *Klin Monatsbl Augenheilkd* 207:239, 1995

Shepler TR, Prieto VG, Diba R *et al.*: Expression of the epidermal growth factor receptor in conjunctival squamous cell carcinoma. *Ophthalm Plast Reconstr Surg* 22:113, 2006

Shields CL, Shields JA, Arbizo V *et al.*: Oncocytoma of the caruncle. *Am J Ophthalmol* 102:315, 1986

Shields CL, Shields JA, Eagle RC Jr: Hereditary benign intraepithelial dyskeratosis. *Arch Ophthalmol* 105:422, 1987

Shields CL, Shields JA, White D *et al.*: Types and frequency of lesions of the caruncle. *Am J Ophthalmol* 102:771, 1986

Shields JA, Demirci H, Mashayekhi A *et al.*: Melanocytoma of optic disc in 115 cases: The 2004 Samuel Johnson Memorial Lecture, Part 1. *Ophthalmology* 111:1739, 2004

Shields JA, Shields CL, Luminais S *et al.*: Differentiation of pigmented conjunctival squamous cell carcinoma from melanoma. *Ophthalmic Surg Lasers Imaging* 34:406, 2003

Slusker-Shternfeld I, Syed NA, Sires BA: Invasive spindle cell carcinoma of the conjunctiva. *Arch Ophthalmol* 115:288, 1997

Stern K, Jakobiec FA, Harrison WG: Caruncular dacryops with extruded secretory globoid bodies. *Ophthalmology* 90:1447, 1983

Streeten BW, Carrillo R, Jamison R *et al.*: Inverted papilloma of the conjunctiva. *Am J Ophthalmol* 88:1062, 1979

Tabin G, Levin S, Snibson G *et al.*: Late recurrences and the necessity for long-term follow-up in corneal and conjunctival intraepithelial neoplasm. *Ophthalmology* 104:485, 1997

Thieblemont C, Berger F, Coiffier B: Mucosa-associated lymphoid tissue lymphomas. *Curr Opin Oncol* 7:415, 1995

Tiemann M, Haring S, Heidemann M *et al.*: Mucosa-associated lymphoid tissue lymphoma in the conjunctiva of a child. *Virchows Arch* 444:198, 2004

Tulvatana W, Bhattarakosol P, Sansopha L *et al.*: Risk factors for conjunctival squamous cell neoplasia: a matched case-control study. *Br J Ophthalmol* 87:396, 2003

uw-Haedrich C, Sundmacher R, Freudenberg N *et al.*: Expression of p63 in conjunctival intraepithelial neoplasia and squamous cell carcinoma. *Graefes Arch Clin Exp Ophthalmol* 244:96, 2006

Weatherhead RG: Wolfring dacryops. *Ophthalmology* 99:1575, 1992

Whittaker KW, Trivedi D, Bridger J *et al.*: Ocular surface squamous neoplasia: report of an unusual case and review of the literature. *Orbit* 21:209, 2002

Widmer S, Tinguely M, Egli F *et al.*: Lethal Epstein–Barr virus associated NK/T-cell lymphoma with primary manifestation in the conjunctiva. *Klin Monatsbl Augenheilkd* 222:255, 2005

Woo JM, Tang CK, Rho MS *et al.*: The clinical characteristics and treatment results of ocular adnexal lymphoma. *Korean J Ophthalmol* 20:7, 2006

Yanoff M: Hereditary benign intraepithelial dyskeratosis. *Arch Ophthalmol* 79:291, 1968

Ye H, Liu H, Attygalle A *et al.*: Variable frequencies of t(11;18)(q21;q21) in MALT lymphomas of different sites: significant association with CagA strains of *H. pylori* in gastric MALT lymphoma. *Blood* 102:1012, 2003

Yeung L, Tsao YP, Chen PY *et al.*: Combination of adult inclusion conjunctivitis and mucosa-associated lymphoid tissue (MALT) lymphoma in a young adult. *Cornea* 23:71, 2004

Young TL, Buch ER, Kaufman LM *et al.*: Respiratory epithelium in a cystic choristoma of the limbus. *Arch Ophthalmol* 108:1736, 1990

8

Cornea and Sclera

CORNEA

NORMAL ANATOMY

I. Introduction
  A. *In vivo* confocal microscopy (CFM) is a valuable tool for the study of corneal diseases. CFM findings complement and corroborate histopathological analyses.
  B. Multiple types of corneal disorders are discussed in this chapter. To appreciate the corneal disease state better, the normal anatomy must be understood.

One indication of the visual significance of each entity is the frequency for which corneal transplantation is required for each disorder. In one large study of 1540 corneal transplants, corneal edema was the most common cause (24.8%), followed by keratitis (24.5%) and corneal dystrophies (24.4%).

  C. The cornea (Fig. 8.1) is a modified mucous membrane (it can also be considered, in part, as modified skin).

It is not surprising, therefore, that the cornea is affected in association with cutaneous disorders. For example, low corneal sensitivity, abnormal tear quality, decreased cellular cohesion, squamous metaplasia of the conjunctiva, and goblet cell loss have been described in the Hallopeau–Siemens subtype of *dystrophic epidermolysis bullosa*. Specific corneal abnormalities in this disorder may include recurrent corneal erosion, and superficial punctate corneal erosions.

---

  1. The cornea is covered anteriorly by a nonkeratinizing squamous epithelium of approximately five layers, representing modified epidermis of skin.

Intermixed within the corneal epithelium are Langerhans' cells (bone marrow-derived, CD la-expressing, dendritic-appearing cells) and occasional dendritic melanocytes. Langerhans' cell histiocytosis has presented as a limbal nodule in an adult.

---

  a. The deepest layer of epithelial cells, the basal layer, is the germinative layer and is attached to its neighboring basal cells and overlying wing cells by desmosomes.
  b. The basal cell layer is also attached by hemidesmosomes to its own secretory product, a somewhat irregular, thin basement membrane.

Three major types of molecules are found in the basement membrane: type IV collagen, heparan sulfate proteoglycans, and noncollagenous proteins (e.g., laminin, nidogen, and osteonectin). The basement membrane represents an important physiologic barrier between the epithelium and the stroma.

---

  c. The flattened, nucleated, superficial epithelial cells desquamate into the overlying trilaminar (mucoprotein, water, lipid) tear film. The mucoprotein layer serves to adhere the tear film to the epithelial microvilli.

Corneal stem cells reside in the transitional epithelium between cornea and conjunctiva (i.e., the limbus). Corneal limbal cells express K3 keratin marker for corneal-type differentiation, in contrast to conjunctival cells. In healing large corneal abrasions that reach the limbus, the stem cells regenerate new corneal epithelium by a process called *conjunctival transdifferentiation*. First, the healing epithelium shows conjunctiva-like

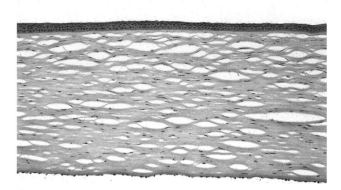

A

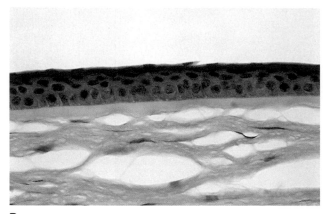

B

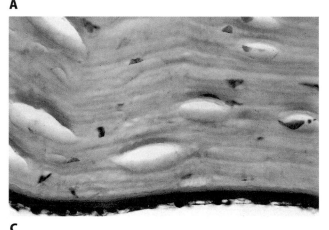

C

Fig. 8.1 Cornea. **A,** The cornea contains five layers: epithelium, Bowman's membrane, stroma, Descemet's membrane, and endothelium. **B,** Increased magnification shows the nonkeratinized, approximately five-layered epithelium, separated from Bowman's membrane (relatively homogeneous) and anterior stroma (numerous large artifactitious clefts) by a thin basement membrane. **C,** Descemet's (basement) membrane and endothelium (a single layer of cuboidal cells) cover the posterior stroma. (**A–C,** Periodic acid–Schiff stain.)

appearance, even to containing goblet cells, but then, slowly, it is transformed into a more cornea-like appearance without goblet cells.

1. Stem cells can become exhausted in multiple conditions that lead to their massive direct injury or to repetitive insults.
2. The *lacrimo-auriculo-dento-digital (LADD) syndrome* is an autosomal-dominant disease with variable expression. Common ocular findings include hypoplasia or aplasia of tear glands, and lacrimal puncta or canaliculi, tear deficiency, recurrent or chronic conjunctivitis, keratoconjunctivitis sicca, and corneal ulceration secondary to sicca. Corneal stem cell deficiency and hypoanesthesia have also been described.
3. Similarly, ocular manifestations of *keratitis–ichthyosis–deafness (KID) syndrome* include lid abnormalities, corneal surface instability, limbal stem cell deficiency with secondary corneal complications, and dry eye.
4. Congenital abnormalities or deficiency of corneal limbal stem cells have been cited as responsible for keratopathy in aniridia, including corneal vascular pannus formation, conjunctival invasion of the corneal surface, corneal epithelial erosions, and epithelial abnormalities. The disorder is secondary to heterozygosity for PAX6 deficiency (PAX6+/−). Other possible causes for these changes include abnormal corneal healing responses secondary to anomalous extracellular matrix metabolism, abnormal corneal epithelial differentiation leading to epithelial cell fragility, reduction in cell adhesion molecules in the heterozygous PAX6 state, and conjunctival and corneal changes leading to the presence of cells derived from conjunctiva on the corneal surface.
5. Idiopathic limbal stem cell deficiency has been reported.

D. Underlying the basal cell basement membrane is a thick, acellular, collagenous layer called *Bowman's membrane* (by light microscopy) or *Bowman's layer* (by transmission electron microscopy).

Abnormalities of corneal epithelium can be demonstrated clinically by the use of fluorescein or rose Bengal. Fluorescein staining is enhanced when disruption of cell–cell junctions occurs, whereas rose Bengal staining is seen with deficiency of protection by the preocular tear film.

E. The bulk of the cornea, the *stroma*, consists of collagen lamellae secreted by fibroblasts called *keratocytes* that lie between the lamellae. The stromal lamellae are arranged much as a collapsed honeycomb with oblique lamellae, the anteriormost lamellae (approximately one third) being the most oblique (i.e., the least parallel), and the posterior (approximately two-thirds) being the least oblique (i.e., the most parallel) to one another.

1. Thy 1 expression is present in cultured corneal fibroblasts and myofibroblasts, but not in fresh keratocytes. Thus, it may be used to differentiate these cell types.

2. The anterior third of the stroma is analogous to a highly modified dermis of the skin, and the posterior two-thirds of the stroma may be usefully considered analogous to a highly modified subcutaneous tissue of the skin.

> The Ocular Hypertension Treatment Study (OHTS) has drawn attention to the importance of variations in corneal thickness relative to the validity of applanation tonometry and the risk of glaucoma, with thin corneas resulting in inappropriately low intraocular pressure measurements and an associated increased risk of glaucoma. Similarly marked increase in central corneal thickness (mean 632 μm) may be associated with aniridia, and may impact the accuracy of intraocular pressure measurements in this disorder. Similar increased corneal thickness has been reported in nevus of Ota. Decreased corneal thickness may result in an inappropriately low intraocular pressure in disorders such as osteogenesis imperfecta, and Down syndrome.

F. An unusually thick basement membrane, *Descemet's membrane*, secreted by the endothelium, lies between the stroma and the endothelial cells.

> Variably pigmented round and reticular posterior intracorneal precipitates have been described at the level of Descemet's membrane in human immunodeficiency virus (HIV)-positive individuals.

G. The posterior surface of the cornea is covered by a single layer of cuboidal cells, the *corneal endothelium* (*mesothelium*); no hemidesmosomes are present along these inverted cells. Endothelial cells decrease progressively with age even in healthy emmetropic eyes. This decrease can be expedited by accompanying disorders such as pseudoexfoliation syndrome. The final common result of endothelial insufficiency is corneal edema.

1. Varying abnormalities in aquaporin distribution have been found in pseudophakic and aphakic bullous keratopathy, and in Fuchs' corneal dystrophy, suggesting the possibility of variations in the mechanism for fluid accumulation in each disorder.

2. Corneal endothelial cell count is reduced and the coefficient of cellular variability is increased in type II diabetes mellitus, but central corneal thickness is not increased.

3. Corneal endothelial cell numbers are decreased, and they express the characteristic mutant DRPLA protein in *dentatorubropallidoluysian atrophy*.

H. The cornea is one of the most unusual structures in the body in that it has no blood vessels and is transparent. Any pathologic lesions, therefore, are easily seen clinically as an opacification in the cornea.

I. The cornea is well innervated.

1. Approximately 20% of corneal nerves respond exclusively to noxious mechanical forces (mechanonociceptors), 70% are stimulated by extreme temperatures, exogenous irritant chemicals, and endogenous inflammatory mediators (polymodal nociceptors), and 10% are cold-sensitive and increase their discharge with moderate cooling of the cornea (cold receptors).

2. Increased tortuosity of corneal nerves as documented by CFM is associated with severity of somatic neuropathy in diabetes mellitus.

J. Although the corneal anatomy may be described as isolated layers for didactic purposes, pathologic conditions affect multiple layers concurrently or sequentially. For example, multiple histologic structures, including corneal nerves, are adversely impacted by Sjögren's syndrome.

CONGENITAL DEFECTS

Absence of Cornea

Absence of the cornea is a very rare condition usually associated with absence of other parts of the eye derived from primitive invaginating ectoderm (e.g., the lens).

Abnormalities of Size

I. Microcornea (<11 mm in greatest diameter; Fig. 8.2)
   A. The eye is usually structurally normal.

> Microcornea may be associated with other ocular anomalies such as are found in microphthalmos with cyst, trisomy 13, and the *Nance–Horan* syndrome (X-linked disorder typified by microcornea, dense cataracts, anteverted and simplex pinnae, brachymetacarpalia, and numerous dental anomalies; there is provisional linkage to two DNA markers—DXS143 at Xp22.3–p22.2 and DXS43 at Xp22.2).

   B. The condition may be inherited as an autosomal-dominant trait.
   C. Histologically, the cornea is usually normal except for its small size.

> A lack of myofilaments and desmin in the cytoplasm of the anterior layer of iris pigment epithelium suggests that congenital microcornea may result from a defect of intermediate filaments.

II. Megalocornea (>13 mm in greatest diameter; see Fig. 8.2)

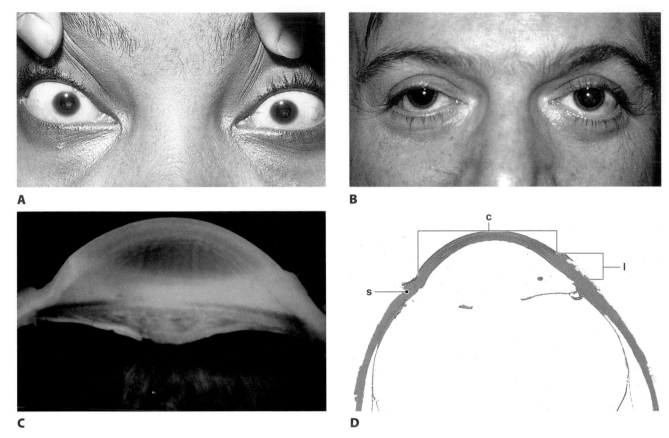

Fig. 8.2 Abnormalities of size. **A,** The patient has bilateral microcorneas. **B,** The patient has bilateral megalocornea, as do other male members of his family. The patient died from metastatic renal cell carcinoma, and the eyes were obtained at autopsy. **C,** Gross examination shows an enlarged cornea and a very deep anterior chamber. **D,** Histologic section shows that the cornea itself (c) is of approximately normal diameter, but the limbal region (l) is elongated and slightly thicker than normal. The patient had had a cataract extraction and a peripheral iridectomy (s, corneal scar of cataract incision). The patient's brother developed renal cell carcinomas. (**C,** Courtesy of Dr. RC Eagle, Jr.)

A. Most megalocorneas present as an isolated finding, are bilateral and nonprogressive, and do not, in themselves, produce symptoms (except for refractive error).

> Cataract and subluxated lens commonly develop in adulthood. Glaucoma may result secondary to the dislocated lens. Rarely, megalocornea is associated with renal cell carcinoma. In some families, renal cell carcinoma also develops in afflicted members.

B. Other ocular findings include arcus juvenilis, mosaic corneal dystrophy, cataracts, and pigmentary glaucoma.

> Megalocornea, usually an isolated finding, may also be associated with ichthyosis, poikiloderma congenitale, Down's syndrome, mental retardation, dwarfism, Marfan's syndrome, craniostenosis, oxycephaly, progressive facial hemiatrophy, osteogenesis imperfecta, multiple skeletal abnormalities, nonketotic hyperglycemia, and tuberous sclerosis.

C. The condition usually has a recessive X-linked (in the region, Xq21–q26) inheritance pattern, but may be autosomal dominant or recessive.

D. Histologically, the cornea is usually normal except for its large size, especially in the limbal region.

Aberrations of Curvature

  I. Astigmatism
 II. Cornea plana
   A. Frequently, cornea plana is associated with other ocular anomalies (e.g., posterior embryotoxon, colobomas of iris and choroid, and congenital cataract).
   B. Both recessive and autosomal-dominant inheritance patterns have been reported, and both map to chromosome 12q21.

> Mutations in keratocan is the probable mechanism of the cornea plana phenotype. Recently, a new point mutation in exon 3 (937C > T) resulting in replacement of arginine by a stop codon at position 313 of keratocan protein has been associated with autosomal-recessive cornea plana, variable anterior-

chamber depths, and short axial lengths. Other mutations have been reported.

C. Histologically, the cornea is usually normal except for its flattened anterior curve.
III. Keratoconus and keratoglobus—see subsection *Endothelial*, section *Dystrophies*, later in this chapter.

Congenital Corneal Opacities

The two main theories of causation are arrested development during embryogenesis and intrauterine inflammation.

Similar changes can also result from trauma or inflammation. In a study of 72 eyes of 47 patients referred for congenital corneal opacities, Peters' anomaly was the most common cause (40.3%), followed by sclerocornea (18.1%), dermoid (15.3%), congenital glaucoma (6.9%), microphthalmia (4.2%), birth trauma and metabolic disease (2.8%). 9.7% were idiopathic. Ten patients had systemic abnormalities associated with the ocular conditions.

Clinicopathologic Types—General

I. Facet
   A. A facet (often the result of an embedded corneal foreign body) is a small, superficial spot seen by focal illumination as a distortion of the corneal light reflex or by slit lamp as a focal increased separation of the anteriormost two lines of corneal relucence.
   B. Histologically, normal epithelium of increased thickness fills in the gap of previously abraded epithelium, focally absent Bowman's membrane, and sometimes the very anteriormost corneal stroma; no scar tissue is present.
II. Nebula (Fig. 8.3)
   A. A nebula is a slight, diffuse, cloudlike opacity with indistinct borders.
   B. Histologically, scar tissue is found predominantly in the superficial stroma.

III. Macula
   A. A macula is a well-circumscribed, moderately dense opacity.
   B. Histologically, the scar is dense and involves the corneal stroma.
IV. Leukoma (Fig. 8.4; see also Fig. 8.10)
   A. A leukoma is a white, opaque scar (e.g., see discussion of Peters' anomaly, later).
   B. Histologically, a large area of stromal scarring is present.

When iris is adherent to the posterior surface of the cornea beneath a region of corneal scarring, the resulting condition is called an *adherent leukoma*.

Clinicopathologic Types—Specific

I. Anterior embryotoxon
   A. Anterior embryotoxon is synonymous with *arcus juvenilis*.
   B. It may be present at birth or develop in early life, and clinically appears identical to an arcus senilis (gerontoxon).
   C. The condition may be associated with elevated serum lipids or cholesterol.
   D. Histology—same as arcus senilis (see Fig. 8.20)
II. Corneal keloid
   A. Corneal keloid presents as a hypertrophic scar involving the entire cornea.

If ectatic and lined by uveal tissue (iris), it is called a *congenital corneal staphyloma*.

   B. Overabundant production of corneal scar tissue after trauma seems to be the cause of corneal keloid.
   C. Although frequently noted at birth, probably secondary to intrauterine trauma, traumatic corneal keloids can occur at any age. They have been associated with Lowe's

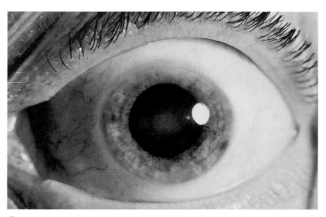

A

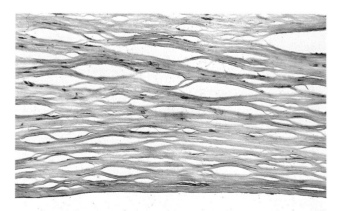

B

Fig. 8.3 Nebula. **A,** Corneal scar appears as diffuse, cloudlike lesion. **B,** Diffuse stromal scarring present in cornea from patient with luetic (congenital) interstitial keratitis. Blood vessel present just anterior to Descemet's membrane.

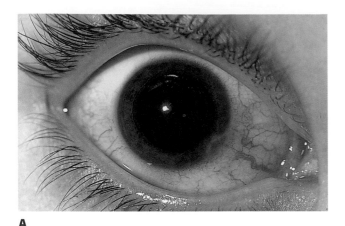

A

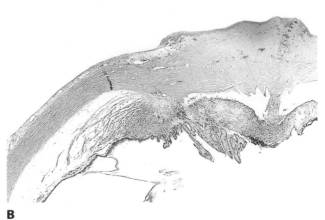

B

Fig. 8.4 Adherent leukoma. **A,** Peripheral adherent leukoma from 4 to 5 o'clock in a 12-year-old girl who had accidental penetration of globe (by scissors) 5 weeks previously; perforation of cornea repaired on the day of injury. Sympathetic uveitis developed 2 days before picture was taken. **B,** Fibroblastic proliferation attaches iris to cornea through gap in Descemet's membrane in 3-week-old wound. Overlying scar present through full thickness of cornea. After organization and shrinkage of fibroblastic membrane, scar will look much like scar of adherent leukoma in **A.**

syndrome, Rubinstein–Taybi syndrome, fibrodysplasia ossificans progressiva, and other developmental ocular disorders.

D. Histologically, abundant scar tissue in disarray replaces most or all of the cornea.

Proliferating myofibroblasts (immunopositivity with alpha-smooth-muscle actin and the intermediate filament vimentin), activated fibroblasts, and haphazardly arranged fascicles of collagen may be seen.

III. *De Barsy syndrome* is characterized by anomalous facial appearance, generalized cutis laxa, mental retardation, hypotonia, hyperreflexia, growth retardation, and corneal opacification and degeneration of Bowman's membrane.

A. Light microscopic examination of representative corneal tissue shows epithelial thickening, absence of Bowman's membrane, and attenuation of stroma, particularly centrally. Hypercellularity and scarring of the anterior superficial stroma may also be seen.

B. Electron microscopy demonstrates replacement of the normal architecture of Bowman's layer with a paucity of longitudinal and oblique collagen fibers. Although elastic fibrils are not usually present in the normal cornea, small bundles of elastic microfibrils are present in amorphous deposits that are immunopositive for elastin. Abnormal banding of Descemet's membrane with normal-appearing endothelium may also be seen.

IV. *Autoimmune polyendocrinopathy–candidiasis–ectodermal dystrophy* (APECED)

A. Seldom described, this is an autoimmune disorder that mainly affects endocrine glands with manifestations such as adrenocortical failure, hypoparathyroidism, insulin-dependent diabetes mellitus, and pernicious anemia. Patients have chronic mucocutaneous candidiasis and ectodermal dystrophies.

B. Ocular manifestations include anterior keratopathy characterized by early epidermalization, destruction of Bowman's membrane and the anterior stroma, which

are replaced by vascularized scarring, proliferating fibroblasts, and chronic inflammation. The deeper stroma, Descemet's membrane, and endothelium are not affected.

V. Central dysgenesis of cornea*

A. Peters' anomaly (Fig. 8.5, see also section *Fetal Alcohol Syndrome* in Chapter 2)

1. Peters' anomaly consists of bilateral central corneal opacities associated with abnormalities of the deepest corneal stromal layers, including local absence of endothelium, and Descemet's and Bowman's membranes. Abnormalities of extracellular matrix may be present.

2. It is associated with anomalies of the anterior-segment structures (corectopia, iris hypoplasia, anterior polar cataract, and iridocorneal adhesions). Congenital corneal staphyloma has been seen.

3. The cause may be a defect of neural crest, ectoderm, and perhaps mesoderm, resulting in failure or delay in separation of the lens vesicle from surface epithelium. The causative event may occur in the migratory neural crest cells between the 4th and 7th weeks of gestation.

4. Associated systemic abnormalities include congenital heart disease, external ear abnormalities, cleft lip and palate, central nervous system abnormalities, hearing loss, and spinal defects.

a. Peters' anomaly may be part of a new syndrome that includes microcephaly with cortical migra-

Corneal endothelial cells, corneal stroma, portions of the trabecular meshwork including endothelial cells, anterior iris stroma, iris melanocytes, ciliary body, sclera, and intraocular vascular pericytes are derived not from mesoderm, as thought previously, but from neural crest. Accordingly, the former term, mesodermal–ectodermal dysgenesis of cornea, now seems best replaced by central dysgenesis of cornea. Similarly, what was formerly termed mesodermal dysgenesis of cornea and iris now seems better termed peripheral dysgenesis of cornea and iris.

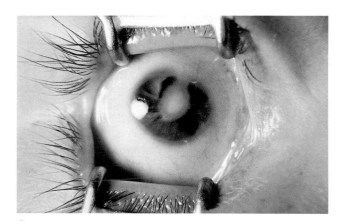

A

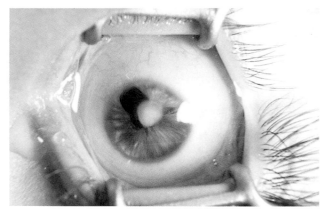

B

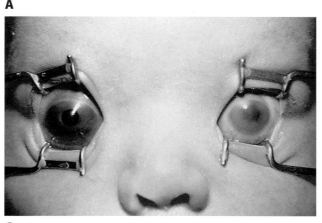

C

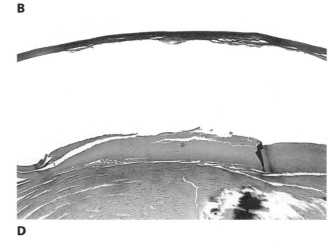

D

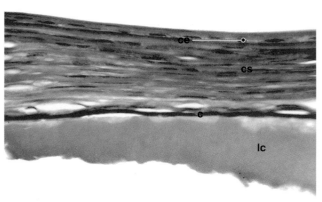

ce

cs

c

lc

E

Fig. 8.5 Peters' anomaly. The right (**A**) and left (**B**) eyes of a patient show bilateral central cornea leukomas and iris anomalies. **C,** In another patient, the right eye shows an enlarged cornea, secondary to glaucoma. The left eye shows a small cornea as part of the anomalous affliction. **D,** Histologic section shows considerable corneal thinning centrally. The space between the cornea and the lens material is artifactitious and secondary to shrinkage of the lens cortex during processing of the eye. **E,** Increased magnification shows lens material attached to the posterior cornea. Centrally, endothelium, Descemet's membrane, and Bowman's membrane are absent. Lens capsule (c) lines the posterior surface of the cornea (ce, corneal epithelium; cs, corneal stroma; lc, lens capsule). (**B** and **C,** Periodic acid–Schiff stain; reported in Scheie HG, Yanoff M: *Arch Ophthalmol* 87:525, 1972. American Medical Association. All rights reserved.)

tion defects, and multiple intestinal atresias. It is believed to be a multiple vascular disruption syndrome.

5. Peters' anomaly is usually inherited as an autosomal-recessive trait, but autosomal dominance or no inheritance pattern may also occur.

Proliferating myofibroblasts (immunopositivity with alpha-smooth-muscle actin and the intermediate filament vimentin), activated fibroblasts, and haphazardly arranged fascicles of collagen may be seen.

Peters' anomaly may be associated with deletion of short arm of chromosome 4 (*Wolf–Hirschhorn syndrome*), partial trisomy 5p, mosaic trisomy 9, deletion of long arm of chromosome 11, deletion of 18q, ring chromosome 21, interstitial deletion 2q14q21, and translocation (2q;15q). It has also been reported in association with ring 20 chromosomal abnormality, trisomy 13, the Walker–Warburg syndrome, and the fetal alcohol syndrome (see Fig. 2.14). Also, in a family that has Axenfeld syndrome and Peters' anomaly, the condition was caused by a point mutation (Phe112Ser) in the *FOXC1* gene

6. *Internal ulcer of von Hippel* is similar to Peters' anomaly in that patients show the typical corneal abnormalities, but differs in that no lens abnormalities are present.

Similar findings have been reported in cerebro-ocular myopathy syndrome.

---

7. Histologically, endothelium, and Descemet's and Bowman's membranes are absent from the cornea centrally, usually along with varying amounts of posterior stroma.
    a. The corneal lamellae are more compact and more irregularly packed than normal corneal lamellae.
    b. Immunohistochemistry shows an increase in fibronectin and collagen type VI.
    c. Lens abnormalities are present (usually an anterior polar cataract); associated abnormalities of the iris and other structures may also be present.

B. Localized posterior keratoconus (Fig. 8.6)
    1. Localized posterior keratoconus consists of a central or paracentral, craterlike corneal depression associated with stromal opacity. The depression involves the posterior corneal surface.
    2. Unlike Peters' anomaly, endothelium and Descemet's membrane are present.
    3. No other ocular anomalies are seen.
    4. Neural crest–mesenchymal maldevelopment, infection, and trauma are proposed causes.
    5. Histologically, the posterior curve of the cornea is abnormal, the overlying collagen of the corneal stroma is in disarray, and Bowman's membrane may be absent centrally.
VI. Peripheral dysgenesis of the cornea and iris*

Peripheral dysgenesis of the cornea and iris includes a wide spectrum of developmental abnormalities, ranging from posterior embryotoxon (Axenfeld's anomaly) to extensive anomalous devel-

---

See footnote on page 260.

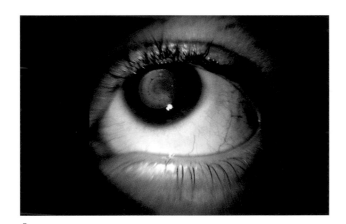

A

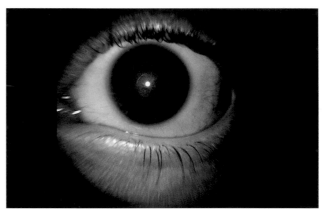

B

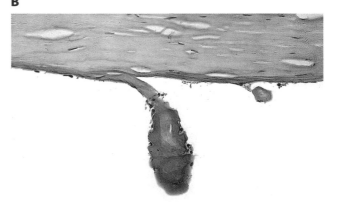

C   **D**

Fig. 8.6 Posterior keratoconus. **A** and **B,** Two views of right eye to show clinical appearance of posterior keratoconus. **C,** Histologic section shows mainly an internal thinning of the central cornea because of a deeper, central posterior curve. Descemet's membrane and endothelium are intact throughout the thinned area. **D,** In the region of the thinned cornea, some Descemet tags are present. Note that Descemet's membrane is continuous. (Courtesy of Dr. BW Streeten.)

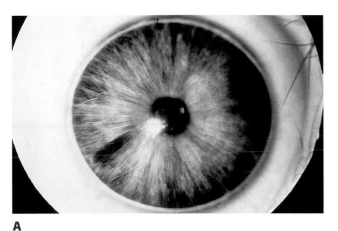

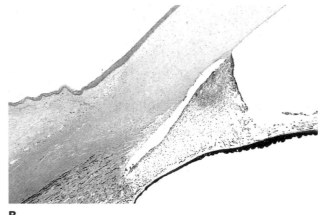

A　　　　　　　　　　　　　　　　　　　　　　　**B**

Fig. 8.7　Axenfeld's anomaly (posterior embryotoxon). **A,** Schwalbe line is anteriorly displaced 360°. **B,** Histologic section of another case shows an iris process attached to the anteriorly displaced Schwalbe ring. (**A,** Courtesy of Dr. WC Frayer; **B,** courtesy of Dr. RY Foos.)

opment of the cornea, iris, and anterior-chamber angle associated with systemic abnormalities (Rieger's syndrome).* An associated congenital glaucoma may occur, but the presence or absence of glaucoma does not necessarily depend on the degree of malformation. The abnormalities may be congenital, noninfectious, and noninherited (e.g., as part of trisomy 13 and partial trisomy 16q); congenital and inherited (e.g., Rieger's syndrome); or congenital and infectious (e.g., rubella syndrome).

A. Posterior embryotoxon or embryotoxon corneae posterius (Axenfeld's anomaly; Axenfeld–Rieger anomaly; Fig. 8.7)
　1. Recognized clinically as a bow- or ring-shaped opacity in the peripheral cornea, posterior embryotoxon is an enlarged ring of Schwalbe located more centrally than normally.
　2. It is often seen in an otherwise normal eye, or one that shows only a few mesodermal strands of iris tissue bridging the chamber angle to attach to the "displaced" Schwalbe ring.
　3. Posterior embryotoxon may be accompanied by glaucoma.
　4. Although most cases are not inherited, dominant and recessive autosomal pedigrees have been reported; the former often has prominent iris involvement.

The differentiation between Axenfeld's anomaly and Rieger's syndrome is one of degree and therefore subject to a host of interpretations and classifications. The classification used here is chosen for its simplicity and because it is as close as possible to what Axenfeld and Rieger described originally. Axenfeld in 1920 described a boy with a white annular corneal line approximately 1 mm from the limbus, at the level of Descemet's membrane. At this level, a semitransparent opacity was observed between the line and the limbus. From the anterior layer of the poorly developed iris stroma (partial iris coloboma), a number of delicate fibrillae traversed the anterior chamber toward this line. He called the abnormality embryotoxon corneae posterius. Axenfeld's patient did not have glaucoma. Rieger in 1935 described a more marked iridocorneal defect in a mother and her two children, showing an autosomal-dominant inheritance pattern. In 1941, Rieger showed an association with dental abnormalities, particularly oligodontia or anodontia.

Axenfeld–Rieger anomaly has been linked to chromosome 6p25 (*FKHL7* gene). Posterior embryotoxon (along with microcornea, mosaic iris stromal hypoplasia, regional peripapillary retinal depigmentation, congenital macular dystrophy, and anomalous optic discs) may be associated with arteriohepatic dysplasia (*Alagille's syndrome*), an autosomal-dominant intrahepatic cholestatic syndrome. Posterior embryotoxon, iris abnormalities, and diffuse fundus hypopigmentation, together with neonatal jaundice, are highly characteristic of *Alagille's syndrome*, which also has a strong association with optic drusen. Another association may be with oculocutaneous albinism.

B. Axenfeld–Rieger syndrome (Rieger's syndrome; Fig. 8.8)
　1. The syndrome includes Axenfeld's anomaly together with more marked anomalous development of the limbus, the anterior-chamber angle, and the iris (ectopia of the pupil, dyscoria, slit pupil, severe hypoplasia of the anterior layer of the iris, iris strands bridging the anterior-chamber angle).

Axenfeld–Rieger's syndrome can be found as part of the SHORT syndrome (short stature, hyperextensibility of joints or hernia, ocular depression, Axenfeld–Rieger's syndrome, and teething delay). Axenfeld–Rieger's syndrome is different from iridogoniodysgenesis, which does not have a linkage to the 4q25 region (see later).

　2. Glaucoma may be present (approximately 60% of cases).
　3. Facial, dental, and osseous abnormalities are present.
　　　Associated neurocristopathy has been reported.
　4. It is inherited as an autosomal-dominant trait, and probably represents abnormal embryonic development of the cranial neural ectoderm.

Genetic causes of Axenfeld–Rieger syndrome include mutations, deletions, or duplications of the forkhead-

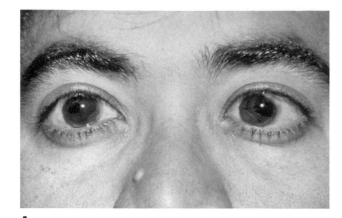

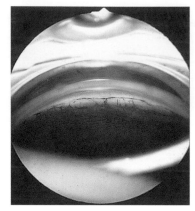

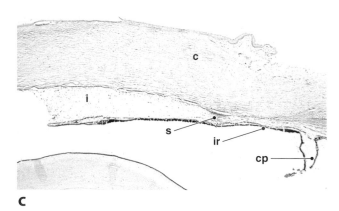

Fig. 8.8 Rieger's syndrome. **A,** The patient has numerous iris abnormalities and bilateral glaucoma. Note the hypertelorism. **B,** The patient's daughter has similar abnormalities. Note the iris processes attached to an anteriorly displaced Schwalbe line (anterior embryotoxon). **C,** Histologic section of an eye from another patient shows an anteriorly displaced Schwalbe ring (s). A diffuse abnormality of the iris stroma is present (c, cornea; i, iris; ir, iris root; cp, ciliary process). (**A** and **B,** Courtesy of Dr. HG Scheie.)

related transcription factor FOXC1, as mutations of the homeodomain (HD) protein PITX2 (*PITX2* gene; chromosome 4q25). Axenfeld–Rieger syndrome caused by a deletion of the paired-box transcription factor *PAX6* has been reported. Finally, a family has been described that has Axenfeld syndrome and Peters' anomaly caused by a point mutation (Phe112Ser) in the *FOXC1* gene

VII. Endothelial dystrophy, iris hypoplasia, congenital cataract, and stromal thinning (EDICT) syndrome

Autosomal-dominant syndrome that has been mapped to chromosome 15q22.1-q25.3.

VIII. An additional familial anterior-segment dysgenesis syndrome includes iris and corneal abnormalities and cataracts.

Histopathologic and electron microscopic examination shows attenuated endothelium with prominent intracellular random aggregates of small-diameter filaments that stained positively for cytokeratin. Other features include abnormal, thickened Descemet's membrane, layered electron-dense material within variably sized vacuoles within and between collagen lamellae and within keratocytes throughout the stroma and Bowman's membrane.

IX. Sclerocornea

A. This condition, usually bilateral, may involve the whole cornea or only its periphery, with superficial or deep vascularization. The cornea appears white and is difficult to differentiate from sclera.

B. Nystagmus, strabismus, aniridia, cornea plana, horizontally oval cornea, glaucoma, and microphthalmos may be present.

C. Congenital cerebral dysfunction, deafness, cryptorchidism, pulmonary disease, brachycephaly, and defects of the face, ears, and skin may also be seen.

D. The condition occurs in three ways: sporadic, isolated cases; familial cases in siblings but without transmission to other generations; and as a dominantly inherited disorder.

Sclerocornea has been described in *Mietens' syndrome.*

E. Histologically, the most frequent findings are increased numbers of collagen fibrils of variable diameters, a decrease in the diameters of collagen fibrils from the anterior to the posterior layers, and a thin Descemet's membrane.

Sclerocornea is mainly a clinical descriptive term, and a distinct clinicopathologic entity of sclerocornea probably does not exist.

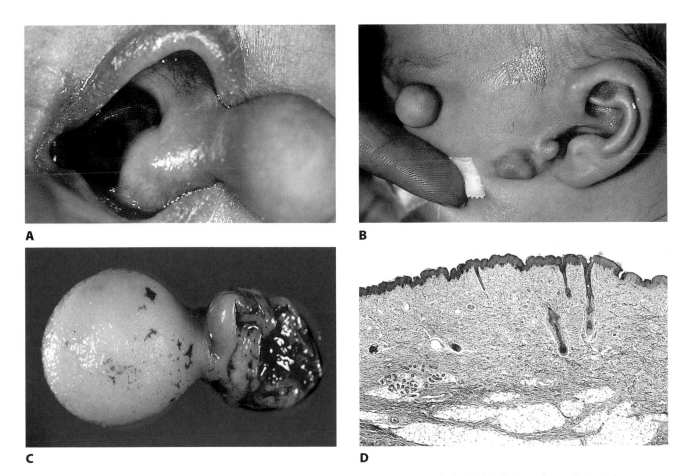

Fig. 8.9 Goldenhar's syndrome. **A,** Pedunculated temporal limbal dermoid present in patient who had Goldenhar's syndrome. **B,** Auricular appendages also present. **C,** Gross specimen of surgically removed pedunculated dermoid. **D,** Histologic section shows epidermis, dermis, epidermal appendages, and adipose tissue. (Case reported in Ziavras E, Farber MG, Diamond G: *Arch Ophthalmol* 108:1032, 1990. © American Medical Association. All rights reserved.)

X. Limbal (corneal; epibulbar) dermoids (Fig. 8.9)
  A. Limbal dermoids are unusual congenital anomalies that contain mesoblastic tissues covered by epithelium.

  > X-linked recessive inheritance has been reported.

  B. They usually occur at the temporal or superior temporal limbal area, but may involve the entire cornea.
     1. Rarely, they may extend through the sclera into the uvea.
     2. Dermoids are choristomas, congenital rests of benign tissue elements in an abnormal location.
        a. Other choristomas in this region include dermolipomas, lacrimal gland choristomas, osseous choristomas, and complex choristomas.
     3. Corneal keloid may mimic dermoid recurrence following surgical excision of the latter lesion.
  C. Histologically, they contain choristomatous tissue (tissue not normally found in the area) such as epidermal appendages, fat, smooth and striated muscle, cartilage, brain, teeth, and bone.
     1. They are covered by corneal or conjunctival epithelium.
     2. They may be cystic or solid.

  D. Goldenhar's syndrome (*Goldenhar–Gorlin* syndrome, oculoauriculovertebral dysplasia; see Fig. 8.9)

  > Goldenhar described the triad of epibulbar dermoids, auricular appendages, and pretragal fistulas in 1952. Gorlin, 11 years later, showed the added association with microtia and mandibular vertebral abnormalities (i.e., oculoauriculovertebral dysplasia).

     1. Goldenhar–Gorlin syndrome is a bilateral condition characterized by epibulbar dermoids, accessory auricular appendages, aural fistulas, vertebral anomalies, and hypoplasia of the soft and bony tissues of the face.

  > Upper-eyelid colobomas commonly occur, but lower-eyelid pseudocolobomas are more often associated with the *Treacher Collins–Franceschetti syndrome*. Epibulbar choristoma, similar to that seen in Goldenhar's syndrome, has been seen in a patient with *nevus sebaceus of Jadassohn*.

     2. Sometimes it is associated with phocomelia and renal malformations.

3. The condition is usually sporadic (frequency approximately 1 : 3000 births), not inherited, and on occasion may be related to first-trimester maternal intake of a teratogenic agent.

4. Histologically, the epibulbar dermoids appear the same as those found elsewhere.

Encephalocraniocutaneous lipomatosis (congenital neurocutaneous syndrome including epibulbar choristomas and connective tissue nevi of the eyelids) should be considered, along with the sebaceous nevus and the Goldenhar–Gorlin syndromes, in the differential diagnosis of epibulbar choristomas.

XI. Dentatorubropallidoluysian atrophy
  A. This neurodegenerative disorder is characterized by choreoathetoid movements, myoclonic seizures, cerebellar ataxia, and dementia.
  B. Decreased corneal endothelial density may be the only ocular finding.
  C. The definitive diagnosis may be made on DNA analysis.
XII. Miscellaneous
  Endothelial abnormalities have been reported in an African American family having a syndrome also characterized by abnormal craniofacial features, and absence of the roof of the sella turcica. Other findings include abnormalities in the maintenance of retinal bipolar cells and of bipolar cells of the auditory system.
  One variation and one mutation of the homeobox transcription factor gene, VSX1 (RINX), characterize this family.

INFLAMMATIONS—NONULCERATIVE

Epithelial Erosions and Keratitis

I. Epithelial erosion may be secondary to traumatic, toxic, radiation-induced (e.g., ultraviolet), or inflammatory (e.g., rubeola) keratitis, or to inherited corneal dystrophies such as lattice and Reis–Bücklers.
  A. The condition is characterized by damage to the corneal epithelial cells, best seen after fluorescein staining of the cornea.
II. Epithelial keratitis may be caused by the same entities that cause epithelial erosions.
  A. It is characterized by large areas of epithelial damage that can be seen grossly without the aid of fluorescein.
  B. *Thygeson's superficial punctate keratitis* is a recurrent corneal disease of unknown cause, characterized by focal epithelial lesions.
    1. The condition is usually bilateral, corneal sensation remains intact, and no accompanying conjunctivitis occurs.
    2. Patients have symptoms of tearing, irritation, and photophobia.

3. The disorder is chronic and may last for 11 years.
  C. (See Chapters 3 and 4.)
    Microsporidial keratitis is usually a disorder of immunocompromised individuals; however, it has been reported to involve apparently immunocompetent patients.
III. Histologically, epithelial erosion and keratitis show prominent basal cell edema of the epithelium, absent hemidesmosomes, and separation of the cells from their basement membrane.

Subepithelial Keratitis

I. Epidemic keratoconjunctivitis (EKC) is a combined epithelial and subepithelial punctate keratitis mainly caused by adenovirus type 8.

The subepithelial opacities, unlike the fine or medium-sized ones with adenoviruses types 3, 4, and 7, tend to be like a cluster of coarse, tiny bread crumbs. The epithelial component is evanescent. Similar findings may be seen with adenovirus type 19. Adenovirus type 8 is the most common cause of EKC. Adenoviruses 3 and 7 are the most common causes of sporadic EKC. Other types (e.g., 1, 2, 4 to 6, 9 to 11, 13 to 15, and 29) may also cause moderate to severe EKC. Among the many other causes of subepithelial keratitis are rosacea, pharyngoconjunctival fever, onchocerciasis, and Crohn's disease. The causes of *nummular keratitis* must also be considered [e.g., Dimmer's (and related processes of Westhoff and of Langraulet) nummular keratitis and the similar interstitial keratitis of Epstein–Barr virus infection, inclusion conjunctivitis (*Chlamydia*), herpes simplex and herpes zoster infection, and brucellosis].

II. Trachoma (see p. 231 in Chapter 7)
III. Leprosy (see p. 81 in Chapter 4)

Superior Limbic Keratoconjunctivitis

I. Superior limbic keratoconjunctivitis (SLK) is characterized by marked inflammation of the tarsal conjunctiva of the upper lid, inflammation of the upper bulbar conjunctiva, fine punctate fluorescein or rose Bengal staining of the cornea at the upper limbus and adjacent conjunctiva above the limbus, and superior limbic proliferation.
II. In approximately one-third of all attacks, filaments occur at the superior limbus or upper cornea.
III. SLK may be associated with thyroid dysfunction and appears to be a prognostic marker for severe Graves' ophthalmopathy.
IV. The cause is unknown.
V. Histology
  A. The conjunctiva shows prominent keratinization of the epithelium with dyskeratosis, acanthosis, cellular infiltration (neutrophils, lymphocytes, and plasma cells), and balloon degeneration of some nuclei.
  B. Electron microscopy shows abnormal distribution and aggregation of nuclear chromatin, filaments in nuclei, dense accumulations of cytoplasmic filaments that surround nuclei and "strangulate" them, and formation of

multilobed nuclei or multinucleated inflammatory cells.

Stromal (Interstitial) Keratitis

I. Viral causes
  A. Herpes simplex virus (HSV; see p. 270 in this chapter)

> It is believed that CD4+ T cells orchestrate the immunologic and inflammatory processes involved in herpes stromal keratitis; however, other variables such as virus replication, cytokine and chemokine production, neovascularization, and contributions from other inflammatory cell types probably set the stage for CD4+ T-cell activities. Conversely, CD8+ T cells reactive to HSV are capable of clearing the virus. Interleukin-17 may play an important role in the induction and/or perpetuation of the immunopathologic processes in human HSV keratitis by modulating the secretion of proinflammatory and neutrophil chemotactic factors by resident corneal fibroblasts. It also probably plays an important role in angiogenesis and tumor growth.

  B. Herpes zoster virus (see p. 78 in Chapter 4)
  C. Epstein–Barr virus (see p. 63 in Chapter 3)

II. Bacterial causes
  A. Syphilis (Fig. 8.10; see also Fig. 8.3B)
    1. Widespread inflammatory infiltrate of the corneal stroma, especially of the deeper layers, is characteristic of luetic keratitis.
    2. An associated anterior uveitis is present in the early stages.
    3. The congenital form
      a. Usually it is bilateral and develops in the second half of the first decade or in the second decade of life.

> It is rare for it to occur before 5 years of age, but the keratitis may be present at birth.

      b. Initially, the cloudy cornea is a result of inflammatory cell infiltration associated with an anterior uveitis that is followed by ingrowth of blood vessels just anterior to Descemet's membrane.

> Sarcoidosis, tuberculosis, leprosy, syphilis, and Cogan's syndrome can all produce a deep interstitial keratitis with deep stromal blood vessels.

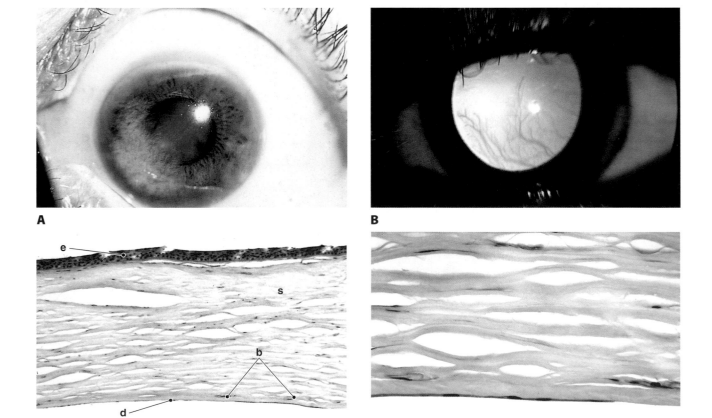

A   **B**

C   **D**

Fig. 8.10 Syphilis. **A,** The cornea shows a range of opacification from a cloudlike nebula, to a moderately dense macula, to a very dense leukoma. **B,** In another case, ghost vessels are easily seen by retroillumination. **C,** The vessels are deep in the corneal stroma (s), just anterior to Descemet's membrane (d). The stroma shows scarring and thinning (e, corneal epithelium; b, blood vessels). **D,** Increased magnification shows blood vessels just anterior to Descemet's membrane (see also Fig. 8.3B). (**A,** Courtesy of Dr. WC Frayer.)

c. The acute inflammation may last 2 to 3 months, followed by a regression over many months.

d. The corneal changes are frequently associated with Hutchinson's teeth and deafness (i.e., *Hutchinson's triad*).

4. The acquired form

a. It is a late manifestation with an average time of appearance of 10 years after the primary luetic infection.

b. It is usually unilateral and often limited to a sector-shaped corneal area.

5. Histology

a. The cornea is edematous and infiltrated by lymphocytes and plasma cells.

1). Blood vessels are present just anterior to Descemet's membrane.

2). With healing, the edema and inflammatory cells disappear, the stroma becomes scarred, and the deep stromal blood vessels persist.

b. In congenital chronic interstitial keratitis, the regenerating corneal endothelium produces excess basement membrane (Descemet's) in a variety of forms.

This produces thickenings of Descemet's membrane, linear cornea guttata, ridges or networks of transparent material (glasleisten), and even networks and strands that project into the anterior chamber.

B. Lyme disease (see p. 83 in Chapter 4)

C. Tuberculosis (see p. 79 in Chapter 4)

III. Parasitic causes

A. Protozoal—leishmaniasis and trypanosomiasis can cause a chronic interstitial keratitis.

B. Nematodal—onchocerciasis (Fig. 8.11)

1. Onchocerciasis is one of the leading causes of blindness in the world, affecting 18 million children and young adults in endemic areas in Africa, and Central and South America.

Uveitis and peripheral anterior and posterior synechiae commonly cause a secondary angle-closure glaucoma. Chorioretinitis secondary to posterior involvement also occurs. The glaucoma and chorioretinitis, along with the keratitis, are common causes of the blindness. The ubiquitous bacteria, *Wolbachia*, colonizes the major pathogenic filarial nematode parasites of humans, including *Onchocerca volvulus*, and may contribute significantly to the inflammatory reaction within the eye.

---

2. Onchocerciasis manifests itself as a severe disease of the skin and eyes (*river blindness*).

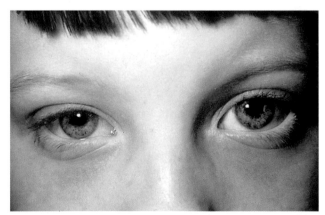

A

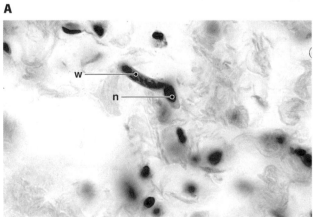

C

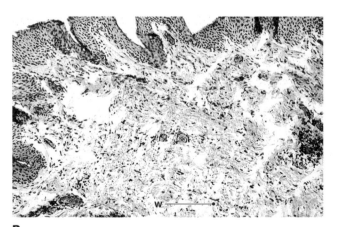

B

Fig. 8.11 Onchocerciasis. **A,** This young girl had just returned from Africa. She had conjunctival infection and small corneal opacities at all levels. During examination at the slit lamp, a tiny, threadlike worm was noted in the aqueous. **B,** Histologic section of a conjunctival biopsy shows a chronic nongranulomatous inflammation and a tiny segment of the worm (w) in the deep substantia propria; this is shown under higher magnification in **C** (w, worm; n, human fibrocyte nucleus). (Case reported in Scheie HG *et al.: Ann Ophthalmol* 3:697, 1971. Reproduced with kind permission of Springer Science and Business Media.)

3. In the acute phase of the infestation, nummular or snowflake corneal opacities form a superficial punctate keratitis.
4. A stromal punctate interstitial keratitis may also occur.

With careful slit-lamp examination, the microfilariae can sometimes be seen in the aqueous fluid in the anterior chamber.

---

5. Healing induces scar tissue to form in the corneal stroma along with a corneal pannus; the cornea can become completely opaque.
6. Optic neuritis and chorioretinitis may also occur and lead to blindness, especially in heavily infested young people.
7. The adult nematode worms, *Onchocerca volvulus*, produce microfilariae that migrate through skin and subcutaneous tissue (not blood) to reach ocular tissue.
   The small black fly, *Simulium* species, ingests the microfilariae from an infected person and transmits them to the next human it bites.

Other filarial nematodes that may involve ocular structures include *Loa loa* and organisms that cause filariasis (e.g., *Wuchereria bancrofti* and *Brugia malayi*).

---

8. Histologically, the tiny worm is found along with an infiltrate of lymphocytes and plasma cells.
   a. Immunologic cross-reactivity of a recombinant antigen of *O. volvulus* to a host ocular component of 44 000 M(r) antigen suggests that intraocular presentation of the cross-reactive parasite antigen by microfilariae is essential for development of the ocular disease.

IV. Other causes
   A. Cogan's syndrome
      1. Cogan's syndrome consists of nonsyphilitic interstitial keratitis and vestibuloauditory involvement.
      2. Patients and their parents have serologies negative for syphilis.
      3. In approximately 70% of cases, an underlying systemic process, often a vasculitis (e.g., periarteritis), occurs.
      4. Atypical presentation of hearing loss may precede corneal symptoms, and result in stromal neovascularization and lipid deposition.
   B. Sarcoidosis (see p. 93 in Chapter 4)
   C. Many other entities, such as atopic keratoconjunctivitis, Hodgkin's disease, lymphogranuloma venereum, hypoparathyroidism, and mycosis fungoides, may cause a secondary stromal keratitis.
   D. Deep stromal keratitis with endothelial involvement and the deposition of polyrefringent crystals may be seen in association with systemic lupus erythematosus. Bilateral corneal immune ring (*Wessely ring*) can occur in Behçet's disease.

Endothelial

Viral
   Endotheliitis may follow mumps parotitis without evidence of epithelial involvement or iridocyclitis.

INFLAMMATIONS—ULCERATIVE*

Peripheral

I. Marginal (catarrhal) ulcer (keratitis; Fig. 8.12)
   A. Marginal ulcer is usually superficial, single, and localized at the limbus or just within the clear cornea.
   B. It may become circumferential to form a superficial marginal keratitis or even a ring ulcer.

An ulcer is characterized by inflammation, necrosis, loss of tissue, progression, and chronicity.

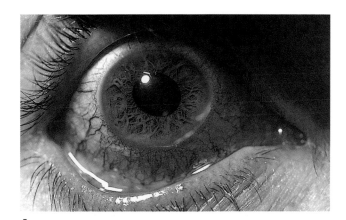

A

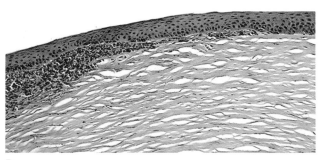

B

Fig. 8.12 Marginal ulcer. **A,** Marginal ulcer (keratitis) present from 3 to 6 o'clock. **B,** Histologic section from another representative case shows a limbal infiltrate of mainly lymphocytes with some plasma cells.

The lesion appears as a gray, crescentic ulcer. It does not spread centrally, but may recur.

C. It is an allergic reaction to toxins or allergens of bacterial conjunctival infections, especially staphylococcal (i.e., an endogenous sensitization to bacterial protein).

D. It may also occur secondary to such systemic diseases as atopy, rheumatoid arthritis, Wegener's granulomatosis, periarteritis nodosa, systemic lupus erythematosus, scleroderma, bacillary dysentery, or Crohn's disease.

E. Histologically, lymphocytes and plasma cells predominate.

II. Phlyctenular ulcer
   A. A phlyctenular ulcer appears early as a small, pinkish-white elevation in a hyperemic limbus; the elevation then develops a central gray crater.

The lesion may remain stationary and evolve through necrosis, shelling out, and healing, or it may travel toward the center of the cornea as a narrow, gray, necrotic, superficial ulcer surrounded by a white infiltrate, having a narrow vascularized scar to mark its path.

   B. It occurs mainly in children, in the first and second decades of life.
   C. It is an allergic reaction to toxins or allergens of conjunctival infections, especially tuberculosis and staphylococcal (i.e., an endogenous sensitization to bacterial protein).
   D. Histologically, lymphocytes and plasma cells predominate.

III. Scleritis-associated peripheral keratopathy
   A. This finding is associated with increased likelihood of necrotizing scleritis, decreased vision, anterior uveitis, impending corneal perforation, and potentially lethal specific-disease association.

IV. Ring ulcer
   A. A ring ulcer (i.e., a superficial ulcer involving the corneal limbus) most often develops in the evolution of superficial marginal keratitis. It may also result from coalescence of several marginal ulcers.
   B. A ring ulcer may be seen with acute systemic diseases such as influenza, bacillary dysentery, ulcerative colitis, acute leukemia, scleroderma, systemic lupus erythematosus, periarteritis nodosa, rheumatoid arthritis, Sjögren's syndrome, Wegener's granulomatosis, midline lethal granuloma syndrome (polymorphic reticulosis), porphyria, brucellosis, gonococcal arthritis, dengue fever, tuberculosis, hookworm infestation, and gold poisoning.
   C. Ischemia, secondary to occlusion of anterior ciliary arteries, may play a major role in its development.
   D. Histologically, the corneal area of involvement is infiltrated with neutrophils, lymphocytes, and plasma cells. Occlusive vasculitis of arteries may be found.

V. Ring abscess (see Fig. 5.23)
   A. Usually, a ring abscess follows trauma to the eye (accidental or surgical).

1. The cornea may not be the initial site of ocular injury.
B. It starts with a 1- to 2-mm, purulent corneal infiltrate in a girdle approximately 1 mm within clear cornea.
   1. A peripheral zone of clear cornea always remains.
   2. The central cornea rapidly becomes necrotic and may slough; a panophthalmitis ensues.
   3. The eye is usually lost.
C. An infectious cause, bacterial or fungal, is most common, but it may also occur with collagen disease.
D. Histologically, the cornea is infiltrated with neutrophils and contains necrotic debris.

Central

I. Viral
   A. HSV (Figs 8.13 and 8.14; see also Fig. 3.6), along with the varicella-zoster viruses, is a member of the subfamily alpha herpesviruses.

The HSV is modest in size, containing only 84 genes (compared with its large relative, the cytomegalovirus, which contains more than 200 genes). HSV consists of a nucleocapsid surrounded by the tegument, a protein compartment, and the envelope. The tegument and the envelope are essential for infectivity.

   1. HSV (see p. 62 in Chapter 3) is the most common cause of central corneal ulcer.
   2. Clinically, it presents as an epithelial infection with a dendritic pattern.
   3. People who have atopic dermatitis are particularly susceptible to HSV infection and may even develop dissemination (eczema herpeticum).

Dendritic keratitis may occur rarely with herpes zoster. Also, *tyrosinemia type II,* an autosomal-recessive disease, is characterized by dendriform keratitis, hyperkeratotic lesions of the palms and soles, and mental retardation (*Richner–Hanhart syndrome*). The corneal pseudodendrites may mimic closely those seen in herpetic keratitis. Dendritic keratitis can also occur with contact lens wear.

   4. A blepharoconjunctivitis associated with HSV may occur in the Wiskott–Aldrich syndrome (see p. 176 in Chapter 6).
   5. HSV that is harbored in neurons in sensory ganglia (mainly trigeminal but possibly also the superior cervical, ciliary, and sphenopalatine) seems to be the main source of recurrent infection at peripheral sites.
      a. A limited transcription of genes is expressed during the latent period.
      b. The virus appears to be transported along the axons.
   6. Complications—spread to stroma, especially with recurrence
      a. Disciform keratitis is a chronic, localized, discoid opacity.

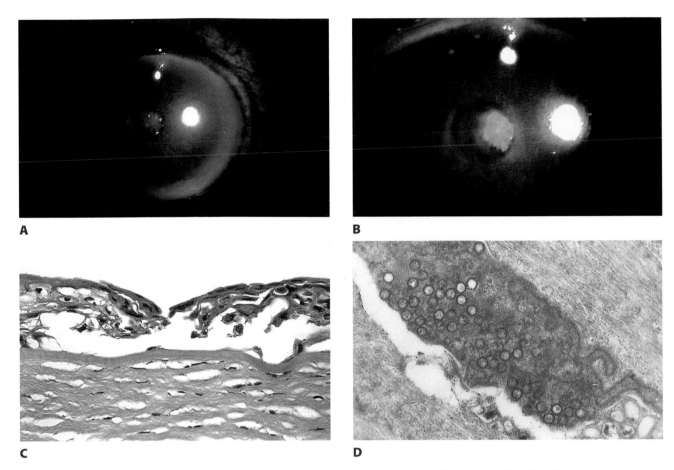

Fig. 8.13 Herpes simplex. Central corneal ulcer (**A**) shows typical dendritic ulcer when stained with fluorescein (**B**). **C,** Many intranuclear inclusions present in corneal epithelium near edge of ulcer. **D,** Virus particles of herpes simplex present in nucleus. Some particles show empty capsids, whereas others are complete, containing nucleoids. (**C** and **D,** Courtesy of Prof. GOH Naumann.)

b. Bullous keratopathy (metaherpetic phase) is associated with stromal involvement and epithelial edema (see Fig. 8.14).

c. HSV antigens have been found in keratocytes, corneal endothelial cells, and foci of epithelioid histiocytes and multinucleated inflammatory giant cells around Bowman's and Descemet's membrane.

Involvement of the corneal endothelium by HSV antigens suggests that the endothelium may play a significant role in chronic ocular herpetic disease.

---

7. Histologically, HSV keratitis is characterized by Cowdry type A epithelial intranuclear inclusion bodies, mainly T lymphocytes, and plasma cells.

a. By electron microscopy, viral particles are found in the epithelial nucleus and cytoplasm.

b. With deep involvement, stromal edema and infiltration with lymphocytes and plasma cells are found.

c. Multinucleated giant cells may be seen, often in association with Bowman's or Descemet's membranes (granulomatous reaction to Descemet's membrane; see p. 97 in Chapter 4), or even in the anterior chamber or iris.

d. Epithelial involvement may be associated with the use of antiglaucoma medications, including latanoprost and topical beta-blocker.

e. Corneal involvement may be associated with endotheliitis. Endotheliitis has been reported in association with other viruses, including vesicular virus (family Rhabdoviridae).

B. Vaccinia

C. Varicella

D. Trachoma (see p. 231 in Chapter 7)

II. Bacterial (Fig. 8.15; see also Fig. 1.1)—these cause a purulent infiltrate of polymorphonuclear leukocytes.

A. *Pneumococcus*

B. β-Hemolytic *Streptococcus*

C. *Pseudomonas aeruginosa*

D. *Klebsiella pneumoniae* (Friedlander)

E. Petit's diplobacillus

F. *Staphylococcus aureus*

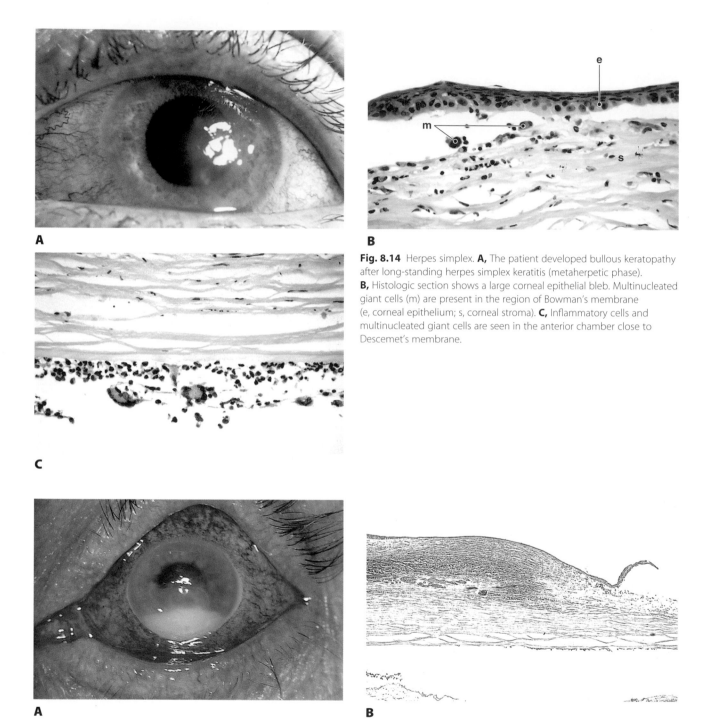

Fig. 8.14 Herpes simplex. **A,** The patient developed bullous keratopathy after long-standing herpes simplex keratitis (metaherpetic phase). **B,** Histologic section shows a large corneal epithelial bleb. Multinucleated giant cells (m) are present in the region of Bowman's membrane (e, corneal epithelium; s, corneal stroma). **C,** Inflammatory cells and multinucleated giant cells are seen in the anterior chamber close to Descemet's membrane.

Fig. 8.15 Bacterial ulcer. **A,** Note central ulcer and large reactive hypopyon. **B,** The right side of the picture shows ulceration. The corneal stroma is infiltrated with polymorphonuclear leukocytes and large, purple, amorphous collections of material. Special stain of the purple areas showed a collection of many Gram-positive bacteria. (**A,** Courtesy of Dr. HG Scheie.)

G. *Haemophilus aphrophilus* and *Streptococcus viridans*, relatively nonvirulent bacteria, may cause a crystalline keratopathy (see subsection *Crystals*, later).

III. Mycotic (Fig. 8.16)

A. Mycotic keratitis is characterized by a "dry" main lesion that may be accompanied by satellite lesions.

   1. Hypopyon is common.

B. Fungus is found most readily in scrapings from viable tissue at the margin and depths of the ulcer rather than in the necrotic central debris.

C. The keratitis may be caused by molds (e.g., *Aspergillus*) or yeasts (e.g., *Candida*).

D. Fungal keratitis is usually a complication of trauma resulting from contamination by plant or animal

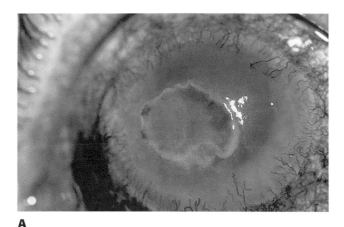

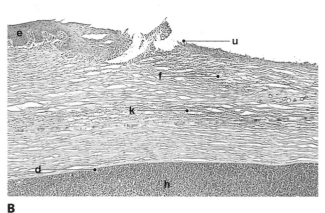

A

B

Fig. 8.16 Mycotic ulcer. **A,** The patient had a central corneal ulcer that was caused by a pigmented fungus. **B,** Histologic section of another case shows ulceration (u) of the corneal epithelium (e) and infiltration of the corneal stroma by polymorphonuclear leukocytes and large fungal elements (f). A hypopyon (h), consisting of polymorphonuclear leukocytes and cellular debris, is seen in the anterior chamber (k, keratitis; d, Descemet's membrane). Often, fungal ulcers have satellite corneal lesions and a hypopyon.

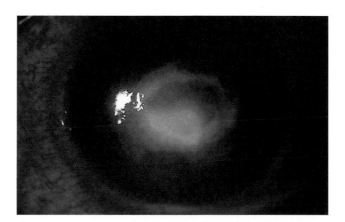

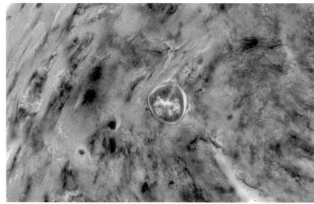

A

B

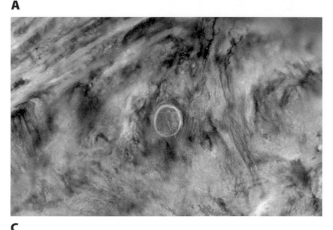

C

Fig. 8.17 *Acanthamoeba.* **A,** Patient was hit in his eye with a stick. Approximately 3 weeks later, the eye became irritated. Note ring infiltrate and central epithelial defect, which stains with fluorescein. Initially he was treated for bacterial ulcer without improvement. A biopsy was performed. **B** and **C,** Note organisms as round cysts of *Acanthamoeba,* one of which contains a nucleus. (**A.** Courtesy of Dr. KF Heffler.)

matter (e.g., as seen in farmers or contact lens wearers).

  E. Histologically, the inflammatory infiltrate may be granulomatous, chronic nongranulomatous, or, rarely, purulent.

  F. Fungal toxins may be important in the pathophysiology of these infections.

IV. Parasitic

  A. *Acanthamoeba* (Fig. 8.17)

    1. Acanthamoebic organisms are ubiquitous, free-living, usually nonparasitic protozoa found in soil, fresh water (e.g., tap water, hot tubs, and swimming pools), and the human oral cavity.

Water storage tanks promote colonization of free-living *Acanthamoeba* and increase the risk of keratitis caused by *Acanthamoeba* in contact lens wearers who use tap water in contact lens care routines.

2. Most cases of acanthamoebic keratitis occur in contact lens wearers.
3. Typically, acanthamoebic keratitis presents with pain, central or paracentral disc-shaped corneal ulcerations, and anterior or mid stromal total or partial ring infiltration.

Rarely, *Acanthamoeba* can cause a chorioretinitis after the keratitis or with prolonged keratitis.

   a. The keratitis has a waxing and waning course, with periods of improvement over days and weeks, but is generally progressive over months, often leading to corneal opacification, ulceration, and even perforation.
   b. Scleral infection may also occur (sclerokeratitis) and may be responsible for much of the pain.
   c. Corneal sensation is often decreased and may lead to the erroneous diagnosis of herpes simplex keratitis.
4. Histologically, numerous acanthamoebic cysts are seen in the corneal stroma by light microscopy and motile trophozoites by culture.
   a. Neutrophils are the most common inflammatory cell.
      1). Confocal microscopy (CFM) can be helpful in the diagnosis. Rarely, a florid granulomatous necrotizing reaction can involve both stroma and anterior chamber.
      2). Impression cytology can also aid in the early diagnosis of the disorder.
   b. Macrophages appear to play an important role in fighting the infestation by acting as a first line of defense in eliminating significant numbers of Acanthamoeba trophozoites.

INFLAMMATIONS—CORNEAL SEQUELAE

   I. Descemetocele
   II. Ectasia (i.e., thinned, protruding area)
   III. Staphyloma (i.e., ectasia lined by uveal tissue)
   IV. Cicatrization (i.e., scarring)
   V. Vascularization (Fig. 8.18)
   VI. Adherent leukoma (i.e., corneal perforating scar with iris adherent to posterior corneal surface; see Fig. 8.4)
   VII. Exposure keratitis (xerosis) (see Fig. 7.11)

INJURIES

See Chapter 5.

DEGENERATIONS

Degenerations (Table 8.1) may be unilateral or bilateral and are secondary phenomena after previous disease (i.e., ocular "fingerprints" of prior disease).

Epithelial

   I. Keratitis sicca
      A. Because the watery part of the tear secretion is lacking, corneal epithelial punctate erosions develop in exposed areas.

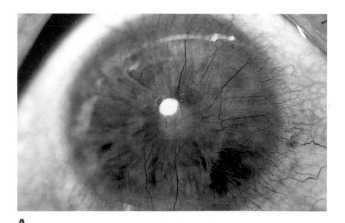

A

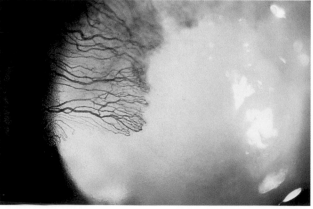

B

Fig. 8.18 Corneal vascularization. **A,** The corneal stroma is vascularized by large trunk vessels. **B,** Another eye shows new blood vessels growing into superficial cornea from the limbus. Corneal vascularization usually occurs in the superficial and mid stromal corneal layers.

An abnormal Schirmer's test result is a universal finding. In addition, approximately 85% of patients show excess ocular tear film mucus, thinned tear film, and decreased marginal tear strip; 80% have corneal and conjunctival staining when tested with rose Bengal (see section *Normal Anatomy*, earlier); and 75% demonstrate an associated conjunctival staphylococcal infection or blepharitis. Corneal mucous plaques of various thicknesses, sizes, and shapes, firmly attached to the corneal epithelium, are also frequently found.

B. Epithelial filaments (filamentary keratitis; Fig. 8.19) may develop.

Filamentary keratitis occurs in approximately 55% of patients. It may also be found in conditions such as Sjögren's syndrome, SLK, viral infections, and after cataract extraction. It is a particu-

lar problem for patients in a chronic vegetative state. A common finding in individuals who develop filamentary keratitis is epithelial edema.

C. Keratitis sicca may be related to *Sjögren's syndrome* (see Fig. 14.8), which consists of keratoconjunctivitis sicca, xerostomia, and rheumatoid arthritis or other connective tissue disease.

D. Corneal melting in Sjögren's syndrome is rare; however, it has occurred as the initial presentation of the disorder.

Epstein–Barr virus may be a risk factor in the pathogenesis of Sjögren's syndrome. Likewise, Sjögren's syndrome (and other chronic autoimmune diseases) constitutes a risk factor for the development of non-Hodgkin's lymphomas.

E. Histologically, filaments are composed of degenerated epithelial cells and mucus.
   1. In Sjögren's syndrome, aside from a mononuclear inflammation, squamous metaplasia of the conjunctival epithelium, extensive goblet cell loss, and mucus aggregates are seen.
   2. Immunocytochemical studies of lacrimal gland biopsies from patients who have Sjögren's syndrome show that the major component of the mononuclear infiltrate consists of B cells and Leu-3+ T-helper cells.

II. Recurrent erosion
A. The epithelium forms small blebs and then desquamates in recurring cycles.

Frequently, the blebs rupture when the eyelids are opened in the morning. This leads to the complaint of sharp, severe pain on awakening with the pain subsiding as the day progresses.

B. The condition usually follows incomplete healing of a traumatic corneal abrasion, most commonly a fingernail, paper, or plant injury.

TABLE 8.1 Degenerations

EPITHELIAL

I. Keratitis sicca
II. Recurrent erosion
III. Keratomalacia
IV. Neuroparalytic keratopathy
V. Exposure keratopathy

STROMAL

I. Arcus senilis
II. Pterygium
III. Terrien's ulcer
IV. Calcific band keratopathy
V. Climatic droplet keratopathy
VI. Salzmann's nodular degeneration
VII. Lipid keratopathy
VIII. Amyloidosis
IX. Limbus girdle of Vogt
X. Mooren's ulcer
XI. Delle
XII. Anterior crocodile shagreen of Vogt

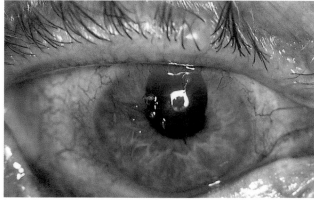

A

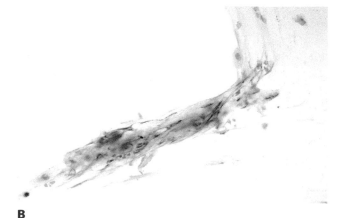

B

Fig. 8.19 Filamentary keratitis. **A,** Numerous filaments in the form of ropy secretions are present on the cornea, mainly superiorly. **B,** Histologic section shows that the filaments are composed of epithelial cells and mucinous material.

C. It may be inherited as an autosomal-dominant trait, but most are not inherited.

Probably at least 50% of recurrent erosions are associated with dot, fingerprint, and geographic patterns (see p. 286 in this chapter).

D. The cause is uncertain but seems to be a defect in the epithelium that produces an abnormal basement membrane.

III. Keratomalacia

A. Keratomalacia, caused by a deficiency of vitamin A, is characterized by diffuse, excessive keratinization of all mucous membrane epithelia, including the cornea and conjunctiva (*xerophthalmia*).

B. The condition occurs most often in children, who characteristically complain of night blindness.

Keratomalacia is caused by vitamin A deficiency itself or in association with kwashiorkor, protein deficiency, cystic fibrosis, or multiple vitamin deficiency, as seen in underdeveloped countries, in people on fad diets, or in the cachectic hospitalized patient. Keratomalacia leading to descemetocele formation may occur in cystic fibrosis. Vitamin A deficiency is a public health problem of great magnitude in underdeveloped countries; it is estimated that xerophthalmia develops in over 5 million children annually, of whom 250000 or more become blind. It is thought to be the leading cause of blindness in children in many underdeveloped countries.

C. It may proceed to hypopyon ulcer, corneal necrosis, panophthalmitis, and even corneal perforation.

Secondary infection by bacteria probably plays a major role in causing the corneal ulceration that may ultimately lead to corneal perforation.

D. Bitot's spot
   1. Bitot's spot is a localized form of keratomalacia, usually involving the limbus, and shows a thickened, bubbly appearance to the involved area.
   2. It is usually associated with, or is a sequela of, vitamin A deficiency.
   3. Young boys are affected most commonly.
   4. *Corynebacterium xerosis* bacteria are found in great numbers on the lesion.

E. Histologically, xerophthalmia shows a thickened and keratinized corneal and conjunctival epithelium associated with loss of conjunctival goblet cells. Extreme cases appear as skin epithelium with rete ridges.

IV. Neuroparalytic keratopathy

A. Early neuroparalytic keratopathy, which may resemble recurrent erosion, often progresses to almost total corneal epithelial desquamation.

B. Frequently, it is complicated by secondary infection that leads to perforation.

C. The condition is caused by a lesion anywhere along the course of the ophthalmic division of the fifth cranial nerve and results in partial or complete loss of corneal sensitivity. It usually runs a chronic, slow course.

Significant neurotrophic corneal disease can occur in diabetic patients. Decreased corneal sensitivity in many patients who have diabetes mellitus is believed to be part of a generalized polyneuropathy.

V. Exposure keratopathy—exposure of the cornea from any cause can lead to epidermidalization (xerosis; see Fig. 7.11) and scarring.

Stromal

I. Arcus senilis (gerontoxon; Fig. 8.20)

A. Lipid deposit is limited to the peripheral cornea and central sclera.
   1. It starts earliest at the inferior pole of the cornea, then involves the superior, becoming annular in the late stage.
   2. The lipid first concentrates in the area of Descemet's membrane, then in the area of Bowman's membrane, forming two apex-to-apex triangles (both clinically and histologically).
   3. Clinically, the extreme anterior peripheral cornea appears free of lipid.

Rarely, lipid accumulates in such large quantities that it may extend into the visual axis (*primary lipidic degeneration of the cornea*). Also rarely, unilateral arcus senilis can occur, usually after blunt trauma or associated with unilateral carotid artery disease.

B. Arcus senilis may have a recessive inheritance pattern.
   1. People younger than 50 years of age who have arcus senilis have a significantly higher incidence of coronary heart disease.
   2. People older than 50 years of age who have arcus senilis have an increased chance of having hypercholesterolemia and hypertriglyceridemia.
   3. Arcus senilis in some patients seems to have an association with alcoholism.

C. Histologically, a narrow peripheral ring of lipid deposit is characteristic.
   1. An anterior stromal triangular lipid deposit is present with its base within Bowman's membrane, near its termination.
   2. A similar stromal triangular lipid deposit is present with its base along and within the periphery of Descemet's membrane.
   3. The peripheral margin of the arcus is sharply defined, whereas the central margin is less discrete.
   4. Histologically (and clinically), it appears identical to an arcus juvenilis.

Histologically, a similar concentration of lipid is demonstrable in the superficial and deep layers of the anterior

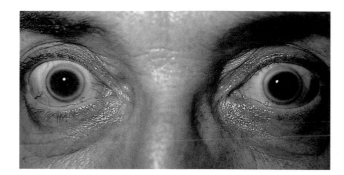

A

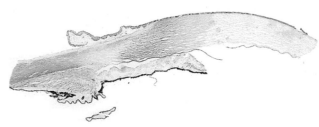

B

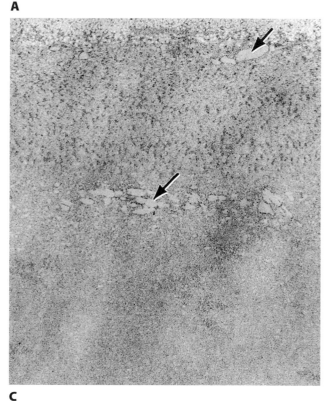

C

Fig. 8.20 Arcus senilis. **A,** A white ring is in the peripheral cornea of each eye. The ring is separated from the limbus by a narrow clear zone. **B,** Histologic section shows that the lipid is concentrated in the anterior and posterior stroma as two red triangles, apex to apex, with the bases being Bowman's and Descemet's membranes, both of which are heavily infiltrated by fat (red staining), as is the sclera. **C,** Arrows indicate sites of lipidic deposits in two planes of Descemet's membrane, as seen by transmission electron microscopy. (**B,** oil red-O stain; **C,** modified from Fine BS *et al.: Am J Ophthalmol* 78:12. Copyright Elsevier 1974.)

sclera posterior to the vascular limbal region, which is free of lipid. Clinically, the lipid is not visible in the opaque, white sclera.

II. Pterygium (Fig. 8.21)
   A. The cause is unknown.

p53 mutations within limbal epithelial cells, probably caused by ultraviolet irradiation, may be an early event in the development of pingueculae, pterygia, and some limbal tumors.

   B. The conjunctival component is identical histologically to pinguecula (see p. 237 in Chapter 7).
   C. Usually it develops nasally, rarely temporally, and is most often bilateral.
   D. Histologically, both pterygia and pingueculae show basophilic degeneration (actinic or senile elastosis) of the subepithelial substantia propria (see Fig. 7.12).

The epithelium overlying a pterygium and a pinguecula may show a variety of secondary changes such as orthokeratosis, acanthosis, and dyskeratosis.

   1. The characteristic that distinguishes a pterygium from a pinguecula is the invasion of superficial cornea preceded by dissolution of Bowman's membrane in pterygia.
   2. Mast cells occur in increased numbers in pterygia.
   3. Deep corneal changes at the level of endothelium and Descemet's membrane may be seen in association with long-standing nasal pterygia in elderly individuals. Endothelial cell density may be reduced in these individuals.
   4. Pterygium cells, which are altered limbal basal epithelial cells, stain positively for multiple types of matrix metalloproteinases, unlike normal conjunctival, limbal, and corneal cells. These cells may con-

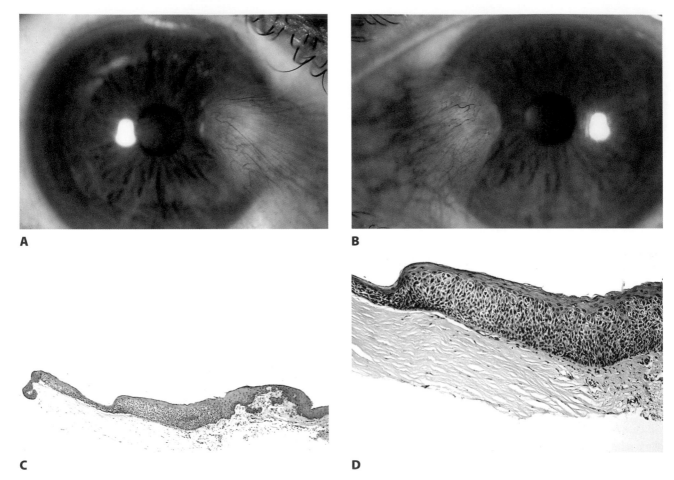

Fig. 8.21 Pterygium. Clinical appearance of typical nasal pterygium in right (**A**) and left (**B**) eyes. **C,** Histologic section of another case shows basophilic degeneration of the conjunctival substantia propria (identical to that seen in a pinguecula) toward the right (shown with increased magnification on the far right side of **D**) and invasion of the cornea with "dissolution" of Bowman's membrane toward the left (shown with increased magnification on the left of **D**); note dysplastic conjunctival epithelium on right. It is the invasion of the cornea that distinguishes a pterygium from a pinguecula (see also Fig. 7.12).

tribute to the dissolution of Bowman's membrane, a characteristic of pterygium. These cells may activate fibroblasts at the head of the pterygium, and may play an important role in the formation and migration of the pterygium.

III. Terrien's ulcer (chronic peripheral furrow keratitis; symmetric marginal dystrophy; gutter degeneration; Fig. 8.22)

   A. The lesion, a limbal depression or gutter, starts as fine, yellow-white, punctate opacities supranasally, usually bilaterally, and spreads circumferentially, rarely reaching inferiorly. It develops slowly, often taking 10 to 20 years.

   B. The peripheral involvement is located similarly to an arcus senilis, so that a clear corneal ring is present between the peripheral margin and the limbus.

   C. The central wall is very steep, and the peripheral wall slopes gradually. The sharp, steep central edge is demarcated by a white-gray line.

   D. The epithelium remains intact, but the underlying stroma thins, and the gutter widens.

    1. The base of the gutter later characteristically becomes vascularized with superficial radial blood vessels that extend across the groove to its anterior extent.

    2. The base also shows scarring and lipid infiltration at the leading edge.

   E. The floor may become so thin that normal intraocular pressure produces an ectasia. Rarely, the lesion may perforate.

   F. The cause is unknown, but degeneration and hypersensitivity have been proposed.

Similar lesions may be seen in rheumatoid arthritis and Sjögren's syndrome, but differ from marginal degeneration in that they are usually located inferiorly, are not vascularized, and rarely encircle the cornea.

   G. Histologically, the main feature is a peripheral corneal stromal thinning.

    1. Fewer than 25% of the resident cells express major histocompatibility complex class II antigens, the

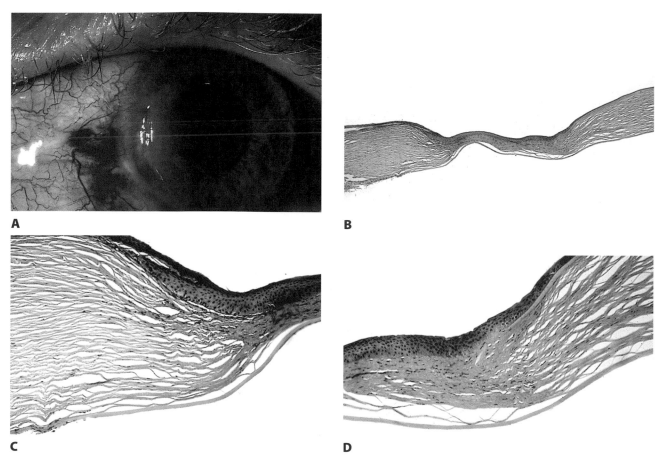

Fig. 8.22 Terrien's ulcer. **A,** Clinical appearance of ulcer. **B,** Histologic section shows limbus on left (iris not present) and central cornea to right. Note marked stromal thinning. Increased magnification shows marked stromal thinning, thickened epithelium, and loss of Bowman's membrane on both limbal side (**C**) and central side (**D**). (Courtesy of Dr. PR Laibson.)

ratio of CD4 cells (T-helper/inducer) to CD8 cells (T-suppressor/cytotoxic) approaches 1 : 1, and fewer than 5% of the infiltrating cells stain positively for CD22 (B cells)—compare with Mooren's ulcer on p. 284 of this chapter.

IV. Calcific band keratopathy (Figs 8.23 through 8.25)

A. Calcific band keratopathy starts in the nasal and temporal periphery with a translucent area at the level of Bowman's membrane; the semiopaque area contains characteristic circular clear areas.

B. The extreme peripheral cornea remains clear, but the central cornea may ultimately become involved.

C. A deposition of calcium salts in and around Bowman's membrane is apparently related to abnormal epithelial activity.

D. Calcific band keratopathy may be secondary to primary hyperparathyroidism; increased vitamin D absorption; chronic renal failure; ocular disease, especially uveitis, and particularly when associated with Still's disease; long-standing glaucoma; local pilocarpine therapy (when pilocarpine contains phenylmercuric nitrate as a preservative); and some forms of nonspecific superficial injury (e.g., from experimental laser).

1. Calcific band keratopathy may develop rapidly in corneas treated with steroid–phosphate drops.

2. Calcific band keratopathy may coexist with climatic droplet keratopathy (CDK; see Fig. 8.25).

3. The degeneration can recur even bilaterally following corneal transplantation.

Superficial reticular degeneration of Kolby is an atypical form of band keratopathy.

E. Histologically, a blue granular material (calcium salts) is seen in and around Bowman's membrane.

V. Climatic droplet keratopathy (CDK Labrador keratopathy; elastotic degeneration; spheroidal degeneration; noncalcific band keratopathy; Bietti's nodular hyaline band-shaped keratopathy; chronic actinic keratopathy; oil droplet degeneration; Nama keratopathy; proteinaceous corneal degeneration; and other designations; see Fig. 8.25)

A. "Oil droplet" or hyaline-like deposits may occur in the superficial corneal stroma, usually bilaterally, in a variety of chronic ocular and corneal disorders having in common a relationship to climate (i.e., outdoor exposure).

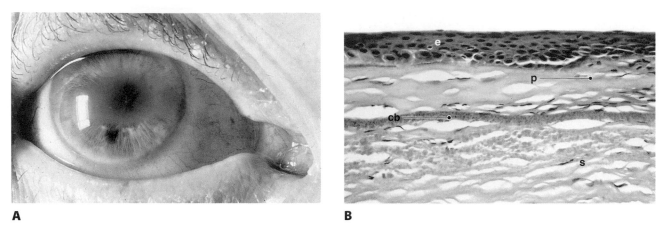

Fig. 8.23 Band keratopathy. **A,** Clinical appearance of the band occupying the central horizontal zone of the cornea and typically sparing the most peripheral clear cornea. **B,** A fibrous pannus (p) is present between the epithelium (e) and a calcified Bowman's membrane (cb). Some deposit is also present in the anterior corneal stroma (s).

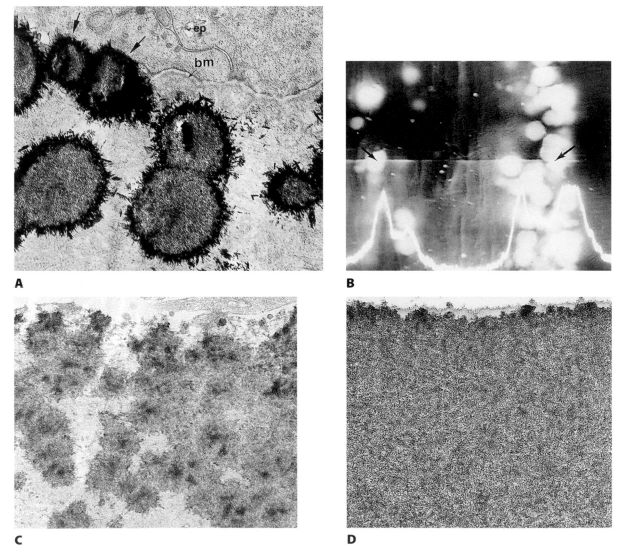

Fig. 8.24 Band keratopathy. **A,** Spherules (*arrows*) in Bowman's layer reach to, but not through, basal plasmalemmas of epithelial basal cells (ep), as seen by transmission electron microscopy. Each spherule consists of a peripheral ring of dense fine crystals surrounding a lucent core. Some spherules fuse together (bm, thin basement membrane of epithelial basal cells). **B,** Calcium line scan across specimen (*arrows*). Concentration of calcium across line scan shown in lower part of figure correlates with calcific spherules. **C,** Moderate-severity calcific band keratopathy. Reversal of spherule density to dense center and lucent periphery (compare with **A**) before fusion of spherules into homogeneous mass of calcium on right. **D,** Late stage of calcific band keratopathy. Homogeneous calcific mass shows no evidence of its formation from calcific spherules.

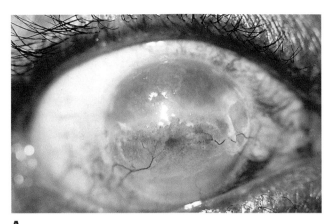

A

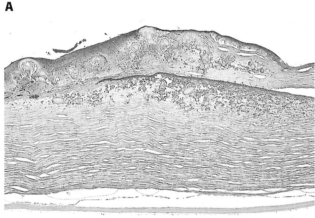

B

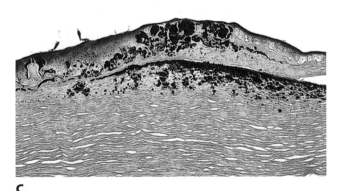

C

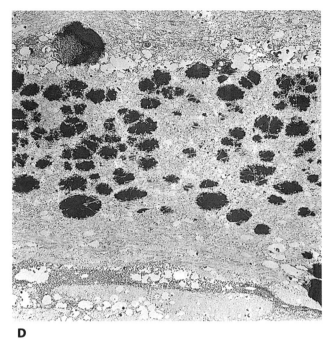

D

Fig. 8.25 Climatic droplet keratopathy. **A,** Band keratopathy contains yellow globules. Eye was enucleated. **B,** Histologic section shows Bowman's membrane as a dark line from the right side, extending two-thirds of the way across the upper quarter of the cornea. Large globules are present in the pannus above Bowman's membrane and in the corneal stroma just below. **C,** Bowman's membrane and the granules stain black with an elastic-tissue stain. **D,** Electron microscopically, small, dense, irregular granules are present in Bowman's layer, many traversed by collagen fibrils. The largest granule shows the characteristic diphasic structure (i.e., lucent or separated macromolecules) coalescing into denser body. Granules are resistant to digestion with elastase.

The droplets usually appear as small, golden-yellow spherules in the subepithelial cornea and conjunctiva. In geographic areas where the eyes are exposed to climatic extremes and to the effects of wind-blown sand or ice, the deposits often occur in a band-shaped pattern across the central cornea. In areas with considerable sunlight but without the traumatic effects of wind-blown sand or ice, pingueculae may also be seen. CDK may occur along with calcific band keratopathy (see earlier discussion).

B. The condition may result from the cumulative effect of chronic actinic irradiation, presumably ultraviolet irra-

diation. Ultraviolet exposure from welding may also contribute to this disorder.

C. Band-shaped, spheroidal keratopathy has been reported in a Chinese family.

Occasionally patients who have corneal elastotic degeneration also show lattice lines in all layers of corneal stroma. Histologically, the lines are positive for amyloid.

D. CDK may be divided into a *primary type* (degenerative, related to aging; or dystrophic in young people) and a *secondary type* (secondary to other ocular disease, e.g., herpetic keratitis and lattice dystrophy, or secondary to the environment, e.g., climatic extremes, wind-blown sand).

    1. CDK is an important cause of blindness in rural populations of the developing world.

E. Histologically, granules and concretions of variable size and shape are located in the superficial stroma and in and around Bowman's membrane.

    1. When extremely small and localized to Bowman's membrane, the granules and concretions are difficult to distinguish from calcium unless special stains are used.

    2. The deposits resemble most the degenerated connective tissue of pingueculae and are considered a form of elastotic degeneration of collagen.

VI. Climatic proteoglycan stromal keratopathy (CPSK)

A. The condition appears mainly in the seventh decade, predominantly in men, and is usually bilateral, although sometimes asymmetric.

B. CPSK occurs in people exposed to the sunny, dry, dusty environment of the Middle East and is thought to be caused by climatic factors.

C. Clinically, CPSK shows a central, horizontally oval corneal stromal haze (ground-glass appearance), of a uniform or lamellar pattern, and occupying 50% to 100% stromal thickness but greatest density in anterior stroma.

D. Histologically, excessive focal intracellular and extracellular proteoglycan deposits are seen.

VII. Salzmann's nodular degeneration (Fig. 8.26)

A. The condition, an elevated white or yellow corneal area, is usually unilateral (but may be bilateral), occurs mainly in women, and is often superimposed on an area of old corneal injury, especially along the edge of an old pannus.

In general, a characteristic history of keratitis is obtained. The keratitis may be phlyctenular, vernal, or secondary to systemic childhood infections such as scarlet fever or measles, or it may be from trachoma. In many cases, however, no previous history of eye disease is obtained.

B. The condition may recur after lamellar excision.

C. Histologically, the epithelium shows areas of both hypertrophy and atrophy, with a marked increase of

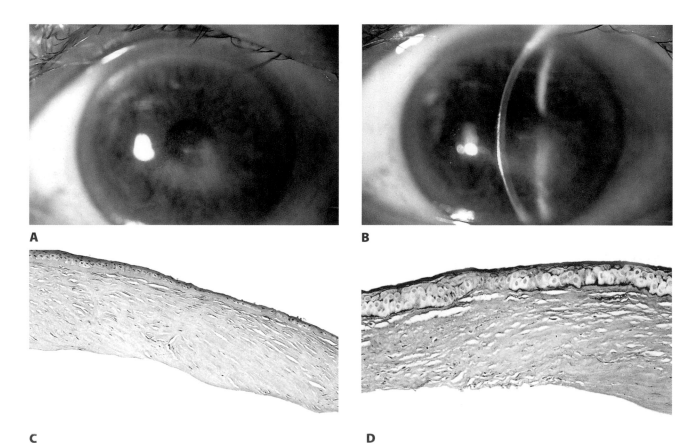

A

B

C

D

Fig. 8.26 Salzmann's nodular degeneration. **A,** Superficial lesion is present in the region of Bowman's membrane in the right eye (slit lamp view in **B**). An almost identical lesion had been removed from the same location 2 years previously. A smaller, similar lesion was present in the inferior central portion of the left eye. **C,** A lamellar biopsy of the first lesion shows marked thinning and basal edema of the epithelium. Bowman's membrane is replaced in many areas by collagen tissue. **D,** Periodic acid–Schiff stain shows irregular thickening of the epithelial basement membrane. (**C** and **D,** Courtesy of Dr. RC Eagle, Jr.)

subepithelial basement membrane material and scar tissue. CFM reveals irregularly shaped basal epithelium with foci of prominent nuclei, and disrupted anterior stromal architecture having an increased reflectivity of the anterior stromal matrix within the nodules.

D. A degeneration characterized by subepithelial fibrosis atypical for Salzmann degeneration is termed "peripheral hypertrophic corneal degeneration."

VIII. Lipid keratopathy (*secondary lipidic degeneration;* Fig. 8.27)

A. Lipid keratopathy may be unilateral or bilateral and follows old injury, especially surgical.

B. Clinically, it appears as a nodular, yellow, often elevated corneal infiltrate.

C. Histologically, the lipid deposition is mainly located in a thick pannus between Bowman's membrane and epithelium.

Lipid keratopathy and primary lipidic degeneration are related. Primary lipidic degeneration seems to be an exaggeration of an arcus senilis, whereas secondary lipidic degeneration follows corneal vascularization.

IX. Amyloidosis (see p. 238 in Chapter 7)

A. Secondary amyloidosis is rarely found as an isolated corneal degeneration.

1. For example, it has been reported in advanced congenital glaucoma.

B. It has been described as secondary to different ocular diseases (e.g., trachoma, interstitial keratitis, retinopathy of prematurity, trichiasis, and penetrating injury).

C. Primary amyloidosis of the cornea may be seen in three forms.

1. Lattice dystrophy (see p. 294 in this chapter)

2. Primary gelatinous droplike dystrophy (see p. 296 in this chapter)

3. Polymorphic amyloid degeneration (polymorphic stromal dystrophy) is characterized by deep, punctate, and filamentous stromal lesions, which resemble crystalline opacities in early lattice corneal dystrophy (LCD).

D. Histology (see Figs 7.13 and 7.14)

X. Limbus girdle of Vogt

A. The limbus girdle of Vogt appears as a symmetric, yellowish-white corneal opacity forming a half-moon-like

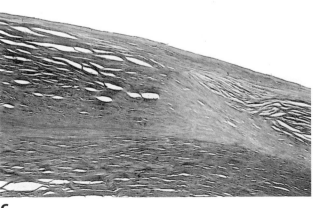

A

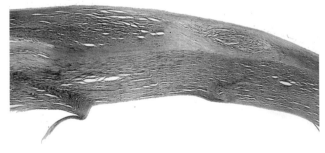

B

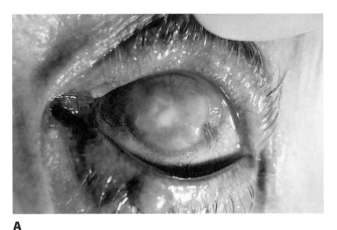

C

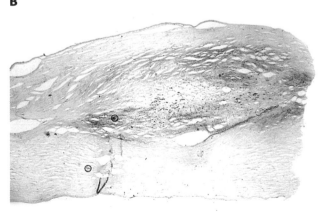

D

Fig. 8.27 Lipid keratopathy. **A,** Both eyes in a patient who had had pterygium surgery approximately 30 years previously developed secondary lipid keratopathy. Corneal graft was performed. **B,** In this acid mucopolysaccharide-stained section of the removed cornea, the pale areas are in a pannus above Bowman's membrane. **C,** Increased magnification shows a linear, deeply stained Bowman's membrane above which is a lipid-containing pannus with a cluster of clefts (which had contained cholesterol crystals) on the far right. **D,** Oil red-O stain is positive (red) for lipid, mainly in pannus.

arc running concentrically within the limbus superficially in the interpalpebral fissure zone, most commonly nasally.

B. Histologically, Bowman's membrane and superficial stroma are largely replaced by basophilic granular deposits.

XI. Mooren's ulcer (chronic serpiginous ulcer; Fig. 8.28)

A. Mooren's ulcer is a chronic, painful ulceration of the cornea. There appear to be two different types.

1. A comparatively benign type, which is usually unilateral, occurs in older people and clears with relatively conservative surgery.

2. A relentlessly progressive type, which is also usually bilateral (approximately 25% of all cases of Mooren's ulcer are bilateral), occurs in younger people and does not clear with any therapy.

B. The ulcer starts in the peripheral cornea and spreads in three directions:

1. Initially, circumferentially

2. Then rapidly, centrally, with the leading edge de-epithelialized, undermined, and often infiltrated with plasma cells and lymphocytes

3. Slowest movement is toward sclera

C. The ulcer may be relentlessly progressive or self-limited.

That inappropriate immunologic responses may be the cause of Mooren's ulcer, or play an important role in the cause, is suggested by: the occasional association of Mooren's-like ulcer with autoimmune disease; the finding of subepithelial tissue from Mooren's ulcer packed with plasma cells and lymphocytes; the demonstration of immunoglobulins and complement bound to conjunctival epithelium and circulating antibodies to conjunctival and corneal epithelium; and, finally, the finding of cellular immunity in the form of positive macrophagic migration inhibition in response to corneal antigen. Bone marrow-derived cells have been noted in Mooren's ulcer as evidenced by immunoreactivity for CD34 (a marker for hematopoietic progenitor cells and endothelium), *c-kit* (a marker for hematopoietic and stromal progenitor cells), and STRO-1 (a differentiation antigen present on bone marrow fibroblast cells and on nonhematopoietic progenitor cells) cells, particularly in the superficial stroma.

D. Histologically, the cornea is infiltrated by lymphocytes and plasma cells.

1. An ulcer undermines the central edge of the stroma and shows a blunt edge peripherally.

2. The inflammation is present primarily at the peripheral edge of the ulcer but is absent centrally. The latter findings are characteristic of a rodent ulcer and can be useful in making the diagnosis. The

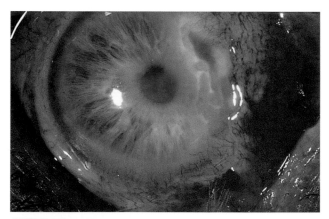

A

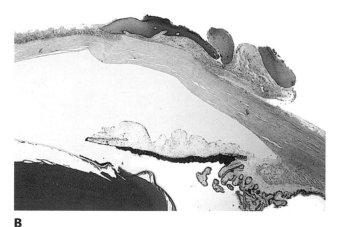

B

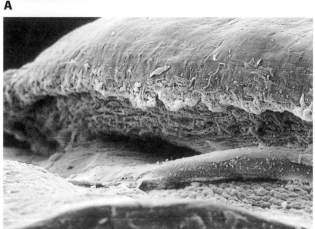

C

Fig. 8.28 Mooren's ulcer. **A,** Clinical appearance of ulcer. **B,** Histologic section of another case shows central absence and peripheral thickening of epithelium. **C,** Scanning electron micrograph of corneal edge of ulcer. Note overhanging lip of epithelium. (**A,** Courtesy of Dr. PR Laibson; **C,** courtesy of Dr. RC Eagle, Jr.)

peripheral portion of the ulcer is characterized by necrobiotic changes and hemorrhage, and absence of overlying epithelium and Bowman's membrane.

3. Approximately 75% to 100% of the resident cells express major histocompatibility complex class II antigens, the ratio of CD4 cells (T-helper/inducer) to CD8 cells (T-suppressor/cytotoxic) approaches 2.4:1, and approximately 25% to 50% of the infiltrating cells stain positively for CD22 (B cells)—compare with Terrien's ulcer on p. 278 of this chapter.

4. On histologic examination, the adjacent conjunctiva has an edematous stroma that is infiltrated primarily by plasma cells and lymphocytes without evidence of vasculitis.

XII. Delle (singular form of *dellen*)

A. A delle is a reversible, localized area of corneal stromal dehydration and corneal thinning owing to a break in the continuity of the tear film layer secondary to elevation of surrounding structures (e.g., with pterygium, filtering bleb, or suture granuloma).

Dellen, also known as *Fuchs' dimples*, may start as early as a few hours after the occurrence of a limbal elevation, but they seldom last longer than 2 days.

B. The histologic picture consists of a partial or full-thickness epithelial defect with the underlying stromal tissues shrinking or even collapsing from dehydration.

XIII. Anterior crocodile shagreen of Vogt (mosaic degeneration of the cornea)

A. The condition consists of a central corneal opacification at the level of Bowman's membrane that presents as a mosaic of polygonal gray opacities separated by clear areas.

1. The condition may occur as a dystrophy with bilaterality and a dominant inheritance pattern.

2. It may also occur as a degeneration after trauma or associated with such conditions as megalocornea, iris malformations, and band keratopathy.

3. A peripheral variety may be seen as an aging change.

B. Histologically, Bowman's membrane is calcified and found in ridges with flattening of the overlying epithelium.

The corneal stroma underlying the ridges is thinned and scarred.

XIV. Microdot stromal degeneration

A. Stromal microdot deposits present in long-term contact lens wearers.

1. It may represent lipofuscin-like material within the stroma secondary to chronic oxygen deprivation and chronic microtrauma.

2. Soft contact lens wear time has the greatest statistical relationship to microdot density and size.

XV. Corneal fibrosis syndrome

A. An unusual, bilateral, superficial, corneal fibrosis has been described in a young woman with homocystinuria.

B. Clinical findings: whitish, elevated, irregular masses accompanied by superficial vascularization were noted in the peripheral cornea of both eyes.

C. Histopathology: variable epithelial thickness is accompanied by melanin pigmentation of the basal epithelium. Fibrovascular pannus with disruption of Bowman's membrane and fibrosis of the anterior stroma is seen. Electron microscopy reveals empty intracytoplasmic vacuoles in the corneal epithelial cells, and intracytoplasmic inclusions incorporating fibrillogranular material in the corneal epithelium and keratocytes.

DYSTROPHIES

These are primary, usually inherited, bilateral disorders with fairly equal involvement of the corneas (Table 8.2). Because of their

---

TABLE 8.2 Dystrophies

EPITHELIAL

I. Heredofamilial—Primary in Cornea
A. Meesmann's (Stocker–Holt)
B. Dot, fingerprint, and geographic map patterns (microcystic dystrophy; epithelial basement membrane dystrophy)

II. Heredofamilial—Secondary to Systemic Disease: Fabry's Disease

SUBEPITHELIAL AND BOWMAN'S MEMBRANE
Subepithelial mucinous corneal dystrophy
Reis–Bücklers dystrophy

STROMAL

I. Heredofamilial—Primary in Cornea
A. Granular
B. Macular
C. Lattice
D. Avellino corneal dystrophy
E. Congenital hereditary stromal dystrophy
F. Hereditary fleck dystrophy
G. Central stromal crystalline corneal dystrophy (Schnyder)
H. Posterior crocodile shagreen
I. Posterior amorphous corneal dystrophy

II. Heredofamilial—Secondary to Systemic Disease
A. Mucopolysaccharidoses
B. Mucolipidoses
C. Sphingolipidoses
D. Ochronosis
E. Cystinosis
F. Hypergammaglobulinemia
G. Lecithin cholesterol acyltransferase deficiency

III. Nonheredofamilial
A. Keratoconus
B. Keratoglobus
C. Pellucid marginal degeneration

ENDOTHELIAL
I. Corneal guttata (Fuchs)
II. Posterior polymorphous dystrophy
III. Congenital hereditary endothelial dystrophy
IV. Nonguttate corneal endothelial degeneration

genetic basis, dystrophies are more likely to recur in the graft following corneal transplantation than other corneal disorders. Bowman's membrane dystrophy has the highest rate of recurrence followed by granular and lattice dystrophies respectively.

Epithelial

I. Heredofamilial—primary in cornea
   A. Meesmann's (Figs 8.29 and 8.30) and Stocker–Holt dystrophy are the same.
      1. The condition is inherited as an autosomal-dominant trait and appears in the first or second year of life.

      > A fragility of the corneal epithelium where K3 and K12 keratins are specifically expressed is found. Dominant-negative mutations in the K3 and K12 keratins (K3 maps to the type II keratin gene cluster on 12q, and K12 to the type I keratin gene cluster on 17q) may be the cause of Meesmann's corneal dystrophy. A clinically similar corneal dystrophy, *Lisch corneal dystrophy*, maps to Xp22.3. A family with a novel missense mutation (423T > G) in exon 1 of the cornea-specific keratin 12 (*KRT12*) gene has been reported.

      2. Myriad, tiny, punctate vacuoles are present in the corneal epithelium that only rarely cause vision problems, and then not until later in life.

> The tiny intraepithelial cysts (vacuoles) appear relatively transparent on retroillumination by slit-lamp examination. Only the cysts that reach the surface and rupture take up fluorescein and stain; those below the surface do not stain.

      3. The involved corneas are prone to recurrent irritations.
      4. Histologically, the characteristic findings consist of a "peculiar substance" in corneal epithelial cells and a vacuolated, dense, homogeneous substance, most commonly in corneal intraepithelial cysts and less commonly in corneal epithelial cells.

> The primary disturbance probably involves the cytoplasmic ground substance of the corneal epithelium and, ultimately, results in complete homogenization of cells and formation of intraepithelial cysts. Thickening of the corneal epithelial basement membrane varies, and is a nonspecific response by the epithelial basal cells.

   B. Dot, fingerprint, and geographic patterns (*microcystic* dystrophy; *epithelial basement membrane* dystrophy; Figs 8.31 through 8.34)
      1. The condition mainly occurs in otherwise healthy people.

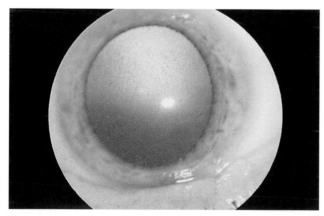

A

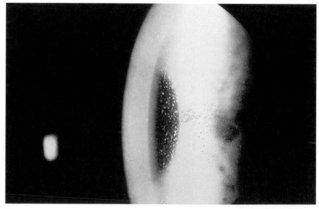

B

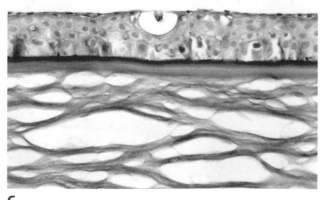

C

Fig. 8.29 Meesmann's dystrophy. **A** and **B** show tiny, fine, punctate, clear vacuoles in the corneal epithelium. **C,** Histologic section shows an intraepithelial cyst that contains debris (called *peculiar substance* in electron microscopy). The epithelial basement membrane is thickened here. (**C,** periodic acid–Schiff stain; case reported in Fine BS *et al.*: *Am J Ophthalmol* 83:633. Copyright Elsevier 1977.)

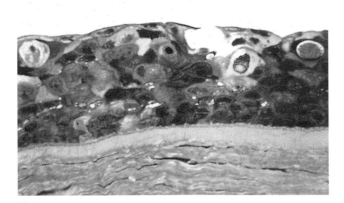

A

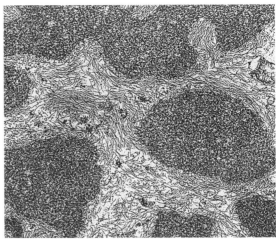

B

Fig. 8.30 Meesmann's dystrophy. **A,** In this thin, plastic-embedded section, numerous tiny cysts of uniform size and one surface pit are present in the epithelium. One cyst to the right of center resembles a cell. **B,** Characteristic intracytoplasmic degeneration—"peculiar substance"—involves cytoplasmic filaments (i.e., "cytoskeleton"). **C,** Cyst contains vacuolated, homogeneous, dense material (i.e., filament-free). (Modified from Fine BS *et al.: Am J Ophthalmol* 83:633. Copyright Elsevier 1977.)

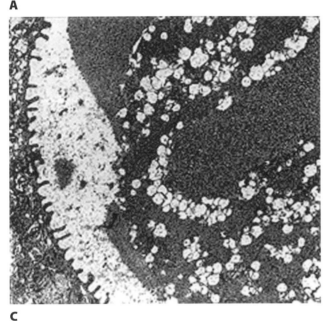

C

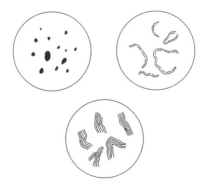

Fig. 8.31 Schematic appearance of dot, map, and fingerprint dystrophies.

Dot, fingerprint, and geographic patterns predispose to sloughing of the corneal epithelium during laser in situ keratomileusis, with subsequent wound healing complications.

2. Clinically, at least three configurations may be found, or any combinations thereof:
   a. Groups of tiny, round or comma-shaped, putty-like grayish-white superficial epithelial opacities of various sizes are seen in the pupillary zones of one or both eyes.
   b. A fingerprint pattern of sinuous, translucent lines, best seen with retroillumination.
   c. A maplike or geographic pattern, best seen on oblique illumination.
3. Inheritance is uncertain.
4. Histologically, three corresponding patterns can be observed:
   a. The grayish dots represent small cystoid spaces in the epithelium into which otherwise normal, superficial corneal epithelial cells desquamate.

Microcystic dystrophy is easily differentiated from Meesmann's dystrophy in that, in the former, the epithelial cells are not morphologically abnormal and contain a normal amount of glycogen.

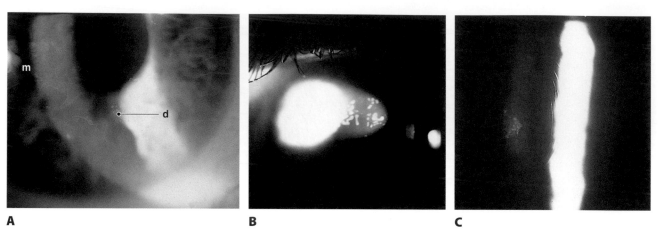

A **B** **C**

Fig. 8.32 Dot, fingerprint, and map patterns. **A,** The dot pattern (d) is shown in the lower central cornea. A map pattern (m) is seen above and to the left of the dot pattern. **B,** The dot pattern resembles "putty" in the epithelium. **C,** The fingerprint pattern, best seen with indirect lighting, is clearly shown. (**B,** Courtesy of Dr. WC Frayer.)

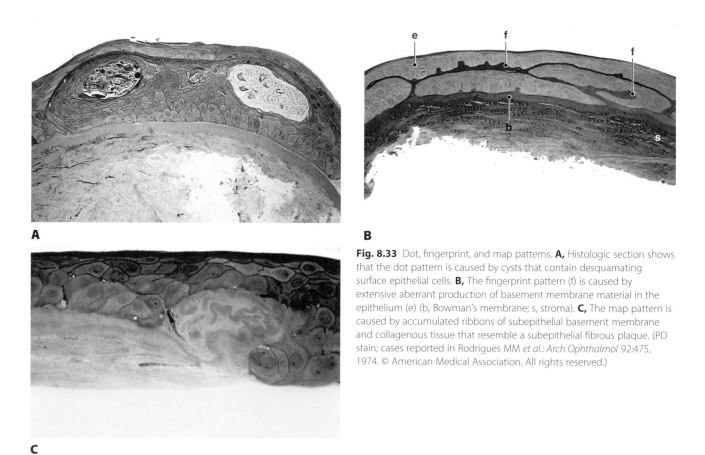

A **B**

C

Fig. 8.33 Dot, fingerprint, and map patterns. **A,** Histologic section shows that the dot pattern is caused by cysts that contain desquamating surface epithelial cells. **B,** The fingerprint pattern (f) is caused by extensive aberrant production of basement membrane material in the epithelium (e) (b, Bowman's membrane; s, stroma). **C,** The map pattern is caused by accumulated ribbons of subepithelial basement membrane and collagenous tissue that resemble a subepithelial fibrous plaque. (PD stain; cases reported in Rodrigues MM *et al.: Arch Ophthalmol* 92:475, 1974. © American Medical Association. All rights reserved.)

b. The fingerprint pattern is formed by both normally positioned and inverted basal epithelial cells producing abnormally large quantities of multilaminar basement membrane. The latter cells have migrated into the epithelial superficial layers.

c. The map pattern is produced beneath the epithelium by basal epithelial cells and possibly a few keratocytes that have migrated from the superficial stroma to elaborate both multilaminar basement membrane and collagenous material.

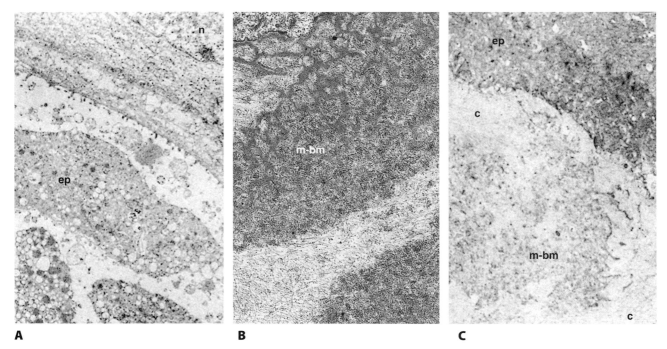

Fig. 8.34 Dot, fingerprint, and map patterns. **A,** Cyst contents consist of almost normal desquamating surface epithelial cells (ep) (n, nucleus of flattened epithelial cell near inverted surface). **B,** Basement membrane consists of two separate multilaminar basement membranes (m-bm) produced by aberrant basal cell. Collagenous filaments separate two basement membranes and epithelial cells from their own multilaminar basement membrane. **C,** Multilaminar nature of irregular whorls of basement membrane (m-bm). Collagenous filaments (c) interspersed between epithelial cells and basement membrane and throughout whorls of poorly formed multilaminar basement membrane (ep, basal cells of epithelium). (**B** and **C,** From Rodrigues MM *et al.: Arch Ophthalmol* 92:475, 1974, with permission. © American Medical Association. All rights reserved.)

> Similar epithelial abnormalities are frequently encountered on routine histopathologic examination of corneal buttons from penetrating keratoplasty surgery for chronic edema and bullous keratopathy.

II. Heredofamilial—secondary to systemic disease: Fabry's disease (angiokeratoma corporis diffusum; see Table 11.5, p. 454)

A. The typical maculopapular skin eruptions (angiokeratoma corporis diffusum) are seen in a girdle distribution and start in early adulthood.

B. Whorl-like (vortex-like) epithelial corneal opacities are seen.

> *Cornea verticillata* (Fleischer–Gruber), the corneal manifestation of Fabry's disease, is the term found in the older literature. Quite similar corneal appearances are seen in chloroquine, amiodarone, indomethacin, atovaquone, and suramin keratopathies.

C. The fundus shows tortuous retinal vessels containing visible mural deposits. The deposits may be so pronounced as partially to occlude the lumen, resulting in sausage-shaped vessels; the blood in the arterioles becomes much darker than normal from stasis.

D. Fabry's disease is caused by a generalized inborn error of glycolipid metabolism wherein α-galactosidase deficiency results in intracellular storage of ceramide trihexoside.

E. Inheritance is X-linked recessive.

> Amniotic fluid can be analyzed during early gestation for levels of α-galactosidase, thereby detecting the condition during early pregnancy.

F. Histologically, lipid-containing, finely laminated inclusions are present in corneal epithelium, lens epithelium, endothelial cells in all organs, liver cells, fibrocytes of skin, lymphocytes, smooth-muscle cells of arterioles, and capillary pericytes.

On light microscopy, material is noted between the epithelium and Bowman's membrane. Oil red-O positive material is present in the subepithelial layer. Duplication of basal lamina is detected on electron microscopic examination.

Subepithelial and Bowman's Membrane (Anterior Limiting Membrane or Layer)

I. Subepithelial mucinous corneal dystrophy (SMCD)

A. SMCD has its onset in the first decade, has an autosomal-dominant inheritance, is characterized by frequent, recurrent corneal erosions, and shows progressive visual loss.

B. The cornea shows bilateral subepithelial opacities and haze that involve the entire cornea but are most dense centrally.

C. Histology

1. An eosinophilic, periodic acid–Schiff (PAS)-positive and Alcian blue-positive, hyaluronidase-sensitive material lies anterior to Bowman's membrane.

2. Immunohistochemical analysis demonstrates chondroitin 4-sulfate and dermatan sulfate in the material.

3. Electron microscopy shows deposition of a fine fibrillar material consistent with glycosaminoglycan.

SMCD resembles *Grayson–Wilbrandt dystrophy*, which differs in having clear intervening stroma, stromal refractile bodies, and Alcian blue negativity, and *honeycomb dystrophy (Thiel–Behnke)*, which differs in having its onset in the second decade, a subepithelial honeycomb opacity, a clear peripheral cornea, and no characteristic histologic staining pattern.

II. Reis–Bücklers corneal dystrophy—see later discussion of granular dystrophies

Stromal (Table 8.3)

I. Heredofamilial–primary in cornea:

A. Genetic overview:

1. Mutations in the transforming growth factor-β-induced gene (*TGFBI: BIGH3*) can produce the granular corneal dystrophy (GCD) phenotype or that of LCD. Mutation of codon 124 of TGFBI from arginine to cysteine (R124C), histidine (R124H), or leucine (R124L) is associated with type I LCD, Avellino dystrophy, and superficial GCD respectively. In one French study, GCD was produced by mutations R124L, R124H, and R124L+delT125-delE126. LCD was produced by mutations R124C, H626R, and A546T. *BIG-h3* genetic analysis may be required to determine the mutation in the keratoepithelin gene in order to diagnose related corneal dystrophies properly.

B. The granular dystrophies (Groenouw type I; Bücklers type I; hyaline; Fig. 8.35; see Table 8.3) can be divided into at least three types: classic, Avellino (see later discussion of LCD), and superficial (Reis–Bücklers and Thiel–Behnke)

1. Classic (CGCD/R555W)

a. Sharply defined, variably sized, white opaque granules are seen in the axial region of the superficial corneal stroma; the intervening stroma is clear.

b. At least two clinical phenotypes exist.

c. Family members with the R555W mutation (C1710T) in exon 12 may present with an unusual vortex pattern of corneal deposits. Another atypical phenotype of GCD demonstrates white dotlike opacities scattered in the anterior and mid-stroma of the central cornea. The mutation resulted in a nucleotide transversion at codon 123 (GAC → CAC), causing Asp → His substitution (D123H); however, there is low penetrance for GCD.

1). An early-onset, superficial variant begins in childhood and is characterized by confluent subepithelial and superficial stromal opacities, frequent attacks of recurrent erosion, and early visual loss.

The peripheral stroma is clear. The variant may be confused histologically with Reis–Bücklers dystrophy. Electron microscopic examination clarifies the diagnosis by demonstrating rod-shaped granules in a plane localized to, or near, Bowman's membrane. The granules may be enveloped by amyloid (9- to 11-nm filaments)

---

2). A milder, late-onset variety is characterized by multiple, crumblike stromal opacities, slow progression, fewer attacks of recurrent erosion, less visual disturbance, and less need for corneal grafting.

The peripheral stroma is clear.

TABLE 8.3 Histopathologic Differentiation of Granular, Macular, and Lattice Dystrophies

Dystrophy	Trichrome	AMP*	Periodic Acid–Schiff	Amyloid†	Birefringence‡	Heredity
Granular	+	–	–	– or +§	–	Dominant
Macular	–	+	+	–	–	Recessive
Lattice	+	–	+	+	+	Dominant

Stains for acid mucopolysaccharides (e.g., Alcian blue and colloidal iron).
†*Stains for amyloid (e.g., Congo red and crystal violet).*
‡*To polarized light.*
§*Periphery of granular lesion (and occasionally within the lesion) stains positively for amyloid.*

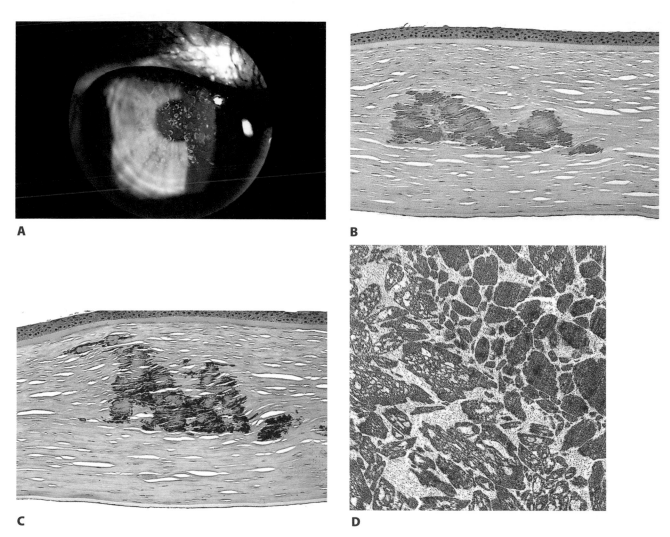

Fig. 8.35 Granular dystrophy. **A,** Clear cornea is present between the small, sharply outlined, white stromal granules. **B,** Histologic section shows that the granules stain deeply with hematoxylin and eosin and (**C**) stain red with the trichrome stain. The periodic acid–Schiff stain and stain for both glycosaminoglycams and amyloids are negative. The condition is inherited as an autosomal-dominant trait. **D,** The granules seen by light microscopy also appear as granules by electron microscopy. Many granules are "apertured."

d. Inheritance is autosomal dominant.

Chromosome linkage analysis shows Reis–Bücklers, Thiel–Behnke, granular, superficial granular, Avellino, and lattice type I dystrophies are linked to a single locus on chromosome 5q31. These dystrophies may represent different clinical forms of the same entity. The severe phenotype of granular dystrophy is caused by homozygous mutations in the keratoepithelin gene (*BIGH3*). In classic granular dystrophy, the specific mutation in the *BIGH3* gene is a R555W mutation. The *TGFBI* gene may also be involved in Reis–Bücklers.

A unique corneal dystrophy involving Bowman's layer and stroma has been reported to be associated with the Gly623Asp mutation in the *TGFBI* gene. Clinical features include findings of LCD and a Bowman's layer dystrophy.

---

e. Histologically, granular, eosinophilic, trichrome red-positive deposits are scattered throughout the stroma.

The periphery of the granule may show positive Congo red staining. Granular dystrophy may recur in otherwise normal donor material after a corneal graft. The recurrence is quite slow and is believed to be caused by the host keratocytes slowly replacing those of the donor. Some recurrences appear more commonly as a localized avascular subepithelial membrane with no involvement of Bowman's membrane or corneal stroma. These superficial membranes can often be stripped away to restore corneal transparency. The deposits may originate in part from the corneal epithelium.

---

1). In addition, unesterified cholesterol is found in the superficial stroma.

2). Electron microscopy shows electron-dense polygonal granules, some of which may be "apertured," scattered throughout the stroma.

2. Reis–Bücklers (Fig. 8.36) and Thiel–Behnke corneal dystrophies
   a. Acute attacks of red, painful eyes caused by recurrent erosions commence in early childhood.
      1). Multiple, minute, discrete opacities are seen early just beneath the epithelium.
      2). These become confluent, often producing the characteristic subepithelial honeycomb pattern.
      3). Usually, by the fifth decade, a marked opacification of the corneas occurs.
   b. Inheritance is autosomal dominant.

Chromosome linkage analysis shows Reis–Bücklers, Thiel–Behnke, granular, superficial granular, Avellino, and lattice type I dystrophies are linked to a single locus on chromosome 5q31. These dystrophies may represent different clinical forms of the same entity. The severe phenotype of granular dystrophy is caused by homozygous mutations in the keratoepithelin

(*BIGH3*) gene. In classic granular dystrophy, the specific mutation in the *BIGH3* gene is a R555W mutation.

1). Reis–Bücklers dystrophy [also known as *superficial variant of corneal granular dystrophy* or *corneal dystrophy of Bowman's layer type 1* (CDB1)] is caused by the R124L mutation of the *BIGH3* gene.
2). Thiel–Behnke dystrophy [also known as *honeycomb-shaped dystrophy* or *corneal dystrophy of Bowman's layer type 2* (CDB2)] is caused by the R555Q mutation of the *BIGH3* gene.

   c. Histology
      1). Epithelial abnormalities may underlie the pathologic process of both conditions.
      2). The corneal changes are limited to levels in and around Bowman's membrane (layer).

The membrane is slowly replaced by scarring or increased layering of collagenous tissue that extends beneath the epithelium. Loss of hemidesmosomes and associated basement membrane appears to lead to the recurrent desquamations or erosions with consequent additional trauma to Bowman's membrane.

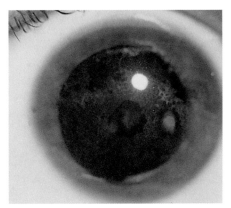

A

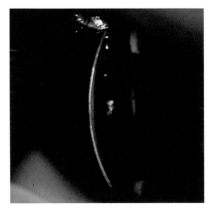

B

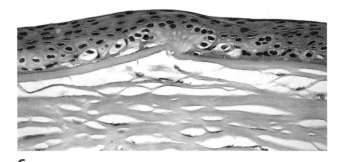

C

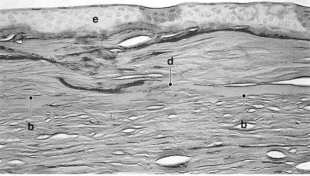

D

Fig. 8.36 Reis–Bücklers dystrophy. **A,** The characteristic honeycomb corneal pattern is seen. **B,** Slit-lamp view shows very superficial location of opacity. **C,** Histologic section in another case shows central degeneration of Bowman's membrane and irregularity of overlying epithelium. **D,** Trichrome stain demonstrates disruption (d) of Bowman's membrane by fibrous tissue, along with a fibrous plaque between Bowman's membrane (b) and epithelium (e). (**A** and **B,** Courtesy of Dr. IM Raber.)

3). Electron microscopy shows involvement in the subepithelial area, Bowman's layer, and anterior stroma. The involvement consists of masses of peculiar curly filaments that have a diameter of approximately 10 nm and indeterminate length.

Reis–Bücklers dystrophy may recur in the donor button of a corneal graft. By both light and electron microscopy, hereditary recurrent erosions may appear similar to Reis–Bücklers dystrophy.

C. Macular (Groenouw type II; Bücklers type II; primary corneal acid mucopolysaccharidosis; Fig. 8.37; see Table 8.3)
1. Macular dystrophy is a localized corneal mucopolysaccharidosis caused by a disorder of keratin sulfate metabolism. Unsulfated keratin sulfate is deposited both within keratocytes and corneal endothelial cells and in the extracellular corneal stroma.

a. A wide range of keratocyte-specific proteoglycan and glycosaminoglycan remodeling processes are activated during degeneration of the stromal matrix in MCD.
2. Diffuse cloudiness of superficial stroma and aggregates of gray-white opacities in the axial region are seen; the intervening stroma is also diffusely cloudy.

A decrease in *N*-acetylglucosamine 6-*O*-sulfotransferase (GlcNAc6ST) activity in the cornea may result in the occurrence of low-sulfate or nonsulfated keratan sulfate and thereby cause the corneal opacity.

The cloudiness usually develops rapidly so that vision in most patients is seriously impaired by 30 years of age, necessitating corneal grafting.

Macular dystrophy may recur in the donor button after corneal graft.

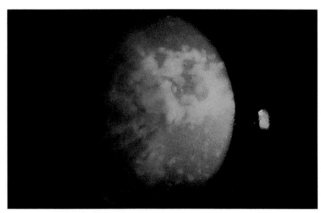

A

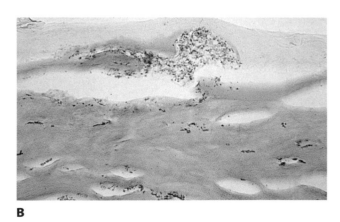

B

C

Fig. 8.37 Macular dystrophy. **A,** The corneal stroma between the opacities is cloudy. **B,** Histologic section shows that keratocytes and vacuolated cells beneath the epithelium (stained yellow) are filled with glycosaminoglycam (stained blue). In this condition, the trichrome stain and stains for amyloid are negative, but the periodic acid–Schiff stain is positive. The condition is inherited as an autosomal-recessive trait. The cornea and serum of most patients who have type I macular dystrophy lack detectable antigenic keratan sulfate, whereas it is present in the cornea and serum in type II. **C,** Keratocyte beneath Bowman's layer (bl) filled with vesicles containing acid mucopolysaccharide (AMP)-positive substance (ep, epithelium; nug, nucleus of keratocyte). (**A,** Courtesy of Dr. JH Krachmer; **B,** AMP stain.)

3. Type I, the most prevalent type, shows a lack of detectable antigenic keratan sulfate in the cornea and serum.

A type IA has been described in which a lack of detectable antigenic keratan sulfate occurs in the corneal stroma and serum, but in which corneal fibroblasts do react with keratan sulfate monoclonal antibody. A further subdivision of this type can be achieved on the basis of reactivity to monoclonal antibody 3D12/H7.

---

4. Type II shows detectable antigenic keratan sulfate in the cornea and serum.
5. Inheritance is autosomal recessive. The gene (*CHST6*) for this dystrophy is located on chromosome 16 (16q22).

Macular dystrophy is thought to result from an inability to catabolize corneal keratan sulfate (keratan sulfate I). Keratan sulfate may be absent from the serum of patients who have macular corneal dystrophy.

---

6. Histologically, basophilic deposits, which stain positively for acid mucopolysaccharides (glycosaminoglycams), are present in keratocytes, in endothelial cells, and in small pools lying extracellularly in or between stromal lamellae.
   a. In addition, unesterified cholesterol is found throughout the stroma and amyloid is sometimes present in the deposits.
   b. Some cases show excrescences of Descemet's membrane.
7. Concomitant keratoconus and macular corneal dystrophy have been reported in two siblings.

D. Lattice (type I, Bücklers type III; Biber–Haab–Dimmer; primary corneal amyloidosis; Figs 8.38 and 8.39; see Table 8.3, and p. 238 in Chapter 7)—six forms exist: (1) LCD type I; (2) LCD type III; (3) LCD type IIIA, (4) gelatinous droplike corneal dystrophy; (5) LCD type II (OMIM 204870); and (6) polymorphic corneal amyloidosis. The R124C mutation frequently accompanies LCD. Two mutations in the *TGFBI* gene have been reported to segregate with LCD in a family having two heterozygous single-nucleotide mutations in exon 12 of the *TGBI* gene (C1637A and C1652A), leading to amino acid substitutions in the encoded TGF-β–induced protein (A546D and P551Q). This family lacked the common R124C mutation. A late-onset

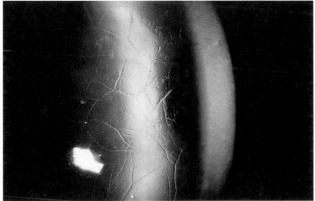

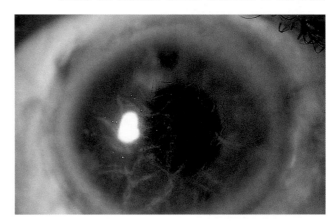

A

B

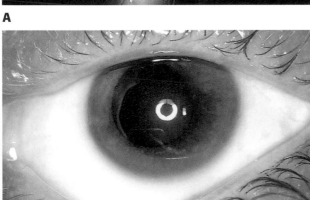

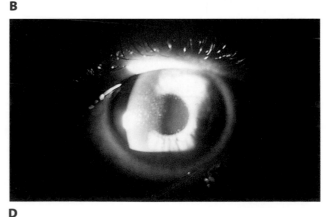

C

D

Fig. 8.38 Lattice dystrophy. **A,** Translucent branching lines of typical lattice dystrophy [lattice corneal dystrophy (LCD type I)] seen best by retroillumination. **B,** Another patient shows an accentuated form of lattice, perhaps LCD type III. **C** and **D,** Corneal deposits appear as granules, similar to granular corneal dystrophy. Histology of cornea, however, is consistent with lattice dystrophy (see Fig. 8.39A). This is the Avellino-type corneal dystrophy. (**A,** Courtesy of Dr. JH Krachmer; **C** and **D,** case reported in Yanoff M *et al.: Arch Ophthalmol* 95:651, 1977. © American Medical Association. All rights reserved.)

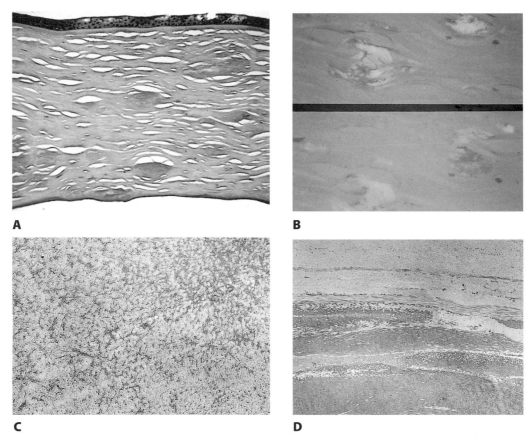

Fig. 8.39 Lattice dystrophy (Avellino type). **A,** Histologic section shows focal areas of "hyalin" irregularities. **B,** Top and bottom taken with both polarizers in place in Congo red-stained section. *Birefringence* is demonstrated by a change in color when the bottom polarizer is turned 90° (when only one polarizer is in place, the corneal amyloid deposit—stained with Congo red—acts as second polarizer and *dichroism* is demonstrated by a change in color when the one polarizer is turned 90°). Electron microscopy shows that lesions are composed of myriad individual filaments either in disarray and therefore nonbirefringent (**C**), or (**D**) highly aligned and therefore birefringent.

form of LCD involved the leu527Arg mutation of the *TGFBI* gene.

Typically, the deposits in LCD are in the mid-stroma, with a mean distance of 79 μm from the epithelium. In contrast, deposits in GCD are mostly superficial, having a mean distance from the epithelium of 28 μm.

1. LCD type I (classic primary LCD) shows corneal lines forming a lattice configuration present centrally in the anterior stroma, leaving the peripheral cornea clear.
   a. The central lattice lines are difficult to visualize with direct illumination.

   > Some authors believe that the lattice lines may represent nerves or nerve degeneration. Proof for this hypothesis is lacking.

   b. LCD type I can progress to involve deeper stromal layers.
   c. Also seen are epithelial abnormalities (e.g., recurrent erosion, band keratopathy, and loss of surface luster), which may be caused by epithelial basement membrane abnormalities.
   d. The autosomal-dominant condition begins in the first decade or early second decade and may progress fairly rapidly; many affected people have marked vision impairment by 40 years of age. LCD is rarely unilateral; however, it may be extremely asymmetrical at the time of presentation.

   > Chromosome linkage analysis shows that Reis–Bücklers, Thiel–Behnke, superficial granular, granular, Avellino, and lattice type I dystrophies are linked to a single locus on chromosome 5q31. These dystrophies may represent different clinical forms of the same entity.

   e. Although lattice lines are typical of LCD type I, presentation as a diffuse opacification of the central corneal stroma without lattice lines may occur. Molecular genetic analysis revealed LCD I-associated heterozygous missense change (C417T) replacing arginine in codon 124 with cysteine (R124C) in the *TGFBI* gene.
   f. Amyloid deposition may recur in a corneal transplant graft. Examination of two grafts 20

years after the original transplants revealed deposits confined to the basement membrane regions in contrast to the initial specimens in which amyloid deposits were present throughout the stroma.

2. LCD type III primary corneal lattice dystrophy has an autosomal-recessive inheritance pattern, has thicker lines extending from limbus to limbus, and has a later onset than type I.

A similar entity, except for an autosomal-dominant inheritance and the presence of corneal erosions, has been called *LCD type IIIA*. Chromosome linkage analysis shows Reis–Bücklers, Thiel–Behnke, granular, superficial granular, Avellino, and lattice type I dystrophies are linked to a single locus on chromosome 5q31. These dystrophies may represent different clinical forms of the same entity. The severe phenotype of granular dystrophy is caused by homozygous mutations in the keratoepithelin [*TGFBI (BIGH3)*] gene. In classic granular dystrophy, the specific mutation in the *TGFBI* gene is an R555W mutation.

---

3. Primary gelatinous droplike dystrophy (familial subepithelial amyloidosis), the third form of *primary* lattice dystrophy, has an autosomal-recessive inheritance pattern, is most common in Japan, and shows a striking corneal picture. It has been divided into four types: band keratopathy type, stromal opacity type, kumquat-like type, and typical mulberry type.
   a. The gene responsible for primary gelatinous droplike dystrophy, *MI1S1*, is localized to chromosome 1p.
   b. The bilateral dystrophy presents in the first decade of life as subepithelial, mulberry-like opacities that grow with age.
   c. The Q118X mutation of the *M1S1* gene can result in a corneal phenotype with either droplike or band-shaped opacities.

4. LCD type II (Meretoja) is a dominantly inherited, familial form of systemic paramyloidosis or *secondary* corneal amyloidosis, mainly in people of Finnish origin, and consists of lattice corneal changes (more peripheral than in LCD type I) plus progressive cranial neuropathy and skin changes. It is also known as gelsolin-related amyloidosis.
   a. Clinical confocal microscopy (CFM) confirms that symptom levels and slit-lamp findings correlate positively with corneal haze intensity, and correlate inversely with visibility of epithelial and stromal nerves. In severe cases, stromal and epithelial nerves are not visible, suggesting progressive neural degeneration.
   b. The lattice lines have been attributed to amyloid deposits and not to corneal nerves based on CFM.
   c. Nerve damage is the probable cause of decreased corneal mechanical and, to a lesser degree, thermal sensitivity.

The disorder is also called *type IV familial neuropathic syndrome, familial amyloid polyneuropathy type IV*, or *amyloidotic polyneuropathy*. Vitreous opacities do not occur. LCD type II is caused by mutations in the gelsolin gene on chromosome 9 (9q32–34).

---

5. Polymorphic corneal amyloidosis is caused by an A546D mutation in the *TGFBI* gene
   a. Multiple polymorphic, polygonal, refractile, chipped ice-appearing gray and white opacities are seen at multiple depths of the cornea.
   b. Occasional deep, filamentous lines that do not form a distinct lattice pattern are noted.
   c. A phenotypic variant of LCD characterized by bilateral, symmetric, radially arranged branching refractile lines within and surrounding an area of central anterior stromal haze accompanied by polymorphic refractile deposits in the mid and posterior stroma may be seen.
      1). Light and electron microscopy demonstrates amyloid and excludes material characteristic of GCD.
      2). Ala546Asp and Pro551Gln missense changes in exon 12 of the *TGFBI* gene may be seen.
   d. Corneal amyloidosis can be associated with lactoferrin, and a Glu561Asp mutation with or without accompanying Aal11Thr and Glu561Asp mutations.

6. Histology
   a. An eosinophilic, metachromatic, PAS-positive and Congo red-positive, birefringent, and dichroic deposit is present in the stroma, mainly superficially.
   b. The epithelium is abnormal and shows areas of hypertrophy and atrophy along with excessive basement membrane production.

It seems that not only keratocytes but, on occasion, corneal epithelial cells have the ability to elaborate the abnormal material considered to be amyloid. LCD may recur in the donor button after corneal graft.

---

   c. In addition, unesterified cholesterol is found in areas corresponding to the Congo red positivity.

The stromal lesions are characteristic of amyloid in all respects. Amyloidosis may be classified into two basic groups: systemic (primary and secondary) and localized (primary and secondary). Secondary systemic amyloidosis, the most frequently encountered type, rarely involves the eyes and is not an important ophthalmologic entity. Lattice dystrophy of the cornea is now considered by many to be a hereditary form of primary localized amyloidosis. The epithelial basement membrane abnormalities are responsible for secondary epithelial erosions and are partially responsible for the vision impairment.

---

d. Electron microscopy shows masses of delicate filaments, many in disarray, whereas others are highly aligned.

   Filaments also infiltrate between collagen fibrils of normal diameter, and alignment is at the edges of lesions.

e. LCD type III shows larger amyloid deposits than types I and II, and contains a ribbon of amyloid between Bowman's membrane and the stroma.

E. Avellino corneal dystrophy (combined granular–lattice dystrophy; see Figs 8.38C and D, and 8.39)

1. Many patients who have granular and lattice dystrophy changes in the same eye can trace their origins to the region surrounding Avellino, Italy.

2. Chromosome linkage analysis shows Reis–Bücklers, Thiel–Behnke, granular, superficial granular, Avellino, and lattice types I and IIIA dystrophies are linked to a single locus on chromosome 5q31 (associated with the R124H mutation of the *BIGH3* gene). These five dystrophies may represent different clinical forms of the same entity.

3. Clinically, well-circumscribed granular lesions are seen along with corneal lesions that are larger than lattice type I opacities and appear snowflake-like.

4. Three signs characterize Avellino corneal dystrophy: anterior stromal discrete, grayish-white deposits; lattice-like lesions located in the mid to posterior stroma; and anterior stromal haze

---

The granular lesions occur early in life, whereas the lattice component appears gradually, maturing later in life.

---

5. Histologically, both eosinophilic, trichrome-positive granular deposits and Congo red-positive fusiform deposits are found.

   Electron microscopy shows discrete, homogeneous, electron-dense deposits and apertured deposits enclosing lacunae of filaments in the superficial stroma.

Loosely arranged fibrils, many of which are oriented randomly, are seen at the periphery of the superficial deposits, as contrasted to the parallel packing of amyloid fibrils seen in the fusiform deposits of deeper stroma.

F. Congenital hereditary stromal dystrophy (Table 8.4)

1. The condition is a congenital, nonprogressive corneal opacification with diffuse and homogeneous small opacities.

2. Inheritance is autosomal dominant.

3. Histologically, the characteristic changes consist of a rather widespread, uniform clefting of the stromal lamellae, composed of collagen filaments of small diameter.

   a. The stroma is thickened.

      1). Electron microscopy demonstrates thickened stroma due to cleaving of the lamellae by alternating layers of small-diameter collagen fibrils arranged in random fashion.

   b. The remaining corneal layers (epithelial, Bowman's, endothelial, and Descemet's membrane) are normal.

G. Hereditary fleck dystrophy (François and Neetens' *hérédodystrophie mouchetée*)

1. Clinically, the condition is characterized by small ringlike or wreathlike opacities that contain clear

TABLE 8.4 Comparison of Features of Congenital Hereditary Endothelial Dystrophy (CHED) and Congenital Hereditary Stromal Dystrophy (CHSD)

	CHED (see p. 308)	CHSD (see p. 297)
CLINICAL CHARACTERISTICS	Bilateral Inherited Present at birth, progressive disease with epithelial changes Thickened cornea	Bilateral Inherited Present at birth, mostly stationary disease with no epithelial changes Cornea of normal thickness
HISTOLOGIC FINDINGS	Thickened cornea (edema) Secondary changes in epithelium and Bowman's membrane Stroma: collagen fibrils of normal or large diameter separated by irregular lakes of fluid; no apparent relationship to keratocytes Secondary changes in Descemet's membrane (thickening); homogeneous or fibrous basement membrane Abnormal endothelium (by function)	Cornea of normal thickness No secondary changes in anterior layers Stroma: uniform distribution of loose and compact lamellae composed of collagen filaments of small diameter; the loose lamellae are always related to a keratocyte Essentially normal Descemet's membrane Normal endothelium (by function)

(From Witschel H et al.: Arch Ophthalmol 96:1043, 1978. © American Medical Association. All rights reserved.)

centers and distinct margins, and are present throughout all layers of the corneal stroma. The opacities vary in size, shape, and depth.

2. Hereditary fleck dystrophy is congenital, bilateral, and nonprogressive with little or no interference with vision.

3. Inheritance is autosomal dominant.

Rarely, affected members of families may also have posterior crocodile shagreen, keratoconus, lens opacities, pseudoxanthoma elasticum, or atopic disease.

---

4. Histologically, the keratocytes are abnormal, and appear swollen and vacuolated. They contain membrane-limited intracytoplasmic vacuoles of a granular to fibrogranular material that stains positively for acid mucopolysaccharides and complex lipids.

H. Schnyder's corneal crystalline dystrophy (central stromal crystalline corneal dystrophy)

1. Clinically, five morphologic phenotypes have been described:
   a. A disc-shaped central opacity lacking crystals
   b. A central crystalline disc-shaped opacity with an ill-defined edge
   c. A crystalline discoid opacity with a garland-like margin of sinuous contour
      1). A central full-thickness disciform lesion having a mosaic pattern instead of the more typical collection of crystals or diffuse haze may also occur.
   d. A ring opacity with local crystal agglomerations with a clear center
   e. A crystalline ring opacity with a clear center

2. The bilateral, symmetric, relatively nonprogressive condition (it may progress significantly over time) is probably not related to blood lipoprotein abnormalities, but occasionally may coexist with a hyperlipoproteinemia.

Rarely, the crystals can regress (e.g., after corneal epithelial erosion).

---

3. Inheritance is autosomal dominant.

4. Histologically, lipids (predominantly phospholipid, unesterified cholesterol, and cholesterol ester) are seen in Bowman's membrane (layer) and corneal stroma.
   a. The deposits stain positively with oil red-O and filipin (a fluorescent probe specific for unesterified cholesterol).
   b. The dystrophy appears to be related to a primary disorder of corneal lipid metabolism.

I. Decorin gene-associated stromal dystrophy
1. Clouded corneas present shortly after birth.
2. No associated systemic or congenital abnormalities.
3. Autosomal-dominant inheritance with linkage to chromosome 12q22, with a maximum logarithm of odds (LOD) score of 4.68 at D12S351 and a

frameshift mutation in the *DCN* gene (c967delT) that encodes for decorin, and predicting a C-terminal truncation of the decorin protein (p.S323fsX5) is seen.

4. Transmission electron microscopy: normal collagen fiber lamellar arrangement separated by abnormal fibrillar layers.

J. Central discoid corneal dystrophy
1. Clinically: bilateral, symmetrical central, discoid, corneal opacification.
2. Symptoms: decreased vision, glare, and photophobia.
3. Histopathology: multiple extracellular vacuoles are located in the anterior one-half of the central corneal stroma.
   a. The material within the vacuoles is intensely positive to Alcian blue and colloidal iron stains, compatible with glycosaminoglycan deposits.
   b. Electron microscopy demonstrates nonmembrane-bound vacuoles in the stroma containing faintly osmophilic matrix and black circular profiles.
4. Chondroitin sulfate is demonstrated on immunohistochemical analysis. Systemic evaluation fails to disclose a systemic storage disorder.
5. Identical clinical findings in other family members suggest dominant inheritance.
6. Genetic analysis does not demonstrate a mutation in the coding region of CHST6.

K. Posterior crocodile shagreen (central cloudy dystrophy of François)
1. It is characterized by large, polygonal gray lesions that are separated by relatively clear lines, seen in the axial two-thirds of the cornea, and most dense in the deep stroma.
2. Inheritance is autosomal dominant.
3. *In vivo* CFM has demonstrated multiple dark striae and abnormal stromal deposits in the disorder.
4. Histologically, an extracellular deposit of mucopolysaccharide and lipid-like material is seen.
5. Electron microscopy shows an irregular, sawtooth-like configuration of the collagen lamellae interspersed with areas of 100-nm spaced collagen, along with extracellular vacuoles, some of which contained fibrillogranular material.

L. Posterior amorphous corneal dystrophy
1. It is characterized by broad, sheetlike opacification, with intervening clear areas, of the posterior stroma associated with corneal flattening and thinning.
2. Inheritance is autosomal dominant.
3. Histologically, by both light and electron microscopy, an irregularity of the stroma is seen just anterior to Descemet's membrane, whereas the endothelium is normal.

II. Heredofamilial—secondary to systemic disease
A. Mucopolysaccharidoses (Fig. 8.40) can be divided into seven major classes (Table 8.5).
1. They all have mucopolysacchariduria.
2. In all but mucopolysaccharidosis IV, degradation of acid mucopolysaccharides is impaired.

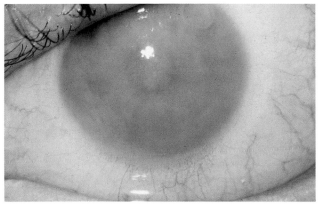

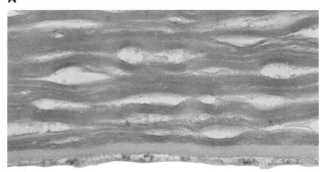

A

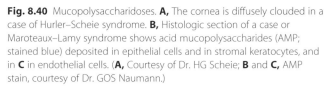

B

Fig. 8.40 Mucopolysaccharidoses. **A,** The cornea is diffusely clouded in a case of Hurler–Scheie syndrome. **B,** Histologic section of a case or Maroteaux–Lamy syndrome shows acid mucopolysaccharides (AMP; stained blue) deposited in epithelial cells and in stromal keratocytes, and in **C** in endothelial cells. (**A,** Courtesy of Dr. HG Scheie; **B** and **C,** AMP stain, courtesy of Dr. GOS Naumann.)

C

3. These genetic mucopolysaccharidoses may be considered as intralysosomal storage diseases with deficiencies of lysosomal hydrolases.
4. Histologically, vacuolated cells (histiocytes, corneal epithelium and endothelium, keratocytes, and iris and ciliary body epithelia) contain acid mucopolysaccharides in the vacuoles. The different classes show varying pathologic findings, fairly consistent within each class.

> In Maroteaux–Lamy syndrome, donor corneal grafts reaccumulate mucopolysaccharides as early as 1 year postgrafting, but some patients may remain clear up to 5 years. Partial clearing of the host cornea may occur after transplantation. Proteoglycans may be present in the corneal epithelium, intercellular spaces, and in swollen desmosomes. Keratocytes may be abnormal. Betaig-h3 labeling is around electron-lucent spaces in the stroma. CFM has detected abnormal keratocytes, particularly in the middle and posterior stroma in this condition in which macular retinal folds are also described.

B. Mucolipidosis (see p. 450 in Chapter 11)
1. An unusual case of mucolipidosis IV affected an African American patient resulting in the formation of intracytoplasmic inclusions in the corneal epithelium and endothelium. Usually, the disorder affects individuals of Jewish descent.
C. Sphingolipidosis (see p. 451 in Chapter 11)
D. Ochronosis (see p. 314 in this chapter)
E. Cystinosis (Lignac's disease; Figs 8.41 and 8.42)

1. The disease, a rare congenital disorder of amino acid metabolism, is characterized by dwarfism and progressive renal dysfunction resulting in acidosis, hypophosphatemia, renal glycosuria, and rickets.

> The precise biochemical defect in cystinosis is not known, but it is believed to be primarily a deficiency of lysosomal enzymes and, hence, a lysosomal disease.

2. Three types of cystinosis are recognized:
   a. Childhood type (nephropathic)—characterized by renal rickets, growth retardation, progressive renal failure, and death usually before puberty; autosomal-recessive inheritance

   > By biomicroscopy, narrowing of the angle and a ciliary body configuration similar to plateau iris may be seen. Also, by gonioscopy, crystals may be seen in the trabecular meshwork.

   The activity of the cystine transport system in patients' leukocytes is deficient.
   b. Adolescent type—onset in the first or second decade, mild nephropathy, diminished life expectancy; probably autosomal-recessive inheritance
   c. Adult (benign) type—onset from late second to sixth decade, typical corneal crystals but no renal disease, normal life expectancy; no known hereditary pattern
3. Patients who have childhood cystinosis may show a retinopathy that does not seem to cause any

TABLE 8.5 Types of Mucopolysaccharidoses (MPS)

	Designation	Clinical Features	Inheritance	Excessive Urinary Mucopolysaccharide	Deficient Substance	OMIM
MPS I H	Hurler's syndrome	Early cloudy cornea, death usually before age 10 years	AR	Dermatan sulfate, heparan sulfate	α-L-Iduronidase (Hurler corrective factor)	252800
MPS I S	Scheie's syndrome	Stiff joints, cloudy cornea, aortic regurgitation, normal intelligence, ? normal life span	AR	Dermatan sulfate, heparan sulfate	α-L-Iduronidase	252800
MPS I H/S	Hurler–Scheie compound	Phenotype intermediate between Hurler's and Scheie's, cloudy cornea	AR	Dermatan sulfate, heparan sulfate	α-L-Iduronidase	—
MPS II A	Hunter's syndrome, severe	Cornea clear, milder course than in MPS I H, but death usually before age 15 years	XL	Dermatan sulfate, heparan sulfate	L-Sulfoiduronate sulfatase	309900
MPS II B	Hunter's syndrome, mild	Survival to 30s–50s, fair intelligence	XL	Dermatan sulfate, heparan sulfate	L-Sulfoiduronate sulfatase	309900
MPS III A	Sanfilippo's syndrome A	Mild somatic, severe central nervous system effects (identical phenotype), clear cornea	AR	Heparan sulfate	Heparan sulfate sulfamidase	252920
MPS III B	Sanfilippo's syndrome B	Mild somatic, severe central nervous system effects (identical phenotype), clear cornea	AR	Heparan sulfate	Heparan sulfate sulfamidase	252920
MPS III C	Sanfilippo's syndrome C	Mild somatic, severe central nervous system effects (identical phenotype), clear cornea	AR	Heparan sulfate	Acetyl-CoA; α-glucosaminide N-acetyltransferase	252930
MPS III D	Sanfilippo's syndrome D	Mild somatic, severe central nervous system effects (identical phenotype), clear cornea	AR	Heparan sulfate	N-acetylglucosamine-6-sulfate sulfatase	252940
MPS IV A	Morquio's syndrome (classic) A	Severe bone changes of distinctive type, cloudy cornea, aortic regurgitation	AR	Keratan sulfate, chondroitin-6-sulfate	Galactose 6-sulfatase, N-acetylgalactosamine-6-sulfatase	253000
MPS IV B	Morquio-like syndrome B	Less severe changes	AR	Keratan sulfate, chondroitin-6-sulfate	β-Galactosidase	253010
MPS VI A	Maroteaux–Lamy syndrome, classic form	Severe osseous and corneal change, normal intellect	AR	Dermatan sulfate	N-acetylgalactosamine-4-sulfatase (arylsulfatase B)	253200
MPS VI B	Maroteaux–Lamy syndrome, mild form	Severe osseous and corneal change, normal intellect	AR	Dermatan sulfate	N-acetylgalactosamine-4-sulfatase (arylsulfatase B)	253200
MPS VII	Sly syndrome	Hepatosplenomegaly, dysostosis multiplex, white cell inclusions, mental retardation, mild cloudy cornea	AR	Dermatan sulfate, heparan sulfate, chondroitin-6-sulfate	β-Glucoronidase	253220

(Modified from Table 11-2 in McMusick VA: Heritable Disorders of Connective Tissue, 4th edn. Copyright Elsevier 1972.)

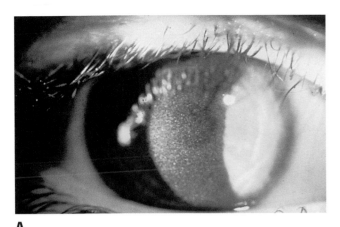

A

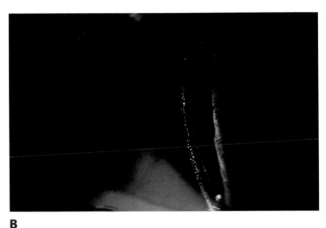

B

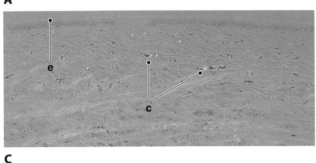

C

Fig. 8.41 Cystinosis. **A,** Myriad tiny opacities give the cornea a cloudy appearance. **B,** Tiny opacities predominantly in corneal epithelium. **C,** Polarization of an unstained histologic section of cornea shows birefringent cystine crystals (c) (e, epithelium). (**A** and **B,** Courtesy of Dr. DB Schaffer.)

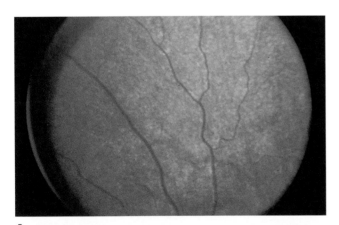

A

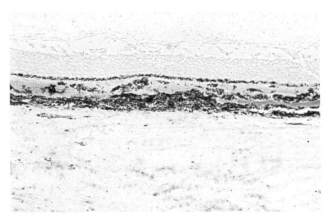

B

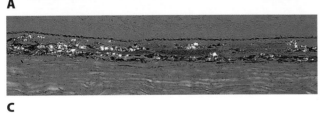

C

Fig. 8.42 Cystinosis. **A,** Myriad tiny crystals seen in retinal fundus. **B,** Unstained histologic section of sclera, choroid, and retina shows abundant gray crystalline bodies throughout the choroid. **C,** The choroidal bodies are birefringent to polarized light. (**B** and **C,** Case presented by Dr. FC Winter to the meeting of the Verhoeff Society, 1975.)

abnormality of retinal function. The retinopathy consists of a very fine pigmentation accompanied by tiny, multiple refractile crystals, probably at the level of retinal pigment epithelium and choroid.

4. Histologically, cystine crystals are deposited in many ocular tissues, including the conjunctiva and cornea.

Cystine can be seen clinically with a slit lamp as tiny, multicolored crystals. Although cystine crystals are stored in the liver, spleen, lymph nodes, bone marrow, eyes (conjunctiva, cornea, retina, and choroid), and kidneys (and probably other organs), they seem to be relatively innocuous. Progressive renal failure starts in the first decade of life with proximal tubular involvement (Toni–

Febré–Fanconi syndrome), but it does not seem to be directly related to renal cystine storage. The underlying enzyme defect is not yet known, but the accumulating cystine is often found in the lysosomal components of the cell.

F. Hypergammaglobulinemia
1. Corneal crystalline deposits (see subsection *Crystals*, later) are a rare manifestation of hypergammaglobulinemic states such as may be found in multiple myeloma, benign monoclonal gammopathy, Hodgkin's disease, and other dysproteinemias.
2. Histologically, positive deposits of immunoglobulin may be seen in corneal stroma (at all levels), conjunctiva, ciliary processes, pars plana, and choroid.
3. The term "immunotactoid keratopathy" has been used to describe corneal immunoglobulin G kappa deposits that appear as tubular, electron-dense, crystalloid deposits having a central lucent core on electron microscopy associated with paraproteinemia.

G. Lecithin cholesterol acyltransferase (LCAT) deficiency
1. LCAT deficiency results from an inborn error of metabolism and consists of a normochromic anemia, proteinuria, renal failure, arteriosclerosis, a high serum level of free cholesterol and lecithin, and greatly reduced esterified cholesterol and lysolecithin.
2. LCAT enzyme is absent.
3. The cornea has a cloudy appearance because of the myriad, tiny, grayish stromal dots, evenly distributed except for being more concentrated near the limbus, where they mimic an arcus.
   a. Vision is not severely affected until late in life.
   b. In addition, retinal hemorrhages, optic disc protrusions, and ruptures in Bruch's membrane may be the result of lipid deposits.
4. Light microscopy shows a vague, mild, diffuse, tiny vacuolation of the corneal stroma.
   a. Electron microscopy strikingly demonstrates myriad tiny vacuoles, many containing membranes and particles, in Bowman's membrane and stroma (larger vacuoles in stroma).
   b. The corneal epithelial basement membrane is thickened.
   c. Amyloid deposition may be found in addition to the other corneal changes.

III. Nonheredofamilial
A. Keratoconus (Figs 8.43 through 8.45)
1. Ectasia of the central cornea usually becomes manifest in youth or adolescence, progresses for 5 to 6 years, and then tends to arrest. Approximately 90% of cases are bilateral.

The condition progresses most rapidly during the second and third decades of life. A high irregular astigmatism is common, an increased incidence of keratoconus occurs in

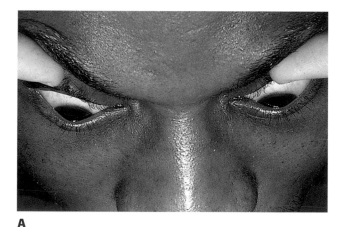

A

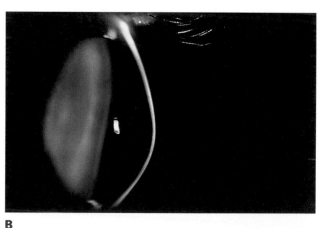

B

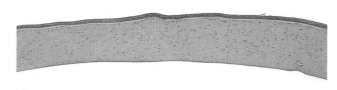

C

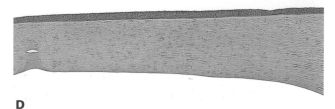

D

Fig. 8.43 Keratoconus. **A,** When patient looks down, the cone in each eye causes the lower lids to bulge (Munson's sign). **B,** Slit-lamp beam passes through apex of cone, which is slightly nasal and inferior to center. Note scarring at apex of cone. **C,** Histologic section through the center of the cone shows corneal thinning, stromal scarring, and breaks in Bowman's membrane. **D,** The thinner peripheral part of the cone is to the left and the more normal-thickness cornea is to the right.

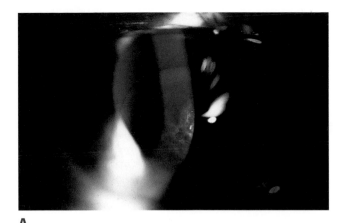

A

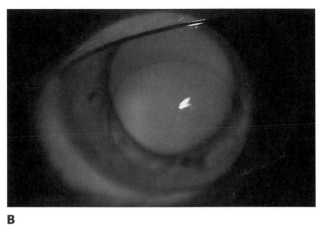

B

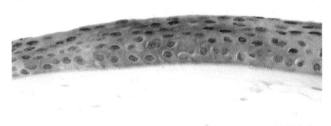

C

Fig. 8.44 Keratoconus—Fleischer ring. **A,** A brown line (i.e., Fleischer ring) is seen in the slit-lamp beam above the apex of the cone. **B,** A cobalt-blue filter shows the Fleischer ring as a black circular line. **C,** Perl's stain for iron demonstrates the epithelial positivity (blue) in the region of the Fleischer ring.

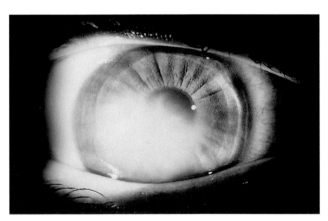

A

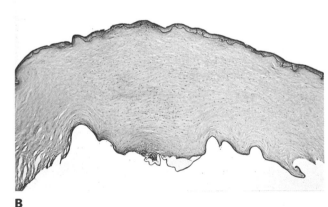

B

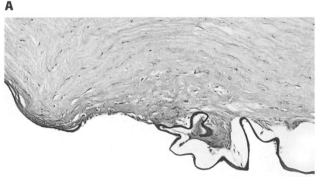

C

Fig. 8.45 Acute hydrops. **A,** Corneal edema developed rapidly in this eye with keratoconus. Penetrating keratoplasty was performed. **B,** Histologic section shows a markedly thickened and edematous cornea. A break has occurred in Descemet's membrane, shown with increased magnification in **C.** (Case courtesy of Dr. RA Levine.)

Down's syndrome (see p. 39 in Chapter 2), and human leukocyte antigen (HLA)-327 may be found. Unilateral keratoconus is rare, and most patients with so-called unilateral keratoconus, if followed long enough, eventually acquire keratoconus in the other eye.

2. Most cases (70%) occur in girls.

It is uncertain if keratoconus is not an inherited condition.

   a. Multiple over- and underexpressed genes have been related to this disorder. The upregulation of keratocan expression may be specific for keratoconus. Keratocan is said to be one of three keratan sulfate proteoglycans important for structure of the stromal matrix and maintenance of corneal transparency.

3. The apex of the cone is usually slightly inferior and nasal to the anterior pole of the cornea and tends to show stromal scarring.

4. *Munson's sign* occurs when the lower lid bulges on downward gaze.

5. *Vogt's vertical lines* are seen in the stroma. CFM suggests that Vogt's striae, which are seen to radiate from the center of the cone, represent stressed collagen lamellae.

6. *Fleischer ring* (see Fig. 8.44) is caused by iron deposition in the epithelium circumferentially around the base of the cone.

   a. It is best seen with the light of the slit lamp through a cobalt-blue filter.

   b. The iron is mainly deposited in the basal layer of epithelium, but is also found in epithelial wing cells.

7. Ruptures in Bowman's membrane (early, giving rise to anterior clear spaces), and in Descemet's membrane (late), and increased visibility of corneal nerves are common.

Ruptures in Descemet's membrane may result in *acute keratoconus* (see Fig. 8.45), a condition characterized by the abrupt onset of severe central corneal edema (hydrops), especially in Down's syndrome. With extreme rarity, the cornea may perforate, which has even occurred bilaterally.

8. Most cases are not inherited, although autosomal-recessive and dominant inheritance patterns may occur.

9. Keratoconus may be associated with, or accompanied by, vernal keratoconjunctivitis, pellucid marginal corneal degeneration, mitral valve prolapse, and, rarely, Fuchs' combined dystrophy. It has also been reported in association with distal arthrogryposis type IIB.

10. Elevated levels of terminal deoxynucleotidyl transferase biotin-dUTP nick end labeling (TUNEL) immunoreactivity suggest that apoptosis may play a role in the pathogenesis of keratoconus.

11. Clinical and histopathologic features compatible with keratoconus have been demonstrated in transplant grafts as long as 40 years after the initial corneal transplant for keratoconus. Population of the graft stroma by host keratocytes and/or aging of the graft has/have been postulated to cause this phenomenon.

12. Protein-related abnormalities are present in keratoconus corneas (e.g., molecular weights of abnormal proteins of 12, 14, and 39 kD); in addition, some normal corneal protein components may be increased, whereas others may be decreased. The level of type XII collagen is reduced in the epithelial basement membrane zone and stromal matrices in keratoconus corneas.

A reduction occurs in highly sulfated keratan sulfate epitopes.

Keratoconus corneas contain a reduced level of α_2-macroglobulin, lending support to the hypothesis that degradation processes may be aberrant in these corneas.

13. Histologically, the central cornea is thinned, the central portion of Bowman's membrane is destroyed, the central stroma is scarred, and the central portion of Descemet's membrane often shows ruptures.

   a. The stromal lamellae have a significant change in their organization, and the collagen fibrillar mass has been demonstrated to be unevenly distributed, particularly at the apex of the cone, indicating inter- and intralamellar slippage and displacement leading to the clinical morphologic changes characteristic of keratoconus.

   b. Guttata may occur.

   c. In the periphery of keratoconic corneas, fine cellular processes of keratocytes can be seen to penetrate Bowman's membrane. These cells may have elevated levels of cathepsins B and G.

   d. CFM has demonstrated a significant reduction in the density of keratocytes in the stroma. Reduced anterior keratocyte density is particularly associated with a history of atopy, eye rubbing, and the presence of corneal staining. CFM has also shown corneal epithelial abnormalities in this disorder, that have been confirmed by light microscopy.

   e. Iron is found in epithelial cells at all levels in the peripheral region of the thinned central cornea (Fleischer ring).

   f. Three acid hydrolases—acid phosphatase, acid esterase, and acid lipase—are significantly elevated in the corneal epithelium, especially in the basal layer.

B. Keratoglobus

1. Keratoglobus is a rare, bilateral, globular configuration of the cornea. The cornea shows generalized thinning from limbus to limbus, but most markedly peripherally.

2. The cornea is transparent, and an iron ring is absent.

3. The condition tends to be stationary, but hydrops can develop.

4. Keratoglobus is probably a variant of keratoconus and may occur in different members of the same family.

> Keratoglobus may be associated with vernal keratoconjunctivitis, idiopathic orbital inflammation, chronic marginal blepharitis with eye rubbing, glaucoma after penetrating keratoplasty, Leber's congenital amaurosis, blue sclera syndrome, and thyroid ophthalmopathy.

C. Pellucid marginal degeneration
1. Pellucid marginal degeneration is a progressive, bilateral, inferior, peripheral thinning of the cornea in a crescentic fashion; rarely, it can occur superiorly.
2. The area of involved cornea is clear with no scarring, infiltration, or vascularization.
3. Protrusion of the cornea occurs above a band of thinning located 1 to 2 mm from the limbus and measuring 1 to 2 mm in width, usually from 4 to 8 o'clock. Acute hydrops may occur.
4. The condition becomes apparent between 20 and 40 years of age; it occurs in both men and women, and results in high irregular astigmatism.

5. Scleroderma has been reported in association with a case of pellucid marginal degeneration.
6. Pellucid marginal degeneration may be an atypical form of keratoconus.
7. Spontaneous hydrops and even perforation may occur rarely.

> It differs from keratoconus in that it has no iron ring; its thinning is in an inferior arc without a cone; and the corneal protrusion is located above (rather than in) the area of thinning; however, it has been reported in association with keratoconus.

Endothelial

I. Cornea guttata (Fuchs' combined dystrophy; Figs 8.46 and 8.47)

> In 1910, Ernst Fuchs described the epithelial component, which is really a degeneration, secondary to the primary endothelial dystrophy (cornea guttata). Koeppe, in 1916, noted the endothelial changes. Vogt coined the term *guttae* in 1921.

A. It occurs predominantly in elderly women and is bilateral.

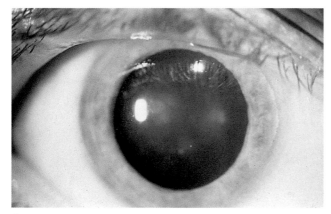

A

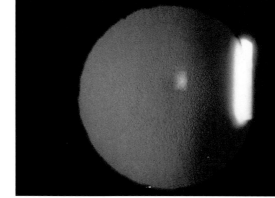

B

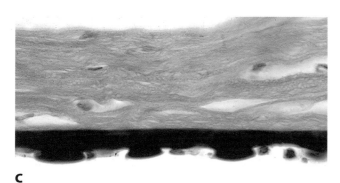

C

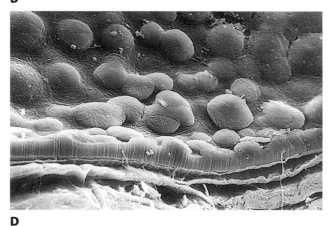

D

Fig. 8.46 Cornea guttata. **A,** The central cornea shows thickening, haze, and distortion of the light reflex. **B,** The typical beaten-metal appearance of the cornea is seen in the fundus reflex. **C,** Periodic acid–Schiff stain demonstrates the characteristic wartlike bumps present in Descemet's membrane, shown better in **D** by scanning electron microscopy. (**D,** Courtesy of Dr. RC Eagle, Jr.)

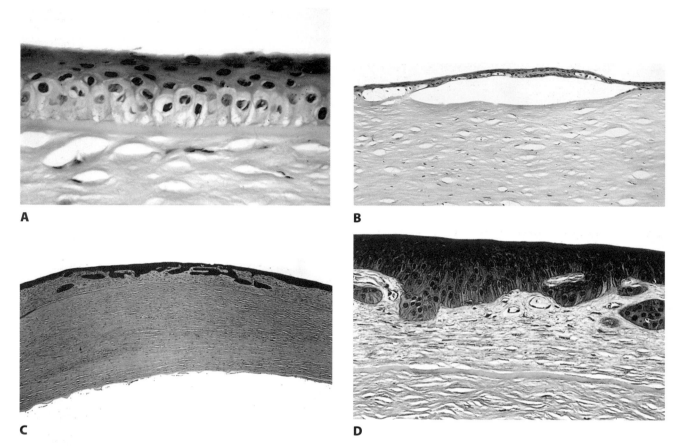

Fig. 8.47 Cornea guttata. **A,** Early cornea guttata causes intracellular edema of the basal layer of epithelium (seen clinically as corneal bedewing). **B,** The edema then spreads intercellularly, and, with increased corneal fluid, collects under the epithelium, leading to bullous keratopathy. **C,** Trichrome stain shows a central subepithelial ingrowth of cells from superficial corneal stroma through Bowman's membrane leading to production of a subepithelial fibrous membrane between epithelium and Bowman's membrane, called a *degenerative pannus,* shown with increased magnification in **D.**

1. Most cases probably have a dominant inheritance pattern.
2. The association of cornea guttata and anterior polar cataract, dominantly inherited in people of Scandinavian origin, has also been reported.
B. Four stages are seen clinically and histologically.
   1. Asymptomatic stage: excrescences resembling Hassall–Henle warts are present centrally.
      a. Electron microscopic studies of cornea guttata demonstrate foci of hyperproduction of Descemet's membrane in an abnormal format.
   2. Stage of painless decrease in vision and symptoms of glare: early changes occur as a mild stromal and intraepithelial edema (mainly the basal layer—*corneal bedewing*) followed by a subepithelial ingrowth of a layer of cells from the superficial stroma through Bowman's membrane, leading to production of a subepithelial fibrous membrane of varying thickness (*degenerative pannus*).
   3. Stage of periodic episodes of pain: a later change is moderate to marked stromal edema and interepithelial edema leading to epithelial bullae (*bullous keratopathy*) that periodically rupture, causing pain.

The corneal epithelium shows areas of atrophy, hypertrophy, and increased basement membrane formation.

   4. Stage of severely decreased vision but no pain: the degenerative pannus thickens so that the resultant scarring decreases vision. The advanced pannus tends to lessen bullae formation greatly.

Other late complications include glaucoma and ruptured bullae that may lead to corneal infection, ulceration, and even perforation.

   5. Oxytalan (oxytalan, elaunin, and elastic fibers are all part of the normal elastic system of fibers), not normally present in the cornea, is found in cornea guttata in the corneal subepithelial tissues and most abundantly deep to the endothelium and surrounding, but not in, the guttate bodies.
   6. Secondary lipid keratopathy is a frequent later finding.
      a. Reticulin fibers are prominent in both the guttate bodies and posterior Descemet's membrane.

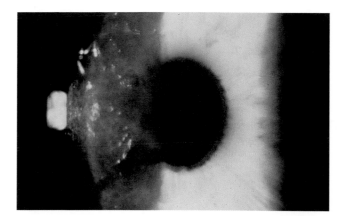

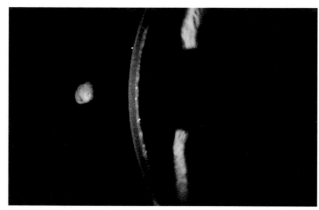

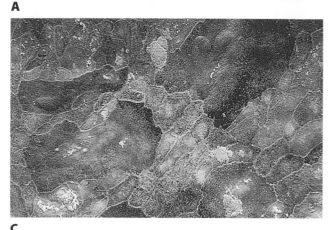

Fig. 8.48 Posterior polymorphous dystrophy. **A** and **B,** Clinical appearance of cornea. **C,** Scanning electron micrograph of posterior surface of cornea shows epithelial-like appearance of endothelium, caused by numerous surface microvilli. (**A** and **B,** Courtesy of Dr. JH Krachmer; **C,** courtesy of Dr. RC Eagle, Jr.)

    b. Disturbance in the regulation of endothelial apoptosis may contribute to the guttata process.

    c. Missense mutations in *COL8A2*, the gene that codes for the alpha-2 chain of type VIII collagen, have been detected in familial and sporadic cases of Fuchs' corneal dystrophy, and in a family with posterior polymorphous corneal dystrophy.

II. Posterior polymorphous dystrophy (PPMD; hereditary deep dystrophy of Schlichting; Fig. 8.48; see Table 16.1)

  A. Irregular, polymorphous opacities and vesicles with central pigmentation and surrounding opacification are seen in the central cornea at the level of endothelium and Descemet's membrane.

    1. CFM has demonstrated craters, streaks, and cracks over the corneal endothelial surface accompanied by endothelial pleomorphism and polymegathism. Wide variation in endothelial cell counts and other abnormalities of Descemet's membrane have also been noted.

The corneal abnormalities may vary greatly, even within the same family. Some individuals show only a few isolated vesicles; others manifest severe secondary stromal and epithelial edema; still others show any stage in

---

between. Posterior corneal vesicles may also occur as an isolated finding unrelated to PPMD.

  B. Ruptures in Descemet's membrane and glaucoma (either open-angle or associated with iridocorneal adhesions) may be associated.

The differential diagnosis between the bandlike structures in PPMD and Haab's striae (see Fig. 16.6) depends on the clinical appearance. The edges of Haab's striae are thickened and curled and contain a secondary hyperproduction of Descemet's membrane; the area between the edges is thin and smooth. PPMD bands are just the opposite.

  C. The condition is inherited as an autosomal-dominant or recessive trait.

PPMD should not be confused with the rare, autosomal-dominant disorder, *posterior amorphous corneal dysgenesis* (dystrophy), which is characterized by gray, sheetlike opacities in the posterior stroma. An association of *Alport's syndrome* and PPMD has been seen in people of Thai origin. The association suggests a common defect in basement membrane formation in the two entities. A mutation in *COL8A2* may cause PPMD in some families.

  D. Histologically, the most posterior layers of stroma demonstrate fracturing, the endothelial cells are attenuated, and Descemet's membrane may be focally or diffusely thickened, or occasionally thinned.

1. Electron microscopically, the posterior stromal lamellae are disorganized and Descemet's membrane is interrupted by bands of collagen resembling stroma.

   a. The posterior surface of the cornea is covered in a geographic pattern by endothelial- and epithelial-like cells with numerous desmosomes, apical villi, and prominent bundles of intracytoplasmic filaments, sometimes creating vesicles and sometimes creating partially detached sheets of cells.

   b. The microvilli-covered cells are present at the onset of the process, and are not a secondary change of long-standing disease.

   c. The total number of endothelial cells is decreased.

2. A layer of cells may be present beneath the corneal epithelium, but epithelial edema is not common.

Although some of the changes may superficially resemble those seen in the iridocorneal endothelial syndrome (see Table 16.1) and in cornea guttata, they are usually easily distinguishable because they result from interstitial keratitis and keratoconus.

III. Congenital hereditary endothelial dystrophy (CHED; Fig. 8.49; see also Table 8.4)

   A. Clinically, a diffuse blue-white opacity (ground-glass appearance) involves the cornea.

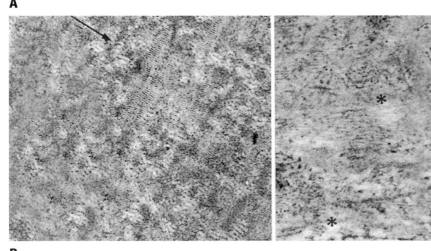
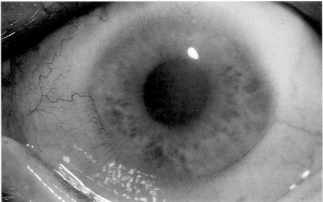
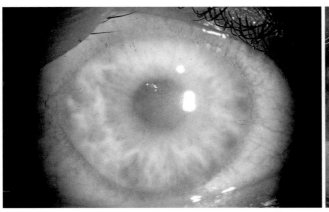
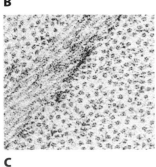
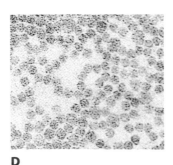

Fig. 8.49 Congenital hereditary endothelial dystrophy (CHED), **A,** Clinical appearance right eye (*left*) and left eye (*right*) of a patient with CHED, previously reported as Hurler's disease (patient #5 in Scheie HG *et al.: Am J Ophthalmol* 53:753, 1962). **B,** Left side shows banded (*arrow*) Descemet's membrane near stroma and thickened posterior layer interspersed with fibrous basement membrane and patches of banded-type basement membrane. Right side shows high magnification of multilaminar patches (*) of homogeneous basement membrane interspersed with multilaminar sheets of fibrous basement membrane. **C,** Collagen fibrils in normal corneal stroma measure approximately 24 nm in diameter. **D,** Stromal collagen fibrils in CHED often measure approximately 48 nm, with some reaching diameters of up to 72 nm. (**B–D**, From Kenyon KR, Maumenee AE: *Invest Ophthalmol* 7:475. Copyright Elsevier 1968.)

B. CHED tends to be bilateral and progressive, and may be associated with nystagmus and glaucoma, or with agenesis of the corpus callosum.

C. The differential diagnosis of CHED includes congenital hereditary stromal dystrophy, congenital glaucoma, cornea guttata, congenital leukoma, hereditary corneal edema, mucopolysaccharidoses, Peters' anomaly, sclerocornea, and stromal dystrophies (e.g., macular corneal dystrophy).

Some cases previously classified as hereditary corneal edema are identical to CHED, whereas others are the same as congenital hereditary stromal dystrophy (see p. 297 in this chapter) and mucopolysaccharidoses.

D. Two modes of inheritance have been reported: an autosomal-recessive and a rarer autosomal-dominant type.
1. In the autosomal-recessive type, corneal clouding is present at birth or within the neonatal period.
2. In the autosomal-dominant type (20q12–q13.1), the cornea is usually clear early in life. Corneal opacification develops slowly and is progressive.

E. Histologically, increased diameter of the stromal collagen fibrils may produce a thick cornea. Spheroidal degeneration may also be present. Descemet's membrane shows fibrous thickening (similar, if not identical to, cornea guttata), implying an endothelial abnormality. Secondary corneal amyloidosis may occur, particularly in association with a subepithelial fibrous pannus.

F. Immunohistochemical staining of corneal endothelium in PPMD and CHED are similar relative to cytokeratins expressed, including CK 7, which is not present in normal endothelium or surface epithelium.

IV. Nonguttate corneal endothelial degeneration
A. The condition is characterized by spontaneous unilateral corneal edema in an otherwise normal eye.

B. Specular microscopy of the nonedematous contralateral cornea reveals endothelial pleomorphism and a cell count reduced to approximately half of normal for the age.

C. Histologically, the edematous cornea shows a Descemet's membrane of variable thickness and composition.
1. Guttata are absent.
2. The endothelium is extremely attenuated or discontinuous.

The remainder of the corneal layers appear normal. Keratocytic invasion of the subepithelial plane has not been observed histologically.

PIGMENTATIONS

Melanin

I. Pigmentation of the basal layer of epithelium, especially in the peripheral cornea, is normally found in dark races (Fig. 8.50A).

II. A posterior corneal membrane may be caused by a proliferation of uveal melanocytes or pigment epithelial cells on to the posterior cornea after an injury.

Lipofuscin pigments, sometimes confused with melanin, may rarely become deposited in the cornea, a condition called corneal lipofuscinosis.

III. Krukenberg's spindle (see Fig. 16.21)

When a Krukenberg's spindle is present unilaterally, ocular trauma is the usual cause.

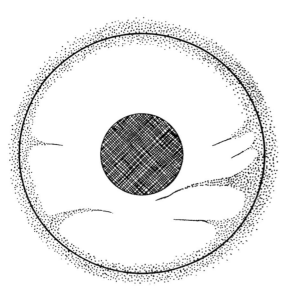
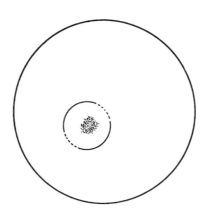

Fig. 8.50 A, Melanin pigment may extend into epithelium of cornea, as depicted in diagram. **B,** Fleischer ring of keratoconus drawn as it would appear in left eye (i.e., slightly nasal and inferior to center of cornea). (**A,** From Gass JDM: *Arch Ophthalmol* 71:348, 1964, with permission. © American Medical Association. All rights reserved.)

A   B

Blood

I. Blood staining of the cornea occurs in the presence of a hyphema when intraocular pressure has been increased for at least 48 hours (see Fig. 5.31).

Staining may occur earlier or even without glaucoma if the endothelium is diseased.

II. Staining of the cornea is due to hemoglobin and other breakdown products of erythrocytes.

The small amount of hemosiderin present is usually contained within keratocytes.

III. The cornea clears first peripherally, and may take several years to clear completely.

IV. Histologically, amorphous extracellular hemoglobin globules, and tiny round spheres and rods (all orange in hematoxylin and eosin-stained sections) are mainly seen between corneal lamellae, but also in keratocytes and in Bowman's membrane.

The extracellular hemoglobin does not stain positive for iron, as does the intracellular oxidized hemoglobin (i.e., hemosiderin) in keratocytes.

Iron Lines

I. Fleischer ring (see Fig. 8.50B; see also Fig. 8.44; see section *Dystrophies*, subsection *Stromal*, earlier)

II. Hudson–Stähli line (Figs 8.51 and 8.52)—deposition of iron in the corneal epithelium in a horizontal line just inferior to the center of the interpalpebral fissure

III. Stocker line (see Fig. 8.51)—deposition of iron in the epithelium at the advancing edge of a pterygium

IV. Ferry line (see Fig. 8.51)—deposition of iron in the corneal epithelium at the corneal margin of a filtering bleb

V. Iron lines may occur in many conditions, such as the annular lines in the donor epithelium of corneal grafts, around old corneal scars, centrally after refractive keratoplasty, and in association with overnight ortho-keratology.

Kayser–Fleischer Ring

I. The Kayser–Fleischer ring (Fig. 8.53) is associated with *hepatolenticular degeneration* (*Wilson's disease*):
A. Increased absorption of copper from gut
B. Decrease in serum ceruloplasmin
C. Usually, an autosomal-recessive inheritance pattern (defect on chromosome 12q14–21), but may have a dominant type

II. The Kayser–Fleischer ring (i.e., copper in Descemet's membrane) is usually apparent by late childhood or early adolescence and may be accompanied by a "sunflower" cataract.

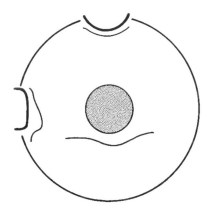

Fig. 8.51 Iron lines. Ferry line depicted at top in front of (i.e., below) filtering bleb; Stocker line depicted on left in front of (to right) of advancing edge of pterygium; Hudson–Stähli line (see also Fig. 8.52) across (horizontal) cornea just below center. All three lines caused by iron in epithelial cells. (Modified with permission from Gass JDM: *Arch Ophthalmol* 71:348, 1964. © American Medical Association. All rights reserved.)

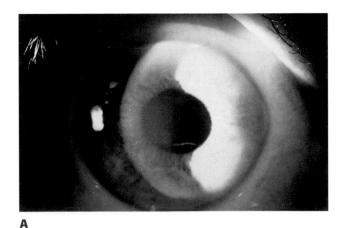

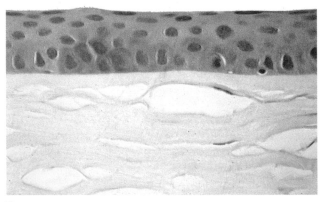

A **B**

Fig. 8.52 Hudson–Stähli line. **A,** A curved horizontal brown line is seen just below the central cornea (lower pupillary space) in the epithelium. **B,** Histologic section shows that the line is caused by iron deposition in the epithelium. The other iron lines (Fleischer, Stocker, and Ferry) have a similar histologic appearance. (**B,** Perl's stain.)

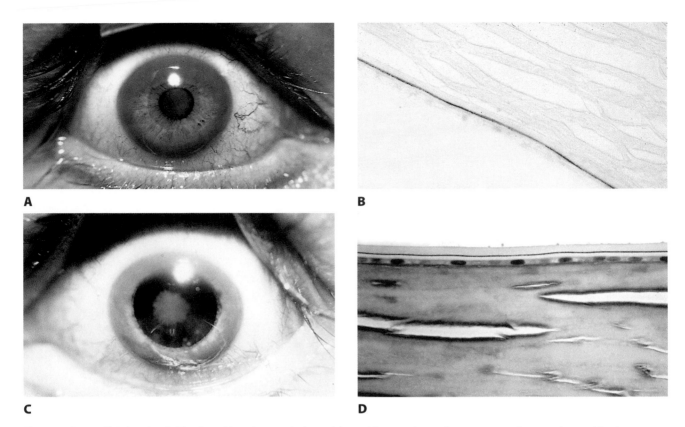

Fig. 8.53 Kayser–Fleischer ring. **A,** The deposition of copper in the periphery of Descemet's membrane, seen as a brown color, partially obstructs the view of the underlying iris, especially superiorly. A "sunflower" (disciform) cataract is present in the lens of this patient with Wilson's disease. **B,** An unstained section shows copper deposition in the inner portion of peripheral Descemet's membrane. **C,** The sunflower cataract is better seen with the pupil dilated. A line of copper is also present deep within the central anterior (**D**) (and posterior) lens capsule and accounts for the clinically observed cataract. (Modified from Tso MOM *et al.: Am J Ophthalmol* 79:479. Copyright Elsevier 1975.)

A. The ring is found in about 63% of children with Wilson's disease, and in all patients with neurologic manifestations of the disease, but in only 58% of patients with only hepatic presentation.

The Kayser–Fleischer ring can be simulated exactly as a result of a retained intraocular copper foreign body. In this event, however, the ring is only present in the eye containing the foreign body. Rarely, a Kayser–Fleischer ring may be the presenting sign of Wilson's disease. Conversely, it may be present in other forms of liver diseases, such as alcoholic liver disease. Ocular deposition of copper involving central Descemet's membrane, iris surface, and lens capsule of both eyes has been reported as the presenting sign of multiple myeloma.

III. Histologically, the copper, bound to sulfur, is deposited in the posterior half of the peripheral portion of Descemet's membrane and in the deeper layers of the central anterior and posterior lens capsule.

Tattoo

I. Corneal tattooing (Fig. 8.54) is usually done to disguise unsightly leukomas.
II. It is performed by chemical reduction of metallic salts (e.g., gold chloride or platinum black).

III. Histologically, the foreign material is seen in the corneal stroma.

Drug-Induced

I. Oxidized epinephrine
II. Chloroquine (see Fig. 11.32)
   A. Long-term chloroquine used systemically causes a decreased corneal sensitivity.
   B. The corneal epithelial deposits vary from diffuse, fine, punctate opacities to focal aggregations arranged in radial, whorling lines that diverge from just below the center of the cornea.

Similar corneal appearances are seen in Fabry's disease, and in amiodarone (Fig. 8.55), suramin, clofazimine and indomethacin keratopathies. These are drug-induced lipidoses.

The deposits may disappear after stoppage of chloroquine.
   C. Confocal microscopy (CFM) demonstrates that the impact of amiodarone on the cornea may extend deeper than the epithelium as, in eyes with advanced keratopathy, microdots can be seen in the anterior and posterior

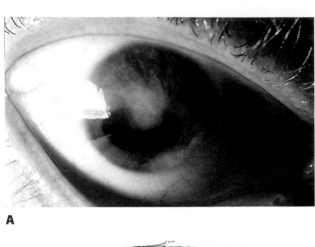

A

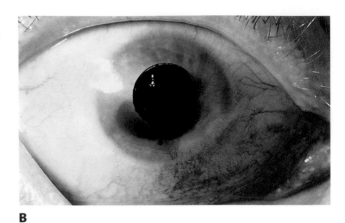

B

Fig. 8.54 Corneal tattoo. Corneal scar before (**A**) and after (**B**) tattooing. **C,** Tattoo in another case is noted histologically as dark black deposits of platinum in the corneal stroma. (**A** and **B,** Courtesy of Dr. JA Katowitz.)

C

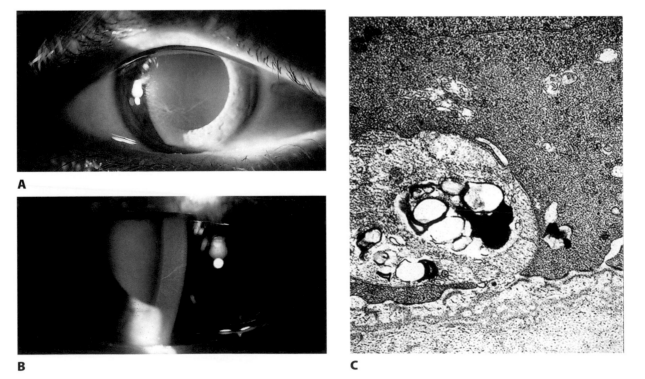

A

B

C

Fig. 8.55 Amiodarone. **A** and **B,** A brown epithelial deposit is seen as radial, whorling, branching lines that diverge from just below the center of the cornea. **C,** Electron microscopy shows electron-dense inclusions in the basal corneal epithelial cell. (**C,** Case presented by Dr. AH Friedman at the meeting of the Verhoeff Society, 1990.)

stroma, and on the endothelial cell layer. Moreover, keratocyte density is decreased.

III. Chlorpromazine

A. The pigmentation (melanin-like) is present immediately under the anterior capsule of the lens in the central (axial) area and in the conjunctival substantia propria in the interpalpebral fissure area.

B. In the area of the interpalpebral fissure, the corneal pigmentation appears as epithelial curvilinear and linear opacifications.

1. In the corneal stroma, it appears as diffuse, granular yellow pigmentations.

2. In the corneal endothelium, it appears as fine deposits.

IV. Other drugs

Other drugs, such as indomethacin, suramin, amiodarone (see Fig. 8.55), and Argyrol (argyrosis; see p. 235 in Chapter 7), can cause a corneal keratopathy. Antimetabolites, such as cytarabine, can result in degeneration of basal cells and secondary epithelial microcyst formation.

INFECTIONS

Keratitis secondary to dematiaceous fungal infection may result in the formation of a pigmented corneal plaque. The fungi are septate and contain brown to black pigment in the cell walls in most cases.

Crystals

I. Infectious crystalline keratopathy (ICK; Fig. 8.56)

A. ICK is a distinctive microbial corneal infection, characterized by fernlike intrastromal opacities without significant inflammation, and most often occurring in donor grafts after penetrating keratoplasty.

B. The most common cause is *Streptococcus* species, but other Gram-positive and Gram-negative bacteria and fungi can cause ICK, such as *Peptostreptococcus*; *Haemophilus aphrophilus*; *Staphylococcus epidermidis*; *Alternaria*; *Pseudomonas aeruginosa*; and *Candida albicans, C. guilliermondi*, and *C. tropicalis*.

C. Histopathologically, the crystalline opacities consist of colonies of microbes insinuated between corneal stromal lamellae.

II. Noninfectious crystalline keratopathy

A. Many causes of noninfectious crystalline keratopathy exist, including Schnyder's corneal dystrophy; lipid keratopathy; Bietti's crystalline retinal and corneal dystrophy; infantile, adolescent, and adult forms of cystinosis; gout; chronic renal failure; hypercalcemia; some familial lipoprotein disorders; dysproteinemias

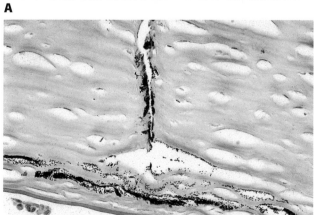

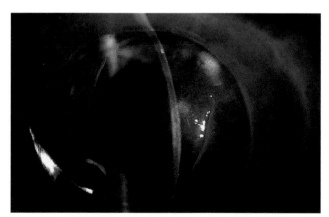

A

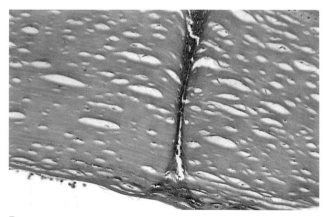

B

C

Fig. 8.56 Infectious crystalline keratopathy. **A,** Patient had "relaxing incisions" to correct postpenetrating keratoplasty astigmatism. Rounded crystallinelike infiltrates developed on both sides of one of the two incisions. **B,** Histologic section shows the posterior aspect of the healing cornea incision. **C,** Brown–Brenn stain shows multiple Gram-positive cocci in the region of the incision. (Case presented by Dr. MC Kincaid at the Eastern Ophthalmic Pathology Society, 1990, and reported by Kincaid MC et al.: *Am J Ophthalmol* 111:374. Copyright Elsevier 1991.)

associated with multiple myeloma, malignant lymphoma, and other lymphoproliferative disorders (gammopathies); *Dieffenbachia* keratitis; and long-term drug therapy with colloidal gold (chrysiasis), chlorpromazine, chloroquine, 5-fluorouracil subconjunctival injection, clofazimine, and immunoglobulin therapy for pyoderma gangrenosum. Gatifloxacin, a fourth-generation fluoroquinolone, may deposit as crystals in the stroma as a result of compromised corneal epithelium. A similar process has been described for ciprofloxacin.
   B. Increasing longevity of patients with nephropathic cystinosis has led to varied anterior-segment manifestations in more mature patients. In addition to classic crystalline deposits, these findings include superficial punctate keratopathy, filamentary keratopathy, severe peripheral corneal neovascularization, band keratopathy, and posterior synechiae with iris thickening and transillumination.
   C. The histologic appearance depends on the cause.

NEOPLASM

I. The cornea is rarely the primary site for neoplasms, but it is frequently involved secondarily in conjunctival tumors such as squamous cell carcinoma and malignant melanoma.
   A. Corneal involvement may occur in 38% of 287 cases of conjunctival squamous cell carcinoma.
   B. Occasionally conjunctival melanoma may present as a corneal mass. Such lesions have been termed "corneally displaced malignant conjunctival melanoma."
II. Myxoma
   A. Myxoma is rarely reported as a corneal tumor in an individual lacking a history of prior corneal disease.
   B. The tumor is composed of spindle-shaped cells in a myxomatous ground substance.
      1. Ultrastructurally, the cellular elements have features characteristic of keratocytes with no basement membrane, much rough endoplasmic reticulum, and vacuoles containing mucoid-like material.
      2. Immunohistopathologic characteristics of the tumor cells are positivity for vimentin, muscle-specific actin, and smooth-muscle antigen.
III. Nevi are rarely diagnosed as primary on the cornea. They were found in 2 eyes of 410 patients having ocular surface nevi in one study.
IV. Juvenile xanthogranuloma has been reported to involve the corneoscleral limbus in a child, and an adult.
V. Primary diffuse neurofibroma may involve the cornea in von Recklinghausen disease.

SCLERA

CONGENITAL ANOMALIES

Blue Sclera

I. Blue sclera may occur alone or with brittle bones and deafness.

> A syndrome of red hair, blue sclera, and brittle cornea with recurrent spontaneous perforation, called *Stein's syndrome* (*brittle cornea syndrome*), has been reported in Tunisian Jewish families. Blue sclera has also been reported in association with Alport's syndrome.

II. There are three types of brittle bones.
   A. Osteogenesis imperfecta—usually apparent at birth and consisting of four types:
      1. Type I is dominantly inherited and is characterized by skeletal osteopenia, fractures, dentinogenesis imperfecta (in some patients), and blue sclera throughout life.
      2. Type II usually results in death in the perinatal period.
      3. Type III is a rare autosomal-recessive disorder in which severe, progressive skeletal deformities occur. The sclera may be blue at birth but becomes normal by adolescence or adulthood.
      4. Type IV is dominantly inherited and is characterized by skeletal osteopenia and blue sclera at birth, which become normal by adulthood.
   B. Osteopsathyrosis—a variant of brittle bones without blue sclera
   C. Osteogenesis imperfecta tarda—delayed onset with levis and gravis forms
III. The sclera retains its normal fetal translucency so that the deep-brown uvea shows through as blue.
IV. In most cases, the disease is inherited as an autosomal-dominant trait, but autosomal-recessive inheritance may occur.
V. Central corneal thickness is reduced in osteogenesis imperfecta, and negatively correlates with the blueness of the sclera in this disorder.
VI. Histologically, the sclera is usually thinner than normal but may be thicker and more cellular than normal. Its collagen fibers are abnormal, being reduced in thickness by approximately 25% in the cornea and more than 50% in the sclera.

Ochronosis (Alkaptonuria)

I. Because the enzyme homogentisic acid oxidase (homogentisate 1,2-dioxygenase) is lacking, homogentisic acid deposits in tissues (especially cartilage, elastic, and collagen, e.g., sclera) and forms a melanin-like substance.
II. The condition is inherited as an autosomal-recessive trait and is caused by mutations in the homogentisate

1,2-dioxygenase gene located to a 16-cM region of the 3q2 chromosome.

III. Histologically, amorphous strands and curlicues are seen in the sclera and overlying substantia propria of the conjunctiva.

INFLAMMATIONS

Episcleritis

I. Episcleritis (Fig. 8.57) involves one eye two-thirds of the time, and is characterized by redness of the eye and discomfort, rarely described as pain.

A. Hyperemia, edema, and infiltration are entirely within the episcleral tissue; the sclera is spared.

B. The episcleral vascular network is congested maximally, with some congestion of the conjunctival vessels and minimal congestion of the scleral vessels.

C. Episcleritis is a benign recurring condition.

> Episcleritis usually resolves without treatment in 2 to 21 days. Episcleritis does not progress to scleritis except in herpes zoster, which sometimes starts as an episcleritis and shows the vesicular stage of the eruption. It reappears approximately 3 months later as a scleritis in the same site.

D. No clear conclusions can be drawn as to the cause of episcleritis.

> Although usually idiopathic, approximately one-third of the cases of episcleritis may be associated with systemic entities such as rheumatoid arthritis, systemic lupus erythematosus, inflammatory bowel disease, relapsing polychondritis, and systemic vasculitic diseases (e.g., Wegener's granulomatosis and Cogan's syndrome); or with local eye diseases such as ocular rosacea, keratoconjunctivitis sicca, and atopic keratoconjunctivitis.

II. Classification

A. Simple episcleritis

1. Redness caused by engorged episcleral vessels that retain their normal radial position and architecture

> In episcleritis, after local instillation of 2.5% phenylephrine, the redness usually mostly disappears, whereas in scleritis, the redness persists.

2. Diffuse edema
3. Sometimes small gray deposits

B. Nodular episcleritis

1. Localized redness and edema
2. An intraepiscleral nodule that is mobile on the underlying sclera

III. Histologically, chronic nongranulomatous inflammation of lymphocytes, plasma cells, and edema is found in the episcleral tissue. Rarely, a chronic granulomatous inflammatory infiltrate may be seen.

Scleritis (Fig. 8.58)

I. Anterior scleritis

A. Diffuse (most benign form)

1. Diffuse anterior scleritis in women is most common in the fourth to seventh decades, with no predilection for any of those decades, whereas in men it is most prevalent in the third to sixth decades and peaks during the fourth.

> Rarely, mucosal-associated lymphoid tissue (MALT) lymphoma can present as a scleritis.

2. Approximately half of the patients have bilateral involvement.
3. Up to 42% of patients who have scleritis have an associated uveitis.

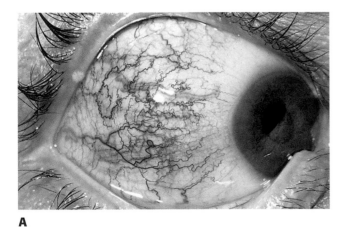
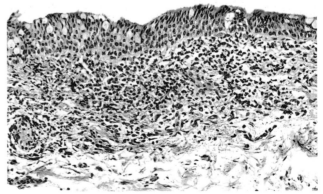

A **B**

Fig. 8.57 Episcleritis. **A,** Clinical appearance. **B,** Biopsy of conjunctiva shows infiltration with lymphocytes and plasma cells.

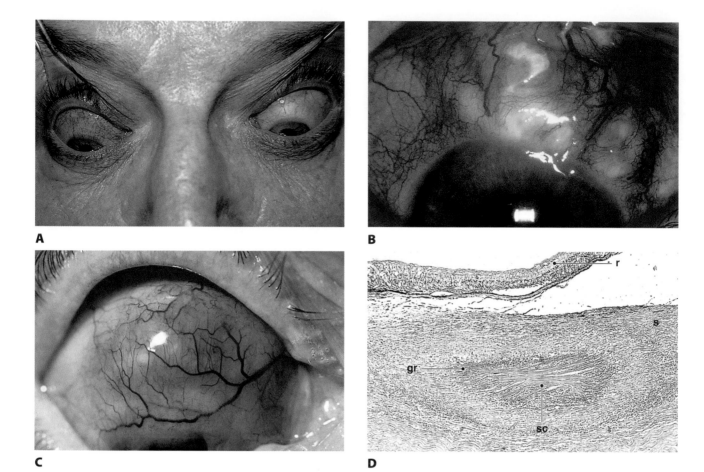

A

B

C

D

Fig. 8.58 Scleritis. Scleritis can go on to (**A**) thickening (brawny scleritis) and (**B**) necrosis. **C,** Healing of the necrotic area leads to scleromalacia perforans. **D,** Histologic section shows a zonal granulomatous reaction (gr) around necrotic scleral collagen (sc) (r, retina; s, sclera). (**D,** Presented by Dr. IW McLean to the meeting of the Armed Forces Institute of Pathology alumni, 1973.)

4. Diffuse anterior scleritis is one of the very few severely painful eye conditions.

The boring pain may be localized to the eye or generalized, usually in the distribution of the second and third branches of the trigeminal nerve.

5. As in all forms of scleritis, scleral edema and inflammation are present.

a. The diagnostic features differentiating it from episcleritis are the outward displacement of the deep vascular network of the episclera and the typical blue-red color.

b. A small area or the whole anterior segment may be involved.

B. Nodular

1. Nodular anterior scleritis is most prevalent in both women and men from the fourth to sixth decades, but in women a noticeable peak occurs in the sixth decade.

Nodular scleritis can be considered of intermediate severity between diffuse and necrotizing disease.

2. Approximately half of the patients have bilateral involvement.

3. The pain is as described in diffuse anterior scleritis.

4. The nodule, unlike the one in nodular episcleritis, is deep red, totally immobile, and quite separate from the overlying congested episcleral tissues.

Rarely, biopsy of such nodule may be diagnostic of sarcoidosis.

C. Necrotizing—with inflammation (most severe form of scleritis)

1. Necrotizing anterior scleritis with inflammation mostly occurs in women.

2. Approximately half of the patients have bilateral involvement.

3. The pain is as described for the diffuse form except that it is the most severe type of ocular pain.

4. It is the most destructive form of scleritis, with over 60% of eyes experiencing complications other than scleral thinning and 40% losing visual acuity.

a. The patients may present with severe edema and acute congestion (*brawny scleritis*) or a patch of avascular episcleral tissue overlying or adjacent to an area of scleral edema.

b. In some cases, the inflammation remains localized to one small area and may result in almost total loss of scleral tissue from that area.

c. Most often, the inflammation starts in one area and then spreads circumferentially around the globe until the whole of the anterior segment is involved.

D. Necrotizing—without inflammation (scleromalacia perforans)

1. Necrotizing anterior scleritis without inflammation mostly afflicts women.

2. Approximately half of the patients have bilateral involvement.

3. Patients rarely complain of pain in scleromalacia perforans and present without subjective symptoms.

4. A grayish or yellowish patch on the sclera, without inflammation, may progress to complete dissolution of sclera and episclera, covered by a thin layer of conjunctiva.

II. Posterior scleritis

A. Posterior scleritis and anterior scleritis are usually associated, and occur most frequently in women in their sixth decade.

Approximately 30% of patients who have a posterior scleritis have an associated systemic disease, such as various types of vasculitis, autoimmune disease, and lymphoma.

B. Most patients have unilateral involvement.

C. The pain is as described for diffuse anterior scleritis.

D. Proptosis, exudative detachment, and other fundus changes such as optic disc edema may be seen in addition to anterior scleritis.

E. Posterior scleritis in a nodular configuration may simulate choroidal neoplasm.

Ultrasonography is most helpful in the diagnosis.

III. Complications

A. A decrease in visual acuity (14%) may result from keratitis, cataract, anterior uveitis, or posterior uveitis.

B. Keratitis (29%)

1. Diffuse anterior scleritis
   a. Localized stromal keratitis
   b. Localized sclerosing keratitis

2. Nodular anterior scleritis
   a. Acute stromal keratitis
   b. Sclerosing keratitis
   c. Corneal gutter

3. Necrotizing scleritis
   a. Sclerosing keratitis
   b. Keratolysis

C. Corneal vascularization (9%)

D. Cataract (7%)

E. Uveitis (30%)

F. Glaucoma (12%)

G. Scleral thinning and scleral defects (perforation of the globe is rare except after subconjunctival steroid injection)

1. Spontaneous rupture of a posterior staphyloma has been reported.

IV. Associated systemic diseases

A. Almost half of the patients with scleritis have a known associated systemic disease, approximately 15% of which represent connective tissue diseases. Almost 80% of the associated systemic diseases are known prior to the onset of the initial scleritis.

Scleromalacia perforans is associated with long-standing rheumatoid arthritis in approximately 46% of patients. The connective tissue diseases are most prevalent in necrotizing anterior scleritis with inflammation. Twenty-one percent of patients with necrotizing anterior scleritis with inflammation, which is probably the malignant phase of systemic connective tissue disease, die within 8 years of diagnosis.

B. Other associated systemic diseases include hypersensitivity disorders (e.g., erythema nodosum, asthma, erythema multiforme, contact dermatitis, Wegener's granulomatosis; Fig. 8.59, and see p. 184 in Chapter 6), polychondritis, Goodpasture's syndrome, granulomatous conditions (e.g., tuberculosis, syphilis), viral and bacterial infection (e.g., herpes zoster, HSV, *Pseudomonas*), porphyria, and metabolic disorders (e.g., gout).

C. Systemic diseases, such as leukemia, may mimic scleritis.

V. Histology—the basic lesion is a granulomatous inflammation surrounding abnormal scleral collagen.

A. Vasculitis with fibrinoid necrosis and neutrophil invasion of the vessel wall are present in 75% of scleral and 52% of conjunctival specimens.

Vascular immunodeposits are present in 93% of scleral and 79% of conjunctival specimens.

B. In the conjunctiva, there are increased T cells of all types, macrophages, and B cells.

C. In the sclera, increased T cells of all types and macrophages are seen.

D. Increased HLA-DR expression is markedly increased in both conjunctiva and sclera.

TUMORS

Fibromas

See discussion of mesenchymal tumors in subsection *Primary Orbital Tumors*, Chapter 14.

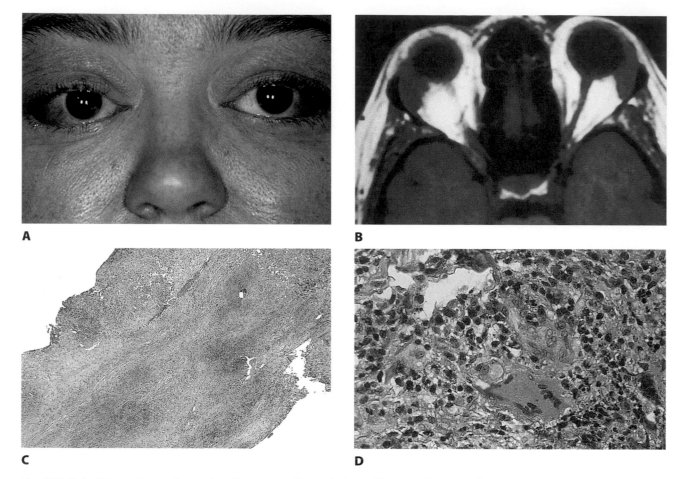

Fig. 8.59 Limited Wegener's granulomatosis. **A,** Recurrent swelling and edema of the upper lids present for approximately 2 months. **B,** Magnetic resonance imaging scan shows bilateral lacrimal gland masses. Antineutrophilic cytoplasmic antibody test was positive. Biopsy was performed. **C,** Histologic section shows a necrotizing granulomatous reaction with epithelioid cells and inflammatory giant cells along with eosinophils and necrotic foci containing neutrophils. **D,** Increased magnification of epithelioid cells and inflammatory giant cells. (Case presented by Dr. ME Smith at the meeting of the Verhoeff Society, 1994.)

Nodular Fasciitis

See discussion of mesenchymal tumors in subsection *Primary Orbital Tumors*, Chapter 14.

Hemangiomas

See discussion of mesenchymal tumors in subsection *Primary Orbital Tumors*, Chapter 14.

Neurofibromas

See discussion of mesenchymal tumors in subsection *Primary Orbital Tumors*, Chapter 14.

Contiguous Tumors

Conjunctival Tumors

   II. Uveal malignant melanoma

Episcleral Osseous Choristoma and Episcleral Osseocartilaginous Choristoma

   I. The tumor (Fig. 8.60) is typically present between the lateral and upper recti.

  II. It is symptomless, is present at birth, and characteristically contains bone.

 III. Histologically, normal-appearing bone is seen in the abnormal episcleral location.

 IV. The differential diagnosis includes classical limbal dermoids, epithelial inclusion cysts, prolapsed orbital fat, papillomas, dermolipomas, and complex choristomas.

Bone formation occurs through the condensation of mesenchyme in two ways: (1) membranous bone forms from mesenchymal condensation directly without first forming cartilage (e.g., many skull bones and intraocular ossification); and (2) bone forms from mesenchymal formation of cartilaginous template (e.g., ribs)—both types of bone formation occur in episcleral osseous choristoma and episcleral osseocartilaginous choristoma.

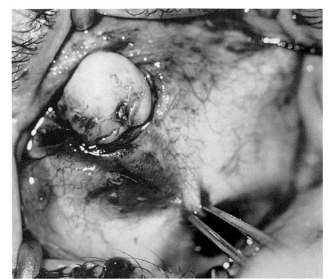

A

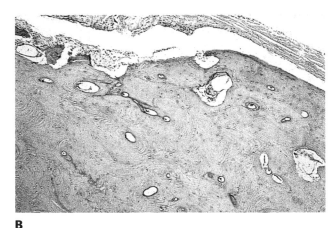

B

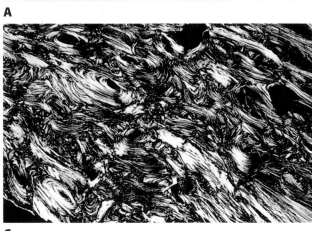

C

Fig. 8.60 Episcleral osseous choristoma. **A,** Clinical appearance of surgically exposed tumor in typical superotemporal location. **B,** Histologic section shows that the tumor is composed of compact bone. **C,** Polarized light demonstrates subunits consisting of concentric osteon lamellae surrounding a central canal (haversian canal). (Modified from Ortiz JM, Canoff M: *Br J Ophthalmol* 63:173, 1979, with permission.)

Ectopic Lacrimal Gland

See p. 543 in Chapter 14.

BIBLIOGRAPHY

Cornea

Normal Anatomy

Belmonte C, Acosta MC, Gallar J: Neural basis of sensation in intact and injured corneas. *Exp Eye Res* 78:513, 2004

Brandt JD, Casuso LA, Budenz DL: Markedly increased central corneal thickness: an unrecognized finding in congenital aniridia. *Am J Ophthalmol* 137:348, 2004

Chu DS, Zaidman GW, Meisler DM *et al.*: Human immunodeficiency virus-positive patients with posterior intracorneal precipitates. *Ophthalmology* 108:1853, 2001

Cortes M, Lambiase A, Sacchetti M *et al.*: Limbal stem cell deficiency associated with LADD syndrome. *Arch Ophthalmol* 123:691, 2005

Diaz-Araya CM, Madigan MC, Provis JM *et al.*: Immunohistochemical and topographic studies of dendritic cells and macrophages in human fetal cornea. *Invest Ophthalmol Vis Sci* 36:644, 1995

Espana EM, Grueterich M, Romano AC *et al.*: Idiopathic limbal stem cell deficiency. *Ophthalmology* 109:2004, 2002

Evereklioglu C, Madenci E, Bayazit YA *et al.*: Central corneal thickness is lower in osteogenesis imperfecta and negatively correlates with the presence of blue sclera. *Ophthalmic Physiol Opt* 22:511, 2002

Evereklioglu C, Yilmaz K, Bekir NA: Decreased central corneal thickness in children with Down syndrome. *J Pediatr Ophthalmol Strabismus* 39:274, 2002

Feenstra RPG, Tseng SCG: Comparison of fluorescein and rose Bengal staining. *Ophthalmology* 99:605, 1992

Fine BS, Yanoff M: *Ocular Histology: A Text and Atlas*, 2nd edn. Hagerstown, Harper & Row, 1979:161–186

Gordon MO, Beiser JA, Brandt JD *et al.*: The Ocular Hypertension Treatment Study: baseline factors that predict the onset of primary open-angle glaucoma. *Arch Ophthalmol* 120:714, 2002

Grupcheva CN, Malik TY, Craig JP *et al.*: Microstructural assessment of rare corneal dystrophies using real-time in vivo confocal microscopy. *Clin Exp Ophthalmol* 29:281, 2001

Inoue K, Kato S, Inoue Y *et al.*: The corneal endothelium and thickness in type II diabetes mellitus. *Jpn J Ophthalmol* 46:65, 2002

Inoue K, Okugawa K, Oshika T *et al.*: Morphological study of corneal endothelium and corneal thickness in pseudoexfoliation syndrome. *Jpn J Ophthalmol* 47:235, 2003

Ito D, Yamada M, Kawai M *et al.*: Corneal endothelial degeneration in dentatorubral-pallidoluysian atrophy. *Arch Neurol* 59:289, 2002

Kallinikos P, Berhanu M, O'Donnell C *et al.*: Corneal nerve tortuosity in diabetic patients with neuropathy. *Invest Ophthalmol Vis Sci* 45:418, 2004

Kenney MC, Atilano SR, Zorapapel N *et al.*: Altered expression of aquaporins in bullous keratopathy and Fuchs' dystrophy corneas. *J Histochem Cytochem* 52:1341, 2004

Kitagawa K, Hayasaka S, Nagaki Y: Falsely elevated intraocular pressure due to an abnormally thick cornea in a patient with nevus of Ota. *Jpn J Ophthalmol* 47:142, 2003

Krause FE, Chen JJY, Tsai RJF *et al.*: Conjunctival transdifferentiation is due to the incomplete removal of limbal basal epithelium. *Invest Ophthalmol Vis Sci* 31:1903, 1990

Ku JY, Grupcheva CN, McGhee CN: Microstructural analysis of Salzmann's nodular degeneration by in vivo confocal microscopy. *Clin Exp Ophthalmol* 30:367, 2002

Lavker RM, Tseng SC, Sun TT: Corneal epithelial stem cells at the limbus: looking at some old problems from a new angle. *Exp Eye Res* 78:433, 2004

Malik RA, Kallinikos P, Abbott CA *et al.*: Corneal confocal microscopy: a non-invasive surrogate of nerve fibre damage and repair in diabetic patients. *Diabetologia* 46:683, 2003

Matsumoto Y, Dogru M, Tsubota K: Ocular surface findings in Hallopeau–Siemens subtype of dystrophic epidermolysis bullosa: report of a case and literature review. *Cornea* 24:474, 2005

McCallum RM, Cobo LM, Haynes BF: Analysis of corneal and conjunctival microenvironments using monoclonal antibodies. *Invest Ophthalmol Vis Sci* 34:1793, 1993

Messmer EM, Kenyon KR, Rittinger O *et al.*: Ocular manifestations of keratitis-ichthyosis-deafness (KID) syndrome. *Ophthalmology* 112:e1, 2005

Miller JK, Laycock KA, Nash MN *et al.*: Corneal Langerhans cell dynamics after herpes simplex virus reactivation. *Invest Ophthalmol Vis Sci* 34:2282, 1993

Paulsson M: Basement membrane proteins: structure, assembly, and cellular interactions. *Crit Rev Biochem Mol Biol* 27:93, 1992

Pei Y, Sherry DM, McDermott AM: Thy-1 distinguishes human corneal fibroblasts and myofibroblasts from keratocytes. *Exp Eye Res* 79:705, 2004

Ramaesh K, Ramaesh T, Dutton GN *et al.*: Evolving concepts on the pathogenic mechanisms of aniridia related keratopathy. *Int J Biochem Cell Biol* 37:547, 2005

Sanchis-Gimeno JA, Lleo-Perez A, Alonso L *et al.*: Corneal endothelial cell density decreases with age in emmetropic eyes. *Histol Histopathol* 20:423, 2005

Saxena T, Kumar K, Sen S *et al.*: Langerhans cell histiocytosis presenting as a limbal nodule in an adult patient. *Am J Ophthalmol* 138:508, 2004

Tuominen IS, Konttinen YT, Vesaluoma MH *et al.*: Corneal innervation and morphology in primary Sjogren's syndrome. *Invest Ophthalmol Vis Sci* 44:2545, 2003

Yanoff M, Fine BS: *Ocular Pathology: A Color Atlas*, 2nd edn. New York, Gower Medical Publishing, 1992:8.1–8.2

Congenital Defects

Akpek EK, Jun AS, Goodman DF *et al.*: Clinical and ultrastructural features of a novel hereditary anterior segment dysgenesis. *Ophthalmology* 109:513, 2002

Aldave AJ, Eagle RC Jr, Streeten BW *et al.*: Congenital corneal opacification in De Barsy syndrome. *Arch Ophthalmol* 119:285, 2001

Alward WLM: Perspective. Axenfeld–Rieger syndrome in the age of molecular genetics. *Am J Ophthalmol* 130:107, 2000

Axenfeld T: Embryotoxon corneae posterius. *Ber Dtsch Ophthalmol Ges* 42:301, 1920

Bourcier T, Baudrimont M, Boutboul S *et al.*: Corneal keloid: clinical, ultrasonographic, and ultrastructural characteristics. *J Cataract Refract Surg* 30:921, 2004

Brodsky MC, Whiteside-Michel J, Merin LM: Rieger anomaly and congenital glaucoma in the SHORT syndrome. *Arch Ophthalmol* 114:1146, 1996

Cibis GW, Waeltermann JM, Hurst E *et al.*: Congenital pupillary-iris-lens membrane with goniodysgenesis (a new entity). *Ophthalmology* 93:847, 1986

deRespinis PA, Wagner RS: Peters' anomaly in a father and son. *Am J Ophthalmol* 104:545, 1987

Dhooge MR, Idema AJ: Fibrodysplasia ossificans progressiva and corneal keloid. *Cornea* 21:725, 2002

Dichtl A, Jonas JB, Naumann GOH: Atypical Peters anomaly associated with partial trisomy 5p. *Am J Ophthalmol* 120:541, 1995

Elliott JH, Feman SS, O'Day DM *et al.*: Hereditary sclerocornea. *Arch Ophthalmol* 103:676, 1985

Emamy H, Ahmadian H: Limbal dermoid with ectopic brain tissue: Report of a case and review of the literature. *Arch Ophthalmol* 95:2201, 1977

Gaviria JG, Johnson DA, Scribbick F III: Corneal keloid mimicking a recurrent limbal dermoid. *J Pediatr Ophthalmol Strabismus* 42:189, 2005

Goldenhar M: Associations malformatives de l'oeil et de l'oreille en particulaire le syndrome dermoide épibulbaire-appendices auriculaires-fistula auris cogenita et ses rélations avec la dysostose mandibulo-faciale. *J Genet Hum* 1:243, 1952

Gorlin RJ, Jue KL, Jacobson V *et al.*: Oculoauriculovertebral dysplasia. *J Pediatr* 63:991, 1963

Hingorani M, Nischal KK, Davies A *et al.*: Ocular abnormalities in Alagille syndrome. *Ophthalmology* 106:330, 1999

Holbach LM, Font RL, Shivitz IA *et al.*: Bilateral keloid-like myofibroblastic proliferations of the cornea in children. *Ophthalmology* 97:1188, 1990

Honkanen RA, Nishimura DY, Swiderski RE *et al.*: A family with Axenfeld–Rieger syndrome and Peters anomaly caused by a point mutation (Phe112Ser) in the *FOCC1* gene. *Am J Ophthalmol* 135:368, 2003

Jensen OA: Arcus corneae chez les jeunes. *Arch Ophthalmol (Paris)* 20:154, 1960

Jun AS, Broman KW, Do DV *et al.*: Endothelial dystrophy, iris hypoplasia, congenital cataract, and stromal thinning (edict) syndrome maps to chromosome 15q22.1-q25.3. *Am J Ophthalmol* 134:172, 2002

Jung DS, Lee JH, Lee JE *et al.*: Corneal endothelial changes as a clinical diagnostic indicator of dentatorubropallidoluysian atrophy. *Cornea* 23:210, 2004

Khan A, Al-Saif A, Kambouris M: A novel KERA mutation associated with autosomal recessive cornea plana. *Ophthalmic Genet* 25:147, 2004

Kodsi SR, Bloom KE, Egbert JE *et al.*: Ocular and systemic manifestations of encephalocraniocutaneous lipomatosis. *Am J Ophthalmol* 118:77, 1994

Lee JS, Lee JE, Shin YG *et al.*: Five cases of microphthalmia with other ocular malformations. *Korean J Ophthalmol* 15:41, 2001

Lee CF, Yue BYJT, Robin J *et al.*: Immunohistochemical studies of Peters' anomaly. *Ophthalmology* 96:958, 1989

Legius E, de Die-Smulders CEM, Verbraak F *et al.*: Genetic heterogeneity in Rieger eye malformation. *J Med Genet* 31:340, 1994

Lehmann OJ, El-Ashry MF, Ebenezer ND et al.: A novel keratocan mutation causing autosomal recessive cornea plana. *Invest Ophthalmol Vis Sci* 42:3118, 2001

Leung ATS, Young AL, Fan DSP et al.: Isolated pedunculated congenital corneal dermoid. *Am J Ophthalmol* 128:756, 1999

Lewis RA, Nussbaum RL, Stambolian D: Mapping X-linked ophthalmic diseases. *Ophthalmology* 97:110, 1990

Lhmann OJ, El-ashry MF, Ebenezer ND et al.: A novel keratocan mutation causing autosomal recessive cornea plana. *Invest Ophthalmol Vis Sci* 42:3118, 2001

Lines MA, Kozlowski K, Kulak SC et al.: Characterization and prevalence of PITX@ microdeletions and mutations in Axenfeld–Rieger malformations. *Invest Ophthalmol Vis Sci* 45:828, 2004

Lucarelli MJ, Ceisler EJ, Talamo JH et al.: Complex choristoma. *Arch Ophthalmol* 114:498, 1996

Mackey DA, Buttery RG, Wise GM et al.: Description of X-linked megalocornea with identification of the gene locus. *Arch Ophthalmol* 109:829, 1991

Mansour AM, Barber JC, Reinecke RD et al.: Ocular choristomas. *Surv Ophthalmol* 33:339, 1989

Mansour AM, Wang F, Henkind P et al.: Ocular findings in the facio-auriculovertebral sequence (Goldenhar–Gorlin syndrome). *Am J Ophthalmol* 100:555, 1985

Matsubara A, Ozeki H, Matsunaga N et al.: Histopathological examination of two cases of anterior staphyloma associated with Peters' anomaly and persistent hyperplastic primary vitreous. *Br J Ophthalmol* 85:1421, 2001

Miller MM, Butrus S, Hidayat A et al.: Corneoscleral transplantation in congenital corneal staphyloma and Peters' anomaly. *Ophthalmic Genet* 24:59, 2003

Mintz-Hittner HA, Semina EV, Frishman LJ et al.: VSX1 (RINX) mutation with craniofacial anomalies, empty sella, corneal endothelial changes, and abnormal retinal and auditory bipolar cells. *Ophthalmology* 111:828, 2004

Mohammad AE, Kroosh SS: Huge corneal dermoid in a well-formed eye: a case report and review of the literature. *Orbit* 21:295, 2002

Mullaney PB, Risco JM, Heinz GW: Congenital corneal staphyloma. *Arch Ophthalmol* 113:1206, 1995

Nischal KK, Hingorani M, Bentley CR et al.: Ocular ultrasound in Alagille syndrome: A new sign. *Ophthalmology* 104:79, 1997

Ohkawa K, Saika S, Hayashi Y et al.: Cornea with Peters' anomaly: perturbed differentiation of corneal cells and abnormal extracellular matrix in the corneal stroma. *Jpn J Ophthalmol* 47:327, 2003

Pe'er J, Ilsar M: Epibulbar complex choristoma associated with nevus sebaceus. *Arch Ophthalmol* 113:1301, 1995

Peters A: Ueber angeborene Defektbildungen der Descemetschen Membran. *Klin Monatsbl Augenheilkd* 44:27, 1906

Rao SK, Padmanabhan P: Posterior keratoconus: An expanded classification scheme based on corneal topography. *Ophthalmology* 105:1206, 1998

Rezende RA, Uchoa UB, Uchoa R et al.: Congenital corneal opacities in a cornea referral practice. *Cornea* 23:565, 2004

Rieger H: Beiträge zur Kenntnis seltener Missbildungen der Iris: I. Membrana iridopupillaris persistens. *Graefes Arch Ophthalmol* 131:523, 1934

Rieger H: Demonstrationen (Gesellschaftsberichte). *Z Augenheilkd* 84:98, 1934

Rieger H: Beiträge zur Kenntnis seltener Missbildungen der Iris: II. Ueber Hypoplasie des Irisvorderblattes mit Verlagerung und Entrundung der Pupille. *Graefes Arch Ophthalmol* 133:602, 1935

Rieger H: Erbfragen in der Augenheilkunde. *Graefes Arch Ophthalmol* 143:227, 1941

Salmon JF, Wallis CE, Murray ADN: Variable expressivity of autosomal dominant microcornea with cataract. *Arch Ophthalmol* 106:505, 1988

Scheie HG, Yanoff M: Peters' anomaly and total posterior coloboma of retinal pigment epithelium and choroid. *Arch Ophthalmol* 87:525, 1972

Shanske AL, Gurland JE, Mbekeani JN et al.: Possible new syndrome of microcephaly with cortical migration defects, Peters anomaly and multiple intestinal atresias: a multiple vascular disruption syndrome. *Clin Dysmorphol* 11:67, 2002

Simpson WAC, Parsons A: The ultrastructural pathological features of congenital microcoria. *Arch Ophthalmol* 107:99, 1989

Snyder AA, Rao NA: Clinicopathological report of cerebroocular myopathy syndrome. *Am J Ophthalmol* 133:559, 2002

Steinsapir DK, Lehman E, Ernest JT et al.: Systemic neurocristopathy associated with Rieger's syndrome. *Am J Ophthalmol* 110:437, 1990

Tarkkanen A, Merenmies L: Corneal pathology and outcome of keratoplasty in autoimmune polyendocrinopathy-candidiasis-ectodermal dystrophy (APECED). *Acta Ophthalmol Scand* 79:204, 2001

Townsend WM, Font RL, Zimmerman LE: Congenital corneal leukomas: 2. Histopathologic findings in 19 eyes with central defect in Descemet's membrane. *Am J Ophthalmol* 77:192, 1974

Townsend WM: Congenital corneal leukomas: 1. Central defect in Descemet's membrane. *Am J Ophthalmol* 77:80, 1974

Townsend WM, Font RL, Zimmerman LE: Congenital corneal leukomas: 3. Histopathologic findings in 13 eyes with noncentral defect in Descemet's membrane. *Am J Ophthalmol* 77:400, 1974

Traboulsi EI, Maumenee IH: Peters' anomaly and associated congenital malformations. *Arch Ophthalmol* 110:1739, 1992

Vesaluoma MH, Sankila E-M, Galler J et al.: Autosomal recessive cornea plana: In vivo corneal morphology and corneal sensitivity. *Invest Ophthalmol Vis Sci* 41:2120, 2000

Walter MA, Mirzayans F, Mears AJ et al.: Autosomal-dominant iridodysgenesis and Axenfeld–Rieger syndrome are genetically distinct. *Ophthalmology* 103:1907, 1996

Yamamoto Y, Hayasaka S, Setogawa T: Family with aniridia, microcornea, and spontaneously resorbed cataract. *Arch Ophthalmol* 106:502, 1988

Ziavras E, Farber MG, Diamond G: A pedunculated lipodermoid in oculoauriculovertebral dysplasia. *Arch Ophthalmol* 108:1032, 1990

Inflammations: Nonulcerative

Adan CB, Trevisani VF, Vasconcellos M et al.: Bilateral deep keratitis caused by systemic lupus erythematosus. *Cornea* 23:207, 2004

Anadakannan K, Gupta CP: *Microfilaria malayi* in uveitis: case report. *Br J Ophthalmol* 61:263, 1977

Banerjee K, Biswas PS, Rouse BT: Elucidating the protective and pathologic T cell species in the virus-induced corneal immunoinflammatory condition herpetic stromal keratitis. *J Leukoc Biol* 77:24, 2005

Biswas PS, Rouse BT: Early events in HSV keratitis—setting the stage for a blinding disease. *Microbes Infect* 7:799, 2005

Burr WE, Brown MF, Eberhard ML: Zoonotic *Onchocerca* (Nematoda: Filaroidea) in the cornea of a Colorado resident. *Ophthalmology* 105:1495, 1998

Buus DR, Pflugfelder SC, Schachter J et al.: Lymphogranuloma venereum conjunctivitis with a marginal corneal perforation. *Ophthalmology* 95:799, 1988

Chan C-C, Nussenblatt RB, Kim MK et al.: Immunopathology of ocular onchocerciasis: 2. Anti-retinal autoantibodies in serum and ocular fluids. *Ophthalmology* 94:439, 1987

Chan CM, Theng JT, Li L, Tan DT: Microsporidial keratoconjunctivitis in healthy individuals: a case series. *Ophthalmology* 110:1420, 2003

Cobo LM, Haynes BF: Early corneal findings in Cogan's syndrome. *Ophthalmology* 91:903, 1984

Cohen S, Kremer I, Tiqva P: Bilateral corneal immune ring opacity in Behcet's syndrome. *Arch Ophthalmol* 109:324, 1991

Contreras F, Pereda J: Congenital syphilis of the eye with lens involvement. *Arch Ophthalmol* 96:1052, 1978

Council on Scientific Affairs: Harmful effects of ultraviolet radiation. *JAMA* 262:380, 1989

Deckard PS, Bergstrom TJ: Rubeola keratitis. *Ophthalmology* 88:810, 1981

Foster CS, Calonge M: Atopic keratoconjunctivitis. *Ophthalmology* 97:992, 1990

Giannini SH, Schittini M, Keithly JS et al.: Karyotype analysis of *Leishmania* species and its use in classification and clinical diagnosis. *Science* 232:762, 1986

Gilbert WS, Talbot FJ: Cogan's syndrome. *Arch Ophthalmol* 82:633, 1969

Hykin PG, Foss AE, Pavesio C et al.: The natural history of recurrent corneal erosion: A prospective randomised trial. *Eye* 8:35, 1994

Kadrmas EF, Bartley GB: Superior limbic keratoconjunctivitis: A prognostic sign for severe Graves ophthalmopathy. *Ophthalmology* 102:1472, 1995

Knox DL, Snip RC, Stark WJ: The keratopathy of Crohn's disease. *Am J Ophthalmol* 90:862, 1980

Kornmehl EW, Lesser RL, Jaros P et al.: Bilateral keratitis in Lyme disease. *Ophthalmology* 96:1194, 1989

Laibson PR, Dhiri S, Oconer J et al.: Corneal infiltrates in epidemic keratoconjunctivitis. *Arch Ophthalmol* 84:36, 1970

Lobos E, Weiss N, Karam M et al.: An immunogenic *Onchocerca* volvulus antigen: A specific and early marker of infection. *Science* 251:1603, 1991

Mabey D, Whitworth JA, Eckstein M et al.: The effects of multiple doses of ivermectin on ocular onchocerciasis: A six-year follow-up. *Ophthalmology* 103:1001, 1996

Maertzdorf J, Osterhaus AD, Verjans GM: IL-17 expression in human herpetic stromal keratitis: modulatory effects on chemokine production by corneal fibroblasts. *J Immunol* 169:5897, 2002

Matoba AY: Ocular disease associated with Epstein–Barr virus infection (review). *Surv Ophthalmol* 35:145, 1990

Matoba AY, Wilhelmus KR, Jones DB: Epstein–Barr viral stromal keratitis. *Ophthalmology* 93:746, 1986

McCarthy JS, Ottesen EA, Nutman TB: Onchocerciasis in endemic and nonendemic populations: Differences in clinical presentation and immunologic findings. *J Infect Dis* 170:736, 1994

McKechnie NM, Braun G, Connor V et al.: Immunologic cross-reactivity in the pathogenesis of ocular onchocerciasis. *Invest Ophthalmol Vis Sci* 34:2888, 1993

Miserocchi E, Baltatzis S, Foster CS: A case of atypical Cogan's syndrome with uncommon corneal findings. *Cornea* 20:540, 2001

Montenegro ENR, Israel CW, Nicol WG et al.: Histopathologic demonstration of spirochetes in the human eye. *Am J Ophthalmol* 67:335, 1969

Nagra PK, Rapuano CJ, Cohen EJ et al.: Thygeson's superficial punctate keratitis: ten years' experience. *Ophthalmology* 111:34, 2004

Naumann G, Gass JDM, Font RL: Histopathology of herpes zoster ophthalmicus. *Am J Ophthalmol* 65:533, 1968

Numasaki M, Fukushi J, Ono M et al.: Interleukin-17 promotes angiogenesis and tumor growth. *Blood* 101:2620, 2003

Pennisi E: New culprit arises in river blindness. *Science* 295:1809, 2002

Pinnolis M, McCulley JP, Urman JD: Nummular keratitis associated with infectious mononucleosis. *Am J Ophthalmol* 89:791, 1980

Saint André A, Blackwell NM, Hall LR et al.: The role of endosymbiotic *Wolbachia* bacteria in the pathogenesis of river blindness. *Science* 295:1892, 2002

Scheie HG, Shannon RE, Yanoff M: Onchocerciasis (ocular). *Ann Ophthalmol* 3:697, 1971

Semba RD, Murphy RP, Newland HS et al.: Longitudinal study of lesions of the posterior segment in onchocerciasis. *Ophthalmology* 97:1334, 1990

Singh K, Sodhi PK: Mumps-induced corneal endotheliitis. *Cornea* 23:400, 2004

Stenson S: Adult inclusion conjunctivitis: Clinical characteristics and corneal changes. *Arch Ophthalmol* 99:605, 1981

Tabbara KF, Ostler HB, Dawson C et al.: Thygeson's superficial punctate keratitis. *Ophthalmology* 88:75, 1981

Thygeson P: Superficial punctate keratitis. *JAMA* 144:1544, 1950

Vollertsen RS, McDonald TJ, Younge BR et al.: Cogan's syndrome: 18 cases and a review of the literature. *Mayo Clin Proc* 61:344, 1986

Waring GO, Font RL, Rodrigues MM et al.: Alterations of Descemet's membrane in interstitial keratitis. *Am J Ophthalmol* 81:773, 1976

Inflammations: Ulcerative

Aitken D, Hay J, Kinnear FB et al.: Amebic keratitis in a wearer of disposable contact lenses due to a mixed *Vahlkampfia* and *Hartmannella* infection. *Ophthalmology* 103:485, 1996

Austin P, Green WR, Sallyer DC et al.: Peripheral corneal degeneration and occlusive vasculitis in Wegener's granulomatosis. *Am J Ophthalmol* 85:311, 1978

Awward ST, Heilman M, Hogan RN et al.: Severe reactive ischemic posterior segment inflammation in *Acanthamoeba* keratitis. *Ophthalmology* 114:313, 2007

Charlton KH, Binder PS, Woziak L et al.: Pseudodendritic keratitis and systemic tyrosinemia. *Ophthalmology* 88:355, 1981

Chynn EW, Lopez MA, Pavan-Langston D et al.: *Acanthamoeba* keratitis: Contact lens and noncontact lens characteristics. *Ophthalmology* 102:1369, 1995

Deai T, Fukuda M, Hibino T et al.: Herpes simplex virus genome quantification in two patients who developed herpetic epithelial keratitis during treatment with antiglaucoma medications. *Cornea* 23:125, 2004

Dougherty PJ, Binder PS, Mondino BJ et al.: *Acanthamoeba* sclerokeratitis. *Am J Ophthalmol* 117:475, 1994

Eiferman RA, Carothers DJ, Yankeelow JA Jr: Peripheral rheumatoid ulceration and evidence for conjunctival collagenase production. *Am J Ophthalmol* 87:703, 1979

Ferry AP, Leopold IH: Marginal (ring) corneal ulcer as presenting manifestation of Wegener's granuloma: Clinicopathologic study. *Trans Am Acad Ophthalmol Otolaryngol* 74:1276, 1970

Foster CS, Kenyon KR, Greiner J et al.: The immunopathology of Mooren's ulcer. *Am J Ophthalmol* 88:149, 1979

Grünewald K, Desai P, Winkler DC et al.: Three-dimensional structure of herpes simplex virus from cryo-electron tomography. *Science* 302:1396, 2003

Gupta K, Hoepner JA, Streeten BW: Pseudomelanoma of the iris in herpes simplex keratoiritis. *Ophthalmology* 93:1524, 1986

Hill VE, Brownstein S, Jackson WB et al.: Infectious crystalline keratopathy: review of light and electron microscopy. *Ophthalmic Pract* 15:31, 1997

Holbach LM, Font RL, Naumann GOH: Herpes simplex stromal and endothelial keratitis: Granulomatous cell reactions at the level of Descemet's membrane, the stroma, and Bowman's layer. *Ophthalmology* 97:722, 1990

Holbach LM, Font RL, Wilhelmus KR: Recurrent herpes simplex keratitis with concurrent epithelial and stromal involvement. *Arch Ophthalmol* 109:692, 1991

Illingworth CD, Cook SD: *Acanthamoeba* keratitis. *Surv Ophthalmol* 42:493, 1998

Kilington S, Gray T, Dart J et al.: *Acanthamoeba* keratitis: the role of domestic tap water contamination in the United Kingdom. *Invest Ophthalmol Vis Sci* 45:165, 2004

Knox DL, Snip RC, Stark WJ: The keratopathy of Crohn's disease. *Am J Ophthalmol* 90:862, 1980

Liesegang TJ: Biology and molecular aspects of herpes simplex and varicella-zoster virus infections. *Ophthalmology* 99:781, 1992

Lindquist TD, Sher NA, Doughman DJ: Clinical signs and medical therapy of early *Acanthamoeba* keratitis. *Arch Ophthalmol* 106:73, 1988

Madhavan HN, Goldsmith CS, Rao SK *et al.*: Isolation of a vesicular virus belonging to the family Rhabdoviridae from the aqueous humor of a patient with bilateral corneal endotheliitis. *Cornea* 21:333, 2002

Margolis TP, Ostler HB: Treatment of ocular disease in eczema herpeticum. *Am J Ophthalmol* 110:274, 1990

Marines HM, Osato MS, Font RL: The value of calcofluor white in the diagnosis of mycotic and *Acanthamoeba* infections of the eye and ocular adnexa. *Ophthalmology* 94:23, 1987

Matherts WD, Sutphin JE, Folberg R *et al.*: Outbreak of keratitis presumed to be caused by *Acanthamoeba*. *Am J Ophthalmol* 121:129, 1996

Matsuo T, Notohara K, Shiraga F *et al.*: Endogenous amoebic endophthalmitis. *Arch Ophthalmol* 119:125, 2001

Meitz H, Font RL: *Acanthamoeba* keratitis with granulomatous reaction involving the stroma and anterior chamber. *Arch Ophthalmol* 115:259, 1997

Miller JK, Laycock KA, Nash MN *et al.*: Corneal Langerhans cell dynamics after herpes simplex virus reactivation. *Invest Ophthalmol Vis Sci* 34:2282, 1993

Mimura T, Amano S, Nagahara M *et al.*: Corneal endotheliitis and idiopathic sudden sensorineural hearing loss. *Am J Ophthalmol* 133:699, 2002

Moshari A, McLean IW, Dodds MT *et al.*: Chorioretinitis after keratitis caused by *Acanthamoeba*: case report and review of literature. *Ophthalmology* 108:2232, 2001

Naiker S, Odhav B: Mycotic keratitis: profile of *Fusarium* species and their mycotoxins. *Mycoses* 47:50, 2004

Pavan-Langston D, McCulley JP: Herpes zoster dendritic keratitis. *Arch Ophthalmol* 89:25, 1973

Perry HD, Donnenfeld ED, Foulks GN *et al.*: Decreased corneal sensation as an initial feature of *Acanthamoeba* keratitis. *Ophthalmology* 102:1565, 1995

Petrelli EA, McKinley M, Troncale FJ: Ocular manifestations of inflammatory bowel disease. *Ann Ophthalmol* 14:356, 1986

Pfister DR, Cameron JD, Krachmer JH *et al.*: Confocal microscopy findings of *Acanthamoeba* keratitis. *Am J Ophthalmol* 121:119, 1996

Rennie AGR, Cant JS, Foulds WS *et al.*: Ocular vaccinia. *Lancet* 2:273, 1974

Rothman RF, Liebmann JM, Ritch R: Noninfectious crystalline keratopathy after postoperative subconjunctival 5-fluorouracil. *Am J Ophthalmol* 128:236, 1999

Sainz de la MM, Foster CS, Jabbur NS *et al.*: Ocular characteristics and disease associations in scleritis-associated peripheral keratopathy. *Arch Ophthalmol* 120:15, 2002

Sawada Y, Yuan C, Huang AJ: Impression cytology in the diagnosis of *Acanthamoeba* keratitis with surface involvement. *Am J Ophthalmol* 137:323, 2004

Sharma S, Srinivasan M, George C: *Acanthamoeba* keratitis in non-contact lens wearers. *Arch Ophthalmol* 108:676, 1990

Sridhar MS, Sharma S, Garg P *et al.*: Epithelial infectious crystalline keratopathy. *Am J Ophthalmol* 131:255, 2001

van Klink F, Taylor WM, Alizadeh H *et al.*: The role of macrophages in *Acanthamoeba* keratitis. *Invest Ophthalmol Vis* Sci 37:1271, 1996

Yanoff M, Allman MI: Congenital herpes simplex virus, type 2 bilateral endophthalmitis. *Trans Am Ophthalmol Soc* 75:325, 1977

Degenerations: Epithelial

Baum JL, Rao G: Keratomalacia in the cachectic hospitalized patient. *Am J Ophthalmol* 82:435, 1976

Brooks HL, Driebe WT, Schemmer GG: Xerophthalmia and cystic fibrosis. *Arch Ophthalmol* 108:354, 1990

Brown N, Bron A: Recurrent erosion of the cornea. *Br J Ophthalmol* 60:84, 1976

Dushku N, Hatcher SLS, Albert DM *et al.*: p53 expression and relation to human papillomavirus infection in pingueculae, pterygia, and limbal tumors. *Arch Ophthalmol* 1117:1593, 1999

Font RL, Yanoff M, Zimmerman LE: Godwin's benign lymphoepithelial lesion of the lacrimal gland and its relationship to Sjögren's syndrome. *Am J Clin Pathol* 48:365, 1967

Hyndiuk RA, Kazarian EL, Schultz RO *et al.*: Neurotrophic corneal ulcers in diabetes mellitus. *Arch Ophthalmol* 95:2193, 1977

Jones DT, Monroy D, Ji Z *et al.*: Sjögren's syndrome: Cytokine and Epstein–Barr viral gene expression within the conjunctival epithelium. *Invest Ophthalmol Vis Sci* 35:3493, 1994

Lavrijsen J, van RG, van den BH: Filamentary keratopathy as a chronic problem in the long-term care of patients in a vegetative state. *Cornea* 24:620, 2005

Mancel E, Janin A, Gosset D *et al.*: Conjunctival biopsy in scleroderma and primary Sjögren's syndrome. *Am J Ophthalmol* 115:792, 1993

Natadisastra G, Wittpenn JR, West KP Jr *et al.*: Impression cytology for detection of vitamin A deficiency. *Arch Ophthalmol* 105:1224, 1987

Nelson JD, Williams P, Lindstrom RL *et al.*: Map-fingerprint-dot changes in the corneal epithelial basement membrane following radial keratotomy. *Ophthalmology* 92:199, 1985

Pepose JS, Akata RF, Pfluglfelder SC *et al.*: Mononuclear cell phenotypes and immunoglobulin gene rearrangements in lacrimal gland biopsies from patients with Sjögren's syndrome. *Ophthalmology* 97:1599, 1990

Pflugfelder SC, Crouse C, Pereira I *et al.*: Amplification of Epstein–Barr virus genomic sequences in blood cells, lacrimal glands, and tears from primary Sjögren's syndrome patients. *Ophthalmology* 97:976, 1990

Pflugfelder SC, Huang AJ, Feuer W *et al.*: Conjunctival cytologic features of primary Sjögren's syndrome. *Ophthalmology* 97:985, 1990

Sommer A: Xerophthalmia, keratomalacia and nutritional blindness. *Int Ophthalmol* 14:195, 1990

Sommer A, Sugana T: Corneal xerophthalmia and keratomalacia. *Arch Ophthalmol* 100:404, 1982

Sommer A, Emran N, Tjakrasudjatma S: Clinical characteristics of vitamin A responsive and nonresponsive Bitot's spots. *Am J Ophthalmol* 90:160, 1980

Sommer A, Green WR, Kenyon KR: Clinicohistopathologic correlations in xerophthalmic ulceration and necrosis. *Arch Ophthalmol* 100:953, 1982

Suan EP, Bedrossian EH, Eagle RC *et al.*: Corneal perforation in patients with vitamin A deficiency in the United States. *Arch Ophthalmol* 108:350, 1990

Tabery HM: Filamentary keratopathy: a non-contact photomicrographic in vivo study in the human cornea. *Eur J Ophthalmol* 13:599, 2003

van der Valk PGM, Hollema H, van Voorst Vander PC *et al.*: Sjögren's syndrome with specific cutaneous manifestations and multifocal clonal T-cell populations progressing to a cutaneous pleomorphic T-cell lymphoma. *Am J Clin Pathol* 92:357, 1989

Vivino FB, Minerva P, Huang CH *et al.*: Corneal melt as the initial presentation of primary Sjogren's syndrome. *J Rheumatol* 28:379, 2001

Wamsley S, Patel SM, Wood MG *et al.*: Advanced keratomalacia with descemetocele in an infant with cystic fibrosis. *Arch Ophthalmol* 123:1012, 2005

Weene LE: Recurrent corneal erosion after trauma: A statistical study. *Ann Ophthalmol* 17:521, 1985

Wilson MR, Mansour M, Atud AE *et al.*: A population-based study of xerophthalmia in the extreme North Province of Cameroon, West Africa. *Arch Ophthalmol* 114:464, 1996

Wood TO: Recurrent erosion. *Trans Am Ophthalmol Soc* 82:850, 1984

Zaidman GW, Geeraets R, Paylor RR *et al.*: The histopathology of filamentary keratitis. *Arch Ophthalmol* 103:1178, 1985

Degenerations: Stromal

Aldave AJ, Principe AH, Lin DY *et al.*: Lattice dystrophy-like localized amyloidosis of the cornea secondary to trichiasis. *Cornea* 24:112, 2005

Barchiesi BJ, Eckel RH, Ellis PP: The cornea and disorders of lipid metabolism. *Surv Ophthalmol* 36:1, 1991

Brown SI, Grayson M: Marginal furrows: Characteristic corneal lesion of rheumatoid arthritis. *Arch Ophthalmol* 79:563, 1968

Brownstein S, Rodrigues MM, Fine BS *et al.*: The elastotic nature of hyaline corneal deposits: A histochemical, fluorescent, and electron microscopic examination. *Am J Ophthalmol* 75:799, 1973

Butrus SI, Ashraf F, Laby DM *et al.*: Increased mast cells in pterygia. *Am J Ophthalmol* 119:236, 1995

Chua BE, Mitchell P, Wang JJ *et al.*: Corneal arcus and hyperlipidemia: findings from an older population. *Am J Ophthalmol* 137:363, 2004

Cogan DG, Kuwabara T: Arcus senilis: Its pathology and histochemistry. *Arch Ophthalmol* 61:353, 1959

Cohen KL, Bouldin TW: Familial, band-shaped, spheroidal keratopathy histopathology in ethnic Chinese siblings. *Cornea* 21:774, 2002

Croxatto JO, Dodds CM, Dodds R: Bilateral and massive lipoidal infiltration of the cornea (secondary lipoidal degeneration). *Ophthalmology* 92:1686, 1985

Cursino JW, Fine BS: A histologic study of calcific and non-calcific band keratopathies. *Am J Ophthalmol* 82:395, 1976

Dushku N, John MK, Schultz GS *et al.*: Pterygia pathogenesis: corneal invasion by matrix metalloproteinase expressing altered limbal epithelial basal cells. *Arch Ophthalmol* 119:695, 2001

Dutt S, Elner VM, Soong HK *et al.*: Secondary localized amyloidosis in interstitial keratitis. *Ophthalmology* 99:817, 1992

Fine BS, Townsend WH, Zimmerman LE *et al.*: Primary lipoidal degeneration of the cornea. *Am J Ophthalmol* 78:12, 1974

Gottsch JD, Liu SH, Stark WJ: Mooren's ulcer and evidence of stromal graft rejection after penetrating keratoplasty. *Am J Ophthalmol* 113:412, 1992

Gray RH, Johnson GJ, Freedman A: Climatic droplet keratopathy. *Surv Ophthalmol* 36:241, 1992

Guyer DR, Barraquer J, McDonnell PJ *et al.*: Terrien's marginal degeneration: Clinicopathologic case reports. *Graefes Arch Clin Exp Ophthalmol* 225:19, 1987

Hidayat AA, Risco J: Amyloidosis of corneal stroma in patients with trachoma. *Ophthalmology* 96:1203, 1989

Kalogeropoulos CD, Malamou-Mitsi VD, Aspiotis MB *et al.*: Bilateral Mooren's ulcer in six patients: diagnosis, surgery and histopathology. *Int Ophthalmol* 25:1, 2004

Krachmer JH, Dubord PJ, Rodrigues MM *et al.*: Corneal posterior crocodile shagreen and polymorphic amyloid degeneration: A histopathologic study. *Arch Ophthalmol* 101:54, 1983

Li DQ, Lee SB, Gunja-Smith Z *et al.*: Overexpression of collagenase (MMP-1) and stromelysin (MMP-3) by pterygium head fibroblasts. *Arch Ophthalmol* 119:71, 2001

Lopez JS, Price FW, Whitcup SM *et al.*: Immunohistochemistry of Terrien's and Mooren's corneal degeneration. *Arch Ophthalmol* 109:988, 1991

Magovern M, Wright JD Jr, Mohammed A: Spheroidal degeneration of the cornea: a clinicopathologic case report. *Cornea* 23:84, 2004

Mannis MJ, Krachmer JH, Rodrigues MM *et al.*: Polymorphic amyloid degeneration of the cornea: A clinical and histopathologic study. *Arch Ophthalmol* 99:1217, 1981

Matta CS, Tabbara KF, Cameron JA *et al.*: Climatic droplet keratopathy with corneal amyloidosis. *Ophthalmology* 98:192, 1991

Maust HA, Raber IM: Peripheral hypertrophic subepithelial corneal degeneration. *Eye Contact Lens* 29:266, 2003

Messmer EM, Hoops JP, Kampik A: Bilateral recurrent calcareous degeneration of the cornea. *Cornea* 24:498, 2005

Mondino BJ, Rabb MF, Sugar J *et al.*: Primary familial amyloidosis of the cornea. *Am J Ophthalmol* 92:732, 1981

Mootha VV, Pingree M, Jaramillo J: Pterygia with deep corneal changes. *Cornea* 23:635, 2004

Naumann GOH, Kuchle M: Unilateral arcus lipoides corneae with traumatic cyclodialysis in two patients. *Arch Ophthalmol* 107:1121, 1989

Ormerod LD, Dahan E, Hagele JE *et al.*: Serious occurrences in the natural history of advanced climatic keratopathy. *Ophthalmology* 101:448, 1994

Perry HD, Leonard ER, Yourish NB: Superficial reticular degeneration of Koby. *Ophthalmology* 92:1570, 1985

Ramsey MS, Fine BS, Cohen SW: Localized corneal amyloidosis: Case report with electron microscopic observations. *Am J Ophthalmol* 73:560, 1972

Rao SK, Krishnakumar S, Sudhir RR *et al.*: Bilateral corneal fibrosis in homocystinuria: case report and transmission electron microscopic findings. *Cornea* 21:730, 2002

Robin JB, Schanzlin DJ, Verity SM *et al.*: Peripheral corneal disorders (review). *Surv Ophthalmol* 31:1, 1986

Santo RM, Yamaguchi T, Kanai A: Spheroidal keratopathy associated with subepithelial corneal amyloidosis. *Ophthalmology* 100:1455, 1993

Savino DF, Fine BS, Alldredge OC: Primary lipidic degeneration of the cornea. *Cornea* 5:191, 1986

Severin M, Kirchhof B: Recurrent Salzmann's corneal degeneration. *Graefes Arch Clin Exp Ophthalmol* 228:101, 1990

Shimazaki J, Hida T, Inoue M *et al.*: Long-term follow-up of patients with familial subepithelial amyloidosis of the cornea. *Ophthalmology* 102:139, 1995

Soong HK, Quigley HA: Dellen associated with filtering blebs. *Arch Ophthalmol* 101:385, 1983

Terrien F: Dystrophie marginale symétrique des deux cornées avec astigmatisme régulier consécutif et guérison par la cautérisation ignée. *Arch Ophthalmol (Paris)* 20:12, 1900

Tripathi RC, Bron AJ: Secondary anterior crocodile shagreen of Vogt. *Br J Ophthalmol* 59:59, 1975

Trittibach P, Cadez R, Eschmann R *et al.*: Determination of microdot stromal degenerations within corneas of long-term contact lens wearers by confocal microscopy. *Eye Contact Lens* 30:127, 2004

Vemuganti GK, Mandal AK: Subepithelial corneal amyloid deposits in a case of congenital glaucoma: a case report. *Cornea* 21:315, 2002

Waring GO, Malaty A, Grossniklaus H *et al.*: Climatic proteoglycan stromal keratopathy, a new corneal degeneration. *Am J Ophthalmol* 120:330, 1995

Ye J, Chen J, Kim JC *et al.*: Bone marrow-derived cells are present in Mooren's ulcer. *Ophthalmic Res* 36:151, 2004

Yoon KC, Park YG: Recurrent Salzmann's nodular degeneration. *Jpn J Ophthalmol* 47:401, 2003

Dystrophies: Epithelial-Heredofamilial (Primary)

Badr IA, Basaffer S, Jabak M *et al.*: Meesmann corneal dystrophy in a Saudi Arabian family. *Am J Ophthalmol* 125:182, 1998

Coleman CM, Hannush S, Covella SP *et al.*: A novel mutation in the helix termination motif of keratin K12 in a US family with Meesmann corneal dystrophy. *Am J Ophthalmol* 128:687, 1999

Eagle RC Jr, Laibson PR, Arentsen JJ: Epithelial abnormalities in chronic corneal edema: A histopathological study. *Trans Am Ophthalmol Soc* 87:107, 1989

Fine BS, Yanoff M, Pitts E *et al.*: Meesmann's epithelial dystrophy of the cornea: Report of two families with discussion of the pathogenesis of the characteristic lesion. *Am J Ophthalmol* 83:633, 1977

Guerry D: Observations on Cogan's microcystic dystrophy of the corneal epithelium. *Trans Am Ophthalmol Soc* 63:320, 1965

Irvine AD, Coleman CM, Moore JE *et al.*: A novel mutation in KRT12 associated with Meesmann's epithelial corneal dystrophy. *Br J Ophthalmol* 86:729, 2002

Irvine AD, Swensson B, Moore JE *et al.*: Mutations in cornea-specific keratins K3 or K12 genes cause Meesmann corneal dystrophy. *Nat Genet* 16:184, 1997

Lisch W, Büttner A, Oeffner F *et al.*: Lisch corneal dystrophy is genetically distinct from Meesmann corneal dystrophy and maps to Xp22.3. *Am J Ophthalmol* 130:461, 2000

Marcon AS, Cohen EJ, Rapuano CJ *et al.*: Recurrence of corneal stromal dystrophies after penetrating keratoplasty. *Cornea* 22:19, 2003

Meesmann A, Wilke F: Klinische und anatomische Utersuchungen über eine bischer unbekannte, dominant vererbte Epitheldystrophie der Hornhaut. *Klin Monatsbl Augenheilkd* 103:361, 1939

Rodrigues MM, Fine BS, Laibson PR *et al.*: Disorders of the corneal epithelium: A clinicopathologic study of dot, geographic and fingerprint patterns. *Arch Ophthalmol* 92:475, 1974

Stocker W, Hot LB: Rare form of hereditary epithelial dystrophy. *Arch Ophthalmol* 53:536, 1955

Dystrophies: Epithelial-Heredofamilial (Secondary)

Chatterjee S, Gupta P, Pyeritz RE *et al.*: Immunohistochemical localization of glycosphingolipid in urinary renal tubular cells in Fabry's disease. *Am J Clin Pathol* 82:24, 1984

Font RL, Fine BS: Ocular pathology in Fabry's disease: Histochemical and electron microscopic observations. *Am J Ophthalmol* 73:419, 1972

Hirano K, Murata K, Miyagawa A *et al.*: Histopathologic findings of cornea verticillata in a woman heterozygous for Fabry's disease. *Cornea* 20:233, 2001

Dystrophies: Bowman's Membrane

Ciulla TA, Tolentino F, Morrow JF *et al.*: Vitreous amyloidosis in familial amyloidotic polyneuropathy: Report of a case with the ValsoMet transthyretin mutation. *Surv Ophthalmol* 40:197, 1995

Dastgheib KA, Clinch TE, Manche EE *et al.*: Sloughing of corneal epithelium and wound healing complications associated with laser in situ keratomileusis in patients with epithelial basement membrane dystrophy. *Am J Ophthalmol* 130:297, 2000

Dighiero P, Valleix S, D'Hermies F *et al.*: Clinical, histologic, and ultrastructural features of the corneal dystrophies caused by the R124L mutation of the BIGH 3 gene. *Ophthalmology* 40:197, 2000

Griffith DG, Fine BS: Light and electron microscopic observations in a superficial corneal dystrophy: Probably early Reis–Bücklers type. *Am J Ophthalmol* 63:1659, 1967

Mashima Y, Yamamoto S, Inoue Y *et al.*: Association of autosomal corneal dystrophies with BIGH3 gene mutations in Japan. *Am J Ophthalmol* 130:516, 2000

Perry HD, Fine BS, Caldwell DR: Reis–Bückler's dystrophy: A study of eight cases. *Arch Ophthalmol* 97:664, 1979

Ridgway AEA, Akhtar S, Munter FL *et al.*: Ultrastructural and molecular analysis of Bowman's layer corneal dystrophies: An epithelial origin? *Invest Ophthalmol Vis Sci* 41:3286, 2000

Dystrophies: Stromal-Heredofamilial (Primary)

Afshari NA, Mullally JE, Afshari MA *et al.*: Survey of patients with granular, lattice, Avellino, and Reis–Bücklers corneal dystrophies for mutations in the *BIGH3* and gelsolin genes. *Arch Ophthalmol* 119:16, 2001

Akhtar S, Meck KM, Ridgeway AEA *et al.*: Deposits and proteoglycan changes in primary and recurrent granular dystrophy of the cornea. *Arch Ophthalmol* 117:310, 1999

Akiya S, Nishio Y, Ibi K *et al.*: Lattice corneal dystrophy type II associated with familial amyloid polyneuropathy type IV. *Ophthalmology* 103:1106, 1996

Aldave AJ, Edward DP, Park AJ *et al.*: Central discoid corneal dystrophy. *Cornea* 21:739, 2002

Aldave AJ, Gutmark JG, Yellore VS *et al.*: Lattice corneal dystrophy associated with the Ala546Asp and Pro551Gln missense changes in the TGFBI gene. *Am J Ophthalmol* 138:772, 2004

Aldave AJ, Rayner SA, King JA *et al.*: A unique corneal dystrophy of Bowman's layer and stroma associated with the Gly623Asp mutation in the transforming growth factor beta-induced (TGFBI) gene. *Ophthalmology* 112:1017, 2005

Aldave AJ, Yellore VS, Hwang DG: Atypical vortex pattern of corneal deposits in granular corneal dystrophy. *Cornea* 22:754, 2003

Aldave AJ, Yellore VS, Thonar EJ *et al.*: Novel mutations in the carbohydrate sulfotransferase gene (CHST6) in American patients with macular corneal dystrophy. *Am J Opthalmol* 137:465, 2004

Ando Y, Nakamura M, Kai H *et al.*: A novel localized amyloidosis associated with lactoferrin in the cornea. *Lab Invest* 82:757, 2002

Bredrup C, Knappskog PM, Majewski J *et al.*: Congenital stromal dystrophy of the cornea caused by a mutation in the decorin gene. *Invest Ophthalmol Vis Sci* 46:420, 2005

Brownstein S, Fine BS, Sherman ME *et al.*: Granular dystrophy of the cornea: Light and electron microscopic confirmation of recurrence in a graft. *Am J Ophthalmol* 77:701, 1974

Chern KC, Meisler DM: Disappearance of crystals in Schnyder's crystalline corneal dystrophy after epithelial erosion. *Am J Ophthalmol* 120:802, 1995

Cursiefen C, Hofmann-Rummelt C, Schlotzer-Schrehardt U *et al.*: Immunohistochemical classification of primary and recurrent macular corneal dystrophy in Germany: subclassification of immunophenotype I A using a novel keratan sulfate antibody. *Exp Eye Res* 73:593, 2001

Dighiero P, Drunat S, Ellies P *et al.*: A new mutation (A546T) of the βig-h3 gene responsible for a French lattice corneal dystrophy type IIIA. *Am J Ophthalmol* 129:248, 2000

Dighiero P, Niel F, Ellies P *et al.*: Histologic phenotype-genotype correlation of corneal dystrophies associated with eight distinct mutations in the TGFBI gene. *Ophthalmology* 108:818, 2001

Dighiero P, Valleix S, D'Hermies F *et al.*: Clinical, histologic, and ultrastructural features of the corneal dystrophies caused by the R124L mutation of the BIGH 3 gene. *Ophthalmology* 40:197, 2000

Dota A, Nishida K, Honma Y *et al.*: Gelatinous drop-like corneal dystrophy is not one of the βig-h3-mutated corneal amyloidoses. *Am J Ophthalmol* 126:832, 1998

Eifrig DE, Afshari NA, Buchanan HW *et al.*: Polymorphic corneal amyloidosis: a disorder due to a novel mutation in the transforming growth factor β-induced (BIGHS) gene. *Ophthalmology* 111:1108, 2004

El-Ashry MF, El-Aziz MMA, Shalaby S *et al.*: Novel CHST6 nonsense znd missense mutations responsible for macular corneal dystrophy. *Am J Ophthalmol* 139:193, 2005

Ellis P, Renard G, Valleix S *et al.*: Clinical outcome of eight BIGH3-linked corneal dystrophies. *Ophthalmology* 109:793, 2002

Endo S, Ha NT, Fujiki K *et al.*: Leu518Pro mutation of the βig-h3 gene causes lattice corneal dystrophy type 1. *Am J Ophthalmol* 128:104, 1999

Feder RS, Jay M, Yue YJT *et al.*: Subepithelial mucinous corneal dystrophy. *Arch Ophthalmol* 3:1106, 1993

Ferry AP, Benson WH, Weinberg RS: Combined granular-lattice ("Avellino") corneal dystrophy. *Trans Am Ophthalmol Soc* 95:61, 1997

Fine BS, Townsend WM, Zimmerman LE *et al.*: Primary lipoidal degeneration of the cornea. *Am J Ophthalmol* 78:12, 1974

Folberg R, Alfonso E, Croxatta O *et al.*: Clinically atypical granular corneal dystrophy with pathologic features of lattice-like amyloid deposits: A study of three families. *Ophthalmology* 95:46, 1988

Folberg R, Stone EM, Sheffield VC *et al.*: The relationship between granular, lattice type 1, and Avellino corneal dystrophies: A histopathologic study. *Arch Ophthalmol* 112:1080, 1994

Fujiki K, Hotta Y, Nakayasu K *et al.*: Six different mutations of TGFBI (betaig-h3) gene found in Japanese corneal dystrophies. *Cornea* 19:842, 2000

Funderburgh JL, Funderburgh ML, Rodrigues MM *et al.*: Altered antigenicity of keratan sulfate proteoglycan in selected corneal diseases. *Invest Ophthalmol Vis Sci* 31:419, 1990

Gupta SK, Hodge WG, Damji KF *et al.*: Lattice corneal dystrophy type 1 in a Canadian kindred is associated with the Arg^{124} → Cys mutation in the kerato-epithelin gene. *Am J Ophthalmol* 125:547, 1998

Ha NT, Cung IX, Chau HM *et al.*: A novel mutation of the TGFBI gene found in a Vietnamese family with atypical granular corneal dystrophy. *Jpn J Ophthalmol* 47:246, 2003

Ha NT, Fujiki K, Hotta Y *et al.*: Q118X mutation of M1S1 gene caused gelatinous drop-like corneal dystrophy: The P501T of BIGH3 gene found in a family with gelatinous drop-like corneal dystrophy. *Am J Ophthalmol* 130:119, 2000

Haddad R, Font RL, Fine BS: Unusual superficial variant of granular dystrophy of the cornea. *Am J Ophthalmol* 83:213, 1977

Hasegawa N, Torii T, Kato T *et al.*: Decreased GlcNAc 6-o-sulfotransferase activity in the cornea with macular corneal dystrophy. *Invest Ophthalmol Vis Sci* 41:3670, 2000

Hida T, Proia AD, Kigasawa K *et al.*: Histopathologic and immunochemical features of lattice corneal dystrophy type III. *Am J Ophthalmol* 104:249, 1987

Hirano K, Hotta Y, Nakamura M *et al.*: Late-onset form of lattice corneal dystrophy caused by leu527Arg mutation of the TGFBI gene. *Cornea* 20:525, 2001

Holland EJ, Daya SM, Stone EM *et al.*: Avellino corneal dystrophy. *Ophthalmology* 99:1564, 1992

Ide T, Nishida K, Maeda N *et al.*: A spectrum of clinical manifestations of gelatinous drop-like corneal dystrophy in japan. *Am J Ophthalmol* 137:1081, 2004

Ingraham HJ, Perry HD, Donnenfeld ED *et al.*: Progressive Schnyder's dystrophy. *Ophthalmology* 100:1824, 1993

Javadi MA, Rafee'i AB, Kamalian N *et al.*: Concomitant keratoconus and macular corneal dystrophy. *Cornea* 23:508, 2004

Johnson AT, Folberg R, Vrabec MP *et al.*: The pathology of posterior amorphous corneal dystrophy. *Ophthalmology* 97:104, 1990

Jonasson F, Oshima E, Thonar EJ-MA *et al.*: Macular corneal dystrophy in Iceland: A clinical, genealogic, and immunohistochemical study of 28 patients. *Ophthalmology* 103:1111, 1996

Jones ST, Zimmerman LE: Histopathologic differentiation of granular, macular and lattice dystrophies of the cornea. *Am J Ophthalmol* 51:394, 1961

Kawasaki S, Nishida K, Quantock AJ *et al.*: Amyloid and Pro501 Thr-mutated βig-h3 gene product colocalize in lattice corneal dystrophy type IIIA. *Am J Ophthalmol* 127:456, 1999

Kivelä T, Tarkkanen A, Frangione B *et al.*: Ocular amyloid deposition in familial amyloidosis, Finnish: An analysis of native and variant gelsolin in Meretoja's syndrome. *Invest Ophthalmol Vis Sci* 35:3759, 1994

Klintworth GK: The molecular genetics of the corneal dystrophies—current status. *Frontiers Biosci* 8:687, 2003

Klintworth GK, Bao W, Afshari NA: Two mutations in the *TGFBI* (*BIGH3*) gene associated with lattice dystrophy in an extensively studied family. *Invest Ophthalmol Vis Sci* 45:1382, 2004

Klintworth GK, Bao W, Afshari NA: Two mutations in the TGFBI (BIGH3) gene associated with lattice corneal dystrophy in an extensively studied family. *Invest Ophthalmol Vis Sci* 45:1382, 2004

Klintworth GK, Oshima E, Al-Rajhi A *et al.*: Macular corneal dystrophy in Saudi Arabia: A study of 56 cases and recognition of a new immunophenotype. *Am J Ophthalmol* 124:9, 1997

Klintworth GK, Valnickova Z, Enghild JJ: Accumulation of βig-h3 gene product in corneas with granular dystrophy. *Am J Pathol* 152:743, 1998

Kobayashi A, Sugiyama K, Huang AJ: In vivo confocal microscopy in patients with central cloudy dystrophy of Francois. *Arch Ophthalmol* 122:1676, 2004

Kocak-Altintas AG, Kocak-Midillioglu I, Akarsu AN *et al.*: BIGH3 gene analysis in the differential diagnosis of corneal dystrophies. *Cornea* 20:64, 2001

Konishi M, Mashima Y, Yamada M *et al.*: The classic form of granular corneal dystrophy associated with R555W mutation in the BIGH3 gene is rare in Japanese patients. *Am J Ophthalmol* 126:450, 1998

Krachmer JH, Dubord PJ, Rodrigues MM *et al.*: Corneal posterior crocodile shagreen and polymorphic amyloid degeneration: A histopathologic study. *Arch Ophthalmol* 101:54, 1983

Küchle M, Cursiefen C, Fischer D-G *et al.*: Recurrent macular corneal dystrophy type II 49 years after penetrating keratoplasty. *Arch Ophthalmol* 117:528, 1999

Lucarelli MJ, Adamis AP: Avallino corneal dystrophy. *Arch Ophthalmol* 112:418, 1994

Mashima Y, Nakamura Y, Noda K *et al.*: A novel mutation at codon 124 (R124L) in the BIGH3 gene is associated with a superficial variant of granular corneal dystrophy. *Arch Ophthalmol* 117:90, 1999

Mashima Y, Yamamoto S, Inoue Y *et al.*: Association of autosomal corneal dystrophies with BIGH3 gene mutations in Japan. *Am J Ophthalmol* 130:516, 2000

Mathew M, Brownstein S, Bao W *et al.*: Unusual superficial variant of granular corneal dystrophy with amyloid deposition. *Arch Ophthalmol* 121:270, 2003

McCarthy M, Innis S, Dubord P *et al.*: Panstromal Schnyder corneal dystrophy: A clinical pathologic report with quantitative analysis of corneal lipid composition. *Ophthalmology* 101:895, 1994

Meisler DM, Tabbara KF, Wood IS *et al.*: Familial band-shaped nodular keratopathy. *Ophthalmology* 92:217, 1985

Morishige N, Chikama T, Ishimura Y *et al.*: Unusual phenotype of an individual with the R124C mutation in the TGFBI gene. *Arch Ophthalmol* 122:1224, 2004

Moshegov CN, Hoe WK, Wiffen SJ *et al.*: Posterior amorphous corneal dystrophy: A new pedigree with phenotypic variation. *Ophthalmology* 103:474, 1996

Nicholson DH, Green WR, Cross HE *et al.*: A clinical and histopathological study of François–Neetens speckled corneal dystrophy. *Am J Ophthalmol* 83:554, 1977

Okada M, Yamamoto S, Tsujikawa M *et al.*: Two distinct kerato-epithelin mutations in Reis–Bücklers corneal dystrophy. *Am J Ophthalmol* 126:535, 1998

Okada M, Yamamoto S, Watanabe H *et al.*: Granular corneal dystrophy with homozygous keratoepithelin mutations. *Invest Ophthalmol Vis Sci* 39:1947, 1998

Owens SL, Sugar J, Edward DP: Superficial granular corneal dystrophy with amyloid deposits. *Arch Ophthalmol* 110:175, 1992

Plaas AH, West LA, Thonar EJ et al.: Altered fine structures of corneal and skeletal keratan sulfate and chondroitin/dermatan sulfate in macular corneal dystrophy. *J Biol Chem* 276:39788, 2001

Rodrigues MM, Kruth HS, Rajagopalan S et al.: Unesterfied cholesterol in granular, lattice and macular dystrophies. *Am J Ophthalmol* 115:112, 1993

Rodrigues MM, Rajagopalan S, Jones K et al.: Gelsolin immunoreactivity in corneal amyloid, wound healing, and macular and granular dystrophies. *Am J Ophthalmol* 115:644, 1993

Rosenberg ME, Tervo TM, Gallar J et al.: Corneal morphology and sensitivity in lattice dystrophy type II (familial amyloidosis, Finnish type). *Invest Ophthalmol Vis Sci* 42:634, 2001

Rosenwasser GOD, Sucheski BM, Rosa N et al.: Phenotypic variation in combined granular-lattice (Avellino) corneal dystrophy. *Arch Ophthalmol* 111:1546, 1993

Rothstein A, Auran JD, Wittpenn JR et al.: Confocal microscopy in Meretoja syndrome. *Cornea* 21:364, 2002

Sandgren O: Ocular amyloidosis with special reference to the hereditary forms with vitreous involvement. *Surv Ophthalmol* 40:1173, 1995

Santo RM, Yamaguchi T, Kanai A et al.: Clinical and histopathologic features of corneal dystrophies in Japan. *Ophthalmology* 102:557, 1995

Seitz B, Behrens A, Fischer M et al.: Morphometric analysis of deposits in granular and lattice corneal dystrophy: histopathologic implications for phototherapeutic keratectomy. *Cornea* 23:380, 2004

Shah GK, Cantrill HL, Holland EJ: Vortex keratopathy associated with atovaquone. *Am J Ophthalmol* 1209:669, 1995

Small KW, Mullen L, Barletta J et al.: Mapping of Reis–Bückler's corneal dystrophy to chromosome 5q. *Am J Ophthalmol* 121:384, 1996

Snead DR, Mathews BN: Differences in amyloid deposition in primary and recurrent corneal lattice dystrophy type 1. *Cornea* 21:308, 2002

Sridhar MS, Laibson PR, Eagle RC Jr et al.: Unilateral corneal lattice dystrophy. *Cornea* 20:850, 2001

Starck T, Kenyon KR, Hanninen LA et al.: Clinical and histopathologic studies of two families with lattice corneal dystrophy and familial systemic amyloidosis (Meretoja syndrome). *Ophthalmology* 98:1197, 1991

Stewart H, Black GCM, Donnai D et al.: A mutation within exon 14 of the TGFBI (BIGH3) gene on chromosome 5q31 causes an asymmetric, late-onset form of lattice corneal dystrophy. *Ophthalmology* 106:964, 1999

Stock EL, Feder RS, O'Grady RB et al.: Lattice corneal dystrophy type III A. *Arch Ophthalmol* 109:354, 1991

Stone EM, Mathers WD, Rosenwasser G et al.: Three autosomal dominant corneal dystrophies map to chromosome 5q. *Nat Genet* 6:47, 1994

Streeten BW, Qi Y, Klintworth GK et al.: Immunolocalization of βigh3 in 5q31-linked corneal dystrophies and normal corneas. *Arch Ophthalmol* 117:67, 1999

Takahashi K, Murakami A, Okisaka S et al.: Kerato-epithelin mutation (R 555 Q) in a case of Reis-Bückler's corneal dystrophy. *Jpn J Ophthalmol* 44:191, 2000

Tasa G, Kals J, Muru K et al.: A novel mutation in the *M1S1* gene responsible for gelatinous corneal dystrophy. *Invest Ophthalmol Vis Sci* 42:2762, 2001

Van GR, De VR, Casteels I et al.: Report of a new family with dominant congenital heredity stromal dystrophy of the cornea. *Cornea* 21:118, 2002

Vance JM, Jonasson F, Lennon F et al.: Linkage of a gene for macular corneal dystrophy to chromosome 16. *Am J Hum Genet* 58:757, 1996

Warren JF, Aldave AJ, Srinivasan M et al.: Novel mutations in the CHST6 gene associated with macular corneal dystrophy in Southern India. *Arch Ophthalmol* 121:1608, 2003

Weiss JS: Schnyder crystalline dystrophy sine crystals. *Ophthalmology* 103:465, 1996

Witschel H, Fine BS, Grützner P et al.: Congenital hereditary stromal dystrophy of the cornea. *Arch Ophthalmol* 96:1043, 1978

Wu CW, Lin PY, Liu YF et al.: Central corneal mosaic opacities in Schnyder's crystalline dystrophy. *Ophthalmology* 112:650, 2005

Yanoff M, Fine BS, Colosi NJ et al.: Lattice corneal dystrophy: Report of an unusual case. *Arch Ophthalmol* 95:651, 1977

Yoshida S, Kumano Y, Yoshida A et al.: Two brothers with gelatinous drop-like dystrophy at different stages of the disease: role of mutational analysis. *Am J Ophthalmol* 133:830, 2002

Yoshida S, Yoshida A, Nakao S et al.: Lattice corneal dystrophy type I without typical lattice lines: role of mutational analysis. *Am J Ophthalmol* 137:586, 2004

Dystrophies: Stromal-Heredofamilial (Secondary)

Ainbinder DJ, Parmley VC, Mader TH et al.: Infectious crystalline keratopathy caused by *Candida guilliermondii*. *Am J Ophthalmol* 125:723, 1998

Akhtar S, Tullo A, Caterson B et al.: Clinical and morphological features including expression of betaig-h3 and keratan sulphate proteoglycans in Maroteaux–Lamy syndrome type B and in normal cornea. *Br J Ophthalmol* 86:147, 2002

Brooks AMV, Grant G, Gillies WE: Determination of the nature of corneal crystals by specular microscopy. *Ophthalmology* 95:448, 1988

Cantor LB, Disseler JA, Wilson FM: Glaucoma in the Maroteaux–Lamy syndrome. *Am J Ophthalmol* 108:426, 1989

Cherry PMH, Kraft S, McGowan H et al.: Corneal and conjunctival deposits in monoclonal gammopathy. *Can J Ophthalmol* 18:142, 1983

Collins MLZ, Traboulsi EI, Maumenee IH: Optic nerve head swelling and optic atrophy in the systemic mucopolysaccharidoses. *Ophthalmology* 97:1445, 1990

Garibaldi DC, Gottsch J, de la CZ et al.: Immunotactoid keratopathy: a clinicopathologic case report and a review of reports of corneal involvement in systemic paraproteinemias. *Surv Ophthalmol* 50:61, 2005

Granek H, Baden HP: Corneal involvement in epidermolysis bullosa simplex. *Arch Ophthalmol* 98:469, 1980

Hambrick GW Jr, Scheie HG: Studies of the skin in Hurler's syndrome. *Arch Dermatol* 85:455, 1962

Katz B, Melles RB, Schneider JA: Recurrent crystal deposition after keratoplasty in nephropathic cystinosis. *Am J Ophthalmol* 104:190, 1987

Lavery MA, Green WR, Jabs EW et al.: Ocular histopathology and ultrastructure of Sanfilippo's syndrome, type III-B. *Arch Ophthalmol* 101:1263, 1983

Levy LA, Lewis JC, Sumner TE: Ultrastructures of Reilly bodies (metachromatic granules) in the Maroteaux–Lamy syndrome (mucopolysaccharidosis VI): A histochemical study. *Am J Clin Pathol* 73:416, 1980

McDonnell JM, Green WR, Maumenee IH: Ocular histopathology of systemic mucopolysaccharidosis, type II-A (Hunter syndrome, severe). *Ophthalmology* 92:1772, 1985

McKusick VA: *Heritable Disorders of Connective Tissue*, 4th edn. St. Louis, CV Mosby, 1972:521

Melles RB, Schneider JA, Rao NA et al.: Spatial and temporal sequence of corneal crystal deposition in nephropathic cystinosis. *Am J Ophthalmol* 104:598, 1987

Mungan N, Nischal KK, Héon E et al.: Ultrasound biomicroscopy of the eye in cystinosis. *Arch Ophthalmol* 118:1329, 2000

Naumann G: Clearing of cornea after perforating keratoplasty in mucopolysaccharidosis type VI (Maroteaux–Lamy syndrome). *N Engl J Med* 312:995, 1985

Naumann GOH, Rummelt V: Aufklaren der transplantatnahen Wirtshornhaut nach perforierender keratoplastik beim Maroteaux–Lamy-Syndrome (Mukopolysaccharidose Typ VI-A). *Klin Monatsbl Augenheilkd* 203:351, 1993

Newman NHJ, Starck T, Kenyon KR *et al.*: Corneal surface irregularities and episodic pain in a patient with mucolipidosis IV. *Arch Ophthalmol* 108:251, 1990

Noffke AS, Feder RS, Greenwald MJ *et al.*: Mucolipidosis IV in an African American patient with new findings on electron microscopy. *Cornea* 20:536, 2001

Ormerod LD, Collins BH, Dohlman CH *et al.*: Paraprotein crystalline keratopathy. *Ophthalmology* 95:202, 1988

Patel DV, Ku JY, Kent-Smith B *et al.*: In vivo microstructural analysis of the cornea in Maroteaux–Lamy syndrome. *Cornea* 24:623, 2005

Richler M, Milot J, Quigley M *et al.*: Ocular manifestation of nephropathic cystinosis. *Arch Ophthalmol* 109:359, 1991

Rummelt V, Meyer HJ, Naumann GOH: Light and electron microscopy of the cornea in systemic mucopolysaccharidosis type I-S (Scheie's syndrome). *Cornea* 2:86, 1992

Scheie HG, Hambrick GW Jr, Barness LA: A newly recognized forme fruste of Hurler's disease (gargoylism). *Am J Ophthalmol* 53:753, 1962

Summers CG, Purple RL, Krivit W *et al.*: Ocular changes in the mucopolysaccharidoses after bone marrow transplantation. *Ophthalmology* 96:977, 1989

Varssano D, Cohen EJ, Nelson LB *et al.*: Corneal transplantation in Maroteaux–Lamy syndrome. *Arch Ophthalmol* 115:428, 1997

Viestenz A, Schlotzer-Schrehardt U, Hofmann-Rummelt C *et al.*: Histopathology of corneal changes in lecithin-cholesterol acyltransferase deficiency. *Cornea* 21:834, 2002

Yassa NH, Font RL, Fine BS *et al.*: Corneal immunoglobulin deposition in the posterior stroma: A case report including immunohistochemical and ultrastructural observations. *Arch Ophthalmol* 105:99, 1987

Zabel RW, MacDonald IM, Mintsioulis G *et al.*: Scheie's syndrome: An ultrastructural analysis of the cornea. *Ophthalmology* 96:1631, 1989

Dystrophies: Stromal-Nonheredofamilial

Aldave AJ, Mabon M, Hollander DA *et al.*: Spontaneous corneal hydrops and perforation in keratoconus and pellucid marginal degeneration. *Cornea* 22:169, 2003

Bourges JL, Savoldelli M, Dighiero P *et al.*: Recurrence of keratoconus characteristics: a clinical and histologic follow-up analysis of donor grafts. *Ophthalmology* 110:1920, 2003

Cheng EL, Maruyama I, SundarRaj N *et al.*: Expression of type XII collagen and hemidesmosome-associated proteins in keratoconus corneas. *Curr Eye Res* 22:333, 2001

Dantas PE, Nishiwaki-Dantas MC: Spontaneous bilateral corneal perforation of acute hydrops in keratoconus. *Eye Contact Lens* 30:40, 2004

Darlington JK, Mannis MJ, Segal WA: Anterior keratoconus associated with unilateral cornea guttata. *Cornea* 20:881, 2001

Edwards M, McGhee CN, Dean S: The genetics of keratoconus. *Clin Exp Ophthalmol* 29:345, 2001

Erie JC, Patel SV, McLaren JW *et al.*: Keratocyte density in keratoconus. A confocal microscopy study (a). *Am J Ophthalmol* 134:689, 2002

Ha NT, Nakayasu K, Murakami A *et al.*: Microarray analysis identified differentially expressed genes in keratocytes from keratoconus patients. *Curr Eye Res* 28:373, 2004

Hollingsworth JG, Bonshek RE, Efron N: Correlation of the appearance of the keratoconic cornea in vivo by confocal microscopy and in vitro by light microscopy. *Cornea* 24:397, 2005

Hollingsworth JG, Efron N: Observations of banding patterns (Vogt striae) in keratoconus: a confocal microscopy study. *Cornea* 24:162, 2005

Hollingsworth JG, Efron N, Tullo AB: In vivo corneal confocal microscopy in keratoconus. *Ophthalmic Physiol Opt* 25:254, 2005

Ihalainen A: Clinical and epidemiological features of keratoconus: Genetic and external factors in the pathogenesis of the disease. *Acta Ophthalmol* 64:5, 1986

Iwamoto T, DeVoe AG: Electron microscopical study of the Fleischer ring. *Arch Ophthalmol* 94:1579, 1976

Kaldawy RM, Wagner J, Ching S *et al.*: Evidence of apoptotic cell death in keratoconus. *Cornea* 21:206, 2002

Kayazawa F, Nishimura K, Kodama Y *et al.*: Keratoconus with pellucid marginal corneal degeneration. *Arch Ophthalmol* 102:895, 1984

Kennedy RH, Bourne WM, Dyer JA: A 48-year clinical and epidemiologic study of keratoconus. *Am J Ophthalmol* 101:267, 1986

Krachmer JH: Pellucid marginal corneal degeneration. *Arch Ophthalmol* 96:1217, 1978

Maruyama Y, Wang X, Li Y *et al.*: Involvement of Sp1 elements in the promoter activity of genes affected in keratoconus. *Invest Ophthalmol Vis Sci* 42:1980, 2001

Meek KM, Tuft SJ, Huang Y *et al.*: Changes in collagen orientation and distribution in keratoconus corneas. *Invest Ophthalmol Vis Sci* 46:1948, 2005

Perry HD, Buxton JN, Fine BS: Round and oval cones in keratoconus. *Ophthalmology* 87:905, 1980

Rabinowitz YS: Keratoconus. *Surv Ophthalmol* 42:297, 1998

Sahni J, Kaye SB, Fryer A *et al.*: Distal arthrogryposis type IIB: unreported ophthalmic findings. *Am J Med Genet A* 127:35, 2004

Sawaguchi S, Twining SS, Yue BYJT *et al.*: Alpha 2-macroglobulin levels in normal and keratoconus corneas. *Invest Ophthalmol Vis Sci* 35:4008, 1994

Shapiro MB, Rodrigues MM, Mandel MR *et al.*: Anterior clear spaces in keratoconus. *Ophthalmology* 93:1316, 1986

Sherwin T, Brookes NH, Loh IP *et al.*: Cellular incursion into Bowman's membrane in the peripheral cone of the keratoconic cornea. *Exp Eye Res* 74:473, 2002

Sii F, Lee GA, Sanfilippo P, Stephensen DC: Pellucid marginal degeneration and scleroderma. *Clin Exp Optom* 87:180, 2004

Sridhar MS, Mahesh S, Bansal AK *et al.*: Pellucid marginal corneal degeneration. *Ophthalmology* 111:1102, 2004

Thalasselis A, Etchepareborda J: Recurrent keratoconus 40 years after keratoplasty. *Ophthalmic Physiol Opt* 22:330, 2002

Tuft SJ, Gregory WM, Buckley RJ: Acute corneal hydrops in keratoconus. *Ophthalmology* 101:1738, 1994

Tuft SJ, Moodaley LC, Gregory WM *et al.*: Prognostic factors for the progression of keratoconus. *Ophthalmology* 101:439, 1994

Wentz-Hunter K, Cheng EL, Ueda J *et al.*: Keratocan expression is increased in the stroma of keratoconus corneas. *Mol Med* 7:470, 2001

Yanoff M: Discussion of Perry HD *et al.*: Round and oval cones in keratoconus. *Ophthalmology* 87:909, 1980

Dystrophies: Endothelial

Abbott RL, Fine BS, Webster RG *et al.*: Specular microscopic and histologic observations in nonguttate corneal endothelial degeneration. *Ophthalmology* 88:788, 1981

Adamis AP, Filatov V, Tripathi BJ *et al.*: Fuchs' endothelial dystrophy of the cornea. *Surv Ophthalmol* 38:149, 1993

Akhtar S, Bron AJ, Meek KM *et al.*: Congenital hereditary endothelial dystrophy and band keratopathy in an infant with corpus callosum agenesis. *Cornea* 20:547, 2001

Akpek EK, tan-Yaycioglu R, Gottsch JD *et al.*: Spontaneous corneal perforation in a patient with unusual unilateral pellucid marginal degeneration. *J Cataract Refract Surg* 27:1698, 2001

Al-Rajhi AA, Wagoner MD: Penetrating keratoplasty in congenital hereditary endothelial dystrophy. *Ophthalmology* 104:930, 1997

Biswas S, Munier FL, Yardley J *et al.*: Missense mutations in COL8A2, the gene encoding the alpha2 chain of type VIII collagen, cause two forms of corneal endothelial dystrophy. *Hum Mol Genet* 10:2415, 2001

Brooks AMV, Grant G, Gillies WE: Differentiation of posterior polymorphous dystrophy from other posterior corneal opacities by specular microscopy. *Ophthalmology* 96:1639, 1989

Cameron JA: Keratoglobus. *Cornea* 12:124, 1993

Cheng LL, Young AL, Wong AK *et al.*: Confocal microscopy of posterior polymorphous endothelial dystrophy. *Cornea* 24:599, 2005

Cibis GW, Tripathi RC: The differential diagnosis of Descemet's tears (Haab's striae) and posterior polymorphous dystrophy bands: A clinicopathologic study. *Ophthalmology* 89:614, 1982

Cockerham GC, Laver NV, Hidayat AA *et al.*: An immunohistochemical analysis and comparison of posterior polymorphous dystrophy with congenital hereditary endothelial dystrophy. *Cornea* 21:787, 2002

Funderburgh JL, Funderburgh ML, Rodrigues MM *et al.*: Altered antigenicity of keratan sulfate proteoglycan in selected corneal diseases. *Invest Ophthalmol Vis Sci* 31:419, 1990

Grimm BB, Waring GO III, Grimm SB: Posterior amorphous corneal dysgenesis. *Am J Ophthalmol* 120:448, 1995

Henriquez AS, Kenyon KR, Dohlman CH *et al.*: Morphologic characteristics of posterior polymorphous dystrophy: A study of nine corneas and review of the literature. *Surv Ophthalmol* 29:139, 1984

Holland DR, Maeda N, Hannush SB *et al.*: Unilateral keratoconus: Incidence and quantitative topographic analysis. *Ophthalmology* 104:1409, 1997

Ingraham HJ, Donnefeld ED, Perry HD: Keratoconus with spontaneous perforation of the cornea. *Arch Ophthalmol* 109:1651, 1991

Johnson AT, Folberg R, Vrabec MP *et al.*: The pathology of posterior amorphous corneal dystrophy. *Ophthalmology* 97:104, 1990

Levy SG, Noble BA, McCartney ACE: Early-onset posterior polymorphous dystrophy. *Arch Ophthalmol* 114:1265, 1996

Li QJ, Ashraf MF, Shen DF *et al.*: The role of apoptosis in the pathogenesis of Fuchs endothelial dystrophy of the cornea. *Arch Ophthalmol* 119:1597, 2001

Lipman RM, Rubenstein JB, Torczynski E: Keratoconus and Fuchs' corneal endothelial dystrophy in a patient and her family. *Arch Ophthalmol* 108:993, 1990

Mandell RB, Polse KA, Brand RJ *et al.*: Corneal hydration control in Fuchs' dystrophy. *Invest Ophthalmol Vis Sci* 30:845, 1989

Moroi SE, Gokhale PA, Schteingart MT *et al.*: Clinicopathologic correlation and genetic analysis in a case of posterior polymorphous corneal dystrophy. *Am J Ophthalmol* 135:461, 2003

Mullaney PB, Risco JM, Teichmann K *et al.*: Congenital hereditary endothelial dystrophy associated with glaucoma. *Ophthalmology* 102:186, 1995

Panjwani N, Drysdale J, Clark B *et al.*: Protein-related abnormalities in keratoconus. *Invest Ophthalmol Vis Sci* 30:2481, 1989

Patel DV, Grupcheva CN, McGhee CN: In vivo confocal microscopy of posterior polymorphous dystrophy. *Cornea* 24:550, 2005

Ross JR, Foulks GN, Sanfilippo FP *et al.*: Immunohistochemical analysis of the pathogenesis of posterior polymorphous dystrophy. *Arch Ophthalmol* 113:340, 1995

Roth SI, Stock EL, Jutabha R: Endothelial viral inclusions in Fuchs' corneal dystrophy. *Hum Pathol* 18:338, 1987

Sawaguchi S, Yue BYT, Sugar J *et al.*: Lysosomal enzyme abnormalities in keratoconus. *Arch Ophthalmol* 107:1507, 1989

Sekundo W, Lee WR, Kirkness CM *et al.*: An ultrastructural investigation of an early manifestation of the posterior polymorphous dystrophy of the cornea. *Ophthalmology* 101:1422, 1994

Stern GA, Knapp A, Hood CI: Corneal amyloidosis associated with keratoconus. *Ophthalmology* 95:52, 1988

Teekhasaenee C, Nimmanit S, Sutthiphan S *et al.*: Posterior polymorphous dystrophy and Alport syndrome. *Ophthalmology* 98:1207, 1991

Threlkeld AB, Green WR, Quigley HA *et al.*: A clinicopathologic study of posterior polymorphous dystrophy: Implications for pathogenetic mechanism of the associated glaucoma. *Trans Am Ophthalmol Soc* 92:133, 1994

Vemuganti GK, Sridhar MS, Edward DP *et al.*: Subepithelial amyloid deposits in congenital hereditary endothelial dystrophy: a histopathologic study of five cases. *Cornea* 21:524, 2002

Wilson SE, Bourne WM, Maguire LJ *et al.*: Aqueous humor composition in Fuchs' dystrophy. *Invest Ophthalmol Vis Sci* 30:449, 1989

Yuen HK, Rassier CE, Jardeleza MS *et al.*: A morphologic study of Fuchs dystrophy and bullous keratopathy. *Cornea* 24:319, 2005

Pigmentations

Ciancaglini M, Carpineto P, Zuppardi E *et al.*: In vivo confocal microscopy of patients with amiodarone-induced keratopathy. *Cornea* 20:368, 2001

Ferry AP: A "new" iron line of the superficial cornea: Occurrence in patients with filtering blebs. *Arch Ophthalmol* 79:142, 1968

Garg P, Vemuganti GK, Chatarjee S *et al.*: Pigmented plaque presentation of dematiaceous fungal keratitis: a clinicopathologic correlation. *Cornea* 23:571, 2004

Gass JE: The iron lines of the superficial cornea. *Arch Ophthalmol* 71:348, 1964

Haug SJ, Friedman AH: Identification of amiodarone in corneal deposits. *Am J Ophthalmol* 3:518, 1991

Hawkins AS, Stein RM, Gaines BI *et al.*: Ocular deposition of copper associated with multiple myeloma. *Am J Ophthalmol* 131:257, 2001

Hidayat AA, Margo CE, Mauriello JA *et al.*: Lipofuscinosis of the cornea. *Ophthalmology* 99:1796, 1992

Hiraoka T, Furuya A, Matsumoto Y *et al.*: Corneal iron ring formation associated with overnight orthokeratology. *Cornea* 23:S78, 2004

Hirst LW, Sanborn G, Green WR *et al.*: Amodiaquine ocular changes. *Arch Ophthalmol* 100:1300, 1982

Holland EJ, Stein CA, Palestine AG *et al.*: Suramin keratopathy. *Am J Ophthalmol* 106:216, 1988

Hollander DA, Aldave AJ: Drug-induced corneal complications. *Curr Opin Ophthalmol* 15:541, 2004

Johnson RE, Campbell RJ: Wilson's disease: Electron microscopic, x-ray energy spectroscopic, and atomic absorption spectroscopic studies of corneal copper deposition and distribution. *Lab Invest* 46:564, 1982

Kaufer G, Fine BS, Green WR *et al.*: Retrocorneal pigmentation with special reference to the formation of retrocorneal membranes by uveal melanocytes. *Am J Ophthalmol* 64:567, 1967

Klingele TG, Newman SA, Burde RM: Accommodation defect in Wilson's disease. *Am J Ophthalmol* 90:22, 1980

Koenig SB, McDonald MB, Yamaguchi T *et al.*: Corneal iron lines after refractive keratoplasty. *Arch Ophthalmol* 101:1862, 1983

Liu M, Cohen EJ, Brewer GJ *et al.*: Kayser–Fleischer ring as the presenting sign of Wilson disease. Am J Ophthalmol 133:832, 2002

Löbner A, Löbner J, Zotter J: The Kayser–Fleischer ring during long-term treatment in Wilson's disease (hepatolenticular degeneration). *Graefes Arch Clin Exp Ophthalmol* 224:152, 1986

Madge GE, Geeraets WJ, Guerry DP: Black cornea secondary to topical epinephrine. *Am J Ophthalmol* 71:402, 1971

Mannis MJ: Iron deposition in the corneal graft: Another corneal iron line. *Arch Ophthalmol* 101:1858, 1983

Orlando RG, Dangel ME, Schaal SF: Clinical experience and grading of amiodarone keratopathy. *Ophthalmology* 91:1184, 1984

Pilger IS: Pigmentation of the cornea: A review and classification. *Ann Ophthalmol* 15:1076, 1983

Prien RF, Cole JO, deLong SL et al.: Ocular effects of long-term chlorpromazine. *Arch Gen Psychiatry* 23:464, 1970

Tso MOM, Fine BS, Thorpe HE: Kayser–Fleischer ring and associated cataract in Wilson's disease. *Am J Ophthalmol* 79:479, 1975

Webber SK, Domniz Y, Sutton GL et al.: Corneal deposition after high-dose chlorpromazine hydrochloride therapy. *Cornea* 20:217, 2001

Williams EJ, Gleeson D, Burton JL et al.: Kayser–Fleischer like rings in alcoholic liver disease: a case report. *Eur J Gastroenterol Hepatol* 15:91, 2003

Yuce A, Kocak N, Demir H et al.: Evaluation of diagnostic parameters of Wilson's disease in childhood. *Indian J Gastroenterol* 22:4, 2003

Crystals

Awwad ST, Haddad W, Wang MX et al.: Corneal intrastromal gatifloxacin crystal deposits after penetrating keratoplasty. *Eye Contact Lens* 30:169, 2004

Budde M, Gusek-Schneider GC, Mayer U et al.: Annular crystalline keratopathy in association with immunoglobulin therapy for pyoderma gangrenosum. *Cornea* 22:82, 2003

Font RL, Sobol W, Matoba A: Polychromatic corneal and conjunctival crystals secondary to clofazimine therapy in a leper. *Ophthalmology* 96:311, 1989

Hunts JH, Matoba AY, Osato MS et al.: Infectious crystalline keratopathy. *Arch Ophthalmol* 3:528, 1993

Khater TT, Jones DB, Wilhelmus KR: Infectious crystalline keratopathy caused by gram-negative bacteria. *Am J Ophthalmol* 124:19, 1997

Kincaid MC, Fouraker BD, Schanzlin DJ: Infectious crystalline keratopathy after relaxing incisions. *Am J Ophthalmol* 111:374, 1991

Lubniewski AJ, Houchin KW, Holland EJ et al.: Posterior infectious crystalline keratopathy with *Staphylococcus epidermidis*. *Ophthalmology* 97:1454, 1990

Matoba AY, O'Brien TP, Wilhelmus KR et al.: Infectious crystalline keratopathy due to *Streptococcus pneumoniae*: Possible association with serotype. *Ophthalmology* 101:1000, 1994

McDonnell PJ, Kwitko S, McDonnell JM et al.: Characterization of infectious crystalline keratitis caused by a human isolate of *Streptococcus mitis*. *Arch Ophthalmol* 109:1147, 1991

McDonnell PJ, Schanzlin DJ, Rao NA: Immunoglobulin deposition in the cornea after application of autologous serum. *Arch Ophthalmol* 106:1423, 1988

Ormerod LD, Ruoff KL, Meisler DM et al.: Infectious crystalline keratopathy. *Ophthalmology* 98:159, 1991

Steuhl KP, Knorr M, Rohrbach JM et al.: Paraproteinemic corneal deposits in plasma cell myeloma. *Am J Ophthalmol* 111:312, 1991

Tsilou ET, Rubin BI, Reed GF et al.: Age-related prevalence of anterior segment complications in patients with infantile nephropathic cystinosis. *Cornea* 21:173, 2002

Wilhelmus KR, Robinson NM: Infectious crystalline keratopathy caused by *Candida albicans*. *Am J Ophthalmol* 112:322, 1991

Neoplasm

Cervantes G, Rodriguez AA Jr, Leal AG: Squamous cell carcinoma of the conjunctiva: clinicopathological features in 287 cases. *Can J Ophthalmol* 37:14, 2002

Hansen LH, Prause JU, Ehlers N et al.: Primary corneal myxoma. *Acta Ophthalmol Scand* 82:224, 2004

Mohamed SR, Matthews N, Calcagni A: Juvenile xanthogranuloma of the limbus in an adult. *Arch Ophthalmol* 120:976, 2002

Park SH, Rah SH, Kim YH: Juvenile xanthogranuloma as an isolated corneoscleral limbal mass: a case report. *Korean J Ophthalmol* 17:63, 2003

Sanchez-Huerta V, Rodriguez-Reyes AA, Hernandez-Quintela E et al.: A corneal diffuse neurofibroma as a manifestation of von Recklinghausen disease. *Cornea* 22:59, 2003

Shields CL, Fasiudden A, Mashayekhi A et al.: Conjunctival nevi: clinical features and natural course in 410 consecutive patients. *Arch Ophthalmol* 122:167, 2004

Tuomaala S, Aine E, Saari KM et al.: Corneally displaced malignant conjunctival melanomas. *Ophthalmology* 109:914, 2002

Wollensak G, Green WR, Seiler T: Corneal myxoma. *Jpn J Ophthalmol* 46:193, 2002

SCLERA

Watson PG, Young RD: Scleral structure, organisation and disease. A review. *Exp Eye Res* 78:609, 2004

Congenital Anomalies

Chan CC, Green WR, de la Cruz ZC et al.: Ocular findings in osteogenesis imperfecta congenita. *Arch Ophthalmol* 100:1459, 1982

Cheskes J, Buettner H: Ocular manifestations of alkaptonuric ochronosis. *Arch Ophthalmol* 118:724, 2000

Ganesh A, Jenny C, Geyer J et al.: Retinal hemorrhages in type I osteogenesis imperfecta after minor trauma. *Ophthalmology* 111:1428, 2004

Kaiser-Kupfer MI, Podgor M, McCain L et al.: Correlation of ocular rigidity and blue sclera in osteogenesis imperfecta. *Trans Ophthalmol Soc UK* 104:191, 1985

Kampik A, Sani JN, Green WR: Ocular ochronosis: Clinicopathological, histochemical, and ultrastructural studies. *Arch Ophthalmol* 98:1441, 1980

Makkar RP, Arora A, Monga A et al.: Alport's syndrome with blue sclera. *J Assoc Physicians India* 51:510, 2003

Odabas AR, Karakuzu A, Selcuk Y et al.: Alkaptonuria: a case report. *J Dermatol* 28:158, 2001

Silence D, Butler B, Latham M et al.: Natural history of blue sclerae in osteogenesis imperfecta. *Am J Med Genet* 45:183, 1993

Ticho U, Ivry M, Merin S: Brittle cornea, blue sclera, and red hair syndrome (the brittle cornea syndrome). *Br J Ophthalmol* 64:175, 1980

Inflammations

Akpek EK, Thorne JF, Qazi FA et al.: Evaluation of patients with scleritis for systemic disease. *Ophthalmology* 111:501, 2004

Akpek EK, Uy HS, Christen W et al.: Severity of episcleritis and systemic disease association. *Ophthalmology* 106:729, 1999

Arevalo JF, Shields CL, Shields JA: Giant nodular posterior scleritis simulating choroidal melanoma and birdshot retinochoroidopathy. *Ophthalmic Surg Lasers Imaging* 34:403, 2003

Benson WE: Posterior scleritis. *Surv Ophthalmol* 32:297, 1988

Burton BJ, Cunningham ET Jr, Cree IA et al.: Eye involvement mimicking scleritis in a patient with chronic lymphocytic leukaemia. *Br J Ophthalmol* 89:775, 2005

de la Maza MS, Foster CS, Jabbur NS: Scleritis associated with systemic vasculitic diseases. *Ophthalmology* 102:687, 1995

de la Maza MS, Foster CS, Jabbur NS: Scleritis-associated uveitis. *Ophthalmology* 104:58, 1997

Fong LP, de la Maza MS, Rice BA et al.: Immunopathology of scleritis. *Ophthalmology* 98:472, 1991

Foster CS, Forstot SL, Wilson LA: Mortality rate in rheumatoid arthritis patients developing necrotizing scleritis or peripheral ulcerative keratitis: Effects of systemic immunosuppression. *Ophthalmology* 91:1253, 1984

Frayer WC: The histopathology of perilimbal ulceration in Wegener's granulomatosis. *Arch Ophthalmol* 64:58, 1960

Hinzpeter EN, Naumann G, Bartelheimer HK: Ocular histopathology in Still's disease. *Ophthalmic Res* 2:16, 1971

Hoang-Xuan T, Bodaghi B, Toublanc M *et al.*: Scleritis and mucosal-associated lymphoid tissue lymphoma: A new masquerade syndrome. *Ophthalmology* 103:631, 1996

Jabs DA, Mudun A, Dunn JP *et al.*: Episcleritis and scleritis: Clinical features and treatment results. *Am J Ophthalmol* 130:469, 2000

Liver-Rallatos C, El-Shabrawi Y, Zatirakis P *et al.*: Recurrent nodular scleritis associated with varicella virus. *Am J Ophthalmol* 126:594, 1998

Mahr MA, Garrity JA, Robertson DM *et al.*: Ocular hypotony secondary to spontaneously ruptured posterior staphyloma. *Arch Ophthalmol* 121:122, 2003

McCluskey PJ, Watson PG, Lightman S *et al.*: Posterior scleritis: Clinical features, systemic associations, and outcome in a large series of patients. *Ophthalmology* 106:2380, 1999

Read RW, Weiss AH, Sherry DD: Episcleritis in childhood. *Ophthalmology* 106:2377, 1999

Riono WI, Hidayat AA, Rao NA: Scleritis: A clinicopathologic study of 55 cases. *Ophthalmology* 106:1328, 1999

Saito W, Kotake S, Ohno S: A patient with sarcoidosis diagnosed by a biopsy of scleral nodules. *Graefes Arch Clin Exp Ophthalmol* 243:374, 2005

Tuft SJ, Watson PG: Progression of scleral disease. *Ophthalmology* 98:467, 1991

Venkatesh P, Garg SP, Kumaran E *et al.*: Congenital porphyria with necrotizing scleritis in a 9-year-old child. *Clin Exp Ophthalmol* 28:314, 2000

Watson PG, Hayreh SS: Scleritis and episcleritis. *Br J Ophthalmol* 60:163, 1976

Watson PG: The diagnosis and management of scleritis. *Ophthalmology* 87:716, 1980

Tumors

Gayre GS, Proia AD, Dutton JJ: Epibulbar osseous choristoma: case report and review of the literature. *Ophthalmic Surg Lasers* 33:410, 2002

Ortiz JM, Yanoff M: Epipalpebral conjunctival osseous choristoma. *Br J Ophthalmol* 63:173, 1979

Santora DC, Biglan AW, Johnson BL: Episcleral osteocartilaginous choristoma. *Am J Ophthalmol* 119:654, 1995

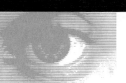

9

Uvea

NORMAL ANATOMY

I. The uvea is composed of three parts: iris, ciliary body, and choroid (Figs 9.1 and 9.2).

A. The iris is a circular, extremely thin diaphragm separating the anterior or aqueous compartment of the eye into anterior and posterior chambers.

1. The iris can be subdivided from pupil to ciliary body into three zones: pupillary, mid, and root; and from anterior to posterior into four zones: anterior border layer, stroma (the bulk of the iris), partially pigmented anterior pigment epithelium (which contains the dilator muscle in its anterior cytoplasm and pigment in its posterior cytoplasm), and completely pigmented posterior pigment epithelium.

2. The sphincter muscle, neuroectodermally derived like the dilator muscle and pigment epithelium, lies as a ring in the pupillary stroma.

B. The ciliary body, contiguous with the iris anteriorly and the choroid posteriorly, is divisible into an anterior ring, the pars plicata (approximately 1.5 mm wide in meridional sections), containing 70 to 75 meridional folds or processes, and a posterior ring, the pars plana (approximately 3.5 to 4 mm wide in meridional sections).

1. The ciliary body is wider on the temporal side (approximately 6 mm) than on the nasal side (approximately 5 mm).

2. From the scleral side inward, the ciliary body can be divided into the suprachoroidal (potential) space, the ciliary muscles (an external longitudinal, meridional, or Brücke's; a middle radial or oblique; and an internal circular or Müller's), a layer of vessels, the external basement membrane, the outer pigmented and inner nonpigmented ciliary epithelium, and the internal basement membrane.

C. The largest part of the uvea, the choroid, extends from the ora serrata to the optic nerve.

1. The choroid nourishes the outer half of the retina through its choriocapillaris and acts as a conduit for major arteries, veins, and nerves.

2. From the scleral side inward, the choroid is divided into the suprachoroidal (potential) space and lamina fusca; the choroidal stroma, which contains uveal melanocytes, fibrocytes, occasional ganglion cells, collagen, blood vessels (outer or Haller's large vessels and inner or Sattler's small vessels), and nerves; the choriocapillaris (the largest-caliber capillaries in the body), and the outer aspect of Bruch's membrane.

3. The choriocapillaris in the posterior region of the eye has a lobular structure, with each lobule fed by a central arteriole and drained by peripheral venules.

CONGENITAL AND DEVELOPMENTAL DEFECTS

Persistent Pupillary Membrane

I. Persistence of a pupillary membrane (Fig. 9.3), a common clinical finding, is caused by incomplete atrophy (resorption) of the anterior lenticular fetal vascular arcades and associated mesodermal tissue derived from the primitive annular vessel.

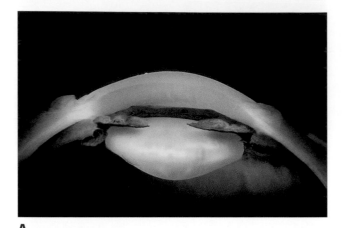

A

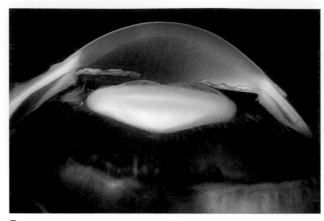

B

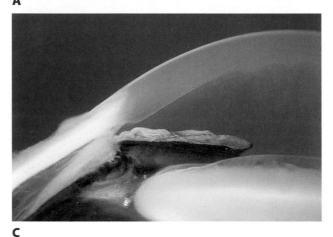

C

Fig. 9.1 Iris and ciliary body. **A** and **B,** The iris is lined posteriorly by its pigment epithelium, and anteriorly by the avascular anterior border layer. The bulk of the iris is made up of vascular stroma. Considerable pigment is present in the anterior border layer and stroma in the brown iris (**A**), as contrasted to little pigment in the blue eye (**B** and **C**). The iris pigment epithelium is maximally pigmented in **A–C**; the color of the iris, therefore, is only determined by the amount of pigment in the anterior border layer and stroma. **A–C**: The ciliary body is wedge-shaped and has a flat anterior end, continuous with the very thin iris root, and a pointed posterior end, continuous with the choroid. (Courtesy of Dr. RC Eagle, Jr.)

Incomplete persistence is the rule. Because the remnants represent fetal mesodermal tissue, they are nonpigmented except when attached to the anterior surface of the lens. The remnants may be attached to the iris alone (invariably to the collarette) or may run from the collarette of the iris to attach on to the posterior surface of the cornea, where occasionally there is an associated corneal opacity. Isolated nonpigmented or pigmented remnants may be found on the anterior lens capsule ("stars") or drifting freely in the anterior chamber. Total persistence of the fetal pupillary membrane is extremely rare and usually associated with other ocular anomalies, especially microphthalmos.

II. Histologically, fine strands of mesodermal tissue are seen, rarely with blood vessels.

Persistent Tunica Vasculosa Lentis

I. Persistence of the tunica vasculosa lentis is caused by incomplete atrophy (resorption) of the fetal tunica vasculosa lentis derived posteriorly from the primitive hyaloid vasculature and anteriorly from the primitive annular vessel posterior to the fetal pupillary membrane.

Persistence of the posterior part of the tunica vasculosa lentis is usually associated with persistence of a hyperplastic primary vitreous, the composite whole being known as *persistent hyper-*

plastic primary vitreous (see Fig. 18.16), and may or may not be associated with persistence of the anterior part of the tunica vasculosa lentis. Persistence of the anterior part of the tunica vasculosa lentis alone probably does not occur. The entire tunica vasculosa lentis may persist without an associated primary vitreous. The condition is extremely rare, however, and is usually associated with other ocular anomalies (e.g., with the ocular anomalies of trisomy 13).

II. Histologically, fine strands of mesodermal tissue, usually with patent blood vessels, are seen closely surrounding the lens capsule.

Persistence and hyperplasia of the primary vitreous may or may not be present.

Heterochromia Iridis and Iridum

Heterochromia iridum (see p. 694 in Chapter 17) is a difference in pigmentation between the two irises (e.g., the involved iris lighter than the uninvolved iris in Fuchs' heterochromic iridocyclitis), as contrasted to *heterochromia iridis*, which is an alteration in a single iris (e.g., ipsilateral heterochromia is occasionally caused by segmental ocular involvement).

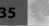

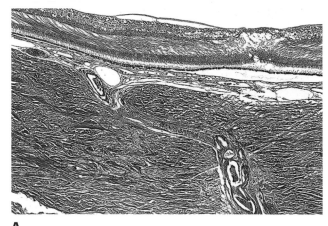

A

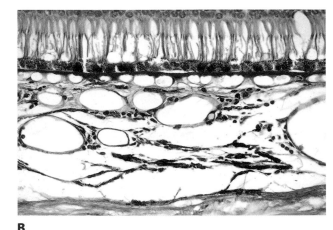

B

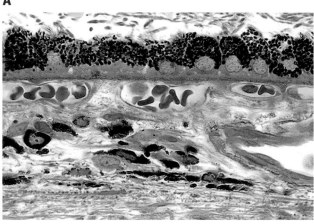

C

Fig. 9.2 Choroid. **A,** The choroid lies between the sclera (blue in this trichrome stain) and the retinal pigment epithelium. Uveal tissue spills out into most scleral canals, as into this scleral canal of the long posterior ciliary artery. **B,** The choroid is composed, from outside to inside, of the suprachoroidal (potential) space and lamina fusca, the choroidal stroma (which contains uveal melanocytes, fibrocytes, collagen, blood vessels, and nerves), the fenestrated choriocapillaris, and the outer aspect of Bruch's membrane. **C,** Whereas the normal capillary in the body is large enough for only one erythrocyte to pass through, the capillaries of the choriocapillaris—the largest capillaries in the body—permit simultaneous passage of numerous erythrocytes. The choriocapillaris' basement membrane and associated connective tissue compose the outer half of Bruch's membrane, while the inner half is composed of the basement membrane and associated connective tissue of the retinal pigment epithelium. Note that the pigment granules are larger in the retinal pigment epithelial cells than in the uveal melanocytes (see also Fig. 17.1C).

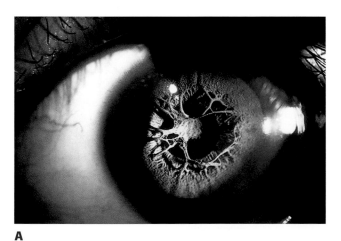

A

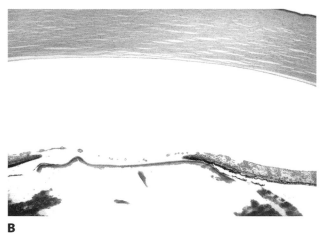

B

Fig. 9.3 Persistent pupillary membrane (PPM). **A,** Massive PPM, extending from collarette to collarette over anterior lens surface. **B,** Photomicrograph shows vascular membrane extending across pupil in 3-day-old premature infant.

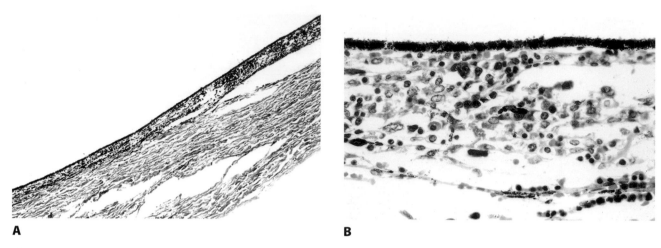

Fig. 9.4 Hematopoiesis. **A,** Infant weighing 1070 g died on the first day of life. Photomicrograph shows choroid thickened by hematopoietic tissue. **B,** Increased magnification demonstrates blood cell precursors.

Hematopoiesis

I. Hematopoiesis in the choroid is a normal finding in premature infants and even in full-term infants for the first 3 to 6 months of life (Fig. 9.4).

> Hematopoietic tissue may occur abnormally in association with intraocular osseous metaplasia (the bone-containing marrow spaces), usually in chronically inflamed eyes in people younger than 20 years of age. A fatty marrow is the rule after 20 years of age. However, hematopoiesis may occur in some cases at any age, especially after trauma.

II. Histologically, hematopoietic tissue containing blood cell precursors is seen in the uvea, especially in the choroid.

Ectopic Intraocular Lacrimal

Gland Tissue

I. Tissue appearing histologically similar to lacrimal gland tissue has been found in the iris, ciliary body, choroid, anterior-chamber angle, sclera, and limbus (Fig. 9.5).
II. Histologically, the tissue resembles normal lacrimal gland tissue.

CONGENITAL AND DEVELOPMENTAL DEFECTS OF THE PIGMENT EPITHELIUM

See pp. 689–692 in Chapter 17.

Aniridia (Hypoplasia) of the Iris

I. Complete absence of the iris, called *aniridia*, is exceedingly rare. In almost all cases, gonioscopy reveals a rudimentary iris in continuity with the ciliary body (i.e., iris hypoplasia; Fig. 9.6; see also Figs 2.18 and 16.5).

> The rudimentary iris may be invisible unless gonioscopy is used. The amount of iris tissue varies in different quadrants.

II. Photophobia, nystagmus, and poor vision may be present.
III. Glaucoma is often associated with hypoplasia of the iris.
IV. Other ocular anomalies such as increased central corneal thickness, dry eyes, cataract, absent fovea, small optic disc, peripheral corneal vascularization, and persistent pupillary membrane may also be present.

> The aniridic eye may show invasion of the cornea by conjunctival epithelium, presumably because of corneal epithelial stem cell deficiency.

V. Aniridia may be associated with Wilms' tumor (see section *Other Congenital Anomalies* in Chapter 2).
VI. The condition may be autosomal dominant or, less commonly, autosomal recessive.

> Aniridia is caused by point mutations or deletions affecting the *PAX6* gene, located on chromosome 11p13.

VII. Histologically, only a rim of rudimentary iris tissue is seen. The iris musculature is usually underdeveloped or absent.

Ectropion Uveae (Hyperplasia of Iris Pigment Border or Seam)

I. Two forms are found: congenital and acquired.
   A. *Congenital ectropion uveae* (Fig. 9.7) results from a proliferation of iris pigment epithelium on to the anterior surface of the iris from the pigment border (seam or ruff), where the two layers of pigment epithelium are continuous.

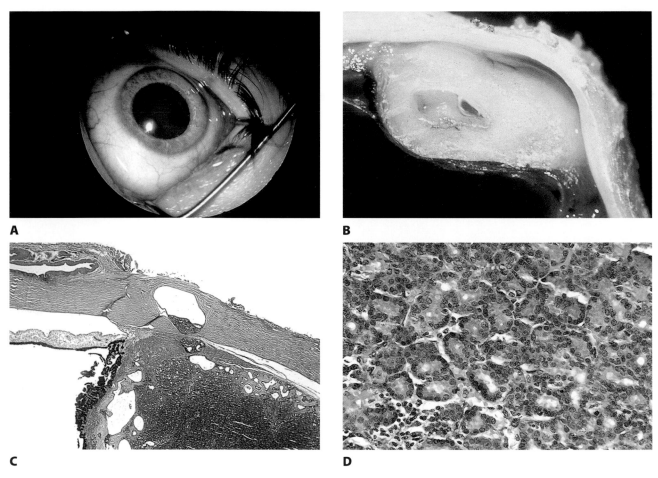

A

B

C

D

Fig. 9.5 Ectopic intraocular lacrimal gland. **A,** Clinical appearance of ciliary body tumor that has caused a sector zonular dialysis. **B,** Grossly, a cystic ciliary body tumor is present. **C,** Histologic section shows an intrascleral and ciliary body glandular tumor. **D,** Increased magnification demonstrates the resemblance to lacrimal gland tissue. (Case presented by Dr. S Brownstein to the meeting of the Eastern Ophthalmic Pathology Society, 1983, and reported by Conway VH *et al.*: adapted and published courtesy of *Ophthalmology* 92:449. Copyright Elsevier 1985.)

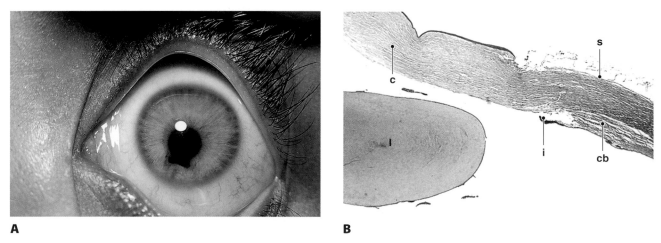

A

B

Fig. 9.6 Hypoplasia of iris. **A,** Clinical appearance of inferior and slightly nasal, partial stromal coloboma. **B,** Histologic section of another case shows marked hypoplasia of the iris (c, cornea; s, sclera; l, lens; i, hypoplastic iris; cb, ciliary body).

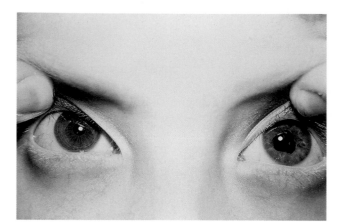

A

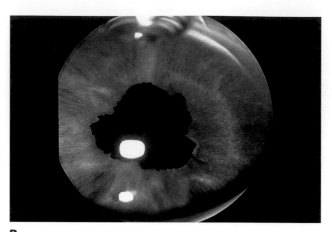

B

Fig. 9.7 Congenital ectropion uveae. **A,** At 6 months of age, infant was noted to have abnormal left eye. Here, at 8 years of age, child has normal right eye, but lighter left eye with ectropion uveae, **B,** and glaucoma. Filtering procedure was performed. **C,** Histologic section of iridectomy specimen shows a pigmented anterior iris surface. Case was previously mistakenly reported as iridocorneal endothelial syndrome. (Case #7 in Scheie HG, Yanoff M: *Arch Ophthalmol* 93:963, 1975. © American Medical Association. All rights reserved.)

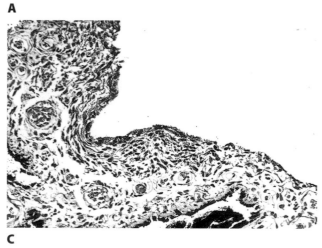

C

1. Glaucoma is often present.
2. The condition may be an isolated finding or may be associated with neurofibromatosis, facial hemihypertrophy, peripheral corneal dysgenesis, or the *Prader–Willi* syndrome (approximately 1% of patients with Prader–Willi syndrome, a chromosome 15q deletion syndrome, have oculocutaneous albinism).

    Histologically, flattened iris pigment epithelium lines the anterior surface of the involved iris, which may show increased neovascularization.

   B. The more common form, *acquired ectropion*, is acquired and progressive, usually a result of iris neovascularization.

Peripheral Dysgenesis of the Cornea and Iris

See pp. 262–264 in Chapter 8.

Coloboma

I. A coloboma (i.e., localized absence or defect) of the iris may occur alone or in association with a coloboma of the ciliary body and choroid (Fig. 9.8; see also Fig. 2.9).

A. Typical colobomas occur in the region of the embryonic cleft, inferonasally, and may be complete, incomplete (e.g., iris stromal hypoplasia; see Fig. 9.6A), or cystic in the area of the choroid.

B. Atypical colobomas occur in regions other than the inferonasal area.

C. Typical colobomas are caused by interference with the normal closure of the embryonic cleft, producing defective ectoderm.

The anterior pigment epithelium seems primarily to be defective. Except in the rare iris bridge coloboma, no tissue spans the defect. Iridodiastasis is a coloboma of the iris periphery that resembles an iridodialysis. In the ciliary body, mesodermal and vascular tissues that fill the region of the coloboma often underlie the pigment epithelial defect. The ciliary processes on either side of the defect, however, are hyperplastic. The mesodermal tissue may contain cartilage in trisomy 13 (see Fig. 2.9). Zonules may be absent so that the lens becomes notched, producing the appearance of a coloboma of the lens. The retinal pigment epithelium (RPE) is absent in the area of a choroidal coloboma but is usually hyperplastic at the edges. The neural retina is atrophic and gliotic and may contain rosettes. The choroid is partially or completely absent. The sclera may be thin or ectatic, sometimes appearing as a large cyst (see subsection *Microphthalmos with Cyst*, p. 531 in Chapter 14).

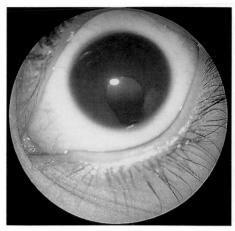
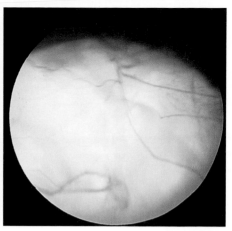

A

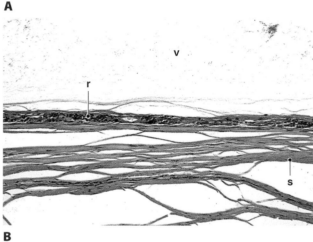

B

Fig. 9.8 Coloboma of iris and choroid. **A,** External and fundus pictures from right eye of same patient show microcornea and iris coloboma (*left*) and choroidal coloboma (*right*) with involvement of optic disc. **B,** Photomicrograph of another case shows an absent retinal pigment epithelium (RPE) and choroid. The atrophic neural retina (r) lies directly on the sclera (s) (v, vitreous). Coloboma (absence) of RPE is the primary cause of coloboma (absence) of choroid. (**A,** Courtesy of Dr. RC Lanciano, Jr.)

II. The extent of a coloboma of the choroid varies.
  A. It may be complete from the optic nerve to the ora serrata inferonasally.
  B. It may be incomplete and consist of an *inferior* crescent at the inferonasal portion of the optic nerve.
  C. It may consist of a linear area of pigmentation or RPE and choroidal thinning in any part of the fetal fissure.
III. Colobomas may occur alone or in association with other ocular anomalies.

About 8% of eyes with congenital chorioretinal coloboma contain a retinal or choroidal detachment.

IV. The condition may be inherited as an irregular autosomal-dominant trait.
V. Histology
  A. The iris coloboma shows a complete absence of all tissue in the involved area; a complete sector from pupil to periphery may be involved, or only a part of the iris.

Iris coloboma is often associated with heterochromia iridum.

  B. The ciliary body coloboma shows a defect filled with mesodermal and vascular tissues (also cartilage in

trisomy 13) with hyperplastic ciliary processes at the edges.
  C. The choroidal coloboma shows an absence or atrophy of choroid and an absence of RPE with atrophic and gliotic retina, sometimes containing rosettes.
    1. The RPE tends to be hyperplastic at the edge of the defect.
    2. The sclera in the region is usually thinned and may be cystic; the cystic space is often filled with proliferated glial tissue.

The proliferated glial tissue may become so extensive (i.e., *massive gliosis*) as to be confused with a glial neoplasm.

Cysts of the Iris and Anterior Ciliary Body (Pars Plicata)

I. Iris stromal cysts (Figs 9.9 and 9.10) resemble implantation iris cysts after nonsurgical or surgical trauma.
  A. The cysts can become quite large and cause vision problems by impinging on the pupil; they may also occlude the angle and cause secondary closed-angle glaucoma.

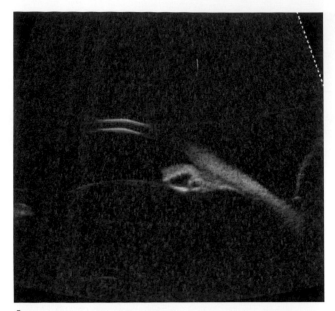

A

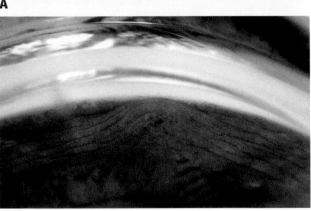

B

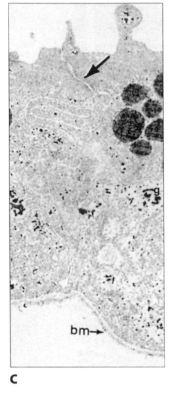

C

Fig. 9.9 Cyst of the iris. **A,** A bulge is present in the iris from the 9 to 10 o'clock position. The stroma in this area is slightly atrophic. **B,** Gonioscopic examination of the region clearly delineates a bulge caused by an underlying cyst of the pigment epithelium of the peripheral iris. **C,** Electron microscopy of iris epithelial cyst shows thin basement membrane (bm), apical adherens junction (*arrow*), and apical villi, which indicate polarization of cells in layer, like that of normal iris pigment epithelium, and presence of glycogen (g), similar to normal iris pigment epithelium.

Echographic evaluation can accurately document the location, size, and internal structure of primary cysts of the iris pigment epithelium. Ultrasonographic biomicroscopy has shown that approximately 54% of "normal" patients may have asymptomatic ciliary body cysts.

B. The origin of the cysts is poorly understood, although evidence suggests a two-part derivation: a component from cells of the iris stroma and an epithelial component from nonpigmented neuroepithelial cells.

Rarely, an occult, intrauterine limbal perforation of the anterior chamber with a needle may occur during amniocentesis.

C. Histologically, the cysts are lined by a multilayered epithelium resembling corneal or conjunctival epithelium, which may even have goblet cells. The cysts usually contain a clear fluid, and may be surrounded by a layer of epithelium.

II. Iris or ciliary body epithelial cysts are associated with the nonpigmented epithelium of the ciliary body or the pigmented neuroepithelium on the posterior surface of the iris or at the pupillary margin.

A. With the possible exception of the development of a secondary closed-angle glaucoma or pupillary obstruction, the clinical course of the pigment epithelial cysts is usually benign.

Multiple iris and ciliary body pigment epithelial cysts may be found in *congenital syphilis*. Secondary closed-angle glaucoma frequently develops in these eyes. Rarely, plateau iris can be caused by multiple ciliary body cysts.

B. The cysts form as the posterior layer of iris pigment epithelium or the inner layer of ciliary epithelium proliferates.

Occasionally, a cyst may break off and float in the anterior chamber. The cyst may then implant in the anterior-chamber

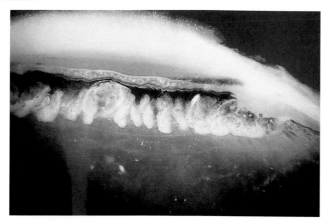

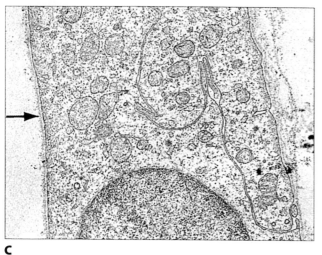

A

B

C

Fig. 9.10 A, Gross specimen shows clear cyst of pars plicata of ciliary body. **B,** Scanning electron micrograph of nonpigmented ciliary epithelial cyst present at anterior margin of pars plicata. **C,** Proliferating nonpigmented epithelial cells in cyst wall. Note thin basement membrane on one side (*arrow*) and poorly formed multilaminar basement membrane on the other. (**A** and **B,** Courtesy of Dr. RC Eagle, Jr.)

angle, where it has on occasion been mistaken for a malignant melanoma. The cyst may also float freely, enlarge, and so obstruct the pupil that surgical removal of the cyst is necessary.

III. Histologically, the pigmented cysts are filled with a clear fluid and are lined by epithelial cells having all the characteristics of mature pigment epithelium.

Cysts of the Posterior Ciliary Body (Pars Plana)

I. Most cysts of the pars plana (Fig. 9.11) are acquired.
II. Pars plana cysts lie between the epithelial layers and are analogous to detachments (separations) of the neural retina.

Clinically, the typical pars plana cysts and those of multiple myeloma appear almost identical. With fixation, however, the multiple myeloma cysts turn from clear to white or milky (see Fig. 9.11E and F), whereas the other cysts remain clear. The *multiple myeloma cysts* contain γ-globulin (immunoglobulin). Cysts similar to the myeloma cysts but extending over the pars plicata

have been seen in nonmyelomatous hypergammaglobulinemic conditions.

III. Histologically, large intraepithelial cysts are present in the pars plana nonpigmented ciliary epithelium.
The nonmyelomatous cysts appear empty in routinely stained sections but are shown to contain a hyaluronidase-sensitive material—hyaluronic acid—when special stains are used to demonstrate acid mucopolysaccharides.

INFLAMMATIONS

See Chapters 3 and 4.

INJURIES

See Chapter 5.

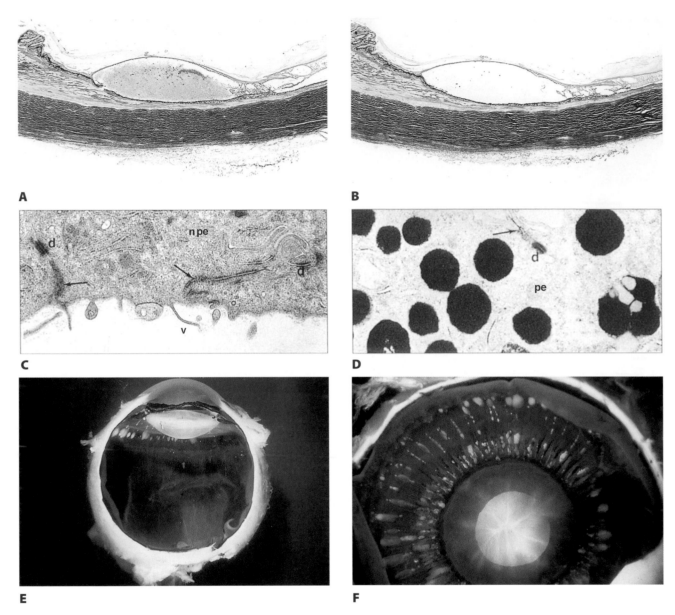

Fig. 9.11 Cyst of the pars plana. **A,** Histologic section shows a large cyst of the pars plana of the ciliary body. A special stain, which stains acid mucopolysaccharides blue, shows that the material in the cyst stains positively. **B,** If the section is first digested with hyaluronidase and then stained as in **A,** the cyst material is absent, demonstrating that the material is hyaluronic acid. **C,** Apical surface of nonpigmented epithelial layer (npe) of pars plana cyst. Note presence of apical microvilli (v), dense apical attachments (*arrows,* zonula adherens prominent), and desmosomes (d) between adjacent cells. **D,** Apical surface of pigment epithelial layer (pe) of pars plana cyst. Note apical villi and apical attachments (*arrow;* d, desmosome). Nonpigmented ciliary epithelial cysts common in region of pars plicata. **E,** Gross, fixed specimen shows milky appearance of multiple myeloma cysts of the pars plicata and pars plana, shown with increased magnification in **F.** (**E** and **F,** Courtesy of Dr. RC Eagle, Jr.)

SYSTEMIC DISEASES

Diabetes Mellitus

See sections *Iris* and *Ciliary Body and Choroid* in Chapter 15.

Vascular Diseases

See section *Vascular Diseases* in Chapter 11.

Cystinosis

See p. 299 in Chapter 8.

Homocystinuria

See p. 385 in Chapter 10.

Amyloidosis

See p. 238 in Chapter 7 and p. 488 in Chapter 12.

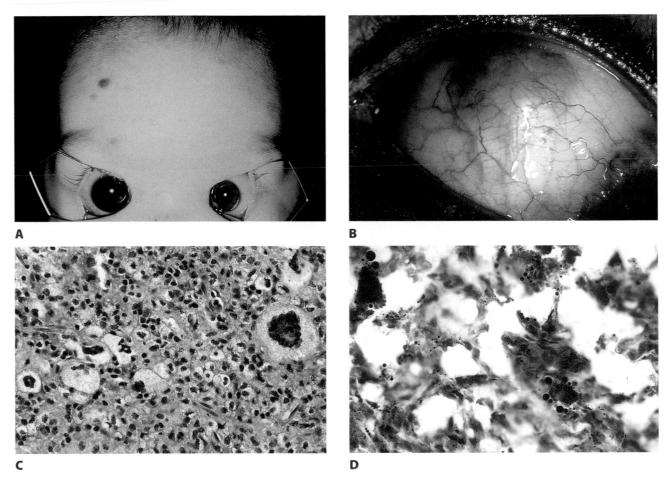

Fig. 9.12 Juvenile xanthogranuloma (JXG). **A,** Patient has multiple orange-skin lesions (biopsy-proved JXG) and involvement of both irises. Hyphema in right eye resulted in glaucoma and buphthalmos. **B,** Another patient shows a superior limbal epibulbar orange mass of the right eye that was sampled for biopsy. **C,** Histologic section shows diffuse involvement of the conjunctival substantia propria by histiocytes and Touton giant cells (see also Fig. 1.20). **D,** Oil red-O shows positive lipid staining of peripheral cytoplasm of Touton giant cell. (**A,** Courtesy of Dr. HG Scheie; case in **B–D** presented by Dr. M Yanoff to the meeting of the Eastern Ophthalmic Pathology Society, 1993, and reported by Yanoff M, Perry HD: *Arch Ophthalmol* 113:915, 1995. © American Medical Association. All rights reserved.)

Juvenile Xanthogranuloma (Nevoxanthoendothelioma)

I. Juvenile xanthogranuloma (JXG), one of the non-Langerhans' cell histiocytoses (Fig. 9.12; see also Fig. 1.18), is a benign cutaneous disorder of infants and young children.

    A. The typical raised orange-skin lesions occur singly or in crops and regress spontaneously.

> Solitary spindle-cell xanthogranuloma (SCXG), another of the non-Langerhans' cell histiocytoses, may involve the eyelids and contains Touton giant cells, but differs from JXG in containing more than 90% spindle cells. SCXG may be an early form of JXG.

    B. The skin lesions may predate or postdate the ocular lesions, or occur simultaneously.

II. Ocular findings include diffuse or discrete iris involvement (most common ocular finding), but occasionally ciliary body and anterior choroidal lesions, epibulbar involvement, corneal lesions, nodules on the lids, and orbital granulomas may be seen.

    A. Most ocular lesions occur unilaterally in the very young, most under 6 months of age.

> Rarely, a limbal nodule can occur in an adult.

    B. The iris lesions are quite vascular and bleed easily.

> When confronted with an infant who has a spontaneous hyphema, the clinician must consider JXG along with retinoblastoma (iris neovascularization here can cause bleeding into the anterior chamber) and trauma (the parents may think that the hemorrhage was spontaneous, but unknown trauma could have caused it).

III. JXG is separate from the group of nonlipid reticuloendothelioses called *Langerhans' granulomatoses* or *histiocytosis X* (eosinophilic granuloma, Letterer–Siwe disease, and Hand–Schüller–Christian disease; see discussion of reticuloendothelial system in subsection *Primary Orbital Tumors* in Chapter 14).

IV. Histologically, a diffuse granulomatous inflammatory reaction with many histiocytes and often with Touton giant cells is seen.

A. Often the lesions are vascular.

B. Touton giant cells may also be found in necrobiotic xanthogranuloma and liposarcoma.

JXG may be confused histologically with necrobiosis lipoidica diabeticorum, granuloma annulare, erythema induratum, atypical sarcoidosis, Erdheim–Chester disease, Rothman–Makai panniculitis, foreign-body granulomas, various xanthomas, nodular tenosynovitis, and the extra-articular lesions of proliferative synovitis.

Langerhans' Granulomatoses (Histiocytosis X)

See discussion of reticuloendothelial system in subsection *Primary Orbital Tumors* in Chapter 14.

Collagen Diseases

See subsection *Collagen Diseases* in Chapter 6.

Mucopolysaccharidoses

See p. 298 in Chapter 8.

ATROPHIES AND DEGENERATIONS

See subsections *Atrophy* and *Degeneration and Dystrophy* in Chapter 1.

Iris Neovascularization (Rubeosis Iridis)

See Figures 9.13 and 9.14; see also Fig. 15.5.

The term *rubeosis iridis* means "red iris" and should be restricted to clinical usage; *iris neovascularization* is the proper histopathologic term.

I. Many causes

A. Vascular hypoxia

1. Central retinal vein occlusion (common)
2. Central retinal artery occlusion (rare)
3. Temporal arteritis
4. Aortic arch syndrome
5. Carotid artery disease

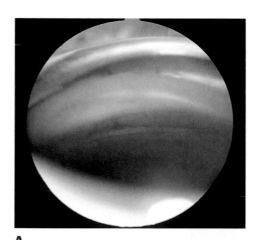

A

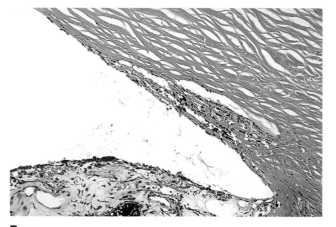

B

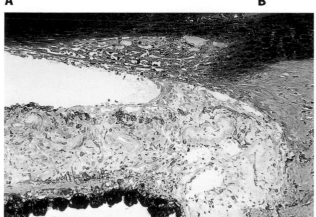

C

Fig. 9.13 Iris neovascularization (IN). **A,** Early stage of IN in partially open angle. **B,** Histologic section of another case that had a central retinal vein oclusion, IN, and secondary glaucoma. Gonioscopy showed angle partially closed. Eye was enucleated. Histologic section shows apparent open angle. Closer examination reveals material in angle and other evidence that the posterior trabecular meshwork had been closed before enucleation, but fixation caused an artifactitious opening of the angle. **C,** The same region shown with a thin plastic-embedded section clearly demonstrates IN and closure of the posterior trabecular meshwork. (**A,** Courtesy of Dr. HG Scheie.)

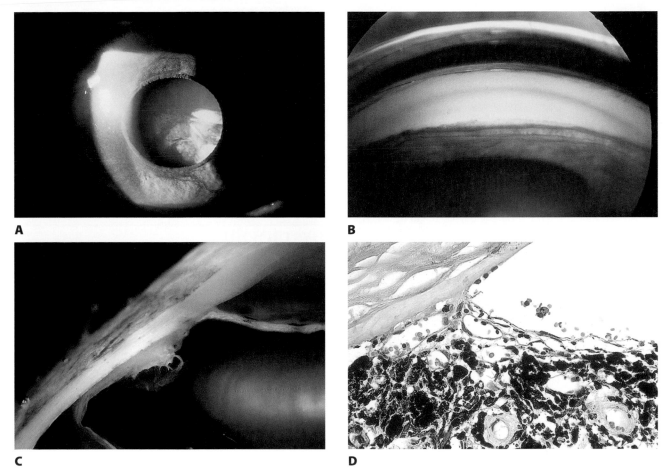

Fig. 9.14 Iris neovascularization (IN). **A,** Significant IN extends to the pupillary margin (and had closed the angle). **B,** Gonioscopy of another case shows vessels climbing angle wall and a red line of vessels on posterior trabecular meshwork. The angle is closed to the left. **C,** Gross specimen of another case shows peripheral anterior synechia (PAS). Translucent tissue in synechia is IN. **D,** Histologic section shows that IN is cause of PAS.

6. Retinal vascular disease
7. Ocular ischemic syndrome

B. Neoplastic
   1. Uveal malignant melanoma
   2. Retinoblastoma
   3. Metastatic carcinoma (uveal)
   4. Embryonal medulloepithelioma
   5. Metastatic tumors

C. Inflammatory
   1. Chronic uveitis (e.g., Fuchs' heterochromic iridocyclitis)
   2. Post retinal detachment surgery
   3. Postradiation therapy
   4. Fungal endophthalmitis
   5. Posttrauma (surgical or nonsurgical)

D. Neural retinal diseases
   1. Diabetes mellitus (usually only in advanced diabetic retinopathy)
   2. Chronic neural retinal detachment
   3. Coats' disease
   4. Chronic glaucoma (almost never with primary chronic open-angle glaucoma unless surgical trauma or central retinal vein occlusion has occurred)

   5. Sickle-cell retinopathy
   6. Retinopathy of prematurity
   7. Eales' disease
   8. Persistent hyperplastic primary vitreous
   9. Leber's miliary microaneurysms
   10. Norrie's disease

II. Iris neovascularization may be induced by hypoxia, by products of tissue breakdown, or by a specific angiogenic factor. Neovascularization of the iris is always secondary to any of a host of ocular and systemic disorders.

III. Neovascularization often starts in the pupillary margin and the iris root concurrently, but can start in either place first; the mid stromal portion is rarely involved early.

Early iris neovascularization in the angle does not cause synechiae and a closed angle but rather a secondary open-angle glaucoma, owing to obstruction of outflow by the fibrovascular membrane. Synechiae are rapidly induced, and chronic secondary closed-angle glaucoma ensues. Rarely, however, the rubeosis iridis involves the angle structures and anterior iris surface without causing synechiae, as may occur in Fuchs' heterochromic iridocyclitis.

IV. A secondary closed-angle glaucoma (called *neovascular glaucoma*) and hyphema are the main complications of iris neovascularization.

> Occasionally, iris neovascularization may be difficult to differentiate from normal iris vessels, especially when iris vessels are dilated secondary to ocular inflammation. Even with such dilatation, however, the normal iris vessels are seen to course radially, in contrast to the random distribution found in iris neovascularization. Fluorescein angiography can be helpful in differentiating normal from abnormal iris vessels by demonstrating leakage from the abnormal vessels.

V. Histologically, fibrovascular tissue is found almost exclusively on the anterior surface of the iris and in the anterior-chamber angle.
  A. The blood vessels, however, are derived initially from the ciliary body near the iris root or from iris stromal blood vessels.
  B. The new vascular growth seems to leave the iris stroma rapidly (most commonly toward the pupil) to grow on and over the anterior surface of the iris.

> With contracture of the myoblastic component of the fibrovascular tissue, the pupillary border of the iris is turned anteriorly (ectropion uveae). Synechiae are characteristically only present in the area of the anterior-chamber angle peripheral to the end of Descemet's membrane. They can be differentiated, therefore, from such broad-based synechiae as may be caused by a persistent flat chamber, chronic closed-angle glaucoma, or iris bombé.

Choroidal Folds

I. The condition consists of lines, grooves, or striae, often arranged parallel and horizontally. Occasionally the folds may be vertical, oblique, or so irregular as to resemble a jigsaw puzzle.

II. The folds appear as a series of light and dark lines, often temporal and confined to the posterior pole, rarely extending beyond the equator.

> Fluorescein angiography shows a series of alternating hyperfluorescent (peaks of folds) and hypofluorescent (valleys of folds) streaks that start early in the arteriovenous (AV) phase, persist through the late venous phase, and do not leak. The hyperfluorescent areas may be the result of RPE thinning or atrophy. The hypofluorescent areas may be caused by an inclination of the RPE in the valleys, which results in increased RPE thickness blocking the choroidal fluorescence, or may be caused by a partial collapse of the choriocapillaris in the valleys. The folds may be bilateral.

III. Causes of choroidal folds include hypermetropia, macular degeneration, neural retinal detachment, hypotony, trauma, orbital tumors, thyroid disease, scleritis, uveitis, and others, including no known cause.

> Choroidal folds are differentiated from neural retinal folds by the latter's finer appearance and normal fluorescein pattern.

IV. Histologically, the choroid and Bruch's membrane are corrugated or folded. RPE involvement seems to be a secondary phenomenon.

Heterochromia

See subsection *Heterochromia Iridis and Iridum*, this chapter, and p. 694 in Chapter 17.

Macular Degeneration

See p. 428 in Chapter 11.

DYSTROPHIES

Iris Nevus Syndrome

See p. 640 in Chapter 16.

Chandler's Syndrome

See p. 640 in Chapter 16.

Essential Iris Atrophy

See p. 641 in Chapter 16.

Iridoschisis

See p. 641 in Chapter 16.

Choroidal Dystrophies

I. Regional choroidal dystrophies
  A. Choriocapillaris atrophy involving the posterior eyegrounds
    1. Involvement of the macula alone—also called *central areolar choroidal sclerosis* (Fig. 9.15), central progressive areolar choroidal dystrophy, and central choroidal angiosclerosis
      a. The condition probably has an autosomal (recessive or dominant) inheritance pattern and is characterized by the onset of an exudative and edematous maculopathy in the third to the fifth decade.

> Autosomal-dominant central areolar sclerosis is caused by an Arg-142-Trp mutation in the peripherin/*RDS* gene. Other mutations that code to the peripherin/*RDS* gene include retinitis pigmentosa, macular dystrophy, pattern dystrophy, and fundus flavimaculatus.

      b. Typical slow progression leads to a sharply demarcated, atrophic appearance involving only the posterior pole area, causing a central scotoma but no night blindness.

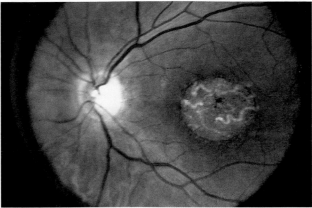

A

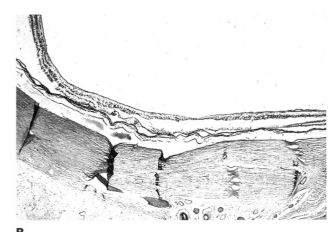

B

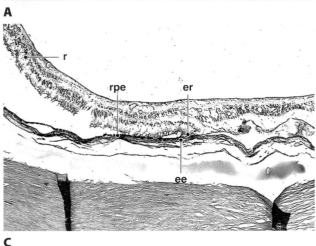

C

Fig. 9.15 Central areolar choroidal sclerosis. **A,** Clinical appearance (left eye) of fundus in patient who had bilateral symmetric macular lesions. **B,** Histologic section of another case shows that the retinal pigment epithelium (RPE) and neural retina, which are relatively normal on the far left, show an abrupt transition to a chorioretinal abnormality that involves the outer neural retinal layers, RPE, and choroid. **C,** Increased magnification of the transition zone shows an intact Bruch's membrane but loss of photoreceptors and RPE and obliteration of the choriocapillaris; no blood-containing vessels seen in remainder of choroid (r, neural retina; rpe, retinal pigment epithelium; ee, end of retinal pigment epithelium; er, end of retinal receptors). (**A,** Courtesy of Dr. WE Benson; **B** and **C,** modified from Ferry AP *et al.: Arch Ophthalmol* 88:39, 1972. © American Medical Association. All rights reserved.)

Clinically, the condition may be indistinguishable from geographic RPE atrophy of age-related macular degeneration.

---

c. Histologically, the area of involvement shows an incomplete or complete loss or degeneration of the choriocapillaris, the RPE, and the outer retinal layers.
2. Involvement of the peripapillary area—peripapillary choroidal sclerosis
   a. The area of involvement, mainly the posterior one-third of the globe surrounding the optic nerve, shows a sharply demarcated atrophic area and easily seen, large choroidal vessels.
   b. Histologically, the area of involvement shows absence of choriocapillaris, RPE, and photoreceptors and a decrease in choroidal arteries and veins.
   Bruch's membrane is intact except for some breaks in the immediate peripapillary region. Angioid streaks may also be found.
3. Involvement of the paramacular area—also called *circinate choroidal sclerosis*
   a. Total choroidal vascular atrophy involving the posterior eye grounds

---

Histologically, the choriocapillaris, the RPE, and the outer neural retinal layers are degenerated and sharply demarcated from adjacent normal chorioretinal areas. Diffuse and focal areas of round cell inflammation (mainly lymphocytes) may be found.

Involvement of the macula alone or throughout most of the posterior eyegrounds—also termed serpiginous choroiditis, serpiginous choroidopathy, serpiginous degeneration of the choroid, geographic helicoid peripapillary choroidopathy, geographic choroiditis, choroidal vascular abiotrophy, and central gyrate atrophy

---

Tuberculous choroiditis may mimic serpiginous choroiditis.

---

b. The dystrophy is characterized by well-defined gray lesions seen initially at the level of the pigment epithelium, usually contiguous with or very close to the optic nerve.
   1). Each new lesion does not change its size or shape.

2). With healing, degeneration of the pigment epithelium, geographic atrophy of the choroid, or even subretinal neovascularization and subretinal scar formation (disciform macular degeneration) may occur.

B. The disease progress is away from the optic disc, with new attacks occurring in areas previously uninvolved.

1. Visual acuity is only affected if the central fovea is involved in an attack.

Rarely, the initial lesion, or the only lesion, may be in the macula.

---

2. Involvement with nasal and temporal foci—also called *progressive bifocal chorioretinal atrophy* (PBCRA)

The gene for PBCRA has been linked to chromosome 6q near the genomic assignment for North Carolina macular dystrophy. The phenotype of PBCRA, although similar to North Carolina macular dystrophy, is quite distinct.

---

3. Involvement of the disc—also called choroiditis areata, circumpapillary dysgenesis of the pigment epithelium, and chorioretinitis striata
4. Malignant myopia (see p. 423 in Chapter 11)

II. Diffuse choroidal dystrophies

A. Diffuse choriocapillaris atrophy—also called *generalized choroidal angiosclerosis, diffuse choroidal sclerosis*, and *generalized choroidal sclerosis*

Histologically, the choriocapillaris, the RPE, and the outer neural retinal layers are degenerated.

B. Diffuse total choroidal vascular atrophy

1. Autosomal-recessive inheritance (carried on chromosome 10q26)—also called *gyrate atrophy of the choroid*
   a. Gyrate atrophy of the choroid is characterized by the development of atrophic chorioretinal patches in the periphery (often with glistening crystals scattered at the equator), progressing more centrally than peripherally, and partially fusing.
   b. Other ocular findings include posterior subcapsular cataracts and myopia, cystoid macular edema, and, rarely, retinitis pigmentosa.

A peripapillary atrophy may develop simultaneously. In the final stage, all of the fundi except the macula may be involved so that the condition may resemble choroideremia.

---

   c. Patients have hyperornithinemia (10- to 20-fold increased ornithine concentration in plasma and other body fluids), caused by a deficiency of the mitochondrial matrix enzyme ornithine-δ-aminotransferase (OAT). They may also show subjective sensory symptoms of peripheral neuropathy.

1). OAT catalyzes the major catabolic pathway of ornithine, which involves the interconversion of ornithine, glutamate, and proline through the intermediate pyrroline-5-carboxylate and requires pyridoxal phosphate (vitamin B_6) as coenzyme.

2). The OAT gene maps to chromosome 10q26, and OAT-related sequences have also been mapped to chromosome Xp11.3–p11.23 and Xp11.22–p11.21.

d. The condition becomes manifest in the second or third decade of life and slowly progresses, causing a concentric reduction of the visual field, leading to tunnel vision, and ultimately to blindness in the fourth to seventh decade of life. Decreasing vision and night blindness are prominent symptoms, along with electrophysiologic dysfunction.

e. An arginine-restricted diet slows the progress of the condition, whereas creatine supplementation appears to have no effect.

f. Histologically, the iris, corneal endothelium, nonpigmented ciliary epithelium, and, to a lesser extent, photoreceptors show abnormal mitochondria.

An abrupt transition occurs between the normal and the involved chorioretinal area; the latter shows near-total atrophy of the neural retina, RPE, and choroid.

2. X-linked inheritance—also called *choroideremia*, progressive tapetochoroidal dystrophy, and progressive chorioretinal degeneration (Fig. 9.16)
   a. This condition is characterized by almost complete degeneration of the retina and choroid (except in the macula) in affected men. It becomes manifest in childhood and progresses slowly until complete at approximately 50 years of age.

The fundus picture in carrier women resembles that seen in the early stages in affected men, namely, degeneration of the peripheral RPE giving a salt-and-pepper appearance. Mutations can cause severe visual loss in female carriers.

---

   b. It is unclear whether the earliest changes are in the choroid or the RPE, or both.
   c. Component A (but not B) of Rab geranylgeranyl transferase appears to be deficient in choroideremia.

Transfer of the Rab geranylgeranyl depends on the participation of Rab escort proteins (REP). REP-1 is produced by a gene on the X chromosome, which is defective in patients who have choroideremia.

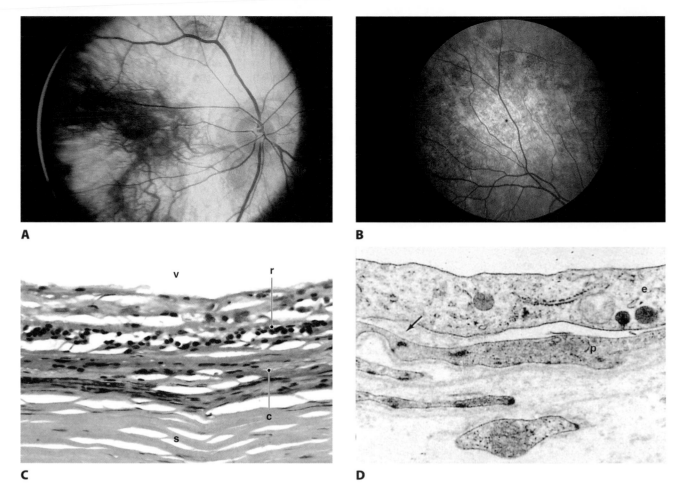

Fig. 9.16 Choroideremia. **A,** Appearance of right eye in male patient who had bilateral choroideremia. **B,** Peripheral fundus of female carrier shows peripheral pigmentation. **C,** Histologic section of another case shows absence of RPE and atrophy of both the overlying neural retina and the underlying choroid (v, vitreous; r, atrophic retina; s, sclera; c, atrophic choroid). **D,** Electron micrograph shows choroidal vessel deep to choriocapillaris. Both endothelial (e) and pericyte (p) basement membranes are absent centrally. A small amount of fragmented basement membrane (*arrow*) persists on the left. (**A,** Courtesy of Dr. WE Benson; **B,** courtesy of Dr. G Lang; **C,** presented by Dr. WS Hunter at the AOA-AFIP meeting, 1969; **D,** modified from Cameron JD *et al.: Ophthalmology* 94:187. Copyright Elsevier 1987.)

    d. Histologically, the choroid and RPE are absent or markedly atrophic, and the overlying outer neural retinal layers are atrophic. Uveal vascular endothelial cell and RPE abnormalities may be found where uveal vessels still persist.

III. All of the aforementioned choroidal entities, although usually called *atrophies*, should more properly be called *dystrophies with secondary retinal changes*; it is likely that the primary dystrophic abnormality resides in the choroidal vasculature or the RPE.

TUMORS

Epithelial

I. Hyperplasias (see p. 22 in Chapter 1 and section *Melanotic Tumors of Pigment Epithelium of Iris, Ciliary Body, and Retina* in Chapter 17)

Occasionally, pseudoadenomatous hyperplasias may become extreme and produce masses that are noted clinically, either localized to the posterior chamber or, rarely, proliferated into the anterior chamber.

II. Benign adenoma of Fuchs (Fuchs' reactive hyperplasia, coronal adenoma, Fuchs' epithelioma, benign ciliary epithelioma; Fig. 9.17)
    A. The small, age-related tumor is present in over 25% of older people, is located in the pars plicata of the ciliary body, is benign, and is usually found incidentally when an enucleated globe is being examined microscopically.
    B. It may rarely cause localized occlusion of the anterior-chamber angle.
    C. The tumor is proliferative rather than neoplastic, i.e, a hyperplasia not an adenoma.
    D. Histologically, it is a benign proliferation of cords of the nonpigmented ciliary epithelium interspersed

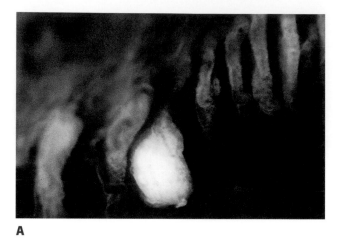

A

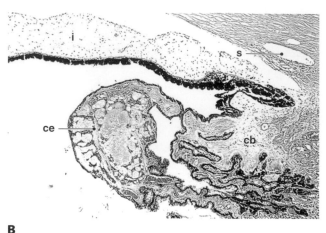

B

Fig. 9.17 Fuchs' adenoma. **A,** The lesion is seen grossly as a white tumor in the pars plicata of the ciliary body. **B,** Histologic section shows a proliferation of nonpigmented ciliary epithelium that is elaborating considerable basement membrane material (i, iris; s, Schlemm's canal, ce, proliferating ciliary epithelium; cb, ciliary body).

with abundant, amorphous, eosinophilic, acellular basement membrane material (type IV collagen and laminin are found immunohistochemically), acid mucopolysaccharides (mainly hyaluronic acid), and glycoproteins.

III. Medulloepithelioma (see p. 686 in Chapter 17)

Muscular

I. Leiomyomas—benign smooth-muscle tumors—may rarely occur in the iris, ciliary body, or choroid.

A. Leiomyomas have a predilection for women.

B. The tumors tend to affect the ciliary body and anterior choroid, unlike melanomas, which favor the posterior choroid.

C. It is difficult to differentiate a leiomyoma from an amelanotic spindle cell nevus and low-grade melanoma without the use of electron microscopy and immunohistochemical studies.

Many cases previously diagnosed as leiomyoma are probably melanocytic, rather than smooth-muscle, lesions.

D. Electron microscopic criteria for smooth-muscle cells include an investing thin basement membrane, plasmalemmal vesicles, plasmalemma-associated densities, and myriad longitudinally aligned, intracytoplasmic filaments with scattered associated densities, characteristics that allow for identification of the cells in less than optimally fixed tissue. In addition, immunohistochemical stains for muscle-specific antigen, smooth-muscle actin, and vimentin are positive in leiomyomas.

E. Mesectodermal leiomyoma (see p. 555 in Chapter 14)

1. This rare variant of leiomyoma, which microscopically resembles a neurogenic tumor more than a myogenic tumor, presumably originates from the neural crest.

2. Histologically (Fig. 9.18), widely spaced tumor cell nuclei are set in a fibrillar cytoplasmic matrix and may show immunoexpression of neural markers.

The tumors resemble ganglionic, astrocytic, and peripheral nerve tumors. The presence of a reticulum differentiates mesectodermal leiomyoma from astrocytic tumors, where the fiber is absent. Immunohistochemistry and electron microscopy are needed to differentiate the tumor from peripheral nerve tumors. If the characteristic immunohistochemical and ultrastructural features of smooth-muscle cells are found, the diagnosis is clear.

F. Leiomyosarcoma has been reported as a rare iris neoplasm.

II. A rhabdomyosarcoma is an extremely rare tumor of the iris and is probably atavistic.

Vascular

I. True hemangiomas of the iris and ciliary body are extremely rare.

A. Presumed iris hemangioma has been reported in association with multiple central nervous system (CNS) cavernous hemangiomas and may represent a distinct form of phakomatosis.

II. Hemangioma of the choroid (Fig. 9.19)

A. Hemangioma of the choroid occurs in two types, circumscibed and diffuse

1. Circumscribed is usually solitary and not associated with any systemic process.

2. Diffuse may rarely occur as an isolated finding but mostly it is part of the Sturge–Weber syndrome (see Fig. 2.2).

B. Over long intervals of observation, choroidal hemangiomas may show slight enlargement.

C. Clinically, it presents as a circumscribed, orange-red mass that shows early fluorescence with fluorecein

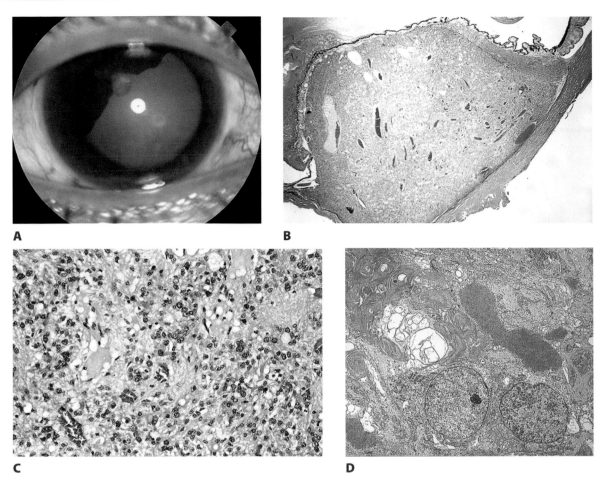

Fig. 9.18 Mesectodermal leiomyoma. **A,** A 47-year-old woman suspected of having a ciliary body melanoma. **B,** Histologic section shows large ciliary body tumor composed of widely spaced tumor cell nuclei in a fibrillar cytoplasmic matrix (shown under increased magnification in **C**). **D,** Electron microscopy shows a dense osmophilic structure called *skeinoid fibers*. (Case presented by Dr. J Campbell at the combined meeting of the Verhoeff and European Ophthalmic Pathology Societies, 1996; case reported by J Campbell *et al.: Ultrastruct Pathol* 28:559, 1997.)

and indocyanine green. Subretinal fluid is quite common

D. Histologically the choroidal tumor shows large, dilated, blood-filled spaces lined by endothelium and sharply demarcated from the normal, surrounding choroid.

III. Hemangiopericytoma
  A. Hemangiopericytomas are much more common in the orbit (see p. 546 in Chapter 14) than intraocularly.
  B. Histologically, well-vascularized spindle cell proliferation is present in the uvea in a sinusoidal pattern.

IV. AV malformation of the iris
  A. AV iris malformation, also called racemose hemangioma, is rare
  B. It consists of a unilateral continuity between an artery and a vein without an intervening capillary bed.
  C. The lesion is benign and stationary.

Osseous

I. Choroidal osteoma (osseous choristoma of the choroid; Fig. 9.20)

A. This benign, ossifying lesion is found mainly in women in their second or third decade of life and is bilateral in approximately 25% of patients.

Bilateral osseous choristoma of the choroid has been reported in an 8-month-old girl.

---

1. Growth may be seen in approximately 51% of cases with long-term follow-up.
2. An associated subretinal fluid, neovascularization, or hemorrhage may be present. Over 10 years about 56% of all patients will have decreased vision to 20/200 or worse.

Choroidal osteomas may follow ocular inflammation, be associated with systemic illness, or be familial. Rarely, they may undergo growth or spontaneous involution.

B. The characteristic clinical findings include:

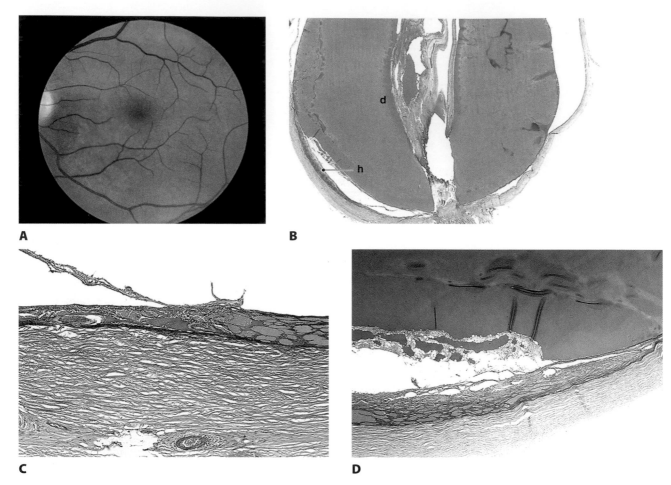

A

B

C

D

Fig. 9.19 Hemangioma of choroid. **A,** An elevated lesion, which shows a characteristic orange color, is seen in the inferior nasal macular region. **B,** A histologic section of another case shows a total retinal detachment (d) and an extensive hemangioma (h) of the choroid in the macular area. **C,** Increased magnification of the temporal edge of the hemangioma shows it is blunted and well demarcated from the adjacent normal choroid to the left. **D,** Similarly, the nasal edge of the hemangioma is blunted and easily demarcated from the adjacent choroid. This hemangioma was not associated with any systemic findings; in Sturge–Weber syndrome, the choroidal hemangioma is diffuse and not clearly demarcated from the adjacent choroid.

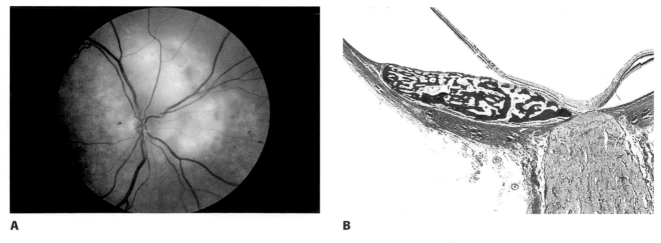

A

B

Fig. 9.20 Choroidal osteoma. **A,** The patient has an irregular, slightly elevated, yellow-white juxtapapillary lesion. Ultrasonography showed the characteristic features of bone in the choroid. **B,** A histologic section of another case shows that the choroid is replaced by mature bone that contains marrow spaces. (**A,** Courtesy of Dr. WE Benson; **B,** presented by Dr. RL Font at the meeting of the Eastern Ophthalmic Pathology Society, 1976.)

1. A slightly irregularly elevated, yellow-white, juxta-papillary choroidal tumor with well-defined geographic borders
2. Diffuse, mottled depigmentation of the overlying pigment epithelium
3. Multiple small vascular networks on the tumor surface

C. The tumor is dense ultrasonically; tissues behind the tumor are silent.

Decalcification occurs over time in almost 50% of patients.

D. Histologically, mature bone with interconnecting marrow spaces is seen sharply demarcated from the surrounding choroid.

Melanomatous

See Chapter 17.

Leukemic and Lymphomatous

I. Acute granulocytic (myelogenous; Fig. 9.21) and lymphocytic leukemias not infrequently have uveal, usually posterior choroidal, infiltrates as part of the generalized disease.

Esterases are enzymes that hydrolyze aliphatic and aromatic esters. Nonspecific esterase activity, as determined by using α-naphthyl acetate as a substrate, is not detectable in granulocytic cells. Specific esterase activity, however, as determined by using naphthol ASD-chloroacetate, is present exclusively in granulocytic cells. By demonstrating specific esterase activity on histologic sections (cytochemical method), acute granulocytic (myelogenous) leukemia can be differentiated from acute lymphocytic leukemia. Demonstrating specific esterase activity histologically is especially helpful in diagnosing leukemic infiltrates [called *myeloid (granulocytic) sarcoma*], particularly in the orbit, where granulocytic leukemic infiltrates may appear greenish clinically because of the presence of the pigment myeloperoxidase, and then are called *chloromas*. In addition, the combined use of the cytochemical

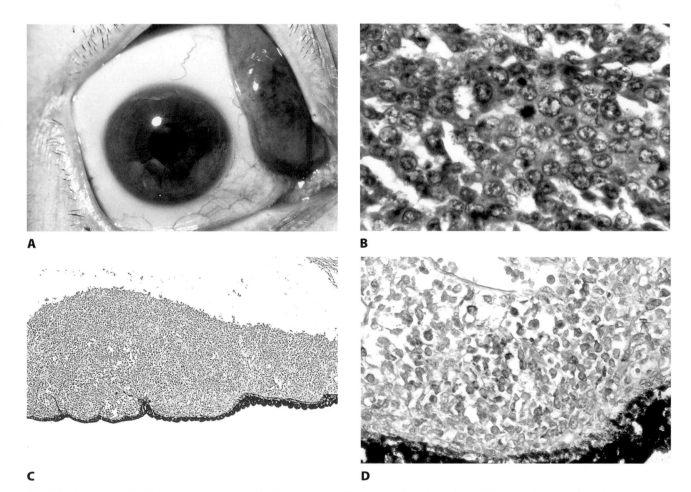

A

B

C

D

Fig. 9.21 Acute leukemia. **A,** A patient presented with a large infiltrate of leukemic cells positioned nasally in the conjunctiva of the right eye, giving this characteristic clinical picture. These lesions look similar to those caused by benign lymphoid hyperplasia, lymphoma, or amyloidosis. **B,** A biopsy of the lesion shows primitive blastic leukocytes. **C,** In another case, the iris is infiltrated by leukemic cells. A special stain (Lader stain) shows that some of the cells stain red, better seen when viewed under increased magnification in **D.** This red positivity is characteristic of myelogenous leukemic cells.

method with immunology (positive for CD43, CD45, antilysozyme, Lader stain) and morphologic study gives the best yield in differentiating the acute blastic leukemias.

A. Approximately 30% of autopsy eyes from fatal leukemic cases show ocular involvement, mainly leukemic infiltrates in the choroid. Also, 42% of newly diagnosed cases of acute leukemia show ocular findings, especially intraretinal hemorrhages, white-centered hemorrhages, and cotton-wool spots.

Rarely, the first sign of granulocytic leukemia relapse is ocular adnexal involvement.

B. Retinal hemorrhages are most likely to occur in patients who have both anemia and thrombocytopenia combined; and when the two are severe (hemoglobin <8 g/100 ml and platelets <100 000/mm), retinal hemorrhages may occur in 70% of patients.

II. Malignant lymphomas (see p. 574 in Chapter 14)—non-Hodgkin's lymphoma of the CNS (NHL-CNS) and systemic non-Hodgkin's lymphoma rarely involve the eye, but do so much more often than Hodgkin's lymphoma.

A. NHL-CNS—old terms—*reticulum cell sarcoma, histiocytic lymphoma, microgliomatosis*

1. NHL-CNS (Fig. 9.22), usually a large B-cell lymphoma, may be associated with similar multifocal neoplastic infiltrates in the vitreous, presenting clinically as uveitis.

Occasionally, NHL-CNS may involve the eye primarily and simulate a chronic uveitis, often with a vitreitis. Concentrations of interleukin-10 from vitreous aspirates may be helpful in making the diagnosis.

a. The retina and choroid may also be involved (oculocerebral non-Hodgkin's lymphoma).

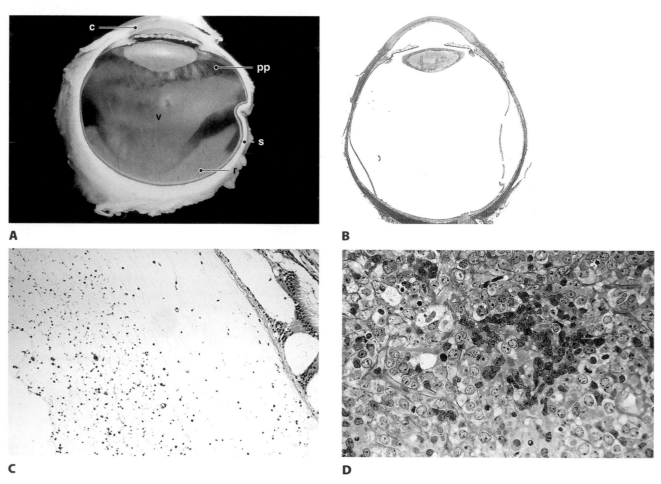

A
B
C
D

Fig. 9.22 Non-Hodgkin's lymphoma of the central nervous system ("reticulum cell sarcoma"). Patient treated for postoperative uveitis of both eyes for over 12 months until central nervous system symptoms developed. **A,** The gross specimen shows a cloudy and prominent vitreous and a partial posterior vitreous detachment (c, cornea; pp, pars plana ciliary body; v, vitreous; s, sclera; r, retina). **B,** The vitreous is partially detached posteriorly and contains many cells (acid mucopolysaccharide stain). **C,** Increased magnification shows non-Hodgkin's malignant lymphoma cells in vitreous. **D,** Plastic-embedded thin section of brain biopsy shows infiltration with non-Hodgkin's malignant lymphoma cells. Malignant cells found only in brain and in vitreous of both eyes; no other tissues (including retina) involved. (Case contributed by Dr. EK Rahn; presented by Dr. M Yanoff at the meeting of the Verhoeff Society, 1974).

b. The neoplasm probably arises in the brain and eye as a result of multicentric origin rather than by metastasis.

> NHL-CNS is composed completely of B lymphocytes 70% of the time, T lymphocytes, 20%, and true histiocytes, less than 10%. When the neoplasm arises multicentrically in subretinal pigment epithelial space, it produces multiple, large, solid detachments of RPE that are characteristic.

   2. Systemic spread outside the CNS and eyes is found in only 7.5% of autopsies.

B. Systemic non-Hodgkin's lymphoma
   1. Systemic non-Hodgkin's lymphoma almost always arises outside the CNS.
   2. Ocular involvement occurs through invasion of choroidal circulation and spreads to the choroid.
   3. Patients who have systemic non-Hodgkin's lymphoma (as well as Hodgkin's lymphoma) often have concurrent signs and symptoms of a systemic lymphoma at the time of ocular involvement and pose less of a diagnostic dilemma than NHL-CNS.
   4. Rarely, adult T-cell lymphoma/leukemia (caused by human T-lymphotropic virus type 1 infection) presents as an intraocular lymphoma.

III. Occasionally, benign lymphoid infiltration (lymphoid tumor), containing lymphocytes, plasma cells, and reticulum cells, may be seen in the uveal tract.
   A. The infiltrates are usually unilateral but may be bilateral. The infiltrates may appear as multifocal, confluent and nonconfluent, creamy choroidal patches that collect fluorescein without leakage into the subneural retinal or subretinal pigment epithelial spaces.
   B. They resemble the inflammatory pseudotumors, especially reactive lymphoid hyperplasia (see p. 574 in Chapter 14), seen in the orbit.

> Probably, uveal lymphoid infiltration (benign lymphoid hyperplasia of the uvea) is a low-grade B-cell lymphoma, which can be associated with episcleral conjunctival nodules.

Other Tumors

I. Neural
   A. Neurofibromas of the uvea occur as part of diffuse neurofibromatosis (see p. 31 in Chapter 2).
   B. Neurilemmomas (see p. 558 in Chapter 14) and glioneuromas (see p. 689 in Chapter 17) are exceedingly rare tumors of the uveal tract.
II. Benign fibrous tumor is exceedingly rare.

Secondary Neoplasms

I. By direct extension:
   A. Squamous (or rarely basal) cell carcinoma of conjunctiva

   B. Malignant melanoma of conjunctiva
   C. Retinoblastoma
   D. Malignant melanoma of uvea (e.g., ciliary body melanoma extending into choroid or iris)
   E. Embryonal and adult medulloepitheliomas
   F. Glioma of optic nerve
   G. Meningioma of optic nerve sheaths

> It is extremely rare for an orbital neoplasm to invade through the sclera into the uvea or through the meninges into the optic nerve.

II. Metastatic—most common adult intraocular neoplasm (Fig. 9.23)

> Although metastatic neoplasms are often considered to be the second most common intraocular neoplasm (second to primary uveal malignant melanomas), clinical and autopsy evidence suggests that metastatic cancer is the most common intraocular neoplasm.

   A. Lung: most common metastatic lesion in men (usually occurs early in the course of the disease and may be the initial finding).

> With increased smoking among women, their frequency of lung carcinoma continues to rise rapidly and now equals the frequency in men.

   B. Breast: most common metastatic lesion in women (usually occurs late in the course of the disease and breast surgery was usually performed previously).
   C. All other primary sites are relatively uncommon as sources of intraocular metastases.
   D. Metastatic intraocular neoplasms are more common in women and are bilateral in approximately 20% to 25% of cases.

> Although metastatic choroidal tumors tend to be oval-shaped clinically, rarely they may be mushroom-shaped and simulate a choroidal melanoma

UVEAL EDEMA (UVEAL DETACHMENT; UVEAL HYDROPS)

Types

I. Uveal effusion syndrome—uveal effusion with choroidal and ciliary body detachment (spontaneous serous detachments)
   A. Uveal effusion is characterized by a slowly progressive, often bilateral neural retinal detachment that shows shifting fluid and is mainly found in middle-aged, otherwise healthy men. Also noted are dilated episcleral vessels, vitreous cells, characteristic "leopard-spot" RPE

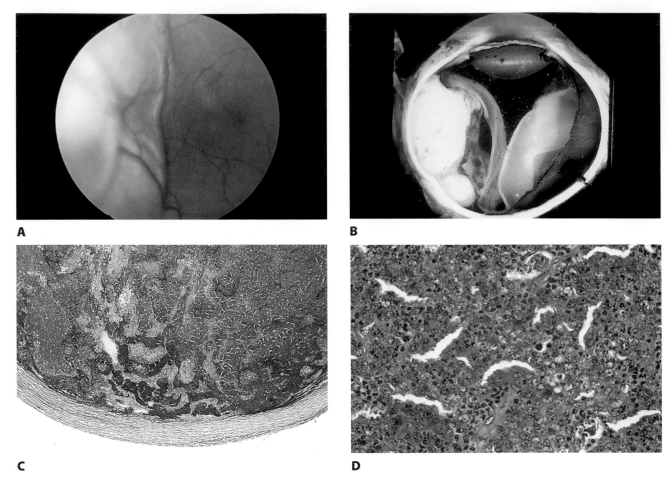

A

B

C

D

Fig. 9.23 Metastatic carcinoma. **A,** Note solid detachment thought to be malignant melanoma. **B,** Opened enucleated eye shows large choroidal tumor on left. **C,** A histologic section shows dark and light areas. The dark areas represent the cellular tumor, and the light areas represent stroma. Even under low magnification, a choroidal malignant melanoma can be ruled out because a melanoma does not have any stroma. **D,** Increased magnification shows the malignant epithelial cells, many of which demonstrate mitotic figures.

changes, and abnormal ultrasonographic and angiographic findings.

> Elevation of cerebrospinal fluid protein occurs in approximately 50% of cases. Although considered idiopathic, it may be caused by a congenital anomaly of the sclera and, in some cases, the vortex veins. The syndrome may also be found in nanophthalmic eyes and in patients who have primary pulmonary hypertension and vomiting.

B. Choroidal effusion is presumably the underlying cause and results from the thickened sclera and vortex vein anomalies.

Signs of uveitis are minimal or absent.

C. Scleral abnormalities, secondary to proteoglycan deposition in the matrix, impede transscleral fluid outflow.

D. The neural retinal detachment may reattach after months or even years, although it may remain permanently detached.

II. Posttrauma—either surgical or nonsurgical trauma

A. Hypotony and vasodilatation after penetration of the globe combine to produce transudation of fluid through uveal vessels, leading to uveal edema.

Clinically, this appears as a combined detachment of uveal tract and retina.

B. Uveal hemorrhage may occur secondary to the trauma and result in uveal detachment.

III. Vascular—malignant hypertension, eclampsia, nephritis, and other conditions that affect the ciliary vessels can lead to uveal edema.

IV. Inflammatory—any type of ocular inflammation (i.e., acute, nongranulomatous, or granulomatous, e.g., Harada's disease) can induce uveal edema.

V. Associated with malignant choroidal tumors

Choroidal detachment can occur in association with metastatic choroidal tumors or choroidal melanomas.

VI. Sequelae—in atrophic eyes with or without shrinkage, secondary to any cause, traction bands and organized scar tissue may induce uveal detachment.

BIBLIOGRAPHY

Normal Anatomy

Fine BS, Yanoff M: *Ocular Histology: A Text and Atlas*, 2nd edn. Hagerstown, Harper & Row, 1979:197–247

Fryczkowski AW, Sherman MD, Walker J: Observations on the lobular organization of the human choriocapillaris. *Int Ophthalmol* 15:109, 1991

Guymer RH, Bird AC, Hageman GS: Cytoarchitecture of choroidal capillary endothelial cells. *Invest Ophthalmol Vis Sci* 45:1796, 2004

Yanoff M, Fine BS: *Ocular Pathology: A Color Atlas*, 2nd edn. New York, Gower Medical Publishing, 1992:9.1–9.3

Congenital and Developmental Defects

Azuara-Blanco A, Spaeth GL, Araujo SV et al.: Plateau iris syndrome associated with multiple ciliary body cysts. *Arch Ophthalmol* 114:666, 1996

Azuma N, Hotta Y, Tanaka H et al.: Missense mutations in the PAX6 gene in aniridia. *Invest Ophthalmol Vis Sci* 39:2524, 1998

Bowman Z, Peiffer RL, Bouldin TW: Pathogenesis of ciliary-body cysts associated with multiple myeloma. *Ann Ophthalmol* 20:292, 1988

Brandt JD, Casuso LA, Budenz DL: Markedly increased central corneal thickness: an unrecognized finding in congenital aniridia. *Am J Ophthalmol* 137:348, 2004

Capo H, Palmer E, Nicholson DH: Congenital cysts of the iris stroma. *Am J Ophthalmol* 116:228, 1993

Daufenbach DR, Ruttman MS, Pulido JS et al.: Chorioretinal colobomas in a pediatric population. *Ophthalmology* 105:1455, 1998

Duke-Elder S: Heterochromia. In Stewart W, ed: *System of Ophthalmology*, vol. 3, part 2. St. Louis, CV Mosby, 1964:813–818

Fine BS: Free-floating pigmented cyst in the anterior chamber. *Am J Ophthalmol* 67:493, 1969

Gupta SK, deBecker I, Tremblay F et al.: Genotype/phenotype correlations in aniridia. *Arch Ophthalmol* 126:203, 1998

Harasymowycz PJ, Papamatheakis DG, Eagle RC Jr et al.: Congenital ectropion uveae and glaucoma. *Arch Ophthalmol* 124:271, 2006

Hoepner J, Yanoff M: Spectrum of ocular anomalies in trisomy 13–15: Analysis of 13 eyes with two new findings. *Am J Ophthalmol* 74:729, 1972

Jastaneiah S, Al-Rajhi AA: Association of aniridia and dry eyes. *Ophthalmology* 112:1535, 2005

Kolin T, Murphee AL: Hyperplastic pupillary membrane. *Am J Ophthalmol* 123:839, 1997

Kuchenbecker J, Motschmann M, Schmitz C et al.: Laser iridectomy for bilateral acute angle-closure glaucoma secondary to iris cysts. *Am J Ophthalmol* 129:390, 2000

Kunimatsu S, Araie M, Ohara K et al.: Ultrasound biomicroscopy of ciliary body cysts. *Am J Ophthalmol* 127:48, 1999

Lee S-T, Nicholls RD, Bundey S et al.: Mutations of the P gene in oculocutaneous albinism, and Prader–Willi syndrome plus albinism. *N Engl J Med* 330:529, 1994

Lois N, Shields CL, Shields JA et al.: Primary iris stromal cysts: A report of 17 cases. *Ophthalmology* 105:1317, 1998

Marsham WE, Lyons CJ, Young DW et al.: Simple choristoma of the anterior segment containing brain tissue. *Arch Ophthalmol* 115:1198, 1997

Nishida K, Kinoshita S, Ohashi Y et al.: Ocular surface abnormalities in aniridia. *Am J Ophthalmol* 120:368, 1995

Onwochei BC, Simon JW, Bateman JB et al.: Ocular colobomata. *Surv Ophthalmol* 45:175, 2000

Rosenthal G, Klemperer I, Zirkin H et al.: Congenital cysts of the iris stroma. *Arch Ophthalmol* 116:1696, 1998

Rowley SA, Wojciech SS: Lacrimal gland choristoma of the ciliary body. *Ophthalmology* 115:1480, 1997

Rummelt V, Rummelt C, Naumann GOH: Congenital nonpigmented epithelial iris cyst after amniocentesis. *Ophthalmology* 100:776, 1993

Scheie HG, Yanoff M: Peters' anomaly and total posterior coloboma of retinal pigment epithelium and choroid. *Arch Ophthalmol* 87:525, 1972

Scheie HG, Yanoff M: Iris nevus (Cogan–Reese) syndrome: A cause of unilateral glaucoma. *Arch Ophthalmol* 93:963, 1975

Sharpe RW, Bethel KJ, Keefe KS et al.: Choroidal hematopoiesis in an adult. *Arch Ophthalmol* 114:1421, 1996

Shields JA, Eagle RC Jr, Shields CL et al.: Natural course and histopathologic findings of lacrimal gland choristoma of the iris and ciliary body. *Am J Ophthalmol* 119:219, 1995

Shields JA, Hogan RN, Shields CL et al.: Intraocular lacrimal gland choristoma involving iris and ciliary body. *Am J Ophthalmol* 129:673, 2000

Sidoti PA, Valencia M, Chen N et al.: Echographic evaluation of primary cysts of the iris pigment epithelium. *Am J Ophthalmol* 120:161, 1995

Thompson WS, Curtin VT: Congenital bilateral heterochromia of the choroid and iris. *Arch Ophthalmol* 112:1247, 1994

Yanoff M, Zimmerman LE: Pseudomelanoma of anterior chamber caused by implantation of iris pigment epithelium. *Arch Ophthalmol* 74:302, 1965

Systemic Diseases

Almanaseer IY, Kosova L, Pellettiere EV: Composite lymphoma with immunoblastic features and Langerhans' cell granulomatosis (histiocytosis X). *Am J Clin Pathol* 85:111, 1986

Ashmore ED, Wilson MW, Morris WR et al.: Corneal juvenile xanthogranuloma in a 4-month-old child. *Arch Ophthalmol* 121:117, 2003

Chaudhry IA, Al-Jishi Z, Shamsi FA et al.: Juvenile xanthogranuloma of the corneoscleral limbus: report and review of the literature. *Surv Ophthalmol* 49:608, 2004

DeStafeno JJ, Carlson A, Myer DR: Solitary spindle-cell xanthogranuloma of the eye lid. *Ophthalmology* 109:258, 2002

Jabs DA, Hanneken AM, Schachat AP et al.: Choroidopathy in systemic lupus erythematosus. *Arch Ophthalmol* 106:230, 1988

Mittleman D, Apple DJ, Goldberg MF: Ocular involvement in Letterer–Siwe disease. *Am J Ophthalmol* 75:261, 1973

Mohamed SR, Matthews N, Calcgni A: Juvenile xanthogranuloma of the limbus in an adult. *Arch Ophthalmol* 120:976, 2002

O'Keefe JS, Sippy BD, Martin DF et al.: Anterior chamber infiltrates associated with systemic lymphoma. Report of two cases and review of the literature. *Ophthalmology* 109:253, 2002

Saxena T, Kumar K, Sen S et al.: Langerhans cell histiocytosis presenting as a limbal nodule in an adult patient. *Am J Ophthalmol* 138:508, 2004

Yanoff M, Perry HD: Juvenile xanthogranuloma of the corneoscleral limbus. *Arch Ophthalmol* 113:915, 1995

Zamir E, Wang RC, Krishnakumar S et al.: Juvenile xanthogranuloma masquerading as pediatric chronic uveitis: A clinicopathologic study. *Surv Ophthalmol* 46:164, 2001

Zimmerman LE: Ocular lesions of juvenile xanthogranuloma: Nevoxanthoendothelioma. *Trans Am Acad Ophthalmol Otolaryngol* 69:412, 1965

Atrophies and Degenerations

Cameron JD, Yanoff M, Frayer WC: Coats' disease and Turner's syndrome. *Am J Ophthalmol* 78:852, 1974

Friberg TR, Grove AS Jr: Choroidal folds and refractive errors associated with orbital tumors: An analysis. *Arch Ophthalmol* 101:598, 1983

John T, Sassani JW, Eagle RC: Scanning electron microscopy of rubeosis iridis. *Trans Pa Acad Ophthalmol Otolaryngol* 35:119, 1982

John T, Sassani JW, Eagle RC: The myofibroblastic component of rubeosis iridis. *Ophthalmology* 90:721, 1983

Patz A: Clinical and experimental studies on retinal neovascularization. *Am J Ophthalmol* 94:715, 1982

Dystrophies

Cameron JD, Fine BS, Shapiro I: Histopathologic observations in choroideremia with emphasis on vascular changes of the uveal tract. *Ophthalmology* 94:187, 1987

Cremers FPM, Armstrong SA, Seabra MC *et al.*: REP-2, a RAB escort protein encoded by the choroideremia-like gene. *J Biol Chem* 269:2111, 1994

Ferry AP, Llovera I, Shafer DM: Central areolar choroidal dystrophy. *Arch Ophthalmol* 88:39, 1972

Flannery JG, Bird AC, Farber DB *et al.*: A histopathologic study of a choroideremia carrier. *Invest Ophthalmol Vis Sci* 31:229, 1990

Godley BF, Tiffin PAC, Evans K *et al.*: Clinical features of progressive bifocal chorioretinal atrophy: A retinal dystrophy linked to chromosome 6q. *Ophthalmology* 103:893, 1996

Gupta V, Gupta A, Arora S *et al.*: Presumed tubercular serpiginous choroiditis: clinical presentations and management. *Ophthalmology* 110:1744, 2003

Hardy RA, Schatz H: Macular geographic helicoid choroidopathy. *Arch Ophthalmol* 105:1237, 1987

Hotta Y, Inana G: Gene transfer and expression of human ornithine aminotransferase. *Invest Ophthalmol Vis Sci* 30:1024, 1989

Hoyng CB, Heutink P, Tester L *et al.*: Autosomal dominant central areolar choroidal dystrophy caused by a mutation in codon 142 in the peripherin/RDS gene. *Am J Ophthalmol* 121:623, 1996

Kaiser-Kupfer MI, Caruso RC, Valle D: Gyrate atrophy of the choroid and retina: Further experience with long-term reduction of ornithine levels in children. *Arch Ophthalmol* 120:146, 2002

Krill AE, Archer D: Classification of the choroidal atrophies. *Am J Ophthalmol* 72:562, 1971

Mashima Y, Shiono T, Inana G: Rapid and efficient molecular analysis of gyrate atrophy using denaturing gradient gel electrophoresis. *Invest Ophthalmol Vis Sci* 35:1065, 1994

Oliveira TL, Andrade RE, Muccioli C *et al.*: Cystoid macular edema of the choroids and retina: a fluorescein angiography and coherence tomography evaluation. *Am J Ophthalmol* 140:147, 2005

Pearlman JT, Heckenlively JR, Bastek JV: Progressive nature of pigment paravenous retinochoroidal atrophy. *Am J Ophthalmol* 85:215, 1978

Peltola KE, Jaaskelainen S, Heinonen OJ *et al.*: Peripheral nervous system in gyrate atrophy of the choroids and retina with hyperornithinemia. *Neurology* 59:735, 2992

Potter MJ, Wong E, Szabo SM *et al.*: Clinical findings in a carrier of a new mutation in the choroideremia gene. *Ophthalmology* 111:1905, 2004

Renner AB, Kellner U, Cropp E *et al.*: Choroideremia: variability of clinical and electrophysiological characteristics and first report of a negative electrortinogram. *Ophthalmology* 113:2066, 2006

Seabra MC, Brown MS, Goldstein JL: Retinal degeneration in choroideremia: Deficiency of Rab geranylgeranyl transferase. *Science* 259:377, 1993

Weiter J, Fine BS: A histologic study of regional choroidal dystrophy. *Am J Ophthalmol* 83:741, 1977

Wilson DJ, Weleber RG, Green WR: Ocular clinicopathologic study of gyrate atrophy. *Am J Ophthalmol* 111:24, 1991

Wu JS, Lewis H, Fine SL *et al.*: Clinicopathologic findings in a patient with serpiginous choroiditis and treated choroidal neovascularization. *Retina* 9:292, 1989

Tumors

Akpek EK, Ahmed I, Hochberg FH *et al.*: Intraocular-central nervous system lymphoma: Clinical features, diagnosis, and outcome. *Ophthalmology* 106:1805, 1999

Aylward GW, Chang TS, Pautler SE *et al.*: A long-term follow-up of choroidal osteoma. *Arch Ophthalmol* 116:1337, 1998

Bardenstein DS, Char DH, Jones C *et al.*: Metastatic ciliary body carcinoid tumor. *Arch Ophthalmol* 108:1590, 1990

Biswas J, Kumar SK, Gopal L *et al.*: Leiomyoma of the ciliary body extending to the anterior chamber: Clinicopathologic and ultrasound biomicroscopic correlation. *Surv Ophthalmol* 44:336, 2000

Bowman CB, Guber D, Brown CH III *et al.*: Cutaneous malignant melanoma with diffuse intraocular metastases. *Arch Ophthalmol* 112:1213, 1994

Britt JM, Karr DJ, Kalina RE: Leukemic iris infiltration in recurrent acute leukemia. *Arch Ophthalmol* 109:1456, 1991

Brown HH, Brodsky MC, Hembree K *et al.*: Supraciliary hemangiopericytoma. *Ophthalmology* 98:378, 1991

Brown HH, Glasgow BJ, Foos RY: Ultrastructural and immunohistochemical features of coronal adenomas. *Am J Ophthalmol* 112:34, 1991

Browning DJ: Choroidal osteoma: observations from a community setting. *Ophthalmology* 110:1327, 2003

Buettner H: Spontaneous involution of a choroidal osteoma. *Arch Ophthalmol* 108:1517, 1990

Campbell RJ, Min K-W, Zolling JP: Skenoid fibers in mesectodermal leiomyoma of the ciliary body. *Ultrastruct Pathol* 21:559, 1997

Chan C-C, Whitcup SM, Solomon D *et al.*: Interleukin-10 in the vitreous of patients with primary intraocular lymphoma. *Am J Ophthalmol* 120:671, 1995

Cheung MK, Martin DF, Chan C-C *et al.*: Diagnosis of reactive lymphoid hyperplasia by chorioretinal biopsy. *Am J Ophthalmol* 118:457, 1994

Cochereau I, Hannouche D, Geoffray C *et al.*: Ocular involvement in Epstein–Barr virus-associated T-cell lymphoma. *Am J Ophthalmol* 121:322, 1996

Cockerham GC, Hidayat AA, Bijwaard KE *et al.*: Re-evaluation of "reactive lymphoid hyperplasia of the uvea": An immunohistochemical and molecular analysis of ten cases. *Ophthalmology* 107:151, 2000

Croxatto JO, D'Alessandro C, Lombardi A: Benign fibrous tumor of the choroid. *Arch Ophthalmol* 107:1793, 1989

Cursiefen C, Holbach LM, Lafant B *et al.*: Oculocerebral non-Hodgkin's lymphoma with uveal involvement. *Arch Ophthalmol* 118:1437, 2000

Del Canizo C, San Miguel JF, Gonzalez M *et al.*: Discrepancies between morphologic, cytochemical, and immunologic characteristics in acute myeloblastic leukemia. *Am J Clin Pathol* 88:38, 1987

DePotter P, Shields JA, Shields CL *et al.*: Magnetic resonance imaging in choroidal osteoma. *Retina* 11:221, 1991

De Rivas P, Marti T, Andreu D *et al.*: Metastatic bronchogenic carcinoma of the iris and ciliary body. *Arch Ophthalmol* 109:470, 1991

Edelstein C, Burnier MN Jr, Gomolin J *et al.*: Choroidal metastasis as the first manifestation of lung cancer. *Ophthalmic Pract* 15:37, 1997

Elsas FJ, Mroczek EC, Kelly DR *et al.*: Primary rhabdomyosarcoma of the iris. *Arch Ophthalmol* 109:982, 1991

El-Zayaty S, Schneider S, Mutema GK *et al.*: Prostatic adenocarcinoma metastatic to the anterior uveal tract. *Arch Ophthalmol* 121:276, 2003

Endo EG, Walton DS, Albert DM: Neonatal hepatoblastoma metastatic to the choroid and iris. *Arch Ophthalmol* 114:757, 1996

Eting E, Savir H: An atypical fulminant course of choroidal osteoma in two siblings. *Am J Ophthalmol* 113:52, 1992

Fan JT, Buettner H, Bartley GB et al.: Clinical features and treatment of seven patients with carcinoid tumor metastatic to the eye and orbit. *Am J Ophthalmol* 119:211, 1995

Finger PT, Warren FA, Gelman YP et al.: Adult Wilms' tumor metastatic to the choroids of the eye. *Ophthalmology* 109:2134, 2002

Foos AJE, Pecorella I, Alexander RA et al.: Are most intraocular "leiomyomas" really melanocytic lesions? *Ophthalmology* 101:919, 1994

George DP, Zamber RW: Chondrosarcoma metastatic to the eye. *Arch Ophthalmol* 114:349, 1996

Gieser SC, Hufnagel TJ, Jaros PA et al.: Hemangiopericytoma of the ciliary body. *Arch Ophthalmol* 106:1269, 1988

Gill MK, Jampol LM: Variations in the presentation of primary intraocular lymphoma: case reports and a review. *Surv Ophthalmol* 45:463, 2001

Grossniklaus HE, Martin DF, Avery R et al.: Uveal lymphoid infiltration: Report of four cases and clinicopathologic review. *Ophthalmology* 105:1265, 1998

Haimovici R, Gragoudas ES, Gregor Z et al.: Choroidal metastases from renal cell carcinoma. *Ophthalmology* 104:1152, 1997

Harbour JW, De Potter P, Shields CL et al.: Uveal metastasis from carcinoid tumor: Clinical observations in nine cases. *Ophthalmology* 101:1084, 1994

Kida Y, Shibuya Y, Oguni M et al.: Choroidal osteoma in an infant. *Am J Ophthalmol* 124:118, 1997

Larson SA, Oetting TA: Presumed iris hemangioma associated with multiple central nervous system cavernous hemangiomas. *Arch Ophthalmol* 120:984, 2002

Leonardy NJ, Rupani M, Dent G et al.: Analysis of 135 autopsy eyes for ocular involvement in leukemia. *Am J Ophthalmol* 109:436, 1990

Mizota A, Tanabe R, Adachi-Usami E: Rapid enlargement of choroidal osteoma in a 3-year-old girl. *Arch Ophthalmol* 116:1128, 1998

Mochizuki M, Watanabe T, Yamaguchi K et al.: Uveitis associated with human T-cell lymphotropic virus type 1. *Am J Ophthalmol* 114:123, 1992

Naumann G, Ruprecht KW: Xanthoma der Iris: Ein klinischpathologischer Befundbericht. *Ophthalmologica* 164:293, 1972

Naumann G, Font RL, Zimmerman LE: Electron microscopic verification of primary rhabdomyosarcoma of the iris. *Am J Ophthalmol* 74:110, 1972

Odashiro AN, Fernandes BF, Al-Kandari A et al.: Report of two cases of ciliary body mesectodermal leiomyoma: unique expression of neural markers. *Ophthalmology* 114:157, 2007

O'Keefe JS, Sippy BD, Martin DF et al.: Anterior chamber infiltrates associated with systemic slymphoma. Report of two cases and review of the literature. *Ophthalmology* 109:253, 2002

Pavan PR, Oteiza EE, Margo CE: Ocular lymphoma diagnosed by internal subretinal pigment epithilium biopsy. *Arch Ophthalmol* 113:1233, 1995

Perri P, Paduano B, Incorvaia C et al.: Mesectodermal leiomyoma exclusively involving the posterior segment. *Am J Ophthalmol* 134:451, 2002

Peterson K, Gordon KB, Heinemann M et al.: The clinical spectrum of ocular lymphoma. *Cancer* 72:843, 1993

Rao NA: HTLV-1 and intraocular lymphoma. Presented at the meeting of the Verhoeff Society, 1993

Read RW, Green RL, Rao NA: Metastatic adenocarcinoma with rupture through the Bruch membrane simulating a choroidal melanoma. *Am J Ophthalmol* 132:943, 2001

Rubenstein RA, Yanoff M, Albert DM: Thrombocytopenia, anemia, and retinal hemorrhage. *Am J Ophthalmol* 65:435, 1968

Schachat AP, Markowitz JA, Guyer DR et al.: Ophthalmic manifestations of leukemia. *Arch Ophthalmol* 107:697, 1989

Schlötzer-Schrehardt U, Jünemann A, Naumann GOH: Mitochondria-rich epithelioid leiomyoma of the ciliary body. *Arch Ophthalmol* 120:77, 2002

Shields CL, Honavar SG, Shields JA et al.: Circumscribed choroidal hemangioma. Clinical manifestations and factors predictive of visual outcome in 200 consecutive patients. *Ophthalmology* 108:2237, 2001

Shields CL, Shields JA, Gross NE et al.: Survey of 520 eyes with uveal metastases. *Ophthalmology* 104:1265, 1997

Shields CL, Shields JA, Varenhorst MP: Transscleral leiomyoma. *Ophthalmology* 98:84, 1991

Shields CL, Sun H, Demirci H et al.: Factors predictive of tumor growth, tumor decalcification, choroidal neovascularization, and visual outcome in 74 eyes with choroidal osteoma. *Arch Ophthalmol* 123:1658, 2005

Shields JA, Shields CA, Eagle RC et al.: Observations on seven cases of intraocular leiomyoma. *Arch Ophthalmol* 112:521, 1994

Shields JA, Shields CL, de Potter P et al.: Progressive enlargement of a choroidal osteoma. *Arch Ophthalmol* 113:819, 1995

Shields JA, Shields CL, Kiratli H et al.: Metastatic tumors to the iris in 40 patients. *Am J Ophthalmol* 119:422, 1995

Shields JA, Stephens RF, Eagle RC et al.: Progressive enlargement of a circumscribed choroidal hemangioma. *Arch Ophthalmol* 110:1276, 1992

Shields JA, Streicher TF, Spirkova JHJ et al.: Arteriovenous malformation of the iris in 14 cases. *Arch Ophthalmol* 124:370, 2006

Velez G, de Smit MD, Whitcup SM et al.: Iris involvement in primary intraocular lymphoma: Report of two cases and review of the literature. *Surv Ophthalmol* 44:518, 2000

Weisenthal R, Brucker A, Lanciano R: Follicular thyroid cancer metastatic to the iris. *Arch Ophthalmol* 107:494, 1989

Whitcup S, de Smet MD, Rubin BI et al.: Intraocular lymphoma. *Ophthalmology* 100:1399, 1993

Wilson DJ, Braziel R, Rosenbaum JT: Intraocular lymphoma. *Arch Ophthalmol* 110:1455, 1992

Yaghouti F, Nouri M, Mannor GE: Ocular adnexal granulocytic sarcoma as the first sign of acute myelogenous leukemia relapse. *Am J Ophthalmol* 127:361, 1999

Yahalom C, Cohen Y, Averbukh E et al.: Bilateral iridociliary T-cell lymphoma. *Arch Ophthalmol* 120:204, 2002

Yanoff M: In discussion of Robb RM, Ervin L, Sallan SE: A pathological study of eye involvement in acute leukemia of childhood. *Trans Am Ophthalmol Soc* 76:100, 1978

Zaidman GW, Johnson BL, Salamon SM et al.: Fuchs' adenoma affecting the peripheral iris. *Arch Ophthalmol* 101:771, 1983

Zaldivar RA, Martin DF, Holden JT et al.: Primary intraocular lymphoma: clinical, and flow ctometric analysis. . *Ophthalmology* 111:1762, 2004

Zimmerman LE: Verhoeff's "terato-neuroma": A critical reappraisal in light of new observations and current concepts of embryonic tumors. *Am J Ophthalmol* 72:1039, 1971

Uveal Edema

Akduman L, Del Priore LV, Kaplan HJ et al.: Uveal effusion syndrome associated with primary pulmonary hypertension and vomiting. *Am J Ophthalmol* 121:578, 1996

Sneed SR, Byrne SF, Mieler WF et al.: Choroidal detachment associated with malignant choroidal tumors. *Ophthalmology* 98:963, 1991

Uyama M, Takahashi K, Kozalki J et al.: Uveal effusion syndrome: Clinical features, surgical treatment, histologic examination of the sclera, and pathophysiology. *Ophthalmology* 107:441, 2000

Yamani A, Wood I, Sugino I et al.: Abnormal collagen fibrils in nanophthalmos: A clinical and histologic study. *Am J Ophthalmol* 127:106, 1999

10

Lens

NORMAL ANATOMY

I. The lens (Fig. 10.1) is a transparent biconvex disc.
   A. The anterior surface of the lens has a radius of curvature greater than that of the posterior surface.
   B. The thickness (anterior to posterior) of the lens is approximately 3.5 to 4 mm at birth and approximately 4.5 to 5 mm after 65 years of age.
   C. The equatorial diameter is about 6 to 6.5 mm at birth and 9 to 9.5 mm after 65 years of age.

> The diameter of the "empty" capsular bag, therefore, is slightly less than 10 mm.

II. The lens is not only transparent but it has an inverted surface epithelium that grows inward at the equator.
   A. New cells are formed constantly during life and are laid down externally to the older cells.
   B. Because the thick epithelial basement membrane (the lens capsule—the thickest basement membrane in the body) completely encloses the lens, the epithelial cells are unable to desquamate or shed, as does corneal or skin epithelium.
   C. The proliferating, elongating lens cells become inwardly compacted with advancing age. The compaction is often accompanied by the formation of an intracellular yellow pigment of varying density.

> On the one hand, accumulating yellow pigment together with increasing cellular compaction decreases the transmission of light and so decreases vision; on the other hand, the same aging changes filter out ultraviolet (UV) light preferentially, which may help protect the foveomacular region of the neural retina from light damage.

   D. Normally, no blood vessels or nerves are present in or attached to the lens.

GENERAL INFORMATION

I. A clinically significant opacity of the lens is called a *cataract*.
II. Cataractous lenses cause light scattering and transmit only a fraction of light at all wavelengths.
III. Cataracts do not cause an afferent pupillary defect.
IV. Risk factors for development of a cataract include heredity, age, diabetes, oral or inhaled steroid therapy, exposure to UV-B radiation, poor nutrition, cigarette smoking, iris color (nuclear cataracts are more likely to develop in eyes with a dark brown iris), and high serum levels of the antioxidant enzymes plasma glutathione peroxidase and erythrocyte superoxide dismutase.
V. Increased intake of protein, vitamin A, niacin, and riboflavin may reduce the risk of nuclear cataract.

CONGENITAL ANOMALIES

Introduction

I. Congenital anomalies of the lens are usually associated with other ocular anomalies.
II. Such entities as coloboma of the lens, spherophakia, and congenital dislocation of the lens may be related to problems of zonular development rather than lenticular development.

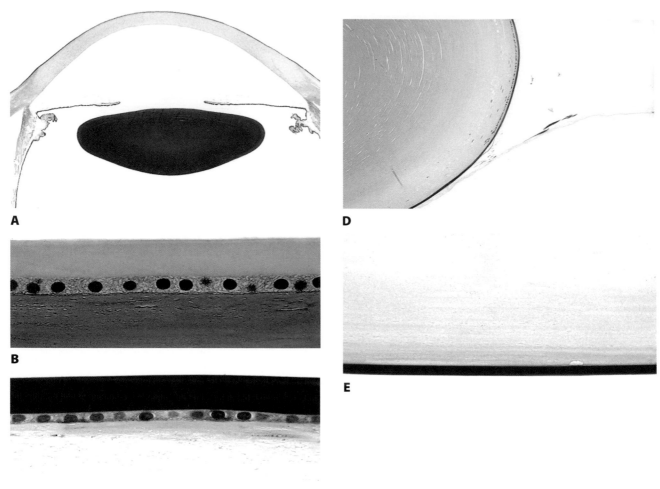

Fig. 10.1 Normal adult lens. **A,** A low-power view shows the biconvex shape of the lens. The anterior lens is less sharply convex than the posterior lens. **B,** The single-layer, anterior, cuboidal, inverted lens epithelium secretes the overlying thick basement membrane, the lens capsule. **C,** The lens capsule is seen better with periodic acid–Schiff (PAS) stain. **D,** The epithelium ends in the lens bow at the equator. The lens cortex and nucleus are composed of layers of lens cells ("fibers") that become more compressed as they move inward. **E,** Posteriorly, no epithelium is present and the lens capsule (stained with PAS), therefore, remains thinner than anteriorly. (**A** and **D,** Courtesy of Dr. MG Farber; **B, C** and **E,** courtesy of Dr. RC Eagle, Jr.)

A true coloboma of the lens probably does not exist. A coloboma of the zonules results in a deformed equator of the lens, simulating a lens coloboma.

Mittendorf's Dot

See p. 481 and Fig. 12.2 in Chapter 12.

Congenital Aphakia

I. Congenital aphakia, a rare anomaly, exists in two forms:
   A. Primary congenital aphakia, in which no lens anlage has developed
   B. Secondary congenital aphakia, in which a lens has developed to some degree but has been resorbed or has been extruded, as through a corneal perforation before or during birth

II. Histologically, primary congenital aphakia is characterized by an absent lens and aplasia of the anterior segment.

Findings in the secondary form depend on the underlying cause.

Congenital Duplication of Lens

I. True duplication of the lens with separate capsules is rare.
II. Associated facial and ocular anomalies (e.g., coloboma of the iris, cornea plana, and hourglass cornea) may be found.

Fleck Cataract

I. Fleck cataract consists of multiple, stationary, tiny anterior subcapsular or anterior and posterior cortical flecks, often associated with adhesions of persistent pupillary membranes.

The flecks tend to occur in the anterior and posterior cortex, are blue instead of white, and are called *cerulean flecks*.

II. Frequently, pigment cells are present on the anterior surface of the lens capsule in the pupillary area at the site of attachment of the pupillary membrane overlying the opacity.

All degrees of changes can be seen (especially with the slit lamp): sometimes only the blue flecks; other times only the membrane adhesions or the pigment cells; or any combination.

III. Most rarely, the same type of fleck cataract can occur in the posterior subcapsular area associated with remnants of the hyaloid vessels or the posterior tunica vasculosa lentis.

Anterior Polar Cataract

I. Anterior polar cataracts (Fig. 10.2) constitute approximately 3% of congenital cataracts.
II. Clinically and histologically, it appears similar to an acquired anterior subcapsular cataract.
III. The cataract is almost always stationary.

Rarely, congenital anterior polar cataract may be secondary to intrauterine keratitis. The capsule of the lens may become adherent to the inflamed cornea, causing lens traction during fetal development. The traction may distort the lens by drawing its axial area out to form an *anterior pyramidal cataract*. Even more rarely, spontaneous anterior capsular rupture may occur.

IV. Often the cause of the cataract is unknown, although occasionally it may be inherited as an autosomal-dominant, autosomal-recessive, or X-linked trait, or may be associated with a reciprocal translocation between chromosomes 2 and 14.
In an autosomal-dominant variant, anterior polar cataract is associated with cornea guttata.

Posterior Polar Cataract

I. Clinically and histologically, a posterior polar cataract appears similar to an acquired posterior subcapsular cataract (PSC: Fig. 10.3; see Fig. 10.2).
II. The cataract, rarer than its anterior counterpart, is usually stationary but may be progressive when associated with persistent hyperplastic primary vitreous (see p. 747 in Chapter 18). When this occurs, a dehiscence in the lens capsule may be seen posteriorly, with fibrovascular tissue within the posterior lens substance.

Anterior Lenticonus (Lentiglobus)

I. The anterior surface of the lens can assume an abnormal conical (lenticonus) or spherical (lentiglobus) shape.

More than 90% of cases of bilateral anterior lenticonus are associated with Alport's syndrome.

II. Either condition predominates in boys, is usually present as the only ocular anomaly, and is usually bilateral.
III. Clinically, an "oil globule" reflex is seen in the pupillary area of the lens.

A similar oil globule reflex may be seen in posterior lenticonus (see later), keratoconus, and, most commonly, nuclear cataract.

IV. The cause is unknown, except rarely it may be inherited as an autosomal-recessive trait.

Anterior lenticonus has been reported in *familial hemorrhagic nephritis* (*Alport's syndrome*). Alport's syndrome is probably inherited as an autosomal-dominant trait, with incomplete penetrance and varying expressivity of the mutant gene. The syndrome shows kidney disease (mild in women and severe in men), perceptive deafness, and ocular lesions. It is much more severe in men, who usually die before 40 years of age. Ocular lesions in addition to anterior lenticonus include spherophakia, anterior polar cataract, anterior lenticonus, posterior cortical cataract, rubeosis iridis, and fundus lesions such as drusen, retinal flecks (macular and mid-periphery) similar to fundus albipunctatus, degeneration of macular pigment epithelium, and retinal neovascularization.

V. Histologically, thinning of the anterior lens capsule, a decreased number of anterior lens epithelial cells, and bulging of the anterior cortex are seen.

Posterior Lenticonus (Lentiglobus)

I. Posterior lenticonus (see Fig. 18.23), more properly called *lentiglobus*, the lenticular abnormality associated with the most common form of unilateral developmental cataract in normal-sized eyes, consists of a spherical elevation or ridge on the posterior surface of the lens and is more common than its anterior counterpart.
II. The condition predominates in girls, occurs sporadically, is usually present as the only ocular anomaly, and is usually, but not always, unilateral.

Sometimes, posterior lenticonus is associated with other congenital anomalies such as microphthalmos, microcornea, iris and retinal pigment epithelial colobomas, anterior-chamber angle anomalies, hyaloid system remnants, axial myopia, and skull deformities.

III. Clinically, an oil globule-like reflex is seen in the pupillary area of the lens.
IV. The cause is unknown; the condition may occur in Lowe's syndrome (see later).
V. Histologically, the capsule is thinned in the central part posteriorly, the lens cortex bulges posteriorly, and often abnormal nuclei, resembling either lens epithelium or pig-

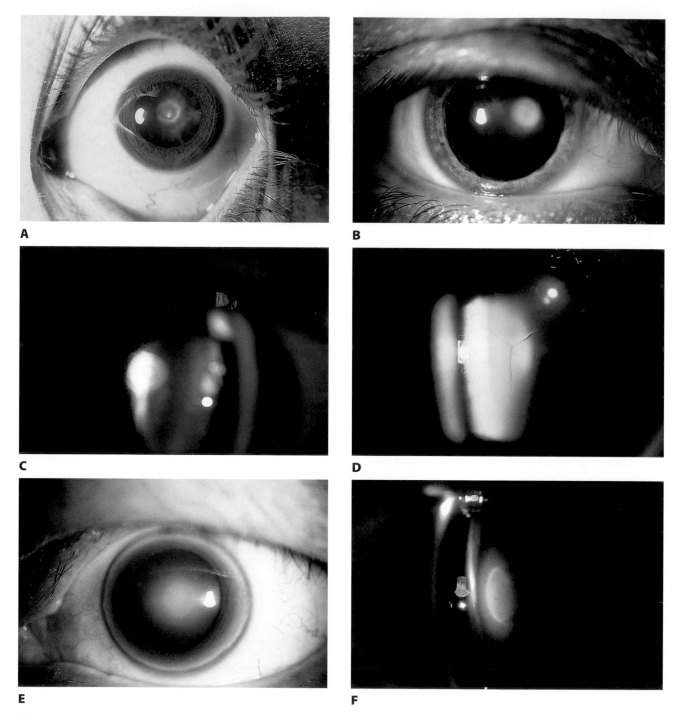

Fig. 10.2 Congenital cataracts. **A,** Congenital anterior and posterior polar cataracts. **B** and **C,** Congenital posterior cataract. **D,** Congenital anterior Y suture. **E** and **F,** Congenital nuclear cataract.

mented and nonpigmented ciliary epithelium, can be seen in the area of the anomaly.

A bulging or umbilicated posterior polar lens abnormality is frequently encountered in enucleated infant eyes. The abnormality is due to a fixation artifact.

Other Congenital Cataracts

I. Autosomal-dominant congenital cataract (ADCC)

Although dominant and recessive autosomal- and X-linked recessive types of congenital cataracts have been described, most

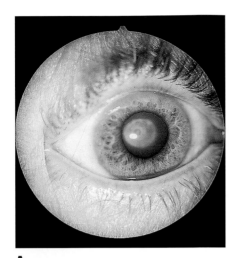

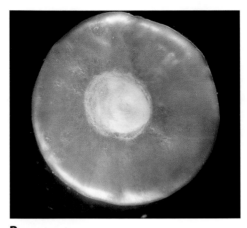

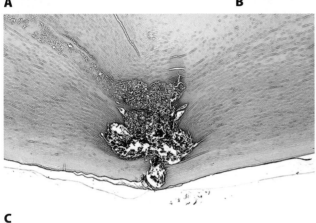

Fig. 10.3 Congenital posterior polar cataract. **A,** Patient had congenital posterior polar cataract. **B,** Gross specimen. **C,** Photomicrograph of another congenital posterior polar cataract shows degeneration of the posterior subcapsular cortex.

familial cataracts are inherited in an autosomal-dominant fashion. At least 15 loci have been reported for various primary forms of ADCC, including on chromosomes 3, 12, and 17.

    A. ADCC is usually bilaterally symmetric but may be unilateral.

    B. The lens opacity may be zonular, fetal nuclear pulverulent, nuclear, or sutural (or any combination; see Fig. 10.2).

  II. Congenital cataracts such as *zonular*, *sutural*, *axial*, *membranous*, and *filiform* types have nonspecific histologic changes.

 III. Cataracts secondary to intrauterine infection

    A. Anterior subcapsular cataract (see p. 373 in this chapter)

    B. PSC (see p. 373 in this chapter)

    C. Rubella cataract (see Fig. 2.12)

 IV. Galactosemia cataract (see p. 381 in this chapter)

  V. Transient neonatal lens vacuoles (Fig. 10.4)

    A. Bilateral, symmetric lens vacuoles are situated predominantly in the posterior cortex near the Y suture close to the lens capsule.

    B. The vacuoles, seen mainly in premature infants, are not present at birth, appear between the 8th and 14th days, and persist for approximately 2 weeks, but may remain up to 9 months before disappearing completely.

    C. Histologically, swelling of lens cortical cells in several lamellae of both anterior and posterior (mainly) cortex is seen.

      1. Large, "watery" cortical vacuoles with a nonstaining content are found.

      2. Lipoidal degenerative products are also seen in the involved areas.

If the vacuoles do not disappear and become exaggerated, they may be responsible for zonular cataracts. The lipoidal degenerative products may cause the punctate opacities seen clinically.

CAPSULE (EPITHELIAL BASEMENT MEMBRANE)

General Reactions

    I. The lens capsule, which is the thickest basement membrane in the body, is elastic, easily molded, and resists rupture (Fig. 10.5). It is impermeable to the passage of particulate matter (e.g., bacteria and inflammatory cells).

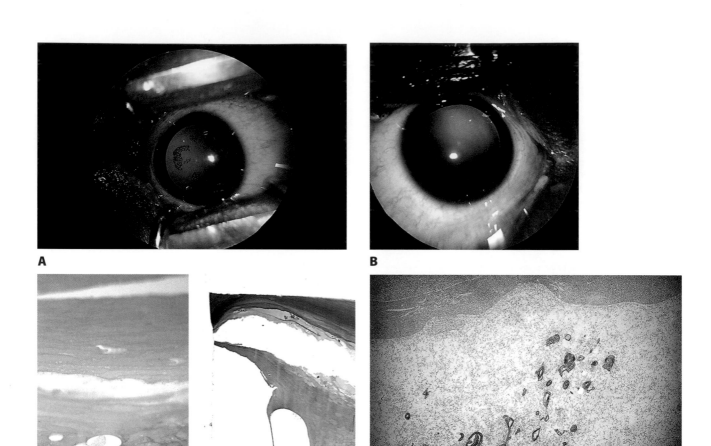

A

B

C

D

E

Fig. 10.4 Transient neonatal lens vacuoles. **A,** Vacuoles in posterior lens of infant. **B,** Vacuoles have disappeared 20 days later. **C,** Periodic acid–Schiff stain shows multiloculated posterior subcapsular cortical cysts. **D,** Plastic-embedded thin section shows swollen lens cortical cells, ruptured artifactitiously, adjacent to edge of cyst. **E,** Electron micrograph shows edematous cortical cells containing dense bodies. Anteriormost cells in figure are relatively normal. (**A** and **B,** Courtesy of Dr. DB Schaffer; **C–E,** modified from Yanoff M *et al.: Am J Ophthalmol* 76:363. Copyright Elsevier 1973.)

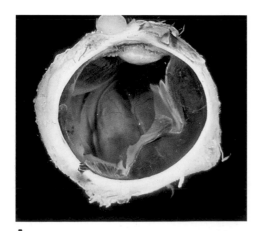

A

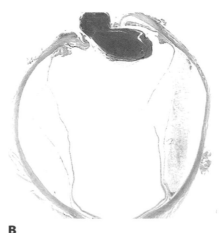

B

Fig. 10.5 Lens capsule elasticity. **A,** This patient had bullous keratopathy secondary to glaucoma. The cornea then became ulcerated and perforated, resulting in an expulsive choroidal hemorrhage. The eye was enucleated. Gross examination shows the massive choroidal hemorrhage and the lens protruding through the ruptured cornea. **B,** Histologic section demonstrates molding of the lens through the corneal opening. The lens capsule is intact.

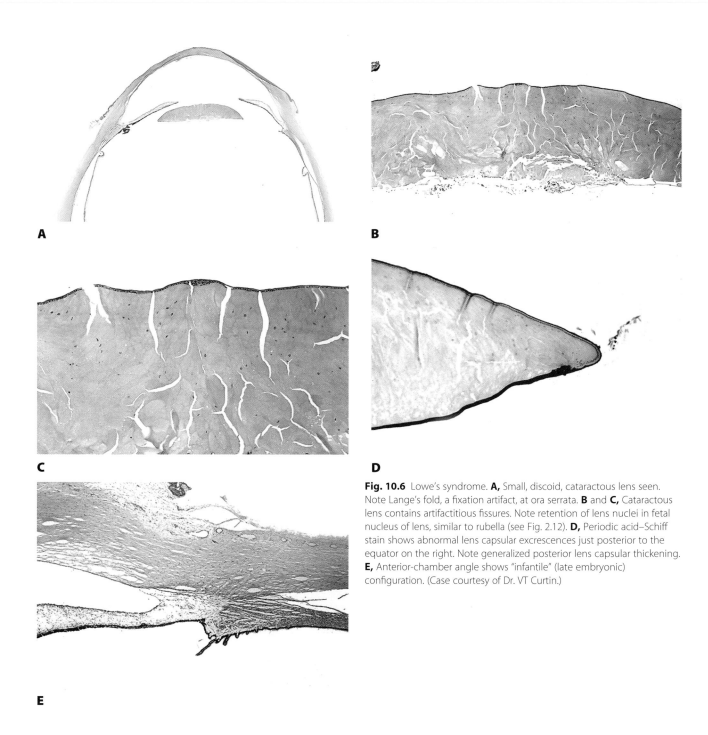

A

B

C

D

Fig. 10.6 Lowe's syndrome. **A,** Small, discoid, cataractous lens seen. Note Lange's fold, a fixation artifact, at ora serrata. **B** and **C,** Cataractous lens contains artifactitious fissures. Note retention of lens nuclei in fetal nucleus of lens, similar to rubella (see Fig. 2.12). **D,** Periodic acid–Schiff stain shows abnormal lens capsular excrescences just posterior to the equator on the right. Note generalized posterior lens capsular thickening. **E,** Anterior-chamber angle shows "infantile" (late embryonic) configuration. (Case courtesy of Dr. VT Curtin.)

E

II. The lens capsule can undergo marked thinning, as in a mature cataract, or focal thickening, as in Lowe's syndrome.

   A. Oculocerebrorenal syndrome of Lowe (Fig. 10.6)

     1. Lowe's syndrome consists of systemic acidosis, organic aciduria, decreased ability to produce ammonia in the kidneys, renal rickets, generalized hypotonia, and buphthalmos.

       a. The syndrome is transmitted as an X-linked recessive trait.

       b. The defect is in the distal long arm of the X chromosome (the *OCRL1* gene) at positions 24 to 26 (Xq24–q26).

       c. Female carriers show characteristic lens opacities—equatorial and anterior cortical clusters of smooth, off-white opacities of various sizes distributed in radial wedges.

     2. Ocular findings include congenital cataract, glaucoma, and miotic pupil.

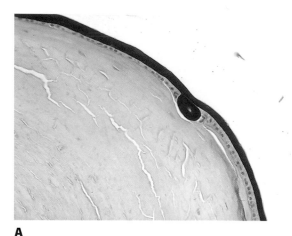

A

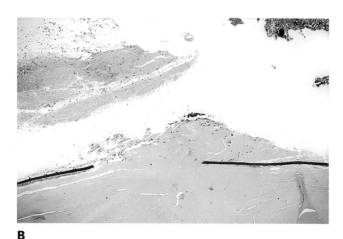

B

Fig. 10.7 Trauma. **A,** Thickened, globular capsule marks site of sealed capsular rent. **B,** Traumatically ruptured lens capsule has allowed lens cortical material to "spill out" into anterior chamber. (**A** and **B,** Periodic acid–Schiff stain.)

Most cases of genetic congenital cataract are not associated with glaucoma and, conversely, most cases of genetic congenital glaucoma are not associated with cataract. The combination of congenital cataract and congenital glaucoma, therefore, is highly suggestive of either Lowe's syndrome or congenital rubella.

   3. Histology
      a. The cataractous lens is small and discoid, frequently containing a posterior lenticonus.
      b. The fetal nucleus may show retention of lens nuclei similar to the cataract in rubella, Leigh's disease, and trisomy 13.
      c. Lens capsular excrescences, similar to those seen in trisomy 21 and Miller's syndrome, may be found.
      d. The anterior-chamber angle resembles that seen in genetic congenital glaucoma.
  III. Rupture of the lens capsule (Fig. 10.7) may be sealed over by the underlying lens epithelium or by the overlying iris, if the rent is small enough.

Most capsular ruptures result from trauma. Rarely, rupture may be spontaneous (e.g., in a hypermature cataract or in lenticonus) or, even more rarely, it may be secondary to a purulent infection.

Exfoliation of the Lens Capsule

   I. True exfoliation of the lens capsule is a rare condition that results from prolonged ocular exposure to infrared radiation (a condition once common in glass and steel workers).

Today, true exfoliation of the lens capsule may be found more frequently as an idiopathic aging change than as a result of long-term exposure to infrared radiation.

  II. The anteriormost layers of the anterior lens capsule split off into one or more sheets that curl into the anterior chamber.

The exfoliated lamellae can be seen clinically waving in the aqueous as a "scroll" on the anterior surface of the lens.

  III. Exfoliation of the lens does not affect the zonules and is not specifically associated with glaucoma.

Pseudoexfoliation Syndrome (Pseudoexfoliation of Lens Capsule, Exfoliation Syndrome, Basement Membrane Exfoliation Syndrome, Fibrillopathia Epitheliocapsularis) (Figs 10.8 to 10.11)

   I. The pseudoexfoliation (PEX) syndrome has a worldwide distribution, but seems to be most common in Scandinavian people (especially in Norway and Finland) and quite rare in black people.
     A. It is probably inherited, possibly as an autosomal-dominant trait with incomplete penetrance and varying expressivity.
     B. The ocular component appears to be the most dramatic part of a systemic disorder (see later).
  II. PEX syndrome occurs mainly in people between 60 and 80 years of age (although rarely it can be seen in young people) and is characterized by a deposition of a peculiar, white, fluffy material on the lens capsule, the zonules, the ciliary epithelium, the iris pigment epithelium, and the trabecular meshwork (i.e., limited to the anterior compartment of the eye).

PEX is a risk factor for cataract development.

     A. Clinically, the anterior surface of the lens shows a characteristic thin, homogeneous white deposit centrally,

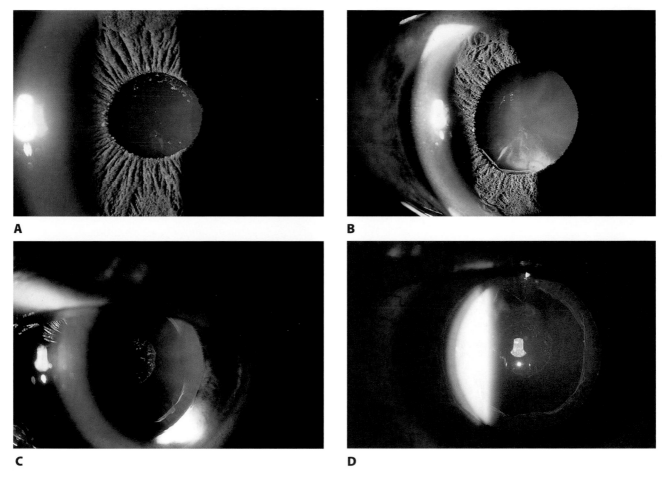

Fig. 10.8 Pseudoexfoliation (PEX) syndrome. **A,** The earliest hint of PEX in the undilated pupil is the presence of dandruff-like material on the pupillary edge of the iris and on the anterior surface of the lens in the region of the pupillary margin. **B,** Partial dilatation shows the beginning (from 6 to 8 o'clock) of the peripheral rim of PEX material. Another case shows the slit-lamp (**C**) and red reflex (**D**) appearance of the central and peripheral deposits.

called the *central disc*, corresponding in extent to the smallest size of the pupil. Often, an inrolled edge defines the end of the central disc, which is surrounded by a relatively clear zone.

The concentration of ascorbic acid, a major protective factor against free radicals, is reduced in the aqueous humor of PEX patients. Free radical action may play a role in the development of PEX. Also, plasma homocysteine, a risk factor for cardiovascular disease, is elevated in PEX with or without glaucoma.

B. On the outer third of the anterior lens surface is a *peripheral band* of a coarse, granular, "hoarfrost" material giving a frosted appearance to the lens surface. The band extends to the lens equator, is not seen unless the iris is dilated, and tends to have radial depressions that correspond to the radial furrows on the posterior surface of the iris.

C. Powdery, dandruff-like particles are commonly seen on the pupillary margin of the iris and occasionally attached to the corneal endothelium.

A consistent finding and essential sign (Naumann's sign) of PEX syndrome are the corneal endothelial changes: small flakes or clumps of pseudoexfoliative material (PEXM) and usually a diffuse, nonspecific melanin pigment deposition on the corneal endothelial surface as observed with the slit lamp; and reduced endothelial density, morphologic changes in cell size (polymegathism) and in cell shape (pleomorphism), endothelial cell damage, cell detritus, intraendothelial inclusions, and retroendothelial accumulations, as observed with specular microscopy. Even with only moderate intraocular pressure elevation, a diffuse corneal decompensation that resembles cornea guttata (Fuchs') may develop in these corneas.

D. The iris tends to be leathery and to dilate poorly because of fusion and atrophy of groups of circumferential ridges on its posterior surface and because of degenerative tissue changes and iris muscle cell atrophy.
   1. Pupillary ruff defects may also be seen.
   2. Iridodonesis and phacodonesis are seen in many patients and, rarely, spontaneous subluxation and dislocation of the lens may occur.

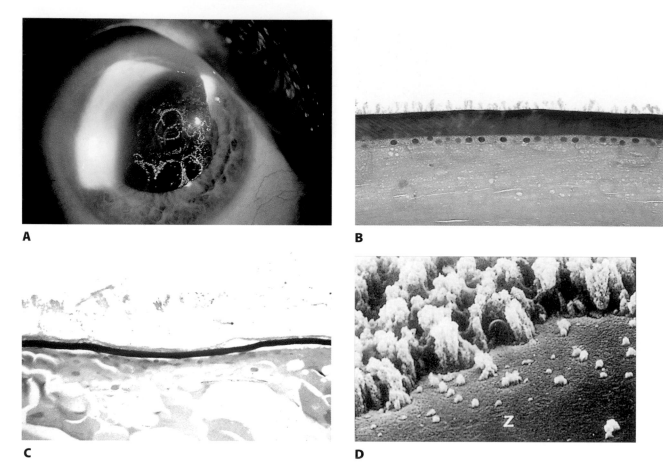

Fig. 10.9 Pseudoexfoliation (PEX) syndrome. **A,** Over the years, PEX material developed on the anterior face of the vitreous in an aphakic patient who did not have PEX syndrome at the time of an intracapsular cataract extraction. **B,** In the central disc area, the PEX material is deposited as small slivers that line up parallel to each other and perpendicular to the lens capsule. **C,** In the peripheral granular area, the material is abundant and has a thick dendritic appearance. **D,** Scanning electron micrograph of anterior lens surface shows a relatively clear zone (z) surrounded by a central edge of peripheral granular area. (**B** and **C,** Periodic acid–Schiff stain; **D,** courtesy of Dr. RC Eagle, Jr.)

Because of zonular weakness, cataract surgery on PEX eyes carries an increased risk of surgical complications. Before surgery, a shallow anterior chamber may be an indicator of zonular instability and should alert the surgeon to possible intraoperative complications.

E. An early sign of the condition is *Sampaoelesi's* line, a pigmented line lying on the corneal side of Schwalbe's line.

III. In slightly more than 50% of people, the condition is bilateral.

The uninvolved eye in patients who have unilateral PEX will develop PEX approximately 38% of the time if followed for 10 years. Although only one eye may seem affected clinically, autopsy analysis has shown that, histologically, the clinically unaffected eye can indeed be affected.

IV. Approximately 8% have glaucoma (glaucoma capsulare), and approximately 12% have ocular hypertension.

A. The cumulative probability of the development of increased intraocular pressure in PEX eyes is approximately 5% in 5 years and 15% in 10 years.

B. Degeneration of iris pigment epithelium and subsequent dense pigmentation of the anterior-chamber angle is often seen.

The picture resembles that of the *pigment dispersion syndrome* (rarely, true pigment dispersion syndrome can coexist with PEX syndrome).

C. The cause of the glaucoma is unknown.
  1. A suggested cause is the accumulation of the PEXM or pigment in the angle.

PEXM is apparently produced locally by trabecular cells and may cause a direct obstruction of aqueous outflow. The severity of glaucoma in PEX syndrome may be related to the amount of PEXM in the middle portion of the trabecular meshwork.

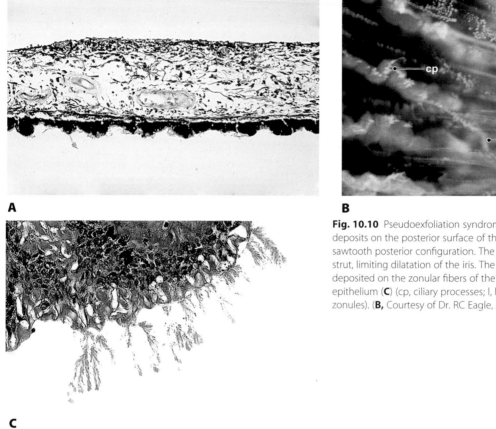

A

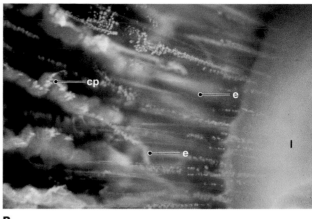

B

C

Fig. 10.10 Pseudoexfoliation syndrome. **A,** The exfoliation material deposits on the posterior surface of the iris, causing the iris to have a sawtooth posterior configuration. The deposited material often acts as a strut, limiting dilatation of the iris. The material can also be seen deposited on the zonular fibers of the lens (**B**) and on the ciliary epithelium (**C**) (cp, ciliary processes; l, lens; e, exfoliation material on zonules). (**B,** Courtesy of Dr. RC Eagle, Jr.; **C,** periodic acid–Schiff stain.)

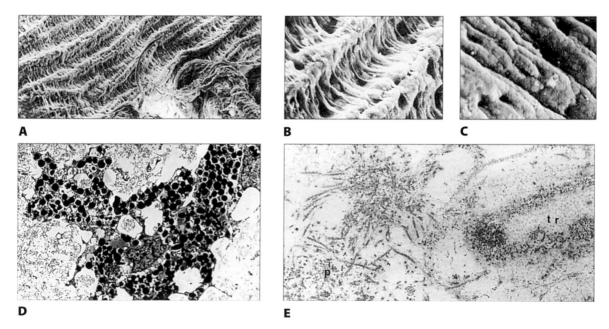

A

B

C

D

E

Fig. 10.11 Pseudoexfoliation (PEX) syndrome. **A,** Scanning electron microscopy shows coarse ridging of posterior iris surface. Encrusted ciliary crests lie below. Compare abnormal iris (**B**) with relatively normal iris (**C**) (same patient). Note compression of several ridges into single coarse ridge in **B. D,** In single coarse ridge, pigment epithelium is compressed into core by accumulating PEX material. **E,** PEX material (p) entering into trabecular (uveal) meshwork (tr).

2. Alternatively, the glaucoma may be caused by a separate gene on a locus close to the gene that causes the other changes, or, conversely, it may be caused by a single gene bearing three characteristics: (1) an abnormality of the aqueous drainage pathways that causes glaucoma; (2) an abnormality that causes production of the PEXM; and (3) an abnormality that causes degeneration of the iris pigment epithelium. Variations in the expressivity of this single gene would explain why the three events are usually found together but sometimes only one or two is present.

Thorleifsson and colleagues have identified two nonsynonymous single nucleotide polymorphisms in exon 1 of the gene, lysyl oxidase-like 1 (*LOXL 1*), located on chromosome 15q24, as associated with pseudoexfoliation and pseudoexfoliation glaucoma in individuals from Iceland and Sweden. About 25% of the general population studied is homozygous for the highest-risk haplotype and the population-attributable risk is more than 99%. Thus, an individual who is homozygous for both of the highest-risk haplotypes is a 700 times more likely than those with the lowest-risk variants to have pseudoexfoliation. The authors further noted that the product of *LOXL 1* catalyzes the formation of elastin fibers, which are a major component of the lesions in pseudoexfoliation.*

---

3. Marked and site-specific elastosis in the lamina cribrosa of patients who have PEX syndrome and glaucoma suggests that an abnormal regulation of elastin synthesis or degradation, or both, occurs in the optic nerves.

V. Cause

A. PEXM is found histologically in the uninvolved fellow eye; in addition, extraocular PEXM has been found in the following sites: around posterior ciliary vessels, palpebral and bulbar conjunctiva of the involved eye, lid and nonlid skin, orbital tissue, lung, heart, liver, gallbladder, kidney, and cerebral meninges.

Elevated plasma homocysteine (a risk factor for cardiovascular disease) is found in patients who have PEX, and increased levels of homocysteine in the aqueous may be involved in the pathogenesis of the glaucoma.

---

1. Almost always, PEXM is found in association with the fibrovascular stroma of these organs, most often adjacent to elastic tissue.
2. PEX syndrome appears to be part of a systemic disorder.

B. Delayed intraocular PEXM development
1. White, fluffy PEXM may appear on the anterior hyaloid and pupillary border years after intracapsu-

lar cataract extraction in eyes where no PEXM had been present before cataract surgery (see Fig. 10.9A).

If, therefore, the lens epithelium is a source of PEXM, it is not the only source.

---

2. PEXM may develop on the anterior vitreous and on the anterior and posterior surfaces of a lens implant after extracapsular cataract extraction and lens implantation.

C. Currently, the most appealing hypothesis is that PEXM is a product of abnormal metabolism of extracellular matrix, in particular abnormal basement membranes and elastic fibers.
1. Chemical analysis indicates that PEXM has a complex carbohydrate composition, with both *O*-linked sialomucin-type and *N*-linked oligosaccharide chains.
2. PEXM reacts with monoclonal antibodies to the HNK-1 epitope. This carbohydrate epitope is characteristic of many extracellular matrix and integral membrane glycoproteins that are implicated in cell adhesion.
3. Whatever the cause, PEXM results in defective or abnormal zonular attachment to the lens capsule so that these patients are in a high-risk group for extracapsular cataract surgery and lens implantation.

Fibrillin appears to be an intrinsic component of pseudoexfoliative fibers, suggesting that enhanced expression of fibrillin or abnormal aggregation of fibrillin-containing microfibrils may be involved in the pathogenesis of PEX syndrome.

VI. Histologically, in the eye, eosinophilic PEXM is found on the anterior surface of the lens, on the zonular fibers, on and in both surfaces of the iris and ciliary body, in the anterior chamber, on the corneal endothelium and incorporated in Descemet's membrane, and in the trabecular meshwork.

A. In the central disc area of the lens, the small, straight, thin PEXM lines up parallel with but perpendicular to the lens (it looks much like iron filings lining up on a magnet).

B. In the area of the peripheral band and on the other ocular structures in the anterior segment, the deposits tend to have a dendritic appearance, usually at right angles to the surface to which they are attached. The deposits are prominent over the free surface of the iris pigment epithelium and are characteristically in atrophic clusters of circumferential ridges.

C. Electron microscopically, a fibrogranular material is found in the deep (posterior) part of the anterior lens capsule.
1. It is most marked toward the equator and in the region of the zonular attachments.

*Damji KF. *Progress in understanding pseudoexfoliation syndrome and pseudoexfoliation-associated glaucoma.* Can J Ophthalmol *42:657, 2007;* Thorleifsson G, Magnusson KP, Sulem P *et al.*: *Common sequence variants in the* LOXL1 *gene confer susceptibility to exfoliation glaucoma.* Science *317:1397, 2007.*

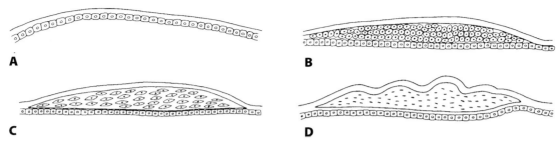

Fig. 10.12 Anterior subcapsular cataract. **A** to **D,** Changes from normal lens epithelium through proliferating epithelial cells to final subcapsular fibrous plaque and formation of new continuous lens capsule.

2. The abnormal material also seems to be present near the underlying lens epithelium.
3. The material is made up of bundles of exceedingly fine filaments that are banded together and have a periodicity of 50 nm—a type of basement membrane.

EPITHELIUM

Proliferation and Migration of Epithelium

Anterior Subcapsular Cataract (Figs 10.12 to 10.15)

I. After an injury (traumatic or noxious, e.g., iritis or keratitis) to the anterior lens, the following sequence of events may take place and result in an anterior subcapsular cataract.
  A. The lens epithelial cells in the region of the anterior pole of the lens become necrotic.
  B. Adjacent cells migrate into the subcapsular area, proliferate, and form an epithelial plaque.
  C. The epithelial cells, except the most posterior layer, undergo fibrous metaplasia to become fibroblasts. They then lay down a connective tissue plaque containing collagen.
  D. With time, the fibroblasts largely disappear and the scar tissue shrinks, wrinkling the overlying lens capsule.
  E. Simultaneously, the remaining epithelial cells, which now line the posterior edge of the fibrous plaque, lay down a new lens capsule (basement membrane). The final result is a fibrous plaque at the anterior pole of the lens between a duplicated lens capsule, called an *anterior subcapsular cataract.*

An anterior subcapsular cataract is rarely seen clinically because an occluded pupil is most often superimposed.

II. Frequently, the same injury that initially caused the damage to the epithelial cells, leading to the previously described anterior subcapsular cataract (the end-stage fibrous plaque between a duplicated capsule), also causes an anterior cortical cataract. The combination of an anterior subcapsular cataract and an anterior cortical cataract is called a *duplication cataract* (see Fig. 10.14).

Posterior Subcapsular Cataract
(Figs 10.16 and 10.17; See Fig. 10.15)

I. The following sequence of events may result in a PSC, either idiopathically (most common) or after an injury to the posterior or equatorial area of the lens (usually noxious, e.g., with choroiditis or retinitis pigmentosa).

Other increased risk factors for a PSC include oral or inhaled steroid therapy, diabetes, and increased UV-B exposure.

  A. In all probability, the subcapsular posterior cortical cells degenerate early.
  B. Later, the lens epithelial cells proliferate and migrate posteriorly, frequently reaching the posterior pole of the lens.

Any lens epithelial cells present between lens capsule and lens cortex posterior to the equator are always in an abnormal location and represent a pathologic change. The epithelial cells may proliferate abnormally until the entire lens capsule appears lined by a continuous layer of cells.

  C. The abnormally positioned epithelial cells enlarge in a grossly aberrant manner and produce large, bizarrely shaped cells that contain abundant, pale-staining, vesicular cytoplasm and small nuclei [i.e., *bladder cells* (of Wedl)].
  D. The changes, mainly bladder cell formation, constitute a PSC.

Pre-age-related PSC is an early finding in *Werner's syndrome,* a rare autosomal-recessive disease that has multiple progeroid characteristics.

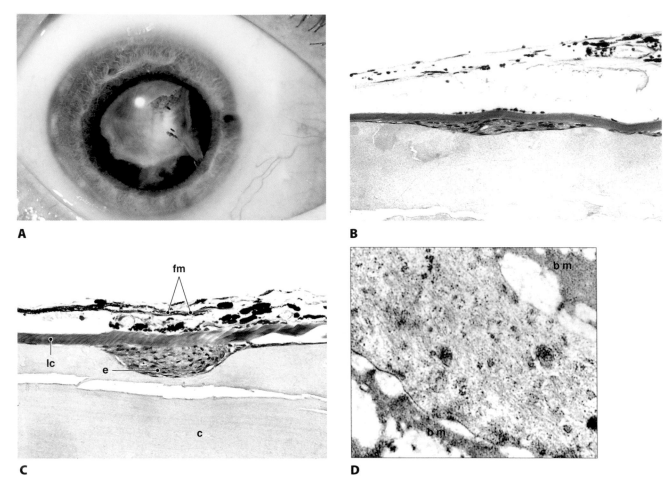

Fig. 10.13 Anterior subcapsular cataract (ASC). **A,** The patient had an anterior subcapsular cataract some years after blunt trauma to the eye. **B,** Histologic section of another case shows early proliferation of the lens epithelium beneath the capsule. **C,** In yet another case, continued proliferation of the lens epithelium has occurred along with fibroblastic metaplasia (fm, pigmented, vascularized fibrous membrane; lc, lens capsule; e, proliferation of the lens epithelium; c, cortex). **D,** Electron micrograph of ASC shows filamentous spindle cell and adjacent irregular patches of basement membrane (bm). (**B** and **C,** Periodic acid–Schiff stain.)

II. The proliferating epithelial cells, including the aberrant forms (bladder cells), may move anteriorly into the posterior cortex and result in a posterior cortical cataract in addition to the PSC.

ELSCHNIG'S PEARLS (See Fig. 5.12)

Degeneration and Atrophy of the Epithelium

I. Degeneration and atrophy of the lens epithelium may occur as the result of aging or secondary to acute or chronic glaucoma, iritis or iridocyclitis, hypopyon, to hyphema, chemical injury (especially alkali burn), noxious products in the aqueous (e.g., with anterior-segment necrosis), or stagnation of the aqueous (e.g., with posterior synechiae and iris bombé).

A. The epithelial damage may be minimal, resulting in no clinically detectable opacity, or it may be extensive, resulting in widespread cortical degeneration and opacification. Between the two extremes, a wide range of abnormalities may occur.

B. Neighboring normal epithelial cells may proliferate to heal a small epithelial defect and sometimes form irregular tufts dipping into the lens substance, or they may overproliferate and form anterior subcapsular or PSC.

C. Localized focal areas of epithelial necrosis, as often occur after an attack of closed-angle glaucoma, may result in multiple, discrete, stationary, permanent subcapsular opacities called *glaukomflecken* (cataracta disseminata subcapsularis glaucomatosa). Undoubtedly, stagnation of aqueous secondary to aqueous outflow blockage, along with a buildup of noxious materials in the aqueous (especially from iris necrosis), plays a role in the development of glaukomflecken (see Fig. 16.8).

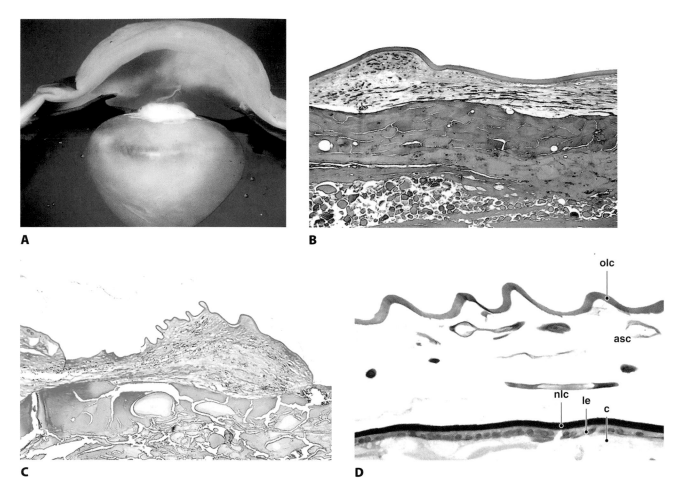

Fig. 10.14 Anterior subcapsular cataract (ASC). **A,** An intumescent cataractous lens shows ASC on its anterior surface. **B,** An anterior subcapsular fibrous plaque and a wrinkled capsule are prominent. The combination of ASC and underlying cortical morgagnian (globular) degeneration is called a *duplication cataract*. **C,** Alizarin red stain demonstrates calcium (red color) in the ASC. **D,** The proliferated epithelium has largely disappeared and has laid down collagen tissue. The original lens capsule is thrown into folds and the original lens epithelium has laid down a new, periodic acid–Schiff-positive lens capsule (olc, original lens capsule; asc, anterior subcapsular cataract; nlc, new lens capsule; le, lens epithelium; c, lens cortex).

CORTEX AND NUCLEUS (LENS CELLS OR "FIBERS")

Cortex ("Soft Cataract")

I. Biochemical changes in the lens cortex from any cause (congenital, inflammatory, traumatic) may result in clinically detectable opacities (i.e., cortical cataracts) (Figs 10.18 to 10.22).

   A. UV irradiation may play a role in the development of cortical cataracts

   B. Matrix metalloproteinase-1 may be upregulated by UV-B light and contribute to cortical cataract formation

II. Many clinical types of cataracts are recognized (e.g., cuneiform, coronal, spokelike), but they do not have well-characterized pathologic counterparts in specific histologic findings.

III. Histologically, the following pathologic changes may be found in cortical cataracts.

   A. *Clefts* seen clinically and histologically are made up of diffuse, watery, or eosinophilic material, probably representing altered or denatured cell proteins.

   B. *Cell fragments* represent pieces of broken-up lens cortical cells.

     1. They are distinguished from artifactitious fragments by the rounding-off of their fractured ends from retraction of the tenacious cytoplasm of the cell.

     2. Cortical fragmentation and rounding, or liquefaction, of their cytoplasm results in the production of morgagnian globules.

   C. *Morgagnian globules* represent small or large fragments of cortical cells that appear rounded from the increased liquidity of the cytoplasm.

     1. They may be present in small or large clefts in otherwise normal-appearing cortex, or they may completely replace the entire cortex.

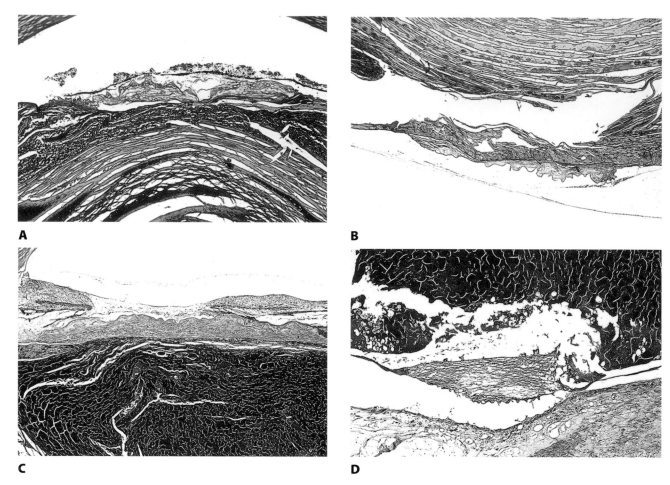

A   **B**   **C**   **D**

Fig. 10.15 Anterior and posterior subcapsular cataract in two different cases. The blue color of the trichrome stain demonstrates the fibrous plaques. **A** and **B,** Anterior and posterior subcapsular cataract in same lens. **C** and **D,** Another case shows the combination of anterior and posterior subcapsular cataract in same lens.

2. As more and more morgagnian globules, together with altered or denatured protein, replace the normal lens cortex, the lens becomes hyperosmolar and absorbs fluid.

3. A swollen (mainly in the anteroposterior diameter) intumescent cataract* results.

4. The globules or abnormal protein may replace the entire cortex and result in a mature (morgagnian or liquefied) cataract. The nucleus then sinks, by gravity, inferiorly (see Fig. 10.20A).

The whole lens looks clinically like a milk-filled sac (the free-floating nucleus cannot usually be seen clearly through an opacified liquid cortex).

During the process of cortical liquefaction, if the fluid is of sufficiently small molecular size, it may escape through the intact capsule and result in a

Clinically, the term mature cataract *refers to the appearance of a swollen (intumescent) lens as well as to the fact that no clear cortex is detectable beneath the anterior capsule. An immature cataract clinically has some clear cortex between the anterior cortical opacity and the lens capsule. The lens may be normal in size or swollen. If swollen, it is an intumescent cataract.*

smaller-than-normal lens with a wrinkled capsule (hypermature cataract; see Fig. 10.20B).

Rarely, the capsule of a mature cataract may rupture spontaneously and spill its contents into the aqueous fluid. In both a mature and a hypermature cataract, the capsule is frequently thinned and the epithelial cells are often degenerated. It is rare to see a hypermature lens in which all of the lens substance has been resorbed, leaving only the capsule.

D. Numerous *crystals*, such as calcium oxalate, cholesterol, and cystine, may become deposited in long-standing cataracts.

A *Christmas-tree cataract* (see Fig. 10.22) consists of highly refractile, multicolored needles throughout the cortex. The needles, previously thought to be cholesterol, are now thought probably to be cystine. Christmas-tree cataract may be associated with *uncombable hair syndrome*, an autosomal-dominant condition.

E. *Calcium salts* may impregnate long-standing cataracts (*cataracta calcarea*). The abnormal calcification of the lens is an example of *dystrophic calcification*.

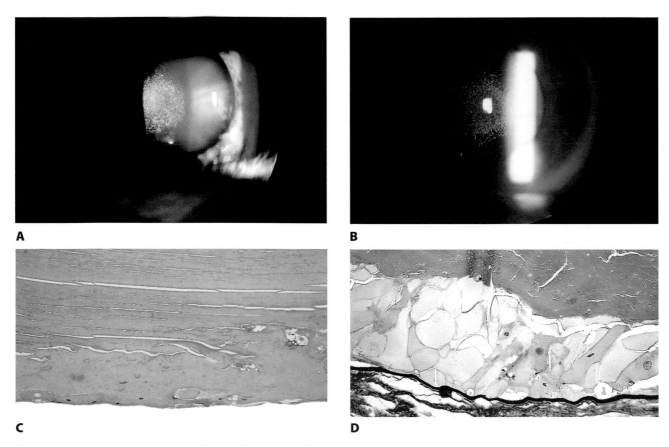

Fig. 10.16 Posterior subcapsular cataract (PSC). **A,** The patient had been on long-term steroid therapy after receiving a renal transplant. PSC developed over many years. **B,** Red reflex view of same case. **C,** Moderate PSC changes in lens from patient with primary retinitis pigmentosa. **D,** Periodic acid–Schiff-stained histologic section shows marked PSC changes, including cortical bladder cell formation (Wedl's cells).

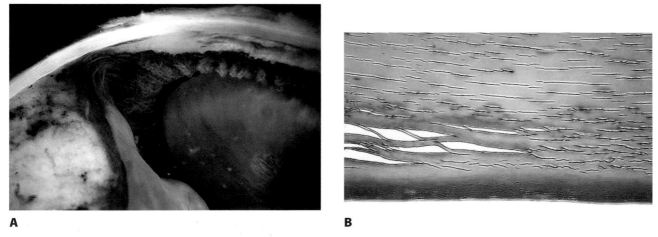

Fig. 10.17 Posterior subcapsular cataract (PSC). **A,** Gross specimen shows early PSC. Eye enucleated because of ciliary body melanoma. **B,** Same case shows posterior migration of lens epithelium and minimal posterior subcapsular cortical degeneration.

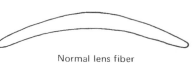

Normal lens fiber

Fig. 10.18 Types of changes that lens "fibers" (i.e., cells) undergo.

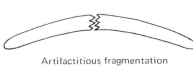

Artifactitious fragmentation

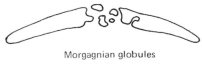

Cataractous fragmentation

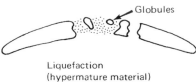

Morgagnian globules

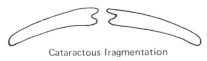

Liquefaction
(hypermature material)

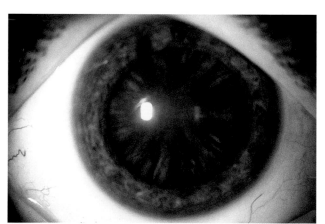

A

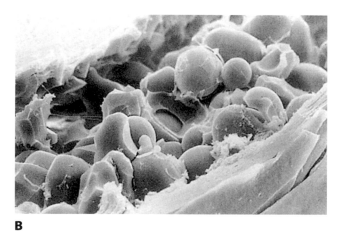

B

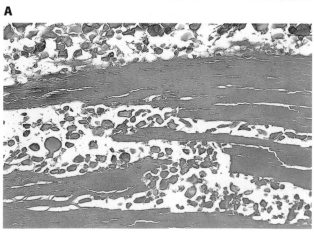

C

Fig. 10.19 Cortical cataract. **A,** Peripheral cataractous clefts, presumably caused by liquefaction of cortex. **B,** Scanning electron microscopic appearance of morgagnian globules in liquefied cortex. **C,** Periodic acid–Schiff-stained histologic section shows morgagnian globules between fragmented lens "fibers" in cortex. (**B,** Courtesy of Dr. RC Eagle, Jr.)

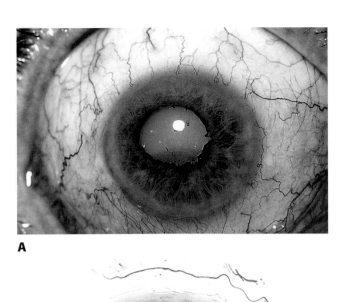

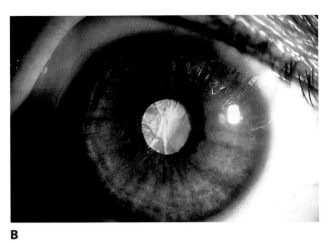

Fig. 10.20 Cortical cataract. **A,** Lens appears white (mature cataract) secondary to complete liquefaction of cortex; no clear cortex is detectable beneath anterior lens capsule. Note gravity has caused brown nucleus to sink inferiorly in liquid cortex. **B,** Liquid cortex has escaped through intact capsule, resulting in a wrinkled capsule, called *hypermature cataract.* **C,** Histologic section of a removed mature lens shows no cortex (except lower right) surrounding the nuclear cataract. The capsular rupture is an artifact of fixation and processing.

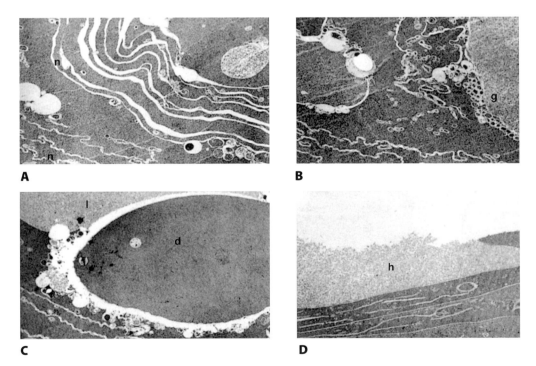

Fig. 10.21 Cortical changes by electron microscopy. **A,** Gross irregularities of cortical cells and few globules above. Normal (n) cells present below. **B,** Cell fragmentation and morgagnian globules (g) present. **C,** Dense (d) and lucent (l) globules present. Lucent globules appear watery. **D,** Watery cell or possibly "hypermature" cell protein (h).

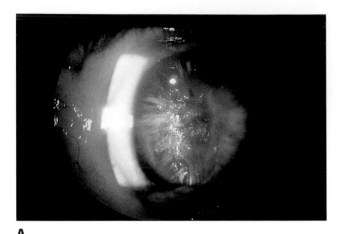

A

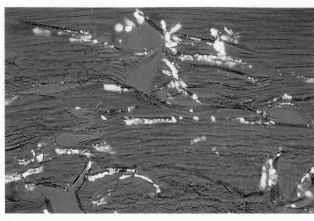

B

Fig. 10.22 Christmas-tree cataract. **A,** Patient had glistening, shimmering crystals in the cortex of both eyes. **B,** Polarization of unstained frozen section of removed lens demonstrates birefringence. Previously thought to be areas of cholesterol, recent evidence suggests that crystals are cystine.

Disruption of the lens capsule can result in intraocular dispersion of calcified lens particles, resulting in a condition called *calcific phacolysis.*

F. A break in the anterior capsule may result in cortical material becoming trapped in the equatorial region of the lens (i.e., a *Soemmerring's ring* cataract; see Fig. 5.12).

   After an acquired break in the lens capsule, or congenitally, mesenchymal tissue may grow into the cataract, leading to bone formation (*cataracta ossea*) or the formation of adipose tissue (*cataracta adiposa* or *xanthomatosis lentis*).

Nucleus ("Hard Cataract")

I. The increasing pressure of cell on cell, the breakdown of intercellular membranes in the lens nucleus, the slow conversion of soluble to insoluble protein, and the dehydration and accumulation of pigment (urochrome) all lead to optical and histologic densification of the nucleus and a nuclear cataract (Figs 10.23 and 10.24; see Fig. 10.20).

Cigarette smokers have an increased risk for development of nuclear lens opacities.

A. With more and more accumulation of pigment in the nucleus, the nuclear color changes from clear to yellow to brown (*cataracta brunescens*) to black (*cataracta nigra*).

B. Both the change in color and the increase in refractive index of the nucleus impede light from entering the eye and cause a decrease in visual acuity.

The increase in index of refraction also causes greater bending of the entering light and results in a lens-induced myopia ("second sight").

II. Histologically, the changes are usually subtle. Disappearance of the usual artifactitious nuclear clefts is noted.

A. The nucleus appears as an amorphous, homogeneous mass, with increased eosinophilia.

Crystals such as calcium oxalate (see Fig. 10.24) may be deposited in the nucleus.

B. As seen by electron microscopy, the cells are very electron-dense, exceedingly folded, and tightly packed, with obliteration of the intercellular spaces.

Age-Related (Senile) Cataracts

I. Age-related cataracts consist of any cataracts without a known cause that develop in elderly people (Fig. 10.25).

A. Clinically, age-related cortical cataracts can be divided into three main types: (1) *cuneiform* (in the peripheral cortex); (2) *punctate perinuclear* (in the cortex next to the nucleus); and (3) *cupuliform* (in the posterior cortex).

B. A nuclear cataract is merely the acceleration of the normal densification process of the innermost lens fibers.

II. Age-related cataracts may subluxate or dislocate spontaneously. The histologic features of cortical and nuclear cataracts were described previously.

SECONDARY CATARACTS

Intraocular Disease

I. Uveitis, malignant intraocular tumors (see Fig. 10.17), glaucoma, and retinitis pigmentosa (see Fig. 10.16C) can cause secondary cataracts.

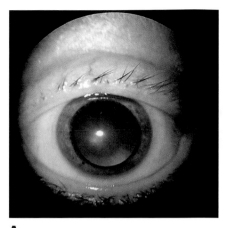

A

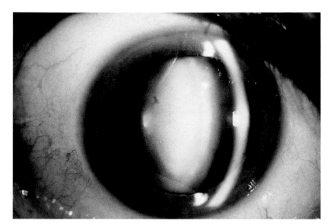

B

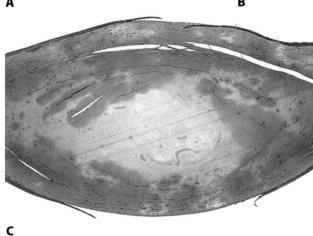

C

Fig. 10.23 Nuclear cataract. **A,** The red reflex shows the "oil droplet" effect of the nuclear cataract. **B,** Slit-lamp examination of another case shows the cataractous yellow pigmented nucleus. **C,** A histologic section of yet another case shows the homogeneous appearance of the compacted cells in the nuclear cataract.

The cataract secondary to intraocular disease has been termed a *complicating cataract* (*cataracta complicata*). Diseases in the anterior part of the eye tend to cause anterior cataract (anterior subcapsular, anterior cortical, or both), whereas diseases in the posterior part of the eye tend to cause posterior cataract (PSC, posterior cortical, or both).

II. Histologically, the lens changes are nonspecific and are the same as those described previously.

Trauma

See p. 115–117 in Chapter 5.

Toxic

I. Drugs such as steroids (topical, inhaled, and systemic), MER 29, phospholine iodide, Myleran, the phenothiazines and dinitrophenol, amiodarone, allopurinol, along with toxic substances such as ergot or metallic foreign bodies [e.g., iron (Fig. 10.26; see also Figs 5.49 and 5.50) or copper (see Fig. 8.53)], can cause cataracts.

II. Histologically, the lens changes are nonspecific except in *siderosis* and *hemosiderosis lentis*, where iron is present in lens epithelial cells (see Fig. 10.26), and in chalcosis, where copper is deposited in the lens capsule.

Endocrine, Metabolic, and Others

I. Cataracts may occur in conditions such as diabetes mellitus (see p. 596 in Chapter 15), galactosemia, hypoparathyroidism, hypothyroidism, aminoacidurias such as Lowe's syndrome (see section *Capsule*, earlier), myotonic dystrophy (see p. 538 in Chapter 14), dermatologic disorders (e.g., atopic dermatitis, chronic eczema, erythema multiforme), and chromosomal abnormalities.

A. Galactosemia

Galactosemia, glucose-6-phosphate dehydrogenase deficiency, and riboflavin deficiency are conditions in which cataracts represent a sensitive indicator of metabolic abnormalities of erythrocytes.

---

1. Galactosemia is an autosomal-recessively inherited condition (homozygous) resulting from a deficiency of the enzyme galactose-1-phosphate uridyl transferase.

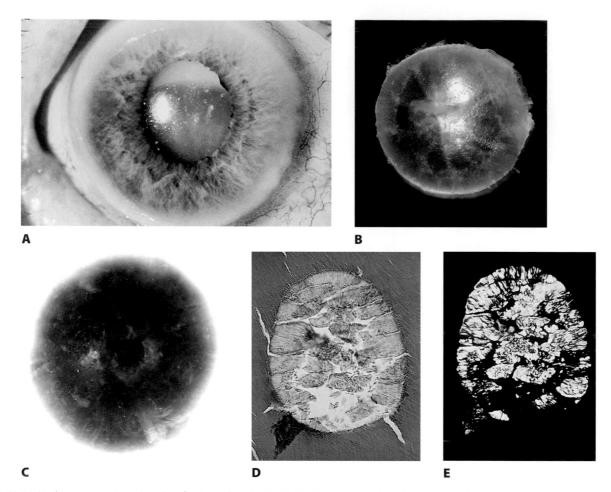

Fig. 10.24 Nuclear cataract. **A,** Dark nucleus floating in liquefied, "milky" cortex (mature cataract) has settled inferiorly because of gravity. Gross appearance of cataracta brunescens (**B**) and cataracta nigra (**C**). **D** and **E,** Calcium oxalate crystal in nucleus before (**D**) and after (**E**) polarization. (**A,** Courtesy of Prof. GOH Naumann.)

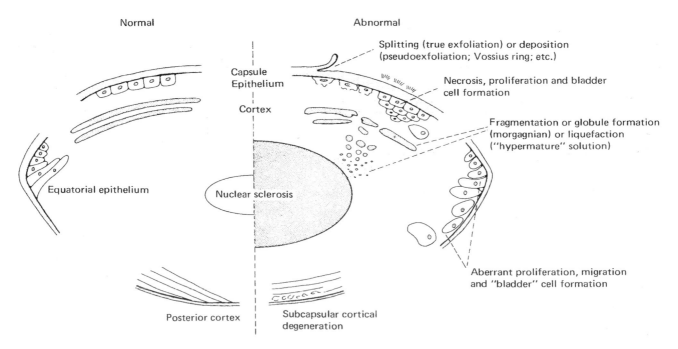

Fig. 10.25 Schematic comparison of histologic features in normal and abnormal lenses. Courtesy of Dr. RC Eagle.

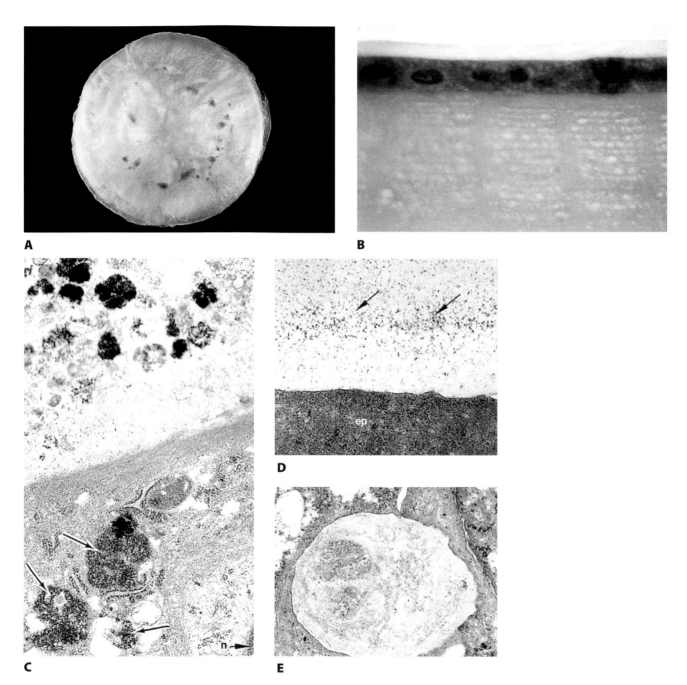

Fig. 10.26 Siderosis lentis (see Figs 5.49 and 5.50). **A,** Gross specimen of cataract caused by intraocular iron foreign body. **B,** Anterior lens nuclei stain blue with Perl's stain for iron. Note lens capsule and cortex do not stain for iron. **C,** Cells in siderotic nodule. Necrotic cell above contains a large number of iron bodies. Cell below viable but iron is accumulating (*arrows*) near segments of granular endoplasmic reticulum (n, nucleus). **D,** Anterior lens capsule and base of epithelial cell (ep). Note line of iron accumulating in capsule (*arrows*). More anteriorly, iron is diffusely distributed throughout lens capsule. However, the iron in the capsule is not concentrated enough to see by light microscopy. **E,** Nodule of basement membrane produced by epithelial cells in epithelial nodule. Basement membrane is mostly homogeneous.

2. The cataract is usually noted a few days to a few months after birth.
   a. In latent galactosemia, however, cataracts may not develop in some patients until they are 1 year of age or even older. In such cases of juvenile cataract, the galactosemia may not be evident and can only be discovered by means of an abnormal galactose loading test result or a raised fasting blood galactose.
   b. Galactosemia may be associated with cataracts that develop in early and middle adulthood in heterozygous patients.

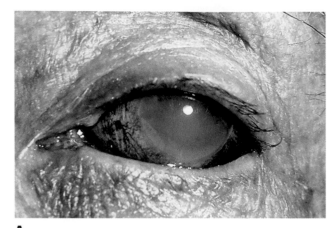

A

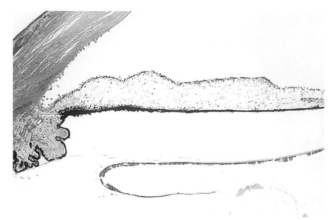

B

Fig. 10.27 Phacolytic glaucoma. **A,** Patient presented with signs and symptoms of acute closed-angle glaucoma. Chalky material seen in anterior chamber. The angle was open. **B,** Histologic section of another case shows hypermature cataract. Most of the cortex has leaked through the intact capsule. Lens-filled macrophages present in anterior chamber, on iris surface, in iris stroma, and clogging anterior-chamber angle, shown at increased magnification in **C.** (**A,** Courtesy of Dr. TR Thorp.)

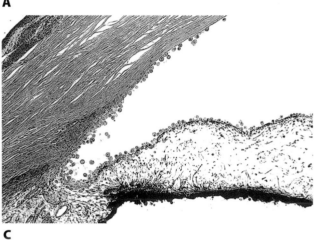

C

B. Clinically and histologically, the lens changes tend to be nonspecific.

COMPLICATIONS OF CATARACTS

Glaucoma

I. Mechanical
  A. An intumescent cataract may cause pupillary block and secondary angle closure.
  B. A cataract may spontaneously dislocate anteriorly and cause a pupillary block directly (see Fig. 5.38), or it may dislocate posteriorly and cause a pupillary block indirectly by prolapsing vitreous into the pupil.

II. Phacolytic glaucoma
  A. Phacolytic glaucoma (Fig. 10.27) is a secondary open-angle glaucoma characterized clinically by signs and symptoms of acute glaucoma, except that the anterior-chamber angle is open, a white cataract is noted, and a milky material may be seen in the anterior chamber. The glaucoma may resemble an open-angle glaucoma secondary to an anterior uveitis, except that keratic precipitates are usually absent.

  B. Phacolytic glaucoma occurs in an eye with a hypermature (white) cataract.
    1. Liquefied, denatured lens material leaks out of the lens through a generally intact lens capsule into the aqueous fluid.

      Often, polychromatic, hyperrefringent crystalline particles are noted on the milky material in the anterior chamber. The particles are presumably composed of cholesterol.

    2. The lens material in the aqueous incites a macrophagic cellular response.

      Liquefied or denatured protein does not seem capable of inciting an antigen–antibody response, only a macrophagic response. Relatively normal lens protein (i.e., not liquefied or denatured), if an abrogation of tolerance to lens protein has occurred, is capable of inciting an antigen–antibody reaction. The result is phacoanaphylactic endophthalmitis (see p. 75 in Chapter 4).

    3. The macrophages engulf the liquefied lens material and obstruct an open anterior-chamber drainage angle, causing an acute rise in the intraocular pressure.

In addition to macrophages filled with denatured lens material, aggregates of high-molecular-weight soluble protein (molecular weight 1.5×10^8) in the anterior-chamber angle may play a role in obstructing aqueous outflow.

C. In 25% of enucleated eyes that show phacolytic glaucoma, a postcontusion deformity of the anterior-chamber angle suggests that trauma may have been the event initiating cataract formation.

D. Histologically, a hypermature cataract is found.
1. Macrophages filled with eosinophilic lens material are seen in the aqueous fluid and on and in the iris, occluding the anterior-chamber angle.
2. The macrophages are not present on the corneal endothelium.

Phacoanaphylactic Endophthalmitis

See p. 75 in Chapter 4.

ECTOPIC LENS

Congenital

I. Congenital ectopia of the lens is usually bilateral and associated with generalized malformations or systemic disease such as *homocystinuria*, *Marfan's syndrome*, or *Weill–Marchesani syndrome*, or less frequently with cutis hyperelastica (Ehlers–Danlos syndrome), proportional dwarfism, oxycephaly, Crouzon's disease, Sprengel's deformity, genetic spontaneous late subluxation of the lens, or Sturge–Weber syndrome. Only the first three are described.
A. Homocystinuria (Fig. 10.28)
1. Homocystinuria is a systemic disease characterized by fair hair and skin, malar flush, poor peripheral circulation, frequent skeletal abnormalities (osteoporosis, arachnodactyly, pectus excavatum, or pectus carinatum), mental retardation, shortening of platelet survival time, and progressive arterial thrombosis.

Thromboembolic phenomena are common in patients who have homocystinuria, especially during or after general anesthesia.

2. Ocular findings include ectopia lentis (often luxated into the anterior chamber or subluxated inferonasally) and peripheral chorioretinal degeneration.
3. The disease, which is caused by a deficiency or absence of cystathionine synthetase, is transmitted by an autosomal-recessive gene. A metabolic block between homocysteine and cystathionine results in the accumulation of homocystine.

4. Histology
a. A thick, periodic acid–Schiff (PAS)-positive, amorphous material overlies the nonpigmented ciliary epithelium.
b. The material is made up of short segments of normal zonules composed of oriented filaments intermingled with myriad short filaments in disarray; the number of abnormal filaments appears to increase with age as the number of normal zonular fiber fragments decreases.

A similar collection or fringe of a mixture of very short, disorganized filaments, together with a few aligned groups of filaments like those present in normal zonules, is found attached to the anterior lens capsule (see Fig. 10.28A). The lens fringe of white zonular remnants is characteristic of homocystinuria. The zonular breakdown and degeneration, even dissolution, result in the ectopic location of the lens.

c. Degeneration of the nonpigmented ciliary epithelium and peripheral neural retina is often present and increases in severity with age.
B. Marfan's syndrome (arachnodactyly, dystrophia mesodermalis hypoplastica; Figs 10.29 and 10.30)
1. Marfan's syndrome consists of ocular, skeletal, and cardiovascular abnormalities.
2. Urinary excretion of hydroxyproline may be present or even excessive, but it may also be normal (i.e., absent).

An attenuation, probably of nonenzymatic steps involved in the maturation of collagen, causes defective collagen organization in the connective tissue of patients. The defect resides on chromosome 15q15–21. The responsible gene is fibrillin-1 (*FBN1*). The estimated prevalence is 2 to 3 per 10 000 individuals.

3. The lens may be subluxated in any direction, but usually superotemporally.
4. Other ocular anomalies include iridodonesis, hypoplasia of the iris, increased positive transillumination of the iris, miosis with decreased ability to dilate, and a fetal anterior-chamber angle.
5. The condition is usually inherited as an autosomal-dominant trait, often with variable degrees of expression.

The condition can also occur de novo, with a mutation rate of 0.7 per 100 000 births.

6. Histology
a. The anterior-chamber angle shows an immature configuration, but this is variable and nonspecific.
b. The iris may show segmental hypopigmentation or absence of pigment from the posterior layer of the pigment epithelium, especially toward the

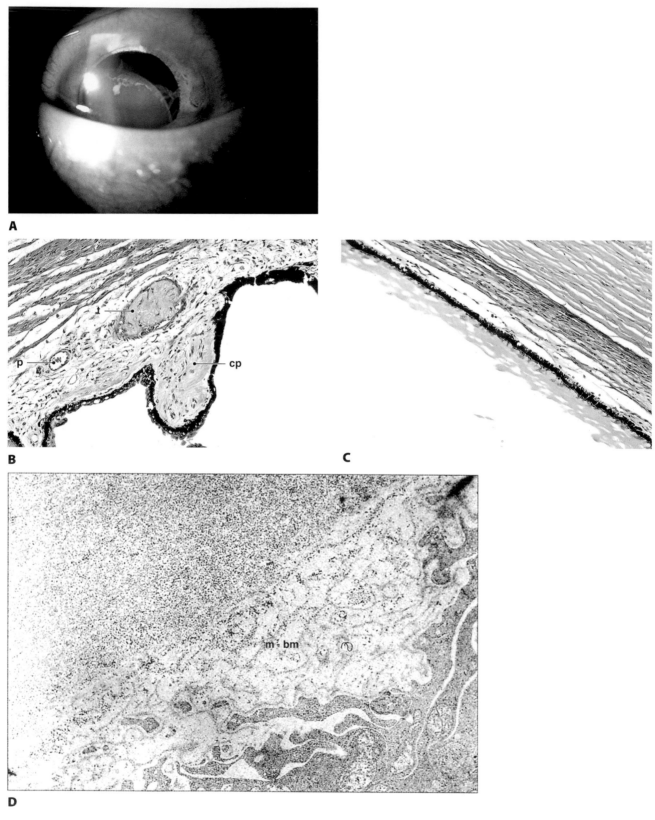

Fig. 10.28 Homocystinuria. **A,** Fringe of white zonular remnants present at equator of lens. These remnants tend to undulate slowly with eye movement. **B,** Histologic section of another case shows a thrombus in the greater arterial circle of the ciliary body. Patient died from a thrombotic episode during general anesthesia (t, thrombus; p, patent blood vessel; cp, ciliary process). **C,** A thick layer of material covers the nonpigmented ciliary epithelium of the pars plana. **D,** Electron micrograph shows a portion of thick, abnormal zonular material lying on normal, multilaminar, internal basement membrane (m-bm) of ciliary epithelium. The abnormal zonular material consists of myriad fragments of zonular filaments. (**A,** From Ramsey MS *et al.: Arch Ophthalmol* 93:318, 1975. © American Medical Association. All rights reserved. **D,** from Ramsey MS *et al.: Am J Ophthalmol* 74:377. Copyright Elsevier 1972.)

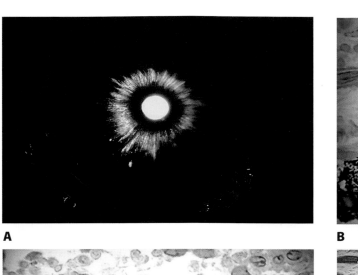

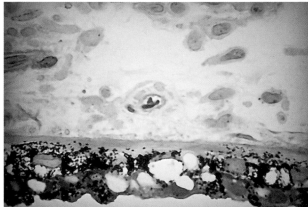

A

B

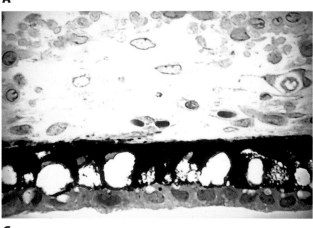

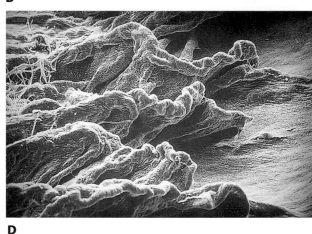

C

D

Fig. 10.29 Marfan's syndrome. **A,** Transillumination of enucleated child's eye shows widespread lucency of most of iris leaf. **B,** Posterior epithelium pigmented slightly and thin dilator muscle present. **C,** Posterior epithelium amelanotic; dilator muscle appears absent. **D,** Scanning electron micrograph of posterior iris near its root. Ciliary crests extend on to peripheral iris. Circumferential ridges and furrows of iris have disappeared and the iris surface has become smooth in its periphery. (**B** and **C,** Plastic-embedded thin sections. From Ramsey MS *et al.: Am J Ophthalmol* 76:102. Copyright Elsevier 1973.)

periphery, with accompanying hypoplasia of the overlying iris dilator muscle.

The hypopigmentation of the posterior iris pigment epithelial layer, when present, is highly characteristic and explains the clinical observation of increased positive retroillumination of the iris diaphragm where stromal pigmentation is not too dense.

---

c. The ciliary body processes or crests may extend sporadically on to the back of the iris and may be maldeveloped.
d. The lens is subluxated in the posterior chamber or dislocated into the anterior chamber or vitreous compartment.

The area of interface between lens capsule and zonular fibers appears abnormal. The zonular attachments seem blunted and rounder than in the normal attachment. It is probably the abnormality of the lens capsule–zonular adhesion area that results in the ectopia of the lens.

---

   e. Qualitative abnormalities in fibrillin-1 staining can be seen in the conjunctiva
C. Weill–Marchesani syndrome
   1. Weill–Marchesani syndrome is a generalized disorder of connective tissues characterized by spherophakia, ectopia lentis, brachymorphism, and joint stiffness.
   2. The spherophakic lens subluxates frequently, usually in a down-and-in direction. High myopia is often present.

Spherophakia may be part of the Weill–Marchesani syndrome and may occur independently, or, rarely, may occur in Marfan's syndrome. The small lens can cause pupillary block glaucoma. Such glaucoma is worsened by miotics but ameliorated by mydriatics. Peripheral anterior synechiae may form secondarily to the pupillary block. The small lens may dislocate into the anterior chamber.

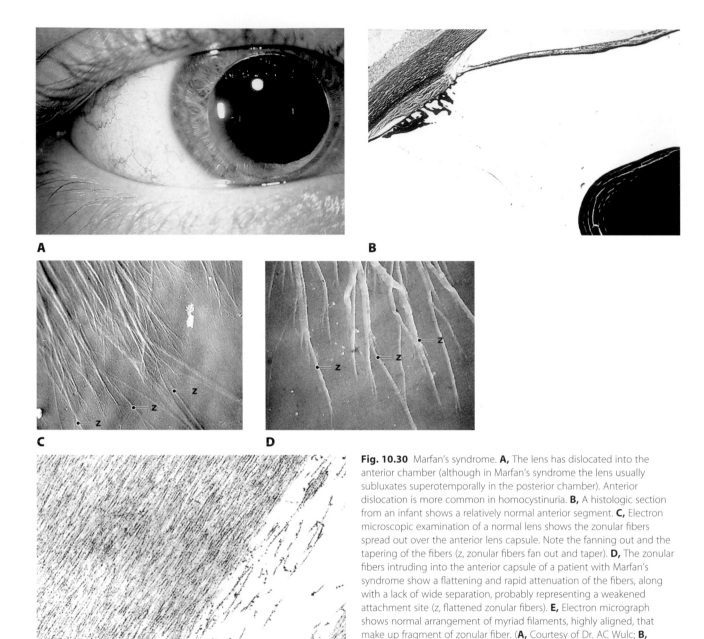

Fig. 10.30 Marfan's syndrome. **A,** The lens has dislocated into the anterior chamber (although in Marfan's syndrome the lens usually subluxates superotemporally in the posterior chamber). Anterior dislocation is more common in homocystinuria. **B,** A histologic section from an infant shows a relatively normal anterior segment. **C,** Electron microscopic examination of a normal lens shows the zonular fibers spread out over the anterior lens capsule. Note the fanning out and the tapering of the fibers (z, zonular fibers fan out and taper). **D,** The zonular fibers intruding into the anterior capsule of a patient with Marfan's syndrome show a flattening and rapid attenuation of the fibers, along with a lack of wide separation, probably representing a weakened attachment site (z, flattened zonular fibers). **E,** Electron micrograph shows normal arrangement of myriad filaments, highly aligned, that make up fragment of zonular fiber. (**A,** Courtesy of Dr. AC Wulc; **B,** reticulum stain; **C** and **D,** scanning electron micrographs; **D** and **E,** from Ramsey MS *et al.: Am J Ophthalmol* 76:102. Copyright Elsevier 1972.)

3. It is inherited as an autosomal-recessive trait.
4. Histologically, a filamentary degeneration of zonular fibers produces a thick PAS-positive layer overlying the ciliary epithelium.

The picture may be almost identical to that seen in homocystinuria.

II. Congenital ectopia of the lens without associated systemic problems
   A. Simple ectopia lentis

1. Simple ectopia lentis is usually bilateral and symmetric, with the lenses subluxated upward and laterally.
2. Iridodonesis is often present.
3. It has an autosomal inheritance pattern, occasionally with decreased penetrance.
4. Associated ocular problems include dislocation of the lens into the anterior chamber, secondary glaucoma, and neural retinal detachment.

B. Ectopia lentis et pupillae is quite similar to simple ectopia lentis, but with the additional feature of ectopia of the pupil.

BIBLIOGRAPHY

Normal Anatomy

Fine BS, Yanoff M: *Ocular Histology: A Text and Atlas*, 2nd edn. Hagerstown, MD, Harper & Row, 1979:149–159

Jaffe NS, Horwitz J: Lens and cataract. In Podos SM, Yanoff M, eds: *Textbook of Ophthalmology*. New York, Gower Medical Publishing, 1992:1.8, 1.9, 2.15–2.19

Taylor VL, Al-Ghoul KJ, Lane CW et al.: Morphology of the normal human lens. *Invest Ophthalmol Vis Sci* 37:1396, 1996

Yanoff M, Fine BS: *Ocular Pathology: A Color Atlas*, 2nd edn. New York, Gower Medical Publishing, 1992:10.1–10.2

General Information

Andley UP, Lewis RM, Reddan JR et al.: Action spectrum for cytotoxicity in the UVA- and UVB-wavelength in cultured lens epithelial cells. *Invest Ophthalmol Vis Sci* 35:367, 1994

Cumming RG: Use of inhaled corticosteroids and the risk of cataracts. *N Engl J Med* 337:8, 1997

Cumming RG, Mitchell P, Lim R: Iris color and cataract: The Blue Mountain Eye Study. *Am J Ophthalmol* 130:237, 2000

Cumming RG, Mitchell P, Smith W: Diet and cataract: The Blue Mountain Eye Study. *Ophthalmology* 107:450, 2000

Delcourt C, Cristol J-P, Léger CL et al.: Association of antioxidant enzymes with cataract and age-related macular degeneration. *Ophthalmology* 106:215, 1999

Fine BS, Yanoff M: *Ocular Histology: A Text and Atlas*, 2nd edn. Hagerstown, MD, Harper & Row, 1979:147–159

Klein BEK, Klein R, Lee KE: Diabetes, cardiovascular disease, selected cardiovascular disease risk factors, and the 5-year incidence of age-related cataract and progression of lens opacities: The Beaver Dam Eye Study. *Am J Ophthalmol* 126:782, 1998

Klein BEK, Klein R, Lee KE et al.: Socioeconomic and lifestyle factors and the 10-year incidence of age-related cataracts. *Am J Ophthalmol* 136:506, 2003

Leske MC, Chylack LT, Wu SY et al.: Risk factors for cataract. *Arch Ophthalmol* 109:244, 1991

Leske MC, Chylack LT, Wu SY et al.: Incidence and progression of cortical and posterior subcapsular opacities. *Ophthalmology* 104:1987, 1997

Mukesch BN, Le A, Dimitrov PN et al.: Development of cataract and associated risk factors. The Visual Impairment Project. *Arch Ophthalmol* 124:79, 2006

Sadun AA, Bassi CJ, Lessell S: Why cataracts do not produce afferent pupillary defects. *Am J Ophthalmol* 110:712, 1990

West S, Munoz B, Emmett E et al.: Cigarette smoking and risk of nuclear cataracts. *Arch Ophthalmol* 107:1166, 1989

Congenital Anomalies

Basti S, Hejtmancik JF, Padma T et al.: Autosomal dominant zonular cataract with sutural opacities in a four-generation family. *Am J Ophthalmol* 121:162, 1996

Bateman JB, Geyer DD, Flodman P et al.: A new βA1-crystalline splice junction mutation in autosomal dominant cataract. *Invest Ophthalmol Vis Sci* 41:3278, 2000

Bateman JB, Johannes M, Flodman P et al.: A new locus for autosomal dominant cataract on chromosome 12q13. *Invest Ophthalmol Vis Sci* 41:2665, 2000

Bleik JH, Traboulsi E, Maumenee IH: Familial posterior lenticonus and microcornea. *Arch Ophthalmol* 110:1208, 1992

Bonneau D, Winter-Fuseau I, Loiseau M-N et al.: Bilateral cataract and high serum ferritin: A new dominant genetic disorder? *J Med Genet* 32:778, 1995

Gaviria JG, Johnson DA, Scribbick FW et al.: Spontaneous anterior capsular rupture associated with anterior capsular rupture. *Arch Ophthalmol* 124:134, 2006

Gehrs KM, Pollock SC, Zilkha G: Clinical features and pathogenesis of Alport retinopathy. *Retina* 15:305, 1995

Haargaard B, Wohlfahrt J, Fledelius HC et al.: A nationwide Danish study of 1027 cases of congenital/infantile cataracts: etiological and clinical classifications. *Ophthalmology* 111:2229, 2004

Hemady R, Blum S, Sylvia BM: Duplication of the lens, hourglass cornea, and cornea plana. *Arch Ophthalmol* 111:303, 1993

Hoepner J, Yanoff M: Craniosynostosis and syndactylism (Apert's syndrome) associated with a trisomy 21 mosaic. *J Pediatr Ophthalmol* 8:107, 1971

Jaafar MS, Robb RM: Congenital anterior polar cataract: A review of 63 cases. *Ophthalmology* 91:249, 1984

Junk AK, Stefani FH, Ludwig K: Bilateral anterior lenticonus: Scheimpflug imaging system documentation and ultrastructural confirmation of Alport syndrome in the lens capsule. *Arch Ophthalmol* 118:895, 2000

Kilty LA, Hiles DA: Unilateral posterior lenticonus with persistent hyaloid artery remnant. *Am J Ophthalmol* 116:104, 1993

Kramer PL, LaMorticella D, Schilling K et al.: A new locus for autosomal dominant congenital cataract. *Invest Ophthalmol Vis Sci* 41:36, 2000

Manschot WA: Primary congenital aphakia. *Arch Ophthalmol* 69:571, 1963

Mohney BG, Parks MM: Acquired posterior lentiglobus. *Am J Ophthalmol* 120:123, 1995

Morrison DA, Fitzpatrick DR, Fleck BW: Iris coloboma with iris heterochromia: A common association. *Arch Ophthalmol* 118:1590, 2000

Salmon JF, Wallis CE, Murray ADN: Variable expressivity of autosomal dominant microcornea with cataract. *Arch Ophthalmol* 106:505, 1988

Shafie SM, von-Bischhoffshausen FRB, Bateman JB: Autosomal dominant cataract: intrafamilial phenotypic variability, interocular asymmetry, and variable progression in four Chilean families. *Am J Ophthalmol* 141:750S, 2006

Scott MH, Hejtmancik F, Wozencraft LA et al.: Autosomal dominant congenital cataract: Interocular phenotypic variability. *Ophthalmology* 101:866, 1994

Seidenberg K, Ludwig IH: A newborn with posterior lenticonus. *Am J Ophthalmol* 115:543, 1993

Traboulsi E, Weinberg RJ: Familial congenital cornea guttata with anterior polar cataracts. *Am J Ophthalmol* 108:123, 1989

Van Setten G: Anterior lenticonus: histologic evaluation and approach for cataract surgery. *J Cataract Refract Surg* 27:1071, 2001

Wheeler DT, Mullaney PB, Awad A et al.: Pyramidal anterior polar cataracts. *Ophthalmology* 106:2362, 1999

Yamamoto Y, Hayasaka S, Setogawa T: Family with aniridia, microcornea, and spontaneously resorbed cataract. *Arch Ophthalmol* 106:502, 1988

Yanoff M, Fine BS, Schaffer DB: Histopathology of transient neonatal lens vacuoles: A light and electron microscopic study. *Am J Ophthalmol* 76:363, 1973

Capsule

Asano N, Schlötzer-Schrehardt U, Naumann GOH: A histopathologic study of iris changes in pseudoexfoliation syndrome. *Ophthalmology* 102:1279, 1995

Bleich S, Roedl J, Schlötzer-Schrehardt U *et al.*: Elevated homocystein levels in aqueous humor of patients with pseudoexfoliation glaucoma. *Am J Ophthalmol* 138:162, 2004

Cashwell LF, Holleman IL, Weaver RG *et al.*: Idiopathic true exfoliation of the lens capsule. *Ophthalmology* 96:348, 1989

Fitzsimon JS, Johnson DH: Exfoliation material on intraocular lens implants. *Arch Ophthalmol* 114:355, 1996

Freissler K, Küchle M, Naumann GOH: Spontaneous dislocation of the lens in pseudoexfoliation syndrome. *Arch Ophthalmol* 113:1095, 1995

Gottanka J, Flügel-Koch C, Martus P *et al.*: Correlation of pseudoexfoliative material and optic nerve damage in pseudoexfoliation syndrome. *Invest Ophthalmol Vis Sci* 38:2435, 1997

Hammer T, Schlötzer-Schrehardt U, Naumann GOH: Unilateral or asymmetric pseudoexfoliation syndrome? An ultrastructural study. *Arch Ophthalmol* 119:1023, 2001

Henry JC, Krupin T, Schmitt M *et al.*: Long-term follow-up of pseudoexfoliation and the development of elevated intraocular pressure. *Ophthalmology* 94:545, 1987

Jehan FS, Mamalis N, Crandall AS: Spontaneous late dislocation of intraocular lens within the capsular bag in pseudoexfoliation patients. *Ophthalmology* 108:1727, 2001

Khalil AK, Kubota T, Tawara A *et al.*: Ultrastructural age-related changes on the posterior iris surface: A possible relationship to the pathogenesis of exfoliation. *Arch Ophthalmol* 114:721, 1996

Kivelä T, Hietanen J, Uusitalo M: Autopsy analysis of clinically unilateral exfoliation syndrome. *Invest Ophthalmol Vis Sci* 38:2008, 1997

Koliakos GG, Konstas AGP, Schlötzer-Schrehardt UM *et al.*: Ascorbic acid concentration is reduced in the aqueous humor of patients with exfoliation syndrome. *Am J Ophthalmol* 134:879, 2002

Konstas AGP, Ritch R, Bufidis T *et al.*: Exfoliation syndrome in a 17-year-old girl. *Arch Ophthalmol* 115:1063, 1997

Kozart DM, Yanoff M: Intraocular pressure status in 100 consecutive patients with exfoliation syndrome. *Ophthalmology* 89:214, 1982

Küchle M, Viestenz A, Martus P *et al.*: Anterior chamber depth and complications during cataract surgery in eyes with pseudoexfoliation syndrome. *Am J Ophthalmol* 129:281, 2000

Lim T, Lewis AL, Nussbaum RL: Molecular confirmation of carriers for Lowe syndrome. *Ophthalmology* 106:119, 1999

Mardin CY, Schötzer-Schrehardt U, Naumann GOH: "Masked" pseudoexfoliation syndrome in unoperated eyes with circular posterior synechiae: Clinical-electron microscopic correlation. *Arch Ophthalmol* 119:1500, 2001

Naumann GOH: Electron-microscopic identification of pseudoexfoliation material in extrabulbar tissue. *Arch Ophthalmol* 109:565, 1991

Naumann GOH: The Bowman Lecture: Corneal transplantation in anterior segment disease. *Eye* 9:395, 1995

Naumann GOH, Schlötzer-Schrehardt UM: Corneal endothelial involvement in PEX syndrome (letter). *Arch Ophthalmol* 112:297, 1994

Naumann GOH, Schlötzer-Schrehardt UM: Keratopathy in pseudoexfoliation syndrome as a cause of corneal endothelial decompensation: A clinicopathologic study. *Ophthalmology* 107:1111, 2000

Naumann GOH, Schlötzer-Schrehardt UM, Küchle M: Pseudoexfoliation syndrome for the comprehensive ophthalmologist: Intraocular and systemic manifestations. *Ophthalmology* 105:951, 1998

Netland PA, Ye H, Streeten BW *et al.*: Elastosis of the lamina cribrosa in pseudoexfoliation syndrome with glaucoma. *Ophthalmology* 102:878, 1995

Puska P: Unilateral exfoliation syndrome: conversion to bilateral exfoliation and to glaucoma. *J Glaucoma* 11:517, 2002

Puska P, Tarkkanen A: Exfoliation syndrome as a risk factor for cataract development. Five-year follow-up of lens opacities in exfoliation syndrome. *J Cataract Refract Surg* 27:1992, 2001

Rich R: Exfoliation syndrome and occludable angles. *Trans Am Ophthalmol Soc* 92:845, 1994

Rich R, Mudumbai R, Liebman JM: Combined exfoliation and pigment dispersion: Paradigm of an overlap syndrome. *Ophthalmology* 107:1004, 2000

Rich R, Schlötzer-Schrehardt UM: Exfoliation syndrome. *Surv Ophthalmol* 45:265, 2001

Rotchford AP, Kirwan JF, Johnson GJ *et al.*: Exfoliation syndrome in black South Africans. *Arch Ophthalmol* 121:863, 2003

Schlötzer-Schrehardt UM, Naumann GOH: Trabecular meshwork in pseudoexfoliation syndrome with and without open-angle glaucoma: A morphometric, ultrastructural study. *Invest Ophthalmol Vis Sci* 36:1750, 1995

Schlöltzer-Schrehardt UM, Dorfler S, Naumann GOH: Corneal endothelial involvement in pseudoexfoliation syndrome. *Arch Ophthalmol* 111:666, 1993

Schlötzer-Schrehardt UM, Koca MR, Naumann GOH *et al.*: Pseudoexfoliation syndrome. *Arch Ophthalmol* 110:1752, 1992

Schlötzer-Schrehardt UM, Küchle M, Naumann GOH: Electron-microscopic identification of pseudoexfoliation material in extrabulbar tissue. *Arch Ophthalmol* 109:565, 1991

Schlötzer-Schrehardt UM, von der Mark K, Sakai LY *et al.*: Increased extracellular deposition of fibrillin-containing fibrils in pseudoexfoliation syndrome. *Invest Ophthalmol Vis Sci* 36:1750, 1997

Silver DN, Lewis RA, Nussbaum RL: Mapping the Lowe oculocerebrorenal syndrome to Xq24–q26 by use of restriction fragment length polymorphisms. *J Clin Invest* 79:282, 1987

Streeten BW, Bookman L, Ritch R *et al.*: Pseudoexfoliative fibrillopathy in the conjunctiva: A relation to elastic fibers and elastosis. *Ophthalmology* 94:1439, 1987

Streeten BW, Dark AJ, Wallace RN *et al.*: Pseudoexfoliative fibrillopathy in the skin of patients with ocular pseudoexfoliation. *Am J Ophthalmol* 110:490, 1990

Streeten BW, Li Z, Wallace RN *et al.*: Pseudoexfoliative fibrillopathy in visceral organs of a patient with pseudoexfoliation syndrome. *Arch Ophthalmol* 110:1757, 1992

Streeten BW, Robinson MR, Wallace R *et al.*: Lens capsule abnormalities in Alport's syndrome. *Arch Ophthalmol* 105:1693, 1987

Tripathi RC, Cibis GW, Tripathi BJ: Pathogenesis of cataracts in patients with Lowe's syndrome. *Ophthalmology* 93:1046, 1986

Uusitalo M, Kivelda T, Tarkkanen A: Immunoreactivity of exfoliation material for the cell adhesion-related HNK-1 carbohydrate epitope. *Arch Ophthalmol* 111:1419, 1993

Vessani RM, Rich R, Lieberman JM *et al.*: Plasma homocysteine is elevated in patients with exfoliation syndrome. *Am J Ophthalmol* 136:41, 2003

Wadelius C, Fagerholm P, Petterson U *et al.*: Lowe oculocerebrorenal syndrome: DNA-based linkage of the gene to Xq24–q26, using tightly linked flanking markers and the correlation to lens examination in carrier diagnosis. *Am J Hum Genet* 44:241, 1989

Yanoff M: Intraocular pressure in exfoliation syndrome. *Acta Ophthalmol* 66(Suppl. 184):59, 1988

Epithelium

Bochow TW, West SK, Azar A *et al.*: Ultraviolet light exposure and risk of posterior subcapsular cataracts. *Arch Ophthalmol* 107:369, 1989

Cumming RG: Use of inhaled corticosteroids and the risk of cataracts. *N Engl J Med* 337:8, 1997

Eagle RC Jr, Yanoff M, Morse PH: Anterior segment necrosis following scleral buckling in hemoglobin SC disease. *Am J Ophthalmol* 75:426, 1973

Font RL, Brownstein S: A light and electron microscopic study of anterior subcapsular cataracts. *Am J Ophthalmol* 78:972, 1974

Jonas JB, Ruprecht KW, Schmitz-Valckenberg P *et al.*: Ophthalmic surgical complications in Werner's syndrome: Report on 18 eyes of nine patients. *Ophthalmic Surg* 18:760, 1987

Sperduto RD, Hiller R: The prevalence of nuclear, cortical, and posterior subcapsular lens opacities in a general population sample. *Ophthalmology* 91:815, 1984

Wedl C: *Atlas der pathologischen Histologie des Auges.* Leipzig, Wigand, 1860–1861:LVIV, 44 and 55

Cortex and Nucleus

Costello MJ, Oliver TN, Cabot LM: Cellular architecture in age-related human nuclear cataracts. *Invest Ophthalmol Vis Sci* 33:3209, 1992

de Jong PTVM, Bleeker-Wagemakers EM, Vrensen GFJM *et al.*: Crystalline cataract and uncombable hair. *Ophthalmology* 97:1181, 1990

Font RL, Yanoff M, Zimmerman LE: Intraocular adipose tissue and persistent hyperplastic primary vitreous. *Arch Ophthalmol* 82:43, 1969

Hiller R, Sperduto RD, Podgor MJ *et al.*: Cigarette smoking and the risk of development of lens opacities: The Framingham studies. *Ophthalmology* 104:1113, 1997

The Italian–American Cataract Study Group: Incidence and progression of cortical, nuclear, and posterior subcapsular cataracts. *Am J Ophthalmol* 118:623, 1994

Sachdev NH, Di Girolamo N, Nolan TM, et al: Matrix metalloporoteinases and tissue inhibitors of matrix metalloporoteinases in the human lens: implications for cortical cataract formation. *Invest Ophthalmol Vis Sci* 45:3863, 2004

Scroggs MW, Proia AD, Charles NC *et al.*: Calcific phacolysis. *Ophthalmology* 100:377, 1993

Shun-Shin GA, Vrensen GFJM, Brown NP *et al.*: Morphologic characteristics and chemical composition of Christmas tree cataract. *Invest Ophthalmol Vis Sci* 34:3489, 1993

Zimmerman LE, Johnson FB: Calcium oxalate crystals within ocular tissue. *Arch Ophthalmol* 60:372, 1958

Secondary Cataracts

Bekhor I, Shi S, Unakar NJ: Aldose reductase mRNA is an epithelial cell-specific gene transcript in both normal and cataractous rat lens. *Invest Ophthalmol Vis Sci* 31:1876, 1990

Cumming RG: Use of inhaled corticosteroids and the risk of cataracts. *N Engl J Med* 337:8, 1997

Garbe E, Suissa S, LeLorier J: Exposure to allopurinol and the risk of cataract extraction in elderly patients. *Arch Ophthalmol* 116:1652, 1998

Orzalesi N, Sorcinelli R, Guiso G: Increased incidence of cataracts in male subjects deficient in glucose-6-phosphate dehydrogenase. *Arch Ophthalmol* 99:69, 1981

Soemmerring W: *Beobachtungen über die Organischen Veränderungen im Auge nach Staaroperationen.* Frankfurt a.M.: Druck und Verlag von Wilhelm Ludwig Wesché, 1828

Stambolian D, Scarpino-Myers V, Eagle RC Jr *et al.*: Cataracts in patients heterozygous for galactokinase deficiency. *Invest Ophthalmol Vis Sci* 27:429, 1986

Toogood JH, Markov AE, Baskerville J *et al.*: Association of ocular cataracts with inhaled and oral steroid therapy during long-term treatment of asthma. *J Allergy Clin Immunol* 91:571, 1993

Complications of Cataracts

Brooks AMV, Grant G, Gillies WE *et al.*: Comparison of specular microscopy and examination of aspirate in phacolytic glaucoma. *Ophthalmology* 97:85, 1990

Flocks M, Littwin CS, Zimmerman LE: Phacolytic glaucoma. *Arch Ophthalmol* 54:37, 1955

Li J, Morlet N, Ng JQ *et al.*: Significant risk factors for endophthalmitis after cataract surgery: EPSWA Fourth Report. Invest Ophthalmol Vis Sci 45:1321, 2004

Smith ME, Zimmerman LE: Contusive angle recession in phacolytic glaucoma. *Arch Ophthalmol* 74:799, 1965

Yanoff M, Scheie HG: Cytology of human lens aspirate: Its relationship to phacolytic glaucoma and phacoanaphylactic endophthalmitis. *Arch Ophthalmol* 80:166, 1968

Ectopic Lens

Farnsworth PN, Burke P, Dotto ME *et al.*: Ultrastructural abnormalities in a Marfan's syndrome lens. *Arch Ophthalmol* 95:1601, 1977

Ganesh A, Smith C, Chan W *et al.*: Immunohistochemical evaluation of conjunctival fibrillin-1 in Marfan syndrome. *Arch Ophthalmol* 124:205, 2006

Gillum WN, Anderson RL: Dominantly inherited blepharoptosis, high myopia, and ectopia lentis. *Arch Ophthalmol* 100:282, 1982

Goldberg MF: Clinical manifestations of ectopia lentis et pupillae in 16 patients. *Trans Am Ophthalmol Soc* 86:158, 1988

Harrison DA, Mullaney PB, Mefer SA *et al.*: Management of ophthalmic complications of homocystinuria. *Ophthalmology* 105:1886, 1998

Jensen AD, Cross HE: Ocular complications in the Weil–Marchesani syndrome. *Am J Ophthalmol* 77:261, 1974

Koenig SB, Mieler WF: Management of ectopic lentis in a family with Marfan syndrome. *Arch Ophthalmol* 114:1058, 1996

Malbran ES, Croxatto O, D'Alessandro C *et al.*: Genetic spontaneous late subluxation of the lens. *Ophthalmology* 96:223, 1989

Razeghinejad MR, Safavian H: Central corneal thickness in patients with Weil–Marchesani syndrome. *Am J Ophthalmol* 142:507, 2006

Ramsey MS, Dickson DH: Lens fringe in homocystinuria. *Br J Ophthalmol* 59:338, 1975

Ramsey MS, Daitz LD, Beaton JW: Lens fringe in homocystinuria. *Arch Ophthalmol* 93:318, 1975

Ramsey MS, Fine BS, Shields JA *et al.*: The Marfan syndrome: A histopathologic study of ocular findings. *Am J Ophthalmol* 76:102, 1973

Ramsey MS, Fine BS, Yanoff M: The ocular histopathology of homocystinuria: A light and electron microscopic study. *Am J Ophthalmol* 74:377, 1972

Taylor RH, Burke J, O'Keefe M *et al.*: Ophthalmic abnormalities in homocystinuria: The value of screening. *Eye* 12:427, 1998

11

Neural (Sensory) Retina

NORMAL ANATOMY

I. The neural retina (Figs 11.1 through 11.3) is a highly specialized nervous tissue, in reality a part of the brain that has become exteriorized.

Although the terms *neural retina* and *sensory retina* are proper, in this chapter, because of "customary" usage, the terms *retina*, *neural retina*, and *sensory retina* are often used interchangeably. The terms refer to all the "layers" of the retina exclusive of its retinal pigment epithelium (RPE), which is discussed separately (see p. 684 in Chapter 17). The term *neurosensory retina* is redundant.

A. Traditionally the retina, from the RPE externally to the internal limiting membrane internally, is divided into 10 layers (see Fig. 11.2B).

B. The neural retina has the equivalent of both white matter (plexiform and nerve fiber layers) and gray matter (nuclear and ganglion cell layers).

C. The glial cells are represented mostly by large, all-pervasive, specialized Müller cells and, less noticeably, by small astrocytes (and possible oligodendrocytes) of the inner neural retinal layers.

D. As in the brain, a vasculature is present in which the endothelial cells possess tight junctions, producing a blood–retinal barrier.

II. Foveomacular region of the neural retina

A. Clinicians often confuse the proper use of the terms *fovea*, *macula*, and *posterior pole* (see Fig. 11.3).

1. For convenience and practicality, the three clinical terms correspond best to the three anatomic terms *foveola*, *fovea* (centralis), and *area centralis* (often called *histologic macula*). The clinical fovea, therefore, equals the anatomic foveola; the clinical macula equals the anatomic fovea; and the clinical posterior pole equals the anatomic area centralis ("histologic macula").

2. The anatomic fovea or fovea centralis (which corresponds to the clinical macula) is a depression or pit in the neural retina that is approximately the same size, especially in horizontal measure, as the corresponding optic disc (i.e., 1.5 mm).

3. The anatomic foveola (which corresponds to the clinical fovea) is a small (~350 μm diameter) reddish disc, the floor of the fovea; it is a major portion of the foveal avascular zone (1500 to 600 μm diameter).

4. The anatomic macula (which corresponds to the clinical posterior pole) comprises an area larger than the anatomic fovea.

   a. The term *macula* is derived from the term *macula lutea*.

   b. It is equated with the histologic appearance of more than a single layer of ganglion cells (i.e., area centralis).

The ganglion cell layer is a continuous, single-cell layer everywhere in the neural retina except in the macular region, where it thickens to form a multilayer.

---

   c. The anatomic macula actually encompasses an area contained just within the optic nerve and the superior and inferior retinal temporal arcades,

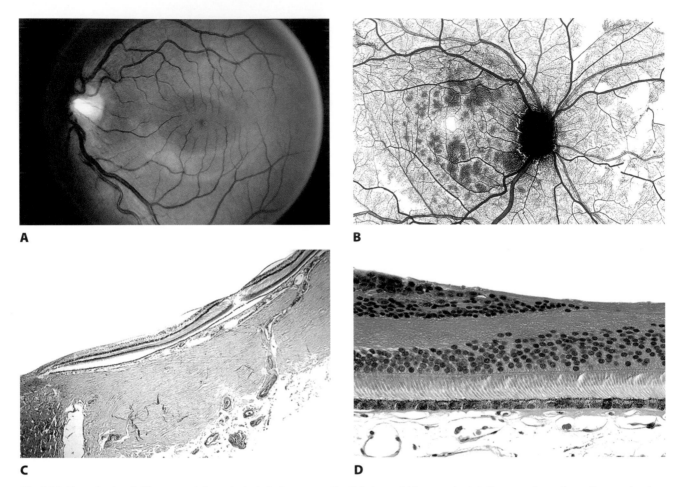

A

B

C

D

Fig. 11.1 Normal retina. **A,** The anatomic fovea (retinal pit, fovea centralis, clinical macula) is approximately the same size as the optic nerve head and is clearly seen in this child's eye as a central, horizontally oval ring reflex. **B,** A retinal trypsin digest preparation shows the dark optic nerve head, the arterioles (which have a small surrounding capillary-free zone and are narrower and darker than the venules), the retinal capillaries, the venules, and the avascular area in the central fovea, the foveal avascular zone. **C,** The ring reflex of the anatomic fovea (clinical macular reflex ring), as seen in **A,** is caused by a change in the light reflex as the retinal internal limiting membrane changes from its normal thickness to a thin basement membrane in the central fovea. **D,** Increased magnification of the anatomic central foveola (clinical fovea) shows, toward the right, the loss of all layers of the neural (sensory) retina except for the photoreceptors, the external limiting membrane, the outer nuclear layer, the outermost portion of the outer plexiform layer, and a thin internal limiting (basement) membrane. (**D,** Courtesy of Dr. RC Eagle, Jr.)

and extends temporally approximately two disc diameters beyond the central fovea.

The darkness of the central area of the anatomic macula as seen in fluorescein angiograms is caused by four factors: (1) the yellow pigment (xanthochrome) present mainly in the middle layers of the central macular retina; (2) the central avascular zone; (3) the taller, narrower RPE cells, which contain more melanin granules per unit than elsewhere; and (4) the increased concentration in the central macular RPE of lipofuscin, which acts as an orange filter in filtering out the fluorescence.

III. The retina is susceptible to many diseases of the central nervous system, as well as to diseases affecting tissues in general. In addition, the highly specialized photoreceptor cells are subject to their own particular disorders.

CONGENITAL ANOMALIES

Albinism (Fig. 11.4)

I. Oculocutaneous albinism (OCA)

A. Three subtypes of tyrosinase-negative (complete universal albinism) OCA: tyrosinase-negative albinism, platinum albinism, and yellow mutant-type albinism

1. Tyrosinase-negative OCA

a. Autosomal-recessive inheritance

b. The condition is characterized by fine white or straw-colored hair; pale, silky skin; pink irides; red pupillary glow; total iris transillumination; poor vision; nystagmus; strabismus; photophobia; hypopigmentation of the uvea; and hypoplasia of the fovea.

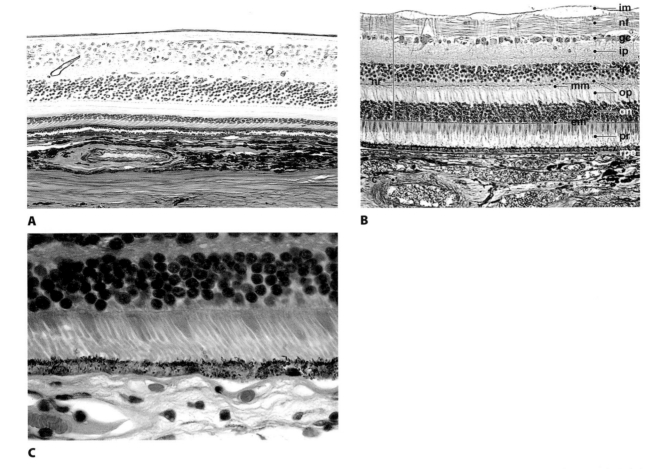

Fig. 11.2 Normal retina. **A,** The anatomic macula (posterior pole) is recognized by the multilayered ganglion cell layer, present between the inferior and superior retinal vascular arcades, and from the optic nerve temporally for a distance of approximately four disc diameters (16 mm). This periodic acid–Schiff stain clearly shows the internal limiting (basement) membrane. **B,** The retina consists of two major parts: the retinal pigment epithelium and the neural (sensory) retina. The latter can be divided into nine layers: (1) photoreceptors (rods and cones); (2) external limiting membrane [terminal bar (zonulae adherentes)—attachment sites of adjacent photoreceptors and Müller cells]; (3) outer nuclear layer (nuclei of photoreceptors); (4) outer plexiform layer (axonal extensions of photoreceptors), which contains the middle limiting membrane (desmosomelike attachments of photoreceptor synaptic expansions); (5) inner nuclear layer (nuclei of bipolar, Müller, horizontal, and amacrine cells); (6) inner plexiform layer (mostly synapses of bipolar and ganglion cells); (7) ganglion cell layer (here a single layer of contiguous cells, signifying a region outside the macula); (8) nerve fiber layer (axons of ganglion cells); and (9) internal limiting membrane (basement membrane of Müller cells) (nr, neural retina; c, choroid; im, internal limiting membrane; nf, nerve fiber layer; gc, ganglion cell layer; ip, inner plexiform layer; in, inner nuclear layer; mm, middle limiting membrane; op, outer plexiform layer; on, outer nuclear layer; em, external limiting membrane; pr, photoreceptors; rpe, retinal pigment epithelium). **C,** Increased magnification of the photoreceptors shows the inner segments to be cone- and rod-shaped. (**B,** Modified with permission from Fine BS, Yanoff M: *Ocular Histology: A Text and Atlas,* 2nd edn. Hagerstown, MD, Harper & Row, 1979:113. © Elsevier 1979. **C,** courtesy of Dr. RC Eagle, Jr.)

1). Optic misrouting, consisting of fewer than normal fibers crossing in the optic chiasm and disorganization of the dorsal lateral geniculate nuclei and their projections to the visual cortex, has been described.

2). A variant, called *minimal-pigment OCA,* differs in that minimal amounts of iris pigment and little hair or skin pigment develop in the first decade of life.

c. Histologically, the foveal pit is absent (foveal aplasia, i.e., no foveal differentiation), ocular structures contain no melanin pigment at all, the photoreceptor terminals show an abnormal synaptic apparatus, retinal pigment epithelial cells have a sparseness of rough endoplasmic reticulum, and the iris and retinal pigment epithelial cells may contain a few nonmembrane-bound, electron-dense lipofuscin granules.

B. At least seven subtypes of tyrosinase-positive (incomplete universal albinism) OCA: tyrosinase-positive albinism, brown albinism, minimal-pigment albinism, Hermansky–Pudlak syndrome (hemorrhagic diathesis), Chédiak–Higashi syndrome, rufous albinism, and autosomal-dominant albinism.

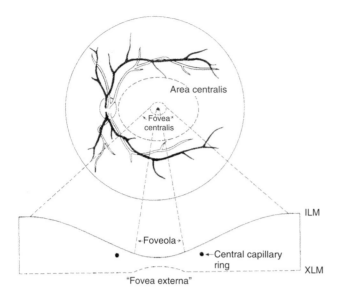

Area centralis

Fovea centralis

ILM

Foveola

Central capillary ring

XLM

"Fovea externa"

Fig. 11.3 Normal retina. Schematic drawing superimposing anatomic terminology on fundus topography. The central capillary ring is also called the *perifoveal capillary ring*. ILM, internal limiting membrane; XLM, external limiting membrane. (Modified with permission from Fine BS, Yanoff M: *Ocular Histology: A Text and Atlas*, 2nd edn. Hagerstown, MD, Harper & Row, 1979:113. © Elsevier 1979.)

In addition, *Cross syndrome* (hypopigmentation, microphthalmos, oligophrenia) and OCA with black lock and congenital sensorineural deafness may be subtypes of tyrosinase-positive (incomplete universal albinism) OCA.

---

1. Tyrosinase-positive albinism
   a. It is an autosomal-recessive inheritance disorder that has been mapped to chromosome segment 15q11–q13.
   b. The condition is more common in blacks than in whites and is characterized by ocular findings similar to those in tyrosinase-negative patients (cutaneous findings, however, are more variable).
   c. Histologically, the foveal pit is absent (foveal aplasia).
   d. A normal number of pigment granules is found, but a deficiency of melanin is present.
2. Chédiak–Higashi syndrome
   a. Inheritance is autosomal recessive.
   b. The condition is one of the immunodeficiency diseases (see p. 21 in Chapter 1) and is associated with a lack of resistance to infection and generalized lymphadenopathy. The condition is fatal from generalized infection, usually during the second decade of life.
   c. Histologically, macromelanosomes may be found in the generally depigmented RPE. The uvea shows decreased pigmentation.

Albinoidism is outlined in Table 11.1.

II. Ocular albinism
   A. Nettleship–Falls
      1. Classic ocular albinism is inherited as an X-linked recessive trait.
      2. In male patients, the condition is characterized by poor visual acuity, nystagmus, photophobia, cartwheel transillumination of the iris, and nonpigmented fundus.

      The skin appears normal clinically, but abnormalities can be seen histologically (see later).

In female carriers, cartwheel transillumination of the iris and pigmentary changes in the fundus may be seen.

---

      3. Histologically, macromelanosomes are present in the pigment epithelium of the retina, ciliary body, and iris.
         a. Fontana-positive and dopa oxidase-positive macromelanosomes are noted in the epidermis and dermis.
         b. The foveal pit is absent (foveal aplasia).

Macromelanosomes may also be found in Chédiak–Higashi syndrome, neurofibromatosis, xeroderma pigmentosum, hypertrophy of the RPE, and grouped pigmentation. Pink or red eyes and translucent irides result from the decreased amount of melanin in the stromal and pigment epithelial cells of the iris. Poor vision is caused by hypoplasia of the foveomacular area of the neural retina. Near vision is often better than distant. Nystagmus and photophobia commonly accompany the defective vision.

   B. Forsius–Erikson syndrome (Åland Island eye disease)

This is probably the same entity as X-linked incomplete congenital stationary blindness.

---

      1. Forsius–Erikson syndrome is a form of congenital night blindness.
      2. X-linked inheritance pattern is similar to the Nettleship–Falls type with the addition of a protanomalous color blindness; deletion of part of band 21 of the short arm of the X chromosome (Xp21) is found.
      3. Macromelanosomes are not found.
   C. Bergsma–Kaiser–Kupfer syndrome (autosomal dominant) is characterized by a diffuse, fine, punctate depigmentation of iris and RPE but without congenital nystagmus and foveal hypoplasia.
   D. Autosomal-recessive type is quite similar to the Nettleship–Falls type, except that it is inherited as an autosomal-recessive trait.

Grouped Pigmentation (Bear Tracks)

I. Grouped pigmentation (see Fig. 17.20) is seen as multiple, discrete, well-circumscribed, flat, uniformly pigmented areas resembling a bear's footprints.

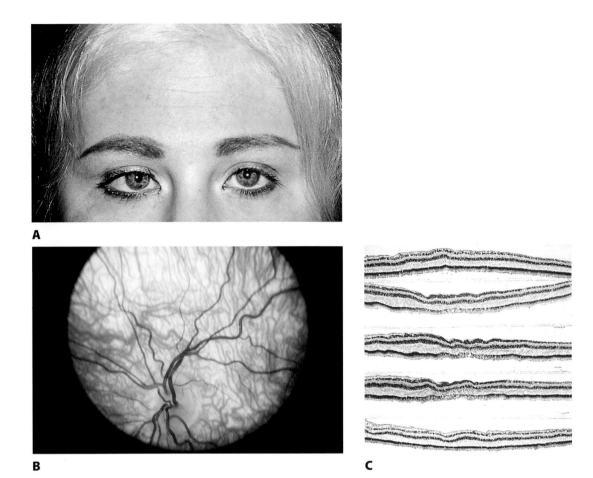

Fig. 11.4 Albinism. **A,** Albino patient uses dark eyelid and eyebrow makeup to cover lack of pigment. **B,** Another patient shows typical albinotic fundus. **C,** Histologic serial sections through the macula of another patient fail to demonstrate any fovea. (**C,** Courtesy of Prof. GOH Naumann.)

TABLE 11.1 Albinoidism

Oculocutaneous or ocular hypopigmentation without nystagmus and photophobia

A. HAIR-BULB TYROSINASE TEST POSITIVE

1.	Autosomal-dominant albinoidism
2.	Punctate oculocutaneous albinoidism
3.	Autosomal-dominant albinoidism and deafness
4.	Ocular depigmentation and Apert's syndrome
5.	Waardenburg-like syndrome
6.	Hypopigmentation–immunodeficiency disease

B. HAIR-BULB TEST NEGATIVE

1.	Menke's syndrome
2.	Prader–Willi syndrome

(Modified from Kinnear PE et al.: Surv Ophthalmol 30:75, 1985.)

II. The condition is unilateral in approximately 85% of cases and is nonprogressive.

III. It affects a single sector-shaped retinal area whose apex points to the optic disc in approximately 60% of cases. It affects several separate sectors in approximately 28% of cases, or is distributed over the entire fundus in approximately 12% of cases.

IV. Histologically, hypertrophy of the RPE and large, football-shaped pigment granules (macromelanosomes) are seen.

   A. The overlying receptors may show degeneration.

   B. The histologic appearance of grouped pigmentation is almost identical to that of congenital hypertrophy of the RPE and probably represents a clinical variant (see p. 689 in Chapter 17).

Coloboma

I. The typical coloboma "of the choroid" (see Fig. 9.8) involves the region of the embryonic cleft (fetal fissure; i.e., inferonasally), and is bilateral in 60% of patients. The coloboma may involve the total region, a large part of it, or one or more small isolated parts.

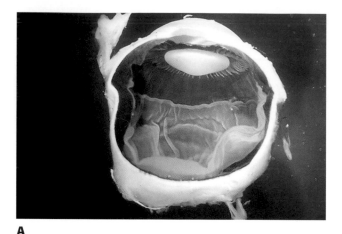

A

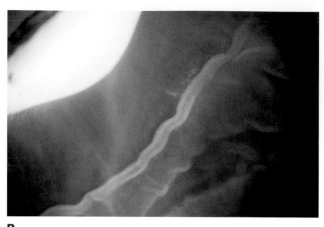

B

Fig. 11.5 Lange's fold. **A,** The inward fold of neural retina at the ora serrata (Lange's fold) is only seen in infants' and children's eyes. The fold is an artifact of fixation (see also Fig. 10.6). **B,** Increased magnification of fold.

II. Histologically, the RPE seems to be primarily involved and is absent in the area of the coloboma.
  A. The neural retina is atrophic and gliotic and may contain rosettes.
  B. The choroid is partially or completely absent.
  C. The RPE is usually hyperplastic at the edge of the coloboma.

The sclera may be thinned or even absent in the area of the coloboma, and the neural retina may herniate through in the form of a cyst (microphthalmos with cyst), undergo massive glial proliferation (massive gliosis), or both (see p. 531 in Chapter 14).

Retinal Dysplasia

See p. 747 in Chapter 18.

Lange's Fold

I. Lange's fold (Fig. 11.5; see also Fig. 10.6) is an inward fold of neural retina at the ora serrata only seen in infants' and children's eyes.
II. The fold is an artifact of fixation. It is not present *in vivo* or in an enucleated, nonfixed eye. However, it is a useful artifact because it helps to identify an eye in tissue section as that of a child.

The consistent axial and forward direction of Lange's fold may be related to the vitreous base–zonular adhesion to the inner neural retinal surface that, in infants, seems to be stronger than the peripheral neural retina–RPE adhesion.

Congenital Nonattachment of the Retina

I. Nonattachment of the neural retina (see Fig. 18.23) is normal in the embryonic eye; persistence after birth is abnormal.

II. The condition is frequently associated with other ocular abnormalities such as microphthalmos, persistent hyperplastic primary vitreous, and colobomas.
III. Histologically, the neural retina and nonpigmented epithelium of the ciliary body are separated from the pigment epithelium of the neural retina and ciliary body.

The neural retina may be normal, completely dysplastic, or anything in between.

The space between the neural retina and the RPE closes progressively during fetal life. If something should happen shortly before birth to reverse this trend and rapidly separate the two layers, a congenital neural retinal detachment, secondary in nature, would result. A *retinal dialysis* (disinsertion), usually located inferotemporally, may develop *in utero* and lead to a secondary congenital or developmental neural retinal detachment.

Neural Retinal Cysts

I. A cyst of the neural retina (see Fig. 11.56) is defined arbitrarily as an intraneural retinal space whose internal–external diameter is greater than the thickness of the surrounding neural retina and of approximately equal dimension in any direction; retinoschisis, on the other hand, is an intraneural retinal space whose internal–external diameter is smaller than the thickness of the surrounding neural retina and much smaller than the width of the space lying parallel to the neural retina.

Cyst is a poor term because a cyst, by definition, is an epithelium-lined space. However, the term (e.g., intraretinal, intracorneal, intrascleral) is frequently used to describe an intratissue space not necessarily lined by epithelium.

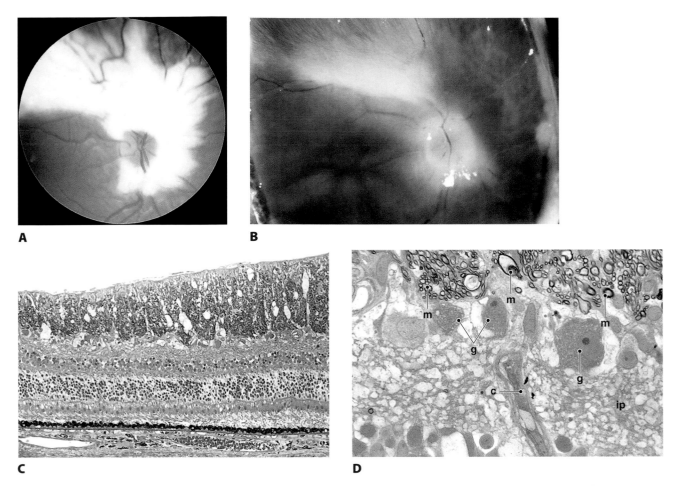

Fig. 11.6 Myelinated nerve fibers. **A,** Child referred by pediatrician because of suspected retinoblastoma. Massive myelinated nerve fibers present. **B,** Gross specimen from another patient shows a patch of myelinated nerve fibers that fan out in an upper temporal direction from the vicinity of the optic disc. Note that the heavily myelinated patch has characteristic feathered edges. **C,** Plastic-embedded thin section shows that the entire nerve fiber layer of the neural retina is thickened by myelination. **D,** Increased magnification shows myelination of nerve fibers (ganglion cell axons) just above ganglion cell layer (m, myelination of nerve fiber layer axons; g, ganglion cells; c, capillary; ip, inner plexiform layer).

II. Congenital neural retinal cysts have been reported in the periphery, usually the inferior temporal region, and in the macula.

> It is not clear if congenital cysts are in fact a manifestation of juvenile retinoschisis (see pp. 437 in this chapter). Secondary neural retinal cysts may occur in congenital nonattachment of the neural retina and in secondary congenital or acquired detachments of the neural retinal.

III. Histologically, the cysts are usually lined by gliotic neural retina and are filled with material that is periodic acid–Schiff (PAS)-positive but negative for acid mucopolysaccharides.

Myelinated (Medullated) Nerve Fibers

I. Myelinated nerve fibers (MNF; Fig. 11.6) usually occur as a unilateral condition, somewhat more common in men than in women.

A. They are seen in approximately 0.5% of eyes. MNF usually appear at birth or in early infancy and then remain stationary.

B. Rarely, MNF occur after infancy and can progress.

II. Clinically, they appear as an opaque white patch or arcuate band with feathery edges.

> The area of myelination clinically is most commonly found continuous with the optic disc, but may be seen in other parts of the neural retina. In autopsy studies, however, only approximately one-third of cases show myelination continuous with the optic nerve; perhaps myelination of the neural retina away from the optic nerve is overlooked clinically. Rarely, the condition may be inherited. The area of myelination may become involved in multiple sclerosis.

III. Histologically, myelin (and possibly oligodendrocytes) is present in the neural retinal nerve fiber layer, but the region of the lamina cribrosa is free of myelination.

Oguchi's Disease

I. Oguchi's disease, inherited as an autosomal-recessive trait, is a form of congenital stationary night blindness (see p. 445 in this chapter).

Forsius–Erikson syndrome (Åland Island eye disease) is also a form of congenital stationary night blindness.

II. The color of the fundus is unusual, varying from shades of gray to yellow; the neural retina may be involved totally or segmentally. Mizuo's phenomenon, a more normal-appearing fundus in the dark-adapted state, is present.

III. Histologically, the cones are more numerous than usual.
  A. Almost no rods are present, especially in the temporal area.
  B. Between the cones and the RPE is a nondescript, amorphous material containing pigment granules.

Foveomacular Abnormalities

I. Hypoplasia
  A. Hypoplasia is characterized by a total or nearly total absence of the clinically seen macular yellow, an absence or irregularity of the foveal reflexes, and an irregular distribution of perifoveal capillaries.
  B. Frequently, it is associated with hereditary anomalies such as aniridia, achromatopsia, X-linked hemeralopia, ocular and systemic complete and incomplete albinism, and microphthalmos.
II. Dysplasia (coloboma of macula)
  A. Many, if not most, of the foveomacular dysplasias or colobomas are secondary to congenital toxoplasmosis (see p. 88 in Chapter 4).
  B. Hereditary forms have been described with both a dominant and recessive autosomal pattern.

Leber's Congenital Amaurosis

I. Leber's congenital amaurosis is a heterogeneous group of infantile tapetoretinal degenerations characterized by connatal blindness, nystagmus, and a markedly reduced or absent response on the electroretinogram (ERG).

The differential diagnosis of connatal blindness includes hereditary optic atrophy, congenital optic atrophy, retarded myelinization of the optic nerve, albinism, aniridia, congenital cataracts, macular "coloboma," and achromatopsia. Only Leber's congenital amaurosis, however, shows an absent or markedly diminished response on ERG.

II. An autosomal-recessive inheritance pattern predominates, although a few cases of dominant transmission have been reported.

Leber's congenital amaurosis has been shown to be associated with at least six gene mutations: *GUCY2D* (encoding retinal guanylate cyclase), *RPE65* (encoding an RPE-specific 65-kD protein); *CRX* (encoding the cone–rod homeobox-containing gene); *TULP1* (encoding the Tubby-like protein 1); *AIPL1* (encoding aryl-hydrocarbon interacting protein-like 1, and the gene product APLI1 is localized exclusively in rod receptors of the adult human retina); and *CRB1*. Rarely, Leber's congenital amaurosis and keratoconus can coexist in the same patients through a genetic linkage to chromosome 17p13.1 (V).

III. The fundus shows a polymorphous picture, including a normal appearance, arteriolar narrowing, optic pallor, granular or salt-and-pepper appearance or bone spicule pigmentation (especially with increasing age), diffuse white spots, a nummular pigmentary pattern, and a local or diffuse chorioretinal atrophy with various pigmentary changes.

A variety of associated ocular findings include ptosis, keratoconus, strabismus, cataract, macular colobomas, and a "bull's-eye" maculopathy. Systemic associations include mental retardation, hydrocephalus, and the *Saldino–Mainzer syndrome* (familial nephronophthisis and cone-shaped epiphyses of the hands).

IV. A low incidence of associated neurologic disease occurs, such as a form of psychomotor retardation and electroencephalographic abnormalities.
V. Histologically, the neural retina appears normal, completely disorganized, or anything in between. In early cases outer segments of the rods and cones are missing, the cones form a monolayer of cell bodies, and the rods tend to cluster in the periphery and sprout neuritis.

Inherited Retinal Arteriolar Tortuosity

I. Inherited retinal arteriolar tortuosity is characterized by spontaneous retinal hemorrhages that resolve without sequelae. The small retinal arterioles show mild to severe tortuosity, especially in the macula.
II. It is inherited as an autosomal-dominant trait.

VASCULAR DISEASES

Definitions

I. The neural retinal circulation is predominantly arteriolar because very shortly after the central retinal artery enters the neural retina (usually by the first intraneural retinal bifurcation), it loses its internal elastic lamina and continuous muscular coat and therefore becomes an arteriole.
II. Similarly, the central retinal vein loses its thick wall and becomes a venule, usually by its first intraneural retinal bifurcation.
III. The inner half of the neural retina (approximately) is supplied by the retinal circulation (retinal capillaries); the

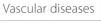

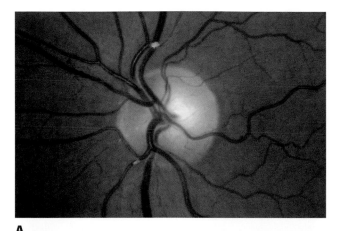

A

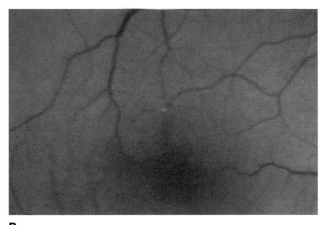

B

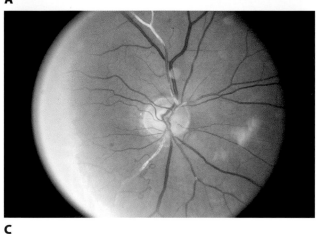

C

Fig. 11.7 Retinal vascular emboli. **A** and **B,** Different fundi with Hollenhorst plaques. **C,** Fundus shows emboli probably originating in ulcerous plaques or thrombosis of the internal carotid arteries.

outer half is supplied by the choroidal circulation (choriocapillaris).

> Clinically, the largest retinal vessels are known by common usage as arteries and veins (rather than arterioles and venules). These terms are carried over into ophthalmic pathology.

Retinal Ischemia

Causes

I. Choroidal vascular insufficiency
  A. Choroidal tumors such as nevus, malignant melanoma, hemangioma, and metastatic carcinoma may "compete" with the outer layers of the neural retina for nourishment from the choriocapillaris.
  B. Choroidal thrombosis caused by idiopathic thrombotic thrombocytopenic purpura, malignant hypertension, collagen diseases, or emboli may occlude the choriocapillaris primarily or secondarily through effects on the choroidal arterioles. Rarely, large areas of choriocapillaris may be occluded chronically by such materials as accumulating amyloid, with surprisingly good preservation of the overlying neural retina.

II. Retinal vascular insufficiency
  A. Large-artery disease anywhere from aortic arch to central retinal artery
    1. Atherosclerosis shows patchy subendothelial lipid deposits and erosion of media.
      a. The ocular manifestations of the aortic arch syndrome are similar to those seen in carotid artery occlusive disease, except that the aortic arch syndrome causes bilateral ocular involvement that tends to be severe.
      b. Embolic manifestations (Figs 11.7 and 11.8; see also Fig. 5.54)

> *Amaurosis fugax* is a common symptom. Preceding this symptom, *Hollenhorst plaques* (cholesterol emboli), less commonly, platelet–fibrin emboli, and, rarely, atrial myxoma emboli, may be observed in retinal arterioles.

  1). Emboli originate in ulcerous plaques or thrombosis of the internal and, rarely, the external carotid arteries. The emboli consist of cholesterol (Hollenhorst plaque), fibrinous, or calcific plaque materials.

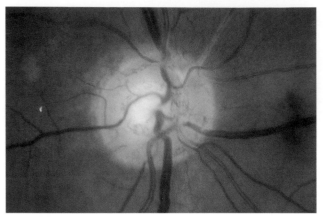

A

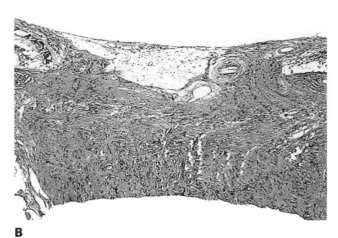

B

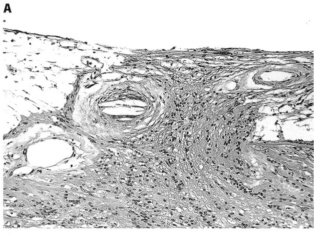

C

Fig. 11.8 Hollenhorst plaque. **A,** Clinical appearance of cholesterol embolus just before enucleation in eye of 67-year-old man who had carotid artery stenosis. **B,** Histologic section of enucleated eye shows cholesterol embolus in retinal artery on right side of optic nerve. **C,** High magnification of embolus. Note foreign-body giant cell reaction around cholesterol clefts.

2). Emboli (e.g., cholesterol, platelet–fibrin emboli, atrial myxoma, talc in drug abusers) to the visual system can cause amaurosis fugax; visual field defects; cranial nerve palsies; central or branch retinal artery occlusion; hypotensive retinopathy (venous stasis retinopathy) and the ocular ischemic syndrome (see later); narrowed retinal arterioles; central retinal vein occlusion (CRVO); and neovascularization of the iris, optic disc, or neural retina.

3). Rarely, ocular emboli cause a condition masquerading as temporal (cranial; giant cell) arteritis.

2. Takayasu's disease usually occurs in young women (frequently Japanese), shows an adventitial giant cell reaction, also involves the media, and produces intimal proliferation with obliteration of the lumen.

Takayasu's syndrome (aortic arch syndrome) occurs in older patients of either sex and differs from the "usual" type of atherosclerosis only in its site of predilection for the aortic arch. Another cause is syphilitic aortitis.

3. Central retinal artery occlusion (CRAO) has many causes, including atherosclerosis, emboli, temporal arteritis, collagen diseases, homocystinuria, and Fabry's disease. Broadly, CRAO can be divided into four types: (1) nonarteritic (NA-CRAO); (2) NA-CRAO with cilioretinal artery sparing; (3) transient NA-CRAO; and (4) arteritic CRAO.

Rarely, bilateral CRAO may occur. It usually involves elderly patients.

4. Collagen diseases, allergic granulomatosis, and midline lethal granuloma syndrome may all involve the larger retinal vessels, causing neural retinal ischemia.

5. Temporal (cranial; giant cell) arteritis (see p. 507 in Chapter 13)

B. Arteriolar and capillary disease of neural retinal vasculature

1. Arteriolosclerosis is associated with hypertension.

2. Branch retinal artery occlusion has many causes, including emboli (see Figs 11.7 and 11.8), arteriolosclerosis, diabetes mellitus, arteritis, dysproteinemias, collagen diseases, and malignant hypertension.

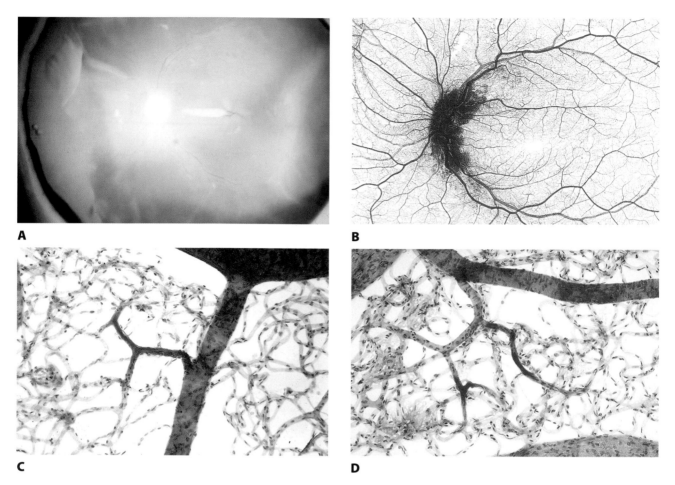

Fig. 11.9 Fatal systemic lupus erythematosus in a 26-year-old woman. **A,** Gross specimen shows numerous cotton-wool spots. **B,** Trypsin digest of retina. Large dark area is optic disc. Retinal arterioles have characteristic capillary-free zone and are darker and slightly narrower than retinal venules. **C** and **D,** Increased magnification of two different areas to show fibrinoid necrosis in transition area between end arteriole and capillary.

3. Diabetes mellitus (see Chapter 15)
4. Malignant hypertension, toxemia of pregnancy, hemoglobinopathies, collagen diseases (Fig. 11.9), dysproteinemias, carbon monoxide poisoning, and blood dyscrasias of many kinds may involve the small retinal vessels and cause neural retinal ischemia.

Leukemic retinopathy commonly occurs in both acute and chronic leukemia. The findings include venous tortuosity and dilatation, perivascular sheathing, retinal hemorrhages (including white-centered hemorrhages, simulating Roth's spots), leukemic infiltrates, cotton-wool spots, optic nerve infiltration, peripheral neural retinal microaneurysm formation, extensive capillary dropout, and even a proliferative retinopathy similar to sickle-cell retinopathy.

Complications of Retinal Ischemia

I. If localized, field defects may result. If massive, complete loss of vision may occur.

II. The ocular ischemic syndrome (OIS; ischemic oculopathy)
A. Ocular ischemia results from chronically reduced ocular blood flow through the ophthalmic artery (or the carotid artery).
1. In the anterior segment, OIS is manifested by aqueous flare, iris neovascularization, secondary angle closure glaucoma, and cataract.

OIS may be the presenting sign of serious cerebrovascular or ischemic heart disease.

---

2. In the posterior segment, OIS is manifested by venous stasis (or hypotensive) retinopathy. *Venous stasis retinopathy* is characterized by narrowed retinal arterioles; dilated, nontortuous, beaded, retinal veins; cystoid macular edema; mid peripheral dot-and-blot neural retinal hemorrhages; optic disc and neural retinal neovascularization; neural retinal detachment; and, ultimately, phthisis bulbi.

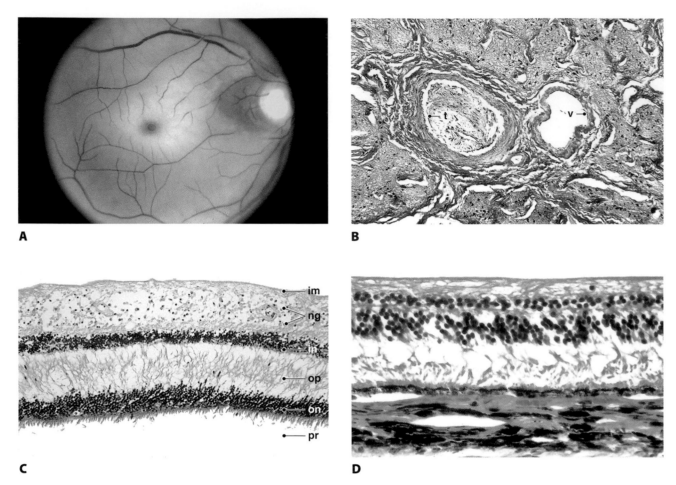

A

B

C

D

Fig. 11.10 Central retinal artery occlusion. **A,** Recent onset shows gray edema of neural retina at posterior pole exaggerating normal redness of foveal disc (i.e., cherry-red spot). Note tiny temporal cilioretinal artery has preserved a small temporal juxtapapillary island of normal neural retina. **B,** Trichrome-stained section shows an organized thrombus (t) occluding the central retinal artery in the optic nerve (v, vein). **C,** Histologic section of early stage shows edema of inner neural retinal layers and ganglion cell nuclei pyknosis. Patient had a cherry-red spot in fovea at time of enucleation (im, inner limiting membrane; ng, swollen nerve fiber and ganglion layers, in, inner nuclear layer; op, outer plexiform layer; on, outer nuclear layer; pr, photoreceptors). **D,** Histologic section of late stage shows a homogeneous, diffuse, acellular zone replacing the inner plexiform, ganglion cell, and nerve fiber layers of the neural retina. Note thin inner nuclear layer.

Unlike what occurs with chronically reduced ocular blood flow, acutely reduced ocular blood flow does not result in venous stasis retinopathy but rather is characterized by 10 or more microinfarcts (cotton-wool spots) of the neural retina.

III. Although the incidence of iris neovascularization is usually thought to be 1% to 5% in eyes after central retinal artery occlusion, some studies have suggested a much higher incidence, in the range of 18%. It is most rare after branch retinal artery occlusion.

Histology of Retinal Ischemia

I. Early (Fig. 11.10; see also Figs 11.9 and 11.15D)
   A. The neural retina shows coagulative necrosis of its inner layers, which are supplied by the retinal arterioles.
      1. The neuronal cells become edematous during the first few hours after occlusion of the artery.

2. The intracellular swelling accounts for the clinical gray neural retinal opacity.
   B. If the area of coagulative necrosis (see p. 23 in Chapter 1) is small and localized, it appears clinically as a cotton-wool spot.
      1. The cotton-wool spot observed clinically (Fig. 11.11; see also Fig. 11.9) is a result of a microinfarct of the nerve fiber layer of the neural retina.
      2. The cytoid body, observed microscopically (see Figs 11.9 and 11.11), is a swollen, interrupted axon in the neural retinal nerve fiber layer.

Histologically, the swollen end-bulb superficially resembles a cell, hence the term *cytoid body*. A collection of many cytoid bodies, along with localized edema, marks the area of the microinfarct. A *cotton-wool* spot represents a localized accumulation of axoplasmic debris in the neural retinal nerve fiber layer. They result from interruption of orthograde or retrograde organelle transport in

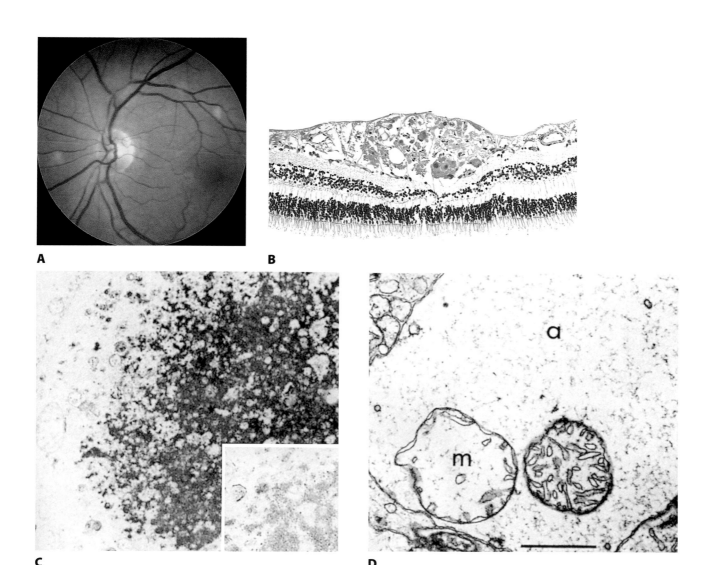

Fig. 11.11 Cotton-wool spots. **A,** Clinical appearance of cotton-wool spots. **B,** Microinfarct of nerve fiber layer produces aggregates of ruptured and enlarged axons (cytoid bodies). Cytoid bodies, observed clinically as cotton-wool spots, lie just under internal limiting membrane. **C,** Nucleoid of cytoid body consists of dense mass of filamentous material, the edge of which is more detailed in inset. **D,** Marked swelling of axon (a) in nerve fiber layer 2 hours after experimental central retinal artery occlusion (m, axonal mitochondrion). (**D,** From Kroll AJ: *Arch Ophthalmol* 79:453, 1968, with permission. © American Medical Association. All rights reserved.)

ganglion cell axons (i.e., obstruction of axoplasmic flow). Ischemia is the most common cause of focal interruption of axonal flow in the neural retinal nerve fiber layer that results in a cotton-wool spot. Any factor, however, that causes focal interruption of axonal flow gives rise to similar accumulations.

C. If the area of coagulative necrosis is extensive, it appears clinically as a gray neural retinal area, blotting out the background choroidal pattern.

The clinically seen gray area is caused by marked edema of the inner half of the neural retina. It is noted several hours after arterial obstruction and becomes maximal within 24 hours. With complete coagulative necrosis of the posterior pole (e.g.,

after a central retinal artery occlusion), the red choroid shows through the central fovea as a cherry-red spot. The foveal retina has no inner layers and is supplied from the choriocapillaris; therefore, no edema or necrosis occurs in the central fovea and the underlying red choroid is seen.

II. Late (see Fig. 11.10)
  A. The outer half of the neural retina is well preserved.
  B. The inner half of the neural retina becomes "homogenized" into a diffuse, relatively acellular zone.
  C. Usually, thick-walled retinal blood vessels are present.

Because the glial cells die along with the other neural retinal elements, gliosis does not occur. The boundaries between the different retinal layers in the inner half of the neural retina

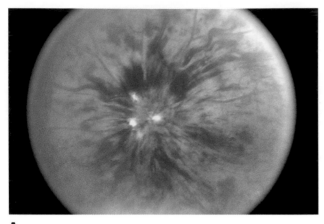

A

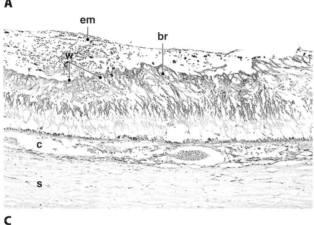

C

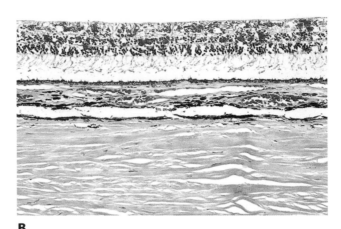

B

Fig. 11.12 Central retinal vein occlusion. **A,** Typically, widespread hemorrhages and sheets of blood are seen in the fundus. **B,** A histologic section shows blood throughout all layers of the neural retina. **C,** With healing, a glial scar is formed. A special stain for iron (Perl's stain) is positive (blue) throughout the retina (em, epiretinal membrane; br, blue staining of retina; w, wrinkled internal limiting membrane; c, choroid; s, sclera). (**A,** Courtesy of Dr. AJ Brucker.)

become obliterated. In central retinal artery occlusion, the inner neural retinal layers become an indistinguishable homogenized zone. In retinal atrophy secondary to glaucoma, to transection of the optic nerve, or to descending optic atrophy, however, the neural retinal layers, although atrophic, are usually identifiable.

Retinal Hemorrhagic Infarction (Fig. 11.12)

Causes and Risk Factors of Hemorrhagic Infarction

I. The many causes (or associations) include chronic primary open-angle glaucoma, atherosclerosis of the central retinal artery, arteriolosclerosis of the retinal arterioles, systemic hypertension, diabetes mellitus, polycythemia vera, mediastinal syndrome with increased venous pressure, dysproteinemias, and collagen diseases.

Arterial vascular disease is commonly present in retinal vein occlusion and is probably related to its cause. Also, CRVO may occur in Reye's syndrome (encephalopathy and fatty degeneration of viscera), which has a typical diphasic course, with a mild viral illness followed by severe encephalitic symptoms, especially coma.

II. Significant risk factors are systemic hypertension, open-angle glaucoma, and male sex. Race, diabetes mellitus, coronary artery disease, and stroke do not appear to be significant risk factors.

Types of Hemorrhagic Infarction

I. Occlusion of central retinal vein, branch retinal vein, or venule
  A. CRVO may be considered to consist of two distinct types.
    1. Nonischemic retinopathy

Approximately one-third of eyes that present with nonischemic retinopathy convert to the ischemic type.

    a. The retinal arterial pressure in CRVO is normal or high, unlike the low arterial pressure found in ocular ischemic syndrome (OIS).

The term *venous stasis retinopathy* is also used for nonischemic retinopathy, but is more appropriately used for the retinopathy of OIS (see earlier).

    b. The condition is probably caused by a reversible, complete occlusion of the central retinal vein, usually behind the lamina cribrosa in the substance of the optic nerve or where the vein enters the subarachnoid space, and is not accompanied by significant hypoxia.

Theoretically, the multiple collaterals available to the central retinal vein behind the lamina cribrosa allow for re-establishment of the venous circulation promptly so that only minimal and transient disturbance of circulation occurs. Perhaps approximately 65% of cases of CRVO fall into the nonischemic retinopathy group. Iris neovascularization rarely develops in nonischemic CRVO. About one-third of a nonischemic CRVO can progress to an ischemic CRVO.

---

  c. Retinal hemorrhages vary from a few, flame-shaped and punctate, to large numbers. Those in the peripheral neural retina tend to be punctate and more numerous than those in the center.

  d. Cotton-wool spots are absent or sparse.

  e. Retinal capillary perfusion is usually normal, so that the choroidal background is easily seen.

    Dilated and leaking retinal capillaries can be seen with fluorescein angiography.

  f. Two subgroups may be identified: one subgroup involves young people in whom some evidence suggests that the condition is most probably inflammatory in origin, caused by phlebitis of the central retinal vein that produces venous thrombosis (see discussion of papillophlebitis, later in this subsection); a second subgroup involves older people who have arteriosclerosis, which probably plays an important role in the venous occlusion.

The second subgroup may consist of two types: one (sometimes called *incomplete occlusion*) shows normal retinal arterial circulation and normal or slightly slowed retinal venous circulation; the other (sometimes called *venous stasis retinopathy*) shows slow retinal arterial and venous circulation. Both show normal capillary perfusion.

---

  g. With time, perhaps one-third of nonischemic types convert to ischemic retinopathy.

2. Ischemic (hemorrhagic) retinopathy

  a. The disease is caused by occlusion of the central retinal vein at, or anterior to, the lamina cribrosa, associated with retinal ischemia that leads to significant retinal hypoxia.

    1). Few venous collateral channels are available to the central retinal vein at, or anterior to, the lamina cribrosa; therefore, severe obstruction of retinal venous flow results.

    2). Perhaps approximately 35% of cases of CRVO fall into the ischemic group. Iris neovascularization occurs in most eyes that have ischemic CRVO.

  b. Neural retinal hemorrhages are usually gross and extensive ("blood and thunder" fundus).

    Cotton-wool spots and retinal capillary nonperfusion are prominent, resulting in partial or complete obscuration of the underlying choroidal pattern. The optic nerve head is usually edematous.

Extensive retinal capillary closure 1 month after vein occlusion (central or branch) or extensive leakage and a broken capillary arcade at the fovea, as determined by fluorescein angiography, indicates a poor visual prognosis. When neovascularization of the neural retina or iris develops, it is invariably in those patients who have extensive retinal capillary closure.

---

3. Eight to 20% of CRVOs occur in patients who already have chronic primary open-angle glaucoma or in whom it will develop.

In at least 80% of eyes that have CRVO uncomplicated by neovascularization of the iris, the intraocular pressure is lower in the eye with the occlusion than in the normal fellow eye. The reduction of intraocular pressure is greater: (1) in those eyes with CRVO than in those with branch-vein occlusion; (2) in those eyes with ischemic retinopathy than in those with nonischemic retinopathy; and (3) in patients who have high pressures in their fellow eyes. The pressure reductions persist for at least 2 years after occlusion.

---

4. Bilateral CRVO may occur as part of the acquired immunodeficiency syndrome (AIDS).

B. Branch retinal vein occlusion

1. Branch retinal vein occlusion occurs approximately three times more frequently than CRVO. In approximately two-thirds of cases, the superior temporal neural retinal vein is involved.

  a. Most of the remaining cases show involvement of the inferior temporal retinal vein.

  b. Rarely, the inferior (or superior) branch of the central retinal vein may be involved, resulting in an inferior (or superior) hemispheric vein occlusion.

  c. A hemispheric vein occlusion behaves like an ischemic CRVO.

2. The occlusion most often occurs in the fifth or sixth decade of life and develops at an arteriovenous crossing.

3. If significant and widespread retinal capillary nonperfusion is present, neovascularization of the optic nerve head, neural retina, or both develops in a high percentage of cases. Iris neovascularization does not occur.

It is important to differentiate retinal venous collaterals from neovascular areas. The former prove to be beneficial, whereas the latter may require photocoagulation therapy.

---

4. Visual acuity may be decreased because of cystoid macular edema (approximately 50% of cases) or foveal hemorrhage.

II. Papillophlebitis (retinal vasculitis, mild and moderate papillary vasculitis, benign retinal vasculitis, optic disc vasculitis)

   A. Papillophlebitis is characterized by a unilateral, partial, reversible central retinal venous occlusion presumably caused by venous inflammation. It usually occurs in young, healthy men and exhibits a benign, somewhat protracted course.

   B. Ophthalmoscopic findings include edema of the optic nerve head, peripapillary neural retina, and sometimes macula; retinal venous dilatation and tortuosity; and scattered, superficial, mid peripheral retinal hemorrhages.

   C. The prognosis for vision is excellent.

      The main sequelae are perivenous sheathing of large veins at the posterior pole and dilated venules over the optic nerve head.

III. Terson's syndrome (see p. 493 in Chapter 12)

Complications of Hemorrhagic Infarction

   I. Macular hemorrhagic infarction may result in permanent loss of vision.

   II. Leakage of fluid into the macula may result in cystoid macular edema.

   III. Iris neovascularization (clinically seen rubeosis iridis)

      A. Iris neovascularization (see Figs 9.13 and 9.14) occurs mainly with ischemic CRVO; it rarely occurs with nonischemic CRVO or occlusion of a branch vein or venule.

      B. Approximately 60% of patients older than 40 years of age have iris neovascularization after ischemic CRVO (rarely after nonischemic CRVO). Iris neovascularization usually does not appear before 6 weeks after occlusion, usually becomes established before 6 months, and, if untreated, causes neovascular glaucoma.

Early, the anterior-chamber angle may show neovascularization for 360° and yet still be open and cause a secondary open-angle glaucoma. This stage tends to be fleeting, peripheral anterior synechiae develop, and a secondary closed-angle glaucoma ensues. The glaucoma is called *neovascular glaucoma.*

      C. Iris neovascularization is rare in people who are younger than 40 years of age at the time of their CRVO.

   IV. Neovascularization of the neural retina (Fig. 11.13) occurs mainly with branch vein or venular occlusion; it rarely occurs with ischemic or nonischemic CRVO.

   V. Neural retinal detachment secondary to branch retinal vein occlusion may occur when the vein occlusion is severe and accompanied by marked capillary nonperfusion and leakage.

   VI. Optociliary shunt vessels (i.e., usually large veins connecting the choroidal and retinal circulations at the optic nerve head) may develop after CRVO.

Optociliary shunt vessels are mainly seen in three clinical situations: as congenital anomalies; as the result of CRVO; and in association with orbital tumors, especially optic nerve sheath meningiomas. The vessels may also be seen in optic nerve juvenile pilocytic astrocytomas (gliomas), arachnoid cysts, optic nerve colobomas and drusen, and with chronic atrophic optic disc edema.

VII. Exudative neural retinal detachment

Histology of Retinal Hemorrhagic Infarction
(See Fig. 11.12)

   I. Early—hemorrhagic necrosis of neural retina

      A. Massive intraneural retinal hemorrhage involves all the neural retinal layers.

         1. The hemorrhage frequently spreads within the nerve fiber layer of the neural retina (see Fig. 15.15) and appears clinically in sheets or flame-shaped.

         2. Rarely, the hemorrhage spreads into the potential submembranous (between the internal limiting membrane and the nerve fiber layer) space and appears clinically as anteriorly placed neural retinal pockets of blood ("subhyaloid" hemorrhage).

      B. Cytoid bodies (see Fig. 11.11) are common histologically, but may be masked by the hemorrhages clinically.

      C. As the hemorrhages resorb, hard, waxy exudates may appear (see p. 606 in Chapter 15, and later).

      D. Optic disc edema usually accompanies the hemorrhagic necrosis of the neural retina in the acute phase.

   II. Late—organization of hemorrhage and gliosis

      A. The architectural pattern of the neural retina, especially the inner neural retinal layers, is frequently disrupted.

      B. Gliosis ("scarring") is usually seen in the inner neural retinal layers.

      C. Hemosiderosis of the retina (see Fig. 11.12C) is present, the hemosiderin often being located in macrophages.

      D. Thick-walled blood vessels are seen in the neural retina.

Hypertensive and Arteriolosclerotic Retinopathy*

   I. Hypertensive retinopathy (Fig. 11.14)

      A. Grade I: a generalized narrowing of the arterioles

      B. Grade II: grade I changes plus focal arteriolar spasms

      C. Grade III: grade II changes plus hemorrhages and exudates

         1. Flame-shaped (splinter) hemorrhages (see Figs 11.12 to 11.14; see also Fig. 15.15) are characteristic in the nerve fiber layer.

         2. Dot-and-blot hemorrhages (see Figs 11.13 and 15.15) may be seen in the inner nuclear layer with spreading to the outer plexiform layer.

         3. Cotton-wool spots (see Figs 11.11 and 11.14; see p. 405 in this chapter) are characteristic and are a result of microinfarction of the nerve fiber layer,

---

It is easier to understand the underlying histopathology if the hypertensive and arteriolosclerotic retinopathies are graded separately.

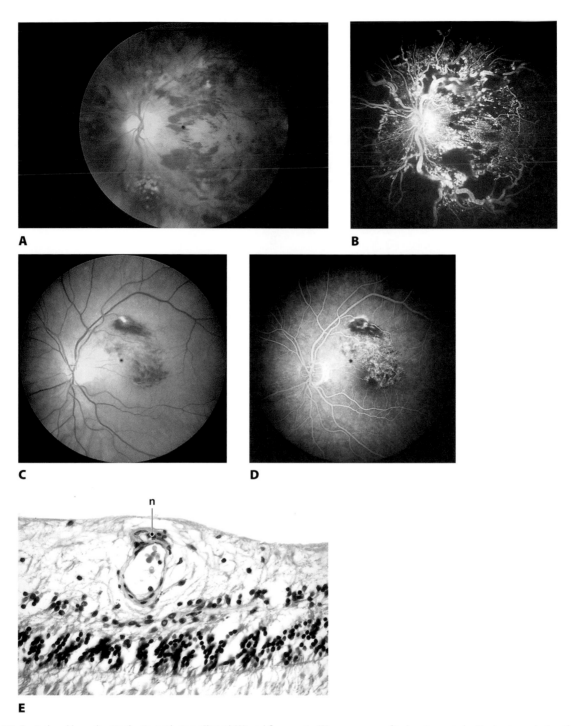

Fig. 11.13 Central and branch retinal vein occlusion. Clinical (**A**) and fluorescein (**B**) appearance of ischemic central retinal vein occlusion. If neovascularization develops (high probability in this case), it will be of the iris. Clinical (**C**) and fluorescein (**D**) appearance of branch retinal vein occlusion. If neovascularization develops, it will be of the neural retina or optic nerve, or both. **E,** Histologic section of new blood vessels (n, neovascularization) budding off from a retinal venule.

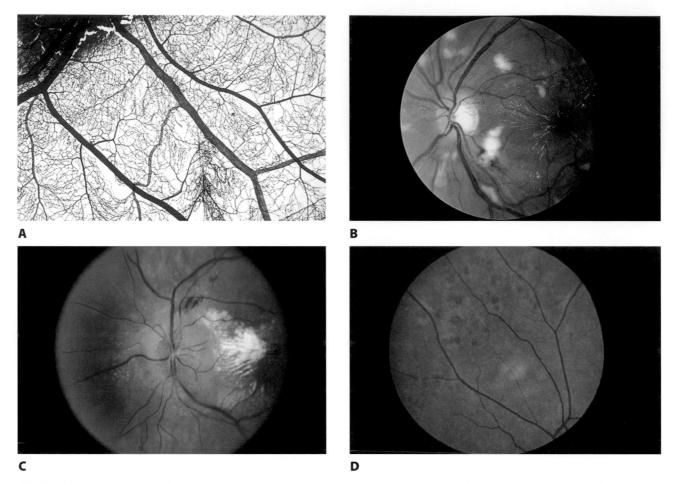

Fig. 11.14 Hypertensive retinopathy. **A,** Trypsin digest preparation of retina from hypertensive patient shows narrowing of arterioles (darker, narrower vessels). **B,** Left eye from patient with marked hypertension and grade III hypertensive retinopathy. Note cotton-wool spots (areas of axoplasmic flow backup) and macular star (exudates in Henle's outer plexiform layer of neural retina). **C,** Grade IV hypertensive retinopathy shows optic disc edema. **D,** The presence of Elschnig's spots is a late manifestation.

which produces aggregates of cytoid bodies (i.e., swollen axons of ganglion cells caused by interruption of axonal flow).

Cotton-wool spots may be seen in many conditions, such as collagen diseases, CRVO, blood dyscrasias, AIDS, and multiple myeloma.

---

4. Hard (waxy) exudates may be seen; these are lipophilic exudates located in the outer plexiform layer (see Figs 11.14, 15.13, and 15.14).

When the exudates are numerous in the macula and lie in the obliquely oriented and radially arranged fiber layer of Henle, they appear as a macular star.

D. Grade IV: all the changes of grade III plus optic disc edema

---

Necrosis, thinning, clumping, and proliferation of the RPE may occur as a result of obliterative changes in the choriocapil-

laris in malignant hypertension. Four types of fundus lesions associated with choroidal vascular changes have been recognized clinically: (1) pale yellow or red patches bordered to a varying extent by pigment deposits; (2) black, isolated spots of pigment with a surrounding yellow or red halo caused by complete obstruction of terminal choroidal arterioles and choriocapillaris by fibrin thrombi (*Elschnig's spots*; see Fig. 11.14D); (3) linear chains of pigment flecks along the course of a yellow-white sclerosed choroidal vessel (*Siegrist's spots*); and (4) yellow or red patches of chorioretinal atrophy.

II. Arteriolosclerotic retinopathy (Fig. 11.15)
   A. Grade I: an increase in the arteriolar light reflex

Subintimal hyalin deposition and a thickened media and adventitia cause the normally transparent arteriolar wall to become semiopaque, producing an increased light reflex.

B. Grade II: grade I changes plus arteriolovenular crossing defects

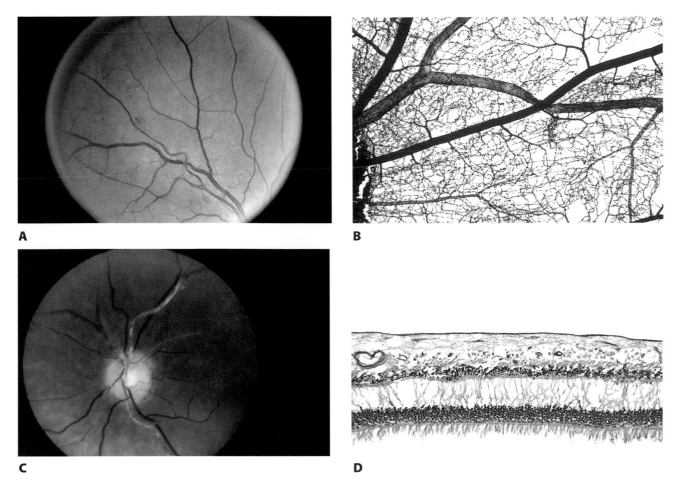

Fig. 11.15 Arteriolosclerotic retinopathy. **A,** Fundus shows grade II hypertensive changes (narrowing and focal spasms of arteriole) and grade II arteriolosclerotic changes [increased arteriolar light reflex and arteriolovenular (AV) crossing defects]. Note dilatation or banking of end of venule distal (to left) of AV defect and narrowing of proximal end. Dilatation caused by backup of venous blood secondary to constriction at crossing by arteriolar adventitia. **B,** Trypsin digest preparation of retina shows AV crossing defect caused by mild arteriolosclerosis involving the common adventitial sheath. **C,** Grade IV arteriolosclerotic changes characterized by silver-wire appearance in superior and inferior retinal arterioles. Other arterioles show grade III arteriolosclerotic changes characterized by copper-wire appearance. **D,** Thickened retinal vessel stained with periodic acid–Schiff (on far left of neural retina) shows arteriolosclerosis. Inner layers of neural retina show marked edema and necrosis of ganglion cells secondary to acute central retinal artery occlusion.

The semiopaque wall of the arteriolosclerotic arteriole, which shares a common adventitia with the venule where they cross, obscures the view of the underlying venule. This results in the clinically seen arteriolovenular crossing defects, or "nicking."

C. Grade III: grade II changes plus "copper-wire" arterioles

The arteriolar wall becomes sufficiently opaque so that the blood column can only be seen by looking perpendicularly through the surface of the wall (i.e., looking through the thinnest area). The arteriole has a burnished or copper appearance owing to reflection of light from the thickened and partially opacified wall.

D. Grade IV: grade II changes plus "silver-wire" arterioles

The wall becomes totally opaque so that the blood column in the lumen cannot be seen. The light is then reflected completely from the surface of the thickened vessel, giving a white or silver appearance. The lumen of the arteriole may or may not be patent. Patency can best be determined by fluorescein angiography.

Hemorrhagic Retinopathy

I. Neural retinal hemorrhages (see Figs 11.12 and 15.15) may be caused by many diseases, such as diabetes mellitus (see Chapter 15), sickle-cell disease, retinal venous diseases, hypertension, blood dyscrasias, leukemias, polycythemia vera, subacute bacterial endocarditis, cytomegalovirus retinitis, acute retinal necrosis (ARN), lymphomas, idiopathic thrombocytopenia, trauma, multiple myeloma, pernicious anemia, collagen diseases, carcinomatosis, anemia, and many others.

Anemia or thrombocytopenia alone rarely causes neural retinal hemorrhages. Anemia and thrombocytopenia combined, however, not infrequently result in neural retinal hemorrhages; when the two are severe (hemoglobin <8 g/100 ml and platelets <100 000/mm), neural retinal hemorrhages may occur in 70% of patients.

II. Histologically, the size and anatomic location of the hemorrhage determine its clinical appearance (see Fig. 15.15).
III. Roth's spots
   A. Roth's spots are a special type of neural retinal hemorrhage characterized by a white center and associated with bacterial endocarditis.

It was Litten who described the association (Litten's sign) and referred to it as *Roth's spots*.

   B. Although the white spots are usually thought to represent septic microabscesses caused by septic microemboli, they probably represent capillary rupture, extravasation, and formation of a central fibrin–platelet plug.

Exudative Retinopathy

I. Retinal exudates (see Figs 11.14, 15.13, and 15.14)
   A. Neural retinal exudates may be caused by the same conditions that cause hemorrhagic retinopathy (see earlier); waxy exudates may occur simultaneously with the hemorrhages, alone, or after the hemorrhage resorbs.
   B. Cotton-wool spots (cytoid bodies), which are not exudates, are usually found in ischemic neural retinal conditions and represent microinfarction of the innermost neural retinal layers, associated with interruption of axoplasmic flow.
II. Circinate retinopathy consists of a circular deposit of masses of hard, waxy exudates around a clear area, often within the anatomic macula.
   A. It is degeneration secondary to ischemic vascular disease (e.g., diabetes mellitus).
   B. Histologically, the exudates are identical to isolated, small, hard, waxy exudates.
III. Histology
   A. Hard, waxy exudates (see p. 606 in Chapter 15)
   B. Cotton-wool spots (cytoid bodies; see p. 404 in this chapter and p. 610 in Chapter 15)

Diabetes Mellitus

See Chapter 15.

Coats' Disease, Leber's Miliary Aneurysms, and Retinal Telangiectasia

See p. 751 in Chapter 18.

Idiopathic Macular Telangiectasia (Idiopathic Juxtafoveolar Retinal Telangiectasis)

See p. 753 in Chapter 18.

Retinal Arterial and Arteriolar Macroaneurysms

I. Macroaneurysms of the retinal arteries and arterioles (Fig. 11.16) may be congenital or acquired.
   A. Congenital entities include angiomatosis retinae and the diseases of Eales, Leber, and Coats.
   B. Acquired macroaneurysms occur in people (most often women) who have hypertension or arteriosclerosis, or both, and less often have diabetic retinopathy, retinal vein occlusion, retinal arteritis, cytomegalovirus retinitis, radiation and sickle-cell retinopathies, hyperviscosity entities, Takayasu's disease, and aortic arch syndromes.
II. Most macroaneurysms involute spontaneously without sequelae.
III. The macroaneurysms may be associated with circinate retinopathy, intraneural retinal hemorrhage, subneural retinal hemorrhage, or even intravitreal hemorrhage.

Hemorrhage in the neural retina along with a subneural retinal hemorrhage ("dumbbell shape") should alert the clinician to the possibility of macroaneurysm.

IV. Histologically, spherical or fusiform aneurysms arise from arterial or arteriolar walls.

Sickle-Cell Disease

I. Sickle-cell disease (Figs 11.17 and 11.18) is caused by a point mutation in the hemoglobin gene.
   A. Polymerization of the abnormal hemoglobin subunits in an anoxic or acidic environment results in the typical sickle configuration of the erythrocytes.
   B. The sickled erythrocytes are much more rigid than normal ones and cause occlusions of small vessels.
II. The retinopathy is most severe with sickle-cell hemoglobin C disease (SC disease) but may also occur in other sickle hemoglobinopathies, including sickle thalassemia, sickle-cell disease, and even in occasional cases of sickle-cell trait.
III. Classification of retinopathy
   A. Stage I: peripheral arteriolar occlusion (between the equator and the ora serrata)
      1. The primary site of occlusion appears to be at the precapillary arteriole level.
      2. The most likely cause of the occlusion is obstruction of the small precapillary arterioles by sickled erythrocytes.
   B. Stage II: peripheral arteriolovenular anastomoses (most commonly in the temporal quadrant)
      1. Arteriolovenular anastomoses appear to be the initial vascular remodeling at the junction of the

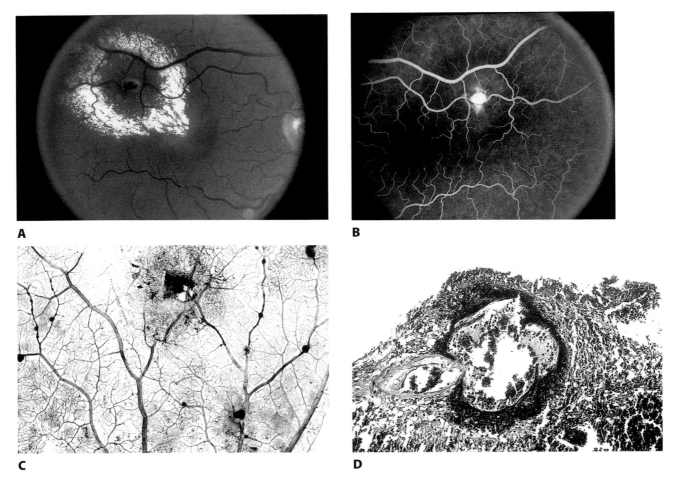

A

B

C

D

Fig. 11.16 Retinal arteriolar macroaneurysm (RAM). **A,** RAM is surrounded by exudation. **B,** RAM shown clearly in fluorescein angiogram. In another case, RAM shown in periodic acid–Schiff-stained trypsin digest preparation (**C**) and in cross-section (**D**). (**C** and **D,** Courtesy of Dr. BW Streeten; case shown in **C** and **D** reported by Fichte C *et al.: Am J Ophthalmol* 85:509. © Elsevier 1978.)

perfused central and nonperfused peripheral neural retina in the region of the equator.

2. The development of arteriolovenular anastomoses most likely is not a neovascular process but rather represents the formation of preferential vascular channels from pre-existing vessels.

C. Stage III: neovascular and fibrous proliferations

1. New vessels arise from pre-existing arteriolovenular anastomoses, on the venular side.

2. When a neovascular patch remains relatively isolated from neighboring patches and coalescence does not occur, the characteristic *sea-fan* anomaly may be observed, most commonly in SC disease.

> The characteristic fibrovascular extraretinal formation is called a *sea fan* because of its resemblance to the marine invertebrate sea fan, *Geogonia flabellum*.

3. Areas of retinal pigment epithelial hypertrophy, hyperplasia, and migration (black sunbursts), which

develop after intraneural and subneural retinal hemorrhage, may occur in all stages, occur posterior to the equator, and may be seen most commonly in sickle-cell disease but also in SC disease.

4. Salmon-patch hemorrhage may occur in sickle-cell disease and SC disease.

a. The salmon-patch hemorrhage, which may be single or multiple, may be seen in all stages of the retinopathy.

b. It is usually found in the mid-periphery adjacent to a retinal arteriole.

c. Initially, the hemorrhages are bright red (but not quite the same red as hemorrhages in a nonsickler), but within a few days become salmon (orange-red)-colored.

d. Within weeks, the lesions evolve into yellow or yellow-white nodules or plaques.

Further resolution results in intraneural retinal retinoschisis, a focal patch of thinned neural retina, or a pigmented scar.

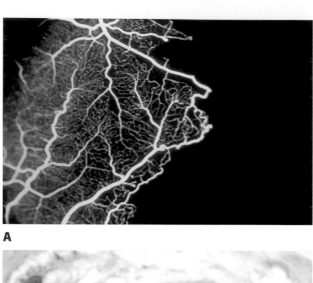

A

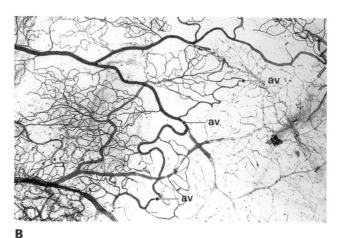

B

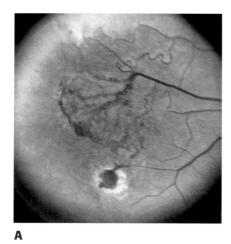

C

Fig. 11.17 Sickle-cell hemoglobin C disease. **A,** The perfusion of the retina stops abruptly at the equator, resulting in nonperfusion of the peripheral retina. **B,** Trypsin digest of the equatorial region of the retina (in this case, of sickle-cell hemoglobin C disease) shows that peripheral blood vessels are devoid of cells and are nonviable. Arteriolovenular collaterals (av) are noted in the equatorial region. **C,** A peripheral arteriole is occluded by sickled red blood cells. (**A-C,** Periodic acid–Schiff stain; case reported by Eagle RC *et al.: Arch Ophthalmol* 92:28, 1974. © American Medical Association. All rights reserved.)

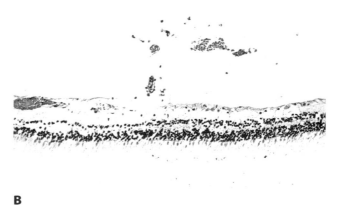

A   **B**

Fig. 11.18 Sickle-cell hemoglobin C disease. **A,** A sea fan is present at the equator and a sunburst is seen below the sea fan. **B,** A histologic section shows that the sea fan lies between the internal surface of the retina and the vitreous body. The neovascularization proceeds from a retinal arteriole into the subvitreal space and then back into a retinal venule. (**A,** Courtesy of Dr. MF Rabb.)

The pigmented scar is called a *black sunburst* (see earlier) and results from the resolution of a salmon patch.

D. Stage IV: vitreous hemorrhage (usually arising from a neovascular patch)

E. Stage V: neural retinal detachment. The detachment of the neural retina may be nonrhegmatogenous (traction) or rhegmatogenous (caused by a neural retinal tear).

IV. The pathogenesis of sickle-cell retinopathy is unknown, but is probably related to local hypoxia (secondary to sickled erythrocytes occluding preretinal arterioles), similar

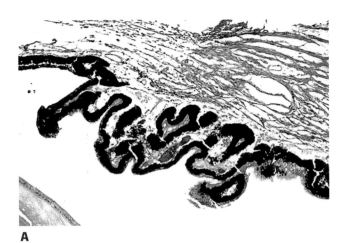
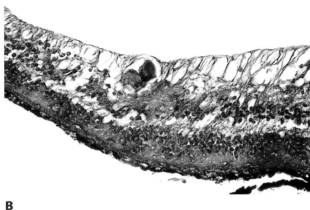

A   **B**

Fig. 11.19 Disseminated intravascular coagulation (DIC). Phosphotungstic acid hematoxylin shows fibrin clot in vessel in pars plicata of ciliary body (**A**) and in retinal arteriole (**B**) in infant who had DIC. (Case reported by Ortiz JM *et al.*: *Arch Ophthalmol* 100:1413, 1982. © American Medical Association. All rights reserved.)

to what occurs in diabetes mellitus, retinopathy of prematurity, carotid occlusive disease, and Takayasu's disease.

Eales' Disease (Primary Perivasculitis of the Retina)

I. Eales' disease occurs typically in young men, usually in their third decade.

It occurs most commonly in the Indian subcontinent.

II. Over 90% of the cases are bilateral.
III. The disease progresses slowly; rapid progression, however, is common as a late event.
   A. Initially, a slight, localized edema of the peripheral neural retina involves only the small venous branches. Exudates around the involved vessels or sheathing of the vessels can be seen.
   B. Next, the larger venules become involved. Neovascularization develops from venules in the neural retina and the new vessels enter the subvitreal space, where they are vulnerable to hemorrhage.
   C. A fibrous membranous component develops (i.e., retinitis proliferans). Shrinkage and traction by the fibrovascular membranes may cause a secondary neural retinal detachment.

The total progression is similar to that in diabetic retinopathy. Rarely, a central form occurs and affects the large central venules. Fluorescein shows obliteration of the venules, producing large areas of capillary nonperfusion toward the neural retinal periphery.

IV. The cause of the disease is unknown.

Retinopathy of Prematurity

See pp. 748–751 in Chapter 18.

Hemangioma of the Retina

I. Hemangioma of the neural retina, a hamartomatous lesion, may be associated with similar cavernous hemangiomas of brain and with angiomatous hamartomas of skin, or it may occur alone.
II. Cavernous hemangioma of the neural retina as an isolated finding is rare.
   A. The hemangioma is congenital, benign, stationary, unilateral, most frequent in women, composed of clusters of dark red saccular aneurysms containing venous blood, and rarely the source of intraocular hemorrhage.
   B. They are not usually discovered before adulthood, when they may be discovered as an incidental finding or may become symptomatic secondary to an overlying serous neural retina detachment.

Rarely, they may be associated with retinal neovascularization.

III. Histologically, a cavernous type of hemangioma of the neural retina is seen.

Hereditary Hemorrhagic Telangiectasia (Rendu–Osler–Weber Disease)

See p. 225 in Chapter 7.

Disseminated Intravascular Coagulation

I. Disseminated intravascular coagulation (DIC; Fig. 11.19) is a syndrome in which a physiologic imbalance occurs between clotting and lysis of clot.
   A. Inappropriate triggers to coagulation result in endothelial injury stimulating the intrinsic cascade, or tissue factor stimulating the extrinsic cascade.

DIC can develop secondary to septicemia in patients who have AIDS.

B. Characteristically, disseminated microthrombi form in small vessels, especially in the kidneys, heart, and brain.

C. Coincident with microthrombi formation, a gradual depletion of coagulation factors, platelets, and fibrin ensues, resulting in a change from a hypercoagulable to a hypocoagulable state.

1. Clinically, gross hemorrhage, thrombosis, or both, or only disordered coagulation parameters, may be found.

2. Detection of the cross-linked fibrin degradation fragment, D-dimer, in patients at risk for DIC is strong evidence for the diagnosis.

a. D-dimer confirms that both thrombin and plasmin generation have occurred.

b. Laboratory D-dimer measurements are less sensitive but highly specific, whereas the fibrinogen degradation product (FDP) test is more sensitive but less specific; performing the two tests in tandem (screening with FDP and confirming with D-dimer) maximizes sensitivity and specificity.

II. Histologically, fibrin thrombi are noted most frequently in the choriocapillaris, often in the macular region with secondary neural retinal detachment. Fibrin may be found in capillaries in the retina, iris, ciliary body, and optic nerve.

INFLAMMATIONS

Nonspecific Retinal Inflammations

Secondary retinitis is usually caused by a vasculitis.

A. It may be secondary to keratitis, iridocyclitis, choroiditis, or scleritis.

B. Perivasculitis occurs around venules with the perivascular infiltrate composed of lymphocytes and plasma cells.

Specific Retinal Inflammations
(See Chapters 2, 3, and 4)

I. A toxic, exudative retinopathy may occur with carbon monoxide intoxication.

II. Septic retinitis of Roth *(Roth's spots)* occurs with a bacteremia, especially with subacute bacterial endocarditis (see p. 412 in this chapter).

III. Endogenous mycotic retinitis (e.g., candidiasis) results from fungus infection.

IV. Viral retinitis

A. Herpes simplex retinitis (see p. 270 in Chapter 8)

1. Type 1 herpes simplex virus produces lesions in nongenital sites, including the mouth, cornea (see Fig. 8.13), skin above the waist, and in the central nervous system.

a. Type 1 virus is a rare cause of retinitis in children and adults.

b. The virus may cause encephalitis.

2. Type 2 herpes simplex virus (see Fig. 3.6) is transmitted as a venereal infection, usually producing lesions below the waist, except in newborns, in whom it may infect any organ. Approximately 20% of neonates infected with type 2 virus have ocular manifestations, including retinitis.

B. Cytomegalic inclusion disease (see p. 77 in Chapter 4)

V. Acute posterior multifocal placoid pigment epitheliopathy (APMPPE), also called *acute multifocal ischemic choroidopathy*, tends to occur in young women and shows multifocal, gray-white placoid lesions at the level of the RPE and involving predominantly the posterior pole, but occurring anywhere in the fundus.

Fluorescein angiography during the acute phase of the disease process shows early blockage of background fluorescence, followed by later staining of the lesions, similar to the findings in Dalen–Fuchs nodules. Cerebral vasculitis may accompany APMPPE. Indocyanine green videoangiopathy suggests choroidal hypoperfusion as the underlying cause.

A. The lesions resolve rapidly, but may leave permanent retinal pigment epithelial alterations.

B. The acute process may result from a primary retinal pigment epithelial inflammation, an acute multifocal choroiditis (choriocapillaris), or random occlusions of the precapillary arterioles feeding the lobules of the choriocapillaris.

C. The histology is unknown.

VI. Acute retinal pigment epitheliitis is characterized by an acute onset, mainly in the posterior pole, that resolves fairly rapidly, usually in 6 to 12 weeks.

A. The acute lesion is a deep, fine, dark gray, sometimes black spot, often surrounded by a halo and that may disappear with healing.

In the choroidal phase, fluorescein angiography shows a window defect of the depigmented halo that surrounds the lesion. The defect does not change in size or shape, nor leak dye, during the later phases of the angiogram.

B. The cause and histology are unknown.

VII. Acute macular neuroretinopathy

A. Acute macular neuroretinopathy, a rare condition, tends to occur bilaterally in young women and shows subtle, reddish-brown, wedge- or tear-shaped (pointing to the fovea) lesions in the fovea.

1. The symptoms are scotomata and minimal depression of visual acuity, which may be transient or permanent. An associated recent systemic immunologic disturbance is common and suggests an immune-based cause.

2. Fluorescein angiography is negative or shows mild dilatation and faint hypofluorescence of the lesion.

Rarely, acute macular neuroretinopathy and multiple evanescent white-dot syndrome (MEWDS; see later) occur in the same patient. Because of overlap and transitional

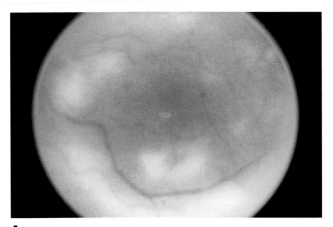

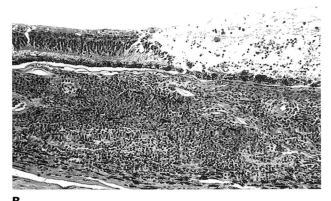

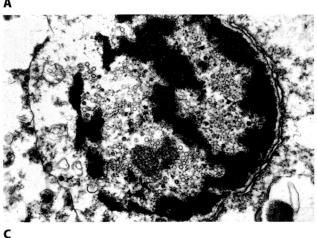

Fig. 11.20 Acute retinal necrosis. **A,** Fundus view is cloudy because of vitreous reaction. **B,** Neural retina shows sharp demarcation from necrotic retina on right and viable retina on left. Intranuclear inclusion bodies found in necrotic retina. **C,** Electron micrograph shows herpeslike virus capsids in nucleus. (Presented by Dr. JDM Gass at the meeting of the Eastern Ophthimic Pathology Society, 1981.)

cases, the idiopathic entities acute macular neuroretinopathy, MEWDS, acute idiopathic blind-spot enlargement syndrome, multifocal choroiditis, or pseudopresumed ocular histoplasmosis syndrome (POHS) may be classified together under the term *acute zonal occult outer retinopathy* (AZOOR).

   B. The cause and histology are unknown.
VIII. Birdshot retinopathy (vitiliginous retinochoroidopathy; diffuse inflammatory salmon-patch choroidopathy)
   A. The condition is characterized by:
     1. A quiet eye (rarely red or injected, but not painful), usually in children or young adults
     2. Minimal, if any, anterior-segment inflammation but chronic inflammation in the vitreous
     3. Usually bilateral, and fairly symmetric, retinal vascular leakage (retinal vasculitis), especially in the macula, so that cystoid macular edema and optic disc edema may result
     4. Distinctive, multiple, cream-colored or depigmented spots, usually discrete, and mostly around the optic disc, radiating out toward the equator
     5. Development of disc pallor, diffuse RPE changes, macular edema, and narrowed retinal arterioles over a period of 6 to 24 months (ERG abnormalities may be found)

A strong association exists with the human leukocyte antigen (HLA)-A29 (especially HLA-A29.2 subtype) *in vitro* (approximately 80% to 90% of patients who have birdshot retinopathy are HLA-A29-positive) and with cell-mediated responses to S-antigen. Also, elevated EA rosettes and C4 complement level may be seen.

---

     6. The ultimate visual prognosis is poor.
   B. This uncommon uveitic syndrome is of presumed autoimmune cause; the histology is unknown.

Patients who have Lyme disease (see p. 83 in Chapter 4) may also carry the HLA-A29 antigen; conversely, patients who have birdshot retinopathy and carry the HLA-A29 antigen may also have antibodies against *Borrelia burgdorferi*. It is still unclear, however, whether this is a cause-and-effect relationship.

IX. Acute retinal nerosis (ARN) (Fig. 11.20)
   A. The condition, which may affect both healthy and immunocompromised people, consists of acute peripheral necrotizing retinitis, retinal arteritis, and vitreitis.

Atypical, severe toxoplasmic retinochoroiditis in the elderly can mimic ARN.

B. After 1 to 3 months, neural retinal detachments develop, followed by proliferative vitreoretinopathy.

C. Approximately 50% of cases are bilateral.

D. The condition is caused most commonly by the varicella-zoster virus (46%) and also by herpes simplex virus types 1 (25%) and 2 (21%).

1. ARN may result from activation of latent, previously acquired infection, usually herpes zoster dermatitis (shingles).

2. Rarely, ARN may develop during the course of primary varicella-zoster (chickenpox) infection.

3. Viral antibodies have been found in intrathecally produced cerebrospinal fluid from patients who have ARN, suggesting central nervous system involvement.

E. Histologically, by light microscopy, Cowdry type A intranuclear inclusions, and by electron microscopy, intranuclear aggregates of viral particles can be seen in the areas of disorganized, necrotic retina.

X. Multiple evaescent white dot syndrome (MEWS)

A. This transient choriorioretinopathy affects young adults, mainly women, is unilateral, and has an acute onset of decreased visual acuity and paracentral scotomas.

B. Multiple, small, white or gray-white dots occur at the level of the superficial choroids–RPE posteriorly to mid peripherally.

C. Vitreal cells, reduced visual acuity, and abnormalities in the ERG and early receptor potential may be found.

1. Fluorescein leakage occurs from optic nerve head capillaries along with late staining of the RPE.

2. Late indocyanine green angiography shows dual-layered highly specific, small, hypofluorescent lesions overlying larger hypofluorescent lesions.

3. Rarely, choroidal neovascularization (CNV) may occur. Also rarely, MEWDS and acute macular neuroretinopathy occur in the same patient.

Acute idiopathic blind-spot enlargement without optic disc edema may be a subset of MEWDS. Because of overlap and transitional cases, the idiopathic entities acute macular neuroretinopathy, MEWDS, acute idiopathic blind-spot enlargement syndrome, multifocal choroiditis, or POHS may be classified together under the term *acute zonal occult outer retinopathy* (AZOOR).

D. The cause and histology are unknown.

XI. Unilateral acute idiopathic maculopathy (UAIM)

A. UAIM occurs in young adults who experience sudden, severe visual loss (to 20/200 or worse), often after a flulike illness, caused by an exudative maculopathy.

1. Initially, an irregular neural retinal detachment overlying a smaller, grayish thickening at the RPE level is noted.

2. Fluorescein angiography shows early irregular hyperfluorescence and hypofluorescence at the RPE level, followed in the late phase by complete staining of the overlying neural retina detachment (similar to the late staining of an RPE detachment).

3. A rapid and complete resolution usually takes place (vision 20/25 or better).

4. Some cases show eccentric macular lesions, subneural retinal exudation, papillitis, and bilaterality; association with pregnancy and human immunodeficiency virus may also occur.

XII. Diffuse unilateral subacute neuroretinitis (see p. 91 in Chapter 4)

XIII. Retinal pigment epitheliopathy associated with the amyotrophic lateral sclerosis/parkinsonism–dementia complex (ALS/PDC) of Guam

A. An extremely high rate of ALS/PDC exists among the native Chamorro population of Guam.

B. Approximately 10% of the Chamorro population have a pigment epitheliopathy that resembles ophthalmomyiasis; the rate is approximately 50% among those who have ALS/PDC.

C. Histologically, focal areas of attenuation of the RPE and a reduced amount of intracellular pigment correlate with the fundus lesions.

1. No larvae are found.

2. The pathogenesis is unknown.

XIV. Acute multifocal retinitis

A. Acute multifocal retinitis usually occurs in otherwise healthy, young to middle-aged adults who experience acute loss of vision, often preceded by a flulike prodrome.

B. The areas of retinitis tend to be posterior and localized to the inner retina, varying in size from 100 to 500 μm in diameter.

The retinal lesions are often multiple and bilateral.

a. Vision usually returns to normal without treatment in 1 to 4 weeks.

b. Optic disc edema may occur.

c. Fluorescein angiography shows early hypofluorescence and late staining of retinal lesions.

d. Occasional patients have a history of a cat scratch and test positively for *Bartonella henselae* antibodies (most patients test negatively).

INJURIES

See Chapter 5.

DEGENERATIONS

Definitions

Degenerations are a result of previous disease (i.e., ocular "fingerprints" left by prior disease).

Microcystoid Degeneration

I. Typical peripheral microcystoid degeneration (Blessig–Iwanoff cysts; Figs 11.21 and 11.22)

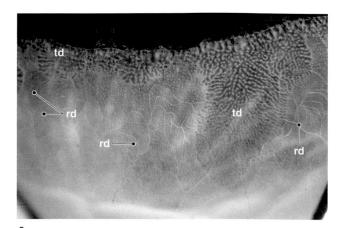

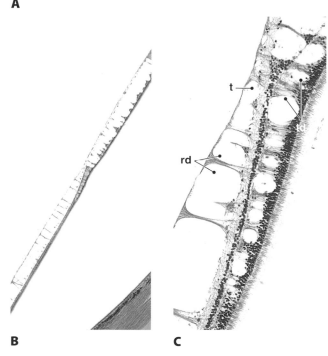

B   **C**

Fig. 11.21 Typical and reticular microcystoid degeneration. **A,** Typical microcystoid degeneration (td) starts just posterior to the ora serrata. Reticular cystoid degeneration (rd) is present just posterior to the typical microcystoid degeneration. **B,** A transitional zone from typical to reticular cystoid degeneration is seen. The typical microcystoid degeneration is to the right (shown under increased magnification in **C;** t, transitional zone; td, middle retinal layers; rd, inner retinal layers). (**B** and **C,** Courtesy of Dr. RY Foos.)

A. Microcystoid peripheral degeneration of the neural retina appears clinically as myriad, tiny, interconnecting channels in the peripheral neural retina, especially temporally.

B. All persons 8 years of age or older show the lesion. It may also be present at birth, with increasing neural retinal involvement up to the seventh decade of life.

C. The tendency is toward relatively equal bilateral involvement.

1. The temporal neural retina is involved more than the nasal, and the superior sectors are affected more than the inferior.
2. Relative neural retinal sparing occurs in the nasal and temporal horizontal meridians (the greatest sparing nasally).

D. The degeneration always seems to begin at the ora serrata. From there, it extends posteriorly and circumferentially.

E. Histologically, spaces within the neural retina (cysts) are located in the outer plexiform and adjacent nuclear layers.

1. Early, the cysts are limited to the middle layers of the neural retina. Later, they may extend to the external and internal limiting membranes of the neural retina.
2. Although they appear empty in hematoxylin and eosin-stained sections, they contain hyaluronic acid, which is best seen with special stains.

   The septa separating the cysts are composed of glial–axonal tissue rich in the cytochrome oxidase enzyme system.
3. As microcysts coalesce, an intraneural retinal macrocyst or retinoschisis cavity is formed when the macrocyst is at least 1.5 mm in length (one average disc diameter).

Pars plana cysts (see Fig. 9.11) are intercellular cysts of the nonpigmented layer of ciliary epithelium and may be filled with hyaluronic acid. They may also contain the protein of multiple myeloma.

II. Reticular peripheral cystoid degeneration (see Fig. 11.21)

A. Reticular peripheral cystoid degeneration appears clinically posterior to typical peripheral microcystoid degeneration. The subsurface retinal vasculature arborizes into fine branches throughout the reticular lesion.

B. The condition is seen in approximately 13% of autopsy eyes and is bilateral in approximately 41%. It can be found in every decade of life without a clear relationship to aging.

C. The inferior and superior temporal regions, each involved to approximately the same extent, are more affected than the inferior and superior nasal regions.

Typical microcystoid peripheral degeneration of the neural retina is always found as an accompanying neural retinal lesion. In some instances, the reticular lesion may become partially surrounded by the posterior extension of typical microcystoid peripheral degeneration. A number of macroscopic features distinguish reticular from typical microcystoid peripheral degeneration. The retinal vasculature, when traced from uninvolved neural retina posteriorly, arborizes into fine branches throughout the reticular lesion, whereas only the larger vessels are apparent in typical lesions. In reticular lesions, the neural retina is less transparent than in typical lesions. The lateral and posterior borders of reticular lesions are linear and angular, often coinciding with the course of large retinal arte-

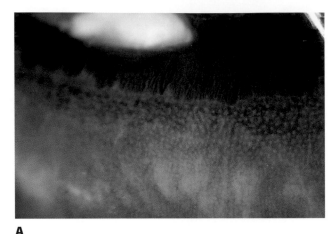

A

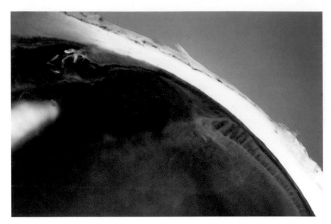

B

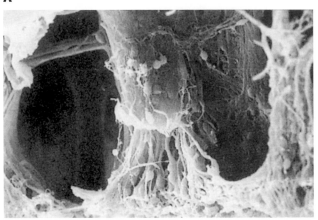

C

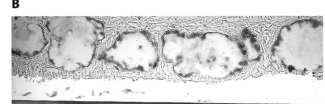

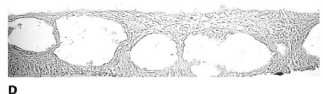

D

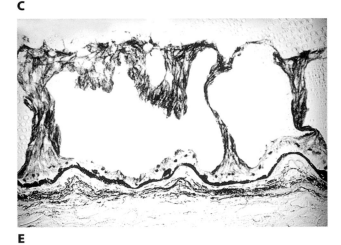

E

Fig. 11.22 Typical microcystoid degeneration. **A,** Gross specimen shows that typical microcystoid degeneration starts just posterior to ora serrata. **B,** Gross appearance in cross-section. **C,** Scanning electron microscopic appearance (receptors at bottom). **D,** Both top and bottom stained for acid mucopolysaccharides; bottom digested with hyaluronidase before staining. Note disappearance of positive staining in microcyst. **E,** Diphosphopyridine nucleotide diaphorase (nitro-blue tetrazolium method). Glial–neuronal columns show dense precipitate of formazan, signifying the presence of the cytochrome oxidase system. (**C,** Courtesy of Dr. RC Eagle, Jr.)

rioles and venules; typical lesions usually have a smoothly rounded margin.

D. Histologically, the neural retinal cysts of reticular peripheral cystoid degeneration are located in the nerve fiber layer of the neural retina.

1. Early, the cysts are located completely within the nerve fiber layer; later, they may extend from the internal limiting membrane to the inner plexiform layer.

2. The cysts contain hyaluronic acid.

3. Similar nerve fiber layer cystic changes can be seen in the neural retina in areas adjacent to the retinoschisis cavity in juvenile retinoschisis (p. 437 in this chapter).

Degenerative Retinoschisis

I. Retinoschisis—typical degenerative senile (adult) type (Fig. 11.23)

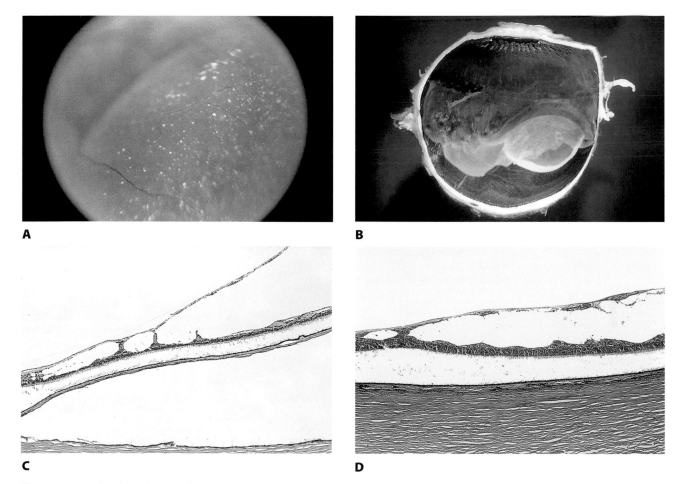

Fig. 11.23 Typical and reticular cystoid degeneration. **A,** A large, dome-shaped retinoschisis is present. Glistening yellow-white dots are seen on its surface. **B,** Gross appearance of retinoschisis. Also note detachment of vitreous base (*upper left*), the result of previous trauma. **C,** Histologic section shows on left-side rupture of middle limiting membrane and of restraining glial–neuronal columns, cleaving neural retina into inner and outer layers (i.e., typical retinoschisis). **D,** Here, on left side, cleaving of the neural retina takes place in the inner layers (i.e., reticular retinoschisis).

Retinoschisis may be defined as an intraneural retinal tissue loss or splitting at least 1.5 mm in length (one disc diameter). It is differentiated from a neural retinal cyst by its configuration—namely, a neural retinal cyst has approximately the same diameter in all directions (and usually a narrow neck), whereas the diameter of retinoschisis parallel to the neural retinal surface is greater than the diameter perpendicular to the surface.

A. Typical retinoschisis is seen in approximately 4% of patients, and is bilateral over 80% of the time.
B. It is most common after the age of 40 and rare before the age of 20 years.
C. Characteristically, it is found in the peripheral inferior temporal quadrant (approximately 70% of cases), with the superior temporal quadrant (approximately 25%) the next most common site; little tendency exists for the retinoschisis to progress posteriorly, but the posterior border is postequatorial in approximately 75% of cases.

The splitting of neural retinal tissue in the area of retinoschisis results in an absolute scotoma. Occasionally, the retinoschisis

involves only the macular area. In most of the macular cases, ocular trauma seems to be the initiating factor.

D. The inner layer of retinoschisis has a characteristic beaten-metal or pitted appearance and frequently has tiny, glistening, yellow-white dots.

The glistening yellow-white dots have been thought to be reflections from the remnants of ruptured glial septa clinging to the internal limiting membrane of the neural retina. However, the dots are not found in all cases, and biomicroscopy shows that they seem to lie internal to the neural retinal internal limiting membrane. Probably, the glial remnants cause an uneven external surface to the inner wall of the retinoschisis cavity and produce the beaten-metal appearance.

E. Neural retinal holes tend to be small and numerous in the inner wall and large and singular in the outer wall (just the reverse of juvenile retinoschisis).

Although retinoschisis can mimic a neural retinal detachment, clinical examination usually shows the difference. In difficult cases, photocoagulation may help to distinguish one from the other. After photocoagulation, a detached neural retina usually shows no blanching effect, but in retinoschisis the outer layer becomes blanched. Rarely, however, blanching can occur with rhegmatogenous neural retinal detachment. Another difference is that retinoschisis shows an absolute scotoma but neural retinal detachment usually shows a relative scotoma.

F. Histologically, a splitting is seen in the outer plexiform layer and adjacent nuclear layers. The cavity is filled with a hyaluronidase-sensitive acid mucopolysaccharide, presumably hyaluronic acid.
   1. As the area of the retinoschisis enlarges, the involved neural retina is destroyed.
   2. The inner wall in advanced retinoschisis is usually made up of the internal limiting membrane, the inner portions of Müller cells (remnants of ruptured glial septa), remnants of the nerve fiber layer, and blood vessels.
   3. The outer wall mainly consists of the outer plexiform layer, the outer nuclear layer, and the photoreceptors.
   4. Bridging the gap between the inner and outer walls are occasional strands or septa composed of compressed and fused remnants of axons, dendrites, and Müller cells.

Senile retinoschisis may develop from a coalescence of the cysts of microcystoid degeneration. Microcystoid degeneration, however, is present in 100% of people older than 8 years of age. Senile retinoschisis is present in approximately 4% of people. Therefore, if senile retinoschisis does arise from peripheral microcystoid degeneration, it does so only in a small number of cases. The cause of the progression to retinoschisis is unknown.

II. Retinoschisis—reticular degenerative (adult) type (see Fig. 11.23)
   A. Reticular retinoschisis is found in approximately 2% of autopsy cases, and is bilateral approximately 16% of the time.
      1. A band of typical microcystoid degeneration always separates the schisis from the ora serrata.
      2. It may occur concomitantly with typical degenerative retinoschisis.
   B. It is most common after the fifth decade and rare before the fourth.
   C. It has a predilection for the inferior temporal quadrant.
   D. Round or oval holes may be present in the outer wall, but rarely in the inner wall.
   E. Histologically, the inner wall of the schisis is composed of the neural retinal internal limiting membrane and minimal remnants of the nerve fiber layer.
      1. The outer wall is made up of receptors and outer nuclear and plexiform layers.
      2. The area of involvement is similar to that found in juvenile retinoschisis (see p. 437 in this chapter).

Secondary Microcystoid Degeneration and Retinoschisis

I. Microcystoid degeneration and retinoschisis have been found in a variety of pathologic conditions such as long-standing neural retinal detachment, choroidal tumors (especially malignant melanomas, hemangiomas, and metastatic carcinomas), age-related macular degeneration (ARMD), retinopathy of prematurity, Coats' disease, retinal angiomatosis, diabetic retinopathy, uveitis, parasitic disease, and aplastic anemia.

II. Histologically, secondary microcystoid degeneration and retinoschisis are similar to the primary typical type, except that in the secondary form the cystoid spaces do not usually contain an acid mucopolysaccharide.

In infants, retinoschisis secondary to trauma may have a cleavage plane much more internal in the neural retina than does the typical senile type or the usual secondary type. This internal cleavage plane resembles the area of involvement in reticular retinoschisis and in hereditary juvenile retinoschisis.

Paving Stone (Cobblestone) Degeneration (Peripheral Chorioretinal Atrophy; Equatorial Choroiditis)

I. The lesions of paving stone degeneration (Fig. 11.24) tend to increase in incidence and in size with age and with axial length of the eye.
   They are present in approximately 25% of autopsy cases and bilateral in approximately 38%.

II. The lesions are located primarily between the ora serrata and equator and are separated from the ora serrata by normal neural retina.
   A. The lesions are nonelevated, sharply demarcated, yellow-white, single or multiple, separate or confluent, and often contain prominent choroidal vessels.
   B. They are most common in the inferior temporal quadrant (approximately 78%), with the inferior nasal quadrant the next most common site (approximately 57%).
   The lesions often coalesce and extend in a band with scalloped borders, from temporal to nasal areas in the inferior neural retina.

III. Histologically, the lesions are characterized by:
   A. Neural retinal thinning in an area devoid of pigment epithelium and an intact Bruch's membrane with the neural retina closely applied to it.

With artifactitious detachment of the neural retina (e.g., after fixation) the neural retina in the area of the paving stone degeneration remains attached. Paving stone degeneration, therefore, is not a predisposing factor for neural retinal detachment and may actually protect against it neural retinal detachment.

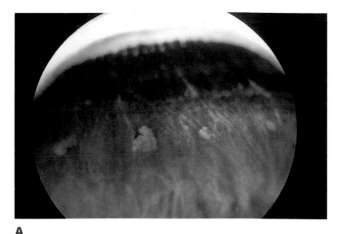

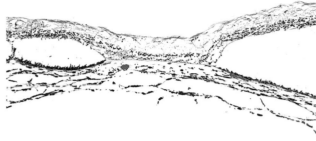

A **B**

Fig. 11.24 Paving stone degeneration. **A,** Typical circumferential lesions near ora serrata. **B,** Retinal pigment epithelium ends abruptly in area of degeneration. Bruch's membrane is intact, but the overlying neural retina (especially outer layers) and the underlying choroid show atrophic changes.

B. An absent choriocapillaris (especially at the center of the lesion) or a partially obliterated choriocapillaris or sometimes only minimal abnormalities such as thickening of the walls of the choriocapillaris; the choroid is otherwise normal
C. Hypertrophy and hyperplasia of the pigment epithelium at the lesion's margin

Peripheral Retinal Albinotic Spots

I. Areas of hypopigmentation in the neural retinal periphery are caused by depigmentation of the RPE.
II. Although the lesions are probably degenerative, a congenital cause cannot be ruled out.

Myopic Retinopathy

I. Myopia of a small or moderate degree is not usually associated with neural retinal degenerative changes.
II. Progressive, pathologic, or "high" myopia (greater than 6 diopters of myopia) affects the neural retina most severely in the posterior pole and in the periphery.
  A. The globe is mainly enlarged in its posterior third, with thinning of the sclera.
  B. Surrounding the optic disc and usually extending temporally (but possibly extending in any direction) to involve the posterior pole, the thinned sclera bulges posteriorly to form a staphyloma that is lined by a thin and atrophic choroid.
  C. Bruch's membrane may develop small breaks (lacquer cracks) through which connective tissue may grow beneath the RPE.

The breaks in Bruch's membrane in the macular region may lead to CNV and a small hemorrhage that later organizes and becomes pigmented. This appears clinically as a small, dark, macular lesion known as *Fuchs' spot* (actually a "mini" exudative macular degeneration).

D. The overlying neural retina in the posterior pole thins and degenerates, affecting mainly the outer layers.
E. The peripheral neural retina also becomes thin and atrophic and, therefore, more susceptible to neural retinal tears.

Macular Degeneration

Idiopathic Serous Detachment of the RPE (Fig. 11.25)

I. The condition occurs mainly in men between the ages of 20 and 55 years.
  A. It is characterized by a sharply demarcated, dome-shaped elevation of the RPE.
  B. Fluorescein angiography shows early and persistent filling of the whole area of detachment.
II. Serous RPE detachments have a good prognosis, and probably are a variant of idiopathic central serous choroidopathy.
  A. Most RPE detachments are between one-fifth and one-half disc diameter, rarely reaching two disc diameters.
  B. Most resorb or flatten, leaving behind a disturbance of pigmentation.

Tears or rips in the RPE result in a profound reduction in vision. When serous RPE detachments occur in patients older than 50 years of age, they may be accompanied by CNV. A flattened or notched border of a detached RPE is an important sign of occult CNV, and may be visualized using indocyanine green angiography. Serous RPE detachments may occur as a component of idiopathic central choroidopathy or in association with entities such as ARMD (dry or exudative types), angioid streaks, or POHS. The detachments should be distinguished from multiple vitelliform lesions, a variant of Best's disease (see p. 442 this chapter).

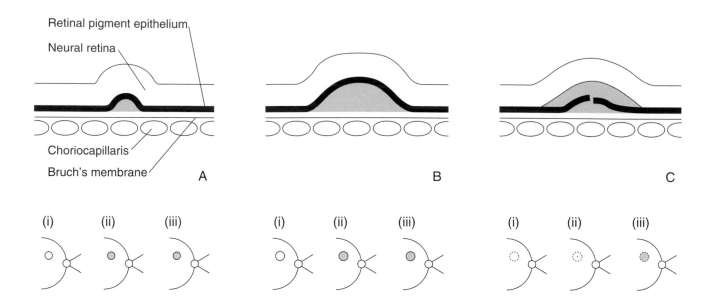

Fig. 11.25 Detachments of the retinal pigment epithelium and neural retina. The schematic histology drawings in the upper panels correspond with the schematic drawings of the fundus in the lower panels. **A,** A small, simple retinal pigment epithelium (RPE) detachment. **B,** A large RPE detachment. **C,** A small RPE detachment with an overlying neural retina (NR) serous detachment. The triple drawings of the fundus represent: (i) before fluorescein injection; (ii) the early fluorescein stage; and (iii) the late fluorescein stage. Note that the RPE detachments are sharply demarcated and completely fill with fluorescein in the late stage, whereas the NR serous detachment has fuzzy borders and does not fill completely in the late stage.

Idiopathic Central Serous Choroidopathy (Central Serous Retinopathy; Central Angiospastic Retinopathy) (See Fig. 11.25)

I. Typically, idiopathic central serous choroidopathy occurs in healthy young adults (most commonly men) between the ages of 20 and 40 years, often after emotional stress.

A positive association exists between central serous retinopathy and gastroesophageal reflux disease (GERD). Also, circulating glucocorticoid and mineralocorticoid levels are abnormal in many patients who have central serous retinopathy and may contribute to its pathogenesis. Other risk factors include systemic steroid use; pregnancy; alcohol, antibiotic, antihistamine, and tobacco uses; autoimmune disease; untreated hypertension; and previous ocular surgery.

II. The symptoms are those of metamorphopsia, positive scotoma, and micropsia.
III. The condition recurs in approximately one-fourth to one-third of patients and occasionally may become bilateral.
IV. Clinically the involved area, most often in the macula, shows fluid under the neural retina. Because the area is not sharply demarcated from normal retina, the borders of the detached neural retina are fuzzy. Often tiny white spots are seen in the area.
V. A localized detachment of the neural retina may be associated with a tiny detachment of the RPE.
   A. Early fluorescein angiography shows a tiny "beacon" of light, which is fluorescein entering the sub-RPE space.

B. Fluorescein then spreads slowly into the large subneural retinal space, classically showing smokestack and umbrella configurations in the early phases. In the late phases, the fluorescein fills the subneural retina space incompletely so that the boundaries of neural retina detachment are not sharply demarcated and show fuzzy borders.

Neural retinal detachments may spread inferiorly, resulting in inferior hemispheric RPE atrophic tracts or gutters.

VI. The basic defect appears to be in Bruch's membrane or the choriocapillaris, or both, but the underlying cause is unknown.
VII. Most cases heal spontaneously with restoration of normal vision.

Sometimes the course is prolonged. Tiny yellow precipitates, probably lipid-filled macrophages, are often seen on the outer surface of the detached neural retina. A chronic course may result in irreversible changes in the RPE and neural retina. Such changes may also result from recurrent attacks. Idiopathic central serous choroidopathy can be simulated by secondary central serous retinopathy, secondary to ocular conditions such as peripheral choroidal malignant melanoma (see Fig. 17.34), choroidal hemangioma, and pars planitis, or such systemic entities as thrombotic thrombocytopenic purpura, malignant hypertension, eclampsia, and Harada's disease. Although idiopathic central serous choroidopathy typically involves the posterior pole, it can occur in any part of the posterior half of the eye, including regions nasal to the optic disc.

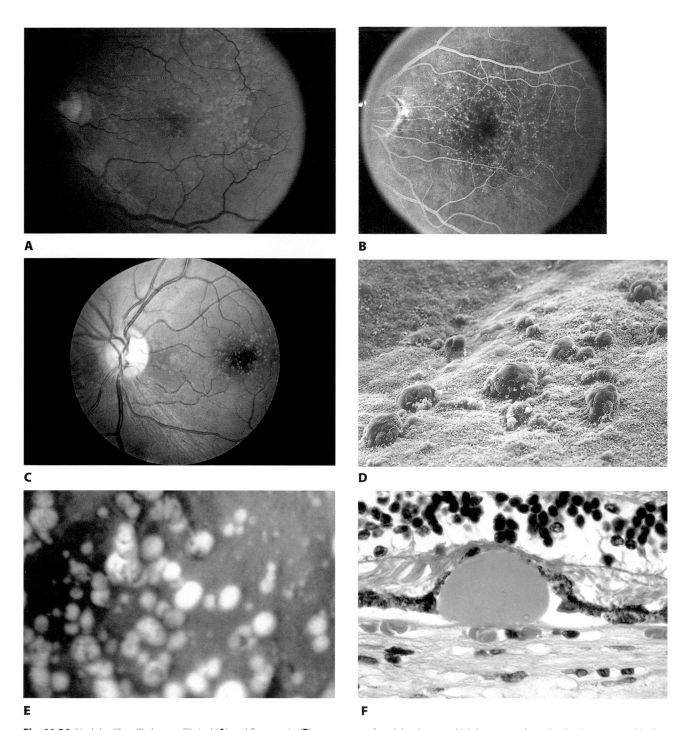

A

B

C

D

E

F

Fig. 11.26 Nodular ("hard") drusen. Clinical (**A**) and fluorescein (**B**) appearance of nodular drusen, which have a random distribution scattered in the posterior pole. **C,** Basal laminar drusen appear in clusters in the posterior pole. Scanning electron microscopic (**D**) and gross (**E**) appearance of nodular drusen. **F,** Histologic section shows an eosinophilic nodular druse external and contiguous to the original thin basement membrane of the retinal pigment epithelium (RPE; i.e., between RPE basement membrane and Bruch's membrane). (**D** and **E,** Courtesy of Dr. RC Eagle, Jr.)

Drusen

I. Drusen (Figs 11.26 and 11.27) are focal or diffuse basement membrane products produced by the RPE and admixed with other materials that may become trapped in the drusen as they pass through them in transit between the RPE and choriocapillaris.

The word *drusen* is plural; *druse* is the singular form—similar to *dellen* (plural) and *delle* (singular).

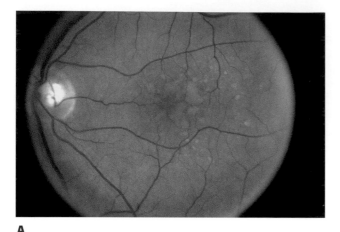

A

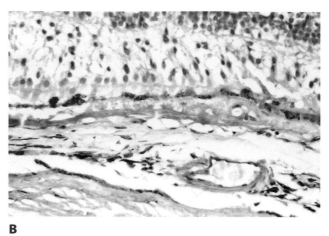

B

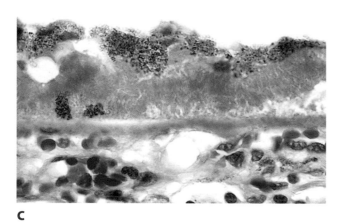

C

Fig. 11.27 Large ("soft") drusen. **A,** Clinical appearance of large drusen scattered in the posterior pole. **B,** An amorphous material is present between retinal pigment epithelium and Bruch's membrane. Note presence of tiny blood vessels in material. **C,** Brushlike appearance helps identify the basal laminar deposit. (**C,** Courtesy of Dr. RC Eagle, Jr.)

A. Drusen tend to be found mainly in four regions of the fundus: (1) in the distribution of the major vascular arcades; (2) in the macular region; (3) a combination of (1) and (2); and (4) in a peripheral distribution.

B. Drusen vary considerably in size (see later), ranging from 30 to 50 μm, or even larger when confluent.

RPE, like other ocular epithelia, may react to a variety of insults or stimuli by producing abnormal quantities of basement membrane. The variable structure of the basement membrane accumulations undoubtedly mirrors the aberrant biochemical activities conducted by the producing cell (e.g., more glycoprotein → more homogeneous or vacuolated basement membrane, more collagen → more filamentous or fibrous basement membrane). The basement membranes so produced are exaggerations of the normal varieties of thin, multilaminar, and thick. In contrast to these exaggerations of the normal or age-related changes, the deposition or addition of materials not normally present in basement membranes (e.g., fibrin, amyloid, or various metals such as silver and copper) would produce more complex pathologic basement membranes. The Bruch's membrane component of RPE, similar to the intima of arteries and arterioles, shows increased deposition of cholesterol with age.

II. Drusen consist of at least two fundamentally different focal types.*

A. The first focal type, nodular ("hard," discrete) drusen, consists of a focal thickening of the RPE basement membrane (see Fig. 11.26).

1. These are congenital or acquired early in life and have a relatively good prognosis. They are small, yellow or yellow-white spots or discrete RPE lesions measuring approximately 50 μm.

2. Nodular drusen have a rather random distribution, appearing as isolated drusen, scattered about in the posterior pole, without a recognizable pattern.

3. When they occur in great numbers, they may, in later life, be associated with the development of the second type of drusen (see later).

4. By fluorescein angiography, some show early fluorescence and late staining.

5. The presence of nodular drusen probably does not represent a high risk factor for the development of exudative (wet) ARMD; it is unclear whether it represents a high risk factor for the development of dry (nonexudative) ARMD.

Personal communication from Dr. JDM Gass.

6. Histologically (see Fig. 11.26), nodular drusen have an eosinophilic, PAS-positive, amorphous appearance and are located external and contiguous to, or replace, the original, thin basement membrane of the RPE (i.e., between RPE basement membrane and Bruch's membrane). The overlying RPE is usually atrophic, whereas the adjacent RPE is frequently hyperplastic.

7. The so-called basal laminar (cuticular) drusen (see Fig. 11.26) are one form of nodular drusen.

Basal laminar *drusen* should not be confused with the electron microscopist's terminology of basal laminar and basal linear *deposits* (confluent drusen or diffuse thickening of the inner aspect of Bruch's membrane), both of which are associated with, or are a form of, large drusen (see later).

---

a. Basal laminar drusen are yellowish, punctiform, and uniform in size.

b. Unlike the aforementioned nodular drusen, basal laminar drusen have a recognizable pattern of distribution, appearing in clusters in the posterior pole.

c. They may appear in early adulthood and occur with equal frequency in black, Hispanic, and white patients.

d. Fluorescein angiography shows focal areas of hyperfluorescence in the early arteriovenous phase, giving a "stars-in-the-sky" or "milky-way" appearance.

e. Patients who have basal laminar drusen may also acquire soft drusen with increasing age; the presence of soft drusen represents a high risk factor for the development of ARMD.

f. Histologically, basal laminar drusen consist of nodular protrusions of the inner side of a thickened RPE basement membrane.

g. Basal laminar (cuticular) drusen phenotype are highly associated with the Tyr402His variant of the complement factor H (*CFH*) gene

8. Nodular drusen may become calcified, lipidized, cholesterolized, or, infrequently, vascularized.

B. The second, focal type is a limited separation of the relatively normal basement membrane of the RPE from its attachment to Bruch's membrane at the inner collagenous zone by a wide variety of materials that differ in consistency from bone to fluid.

1. These usually are acquired at 50 years of age or later and represent the earliest sign of ARMD.

2. The second type of drusen may be impossible to differentiate by clinical methods or by light microscopy from small detachments of the RPE.

3. One form of this second type is large ("soft," exudative, fluffy) drusen (see Fig. 11.27).

a. Large drusen are bigger than nodular drusen, appear less dense and more fluffy, and when quite large are indistinguishable from small detachments of the RPE.

A subset of large drusen are *confluent drusen* ("diffuse" drusen), which appear clinically as diffuse yellow deposits and histopathologically as confluent large drusen.

---

b. Large drusen may develop under, and engulf or encompass, nodular drusen.

c. Fluorescein angiography usually shows staining of the drusen, although some may appear hypofluorescent, presumably because of lipid accumulation.

d. The presence of large drusen represents a high-risk factor for the development of dry (atrophic) and exudative (wet) ARMD.

4. Histologically, large drusen consist of an amorphous, PAS-positive material, which is indistinguishable from an RPE detachment.

a. *Basal laminar deposits* consist of banded basement membrane ("wide-spaced collagen") material located between (external to) the basal plasmalemma of the RPE and the internal surface of Bruch's membrane.

PAS stains basal laminar deposits as brush-like deposits along the inner aspect of the RPE basement membrane.

b. *Basal linear deposits* refer to material located external to the basement membrane of the RPE (i.e., in the innermost layer of Bruch's membrane).

Large drusen may result from localized detachments of basal laminar deposits (localized small detachments may appear clinically as large drusen and large detachments as serous RPE detachments), from localized detachments of basal linear deposits (confluent drusen—often appear clinically as a serous RPE detachment), or from localized accumulations of basal linear deposits (appear clinically as large drusen). Basal laminar and basal linear deposits, both of which are often present in the same eye, may be difficult to differentiate clinically and by light microscopy, although by light microscopy, the PAS-positive brushlike appearance of the basal laminar deposit (see Fig. 11.27C) is helpful in making the distinction. The amount of basal laminar deposit correlates strongly with the histologic presence of ARMD.

---

c. Large drusen may become calcified, lipidized, cholesterolized, or, infrequently, vascularized.

C. Reticular pseudodrusen

1. Reticular pseudodrusen appear as a yellow, interlacing network 125 to 250 μm wide, appearing first in the superior outer macula, and then extending circumferentially and beyond.

2. They do not fluoresce with fluorescein or indocyanine green angiography.

a. They are best seen with red-free light or the He-Ne laser of the scanning laser ophthalmoscope.

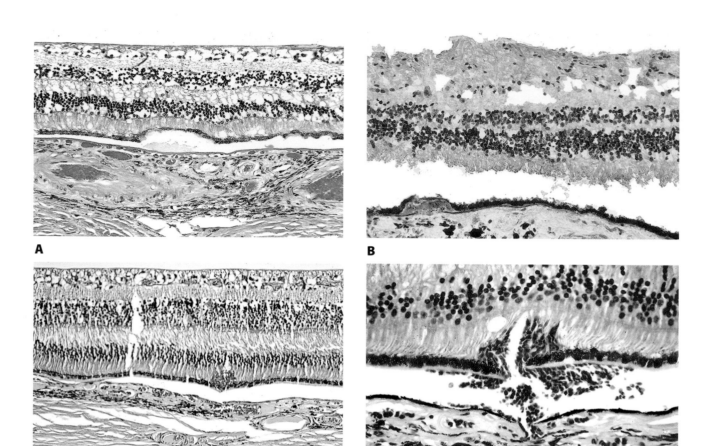

Fig. 11.28 Dry, age-related macular degeneration. **A,** Basophilia in region of Bruch's membrane commonly found as an aging change. Note choriocapillaris partially obliterated and small "detachment" of neural retina from retinal pigment epithelium, which is impossible to differentiate from a large druse. Such changes may be precursors to some senile degenerations in macular region. **B,** An oil red-O stain is positive for fat in another druse. **C,** Another case shows basophilia of Bruch's membrane and a probable artifactitious hemorrhage into neural retina. **D,** A von Kossa stain is strongly positive for calcium in Bruch's membrane (note "crack" in the fragile Bruch's membrane).

    b. They may be an important risk factor for the development of exudative ARMD.

  3. Histologically, the changes are choroidal and do not represent an accumulation of basal laminar and linear deposits or drusen.

    An almost total absence of the small vessels that normally occupy the middle choroidal layers and that also lie between the large choroidal veins seems to cause the clinically seen reticular pattern.

The photoreceptor gene, *ABCR* (ATP-binding cassette transporter-retina; also known as *STGD1*) on chromosome 1p21 is mutated in Stargardt's disease. Approximately 18.7% of cases of dry ARMD also have mutations in the *ABCR* gene. In one large family, which had mainly dry ARMD, the ARMD segregated as an autosomal-dominant trait localized to chromosome 1q25–q31. A small fraction of patients with ARMD may actually have a late-onset variant of Best's disease. The alleles of the apolipoprotein (apoE) gene are the most consistently associated with ARMD. The ε4 allele seems to be protective or delaying and the ε2 allele seems to accelerate the course of ARMD. Autosomal-dominant ARMD can be caused by mutations (e.g., 208delG mutation) in the *FSCN2* gene, as may autosomal-dominant retinitis pigmentosa (RP).

Age-Related Dry Macular Degeneration (Dry, Atrophic, or Senile Atrophic Macular Degeneration)

  I. Dry ARMD (Figs 11.28 and 11.29) is characterized by a gradual reduction of central vision.

    A. The cause is unknown.

B. The risk increases with age, especially 75 years and older, and in women.

In first-degree relatives of patients who have "late" ARMD, ARMD develops at an increased rate at a relatively young age. Perhaps 25% of all late ARMD is genetically determined.

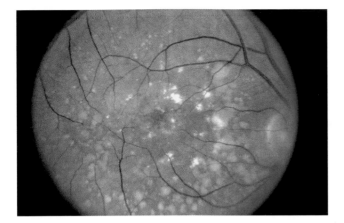

A

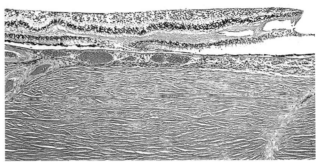

B

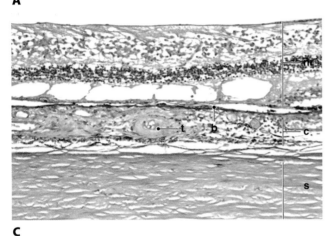

C

Fig. 11.29 Dry, age-related macular degeneration. **A,** The patient showed drusen and other abnormalities of the retinal pigment epithelium (RPE) in the form of increased translucency, pigment mottling, and pigment loss. No subretinal choroidal neovascularization (CNV) was present in this eye. However, CNV was present in the other eye. **B,** A histologic section of another eye shows irregular degeneration of the RPE and the outer retinal layers, as well as cystic changes in the outer plexiform layer. **C,** Another level of the same eye shows similar retinal changes along with a thrombus (t) in a choroidal artery. Whether the choroidal thrombosis is related to the retinal changes in atrophic macular degeneration is unknown (nr, neural retina; c, choroid; s, sclera; b, Bruch's membrane).

1. Risk factors:
   a. High intake of saturated fat and cholesterol
   b. Exposure to sunlight
   c. Soft and perhaps hard drusen
   d. A dose-related relationship exists between smoking and ARMD, especially the exudative form
   e. Both blue iris color and abnormal skin sun sensitivity
   f. A modest association exists between increased systolic blood pressure and pulse pressure and increased 10-year incidence of ARMD
   g. Elevated C-reactive protein and hyperhomocysteinemia are independent risk factors.
   h. Smoking (10 pack-years or more)
   i. Presence of *CFH CC* genotype

   The use of statins and vitamin supplements may be positive risk factors in preventing or delaying ARMD.

II. Clinically, the retinal damage is limited to the foveomacular area and causes a gradual and subtle visual loss (never sudden or dramatic, as in exudative ARMD).

The complaint of abrupt loss of vision in a patient who has dry ARMD should alert the clinician to the possibility of the development of superimposed subneural retinal neovascularization. Patients who have dry ARMD do not complain of visual distortion, as do those who have acute neural retinal detachments.

A. Pigment disturbances (e.g., increased and decreased pigmentation) are seen in the macula.

Pigmentary macular changes may also be seen in inherited diseases such as Bardet–Biedl syndrome, Bassen–Kornzweig syndrome, Batten–Mayou disease, central RP, Cockayne's syndrome, cone–rod dystrophy, familial hypobetalipoproteinemia, Hallervorden–Spatz syndrome, Hallgren's syndrome, Hooft's syndrome, patterned dystrophy of the RPE, Pelizaeus–Merzbacher disease, Refsum's disease, Stargardt's disease, and others.

B. The RPE atrophy tends to spread and form well-demarcated borders, called *geographic atrophy.*
   1. The atrophic areas, which are often bilateral and relatively symmetric, are multifocal in approximately 40% of eyes.

2. The atrophic areas tend to follow the disappearance or flattening of soft drusen, RPE detachment, or reticular mottling of the RPE.

3. The underlying choriocapillaris is atrophic.

III. The changes are usually bilateral and found in people older than 50 years of age. The rate of significant visual loss is approximately 8% per year.

IV. Histologically, the following changes may be seen.

A. The choriocapillaris may be partially or completely obliterated.

B. Bruch's membrane may be thickened and may show basophilic changes.

C. The RPE may show atrophy with depigmentation, hypertrophy, or even hyperplasia.

In both dry and wet ARMD, RPE, photoreceptors, and inner nuclear cells die by apoptosis.

D. The neural retina often shows microcystoid or even macrocystoid (retinoschisis) degeneration.

1. Hole formation may occur in the inner wall of the macrocyst.

2. Rarely, total hole formation may occur, leaving the macular retinal ends with rounded, smooth edges.

The aforementioned changes, characterized as *age-related macular choroidal degeneration* and often noted clinically by the presence of drusen (see earlier), also occur in, and are related to the cause of, idiopathic serous detachment of the RPE, idiopathic central serous choroidopathy, and exudative ARMD. Soft or hard drusen may predispose the eye to the development of dry ARMD. Each year 16 000 people in the United States become blind from ARMD. ARMD is the most prevalent cause of legal blindness in white adults in the United States (a similar frequency of blindness is seen in the dry and exudative forms, but the blindness tends to be more profound in the exudative form).

---

3. The normal aging phenomenon of slow, steady rod loss is accompanied in ARMD by cone degeneration, so that eventually only degenerative cones remain; ultimately all photoreceptors may disappear.

4. The RPE and Bruch's membrane in postmortem eyes containing nonexudative and exudative AMD have increased iron content, some of which is chelatable.

The iron may generate highly reactive hydroxyl radicals that may contribute to the development of AMD.

E. In addition to the well-known aging changes of the RPE, including drusen and an increase in cell lipofuscin, the cell, *in situ*, can also undergo a change known as *lipidic degeneration*, the noxious stimulus for which is unknown (see Fig. 17.41).

F. With aging, Bruch's membrane shows, in addition to drusen, increased amounts of calcium and lipid.

Age-Related Exudative Macular Degeneration (Exudative, Wet, or Senile Disciform Macular Degeneration; Kuhnt–Junius Macular Degeneration)

I. Typically, exudative ARMD (Fig. 11.30) rarely occurs in people younger than 60 years of age.

The complaint of abrupt loss of vision in a patient who has dry ARMD should alert the clinician to the possibility of the development of superimposed subneural retinal vascularization. Exudative ARMD in patients younger than 60 years of age most commonly is caused by, in decreasing frequency: high myopia; POHS; angioid streaks; and miscellaneous hereditary, traumatic, or inflammatory disorders.

A. The cause is unknown.

The photoreceptor gene, *ABCR* (also known as *STGD1*) on chromosome 1p21 is mutated in Stargardt's disease. Approximately 3% of cases of wet ARMD also have mutations in the *ABCR* gene.

B. The risk increases with age, especially 75 years and older, and in women.

The 3-year incidence of wet ARMD is about 10 per 1000 Americans 65 years and older.

C. No sex predilection exists and the degeneration is often bilateral.

D. The main risk factor is age-related macular choroidal degeneration (soft drusen, pigment epithelial disturbances, and loss of foveal reflex).

E. High intake of saturated fat and cholesterol is also associated with an increased risk for early ARMD.

Consumption of foods rich in certain carotenoids (e.g., dark-green leafy vegetables) may decrease the risk for development of ARMD.

---

1. Exudative ARMD may be associated with moderate to severe hypertension, particularly among patients receiving antihypertensive therapy.

A modest association exists between increased systolic blood pressure and pulse pressure and increased 10-year incidence of ARMD.

---

2. Hyperopia may also be a risk factor.

F. A dose-related relationship between smoking and ARMD, especially the exudative form and smoking 10 pack-years or more, has been found.

Patients who have unilateral exudative ARMD have a 12% to 15% chance every year for development of exudative ARMD in the other eye. Patients who have large, soft, confluent drusen

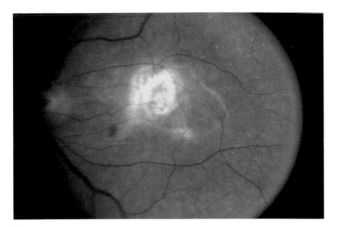

A

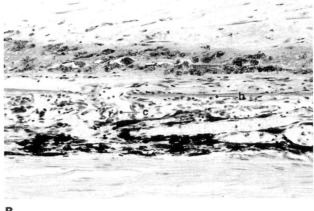

B

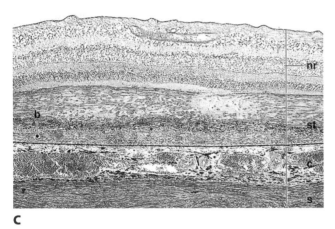

C

Fig. 11.30 Exudative age-related macular degeneration. **A,** The patient had subretinal neovascularization followed by numerous episodes of hemorrhage, resulting in an organized scar. **B,** A small vessel (c, capillary) has grown through Bruch's membrane (b) into the subretinal pigment epithelial space, resulting in hemorrhage and fibroplasia. **C,** The end stage of the process shows a thick fibrous scar between the choroid and the outer retinal layers (trichrome stain). Note the good preservation of the retina, except for the complete degeneration of the photoreceptors (nr, neural retina; st, scar tissue; c, choroid; s, sclera; b, Bruch's membrane). (Case in **B** reported in Frayer WC: *Arch Ophthalmol* 53:82, 1955. © American Medical Association. All rights reserved.)

are at the greatest risk for development of exudative ARMD in the second eye. Systemic hypertension is another risk factor for the development of subneural retinal (choroidal) neovascularization.

G. A high serum level of the antioxidant enzyme plasma glutathione peroxidase is associated with a significant increase in late ARMD prevalence.

H. About a fivefold risk for late-stage ARMD (especially exudative ARMD) exists in eyes that have previously had cataract surgery.

I. Presence of *CFH CC* genotype increases the risk 144-fold.

J. Possessing the *LOC387715* (rs 10490924) variant may increase the risk (if homozygous for both variants, an earlier development of neovascular AMD may occur).

II. Evolution of exudative ARMD

A. Early degenerative changes are seen in the choriocapillaris and in Bruch's membrane in the macular area, manifested clinically as drusen, especially soft drusen; collectively these changes are called *age-related macular choroidal degeneration.*

1. Large, soft drusen seem to predispose the eye to exudative ARMD.

2. Each year, 16 000 people in the United States become blind from ARMD.

The age-related macular choroidal degenerative changes may remain stationary or lead to idiopathic serous detachment of the RPE, idiopathic central serous choroidopathy, or dry or exudative ARMD.

3. ARMD is the most prevalent cause of legal blindness in the United States; a similar frequency of blindness is seen in the dry and the exudative forms.

B. The age-related macular choroidal degeneration becomes complicated by neovascular invasion.

1. The new vessels grow from the choroid (from the choriocapillaris) through Bruch's membrane, usually under the RPE, rarely between the RPE and neural retina, or in both regions.

Sub-RPE neovascularization is characteristic of age-related "wet" macular degeneration, whereas subneural retinal neovascularization (CNV) is characteristic of POHS. CNV, also called *subretinal neovascularization* (i.e., neovascularization under the RPE, between the RPE and neural retina, or in both regions), may also develop from new vessels growing from the choroid around the end of Bruch's membrane in the juxtapapillary region. CNV may occasionally occur in the periphery. Granulomatous reaction to Bruch's membrane, with multiple multinucleated giant cells, may play a role in the breakdown of Bruch's membrane and be a stimulus for neovascularization in some cases.

2. Two fundamentally different types of CNV arise from the choroid: types 1 and 2.
   a. Type 1, the most common type, consists of subretinal pigment epithelial neovascularization—it occurs primarily in people older than 50 years of age, often in association with ARMD.

      The CNV develops in eyes that show diffuse, age-related macular choroidal degeneration in the choriocapillaris–Bruch's membrane–RPE complex.
   b. Type 2 consists of subneural retinal neovascularization—it occurs primarily in people younger than 50 years of age, POHS being the prototype.

   The CNV develops in an area of focal scarring, the choriocapillaris–Bruch's membrane–RPE complex being normal elsewhere.
C. All of the aforementioned factors produce an altered state of the internal choroid and external retina, predisposing the eye to the development of serous and hemorrhagic phenomena.
D. Finally, a hemorrhage between Bruch's membrane and RPE occurs (hematoma of the choroid).
E. Although the hemorrhage may remain localized, it usually breaks through the RPE under the neural retina; rarely it may extend into the choroid, the neural retina, or even the vitreous.
F. Organization of the hemorrhage is accompanied by RPE proliferation and fibrous metaplasia.
   1. Ingrowth of mesenchymal tissue forms granulation tissue.
   2. A disciform fibrovascular scar forms in the macular region, causing degeneration of the macular RPE and neural retina.
   3. Central vision is irreversibly impaired.
G. Retinal angiomatous proliferation (RAP)
   1. RAP is a distinct form of occult CNV associated with proliferation of intraneural retinal capillaries in the paramacular neural retina and a contiguous telangiectatic response that has a progressive vasogenic sequence.
   2. RAP is an "upside-down" form of exudative ARMD, starting initially in the neural retina and ultimately connecting to subneural CNV.

3. Three stages have been described:
   a. Stage I—intraretinal neovascularization (IRN) originating from the deep capillary plexus in the paramacular neural retina.
   b. Stage II—the IRN extends posteriorly into the subneural space (subneural retinal neovascularization).
   c. Stage III—IRN anastamosing with CNV.
III. Histologically, the following features are noted:
   A. Age-related choroidal macular degenerative changes, as described previously, are seen.

In both dry and wet ARMD, RPE, photoreceptors, and inner nuclear cells die by apoptosis.

   B. The subretinal (sub-RPE or subneural retinal) membranes consist of a cellular and an extracellular matrix component.
   1. The cellular component contains RPE, inflammatory cells (mainly lymphocytes, plasma cells, and macrophages), vascular endothelium, glial cells, myofibroblasts, photoreceptor cells, fibrocytes, and erythrocytes.
   2. The extracellular matrix component contains fibrin; collagen types I, III, IV, and V; fibronectin; laminin; acid mucopolysaccharides; and lipid.
   3. Transforming growth factor-β_1 (TGF-β_1) and basic growth factor are present in the major cell types (vascular endothelium, fibroblasts, RPE cells) and possibly may play a role in the development of the neovascular complex.

Surgically excised human subfoveal fibrovascular membranes have been shown to express vascular endothelial growth factor (VEGF), both VEGF mRNA and protein.

   4. The RPE and Bruch's membrane in postmortem eyes containing nonexudative and exudative AMD have increased iron content, some of which is chelatable.

The iron may generate highly reactive hydroxyl radicals that may contribute to the development of AMD.

   C. Basically, the pathologic process is that of a localized granulation tissue associated with diffuse, soft drusen.

Rarely the CNV is in the choroid (i.e., intrachoroidal neovascularization).

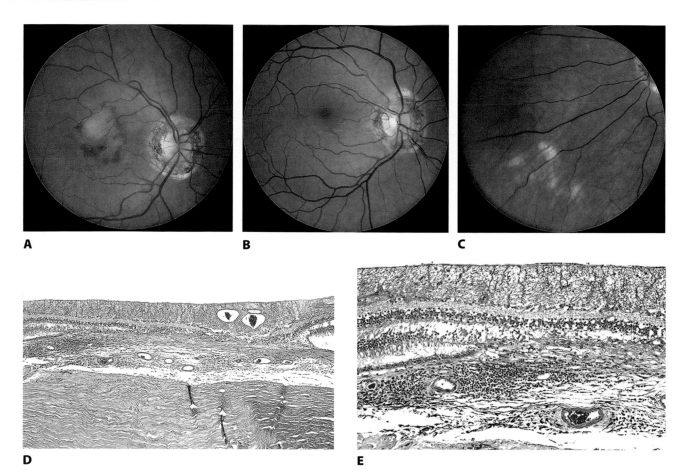

Fig. 11.31 Presumed histoplasmic choroiditis. **A** and **B,** An irregular area of peripapillary degeneration of the choroid is seen in each eye. The right eye shows subneural retinal neovascularization. **C,** Peripheral, tiny, sharply circumscribed, punched-out lesions are seen. **D,** Histologic section shows a chorioretinal granulomatous inflammation along with scarring. **E,** Increased magnification of chorioretinal inflammation. (Case presented by Dr. TA Makley, Jr. at the meeting of the Verhoeff Society, 1983.)

Exudative Macular Degeneration Secondary to Focal Choroiditis (Juvenile Disciform Degeneration of the Macula)

I. Most patients with this degeneration are younger than 50 years of age, have over 50% bilateral involvement, show a high incidence of macular hemorrhagic phenomena, and usually have irreversibly damaged central vision; both sexes are affected equally.

II. Most cases probably occur secondary to focal inflammatory cell infiltration of the choroid.

III. Five subdivisions have been identified:

    A. Exudative (wet) macular detachment secondary to multifocal choroiditis (POHS; Fig. 11.31)—the most common type

        1. Presumed ocular histoplasmosis syndrome (POHS) occurs in otherwise healthy young adults, with the initial symptom being sudden blurring of vision in one eye.

Although most patients in the United States who have POHS show a positive skin reaction to intracutaneous injection of 1:1000 histoplasmin and chest radiographic evidence of healed pulmonary histoplasmosis, the fungal organism has never been cultured or demonstrated satisfactorily in a histologic section from a typical retinal lesion in a nonimmunologically deficient patient. The cause, therefore, remains open to question. In Germany, where histoplasmosis is extremely rare, a condition called *focal hemorrhagic chorioretinopathy* is not uncommon. It is indistinguishable clinically from presumed histoplasmic choroiditis found in the United States, where almost all the patients have negative skin tests for histoplasmosis.

        2. Early, a yellowish-white or gray, circumscribed, slightly elevated area of choroidal infiltration is present in the macular region.

           Overlying RPE disturbances soon appear, resulting in a small, dark greenish macular ring.

        3. CNV develops.

CNV is characteristic of POHS, whereas sub-RPE neovascularization is characteristic of "wet" ARMD.

4. Serous and hemorrhagic disciform detachment of the neural retina may ensue.

5. Multiple, small to tiny, sharply circumscribed, punched-out white defects are scattered about the fundus.

6. An irregular area of peripapillary degeneration of the choroid and RPE is frequently seen.

7. HLA-B7 is found in association with POHS.

8. Histologically, the peripheral lesions show either a chronic nongranulomatous or granulomatous inflammatory infiltrate in the choroid.

   a. Overlying Bruch's membrane and RPE may or may not be involved.

   b. The typical acute macular lesions have not been examined histologically.

   c. Excised subretinal membranes are composed of fibrovascular tissue between Bruch's membrane and RPE and probably represent nonspecific granulation tissue.

      1). The cellular component contains RPE, inflammatory cells (mainly lymphocytes, plasma cells, and macrophages), vascular endothelium, glial cells, myofibroblasts, photoreceptor cells, fibrocytes, smooth-muscle cells, and erythrocytes.

      2). The extracellular matrix component contains 20- to 25-nm collagen fibrils, 10-nm collagen fibrils, and fibrin.

      3). TGF-β_1 and basic growth factor are present in the major cell types (vascular endothelium, fibroblasts, RPE cells) and may possibly play a role in the development of the neovascular complex.

B. Idiopathic subretinal (choroidal) neovascularization

   1. Idiopathic subretinal neovascular membranes occur in the absence of any associated disorder, tend to occur in younger people, and may regress spontaneously.

   2. The cellular component contains RPE, macrophages, vascular endothelium, glial cells, myofibroblasts, photoreceptor cells, and erythrocytes.

   3. The extracellular matrix component contains 20- to 25-nm collagen fibrils, 10-nm collagen fibrils, and fibrin.

C. Exudative macular detachment secondary to focal peripapillary choroiditis—the patients have negative histoplasmin skin tests and no peripheral fundus lesions. Their macular lesions are probably caused by an underlying peripapillary choroiditis.

D. Exudative macular detachment secondary to focal macular choroiditis—the patients have negative histoplasmin skin tests, no peripheral fundus lesions, and no peripapillary choroiditis. Their macular lesions are probably caused by an underlying, focal, macular choroiditis.

E. Exudative macular detachment secondary to *Toxocara canis* (see p. 90, Chapter 4).

Idiopathic Polypoidal Choroidal Vasculopathy

I. Idiopathic polypoidal choroidal vasculopathy (IPCV) has a predilection for members of darkly pigmented races (rarely, it may be associated with sickle-cell retinopathy).

II. Clinical characteristics

   A. Reddish-orange, spheroidal, polyp-like structures, presumably aneurysmal dilatations of the inner choroidal vascular network

   B. Multiple, recurrent, serosanguineous detachments of the RPE and neural retina, secondary to leakage and bleeding from the peculiar choroidal vascular lesions

---

IPCV can resemble ARMD. The former, however, is more common in the peripapillary area, usually has no associated drusen, and is most common in nonwhite patients.

   C. Occasional vitreous hemorrhage and relatively minimal fibrous scarring

III. Histopathology

   A. The network of peripapillary vessels seen on fluorescein angiography and indocyanine green angiography correspond to branches of the short posterior ciliary arteies

   B. The elevated polypoidal and tubular lesions correspond to large, thin-walled cavernous vascular channels and choroidal

   C. Intra-Bruch's membrane neovascularization is in continuity with the vascular channels.

Cystoid Macular Edema (Irvine–Gass Syndrome)

See pp. 122–123 in Chapter 5 and p. 606 in Chapter 15.

Toxic Retinal Degenerations

I. Chloroquine (Fig. 11.32) and hydroxychloroquine

   A. The characteristic but nonspecific "bull's-eye" macular degeneration appears to be directly related to the total dosage of chloroquine.

      1. The bull's-eye macular degeneration indicates advanced, irreversible damage.

      2. Other causes of bull's-eye macula include ARMD, chronic macular hole, Bardet–Biedl syndrome, benign concentric annular macular dystrophy, clofazimine toxicity, cone–rod dystrophy, dominant cystoid macular dystrophy, fenestrated sheen macular dystrophy, fucosidosis, Hallervorden–Spatz syndrome, hereditary ataxia, neuronal ceroid lipofuscinosis (Batten's disease), olivopontocerebellar atrophy, quinacrine therapy for malaria, RP, Sjögren–Larsson syndrome, Stargardt's disease, UAIM, and uvi ursi herbal toxicity.

         a. Serious vision impairment rarely occurs if the daily dose of chloroquine does not exceed 250 mg (and 6.5 mg/kg of body weight for hydroxychloroquine).

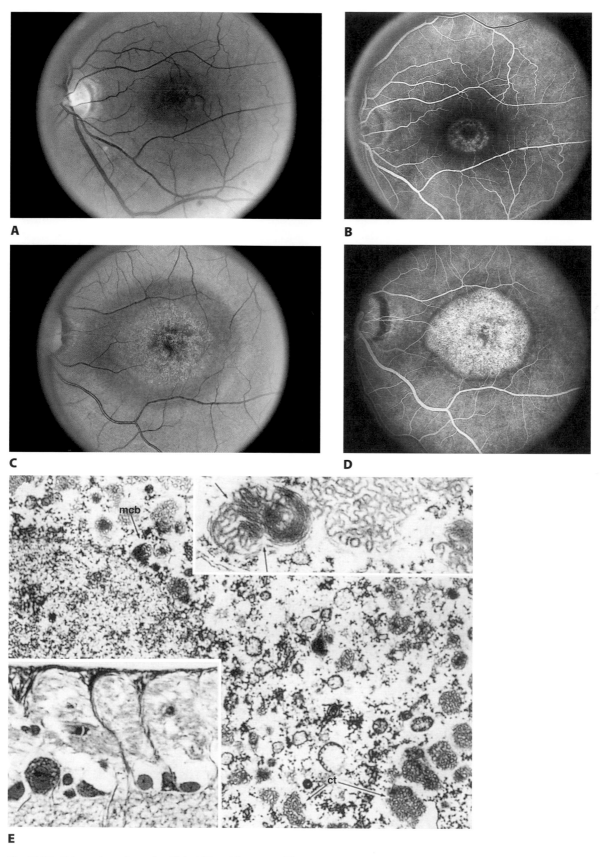

Fig. 11.32 Chloroquine retinopathy. Clinical (**A**) and fluorescein (**B**) appearance of left eye. **C** and **D,** Another patient more severely afflicted. **E,** Cytoplasm of retinal ganglion cell contains myriad clusters of curvilinear structures (ct) and membranous cytoplasmic bodies (mcb). Bodies better seen in top inset **B,** probable continuity of curvilinear structure with membraneous body seen at free (*arrows*). Bottom inset shows retinal ganglion cell by light microscopy. (**C** and **D,** Courtesy of Dr. AJ Brucker; **E,** from Ramsey MS, Fine BS: *Am J Ophthalmol* 73:229. © Elsevier 1972.)

In following patients, examination every 3 months is recommended (probably less frequent examinations would suffice, i.e., first follow-up in 6 months and then annually). At the initial examination, the patient is given a color vision test and instructed in the use of the Amsler grid. At subsequent visits, color vision testing is performed, and confirmation of the proper use of the Amsler grid is obtained.

  b. Corneal deposition of drug is seen in 90% of patients who use chloroquine, but in less than 5% who use hydroxychloroquine.
 B. Night blindness is usually the first symptom.
  1. Patients may show extinguished ERGs but have normal or minimally abnormal final dark adaptation thresholds, differentiating advanced chloroquine retinopathy from RP.
  2. After chloroquine is stopped, the degree of retinopathy and its rate of progression are determined by the total dose of the drug and the patient's susceptibility to it.
 C. Histologically, RPE abnormalities, destruction of receptors and ganglion cells, and pigment migration into the macular neural retina are seen.

As seen by electron microscopy, degenerative changes occur in most of the ocular tissues in the human eye. The changes are prominent in the neural retinal neurons, where they appear as curvilinear structures and membranous cytoplasmic bodies.

II. Many other drugs, such as canthaxanthin, chlorpromazine, chloramphenicol, deferoxamine, indomethacin, quinine, sparsomycin, thioridazine, and vitamin A, may cause a retinopathy, usually of a secondary pigmentary type.

Postirradiation Retinopathy

 I. Postirradiation retinopathy may occur months to years after irradiation of the eye, usually for cure or control of retinoblastoma, malignant melanoma, or lid, orbital, or sinus neoplasm.

The irradiation source may be X-rays, ^{60}Co, or radon seeds. Usually, a latent period of 12 months or more elapses before a retinopathy develops.

II. The neural retina may show capillary occlusion and capillary microaneurysms, telangiectatic vessels, neovascularization, hard exudates, cotton-wool spots, hemorrhages, and signs of arteriolar or venular occlusion—all caused by retinal vascular obliteration secondary to the irradiation.

Bone Marrow Transplant Retinopathy

 I. A retinopathy develops in perhaps 60% of patients who survive at least 6 months after bone marrow transplantation for the therapy of acute leukemia.

An optic neuropathy also develops in many of these patients.

II. The main finding is an occlusive microvascular retinopathy that can cause macular edema and proliferative retinopathy.

Cancer-Associated Retinopathy (Paraneoplastic Syndrome; Paraneoplastic Retinopathy; Paraneoplastic Photoreceptor Retinopathy; Melanoma-Associated Retinopathy)

 I. The paraneoplastic syndrome (PNS) is a consequence of remote effects of tumors on different organ systems, sometimes years before the tumor is apparent.
 A. The neurologic PNS may involve any site (e.g., myasthenic syndrome associated with lung carcinoma or other malignant neoplasms (Lambert–Eaton syndrome), myasthenia gravis associated with thymoma, opsoclonus associated with neuroblastoma, cancer-associated retinopathy (CAR) in the face of a distant carcinoma or lymphoma, and melanoma-associated retinopathy (MAR) associated with a cutaneous melanoma.
 B. Histologically, the inner nuclear and ganglion cell layers of the neural retina show a reduced thickness, whereas the photoreceptors appear preserved.
II. CAR is most commonly associated with small cell lung carcinoma, but many other carcinomas and lymphomas can cause it.

Rarely, PNS, rather than causing eye involvement, can cause orbital involvement in the form of an orbital myositis.

 A. Visual loss may predate the discovery of the distant cancer.
 B. Typically, the visual loss is progressive and evolves over weeks to months.
 C. Clinical, ERG, and histopathologic evidence shows dysfunction and death of neural retinal photoreceptors.
 D. Sera of patients with CAR may contain antibodies that react with photoreceptors and ganglion cell antigen (e.g., recoverin).
 E. It is thought that autoantibodies developed against a cancer cell antigen cross-react with certain components of neural retinal cells and cause CAR.
III. MAR is associated with cutaneous malignant melanoma.
 A. Usually, a relatively acute onset of night blindness occurs months to years after a diagnosis of cutaneous malignant melanoma has been made.
 B. The patients typically have a sensation of shimmering lights, elevated dark-adapted thresholds, and an ERG resembling that found in some forms of stationary night blindness.
 C. Unlike CAR, photoreceptor function is intact, but the signal between photoreceptors and second-order neural retinal interneurons is defective.

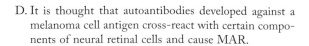

D. It is thought that autoantibodies developed against a melanoma cell antigen cross-react with certain components of neural retinal cells and cause MAR.

The identity of the retinal bipolar antigen recognized by MAR autoantibodies helps to make the diagnosis of MAR.

Idiopathic Macular Holes

I. The pathogenesis of idiopathic macular holes (IMH) is not known.

A. IMH may be bilateral and tend to occur in eyes that do not have a posterior vitreous detachment.

1. Given a full-thickness macular hole in one eye, a 13% chance exists for development of a full-thickness hole in the other eye.

2. If the first eye has an incomplete hole, a 19% chance exists of bilaterality in 48 months.

Patients who have a unilateral macular hole and a normal fellow eye that does not have a posterior vitreous detachment have a 16% 5-year incidence of full-thickness hole formation in the fellow eye.

B. It appears that vitreous contraction or separation may play an important role in the development of IMH.

1. The primary mechanism is postulated to be a spontaneous, usually abrupt, focal contraction of the prefoveal cortical vitreous, which elevates the neural retina in the central foveal region.

2. Spontaneous complete vitreous separation from the fovea could reverse the process.

Although the vitreous seems to play a role, some studies suggest that most IMH develop in the absence of posterior vitreous detachment and that the pathogenesis of IMH may be independent of posterior vitreous detachment.

II. The development of IMH can be divided into three stages:

A. Stage 1: tractional detachment or impending macular hole

1. Stage 1-A has a characteristic biomicroscopic appearance of a yellow spot (increased visibility of the neural retinal pigment xanthophyll), and stage 1-B of a yellow ring and loss of the foveolar depression in the absence of a posterior vitreous detachment.

A hole may be covered by semiopaque contracted prefoveal cortical vitreous bridging the yellow ring (stage 1-B occult hole). Stage 1-B occult holes become manifest (stage 2 holes) either after separation of the contracted prefoveal cortical vitreous from the retina surrounding a small hole or as an eccentric can-opener-like tear in the contracted prefoveal cortical vitreous, at the edge of larger stage 2 holes.

B. Stage 2: small hole formation

1. Increased traction causes a tangential tear, usually at the foveal edge.

2. Tractional elevation of Henle's nerve fiber layer along with intraneural retinal central foveal cyst formation is the initial feature of macular hole formation.

Most (approximately 75%) stage 2 macular holes, both centric and eccentric, especially when they show pericentral hyperfluorescence, progress to stage 3 or 4.

C. Stage 3: large hole formation

Over several months or longer, the tear enlarges to a fully developed, one-third disc diameter-sized hole.

III. Histologically, in membranes stripped out during vitrectomy for stage 1 IMH, an acellular collagenous tissue layer is found.

A. Membranes from stages 2 and 3 IMH show an increased number of glial cells (fibrous astrocytes) and other cells such as RPE (often the predominant cell), fibrocytes, and myofibroblasts.

B. Depending on the constituents of the membrane, immunohistochemical staining is positive for cytokeratin, glial fibrillary acidic protein, vimentin, actin, and fibronectin.

Light Energy Retinopathy

See pp. 155 in Chapter 5.

Traumatic Retinopathy

See pp. 144–145 in Chapter 5.

HEREDITARY PRIMARY RETINAL DYSTROPHIES

Definitions

I. Dystrophies are primary phenomena that are inherited and tend to be bilateral and symmetric.

II. They may remain stationary or be slowly progressive.

III. Many retinal dystrophies may be genetically determined by the process of apoptosis (see p. 23 in Chapter 1).

Juvenile Retinoschisis (Vitreous Veils; Congenital Vascular Veils; Cystic Disease of the Retina; Congenital Retinal Detachment)

I. Juvenile retinoschisis (Fig. 11.33) is a bilateral condition, tends to be slowly progressive, and often culminates

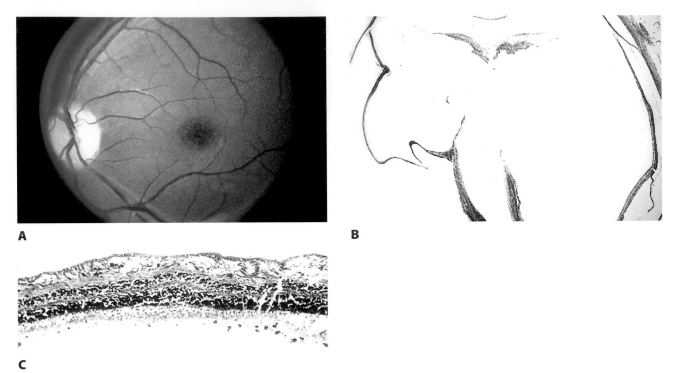

A

B

C

Fig. 11.33 Juvenile retinoschisis. **A,** The characteristic foveal lesion, resembling a polycystic fovea, is shown. Typically, no leakage is present when fluorescein angiography is performed. **B,** A histologic section of another eye shows a large temporal peripheral retinoschisis cavity. **C,** A histologic section of another area of the same eye shows a splitting in the ganglion and nerve fiber layers of the retina—the earliest finding in juvenile retinoschisis. The area of pathology is the same as that seen in reticular microcystoid degeneration and retinoschisis. (**A,** Courtesy of Dr. AJ Brucker; **B** and **C,** case reported by Yanoff M *et al.: Arch Ophthalmol* 1968. © American Medical Association. All rights reserved.)

in extensive chorioretinal atrophy with macular involvement.

Retinoschisis may be defined as an intraneural retinal tissue loss or splitting at least 1.5 mm in length (one average disc diameter). It is differentiated from a neural retinal cyst by its configuration; that is, a neural retinal cyst has approximately the same diameter in all directions (and usually a narrow neck), whereas the diameter of retinoschisis parallel to the neural retinal surface is greater than the diameter perpendicular to the surface.

II. Most often it is inherited as an X-linked recessive trait, but occasionally it occurs as an autosomal-recessive trait and then usually without macular involvement, or as an autosomal-dominant trait, often with macular involvement.

Genetic linkage studies have localized the retinoschisis gene to the p22.2 region of the X chromosome (Xp22), designated the *XRLS1* gene.

III. Ophthalmoscopic appearance
A. Approximately 50% of patients have a translucent, veil-like membrane that bulges into the vitreous, has a neural retinal origin, and usually occurs in the inferior temporal quadrant.

This membrane, really a retinoschisis cavity, has retinal vessels coursing over its inner wall, which frequently contains large round or oval holes. The outer wall of the cavity may contain small holes.
B. Foveal retinoschisis is present in almost all cases. It appears clinically much like the polycystic fovea seen in Irvine–Gass syndrome, but without fluorescein leakage.

Infantile cystoid maculopathy has been reported in infants; the findings are indistinguishable ophthalmoscopically from the macular lesions of juvenile retinoschisis.

Foveal and peripheral retinoschisis have been seen in a woman who has homozygous, X-linked retinoschisis. Familial foveal retinoschisis is similar to juvenile retinoschisis in the foveal appearance and has an autosomal-recessive inheritance pattern, but does not show typical peripheral retinoschisis. Cone–rod dystrophy may be associated with familial foveal retinoschisis.

IV. Histologically, in the region of the retinoschisis, the neural retina shows a cleavage at the level of the nerve fiber and ganglion cell layers; in areas away from the schisis, the neural retina shows a "looseness" or microcystic degeneration that mainly involves the nerve fiber layer and, to a lesser extent, the ganglion cell layer.

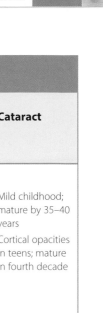

TABLE 11.2 Clinical Findings in Syndromes with Wagner-Like Vitreoretinal Degenerations

Disease	Systemic Findings	Refractive Error	Vitreous Veils and Perivascular Lattice	Retinal Detachments	Cataract
A. WITH OCULAR SYMPTOMATOLOGY ONLY					
1. Wagner's syndrome	Normal	Moderate myopia; occasionally severe myopia	Yes	None	Mild childhood; mature by 35–40 years
2. Jansen's syndrome	Normal	Low hypermetropia or moderate myopia; occasionally severe myopia	Yes	Yes	Cortical opacities in teens; mature in fourth decade
B. WITH ASSOCIATED SYSTEMIC ANOMALIES					
1. Hereditary arthro-ophthalmopathy with marfanoid habitus (Stickler's syndrome)	Micrognathia, cleft palate, joint laxity, epiphyseal dysplasia	Moderate to severe myopia; occasionally mild myopia	Yes	Yes	Common
2. Hereditary arthro-ophthalmopathy with Weill–Marchesani-like habitus	Low normal stature, cleft palate, joint stiffness, epiphyseal dysplasia, deafness	Moderate to severe myopia; occasionally mild myopia	Yes	Occasional	Common
3. Short stature, type undetermined	Below third percentile in stature, cleft palate, epiphyseal dysplasia, deafness	Severe myopia	Yes	None	No
4. Kniest's syndrome	Adult height 106–145 cm, abnormal facies, cleft palate, joint limitation, epiphyseal dysplasia, deafness	Severe myopia	Yes	Occasional	Occasional
5. Diastrophic variant	Adult height 102 cm, bifid uvula, torus planitus, loose joints, epiphyseal dysplasia, deafness	Severe myopia	Yes	Yes	Yes
6. Spondyloepiphyseal dysplasia congenita	Adult height 84–128 cm, loose joints, epiphyseal dysplasia	Mild hypermetropia to severe myopia	Yes	None	No

(Modified from Maumenee IH: Am J Ophthalmol *88:432. Copyright Elsevier 1979.)*

A. Mutation of the *RS1* gene appears to give rise to a dysfunctional adhesive protein, resulting in defective cellular adhesion that eventually leads to schisis formation.

B. The area of neural retinal involvement is similar to that found in reticular peripheral cystoid degeneration and retinoschisis, but different from the middle-layer neural retinal involvement of typical microcystoid peripheral neural retinal degeneration and retinoschisis.

C. In juvenile retinoschisis, the neural retinal spaces appear empty and do not stain for acid mucopolysaccharides.

V. Goldmann–Favre vitreoretinal dystrophy consists of juvenile retinoschisis and the following:

A. Vitreous degeneration and liquefaction and the formation of preretinal strands and cords

B. Secondary pigmentary and degenerative changes of the retina resembling RP

C. Leakage of fluorescein from retinal vessels

D. Hemeralopia with abolition of the ERG response and a progressive decrease in vision function

E. Cataracta complicata lens opacities

F. An autosomal-recessive heredity

VI. Wagner's vitreoretinal dystrophy (Table 11.2) consists of:

A. Juvenile retinoschisis plus marked vitreous syneresis

B. No posterior pole involvement

C. Normal dark adaptation but a subnormal ERG

D. Cataracta complicata lens opacities

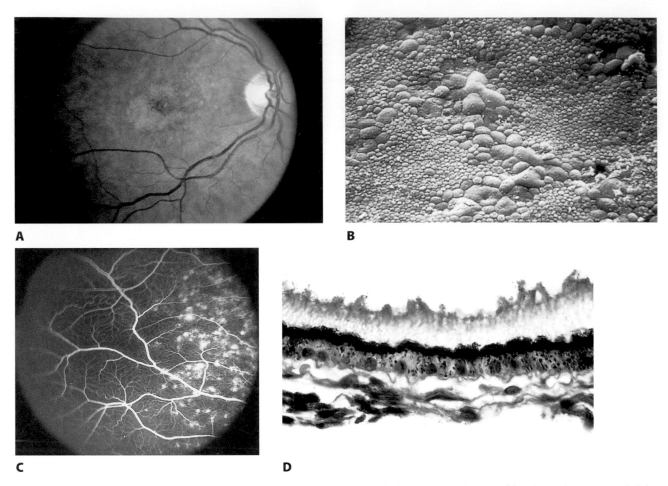

Fig. 11.34 Stargardt's disease (fundus flavimaculatus). **A,** Characteristic yellow-white flecks and an annular zone of foveal retinal pigment epithelial atrophy ("bull's-eye" maculopathy) are present. **B,** A scanning electron micrograph of an enucleated eye from the brother of the woman whose eye is shown in **A** demonstrates that the yellow-white flecks are caused by irregular pisciform aggregates of enormous retinal pigment epithelium (RPE) cells, surrounded by a mosaic of smaller, relatively normal RPE cells. **C,** Fluorescein angiography performed on the patient shown in **A** reveals a characteristic damping-out of the background choroidal fluorescence (dark fundus). **D,** A histologic section of the eye of the patient in **B** shows that the fluorescein effect is caused by enlarged lipofuscin-containing RPE cells, which act as a fluorescent filter. (**B** and **D,** Case reported by Eagle RC Jr *et al.: Ophthalmology* 7:1189. Copyright Elsevier 1980.)

The polymorphous ocular signs of this disease may also include myopia, retinal pigmentation, neural retinal breaks, patchy areas of thinned RPE, chorioretinal atrophy, narrowing and sheathing of retinal vessels, extensive neural retinal areas of white with pressure, lattice degeneration of the neural retina, marked neural retinal meridional folds, and optic atrophy. The condition should be differentiated from *snowflake vitreoretinal degeneration* (SVD), a hereditary vitreoretinal degeneration characterized by multiple, minute, whitish-yellow dots in the peripheral neural retina. The genetic locus for SVD is in a region of chromosome 2q36, flanked by D28S2158 and D2S2202.

E. An autosomal-dominant heredity—mutations that cause Wagner's disease (and also erosive vitreoretinopathy) type I are linked to markers on the long arm of chromosome 5 (5q13–14) and type II the *COL2A1* gene on locus 12q13–14.

Many cases previously reported as Wagner's syndrome (and also Pierre Robin syndrome) probably represent Stickler's syn-

drome (hereditary progressive arthro-ophthalmopathy). *Stickler's syndrome* (see Table 11.2), which has an autosomal-dominant inheritance pattern and shows ocular, orofacial, and skeletal abnormalities, can be divided into thre types: type I is caused by mutations in the *COL2A1* gene on chromosome 12q13–14 in the nonhelical 3' end of the type II procollagen gene; type II *COL11A1* gene on locus 1p21; and type III *COL11A2* gene on 6p22–23.

Choroidal Dystrophies

See pp. 346 in Chapter 9.

Stargardt's Disease (Fundus Flavimaculatus)

I. Stargardt's disease (Fig. 11.34) is inherited as an autosomal-recessive trait [the photoreceptor gene, *ABCR* or *ABCA4* (also known as *STGD1*) on chromosome 1p21 is mutated in Stargardt's disease].

The mechanism involved in the loss of vision is not known, although all-*trans*-retinol dehydrogenase, a photoreceptor outer-segment enzyme, may be defective in Stargardt's disease. Rarely, Stargardt's disease is inherited as an autosomal-dominant trait. Linkage analysis of families with autosomal-dominant Stargardt-like macular dystrophy has shown the disease gene in one family on 13q34 and on 6q14 in other families. The gene responsible for dominant Stargardt macular dystrophy is a retinal photoreceptor-specific gene, *ELOVL4*.

II. Stargardt's disease consists of two parts that may occur simultaneously or independently: a macular dystrophy and a flecked neural retina (*fundus flavimaculatus*).
   A. The macular dystrophy component
     1. Initially, it is confined to the posterior pole, eventually leading to loss of central vision.
     2. Reduced visual acuity is the initial symptom, and is usually first noted between the ages of 8 and 15 years.
     3. In the early stages of reduced visual acuity, the macula may appear normal. Later, a horizontally oval area of atrophy and pigment dispersal develops in the fovea.
     4. Ophthalmoscopically, the macula takes on a "beaten-bronze atrophy" caused by a sharply defined RPE atrophy.
       a. The macula also shows a bull's-eye configuration (see p. 434 in this chapter for differential diagnosis of bull's-eye macula).
       b. The peripheral neural retina may show areas that resemble RP.

> Stargardt's original report described numerous shark-fin-shaped spots around the papillofoveal area characteristic of fundus flavimaculatus (see later). Fundus flavimaculatus and Stargardt's disease represent different ends of a spectrum of the same disease, the former in its pure form consisting of a pericentral tapetoretinal dystrophy and the latter in its pure form consisting of a central tapetoretinal dystrophy, but usually showing considerable overlap.

     5. Dark adaptation and ERG are normal or only mildly abnormal in the purely central type, but are subnormal in the perifoveal and peripheral neural retinal type.
     6. Fluorescein angiography shows fluorescence of the central fovea without leakage, often in a bull's-eye configuration, suggesting defects in the RPE but an intact Bruch's membrane.
       a. In addition, in approximately 86% of cases, fluorescein angiography shows a dark fundus picture with a generalized diminution of background fluorescence.
       b. An increased amount of lipofuscin-like material in the RPE causes the decreased fluorescence.
     7. Histologically, there is a complete disappearance of the RPE and of the visual elements in the macular area.

The inner layers of the neural retina may show cystoid degeneration and calcium deposition.
   B. The flecked neural retina (fundus flavimaculatus) component

> The differential diagnosis of flecked neural retina includes ARMD, autosomal-dominant central pigmentary sheen dystrophy, crystalline dystrophy, benign familial fleck neural retina, Bietti's crystalline dystrophy, canthaxanthine (skin-tanning agent), central and peripheral drusen retinopathy, cystinosis, dominant drusen of Bruch's membrane (Doyne's honeycomb dystrophy), familial flecked retina with night blindness, flecked retina of Kandori, fundus flavimaculatus, glycogen storage disease (GSD), gyrate atrophy, Hollenhorst plaques, Kjellin's syndrome, juxtafoveal telangiectasis, oxylosis (primary, or secondary to long-standing neural retinal detachment, methoxyflurane general anesthesia, or ingestion of an oxalate precursor such as ethylene glycol, i.e., antifreeze), retinitis punctata albescens, ring 17 chromosome, Sjögren–Larsson syndrome, Sorsby's pseudoinflammatory macular dystrophy, talc retinopathy (intravenous drug abusers), tamoxifen (antiestrogen medication), and nitrofurantoin medications.

     1. Fundus flavimaculatus shows ill-defined, yellowish spots shaped like crescents, shark fins, fishtails, fish, or dots located at the level of the RPE.
     2. Approximately 50% of eyes show a Stargardt-type macular dystrophy with a decrease in visual acuity.
     3. The peripheral neural retina may show areas that resemble RP.
     4. Dark adaptation and ERG are usually normal but may be subnormal.
     5. Fluorescein angiography does not cause fluorescence of the spots in early lesions, and not all the spots fluoresce in late lesions.
       a. The fluorescein shapes are irregular, soft, and fuzzy and show a marked tendency for confluence.
       b. The fluorescein pattern clearly differentiates the spots from drusen.
       c. Fluorescein angiography shows a dark fundus (see earlier).
     6. Histologically, the RPE is solely involved—hence the abnormal electro-oculogram (EOG)—and shows:
       a. PAS positivity and increased autofluorescence
       b. Displacement of the nucleus from near the base of the cell to the center or apical surface
       c. An increased amount of pigment granules, most of which are lipofuscin-like, in the center or near the apical surface of the cell, often at the level of the displaced nucleus
       d. Great variation in RPE cell size, from much larger than normal to normal

Dominant Drusen of Bruch's Membrane

Doyne's Honeycomb Dystrophy; Malattia Lèventinese; Hutchinson–Tay Choroiditis; Guttate Choroiditis; Holthouse–Batten Superficial Choroiditis; Family Choroiditis; Crystalline Retinal Degeneration; Iridescent Crystals of the Macula; Hyaline Dystrophies

I. Dominant drusen of Bruch's membrane is a bilateral, symmetric, progressive disease whose onset is usually between 20 and 30 years of age.
 A. It involves the posterior pole predominantly and results in loss of vision.
  1. The posterior polar lesion consists of moderate- to large-sized drusen, resembling soft drusen.

Although there may be subtle differences, dominant drusen can be considered to be synonymous with Doyne's honeycomb dystrophy and malattia lèventinese.

 B. It is inherited as an autosomal-dominant trait.

The gene responsible has been mapped to the short arm of chromosome 2 (2p16–21) in both dominant drusen and malattia lèventinese. Other families map to 1q25–q31 and 6q14.

II. Dark adaptation and ERG are normal.
III. Fluorescein angiography shows multiple, sharply defined fluorescent spots or flecks (see p. 441 in this chapter for differential diagnosis of fleck retina) corresponding to the clinically seen lesions; some confluence of fluorescent areas occurs, but there is no leakage of dye.
IV. Histologically, the lesions appear as large, soft drusen between the RPE and Bruch's membrane.

The predominant ultrastructural features include deposition of a material composed of tubelike structures, vesicles, and membranous material between the basement membrane of the RPE and the inner collagenous layer of Bruch's membrane.

Best's Disease

Vitelliform Foveal Dystrophy; Vitelliform Macular Degeneration; Vitelliruptive Macular Degeneration; Exudative Central Detachment of the Retina—Macular Pseudocysts; Cystic Macular Degeneration; Exudative Foveal Dystrophy

I. Best's disease (Fig. 11.35) is a bilateral, symmetric, progressive disease involving the RPE of the macular area with resultant loss of vision.
 A. Its onset is usually before 15 years of age.
 B. It has an autosomal-dominant mode of transmission with diminished penetrance and a highly variable expression. The Best's disease gene lies on the long arm of chromosome 11 (11q13), the *VMD2* gene.
 C. Only approximately 1% of all cases of macular degeneration are attributable to Best's disease.
II. Ophthalmoscopically, the central macula takes on an early egg-yolk appearance (the color is probably caused by lipofuscin pigment) that later becomes "scrambled" and pigmented.

The egg-yolk appearance of the macula is not always present and sometimes may never occur. The fundus may show only very slight changes or resemble the terminal stage of extensive central inflammatory chorioretinitis, or any stage in between.

III. Dark adaptation and ERG are usually normal.
 A. EOG shows an abnormal light-peak/dark-trough ratio in affected patients as well as in carriers.
 B. Fluorescein angiography shows no leakage into the yellow deposits, but rather a transmission (window) defect in the area.

Multiple vitelliform cysts, macular and extramacular, may develop in patients who have Best's disease. The cysts typically obstruct choroidal fluorescence and do not stain during the early phases, thus differentiating them from idiopathic serous detachment of the RPE.

IV. Histologically, RPE cells show a generalized enlargement, flattening, and engorgement by abnormal lipofuscin and pleomorphic melanolipofuscin granules, most pronounced in the fovea. The outer nuclear layer attenuation is prominent.
V. Lesions similar to those seen in Best's disease may occur in patients without Best's disease as part of ARMD, a condition called *pseudovitelliform* or *adult vitelliform macular degeneration*.
 A. Pseudovitelliform macular degeneration can occur with nonspecific RPE changes, cuticular or basal laminar drusen, detachment of the RPE, and perifoveal retinal capillary leakage.
 B. The visual acuity is decreased but usually stabilizes.
 C. Dry ARMD may develop in some cases and, rarely, some of these pseudovitelliform lesions develop full-thickness holes.

Dominant Progressive Foveal Dystrophy

I. The clinical picture of dominant progressive foveal dystrophy is quite similar to Stargardt's disease (which has a recessive inheritance) except that it tends less toward involvement of the peripheral neural retina, occurs at a later age, and usually takes a less progressive course. It is inherited as an autosomal-dominant trait.
II. The one histologic study in a 78-year-old woman showed disappearance of the outer nuclear layer and receptors and pronounced changes in the RPE.

A similar entity, *dominant slowly progressive macular dystrophy*, differs only slightly from dominant progressive foveal dystrophy.

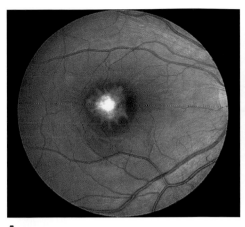
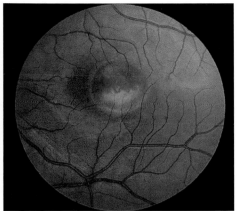

A

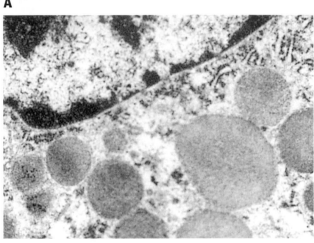

B

Fig. 11.35 Best's disease (vitelliform foveal dystrophy). **A,** Fundus picture of a patient with Best's disease shows a "scrambled-egg" appearance of the fovea in the right eye (*left*) and a typical "egg yolk" appearance in the left eye (*right*). **B,** Another eye from a 28-year-old man with Best's disease was enucleated after an accidental death. Electron micrograph shows cells of retinal pigment epithelium in the involved area are engorged by abnormal lipofuscin granules. (**B,** Adapted from Weingeist TA *et al.: Arch Ophthalmol* 100:1108, 1982. © American Medical Association. All rights reserved.)

Dominant Cystoid Macular Dystrophy

I. Dominant cystoid macular dystrophy consists of macular cystoid edema with central bull's-eye (see p. 434 in this chapter for differential diagnosis of bull's-eye macula) and peripheral neural retinal pigmentary disturbance, cells in the vitreous body, wrinkling of the internal limiting membrane, and axial hypermetropia.

  A. It is inherited as an autosomal-dominant trait.

  B. Fluorescein angiography shows the changes typical of cystoid macular edema in some, but not all, cases.

  C. Sometimes a lamellar macular hole may develop.

II. The histology is unknown.

Fenestrated Sheen Macular Dystrophy

I. This autosomal-dominant condition starts in childhood as a yellowish, refractile sheen that contains red fenestrations in the macular neural retina.

  A. In the early stage small, red, demarcated lesions deep in the nonthickened neural retina have been called *fenestrations.*

  B. By the third decade, an annular zone of hypopigmentation of the RPE appears and then progressively enlarges around the area of the sheen.

  C. The hypopigmented area is surrounded by an area of hyperpigmentation (bull's-eye appearance—see p. 434 in this chapter for differential diagnosis of bull's-eye macula).

II. Fluorescein angiography shows no abnormalities in the neural retina and an intact choriocapillaris perfusion.

III. The histology is unknown.

North Carolina Macular Dystrophy

I. North Carolina macular dystrophy is an autosomal-dominant, slowly progressive macular dystrophy, fully penetrant, with highly variable expressivity.

  The chromosomal locus for this retinal macular dystrophy gene (*MCDR1*) is found on the long arm of chromosome 6 (6q14–q16.2)

II. In younger people, the characteristic fundus abnormalities consist of numerous drusen-like deposits mainly in the macula, and in older people, geographic atrophy in the macula.

III. Affected individuals show a light iris and choroid, prolonged dark adaptation, and increased light sensitivity.

IV. Histopathology

A. Discrete macular lesion characterized by focal absence of photoreceptor cells and RPE

B. Bruch's membrane is attenuated and the choriocapillaris is focally atrophic.

Familial Internal Limiting Membrane Dystrophy

I. Familial internal limiting membrane dystrophy, a type of sheen retinal dystrophy, is probably inherited as an autosomal-dominant trait.

A. The characteristic fundus finding is a glistening inner retinal surface throughout the posterior pole.

B. ERG demonstrates a selective diminution of the b wave.

II. Histologically, the internal limiting membrane of the neural retina shows areas of diffuse, irregular thickening and undulation.

A. Inner schisis cavities and cystoid spaces in the inner nuclear layer are also seen.

B. Electron microscopy of the retinal capillaries shows endothelial cell swelling, pericyte degeneration, and basement membrane thickening.

Central Pigmentary Sheen Dystrophy

I. Central pigmentary sheen dystrophy is a familial (probably autosomal-dominant), bilateral, symmetric, mild pigmentary maculopathy involving the posterior pole that has a variable effect on visual acuity.

A. The posterior pole shows a diffuse yellowish sheen associated with yellow dots or flecks (see p. 441 in this chapter for differential diagnosis of fleck retina).

B. The peripheral fundus is normal.

II. Fluorescein angiography shows a transmitted hyperfluorescence without leakage.

Cone–Rod Dystrophy

I. Cone–rod dystrophy (also called *cone dystrophy*) represents a clinically heterogeneous group of disorders, characterized by a decrease in previously normal vision usually in the first two decades of life, with normal or only minimally abnormal fundi.

A. It is most often inherited as an autosomal-dominant trait, although autosomal-recessive and X-linked inheritance patterns have been reported.

Autosomal-dominant cone–rod dystrophy has been localized to chromosomes 1q12–q24, 6p21.1, 19q13.3, and 17p12–. At least nine genes have been identified: *CRX, GUCY2D, AIPL1, GUCA1A, GCAP1, RIMS1,* and *UNC119.* The autosomal-recessive cone–rod dystrophy locus is 1p21–p13; *ABCA4* and *RDH5* are causative genes. *RPGR* is the causative gene for the X-linked recessive form.

B. At least four functionally distinct subtypes of cone–rod dystrophy exist.

C. Ophthalmoscopically, the fundus may be normal, show nonspecific foveal RPE changes (hypopigmentation, mottling, atrophic appearing), a bull's-eye macula (see p. 434 in this chapter for differential diagnosis of bull's-eye macula), or peripheral hypopigmentation and hyperpigmentation.

Alström's syndrome, an autosomal-recessive, congenital, progressive cone–rod retinal degeneration associated with infantile-onset obesity, can be confused with cone–rod dystrophy.

II. Histologically, a loss of photoreceptors occurs mainly in the central macula, along with attenuation of the RPE.

A. Reduced numbers of cones occur to a lesser extent around the macula and in the periphery of the neural retina.

B. Electron microscopy shows an accumulation of abnormal lipofuscin granules in the RPE and marked enlargement and distortion of the cone photoreceptor pedicles.

Annular Macular Dystrophy (Benign Concentric Annular Macular Dystrophy)

I. Annular macular dystrophy is characterized by a depigmented ring around an intact central macular area.

With time, the dystrophy, which is inherited as an autosomal-dominant trait, takes on the functional characteristics of a cone–rod dystrophy.

II. The dystrophy locus maps to the BCAMID defect with chromosome 6, region p12.3-q16. A leu579Pro mutation in the *IMPGI* gene may play a causal role.

III. The histology is unknown.

Retinitis Punctata Albescens (Albipunctate Dystrophy; Fundus Albipunctatus; Panretinal Degeneration)

I. Retinitis punctata albescens is a bilateral, symmetric disease that may extend to the peripheral neural retina, characterized by flecks (flecked neural retina) and white-dot or punctate lesions with maximum density in the equatorial region; see p. 441 in this chapter for differential diagnosis of fleck neural retina.

The hereditary pattern is not clear; both dominant and recessive forms may exist.

Mutations of the 11-*cis* retinal dehydrogenase (*RDH5*) gene cause retinitis punctata albescens, and probably also cause a progressive cone dystrophy.

II. Two types have been described.

A. Stationary retinitis punctata albescens (fundus albipunctatus) shows little or no constriction of visual fields, normal or mildly subnormal ERG, good central vision, white dots in the fundus, and no pigmentary changes.

    1. Although the physiologic (functional) defects appear to be stable, the fundus lesions can evolve from flecks in childhood to relatively permanent punctate dots that increase in number over the years.

    2. Fundus albipunctatus is a form of *congenital stationary night blindness.*

       Congenital stationary night blindness is most often caused by a primary defect of the rod system. Autosomal-dominant and recessive (*RDH5*; 12q13-q14) and X-linked inheritance patterns of the disease have been described. Most cases of congenital stationary night blindness have normal fundi; two with abnormal fundi are fundus albipunctatus and Oguchi's disease.

  B. Progressive retinitis punctata albescens (also called *retinitis punctata albescens*) shows increasing constriction of visual fields, deterioration of central vision, anomalies of color vision, night blindness, extinguished ERG, mild to moderate optic atrophy, and occasionally some retinal pigmentary changes and is a variant of RP.

  III. Fluorescein shows multiple areas of fluorescent staining without leakage, corresponding to the dot lesions.

  IV. No pathologic specimens have been studied histologically, but the defect is suspected of being at the level of the RPE, probably similar to drusen.

Central Retinitis Pigmentosa (Central Retinopathia Pigmentosa; Retinopathia Pigmentosa Inversa; Retinitis Pigmentosa Inversa; Pericentral Pigmentary Retinopathy)

  I. Central RP shows the changes of classic RP but is confined to the posterior pole.

    A. It is presumably inherited as an autosomal-recessive trait.

    B. It may have a pericentral location.

  II. Dark adaptation and ERG are normal or only minimally subnormal.

  III. Histologically, the changes are the same as those of classic RP.

    Pigmentary macular changes may also be seen in ARMD, and inherited diseases such as Bardet–Biedl syndrome, Bassen–Kornzweig syndrome, Batten–Mayou disease, Cockayne's syndrome, familial hypobetalipoproteinemia, Hallervorden–Spatz syndrome, Hallgren's syndrome, Hooft's syndrome, patterned dystrophy of the RPE, Pelizaeus–Merzbacher disease, Refsum's disease, Stargardt's disease, and others.

Retinitis Pigmentosa (Retinopathia Pigmentosa; Pigmentary Degeneration of the Retina)

  I. RP (Fig. 11.36) is a bilateral, symmetric, progressive disease whose onset is in early adult life.

    A. It starts in the equatorial area of the retina and spreads centrally and peripherally, but more rapidly in the latter direction.

    B. The inheritance pattern may be autosomal-dominant or recessive (about 40% of patients), X-linked, digenic, mitochondrial, or sporadic.

Autosomal-dominant RP loci have been mapped on chromosomes 3q (*rhodopsin*), 6p (*peripherin/RDS*), 7p, 7q, 8cen, 17p, 17q, and 19q. Evidence suggests that at least 11 diffferent genes can cause dominant RP but only four have been identified: rhodopsin (*RHO*), retinal degeneration slow (*RDS*), neural retinal leucine zipper (*NRL*), and *RP1*. Autosomal-recessive RP loci have been mapped on chromosomes 1q, 3q, 4p, 4cen, 5q, 6p, 11p, 11q, 14q, 15q, and 16q. Digenic RP loci have been mapped on chromosomes 6p and 11q. The *rhodopsin* and the *peripherin*/RDS genes account for perhaps 25% of all cases of autosomal-dominant RP. In fact, over 70 different mutations in the rhodopsin gene have been shown to cause RP. The gene for X-linked RP, the most severe form of the disease, has been localized within a 1/cM region at Xp21. At least two loci exist on the X chromosome: *RP2* at the proximal (Xp11) region of the short arm; and *RP3* distal to *RP2*. The degree of central vision loss is mildest in cases of autosomal-dominant inheritance and most severe in X-linked recessive inheritance. Most, if not all, adult heterozygous (X-linked type) women have detectable degenerative changes in the fundus, mainly peripheral atrophy of the RPE.

    C. The primary defect (a form of apoptosis) appears to be in the receptors and is gene-determined (see p. 23 in Chapter 1).

  II. Night blindness is an early symptom and marked vision impairment a late symptom.

    A. The tetrad of bone–corpuscular neural retinal pigmentation; pale, waxy optic disc; attenuation of retinal blood vessels; and posterior subcapsular cataract (see Fig. 10.16C) is characteristic.

    B. Some degree of vitreous degeneration is found in almost all patients.

    C. Three types of central macular lesion may be seen:

      1. Atrophy with RPE thinning (hypopigmentation) and mottled transmission on fluorescein angiography (most common, approximately 58%)

Blacks who have RP are approximately twice as likely as whites to have an atrophic-appearing macular lesion.

---

      2. Cystoid macular edema and leakage of fluorescein from foveal retinal capillaries (approximately 23%)

      3. Cystic macular lesions with radial, inner neural retinal traction lines, often associated with epiretinal membranes which cause a surface wrinkling (approximately 19%)

    D. RP may be associated with an exudative vasculopathy that may be derived from abnormal retinal blood vessels (resembling Coats' disease) or from abnormal choroidal blood vessels.

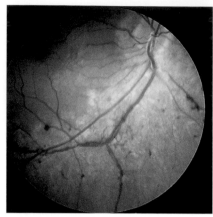

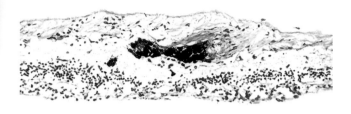

A B

C

Fig. 11.36 Retinitis pigmentosa. **A,** The fundus picture shows a characteristic sharp demarcation from the relatively normal posterior pole to the "moth-eaten" appearance of the retina that extends out to the equator. Bone–corpuscular retinal pigmentation is present. **B,** A histologic section of another case shows melanin-filled macrophages and retinal pigment epithelium cells in the neural retina, mainly around blood vessels, resulting in the clinically seen bone–corpuscular retinal pigmentation. **C,** A histologic section of the posterior pole shows loss of photoreceptors and atrophy of the choriocapillaris. (See Fig. 10.16C for picture of cataract in retinitis pigmentosa.)

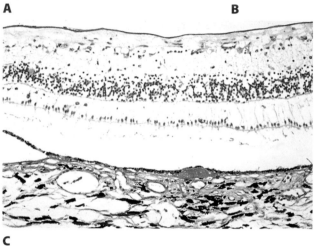

E. Mulberry drusen of the optic nerve or peripapillary neural retina may be seen in approximately 20% of cases, regardless of genetic subtype.

III. Dark adaptation is markedly abnormal, as is the ERG, which is usually extinguished.

Fluorescein study shows a mottled hyperfluorescence involving the posterior and pre-equatorial eyegrounds, even when minimal ophthalmoscopic changes are present.

In most cases of secondary RP, fluorescein shows a mottled hyperfluorescence only in areas of abnormal pigmentation, thereby differing from primary RP.

IV. Histologically, the earliest changes are in the RPE and rods and cones, mainly in the equatorial region.
  A. With progression, all rods and cones disappear except for rods in the far periphery and cones in the fovea.
  B. The RPE undergoes both degeneration and proliferation, most marked from the equator posteriorly almost to the posterior pole.

1. Intrasensory neural retinal migration of pigment-filled macrophages and of RPE occurs.
2. The pigment tends to collect and remain around blood vessels, which accounts for the clinical bone–corpuscular appearance.

C. Bruch's membrane remains intact, even in the latest stages of the disease.

D. An epiretinal glial membrane may be present on the peripapillary neural retina and also over the optic disc.

Traumatic chorioretinopathy, which can resemble primary RP to a marked degree both clinically and histologically, is usually accompanied by interruptions of Bruch's membrane and true chorioretinal scars. If no chorioretinal scars are present histologically, the diagnosis of primary RP may be made. If chorioretinal scars are present histologically, however, the diagnosis remains uncertain because eyes blind from primary RP are often also traumatized and, therefore, have secondary chorioretinal scars.

V. Secondary RP (Table 11.3).

TABLE 11.3 Causes of Secondary Retinitis Pigmentosa

Cause	Major Findings	Inheritance
Älstrom's syndrome	Obesity, diabetes mellitus, nystagmus	Autosomal-recessive
Arteriohepatic dysplasia	Intrahepatic cholestatic syndrome	Autosomal-dominant
Bacterial or protozoal retinitis (e.g., congenital or acquired syphilis or toxoplasmosis)	According to specific agent	—
Bardet–Biedl syndrome	Mental retardation, obesity, hypogenitalism, polydactyly	Autosomal-recessive
Bassen–Kornzweig syndrome (abetalipoproteinemia)	Acanthocytosis, heredodegenerative neuromuscular disease, abetalipoproteinemia	Autosomal-recessive
Boucher–Neuhäuser syndrome	Cerebellar ataxia, hypogonadotropic hypogonadism, chorioretinal dystrophy	Autosomal-recessive
Cockayne's syndrome	Progressive infantile deafness, dwarfism, progeria, oligophrenia, changes in Bowman's membrane	Autosomal-recessive
Cystinosis	Polyuria, growth retardation, rickets, progressive renal failure	Autosomal-recessive
Drug-induced retinopathy (e.g., vitamin A, chloroquine, or chlorpromazine intoxication)	According to specific agent	—
Familial juvenile nephronophthisis (Senioz's syndrome)	Interstitial nephritis, hepatic fibrosis	Autosomal-recessive
Flynn–Aird syndrome	Cataracts, ataxia, dementia, epilepsy, cutaneous changes	Autosomal-dominant
Friedreich's ataxia	Posterior column disease, nystagmus, ataxia	Autosomal-recessive
Goldmann–Favre disease	Vitreous degeneration, preretinal strands, juvenile retinoschisis	Autosomal-recessive
Hallervorden–Spatz syndrome	Extrapyramidal signs related to changes in the basal ganglia, which are rust-brown at autopsy	Autosomal-recessive
Hallgren's syndrome	Congenital deafness, vestibulocerebellar ataxia, mental deficiency, psychoses, nystagmus, cataract	Autosomal-recessive
Hereditary olivopontocerebellar degeneration	Ataxia of all extremities, slurred speech, writhing athetosis	Autosomal-dominant
Imidazole aminoaciduria	Seizures, mental deterioration, excess carnosine and anserine excretions	Autosomal-recessive
Infantile phytanic acid storage disease	Hypotonia, hearing loss, hepatic dysfunction	Autosomal-recessive
Jeune's asphyxiating thoracic dystrophy	Respiratory insufficiency, hepatic fibrosis, interstitial nephritis	Autosomal-recessive
Juvenile familial nephrophthisis	Cystic disease of the renal medulla	Autosomal-recessive
Kartagener's syndrome	Dextrocardia, bronchiectasis, sinusitis	Autosomal-recessive
Kearns–Sayre's syndrome (mitochondrial myopathy)	Progressive external ophthalmoplegia, heart blocks	—
Laurence–Moon–Biedl (Bardet–Biedl) syndrome	Mental retardation, hypogenitalism, spastic paraplegia	Autosomal-recessive
Leber's congenital amaurosis of retinal origin	Nystagmus, zonular cataracts, keratoconus and keratoglobus, mental retardation	Usually autosomal-recessive but rarely autosomal-dominant
Lignac–Fanconi syndrome	Renal dwarfism, osteoporosis, chronic nephritis	Autosomal-recessive
Mucopolysacchiridoses	See p. 298, Chapter 8	—
Myotonic dystrophy	Myotonia, frontal baldness, endocrinopathy, cataracts	Autosomal-dominant
Neonatal adrenoleukodystrophy	Severe neurologic involvement	Autosomal-recessive
Neuronal ceroid lipofuscinosis	Late infantile (Hagberg–Santavuori) and juvenile (Batten–Spielmeyer–Vogt) forms of amaurotic idiocy	Autosomal-recessive
Organization of retinal hemorrhages	—	—
Pelizaeus–Merzbacher disease	Diffuse cerebral sclerosis, extrapyramidal signs, mental deterioration	X-linked recessive
Pigmented paravenous chorioretinal atrophy	Bilateral, bone–corpuscular pigmentation along veins	—
Refsum's disease	Chronic polyneuritis, cardiac abnormalities, α-hydroxylase lacking, phytanic acid stored in tissues	Autosomal-recessive
Trauma	—	—
Turner's syndrome	Infertility, short stature, shield chest, low hairline, 45,XO	—
Usher's syndrome	Familial congenital deafness	Autosomal-recessive
Viral retinitis (e.g., congenital rubella)	According to specific agent	—
Zellweger's (cerebrohepatorenal) syndrome	Severe neurologic involvement	Autosomal-recessive

Clumped Pigmentary Retinal Dystrophy (Clumped Pigmentary Retinal Degeneration)

I. Clumped pigmentary retinal dystrophy is characterized by numerous clumped pigment deposits throughout the mid peripheral fundus.
   A. The onset of night blindness varies from the first to the sixth decade of life.
   B. The ERG amplitude is reduced.
   C. Peripheral visual field loss is present.
II. An autosomal-recessive mode of inheritance is suggested.
III. Histologically, the clinically observed clumped pigmentation is caused by the accumulation of melanin granules in RPE cells.

The photoreceptors in the areas of clumped pigmentation show considerable generation.

Hereditary Pigmented Paravenous Chorioretinal Atrophy

I. Hereditary pigmented paravenous chorioretinal atrophy is characterized by bone spicule pigment accumulation in a paravenous distribution.
II. The abnormal ERG suggests a localized dystrophy and the abnormal EOG suggests a more widespread phenomenon.
III. The condition can be inherited, but the inheritance pattern is uncertain.

Pigment Epithelial Dystrophy

I. The condition, which occurs at birth or shortly thereafter, consists of myopia, nystagmus, and an RPE dystrophy that appears to be stationary or slowly progressive.
   It is inherited as an autosomal-dominant trait.
II. Ophthalmoscopically, the RPE shows changes from a mild peripapillary sheen often associated with an irregularity of foveal reflex, or a loss of it, to an advanced stage that shows a geographic loss of RPE, increased visibility of choroidal vasculature, and pigment clumping.
III. Tests of visual function (visual acuity, perimetric fields, ERG, and EOG) tend to be altered in proportion to the retinal dystrophy.
IV. The histologic lesion is unknown but presumed to be at the level of the RPE.

Central Areolar Pigment Epithelial Dystrophy

I. Central areolar pigment epithelial dystrophy is characterized by childhood onset, good visual acuity, and nonprogression.
   It has an autosomal-dominant inheritance pattern with a late onset and variable expressivity.
II. Ophthalmoscopically, a central, areolar, depigmented, sharply demarcated area is noted that involves the RPE.

III. Retinal function studies are negative. Fluorescein angiography shows a transmission (window) defect.
IV. The histologic lesion is unknown, but it is presumed to be at the level of the RPE.

Patterned Dystrophies of the Retinal Pigment Epithelium (Reticular Dystrophy or Sjögren Dystrophia Reticularis Laminae Pigmentosae Retinae; Butterfly-Shaped Pigment Dystrophy of the Fovea; Macroreticular or Spider Dystrophy)

I. Patterned dystrophies of the RPE are bilateral and symmetric, characterized by foveal involvement with preservation of good vision, and have an autosomal-recessive inheritance pattern.

Mutations of the *peripherin/RDS* gene may be associated with patterned dystrophies of the RPE, autosomal-dominant RP, and fundus flavimaculatus. Macroreticular (macular) pattern dystrophy may be associated with maternally inherited diabetes and deafness, associated with a mutation of mitochondrial DNA [the substitution of guanine for adenine (A–G) at position 3243 of leucine transfer RNA]. Different members of the same family may show the three varieties (i.e., reticular dystrophy, butterfly-shaped foveal pigment dystrophy, and macroreticular or spider dystrophy). Patients who have adult-onset foveomacular dystrophy (AOFMD) may show a frameshift null mutation in the RDS/peripherin gene on chromosome 6p21. A rare case of patterned dystrophy has been reported to be associated with McArdle's disease, a type V GSD.

II. Ophthalmoscopic appearance
   A. Reticular dystrophy—the macula shows a fishnet-like pattern with an accumulation of dark pigment, surrounded by a finely meshed network of polygonally arranged pigment with densification at the sites of the knots of the network.
   B. Butterfly-shaped foveal pigment dystrophy—the fovea shows a small, delicate pigmentary pattern, resembling a butterfly, at the level of the RPE.
   C. Macroreticular or spider dystrophy—the macula shows a branching pigmentary pattern, resembling a spider, at the level of the RPE.
III. Retinal function test results are normal, except for a subnormal EOG in the butterfly-shaped pigment dystrophy of the fovea.
IV. Fluorescein angiography is similar in all three varieties, showing nonfluorescent bands or segments surrounded by areas of nonleaking hyperfluorescence.
V. Histologic study shows focal, abrupt transition from intact retina to a small area of RPE hypertrophy to photoreceptor and RPE atrophy.

Bietti's Crystalline Dystrophy (Bietti's Tapetoretinal Degeneration with Marginal Corneal Dystrophy, Crystalline Retinopathy)

I. Bietti's crystalline dystrophy (Fig. 11.37) consists of small, yellow-white, glistening intraretinal crystals in the poste-

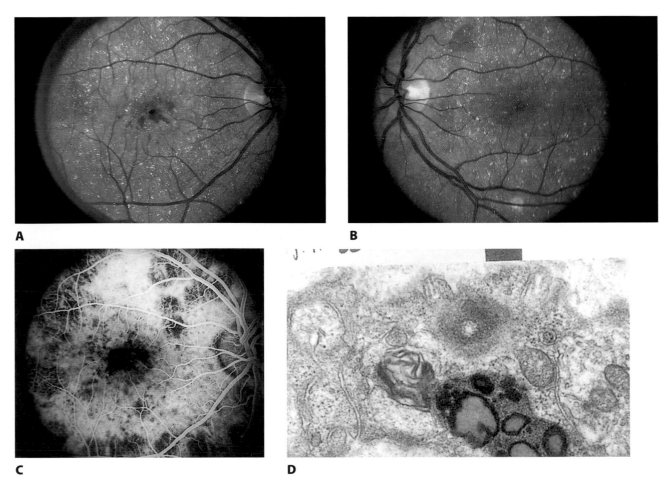

Fig. 11.37 Crystalline retinopathy of Bietti. Clinical appearance of glistening, intraretinal crystals in right (**A**) and left (**B**) eyes. **C,** Fluorescein angiography shows atrophy of choriocapillaris in areas of geographic atrophy of retinal pigment epithelium. **D,** Electron microscopy of conjunctival biopsy from another patient with crystalline retinopathy of Bietti shows dark lipid material in subepithelial fibroblasts. (**D,** Republished from Welch RB: *Trans Am Ophthalmol Soc* 75:164, 1977.)

rior pole, tapetoretinal degeneration with atrophy of the RPE and "sclerosis" of the choroid, and, in many patients, sparkling yellow crystals in the superficial marginal cornea.

It is inherited as an autosomal-recessive trait (4q35-tel) and usually has its onset in the third decade of life.

A closely related entity, including clinical, systemic, and pathologic findings (crystals and granular dense material—similar to that found in cholesterol storage disease—in abnormal lysosomes of circulating lymphocytes, but not in cornea) but with an autosomal-dominant inheritance pattern, a limited expression of the disease, no corneal involvement, a female preponderance, and a later age at onset, has been named *autosomal-dominant crystalline dystrophy.*

II. Ophthalmoscopically, many fine, dotlike crystalline opacities are present at the level of the RPE along with scattered aggregates of retinal pigment (see p. 441 in this chapter for differential diagnosis of fleck neural retina).

The corneal involvement consists of tiny crystals deposited in the peripheral cornea and the superficial layers of the limbal conjunctival substantia propria.

III. Both the ERG and EOG may be abnormal.
   A. Fluorescein angiography shows atrophy of the choriocapillaris confined to the areas of geographic atrophy of the RPE.
   B. Central or paracentral scotomas can be demonstrated on visual field testing.
IV. Histology
   A. The peripheral corneal and limbal conjunctiva deposits are lipid and contained in fibroblasts.
      1. Although the deposits resemble cholesterol (or cholesterol ester) and complex lipid inclusions, their exact nature is unknown.
      2. Biochemical studies have shown that the crystalline liposomal material is not cholesterol.
   B. Similar lipid inclusions may be found in circulating lymphocytes, suggesting that a systemic abnormality of lipid metabolism is the cause.

C. The globe may show advanced panchorioretinal atrophy.

Crystals and complex lipid inclusions are found in choroidal fibroblasts.

Sorsby Fundus Dystrophy (Sorsby's Pseudoinflammatory Macular Dystrophy; Hereditary Macular Dystrophy)

I. Sorsby fundus dystrophy (SFD) is a bilateral, symmetric disease with a late onset, usually in the fifth decade, and an autosomal-dominant or, rarely, recessive inheritance pattern.

The autosomal-dominant variety seems to be related to a Ser-181Cys mutation in chromosome 22 of exon 5 of the gene coding for the tissue inhibitor of metalloproteinases 3 (*TIMP3*) .SFD is caused by mutations in the gene-encoding tissue inhibitor of metalloproteinases-3 (an extracellular matrix protein), the *TIMP3* gene.

II. Onset is acute with loss of central vision and an inflammatory-like macular lesion showing edema, hemorrhages (sometimes in the macula of both eyes), and exudates.
  A. Often, white to yellow spots at the level of Bruch's membrane are present early in the course of the condition (see p. 441 in this chapter for differential diagnosis of fleck neural retina).
  B. Healing takes place slowly; CNV is a rare occurrence.
  C. Over a few decades, the process extends slowly toward the periphery, leaving a spreading area of choroidal atrophy and some pigment deposition.

III. Early, dark adaptation and ERG are normal, but later the ERG becomes subnormal. Fluorescein early in the course of the condition shows delayed filling of the central choriocapillaris; later, extensive defects in the RPE are noted.

IV. Histology
  A. Marked atrophy of the outer neural retina occurs along with a discontinuous RPE and atrophy of the choriocapillaris and choroid.
  B. A 3-μm-thick deposit is seen in Bruch's membrane.

The deposits resemble those found in *late-onset retinal degeneration*, an autosomal-dominant disorder characterized by onset of night vision problems in midlife, and in ARMD.

HEREDITARY SECONDARY RETINAL DYSTROPHIES

Angioid Streaks

I. Angioid streaks (Fig. 11.38) may be found most often in pseudoxanthoma elasticum (Grönblad–Stranberg syndrome) and idiopathically.

A. The streaks may also be found in acromegaly, Bassen–Kornzweig syndrome (abetalipoproteinemia), choriocapillaris atrophy involving the posterior eyegrounds, chromophobe adenoma, diffuse lipomatosis, dwarfism, epilepsy, facial angiomatosis, fibrodysplasia hyperelastica (Ehlers–Danlos syndrome), hemoglobinopathies, hereditary spherocytosis, hyperphosphatemia, idiopathic thrombocytopenic purpura, lead poisoning, neurofibromatosis, osteitis deformans (Paget's disease), and trauma.

The hemoglobinopathies include sickle-cell HbSS, HbSC, HbS (thalassemia), and HbAS (trait) diseases; hemoglobin H disease (HgH); and β-thalassemia major (homozygous), intermedia, and minor.
  B. The mode of hereditary transmission depends on the primary cause.

II. CNV and hemorrhages in and around the macula frequently complicate the condition and may lead to exudative (disciform) macular degeneration.

III. Histologically, Bruch's membrane shows basophilia and is broken and interrupted at the sites of the "streaks."
  A. Fibrovascular tissue usually fills the break.
  B. The contiguous RPE may be abnormal.

Sjögren–Larsson Syndrome

I. Sjögren–Larsson syndrome consists of congenital, low-grade, stationary mental deficiency, congenital ichthyosis, and symmetric spastic paresis of the extremities that tends to involve the legs more than the arms.
  A. It is inherited as an autosomal-recessive trait.
  B. The syndrome is caused by deficient activity of fatty aldehyde dehydrogenase, a transmembrane protein that is part of the microsomal enzyme complex fatty alcohol–nicotinamide adenine oxidoreductase.

II. Approximately 20% to 30% of patients have fundus abnormalities consisting predominantly of depigmented, pale areas in the macular region and neural retinal flecks (see p. 441 in this chapter for differential diagnosis of fleck neural retina).

III. No histologic studies have been done, but the pathologic process is presumed to be at the level of the RPE.

Mucopolysaccharidoses

See p. 298 in Chapter 8; RP-like fundus changes may be found in approximately 20% of the patients. Types IV (Morquio) and VI (Maroteaux–Lamy) are usually excepted.

Mucolipidoses

I. The mucolipidoses are a group of storage diseases (Hurler variants) that exhibit signs and symptoms of both the mucopolysaccharidoses and sphingolipidoses (Table 11.4).

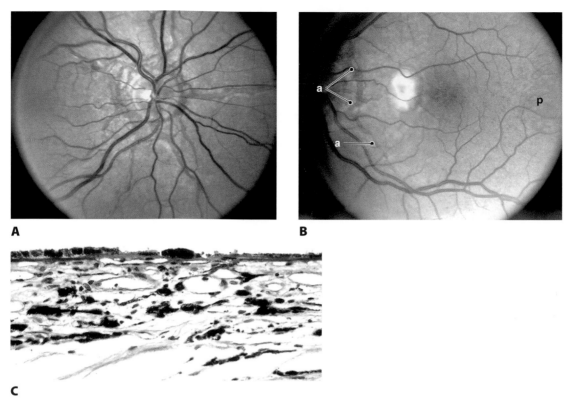

Fig. 11.38 Angioid streaks. **A,** This patient with angioid streaks also had pseudoxanthoma elasticum. Breaks in Bruch's membrane around the optic nerve resulted in angioid streaks. **B,** Similar breaks away from the optic nerve have resulted in "peau d'orange" appearance (a, angioid streaks; p, peau d'orange). The yellow area just temporal to the optic nerve represents subretinal neovascularization. **C,** A histologic section of another case, from a patient with Paget's disease, also shows streaks caused by an interruption (break) in Bruch's membrane. Other causes of angioid streaks include acromegaly, Bassen–Kornzweig syndrome, chromophobe adenoma, diffuse lipomatosis, dwarfism, Ehlers–Danlos syndrome, epilepsy, facial angiomatosis, hemoglobinopathies, hyperphosphatemia, idiopathic thrombocytopenic purpura, lead poisoning, neurofibromatosis, and trauma. Approximately half of angioid streak cases are idiopathic.

II. With the exception of Austin-type sulfatidosis, renal excretion of uronic acid-containing mucopolysaccharides is normal.

> One important feature that differentiates mucolipidoses from mucopolysaccharidoses is that the conjunctival cells in the former group contain single membrane-limited vacuoles filled with fibrillogranular material as well as lamellar bodies, whereas in the latter group lamellar bodies are only occasionally observed. Membranous inclusion bodies are the most characteristic neuronal cellular abnormality in the sphingolipidoses, and similar lamellar storage bodies have been noted in Fabry's disease. Thus, the accumulation of both membranous and fibrillogranular inclusion bodies, suggestive of defects in the degradation of both lipids and complex carbohydrates, is the hallmark of the ultrastructural lesion in the mucolipidoses.

Sphingolipidoses

I. The sphingolipidoses (Fig. 11.39 and Table 11.5) are a group of diseases that have in common the storage of a complex lipid called *ceramide*.

> Ceramide is the long-chain amino alcohol called *sphingosine* to which a long-chain fatty acid is joined by an amide bond to the nitrogen atom on carbon 2 of sphingosine.

A. The stored portion is characteristic for each separate disease.

B. Tay–Sachs disease
  1. Tay–Sachs disease is the prototypical lysosomal sphingolipid storage disease.
  2. Tay–Sachs disease is a uniformly fatal (by 3 to 5 years of age), inherited (autosomal-recessive), neurodegenerative disease found in infants of Central or East European Jewish ancestry, caused by a profound disturbance of the lysosomal hydrolase β-hexosaminidase A (HEX A or GM_2-gangliosidase).
  3. Clinically, the hallmark is a cherry-red spot in the central fovea.

> The ganglion cells, enlarged by storage material, render the neural retina relatively opaque, especially in the posterior pole (anatomic macula) where the ganglion cells are multilayered, giving the neural retina a milky orange

TABLE 11.4 Mucolipidoses (an Arbitrary Classification Subject to Change as New Knowledge Accumulates Rapidly in This Area)

Disease	Eponym/Alternate Name	Enzyme Defect	Tissue Storage	Ocular Signs	Inheritance
GM$_1$-gangliosidosis, type I	Generalized gangliosidosis; Norman–Landing disease	β-Galactosidase	Keratan sulfate (cornea); GM$_1$-ganglioside in retinal ganglion cells and elsewhere	Corneal clouding; macular cherry-red spot	Autosomal-recessive
GM$_1$-gangliosidosis, type II	Late-onset GM$_1$-gangliosidosis	β-Galactosidase	Keratan sulfate (viscera); GM$_1$-ganglioside (brain only)	Not important	Autosomal-recessive
Fucosidosis	—	α-L-Fucosidase	Fucose-containing glycolipids	Bull's-eye maculopathy	Autosomal-recessive
Mannosidosis	—	α-Mannosidases A and B	Mannose-containing glycolipids	Corneal and lenticular opacities; pale optic disc	Autosomal recessive
Juvenile sulfatidosis, Austin type	—	Arylsulfatases A, B, and C	Sulfated mucopolysaccharides (Alder–Reilly granules in leukocytes and Buhot cells in bone marrow)	Pale optic disc; retinal hypopigmentation	Autosomal-recessive
Mucolipidosis I	Lipomucopolysaccharidosis	α-N-acetyl neuraminidase	Acid mucopolysaccharides and glycolipids	Corneal opacities; macular cherry-red spot	Autosomal-recessive
Mucolipidosis II	I-cell disease	β-Galactosidase	Acid mucopolysaccharides and glycolipids; peculiar fibroblast inclusions	Corneal opacities; macular cherry-red spot	Autosomal-recessive
Mucolipidosis III	Pseudo-Hurler's polydystrophy	N-acetylglucosaminyl phosphotransferase	Acid mucopolysaccharides and glycolipids	Corneal clouding	Autosomal-recessive
Mucolipidosis IV	Berman	Ganglioside neuraminidase	Acid mucopolysaccharides and glycolipids	Corneal clouding	Autosomal-recessive
Mucolipidosis V	Newell	Not known	Acid mucopolysaccharides and glycolipids	Corneal clouding; retinal degeneration	Not known
Disseminated lipogranulomatosis	Farber's disease	Ceramidase	Ceramide and glycolipid	Macular cherry-red spot	Autosomal-recessive

appearance. The foveal retina, however, has no inner layers, and therefore no ganglion cells, so that the underlying normal red choroid is seen as a cherry-red spot.

4. Histologically, the ganglion cells become "ballooned" by the massive intralysosomal accumulation (storage) of lipophilic membranous bodies consisting of the sphingolipid GM$_2$-ganglioside.

II. To detect patients and carriers, assay procedures are available for all the sphingolipidoses.

Other Lipidoses

I. Schilder's disease and the Pelizaeus–Merzbacher syndrome—these primarily affect the white matter (optic nerve) with secondary degeneration of the neural retina (see Chapter 13).

II. Late infantile-type galactosialidosis—macular cherry-red spot, corneal clouding, and β-galactosidase and sialidase deficiency characterize the disease, which is a syndrome that combines clinical features of several storage diseases (mucopolysaccharidoses, sphingolipidoses, and mucolipidoses) and is inherited as an autosomal-recessive trait.

III. Wolman's disease

A. Although similar to Niemann–Pick disease clinically, Wolman's disease differs in that it has cholesterol and triglycerides rather than phospholipids deposited in foam cells.

1. Wolman's disease has an autosomal-recessive inheritance pattern and is characterized by hepatospleno-

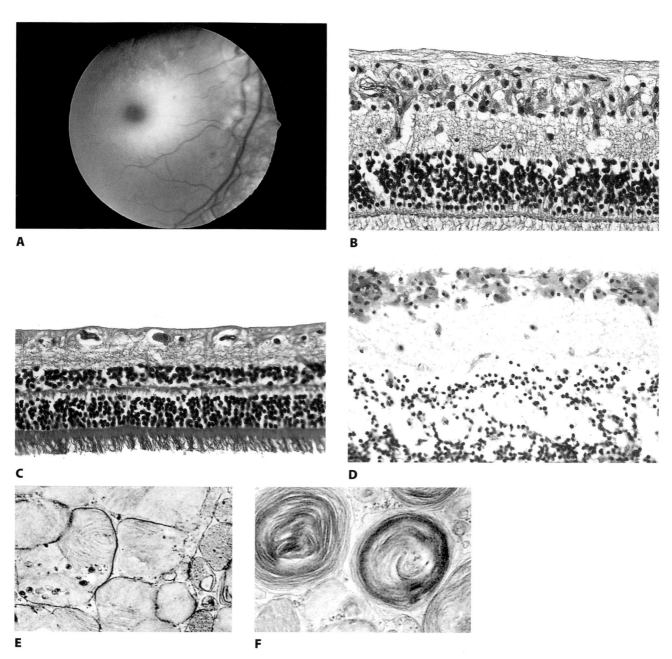

Fig. 11.39 Tay–Sachs disease (histologic findings identical in Sandhoff's disease). **A,** A characteristic cherry-red spot is present in the central macula. **B,** A histologic section shows a normal macular retina, except for ganglion cells that are swollen by periodic acid–Schiff (PAS)-positive material (sphingolipid). **C,** The peripheral retina also shows ganglion cells whose cytoplasm is swollen by PAS-positive material. **D,** Another case shows extensive involvement of ganglion cells. **E,** Electron micrograph shows ganglion cell cytoplasm filled with fine, laminated bodies. Accumulated ganglioside produces opacification of retina, most prominent in foveomacular area. **F,** Another area shows dense lamination in accumulating substance. In other eyes more variegated appearance can be found. (**B–D,** PAS stain.)

megaly, malabsorption, adrenal calcification, and death in early infancy.

2. The cause is a deficiency of a lysosomal acid esterase.

B. Histologically, neural retinal ganglion cells are swollen and contain foamy cytoplasm. Sudanophilic droplets, both free and in macrophages, are found in the sclera, cornea, and ciliary body.

IV. Primary familial hyperlipoproteinemia

A. Five types of hyperlipoproteinemia may be distinguished by paper electrophoresis.

B. The main ocular findings include eruptive xanthomas, conjunctival xanthomas, arcus juvenilis and senilis, lipid keratopathy, iris xanthomas, choroidal xanthomas, lipemia retinalis, retinal hemorrhages, and adult-onset Coats' disease.

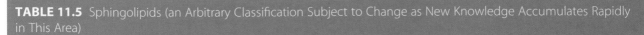

TABLE 11.5 Sphingolipids (an Arbitrary Classification Subject to Change as New Knowledge Accumulates Rapidly in This Area)

Disease	Eponym/Alternate Name	Enzyme Defect	Tissue Storage	Ocular Signs	Inheritance
GM$_2$-gangliosidosis, type I	Tay–Sachs disease	Hexosaminidase A	GM$_2$-ganglioside and ceramide trihexoside	Macular cherry-red spot	Autosomal-recessive
GM$_2$-gangliosidosis, type II	Sandhoff's disease	Hexosaminidase A and B	GM$_2$-ganglioside	Macular cherry-red spot	Autosomal-recessive
GM$_2$-gangliosidosis, type III	Late-onset GM$_2$-gangliosidosis; late infantile or juvenile amaurotic idiocy	Partial deficiency hexosaminidase A	GM$_2$-ganglioside	Not important	Autosomal-recessive
GM$_2$-gangliosidosis, type IV	Type AB	Hexosaminidase A and B	GM$_2$-ganglioside	Macular cherry-red spot	Autosomal-recessive
GM$_3$-gangliosidosis	Max	UDP-GalNAc: GM$_3$ N-acetyl-galactose-aminyl-transferase	GM$_3$-ganglioside in brain and liver	None	Autosomal-recessive
Neuronal ceroid lipofuscinosis (lipopigment storage disorders)	Infantile (Hagberg–Santavuori), late infantile (Jansky–Bielschowsky), juvenile (Spielmeyer–Vogt) and adult (Kufs) forms found	Peroxidase deficiency	Lipofuscin	Macular abnormalities (*not* cherry-red spot), optic atrophy, secondary retinitis pigmentosa	Autosomal-recessive
Essential lipid histiocytosis	Infantile Niemann–Pick disease—type A*	Sphingomyelinase	Sphingomyelin and cholesterol	Macular cherry-red spot	Autosomal-recessive
Lactosyl ceramidosis†	—	Lactosyl ceramide β-galactosidase	Lactosyl ceramide	None	—
Primary splenomegaly‡	Gaucher's disease (infantile neuropathic form)	β-Glucosidase (glucocerebrosidase)	Ceramide glucoside (glucocerebroside)	Pinguecula, cranial nerves involvement	Autosomal-recessive
Angiokeratoma corporis diffusum universale	Fabry's disease	α-Galactosidase	Ceramide trihexoside	Corneal lesions; tortuous retinal blood vessels containing lipid deposits	Sex-linked recessive
Globoid leukodystrophy	Krabbe's disease; infantile diffuse cerebral sclerosis	Galactocerebroside β-galactosidase	Ceramide galactoside (galactocerebroside)	Optic atrophy; nystagmus	Autosomal-recessive
Infantile metachromatic leukodystrophy	Sulfatide lipidosis	Arylsulfatase A	Sulfated glycolipids; metachromatic granules in retinal ganglion cells (mainly the large ones)	Grayness of macula; macular cherry-red spot; optic atrophy	Autosomal-recessive

*Types B, C, D, and E also present. B shows sphingomyelinase deficiency and is a chronic form with no central nervous system involvement. Macular halos may be present. C, D, and E show no sphingomyelinase deficiency; only E shows ocular (macular) involvement as a cherry-red spot.
†Lactosyl ceramidosis shows a partial deficiency of sphingomyelinase and is probably a variant of Niemann–Pick disease.
‡An adult type (nonneuropathic form) may also have an autosomal-dominant mode of inheritance.

Disorders of Carbohydrate Metabolism

I. Diabetes mellitus (see Chapter 15)
II. Lafora's disease (Fig. 11.40)
  A. Lafora's disease is caused by a deficiency of an unknown enzyme.
    1. As a result, polyglucosans are stored in the tissues in different stages of aggregation.
    2. The disease is inherited as an autosomal-recessive trait.
  B. The disease starts in preadolescence or early adolescence and is characterized by Unverricht's syndrome, which consists of myoclonic seizures, grand mal attacks, pro-

gressive ataxia, dysarthria, dyskinesia, amaurosis, and dementia. The disease is relentlessly progressive, with death occurring 4 to 10 years after its onset.
  C. Histologically, basophilic, spherical, laminated deposits (Lafora bodies) are found in the ganglion cells and inner nuclear layer of the neural retina, in the optic nerve, and in the brain. An amorphous, basophilic deposit is found in heart, striated muscle, and liver cells.

Lafora bodies consist of a long-chain polysaccharide amylo-pectin-like material, similar to that found in type IV glycogenosis (Anderson).

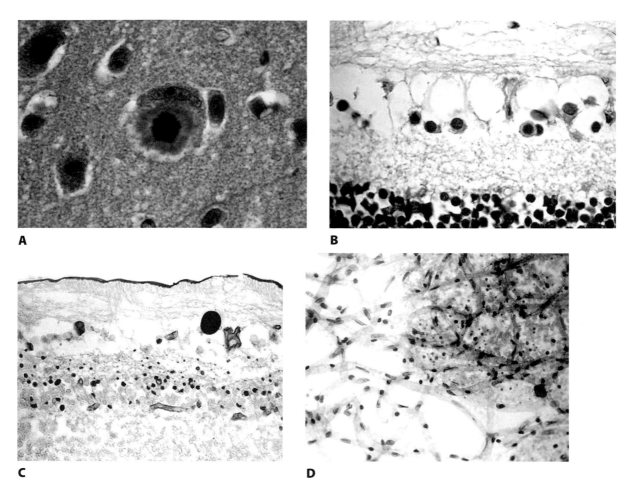

Fig. 11.40 Lafora's disease. Laminated Lafora body seen within neuron in brain (**A**) and within ganglion cell in neural retina (**B**). **C,** Periodic acid–Schiff (PAS) stain without counterstain shows PAS-positive (red) Lafora bodies in neurons of the inner nuclear layer and in ganglion cells. **D,** Lafora bodies seen as small, red, PAS-positive bodies in areas of incomplete digestion on right half of retinal trypsin digest preparation.

III. Glycogen storage disease
   A. Type I GSD (von Gierke's disease) is inherited as an autosomal-recessive trait and caused by a deficiency of the enzyme glucose-6-phosphatase, which results in glycogen storage in the tissues.
      1. Bilateral, symmetric, yellowish, nonelevated, discrete, paramacular neural retinal lesions resembling drusen are found (see p. 441 in this chapter for differential diagnosis of fleck neural retina).
      2. No histopathologic data are available, but the lesions are presumed to be at the level of the RPE.
   B. Type II GSD (Pompe) is caused by a deficiency of the enzyme α-1,4-glucosidase (acid maltase).
      1. As a result, glycogen is stored in the tissue.
      2. The disease is inherited as an autosomal-recessive trait.

More than 70 mutations have been identified in tha α-glucosidase gene.

3. No clinical ocular signs are present.
4. Histologically, lysosomal glycogen is found in neural retinal ganglion cells and pericytes and in smooth and striated ocular muscles.

Type III GSD (Forbes) is caused by amylo-1,6-glucosidase (debrancher) deficiency; type IV GSD (Anderson) is caused by α-1,-4-glucan: α-1,4-glucan 6-glucosyl transferase (brancher) deficiency; type V GSD (McArdle–Schmid–Pearson) is caused by muscle phosphorylase (myophosphorylase) deficiency; type VI GSD (Hers) is caused by hepatic phosphorylase deficiency; type VII GSD is caused by phosphoglucomutase deficiency; type VIII GSD is caused by hepatic phosphorylase deficiency (normal after glucagon or epinephrine administration); type IX GSD is caused by hepatic phosphorylase deficiency (no change after glucagon or epinephrine administration). Types III, IV, and VI through IX have no known ocular findings.

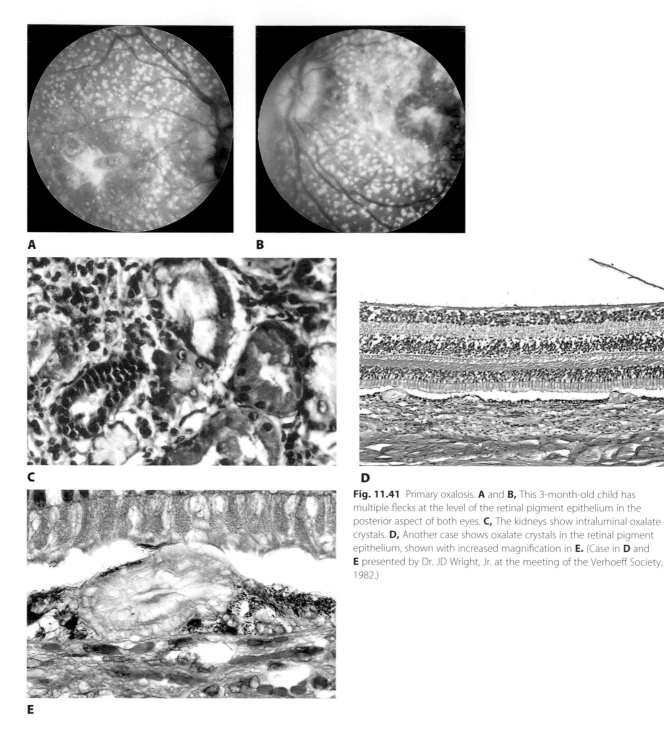

Fig. 11.41 Primary oxalosis. **A** and **B,** This 3-month-old child has multiple flecks at the level of the retinal pigment epithelium in the posterior aspect of both eyes. **C,** The kidneys show intraluminal oxalate crystals. **D,** Another case shows oxalate crystals in the retinal pigment epithelium, shown with increased magnification in **E.** (Case in **D** and **E** presented by Dr. JD Wright, Jr. at the meeting of the Verhoeff Society, 1982.)

Primary Oxalosis (Fig. 11.41)

I. The condition is inherited as an autosomal-recessive trait, is characterized by hyperoxaluria, is usually fatal (renal failure) before the third decade of life, and has two variants.

    A. Type I is caused by a deficiency of the cytoplasmic enzyme α-ketoglutarate glyoxylate carboligase.

    B. Type II is caused by a deficiency of δ-glyceric dehydrogenase.

C. Clinically a maculopathy, often large, pigmented, and geographic, occurs along with RPE flecks (see p. 441 in this chapter for differential diagnosis of fleck neural retina).

Secondary oxalosis may be caused by ingestion of an oxalate precursor such as oxalic acid, ethylene glycol (antifreeze), or rhubarb; hyperabsorption of oxalate after small-bowel resection; renal failure; sarcoidosis; chronic renal failure; cirrhosis of the liver; or after general anesthesia with the anesthetic agent methoxyflurane.

II. Histologically, in primary oxalosis, oxalate crystals are found in the RPE.

The crystals correspond to the clinically seen flecked neural retina. In secondary oxalosis, the oxalate crystals can be found in the walls of retinal blood vessels.

Osteopetrosis

I. Osteopetrosis, caused by an inborn error of metabolism in which the basic metabolic defect is unknown, has infantile (juvenile) and adult forms.
   A. In the infantile form (which is lethal in the first decade if not treated by bone marrow transplantation), visual loss, pendular nystagmus, ptosis, squint, optic disc edema, optic atrophy, and exophthalmos may be seen.

A dysfunction of the monocyte–macrophage system-derived osteoclast leads to failure of cartilage and bone resorption so that the primary spongiosa cannot be removed and converted to more mature bone. New bone formation continues and mineralization of persisting cartilage occurs (endochondral ossification). Spread of abnormal bone into the marrow spaces leads to lethal failure of hematopoiesis.

   An autosomal-recessive inheritance pattern is seen.
   B. In the adult form, a good prognosis exists without treatment.
   An autosomal-dominant inheritance pattern is seen.
II. Histologically, in the infantile form, degeneration of rods, cones, and the outer nuclear layer may be found as well as atrophy and gliosis of the neural retinal ganglion cell and nerve fiber layers and of the optic nerve.

Neural retinal degeneration may occur in the absence of any bone pressure on the optic nerves. The degeneration therefore is probably a primary dystrophy and an integral part of the disease.

Homocystinuria

I. Homocystinuria (see p. 385 in Chapter 10) is an autosomal-recessive disease caused by a deficiency in the enzyme cystathionine synthetase, resulting in an increased concentration of homocysteine, homocystine, or a derivative of homocysteine.
II. A peripheral neural retinal pigmentary dystrophy may be seen ophthalmoscopically in the far periphery near the equator.
III. Histologically, the peripheral retina may show atrophy of its outer layers with inward migration of pigment-filled macrophages.

SYSTEMIC DISEASES INVOLVING THE RETINA

Hereditary Secondary Retinal Dystrophies

See pp. 450–454 in this chapter.

Diabetes Mellitus

See pp. 602–618 in Chapter 15.

Hypertension and Arteriolosclerosis

See pp. 408–411 in this chapter.

Collagen Diseases

See pp. 182–184 in Chapter 6. Rheumatoid arthritis, scleroderma, periarteritis nodosa, systemic lupus erythematosus, dermatomyositis, and temporal arteritis can all cause retinal vasculitis with secondary retinal hemorrhages and exudates.

Blood Dyscrasias

Leukemia (Fig. 11.42), lymphoma, aplastic anemia, sickle-cell anemia, and macroglobulinemia can all cause retinal vascular problems or infiltrates.

Demyelinating Diseases

See pp. 510–511 in Chapter 13. Primary white matter (optic nerve) disease followed by secondary retinal atrophy may be found in multiple sclerosis, neuromyelitis optica, and diffuse cerebral sclerosis (Schilder's, Krabbe's, and Pelizaeus–Merzbacher diseases, and metachromatic leukodystrophy).

Many systemic diseases may also have retinal manifestations.

TUMORS

Glia

I. Ordinary neural retinal gliosis
   A. The disorder may be intraneural retinal, epiretinal (Figs 11.43 to 11.45), preretinal (see Fig. 11.53C), or postretinal (subneural retina; see Figs 11.45 and 11.53C).

Preretinal or epiretinal membranes* may be composed of glia (astrocytes as well as Müller cells), RPE, fibrous or myofibroblas-

---

*Preretinal *actually refers to all membranes lying anterior to the neural retinal surface, whereas* epiretinal *refers specifically to membranes lying on the surface of the neural retina. Most ophthalmologists refer to elevated membranes as* preretinal membranes *and to closely applied membranes as* epiretinal membranes. Epiretinal membranes *affect approximately 12% of the population.*

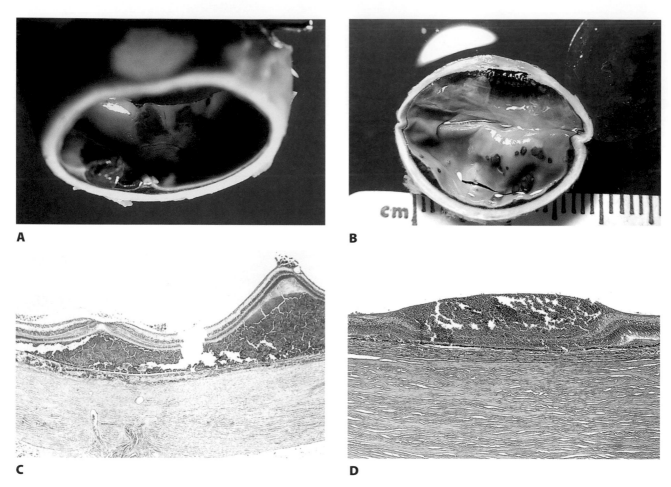

A

B

C

D

Fig. 11.42 Leukemic retinopathy. Gross specimen from patient who died from acute leukemia shows large hemorrhages in the posterior pole (**A**) and in the periphery (**B**). Some of the peripheral hemorrhages have white centers, simulating Roth spots. **C,** The central macular area shows mainly subneural retinal hemorrhages. **D,** A large subinternal limiting membrane hemorrhage is seen in the periphery.

tic tissue, fibroinflammatory tissue, cortical vitreous, or any combination of these; all are nonvascular membranes—if they have a vascular component, they are called *neovascular* (preretinal or epiretinal) membranes. Nonvascular membranes may grow in the macular area and surround, but spare, the fovea, thus simulating a foveal hole (i.e., pseudolamellar hole; see Fig. 11.43A).

B. It is found in such diverse conditions as otherwise normal eyes, chronic neural retinal detachment, most types of chronic secondary glaucoma, chronic retinitis or chorioretinitis, CRVO, diabetic retinopathy, and

after several surgical procedures such as scleral buckling, cataract extraction, retinal cryopexy, and laser retinal photocoagulation.

Epiretinal macular membranes that occur after retinal surgery are commonly called *macular pucker.*

The early form of epiretinal membranes "cellophane macular reflex" is more common in Latinos than in whites. The more severe form "preretinal macular fibrosis" (macular pucker) occurs equally in Latinos and whites.

Fig. 11.43 Epiretinal (flat) gliosis. **A,** Membrane on surface of retina, noted clinically as "cellophane" retina, spares the central fovea, giving the appearance of a retinal hole (pseudolaminar hole). **B,** Histologic section of another case shows nuclei of a fine glial membrane on the internal surface of the internal limiting membrane, shown with increased magnification in **C** (em, epiretinal membrane). **D,** Electron micrograph shows Müller cell (mc) passing through (*arrows*) thin basement membrane of foveola. **E,** Filament (fil)- and nonfilament-containing cells indicate fibrous and protoplasmic-type glial cells, respectively. Dense, maculalike attachments (*arrows*) present between cell villi suggest Müller cell origin (ilm, internal limiting membrane; mc, basal footplates of Müller cells).

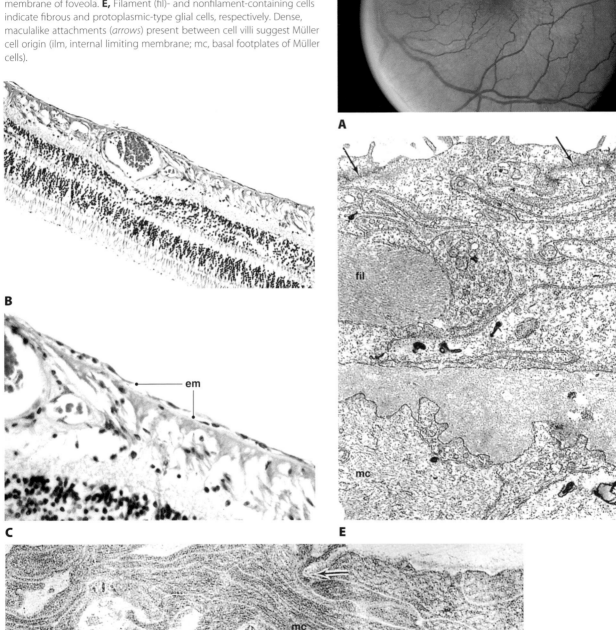

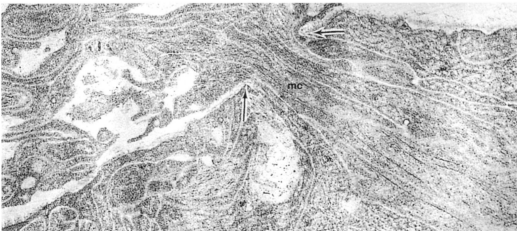

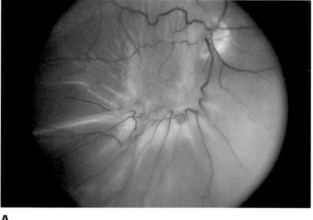

A

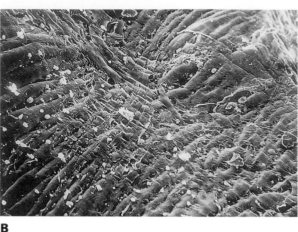

B

C

Fig. 11.44 Epiretinal (flat) gliosis. Light (**A**) and scanning electron (**B**) micrographs show that shrinkage of fine glial membranes produces multiple, tiny folds of internal neural retina, appearing clinically as "cellophane" retina. **C,** Increased magnification shows glial cells on internal limiting membrane. (**B** and **C,** Courtesy of Dr. RC Eagle, Jr.)

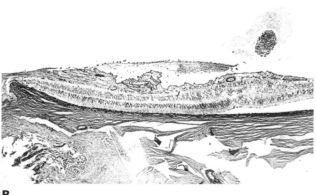

A

B

Fig. 11.45 Fixed folds. **A,** Clinical appearance of fixed folds. **B,** Both epiretinal and postretinal (subneural retinal) membranes are present, causing fixed folds of the atrophic neural retina. Membranes on outer surface (postretinal) of neural retina may be glial or retinal pigment epithelial in origin.

C. Preretinal macular fibrosis/idiopathic premacular gliosis (macular pucker, idiopathic premacular gliosis, idiopathic premacular fibrosis)

    1. An epiretinal membrane that occurs in the macular region without apparent cause is called idiopathic macular pucker, idiopathic preretinal macular fibrosis cellophane or surface wrinkling retinopathy, or idiopathic premacular gliosis.

        a. The 5-year incidence in an older white population is around 5%.

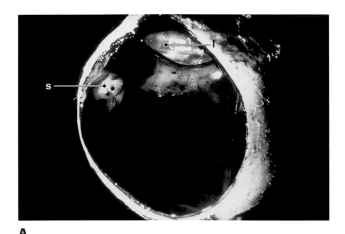

A

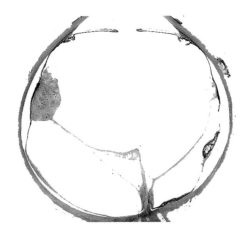

B

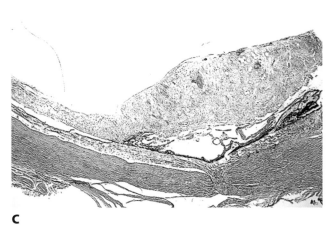

C

Fig. 11.46 Massive gliosis. **A,** Segmental thickening of the peripheral neural retina is seen in this gross specimen. The lesion was mistaken for a malignant melanoma and the eye was enucleated (s, segmental thickening of retina, forming a tumor nodule; l, lens). **B,** A histologic section of another case shows a sudden transition peripherally from a retina of normal thickness to a thickened, abnormal one. **C,** Massive gliosis is characterized histologically by total replacement and thickening of the retina by glial tissue and abnormal blood vessels. Frequently, calcium and even inflammatory round cells are present within the tumor. (Cases reported by Yanoff M *et al.: Int Ophthalmol Clin* 11:211, 1971.)

b. Five-year cumulative incidence rates in an older white population for preretinal macular fibrosis is 1.5% and for cellophane macula is 3.8%.

2. Most affected patients have only mild visual disturbances.

a. Histologically, in both the idiopathic and the secondary varieties of epiretinal membranes, although there is an increased number of glial cells (fibrous astrocytes), with or without preservation of the normal neural retinal architecture, other cells such as RPE (often the predominant cell), fibrocytes, and myofibroblasts can be found. Depending on the composition of the membrane, immunohistochemical staining is positive for cytokeratin, glial fibrillary acidic protein, vimentin, actin, and fibronectin.

If the neural retina becomes atrophic and the normal retinal architecture becomes totally replaced by glial cells (e.g., in toxoplasmosis, where there may be complete replacement of a neural retinal segment by glial tissue), the neural retina becomes thinned. Conversely, with massive gliosis (see later) the neural retina becomes thickened.

II. Massive gliosis (Fig. 11.46; see also Fig. 18.11)

A. Criteria for massive gliosis are:

1. Segmental or total replacement of the neural retina by a mass of glial tissue

2. Abnormal blood vessels in the mass

3. A resultant thickening of the neural retina in the involved area

B. Massive gliosis is a benign, nonneoplastic proliferation of neural retinal glia either as an idiopathic, isolated finding or in response to diverse pathologic states initiated by a variety of factors (e.g., chronic inflammatory processes resulting in atrophia bulbi, congenital malformations, retinal vascular disorders, and trauma).

C. Histologically, the tumors are composed of: (1) interweaving groups of large, pale spindle cells that have rather uniform nuclei, abundant, faintly eosinophilic, fibrillated cytoplasm, and indistinct cell borders; (2) dilated, large, abnormal blood vessels with thin walls and an anastomotic pattern; and (3) frequently calcium deposits in blood vessel walls and in the tumor.

1. Immunohistochemical staining is positive for S-100 protein and glial fibrillary acidic protein.

2. Electron microscopy confirms the glial origin of the cells.

The proliferating cells are probably Müller cells. Rarely, massive gliosis can clinically mimic a choroidal malignant melanoma. Vasoproliferative retinal tumors (reactionary retinal glioangiosis; gliosis; see later) are most probably a form of massive gliosis.

3. True glioma—true gliomas of the neural retina are exceedingly rare and behave much like juvenile pilocytic astrocytomas of the optic nerve (see pp514–518 in Chapter 13).

Rarely, an oligodendroglioma can arise from retinal accessory glia.

III. Vasoproliferative retinal tumors (reactionary retinal glioangiosis)
   A. Idiopathic
      1. Usually solitary but may be multiple, diffuse, and even bilateral
      2. Average age at onset 40 years, but with a range of 11 to 76 years
   B. Secondary
      1. Usually solitary or multiple, but may be diffuse and even bilateral
      2. Secondary to such pre-existing entities as pars planitis, RP, and toxoplasmic retinitis
      3. Average age at onset 36 years, but with a range of 2 to 75 years
   C. Histology
      1. Full-thickness neural retina is replaced by benign glial cell proliferation, vasoproliferation, and a sprinkling of round inflammatory cells (mainly lymphocytes).
      2. The lesion is most probably a form of massive gliosis (see earlier).

Phakomatoses

See Chapter 2.

Retinal Pigment Epithelium

See Chapter 17.

Retinoblastoma and Pseudogliomas

See Chapter 18.

Neural Retinal Metastases (Fig. 11.47)

I. It seems paradoxical that choroidal metastases are common yet neural retinal metastases are rare.
II. Most neural retinal metastases are carcinomas (approximately half of these from lung), whereas the remainder are mainly metastases from cutaneous malignant melanomas.

Retinal metastasis (adenocarcinoma) has been reported in the Muir–Torre syndrome (sebaceous gland tumor and internal malignancy).

III. In the early stages, neural retinal metastasis may mimic an ischemic neural retinal infarction. As the tumor enlarges, it can simulate an inflammatory process.
IV. The histologic picture depends on the primary tumor.

NEURAL RETINAL DETACHMENT

Definitions

I. A neural retinal detachment is a separation between the neural retina and the RPE rather than a "true" neural retinal detachment (i.e., a separation of both neural retina and RPE from Bruch's membrane).
II. An artifactitious neural retinal detachment (Fig. 11.48), a common finding after formaldehyde fixation, can be differentiated histologically from a true neural retinal detachment by the following:
   A. An "empty" subneural retinal space
   B. Good preservation of rods and cones
   C. Pigment granules (derived from apices of RPE cells) adherent to the external ends of the rods and cones

Major Causes

I. Accumulation of fluid beneath an intact neural retina (e.g., in Harada's disease, Coats' disease, malignant hypertension, eclampsia, choroidal malignant melanomas, or subneural retinal hemorrhages)
II. Traction bands in the vitreous from many causes [e.g., vitreous bands in diabetes mellitus, posttraumatic vitreous condensation and fibrosis, and complications after cataract extraction (especially with vitreous loss).]
III. Accumulation of fluid beneath a broken neural retina associated with vitreous traction (e.g., a rhegmatogenous neural retinal detachment)

Classification of Neural Retinal Detachment

I. Rhegmatogenous: caused by a neural retinal hole usually associated with vitreous traction
   A. Equatorial type (mainly in age group older than 40 years): pathologic cause occurs at the equatorial area.
      1. Myopia—approximately one-third of all nontraumatic neural retinal detachments occur in myopic patients, and approximately 1% to 3% of all patients who have high myopia experience a neural retinal detachment.
      2. Secondary to lattice degeneration (see later)
      3. Secondary to other perivascular degenerations
      4. Secondary to neural retinal horseshoe tears (Fig. 11.49) or round holes (Fig. 11.50)

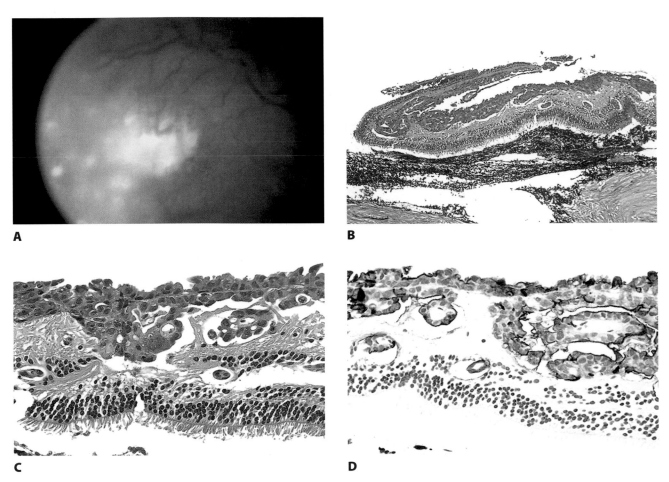

A

B

C

D

Fig. 11.47 Retinal metastasis. **A,** Patient presented with metastatic retinal lesions of unknown origin. **B,** Histologic section shows metastatic, carcinomatous cords and sheets infiltrating the inner neural retina, shown with increased magnification in **C. D,** Immunohistochemical stains for epithelial membrane antigen (this figure) and cytokeratin are positive and demonstrate the epithelial origin of the carcinoma. (Case presented by Dr. RC Eagle Jr. at the meeting of the Eastern Ophthalmic Pathology Society, 1989; case contributed by Dr. RC Kleiner.)

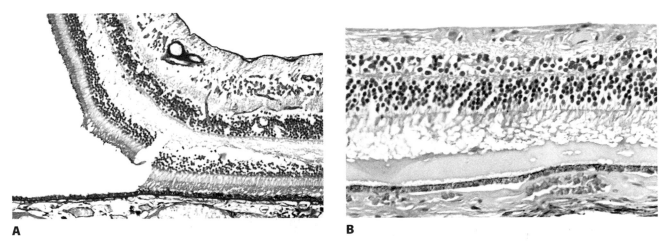

A

B

Fig. 11.48 Retinal detachment. **A,** An artifactitious neural retinal detachment (RD) shows no fluid in the subneural retinal space, pigment adherent to the tips of the photoreceptors, and good preservation of the normal retinal architecture in all layers. **B,** A true RD shows material in the subneural retinal spaces and degeneration of the outer retinal layers.

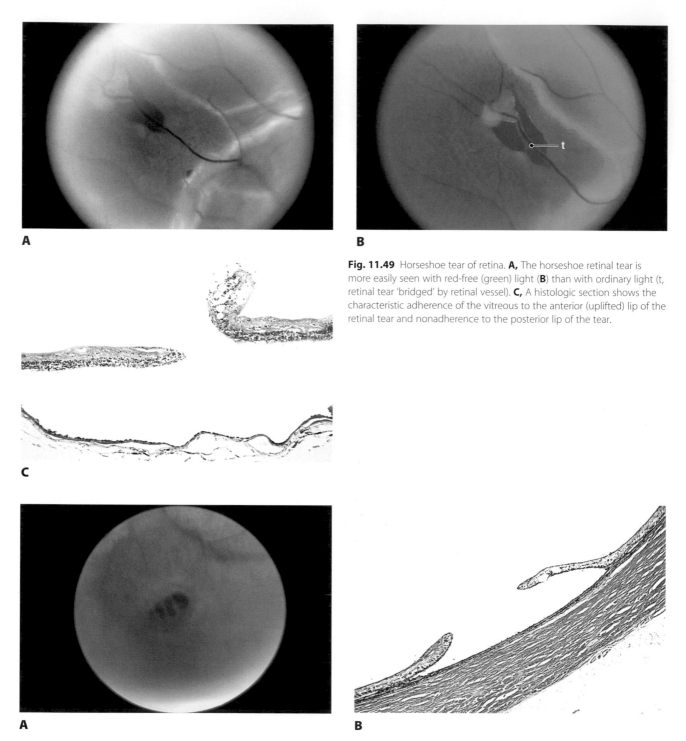

A

B

Fig. 11.49 Horseshoe tear of retina. **A,** The horseshoe retinal tear is more easily seen with red-free (green) light (**B**) than with ordinary light (t, retinal tear 'bridged' by retinal vessel). **C,** A histologic section shows the characteristic adherence of the vitreous to the anterior (uplifted) lip of the retinal tear and nonadherence to the posterior lip of the tear.

C

A

B

Fig. 11.50 Round retinal tear. **A,** A round retinal tear is surrounded by a small retinal detachment in the inferior retina. **B,** A histologic section shows that, in a round retinal tear, vitreous is not adherent to the edge of the tear. Note the round, smooth edges of the tear. An artifactitious retinal tear has sharp edges. (**B,** Courtesy of Dr. WR Green.)

5. Secondary to uveitis—about 3% of patients who have uveitis will develop a rhegmatogenous retinal detachment

B. Oral type (mainly in age group older than 40 years, but somewhat younger than equatorial type): pathologic cause occurs at the ora serrata area.

1. Aphakic—before the era of extracapsular cataract extraction and lens implantation, approximately 20% of all neural retinal detachments occurred in aphakes, and a neural retinal detachment developed in approximately 2% to 5% of all aphakes.

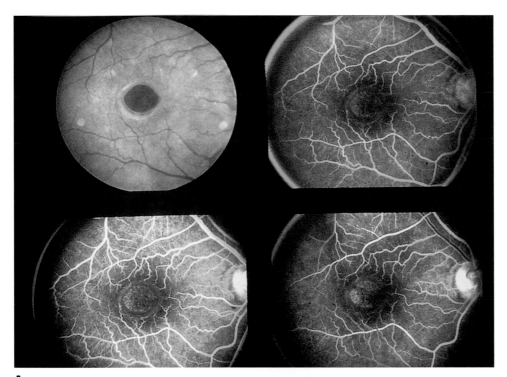

A

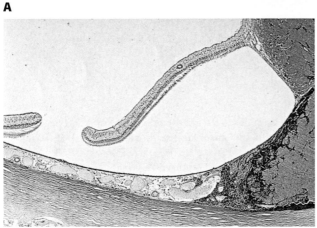

B

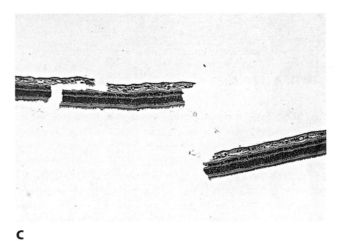

C

Fig. 11.51 Macular hole. **A,** Clinical appearance of hole in central macula (fovea). Fluorescein angiography shows staining of base of hole. **B,** Periodic acid–Schiff-stained histologic section shows macular hole in melanoma-containing eye. Origin of hole not clear but thought to be secondary to intraretinal edema somehow caused by, or related to, the melanoma. Note rounded edges of macular hole, demonstrating that this is a true hole, as compared with an artifactitious tear, **C,** which has sharp, jagged edges. (**A,** Courtesy of Dr. H Schatz.)

Now, extracapsular cataract extraction is followed by neural retinal detachment in fewer than 1% of cases.

---

2. Dialysis in young—congenital and usually located inferotemporally

---

The congenital neural retinal disinsertion syndrome refers to cases of nonattachment of the neural retina with retinal dialysis (disinsertion).

---

3. Traumatic dialysis—usually superonasally

4. Giant neural retinal break (a neural retinal break greater than 90°)

C. Macular type (Fig. 11.51; rarest): pathologic cause occurs at the macula
   1. High myopia
   2. Posttraumatic

Causes of macular holes include trauma, cystoid macular edema, intraocular inflammation, vitreous traction, myopia, ARMD, and solar retinopathy. The pathogenesis of another cause, IMH, is not clear (see p. 437 in this chapter).

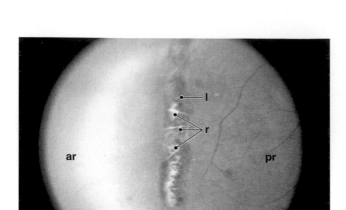

A

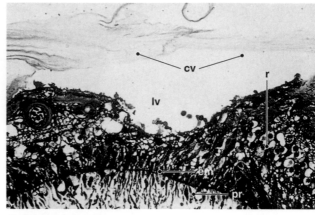

B

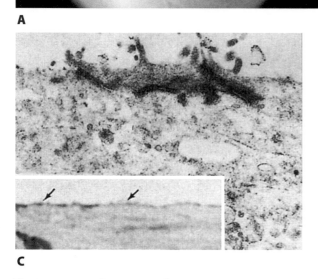

C

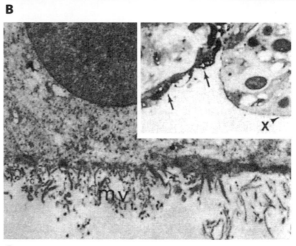

D

Fig. 11.52 Lattice degeneration of retina. **A,** Heavy pigmentation and thinning of the neural retina are present circumferentially in an oval area [l, lattice lesion; r, white retinal vessels ("lattice work"); ar, anterior retina; pr, posterior retina]. **B,** The internal layers of the neural retina, including the internal limiting membrane, are not present. The overlying formed vitreous is split (vitreoschisis) or separated from the neural retina by fluid (cv, condensed cortical vitreous; lv, "liquid vitreous"; r, retina; em, external limiting membrane; pr, receptors). **C,** *Inset*: Periodic acid–Schiff stain shows glia proliferating along "opened" inner surface of lesion. Note formation of surface membrane beyond which delicate villi (*arrows*) project. Electron micrograph shows glial cells, their characteristic dense attachments (see also Fig. 11.43), and their villous projections. **D,** *Inset*: Outer neural retinal surface approximately at mid-lesion. Note loss of photoreceptors. External limiting membrane (x) of neural retina interrupted by ingrowing, proliferating pigment epithelial cells (*arrows*). Electron micrograph illustrates terminal barlike arrangement of external glial (i.e., Müller) cells. Glial microvilli (mv) project into subneural retinal space.

II. Nonrhegmatogenous: may be transudative, exudative, or hemorrhagic
    A. Uveitis (e.g., pars planitis, sympathetic uveitis, Harada's disease, posttraumatic, eclampsia, or Goodpasture's syndrome)

Goodpasture's syndrome is characterized by the onset of hemorrhagic pulmonary disease with glomerulonephritis, leading to progressive pulmonary and renal failure. The hallmark of the disease is linear deposition of antibasement membrane immunoglobulin G in the basement membranes of the kidneys, lungs, Bruch's membrane, and choroidal vessels. Other ocular findings include choroidal infarction and macular edema.

    B. Scleritis, especially posterior scleritis
    C. Choroidal tumor: approximately 75% of uveal malignant melanomas have an associated neural retinal detachment, most of which (approximately 83%) are segmental.
    D. Traction of vitreous bands [e.g., with retinopathy of prematurity, diabetic retinopathy (see Fig. 11.53C), sickle-cell retinopathy, or posttraumatic].

Predisposing Factors to Neural Retinal Detachment

    I. Juvenile and senile retinoschisis
    II. Lattice (palisade) degeneration (Fig. 11.52)

A. Lattice degeneration may occur in any decade of life, with the average age between 40 and 50 years, affects the sexes equally, is usually bilateral, and involves the neural retina circumferentially between the equator and the ora serrata.

In approximately 7% of cases, lattice degeneration occurs at an angle of 61° to 90° from the ora serrata, sometimes posterior to the equator, and often associated with a paraxial vessel. It is called *radial perivascular lattice degeneration*. An increased incidence of lattice degeneration is seen in patients who have retinopathy of prematurity.

B. Lattice degeneration consists of criss-crossing white lines (latticework) representing the branching pattern of thickened, hyalinized, retinal blood vessels. Pigmentation and depigmentation are common in the involved area, and the overlying vitreous is liquefied.
C. Vitreous condensations adhere to the edges or margins of the area of lattice; subsequent shrinkage or vitreous detachment may cause neural retinal tears.
D. In 20% to 30% of patients with neural retinal detachment, lattice degeneration is the cause; however, a neural retinal detachment develops in only approximately 1% of patients and 0.7% of eyes that have lattice degeneration.

Although approximately 99% of patients who have lattice degeneration never have a neural retinal detachment, an accompanying myopia exceeding 5 diopters puts these patients at a high risk for development of a detachment during their lifetime.

E. Histologically, the neural retina is thinned and gliosed (especially the inner layers), and thick, hyalinized blood vessels are present.
  1. No basement membrane (internal limiting membrane of the neural retina) exists over the area of lattice.
     Vitreoretinal adhesions are mainly seen on the anterior side of the area of lattice degeneration.
  2. The defect in the neural retinal basement membrane (internal limiting membrane) may be congenital and primary in causing lattice degeneration, or secondary to a tear or schisis in the adjacent vitreous body.
III. Retinal pits
  A. Retinal pits, most often found in the peripheral neural retina, are small defects in the inner neural retinal layers.
  B. They are probably caused by minute vitreoretinal adhesions adjacent to sclerotic blood vessels.
     1. The adhesions may tear off a partial-thickness piece of neural retina at the time of a vitreous detachment.

  2. Alternatively, the pit may be formed initially by focal atrophy of the Müller cells in the paravascular regions.
  C. Histologically, a small, funnel-shaped defect occupies most of the thickness of the inner neural retina, often leaving only the receptors and the external part of the outer nuclear layer remaining.
IV. Vitreoretinal adhesions (see p. 483 in Chapter 12)
V. Trauma and cataract surgery (see p. 115–117 in Chapter 5)

Schwartz's syndrome, which often follows trauma and is prevalent in male patients in their second or third decades, consists of rhegmatogenous neural retinal detachment, secondary aqueous cells (actually, not always cells, but photoreceptor outer segments), and increased intraocular pressure (instead of the usual decreased pressure associated with rhegmatogenous detachment).

VI. Myopia (see p. 423 in this chapter and p. 504 in Chapter 13)
VII. Paving stone degeneration (probably not a predisposing factor to neural retinal detachment; see p. 422 in this chapter)

Pathologic Changes After Neural Retinal Detachment

I. Neural retinal atrophy (see Figs 11.48 and 11.53C)—the outer neural retinal layers are mainly affected because they are removed from their source of nourishment (i.e., the choriocapillaris), whereas the inner neural retinal layers retain their blood supply from the central retinal artery.

Apoptosis is an important mechanism of photoreceptor cell degeneration in the early stage after traumatic neural retinal detachment.

II. The subneural retinal space is filled with material [e.g., serous fluid (see Fig. 11.48), blood, inflammatory cells, or neoplasm].

The material may be quite watery so that it runs out of the tissue during processing; the subneural retinal space then appears empty histologically.

III. Glial or RPE membranes can occur on the internal or external surface of the neural retina (Fig. 11.53) as well as in the neural retina (proliferative vitreoretinopathy—see p. 494 in Chapter 12). Shrinkage of these membranes causes fixed neural retinal folds (see Figs 11.45 and 11.53).
IV. RPE may proliferate at the anterior (usually ora serrata) or posterior edge of a detached neural retina.
  A. The proliferated RPE at the posterior edge may lay down considerable amounts of basement membrane* and is seen clinically and pathologically as a *demarcation line* (Fig. 11.54).

Clinically, the basement membrane material should be clear or white. The proliferated RPE cells may accentuate the demarcation line by giving it a brown color.

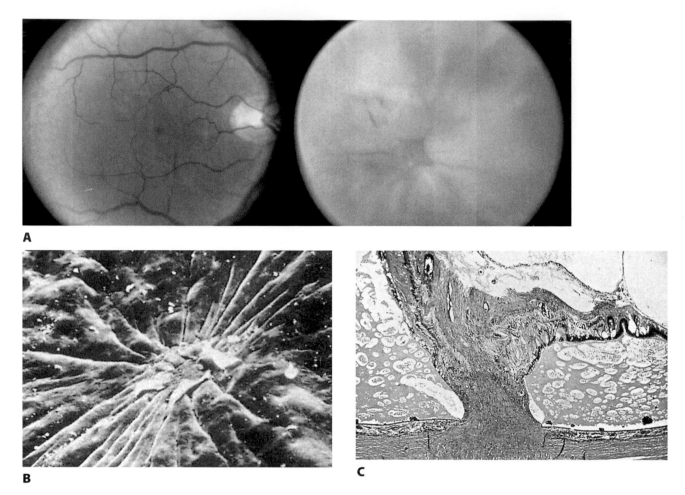

A

B

C

Fig. 11.53 Fixed folds. **A,** Eye containing neural retinal detachment before surgery (*left*); eye 1 year later (*right*). Total neural retinal detachment caused by proliferative vitreoretinopathy. **B,** Scanning electron micrograph of fixed folds on internal surface of neural retina. **C,** Preneural and postneural retinal fixed folds, along with an elevated preneural retinal membrane, have caused a traction detachment of the atrophic neural retina in this diabetic patient's eye. (**B,** Courtesy of Dr. RC Eagle, Jr.)

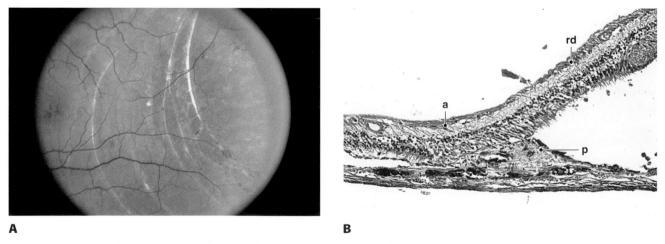

A

B

Fig. 11.54 Demarcation line. **A,** Concentric yellow-white lines are present at the edge of a neural retinal detachment. Some pigment is also present. **B,** A histologic section shows the region of transition between neural retinal detachment (rd) and attachment (a). The retinal pigment epithelium (RPE) has undergone proliferation (p) and the thickness of the basement membrane has increased. The yellow-white appearance of the demarcation lines is presumably due to the basement membrane material. When the RPE cells are sufficiently pigmented, the demarcation lines will also be pigmented. (**B,** Courtesy Dr. WR Green.)

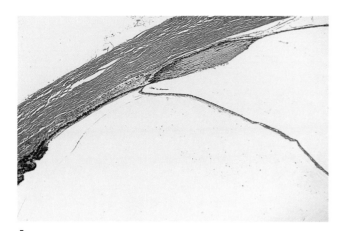

A

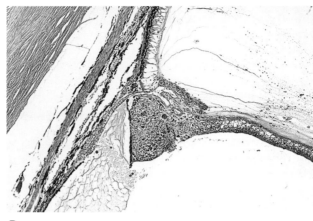

B

Fig. 11.55 Ringschwiele. **A,** Ringschwiele caused by retinal pigment epithelium (RPE) proliferation at ora serrata where detached neural retina "tugs" on RPE. **B,** Periodic acid–Schiff-stained histologic section of another case with a ringschwiele shows a break in RPE caused by traction. Material in sub-RPE and subneural retinal spaces shows that break is probably not artifactitious. Note blood vessel extending from choroid, through RPE, just posterior to ora serrata, into upper aspect of ringschwiele.

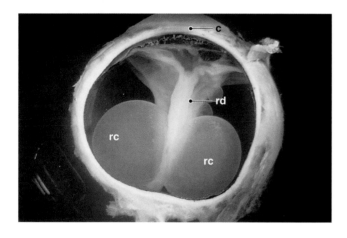

Fig. 11.56 Retinal cysts. This gross specimen shows numerous large retinal cysts (rc) from a case of long-standing retinal detachment (rd) (c, cornea).

V. Large, PAS-positive but acid mucopolysaccharide-negative intraneural retinal cysts may form.

> A neural retinal cyst (Fig. 11.56) is defined as an intraneural retinal space with a "neck" of smaller diameter than the largest diameter of the cyst. If there is no neck, then the space is called *microcystic* if small (<1.5 mm) and *retinoschisis* if large (1.5 mm or greater). With reattachment of the neural retina, the cysts may resorb rapidly.

VI. Calcium oxalate crystals may form in the neural retina (Fig. 11.57).

Pathologic Complications after Neural Retinal Detachment Surgery

See section *Complications of Neural Retinal Detachment and Vitreous Surgery* in Chapter 5.

B. A similar proliferation of the RPE at the anterior edge just posterior to the ora serrata is known as a *ringschwiele* (Fig. 11.55).

> Approximately 17% of phakic and 14% of aphakic neural retinal detachments show demarcation lines. Most neural retinal detachments with demarcation lines are of at least 3 months' duration.

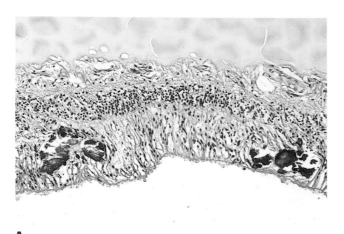

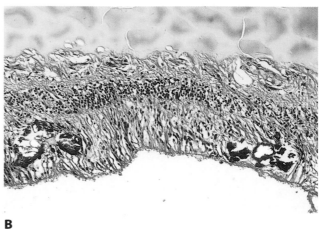

A

B

Fig. 11.57 Calcium oxalate crystals. **A,** Calcium oxalate crystals have formed in the outer layers of the long-standing detached neural retina. **B,** Polarization shows that the crystals are birefringent to polarized light.

BIBLIOGRAPHY

Normal Anatomy

Federman JL, Gouras P, Schubert H *et al.*: Retina and vitreous. In Podos SM, Yanoff M, eds: *Textbook of Ophthalmology*, vol. 9. London, Mosby, 1994:1.2–1.8, 2.1–2.15

Fine BS, Yanoff M: *Ocular Histology: A Text and Atlas*, 2nd edn. Hagerstown, MD, Harper & Row, 1979:61–127

Yanoff M, Fine BS: *Ocular Pathology: A Color Atlas*, 2nd edn. New York, Gower Medical Publishing, 1992:11.1–11.2

Congenital Anomalies

Abramov I, Gordon J, Hendrickson A *et al.*: The retina of the newborn infant. *Science* 217:265, 1982

Akeo K, Shirai S, Okiska S *et al.*: Histology of fetal eyes with oculocutaneous albinism. *Arch Ophthalmol* 114:613, 1996

Creel DJ, Summers CG, King RA: Visual anomalies associated with albinism. *Ophthalmic Paediatr Genet* 11:193, 1990

Dryja TP: Molecular genetics of Oguchi disease, fundus albipunctatus, and other forms of stationary night blindness: LVII Edward Jackson Memorial Lecture. *Am J Ophthalmol* 130:547, 2000

Fine BS, Yanoff M: *Ocular Histology: A Text and Atlas*, 2nd edn. Hagerstown, MD, Harper & Row, 1979:68

Hameed A, Khaliq S, Ismail M *et al.*: A novel locus for Leber congenital amaurosis (LCA4) with anterior keratoconus mapping to chromosome 17p13. *Invest Ophthalmol Vis Sci* 41:629, 2000

Iwata F, Reed GF, Caruso RC *et al.*: Correlation of visual acuity and ocular pigmentation with the 16bp duplication in the HPS-1 gene of Hermansky–Pudlak syndrome, a form of albinism. *Ophthalmology* 107:783, 2000

Lee S-T, Nicholls RD, Bundey S *et al.*: Mutations of the P gene in oculocutaneous albinism, and Prader–Willi syndrome plus albinism. *N Engl J Med* 330:529, 1994

Lotery AJ, Jacobson SG, Fishman GA *et al.*: Mutations in the *CRB1* gene cause Leber congenital amaurosis. *Arch Ophthalmol* 119:415, 2001

Lotery AJ, Namperumalsamy P, Jacobson SG *et al.*: Mutation of 3 genes in patients with Leber congenital amaurosis. *Arch Ophthalmol* 118:538, 2000

Mietz H, Green WR, Wolff SM *et al.*: Foveal hypoplasia in complete oculocutaneous albinism. *Retina* 12:254, 1992

Milman AH, Barakat MR, Gupta N *et al.*: Clinicopathologic effects of mutant *GUCY2D* in Leber congenital amaurosis. *Ophthalmology* 110:549, 2003

Nakamachi Y, Nakamura M, Fujii S *et al.*: Oguchi disease with sectorial retinitis pigmentosa harboring adenine deletion at position 1147 in the arrestin gene. *Am J Ophthalmol* 125:182, 1998

Regillo CD, Eagle RC Jr, Shields JA *et al.*: Histopathologic findings in congenital grouped pigmentation of the retina. *Ophthalmology* 100:400, 1993

Rosen B, Barry C, Constable IJ: Progression of myelinated retinal nerve fibers. *Am J Ophthalmol* 127:471, 1999

Ruttum MS, Poll J: Unilateral retinal nerve fiber mylination with contralateral amblyopia. *Arch Ophthalmol* 124:128, 2006

Scheie HG, Yanoff M: Peters' anomaly and total posterior coloboma of retinal pigment epithelium and choroid. *Arch Ophthalmol* 87:525, 1972

Van der Spuy J, Chapple JP, Clark BJ *et al.*: The Leber congenital amaurosis gene product AIPL1 is localized exclusively in rod receptors of the adult human retina. *Hum Mol Genet* 11:823, 2002

Straatsma BR, Foos RY, Heckenlively JR *et al.*: Myelinated retinal nerve fibers. *Am J Ophthalmol* 91:25, 1981

Summers CG, Knobloch WH, Witkop CJ Jr *et al.*: Hermansky–Pudlak syndrome: Ophthalmic findings. *Ophthalmology* 95:545, 1988

Valenzuela R, Morningstar WA: The ocular pigmentary disturbance of human Chediak–Higashi syndrome: A comparative light- and electron-microscopic study and review of the literature. *Am J Clin Pathol* 75:591, 1981

Verdaguer TJ: Juvenile retinal detachment. *Am J Ophthalmol* 93:145, 1982

Wack MA, Peachey NS, Fishman GA: Electroretinographic findings in human oculocutaneous albinism. *Ophthalmology* 96:1778, 1989

Weleber RG, Pillers DM, Powell BR *et al.*: Aland island eye disease (Forsius–Eriksson syndrome) associated with contiguous deletion syndrome at Xp21. *Arch Ophthalmol* 107:1170, 1989

Vascular Disease

Aisen ML, Bacon BR, Goodman AM *et al.*: Retinal abnormalities associated with anemia. *Arch Ophthalmol* 101:1049, 1983

Asdourian G, Nagpal KC, Goldbaum M *et al.*: Evolution of the retinal black sunburst in sickling haemoglobinopathies. *Br J Ophthalmol* 59:710, 1975

Biswas J, Sharma T, Gopal L *et al.*: Eales disease—an update. *Surv Ophthalmol* 47:197, 2002

The Central Retinal Vein Occlusion Study Group: Natural history and clinical management of central retinal vein occlusion. *Arch Ophthalmol* 115:486, 1997

Downes SM, Hambleton IR, Chuang EL *et al.*: Incidence and natural history of proliferative sickle cell retinopathy. *Ophthalmology* 112:1896, 2005

Duker JS, Magargat LE, Stubbs GW: Quadrantic venous-stasis retinopathy secondary to an embolic branch retinal artery obstruction. *Ophthalmology* 97:167, 1990

Eagle RC, Yanoff M, Fine BS: Hemoglobin SC retinopathy and fat emboli to the eye: A light and electron microscopical study. *Arch Ophthalmol* 92:28, 1974

The Eye Disease Case-Control Study Group: Risk factors for central retinal vein occlusion. *Arch Ophthalmol* 114:545, 1996

Fichte C, Streeten BW, Friedman AH: A histopathologic study of retinal arterial aneurysms. *Am J Ophthalmol* 85:509, 1978

Font RI, Naumann G: Ocular histopathology in pulseless disease. *Arch Ophthalmol* 82:784, 1969

Gagliano DA, Goldberg MF: The evolution of salmon-patch hemorrhages in sickle cell retinopathy. *Arch Ophthalmol* 107:1814, 1989

Gass JDM: A fluorescein angiographic study of macular dysfunction secondary to retinal vascular disease: I. Embolic retinal artery obstruction. II. Retinal vein occlusion. III. Hypertensive retinopathy. IV. Diabetic retinal angiopathy. V. Retinal telangiectasis. VI. X-ray irradiation, carotid artery occlusion, collagen vascular disease, and vitritis. *Arch Ophthalmol* 80:535, 550, 569, 583, 592, 606, 1968

Gass JD, Braunstein R: Sessile and exophytic capillary angiomas of the juxtapapillary retina and optic nerve head. *Arch Ophthalmol* 98:1790, 1980

George RK, Walton RC, Whitcup SM *et al.*: Primary retinal vasculitis: Systemic associations and diagnostic evaluation. *Ophthalmology* 103:384, 1996

Glacet-Bernard A, Coscas G, Chabanel A *et al.*: Prognostic factors for retinal vein occlusion: A prospective study of 175 cases. *Ophthalmology* 103:551, 1996

Goldberg MF: Classification and pathogenesis of proliferative sickle retinopathy. *Am J Ophthalmol* 71:649, 1971

Harino S, Motokura M, Nishikawa N *et al.*: Chronic ocular ischemia associated with the Eisenmenger's syndrome. *Am J Ophthalmol* 117:302, 1994

Hayreh SS, Zimmerman B: Central retinal artery occlusion: visual outcomes. *Am J Ophthalmol* 140:376, 2005

Hayreh SS, Zimmerman B, McCarthy MJ *et al.*: Systemic diseases associated with various types of central retinal vein occlusion. *Am J Ophthalmol* 131:61, 2001

Hayreh SS, Zimmerman MB, Podhajsky P: Incidence of various types of retinal vein occlusion and their recurrence and demographic characteristics. *Am J Ophthalmol* 117:429, 1994

Irvine AR, Shorb SR, Morris BW: Optociliary veins. *Trans Am Acad Ophthalmol Otolaryngol* 83:541, 1977

Jacobson DM: Systemic cholesterol microembolization syndrome masquerading as giant cell arteritis. *Surv Ophthalmol* 35:23, 1991

Klein R, Klein BEK, Moss SE *et al.*: Hypertension and retinopathy, arteriolar narrowing, and arteriovenous nicking in a population. *Arch Ophthalmol* 112:92, 1994

Kozak I, Bartsch D-U, Cheng L *et al.*: In vivo histology of cotton-wool spots using high-resolution optical coherence tomography. *Am J Ophthalmol* 141:748, 2006

Kushner MS, Jampol LM, Haller JA: Cavernous hemangioma of the optic nerve. *Retina* 14:359, 1994

Lang GE, Lang GK: Ocular manifestations of carotid artery disease. *Curr Opin Ophthalmol* 1:167, 1990

Lertsumitkul S, Whitcup SM, Chan C-C: Ocular manifestations of disseminated intravascular coagulation in a patient with the acquired immunodeficiency syndrome. *Arch Ophthalmol* 115:676, 1997

Leys AM, Bonnet S: Case report: Associated retinal neovascularization and choroidal hemangioma. *Retina* 13:22, 1993

McLeod DS, Goldberg MF, Lutty GA: Dual-perspective analysis of vascular formations in sickle cell retinopathy. *Arch Ophthalmol* 111:1234, 1993

McLeod DS, Merges C, Fukushima A *et al.*: Histopathologic features of neovascularization in sickle cell retinopathy. *Am J Ophthalmol* 124:455, 1997

Mizener JB, Podhajsky P, Hayreh SS: Ocular ischemic syndrome. *Ophthalmology* 104:859, 1997

Morse PH: Elschnig's spots and hypertensive choroidopathy. *Am J Ophthalmol* 66:844, 1968

Ohara K, Okuba A, Sasaki H *et al.*: Branch retinal vein occlusion in a child with ocular sarcoidosis. *Am J Ophthalmol* 119:806, 1995

Om A, Ellahham S, Disciascio G: Cholesterol embolism: An underdiagnosed clinical entity. *Am Heart J* 124:1321, 1991

Ortiz JM, Yanoff M, Cameron JD *et al.*: Disseminated intravascular coagulation in infancy and in the neonate: Ocular findings. *Arch Ophthalmol* 100:1413, 1982

Peachey NMS, Gagliano DA, Jacobson MS: Correlation of electroretinographic findings and peripheral retinal nonperfusion in patients with sickle cell retinopathy. *Arch Ophthalmol* 108:1106, 1990

Pomeranz HD: Roth spots. *Arch Ophthalmol* 120:1596, 2002

Rabb MF, Gagliano DA, Teske MP: Retinal arterial macroaneurysms. *Surv Ophthalmol* 33:73, 1988

Recccchia FM, Carvalho-Recchia CA, Hassan TS: Clinical course of younger patients with central retinal vein occlusion. *Arch Ophthalmol* 122:317, 2004

Rubenstein RA, Yanoff M, Albert DM: Thrombocytopenia, anemia, and retinal hemorrhage. *Am J Ophthalmol* 65:435, 1968

Tanaka T, Shimizu K: Retinal arteriovenous shunts in Takayasu disease. *Ophthalmology* 94:1380, 1987

Tso MOM, Bettman JW: Occlusion of choriocapillaris in primary nonfamilial amyloidosis. *Arch Ophthalmol* 86:281, 1971

Inflammation

Chittum ME, Kalina RE: Acute retinal pigment epitheliitis. *Ophthalmology* 94:1114, 1987

Culbertson WW, Brod RD, Flynn HW *et al.*: Chickenpox-associated acute retinal necrosis syndrome. *Ophthalmology* 98:1641, 1991

Cunningham ET Jr, Schatz H, McDonald HR *et al.*: Acute multifocal retinitis. *Am J Ophthalmol* 123:347, 1997

de Boer JH, Luyendijk L, Rothova A *et al.*: Detection of intraocular antibody production to herpesviruses in acute retinal necrosis syndrome. *Am J Ophthalmol* 117:201, 1994

Ferguson LS, Burke MJ, Choromokos EA: Carbon monoxide retinopathy. *Arch Ophthalmol* 103:66, 1985

Freund KB, Yannuzzi LA, Barile GR *et al.*: The expanding clinical spectrum of unilateral acute idiopathic maculopathy. *Arch Ophthalmol* 114:555, 1996

Ganatra JB, Chandler D, Santos C *et al.*: Viral causes of the acute retinal necrosis syndrome. *Am J Ophthalmol* 129:166, 2000

Grevin CM, Ford J, Stanton M et al.: Progressive outer retinal necrosis syndrome secondary to varicella zoster virus in acquired immune deficiency syndrome. *Retina* 15:14, 1995

Gross NE, Yannuzzy LA, Freund KB et al.: Multiple evanescent white dot syndrome. *Arch Ophthalmol* 124:493, 2006

Jacobson SG, Morales DS, Sun XK et al.: Pattern of retinal dysfunction in acute zonal occult outer retinopathy. *Ophthalmology* 102:1187, 1995

Jampol LM, Becker KG: White spot syndromes of the retina: a hypothesis based on the common genetic hypothesis of autoimmune/inflammatory diease. *Am J Ophthalmol* 135:376, 2003

Johnson MW, Greven CM, Jaffe GJ et al.: Atypical, severe toxoplasmic retinochoroiditis in elderly patients. *Ophthalmology* 104:48, 1997

Kezuka T, Sakal J-I, Usui N et al.: Evidence for antigen-specific immune deviation in patients with acute retinal necrosis. *Arch Ophthalmol* 119:1044, 2001

Khurana RN, Albini T, Dea MK et al.: Atypical presentgation of multiple evanescent white dot syndrome involving granular lesions of varying size. *Am J Ophthalmol* 139:935, 2005

Lardenoye CWTA, van der Lelij A, de Loos WS et al.: Peripheral multifocal chorioretinitis: A distinct entity. *Ophthalmology* 104:1820, 1997

Monnet D, Brèzin AP, Holland GN et al.: Longitudinal cohort study of patients with birdshot chorioretinopathy. I. Baseline clinical caracteristcs. *Am J Ophthalmol* 141:135, 2006

Nelson DA, Weiner A, Yanoff M et al.: Retinal lesions in subacute sclerosing panencephalitis. *Arch Ophthalmol* 84:613, 1970

Oh KT, Christmas NJ, Folk JC: Birdshot retinochoroiditis: longterm follow-up of a chronically progressive disease. *Am J Ophthalmol* 133:622, 2002

O'Halloran HS, Berger JR, Lee WB et al.: Acute multifocal placoid pigment epitheliopathy and central nervous system involvement: nine new cases and a review of the literature. *Ophthalmology* 108:861, 2001

Rahhal FM, Siegel LM, Russak V et al.: Clinicopathologic correlations in acute retinal necrosis caused by herpes simplex virus type 2. *Arch Ophthalmol* 114:1416, 1996

Rothova A, Berendschot TTJN, Probst K et al.: Birdshot chorioretinopathy. Long-term manifestations and visual prognosis. *Ophthalmology* 111:954, 2004

Slakter JS, Giovannini A, Yannuzzi LA et al.: Indocyanine green angiography of multifocal choroiditis. *Ophthalmology* 104:1813, 1997

Thorne JE, Jabs DA, Peters GB et al.: Birdshot retinochoroidopathy: ocular complications and visual impairment. *Am J Ophthalmol* 140:45, 2005

Tsai L, Jampol LM, Pollock SC: Chronic recurrent multiple evanescent white dot syndrome. *Retina* 14:160, 1994

Turbeville SD, Cowan LD, Gass JDM: Acute macular neuroretinopathy: a review of the literature. *Surv Ophthalmol* 48:1, 2003

Yanoff M, Allman MI, Fine BS: Congenital herpes simplex virus, type 2, bilateral endophthalmitis. *Trans Am Ophthalmol Soc* 75:325, 1977S

Degenerations

Abdelsalam A, Del Priore L, Zabin MA: Drusen in age-related macular degeneration: Pathogenesis, natural course, and laser photocoagulation-induced regression. *Surv Ophthalmol* 44:1, 1999

Age-Related Eye Disease Study Research Group: Risk factors associated with age-related macular degeneration: A case-control study in the Age-Related Eye Disease Study. Age-Related Eye Disease Study report number 3. *Ophthalmology* 107:2224, 2000

Age-Related Eye Disease Study Research Group: A randomized, placebo-controlled, clinical trial of high-dose supplementation with vitamins C and E, beta carotene and zinc for age-related macular degeneration and vision loss: AREDS Report No. 9. *Arch Ophthalmol* 119:1417, 2001

Aiello LP, Arrig PG, Shah ST et al.: Solar retinopathy associated with hypoglycemic insulin reaction. *Arch Ophthalmol* 112:982, 1994

Akiba J, Quiroz MA, Trempe CL: Role of posterior vitreous detachment in idiopathic macular holes. *Ophthalmology* 97:1610, 1990

Ambati J, Ambati BK, Yoo SH et al.: Age-relatedmacular degeneration: etiology, pathogenesis, and therapeutic strategies. *Surv Ophthalmol* 48, 257, 2003

Arnold JJ, Quaranta M, Soubrane G et al.: Indocyanine green angiography of drusen. *Am J Ophthalmol* 124:344, 1997

Arnold JJ, Sarks SH, Killingsworth MC et al.: Reticular pseudodrusen: A risk factor in age-related maculopathy. *Retina* 15:183, 1995

Augood CA, Vingerling JR, de Jong PTVM et al.: Prevalence of age-related maculopathy in older Europeans. The European Eye Study (EUREYE). *Arch Ophthalmol* 124:529, 2006

Axer-Siegel R, Bourla D, Ehrlich R et al.: Association of neovascular age-related macular degeneration and hyperhomocysteinemia. *Am J Ophthalmol* 137:84, 2004

Baird PN, Guida E, Chu DT et al.: The ε2 and ε4 alleles of the apolipoprotein gene are associated with age-related macular degeneration. *Invest Ophthalmol Vis Sci* 45:1311, 2004

Borkowski LM, Grover S, Fishman GA et al.: Retinal findings in melanoma-associated retinopathy. *Am J Ophthalmol* 132:273, 2001

Bressler NM, Silva JS, Bressler SB et al.: Clinicopathologic correlation of drusen and retinal pigment epithelial abnormalities in age-related macular degeneration. *Retina* 14:130, 1994

Brown GC, Shields JA: Choroidal melanomas and paving stone degeneration. *Ann Ophthalmol* 15:705, 1983

Browning DJ: Bull's-eye maculopathy associated with quinacrine therapy for malaria. *Am J Ophthalmol* 137:577, 2004

Byer NE: Long-term natural history study of senile retinoschisis with implications for management. *Ophthalmology* 93:1127, 1986

Chan JW: Paraneoplastic retinopathies and optic neuropathies. *Surv Ophthalmol* 48:12, 2003

Chang TS, Aylward GW, Clarkson JG et al.: Asymmetric canthaxanthin retinopathy. *Am J Ophthalmol* 119:801, 1995

Chen JC, Fitzke FW, Pauleikhoff D et al.: Functional loss in age-related Bruch's membrane change with choroidal perfusion defect. *Invest Ophthalmol Vis Sci* 33:334, 1992

Cheng L, Freeman WR, Ozerdem U et al.: Prevalence, correlates, and natural history of epiretinal membranes surrounding idiopathic macular holes. *Ophthalmology* 107:853, 2000

Chew EY, Sperduto RD, Hiller R et al.: Clinical course of macular holes: The Eye Disease Case-Control Study. *Arch Ophthalmol* 117:242, 1999

Cohen SY, Laroche A, Leguen Y et al.: Etiology of choroidal neovascularization in young patients. *Ophthalmology* 103:1241, 1996

Coskuncan NM, Jabs DA, Dunn JP et al.: The eye in bone marrow transplantation. *Arch Ophthalmol* 112:372, 1994

Cruickshanks KJ, Klein R, Klein BEK: Sunlight and age-related macular degeneration. *Arch Ophthalmol* 111:514, 1993

Curcio CA, Medeiros NE, Millican CL: Photoreceptor loss in age-related macular degeneration. *Invest Ophthalmol Vis Sci* 37:1236, 1996

Curcio CA, Millican CL: Basal linear deposit and large drusen are specific for early age-related maculopathy. *Arch Ophthalmol* 117:329, 1999

Curcio CA, Millican CL, Bailey T et al.: Accumulation of cholesterol with age in human Bruch's membrane. *Invest Ophthalmol Vis Sci* 42:265, 2001

Dastrgheib K, Green WR: Granulomatous reaction to Bruch's membrane in age-related macular degeneration. *Arch Ophthalmol* 112:813, 1994

DeAngelis MM, Kim IK, Adams S et al.: Cigarette smoking, *CFH, APOE, ELOVL4*, and risk of neovascular age-related macular degeneration. *Arch Ophthalmol* 125:49, 2007

Delcourt C, Cristol J-P, Léger CL et al.: Association of antioxidant enzymes with cataract and age-related macular degeneration. *Ophthalmology* 106:215, 1999

Delcourt C, Diaz J-L, Ponton-Sanchez A et al.: Smoking and age-related macular degeneration: The POLA study. *Arch Ophthalmol* 116:1031, 1998

Dunaif JL, Dentchez T, Ying G-S et al.: The role of apoptosis in age-related macular degeneration. *Arch Ophthalmol* 120:1435, 2002

Espaillar A, Aiello LP, Arrigg PG et al.: Canthaxanthine retinopathy. *Arch Ophthalmol* 117:412, 1999

Ezra E, Wells JA, Gray RH et al.: Incidence of idiopathic full-thickness macular holes in fellow eyes: A 5-year prospective natural history study. *Ophthalmology* 105:353, 1998

Fine BS: Retinal structure: Light- and electron-microscopic observations. In McPherson A, ed: *New and Controversial Aspects of Retinal Detachment.* New York, Harper & Row, 1968:16

Fine BS: Lipoidal degeneration of the retinal pigment epithelium. *Am J Ophthalmol* 91:469, 1981

Foos RY, Feman SS: Reticular cystoid degeneration of the peripheral retina. *Am J Ophthalmol* 69:392, 1970

Frank KE, Purnell EW: Subretinal neovascularization following rubella retinopathy. *Am J Ophthalmol* 86:462, 1978

Fraser-Bell S, Guzowski M, Rochtchina E et al.: Five-year cumulative incidence and progression of epiretinal membranes: the Blue Mountain Eye Study. *Ophthalmology* 110:34, 2003

Frayer WC: Elevated lesions of the macular area: A histopathologic study emphasizing lesions similar to disciform degeneration of the macula. *Arch Ophthalmol* 53:82, 1955

Fukushima I, McLeod DS, Lutty GA: Intrachoroidal microvascular abnormality: A previously unrecognized form of choroidal neovascularization. *Am J Ophthalmol* 124:473, 1997

Gass JDM: Pathogenesis of disciform detachment of the neuroepithelium: I. General concepts and classification. II. Idiopathic central serous choroidopathy. III. Senile disciform macular degeneration. V. Disciform macular degeneration secondary to focal choroiditis. VI. Disciform detachment secondary to heredodegenerative, neoplastic and traumatic lesions of the choroid. *Am J Ophthalmol* 63:573, 587, 617, 661, 689, 1967

Gass JDM: Reappraisal of biomicroscopic classification of stages of development of a macular hole. *Am J Ophthalmol* 119:752, 1995

Göttinger W: Senile retinoschisis: Morphological relationship of the intraretinal spaces of retinal periphery with senile retinoschisis and schisis-detachment. *Ophthalmologia* 1:312, 1989

Grassi MA, Folk JC, Scheetz TE et al.: Complement factor polymorphism p.Tyr402His and cuticular drusen. *Arch Ophthalmol* 125:93, 2007

Green WR: The macular hole. Histopathologic studies. *Arch Ophthalmol* 124:317, 2006

Green WR, Enger C: Age-related macular degeneration histopathologic studies. *Ophthalmology* 100:1519, 1993

Grossniklaus HE, Gass JDM: Clinicopathologic correlations of surgically excised type 1 and type 2 submacular choroidal neovascular membranes. *Am J Ophthalmol* 126:59, 1998

Grossniklaus HE, Green WR: Pathologic findings in pathologic myopia. *Retina* 12:127, 1992

Grossniklaus HE, Green WR: Histopathologic and ultrastructural findings of surgically excised choroidal neovascularization. *Arch Ophthalmol* 116:745, 1998

Hageman GS, Mullins RF: Molecular composition of drusen as related to substructural phenotype. *Mol Vis* 5:28, 1999

Hahn P, Hamilton AH, Dunaief JL: Maculas affected by age-related macular degeneration contain increased chelatable iron in the retinal pigment epithelium and Bruch's membrane. *Arch Ophthalmol* 121:1099, 2003

Haimovici R, Koh S, Gagnon DR et al.: Risk factors for central serous chorioretinopathy. A case-control study. *Ophthalmology* 111:244, 2004

Harris GJ, Murphy ML, Schmidt EW et al.: Orbital myositis as a paraneoplastic syndrome. *Arch Ophthalmol* 112:380, 1994

Ho AC, Guyer DR, Fine SL: Macular hole. *Surv Ophthalmol* 42:393, 1998

Ho AC, Yannuzzi LA, Pisicano K et al.: The natural history of idiopathic subfoveal choroidal neovascularization. *Ophthalmology* 102:782, 1995

Hyman L, Schachat AP, He Q et al.: Hypertension, cardiovascular disease, and age-related macular degeneration. *Arch Ophthalmol* 118:351, 2000

Javitt JC, Zhou Z, Maguire MG et al.: Incidence of exudative age-related macular degeneration among elderly Americans. *Ophthalmology* 110:1534, 2003

Khawly JA, Rubin P, Petros W et al.: Retinopathy and optic neuropathy in bone marrow transplantation for breast cancer. *Ophthalmology* 103:87, 1996

Kim JW, Freeman WR, El-Haig W et al.: Baseline characteristics, natural history, and risk factors to progression in eyes with stage 2 macular holes: Results from a prospective randomized clinical trial. *Ophthalmology* 102:1818, 1995

Kinyoun JL, Lawrence BS, Barlow WE: Proliferative radiation retinopathy. *Arch Ophthalmol* 114:1097, 1996

Klaver CCW, Wolfs RCW, Assink JJM et al.: Genetic risk of age-related maculopathy: Population-based aggregation study. *Arch Ophthalmol* 116:1646, 1998

Klein RM, Green S: The development of lacquer cracks in pathologic myopia. *Am J Ophthalmol* 106:282, 1988

Klein ML, Mauldin WM, Stoumbos VD: Heredity and age-related macular degeneration: Observations in monozygomatic twins. *Arch Ophthalmol* 112:932, 1994

Klein ML, Schultz DW, Edwards A et al.: Age-related macular degeneration: Clinical features in a large family and linkage to chromosome 1q. *Arch Ophthalmol* 116:1082, 1998

Klein R, Klein BEK, Jensen SC et al.: The five-year incidence and progression of age-related maculopathy: The Beaver Dam Eye Study. *Ophthalmology* 104:7, 1997

Klein R, Peto T, Bird A et al.: The epidemiology of age-related macular degeneration. *Am J Opthalmol* 137:486, 2004

Klein RM, Wany Q, Klein BE et al.: The relationship of age-related maculopathy, cataract, and glaucoma to visual acuity. *Invest Ophthalmol Vis Sci* 36:182, 1995

Kozy D, Doft BH, Lipkowitz J: Nummular thioridazine retinopathy. *Retina* 4:253, 1984

Krill AE, Deutman AE: Dominant macular degeneration. *Am J Ophthalmol* 73:352, 1972

Kvanta A, Algvere P, Berglin L et al.: Subfoveal fibrovascular membranes in age-related macular degeneration express vascular endothelial growth factor. *Invest Ophthalmol Vis Sci* 37:1928, 1996

Lafaut BA, Bartz-Schmidt KU, Broecke V et al.: Clinicopathological correlation in exudative age related macular degeneration: Histological differentiation between classical and occult choroidal neovascularization. *Br J Ophthalmol* 84:239, 2000

Lakhanpal V, Schocket SS, Jiji R: Deferoxamine (Desferal) induced toxic retinal pigmentary degeneration and presumed optic neuropathy. *Ophthalmology* 91:443, 1984

Lambert SR, High KA, Cotlier E *et al.*: Serous retinal detachments in thrombotic thrombocytopenic purpura. *Arch Ophthalmol* 103:1172, 1985

Lewis ML, Cohen SM, Smiddy WE *et al.*: Bilaterality of idiopathic macular holes. *Graefes Arch Clin Exp Ophthalmol* 234:241, 1996

Lincoff H, Lopez R, Kreissig I *et al.*: Retinoschisis associated with optic nerve pits. *Arch Ophthalmol* 106:61, 1988

Lotery AJ, Munier FL, Fishman GA *et al.*: Allelic variation in the VMD2 gene in Best disease and age-related macular degeneration. *Invest Ophthalmol Vis Sci* 41:1291, 2000

Macular Study Group: Risk factors for choroidal neovascularization in the second eye of patients with juxtafoveal or subfoveal choroidal neovascularization secondary to age-related macular degeneration. *Arch Ophthalmol* 115:741, 1997

Madjarov B, Hilton GF, Brinton DA *et al.*: A new classification of the retinoschises. *Retina* 15:282, 1995

Mansuetta CC, Mason JO III, Swanner J *et al.*: An association between central serous chorioretinopathy and gastroesophageal reflux disease. *Am J Ophthalmol* 137:1096, 2004

Mares-Perlman JA, Brady WE, Klein R *et al.*: Dietary fat and age-related macular degeneration. *Arch Ophthalmol* 113:743, 1995

Marmour MF, Carr RE, Easterbrook M *et al.*: Recommendations on screening for chloroquine and hydroxychloroquine retinopathy. *Ophthalmology* 109:1377, 2002

McCarty CA, Mukesh BN, Fu CL *et al.*: Risk factors for age-related maculopathy: The visual impairment project. *Arch Ophthalmol* 119:1455, 2001

McFarlane JR, Yanoff M, Scheie HG: Toxic retinopathy following sparsomycin therapy. *Arch Ophthalmol* 76:532, 1966

McGwin Jr G, Owsley C, Curcio CA *et al.*: The association of statin use and age related maculopathy. *Br J Ophthalmol* 87:1121, 2003

Michael JC, de Venecia G: Retinal trypsin digest study of cystoid macular edema associated with choroidal melanoma. *Am J Ophthalmol* 119:152, 1995

Mitchell P, Smith W, Wang JJ: Iris color, skin sun sensitivity, and age-related maculopathy: The Blue Mountains Eye Study. *Ophthalmology* 105:1359, 1998

Niwa H, Terasaki H, Ito Y *et al.*: Macular hole development in fellow eyes of patients with unilateral macular hole. *Am J Ophthalmol* 140:370, 2005

Ohguro H, Yokoi Y, Ohguro I *et al.*: Clinical and immunologic aspects of cancer-associated retinopathy. *Am J Ophthalmol* 137:1117, 2004

O'Malley PF, Allen RA: Peripheral cystoid degeneration of the retina: incidence and distribution in 1000 autopsy eyes. *Arch Ophthalmol* 77:769, 1967

O'Malley PF, Allen RA, Straatsma BR *et al.*: Paving stone degeneration of the retina. *Arch Ophthalmol* 73:169, 1965

Ramrattan RS, van der Schaft TL, Mooy CM *et al.*: Morphometric analysis of Bruch's membrane, the choriocapillaris, and the choroid in aging. *Invest Ophthalmol Vis Sci* 35:2857, 1994

Ramsey MS, Fine BS: Chloroquine toxicity in the human eye: Histopathologic observations by electron microscopy. *Am J Ophthalmol* 73:229, 1972

Reddy VM, Zamora RL, Kaplan HJ: Distribution of growth factors in subfoveal neovascular membranes in age-related macular degeneration and presumed ocular histoplasmosis syndrome. *Am J Ophthalmol* 120:291, 1995

Rosa RH Jr, Davis JL, Eifrig CWG: Clinicopathologic correlation of idiopathic polypoidal choroidal vasculopathy. *Arch Ophthalmol* 120:502, 2002

Rosa RH, Thomas MA, Green WR: Clinicopathologic correlation of submacular membranectomy with retention of good vision in a patient with age-related macular degeneration. *Arch Ophthalmol* 114:480, 1996

Roth AM: Gyrate-like atrophy and colon cancer. Presented at the meeting of the Verhoeff Society, April 6–8, 1990

Russell SR, Mullins RF, Schneider BL *et al.*: Location, substructure, and composition of basal laminar drusen compared with drusen associated with aging and age-related macular degeneration. *Am J Ophthalmol* 129:205, 2000

Saito W, Kase S, Yoshida K *et al.*: Bilateral diffuse melanocytic proliferation in a patient with cancer-associated retinopathy. *Am J Ophthalmol* 140:942, 2005

Sandberg MA, Gaudio AR, Miller S *et al.*: Iris pigmentation and extent of disease in patients with neovascular age-related macular degeneration. *Invest Ophthalmol Vis Sci* 35:2734, 1994

Sandberg MA, Tolentino MJ, Miller S *et al.*: Hyperopia and neovascularization in age-related macular degeneration. *Ophthalmology* 100:1009, 1993

Sarks SH, Arnold JJ, Killingsworth MC: Early drusen formation in the normal and aging eye and their relation to age related maculopathy: A clinicopathologic study. *Br J Ophthalmol* 83:358, 1999

Schatz H, McDonald HR, Johnson RN *et al.*: Subretinal fibrosis in central serous chorioretinopathy. *Ophthalmology* 102:1077, 1995

Schlernitzauer DA, Green WR: Peripheral retinal albinotic spots. *Am J Ophthalmol* 72:729, 1971

Scholz R, Green WR, Kutys R *et al.*: *Histoplasma capsulatum* in the eye. *Ophthalmology* 91:1100, 1984

Scott IU, Flynn HW Jr, Smiddy WE: Bull's-eye maculopathy associated with chronic macular hole. *Arch Ophthalmol* 116:1116, 1998

Seddon JM, Afshari MA, Sharma S *et al.*: Assessment of mutations in the Best macular dystrophy (VMD2) gene in patients with adult-onset foveomacular vitelliform dystrophy, age-related maculopathy, and bull's-eye maculopathy. *Ophthalmology* 108:2060, 2001

Seddon JM, Gensler G, Milton RC *et al.*: Association between c-reactive protein and age-related macular degeneration. *JAMA* 291:704, 2004

Shuler RK, Hauser MA, Caldwell J *et al.*: Neovascular age-related macular degeneration and its association with *LOC*#387715 and complement factor H polymorphism. *Arch Ophthalmol* 125:63, 2007

Slakter JS, Yannuzzi LA, Schneider U *et al.*: Retinal choroidal anastomosis and occult choroidal neovascularization in age-related macular degeneration. *Ophthalmology* 107:742, 2000

Smith RE, Wise K, Kingsley RM: Idiopathic polypoidal choroidal vasculopathy and sickle cell retinopathy. *Am J Ophthalmol* 129:544, 2000

Spraul CW, Grossniklaus HE: Characteristics of drusen and Bruch's membrane in postmortem eyes with age-related macular degeneration. *Arch Ophthalmol* 115:267, 1997

Spraul CW, Lang GE, Grossniklaus HE: Morphometric analysis of the choroid, Bruch's membrane, and retinal pigment epithelium in eyes with age-related macular degeneration. *Invest Ophthalmol Vis Sci* 37:2724, 1996

Straatsma BR, Foos RY: Typical and reticular degenerative retinoschisis. *Am J Ophthalmol* 75:551, 1973

Suhler EB, Chan C-C, Caruso RC *et al.*: Presumed teratoma-associated retinopathy. *Arch Ophthalmol* 121:33, 2003

To KW, Thirkill CE, Jakobiec FA *et al.*: Lymphoma associated retinopathy. *Ophthalmology* 109:2149, 2002

Tomany SC, Wang JJ, van Leeuwen R *et al.*: Risk factors for incident age-related macular degeneration. . *Ophthalmology* 111:1280, 2004

Toth CA, Pasquale AC, Graichen DF: Clinicopathologic correlation of spontaneous retinal pigment epithelial tears with choroidal neovascular membranes in age-related macular degeneration. *Ophthalmology* 102:272, 1995

Tsujikawa A, Sashara M, Otani A *et al.*: Pigment epithelial detachment in polypoid choroidal vasculopathy. *Am J Ophthalmol* 143:102, 2007

Uyama M, Matsubara T, Fukushima I et al.: Idiopathic polypoidal choroidal vasculopathy in Japanese patients. *Arch Ophthalmol* 117:1034, 1999

Uyama M, Wada M, Nagai Y et al.: Polypoidal choroidal vasculopathy: natural history. *Am J Ophthalmol* 133:639, 2002

van der Schaft TL, de Bruijn WC, Mooy CM: Is basal laminar deposit unique for age-related macular degeneration? *Arch Ophthalmol* 109:420, 1991

Van Leeuwen R, Klaver CCW, Vingerling JR et al.: The risk and natural course of age-related maculopathy. Follow-up at 6½ years in the Rotterdam study. *Arch Ophthalmol* 121:519, 2003

Vingerling JR, Hofman A, Grobbee DE et al.: Age-related macular degeneration and smoking: The Rotterdam Study. *Arch Ophthalmol* 114:1193, 1996

Wada Y, Abe T, Sato H et al.: Autosomal dominant macular degeneration associated with 208delG mutation in the *FSCN2* gene. *Arch Ophthalmol* 121:1613, 2003

Wang L, del Priore LV: Bull's-eye maculopathy secondary to herbal toxicity from uva ursI. *Am J Ophthalmol* 137:1135, 2004

Wang JJ, Klein R, Smith W et al.: Cataract surgery and the 5-year incidence of late-stage age-related maculopathy: pooled findings from the Beaver Dan and Blue Mountains Eye Studies. *Ophthalmology* 110:1960, 2003

Wang Q, Chappell RJ, Klein R et al.: Pattern of age-related maculopathy in the macular area: The Beaver Dam Eye Study. *Invest Ophthalmol Vis Sci* 37:2234, 1996

Weleber RG, Watzke RC, Shults WT et al.: Clinical and electrophysiologic chacterization of paraneoplastic and autoimmune retinopathies associated with antienolase antibodies. *Am J Ophthalmol* 139:780, 2005

Whitcup SM, Vistica BP, Milam AH et al.: Recoverin-associated retinopathy: A clinically and immunologically distinctive disease. *Am J Ophthalmol* 126:230, 1998

Yannuzzi LA: Retinal angiomatous proliferation in AMD. *Rev Ophthalmol* 10:30, 2003

Yanoff M: Macular pathology. In Yanuzzi LA, Gitter KA, Schatz H, eds: *The Macula: A Comprehensive Text and Atlas.* Baltimore, Williams & Wilkins, 1979:3

Yanoff M, Rahn EK, Zimmerman LE: Histopathology of juvenile retinoschisis. *Arch Ophthalmol* 79:49, 1968

Yanoff M, Tsou K-C: Demonstration of ocular reduced diphosphopyridine nucleotide (DPNH) and triphosphopyridine nucleotide (TPNH) diaphorases using tetrazolium salts. *Am J Ophthalmol* 60:312, 1965

Yanoff M, Tsou K-C: Tetrazolium studies of the whole eye: Effect of chloroquine in the incubation medium. *Am J Ophthalmol* 59:808, 1965

Yuzawa M, Watanabe A, Takahashi Y et al.: Observation of idiopathic full-thickness macular holes: Follow-up observations. *Arch Ophthalmol* 112:1051, 1994

Zimmerman LE, Naumann G: The pathology of retinoschisis. In McPherson A, ed: *New and Controversial Aspects of Retinal Detachment.* St. Louis, CV Mosby, 1968:400

Hereditary Primary Retinal Dystrophies

Ali A, Feroze AH, Rizvi ZH et al.: Consanguinous marriage resulting in homozygous occurrence of X-linked retinoschisis in girls. *Am J Ophthalmol* 136:767, 2003

Andréasson S, Ponjavic V, Abrahamson M et al.: Phenotypes in three Swedish families with X-linked retinitis pigmentosa caused by different mutations in the RPGR gene. *Am J Ophthalmol* 124:95, 1997

Bastek JV, Foos RY, Heckenlively J: Traumatic pigmentary retinopathy. *Am J Ophthalmol* 92:624, 1981

Berson E: Retinitis pigmentosa. *Invest Ophthalmol Vis Sci* 34:671, 1993

Berson EL, Adamian M: Ultrastructural findings in an autopsy eye from a patient with Usher's syndrome type 11. *Am J Ophthalmol* 114:748, 1992

Betten MG, Bilchik RC, Smith ME: Pigmentary retinopathy of myotonic dystrophy. *Am J Ophthalmol* 72:720, 1971

Billimoria JD, Clemens ME, Gibberd FB et al.: Metabolism of phytanic acid in Refsum's disease. *Lancet* 1:194, 1982

Bird AC: Retinal photoreceptor dystrophies: LI Edward Jackson Memorial Lecture. *Am J Ophthalmol* 119:543, 1995

Birnbach CD, Järveläinen M, Possin DE et al.: Histopathology and immunocytochemistry of the neurosensory retina in fundus flavimaculatus. *Ophthalmology* 101:1211, 1994

Briggs CE, Rucinbski D, Rosenfeld PJ et al.: Mutations in *ABCR* (*ABCR4*) in patients with Stargardt macular degeneration or cone-rod degeneration. *Invest Ophthalmol Vis Sci* 42:2229, 2001

Brown DM, Kimura AE, Gorin MB: Clinical and electroretinographic findings of female carriers and affected males in a progressive X-linked cone-rod dystrophy (COD-1) pedigree. *Ophthalmology* 107:1104, 2000

Campo RV, Aaberg TM: Ocular and systemic manifestations of the Bardet–Biedl syndrome. *Am J Ophthalmol* 94:750, 1982

Carr RE, Noble KG: Juvenile macular degeneration. *Ophthalmology* 87:83, 1980

Carrero-Valenzuela RD, Klein ML, Weleber RG et al.: Sorsby fundus dystrophy: A family with the Ser181Cys mutation of the tissue inhibitor of metalloproteinases 3. *Arch Ophthalmol* 114:737, 1996

Chen JC, Fitzke FW, Bird AC: Long-term effect of acetazolamide in a patient with retinitis pigmentosa. *Invest Ophthalmol Vis Sci* 31:1914, 1990

Condon GP, Brownstein S, Wang N-S et al.: Congenital hereditary (juvenile X-linked) retinoschisis: Histopathologic and ultrastructural findings in three eyes. *Arch Ophthalmol* 104:576, 1986

DeAngelis MA, Grimsby JL, Sandberg MA et al.: Novel mutations in the *NRL* gene and associated clinical findings in patients with retinitis pimentosa. *Arch Ophthalmol* 120:369, 2002

Donoso LA, Frost AT, Stone EM et al.: Autosomal dominant Stargardt-like macular dystrophy. *Arch Ophthalmol* 119:564, 2001

Downes SM, Holder GE, Fitzke FW et al.: Autosomal dominant cone and cone-rod dystrophy with mutations in the guanylate cyclase activator 1A gene-encoding guanylate cyclase activating protein-1. *Arch Ophthalmol* 119:96, 2001

Driessen CAGG, Janssen BPM, Winkens HJ et al.: Null mutation in the human 11-cis retinol dehydrogenase gene associated with fundus albipunctatus. *Ophthalmology* 108:1479, 2001

Dryja TP: Molecular genetics of Oguchi disease, fundus albipunctatus, and other forms of stationary night blindness: LVII Edward Jackson Memorial Lecture. *Am J Ophthalmol* 130:547, 2000

Eagle RC Jr, Hedges TR, Yanoff M: The atypical pigmentary retinopathy of Kearns–Sayre syndrome: A light and electron microscopic study. *Ophthalmology* 89:1433, 1982

Eagle RC Jr, Lucier AC, Bernardino VB et al.: Retinal pigment epithelial abnormalities in fundus flavimaculatus: A light and electron microscopic study. *Ophthalmology* 7:1189, 1980

Edwards AO, Donosa LA, Ritter R III: A novel gene for autosomal dominant Stargardt-like macular dystrophy with homology to the SUR4 protein family. *Invest Ophthalmol Vis Sci* 42:2652, 2001

Edwards AO, Klein ML, Berselli CB et al.: Malattia leventinese: Refinement of the genetic locus and phenotypic variability in autosomal dominant macular drusen. *Am J Ophthalmol* 126:417, 1998

Edwards AO, Miedziak A, Vrabec T et al.: Autosomal dominant Stargardt-like macular dystrophy: I. Clinical characterization, longitudinal follow-up, and evidence for a common ancestry in families linked to chromosome 6q14. *Am J Ophthalmol* 127:426, 1999

Eksandh LC, Ponjavic V, Ayyagari R *et al.*: Phenotypic expression of juvenile X-linked retinoschisis in Swedish families with different mutations in the XLRS1 gene. *Arch Ophthalmol* 118:1098, 2000

Eshaghian J, Rafferty NS, Goossens W: Ultrastructure of human cataract in retinitis pigmentosa. *Arch Ophthalmol* 98:2227, 1980

Evans K, Gregory CY, Wijesurya SD *et al.*: Assessment of the phenotypic range seen in Doyne honeycomb retinal dystrophy. *Arch Ophthalmol* 115:904, 1997

Fish G, Grey R, Shemi KS *et al.*: The dark choroid in posterior retinal dystrophies. *Br J Ophthalmol* 65:359, 1981

Fishman GA, Anderson RJ, Lam BL *et al.*: Prevalence of foveal lesions in type 1 and type 2 Usher's syndrome. *Arch Ophthalmol* 113:770, 1995

Fishman GA, Lam BL, Anderson RJ: Racial differences in the prevalence of atrophic-appearing macular lesions between black and white patients with retinitis pigmentosa. *Am J Ophthalmol* 118:33, 1994

Fishman GA, Stone EM, Eliason DA *et al.*: ABCA4 gene sequence variations in patients with autosomal recessive cone-rod dystrophy. *Arch Ophthalmol* 121:851, 2003

Fishman GA, Stone EM, Grover S *et al.*: Variation of clinical expression in patients with Stargardt dystrophy and sequence variations in the ABCR gene. *Arch Ophthalmol* 117:504, 1999

Fossarello M, Bertini C, Galantuoma MS *et al.*: Deletion in the peripherin/RDS gene in two unrelated Sardinian families with autosomal dominant butterfly-shaped dystrophy. *Arch Ophthalmol* 114:448, 1996

Frangieh GT, Green WR, Fine SL: A histopathologic study of Best's macular dystrophy. *Arch Ophthalmol* 100:1115, 1982

Frisch IB, Haag P, Steffen H *et al.*: Kjellin's syndrome: fundus autofluorescence, angiographic, and electrophysiologic findings. *Ophthalmology* 109:1484, 2002

Gass JD, Taney BS: Flecked retina associated with café au lait spots, microcephaly, epilepsy, short stature, and ring 17 chromosome. *Arch Ophthalmol* 112:738, 1994

Gass JD, Jallow S, Davis B: Adult vitelliform macular detachment occurring in patients with basal laminar drusen. *Am J Ophthalmol* 99:445, 1985

George NDL, Yates JRW, Moore AT: Clinical features in affected males with X-linked retinoschisis. *Arch Ophthalmol* 114:274, 1996

Gomolin JES, Lucchese NJ, Bresnick GH: Autosomal dominant peripheral preretinal deposits. *Arch Ophthalmol* 102:74, 1984

Gorin MB, Jackson KE, Ferrell RE *et al.*: A peripherin/retinal degeneration slow mutation (Pro-210-Arg) associated with macular and peripheral retinal degeneration. *Ophthalmology* 102:246, 1995

Graemiger RA, Niemeyer G, Schneeberger SA *et al.*: Wagner vitreoretinal degeneration: Follow-up of the original pedigree. *Ophthalmology* 102:1830, 1995

Green JS, Parfrey PS, Harnett JD *et al.*: The cardinal manifestations of Bardet–Biedl syndrome, a form of Laurence–Moon–Biedl syndrome. *N Engl J Med* 321:1002, 1989

Grover S, Fishman GA, Brown J Jr: Frequency of optic disc or parapapillary nerve fiber drusen in retinitis pigmentosa. *Ophthalmology* 104:295, 1997

Gupta SK, Leonard BC, Damji KF *et al.*: A frame specific mutation in a tissue-specific alternatively spliced exon of collagen 2A1 in Wagner's vitreoretinal drgeneration. *Am J Ophthalmol* 133:203, 2002

Guymer RH, Héon, Lotery AJ *et al.*: Variation of codons 1961 and 2177 of the Stargardt disease gene is not associated with macular degeneration. *Arch Ophthalmol* 119:745, 2001

Hamidi-Toosi S, Maumenee IH: Vitreoretinal degeneration in spondyloepiphyseal dysplasia congenita. *Arch Ophthalmol* 100:1104, 1982

Harrison TJ, Boles RG, Johnson DR *et al.*: Macular pattern retinal dystrophy, adult-onset diabetes, and deafness: A family study of A3243G mitochondrial heteroplasmy. *Am J Ophthalmol* 124:217, 1997

Heher KL, Johns DR: A maculopathy associated with the 15257 mitochondrial DNA mutation. *Arch Ophthalmol* 111:1495, 1993

Héon E, Piguet B, Munier F *et al.*: Linkage of autosomal dominant radial drusen (malattia leventinese) to chromosome 2p16–21. *Arch Ophthalmol* 114:193, 1996

Hirose E, Inoue Y, Morimura H *et al.*: Mutations in the 11-cis retinal dehydrogenase gene in Japanese patients with fundus albipunctatus. *Invest Ophthalmol Vis Sci* 41:3733, 2000

Holz FG, Owens SL, Marks J *et al.*: Ultrastructural findings in autosomal dominant drusen. *Arch Ophthalmol* 115:788, 1997

Ibanez HE, Williams DF, Boniuk I: Crystalline retinopathy associated with long-term nitrofurantoin therapy. *Arch Ophthalmol* 112:304, 1994

Inoue Y, Yamamoto S, Inoue T *et al.*: Two novel mutations of the XLRS1 gene in patients with X-linked juvenile retinoschisis. *Am J Ophthalmol* 134, 622, 2002

Ito S, Nakamura M, Nuno Y *et al.*: Novel complex *GUCY2D* mutation in Japanese family with cone-rod dystrophy. *Invest Ophthalmol Vis Sci* 45:1480, 2004

Jacobson SG, Cideciyan AV, Bennett J *et al.*: Novel mutation in the *TIMP3* gene causes Sorsby fundus dystrophy. *Arch Ophthalmol* 120:376, 2004

Jaffe GJ, Schatz H: Histopathologic features of adult-onset foveomacular pigment epithelial dystrophy. *Arch Ophthalmol* 106:958, 1988

Jiao X, Ritter R III, Hejtmancik JF *et al.*: Genetic linkage of snowflake vitreoretinal degeneration to chromosome 2q36. *Invest Ophthalm Vis Sci* 45:4498, 2004

Kaiser-Kupfer MI, Chan C-C, Markello TC *et al.*: Clinical biochemical correlations in Bietti's crystalline dystrophy. *Am J Ophthalmol* 118:569, 1994

Kaliq S, Hameed A, Ismail M *et al.*: Novel locus for mapping autosomal recessive cone-rod dystrophy CORD8 mapping to chromosome 1q12-Q24. *Invest Ophthalmol Vis Sci* 41:3709, 2000

Kandori F, Tamai A, Kurimoto S *et al.*: Fleck retina. *Arch Ophthalmol* 73:673, 1972

Keithahn MAZ, Huang M, Keltner JL *et al.*: The variable expression of a family with central areolar pigment epithelial dystrophy. *Ophthalmology* 103:406, 1996

Khouri G, Mets MB, Smith VC *et al.*: X-linked congenital stationary night blindness: Review and report of a family with hyperopia. *Arch Ophthalmol* 106:1417, 1988

Kniazeva M, Traboulsi EI, Yu Z *et al.*: A new locus for dominant drusen and macular degeneration maps to 6q14. *Am J Ophthalmol* 130:197, 2000

Krill AE, Archer D: Classification of the choroid atrophies. *Am J Ophthalmol* 72:562, 1971

Lazaro RP, Dentinger MP, Rodichok LD *et al.*: Muscle pathology in Bassen–Kornzweig syndrome and vitamin E deficiency. *Am J Clin Pathol* 86:378, 1986

Lee MM, Ritter R, Hirose T *et al.*: Snowflake vitreoretinal degeneration: follow-up of the original family. *Ophthalmology* 110:2418, 2003

Levin PS, Green WR, Victor DI *et al.*: Histopathology of the eye in Cockayne's syndrome. *Arch Ophthalmol* 101:1093, 1983

Li Z-Y, Possin DE, Milam AH: Histopathology of bone spicule pigmentation in retinitis pigmentosa. *Ophthalmology* 102:805, 1995

Lim JI, Enger C, Fine S: Foveomacular dystrophy. *Am J Ophthalmol* 117:1, 1994

Lines MA, Hébert M, McTaggart KE *et al.*: Electrophysiologic and phenotypic features of an autosomal cone-rod dystrophy caused by a novel *CRX* mutation. *Ophthalmology* 109:1862, 2002

Lois N, Holder GE, Bunce C *et al.*: Phenotypic subtypes of Stargardt macular dystrophy—fundus flavimaculatus. *Arch Ophthalmol* 119:359, 2001

Lotery AJ, Munier FL, Fishman GA *et al.*: Allelic variation in the VMD2 gene in Best disease and age-related macular degeneration. *Invest Ophthalmol Vis Sci* 41:1291, 2000

Luckenbach MW, Green WR, Miller NR *et al.*: Ocular clinicopathologic correlation of Hallervorden–Spatz syndrome with acanthocytosis and pigmentary retinopathy. *Am J Ophthalmol* 95:369, 1983

Madjarov B, Hilton GF, Brinton DA *et al.*: A new classification of the retinoschises. *Retina* 15:282, 1995

Marmor MF, McNamara JR: Pattern dystrophy of the retinal pigment epithelium and geographic atrophy of the macula. *Am J Ophthalmol* 122:382, 1996

Matsumoto M, Traboulsi EL: Dominate radial drusen and Arg345Trp *EFEMP1* mutation. *Am J Ophthalmol* 131:810, 2001

Maugeri A, Meire F, Hoyng CB *et al.*: A novel mutation in the *ELOVL4* gene causes autosomal Stargardt-like macular dystrophy. *Invest Ophthalm Vis Sci* 45:4263, 2004

Michaelides M, Holder GE, Bradshaw K *et al.*: Cone-rod dystrophy, intrafamilial variability, and incomplete penetrance associated with the R172W mutation in the peripherin/*RDS* gene. *Ophthalmology* 112:1592, 2005

Milam AH, Curcio CA, Cideciyan AV *et al.*: Dominant late-onset retinal degeneration with regional variation of sub-retinal pigment epithelium deposits, retinal function, and photoreceptor degeneration. *Ophthalmology* 107:2256, 2000

Milam AH, Li Z-Y, Cideciyan AV *et al.*: Clinicopathologic effects of the Q64ter rhodopson mutation in retinitis pigmentosa. *Invest Ophthalmol Vis Sci* 37:753, 1996

Moy CM, van den Born LI, Paridaens DA *et al.*: Hereditary X-linked juvenile retinoschisis: a review of the role of müller cells. *Arch Ophthalmol* 120:979, 2002

Mullins RF, Oh KT, Heffron E *et al.*: Late development of vitelliform lesions and flecks in a patient with Best disease. *Arch Ophthalmol* 123:1588, 2005

Nakamachi Y, Nakamura M, Fujii S *et al.*: Oguchi disease with sectorial retinitis pigmentosa harboring adenine deletion at position 1147 in the arrestin gene. *Am J Ophthalmol* 125:182, 1998

Nakamura M, Hotta Y, Tanikawa A *et al.*: A high association with cone dystrophy in fundus albipunctatus caused by mutations of the *RDH5* gene. *Invest Ophthalmol Vis Sci* 41:3725, 2000

Nakazawa M, Xu S, Gal A *et al.*: Variable expressivity in a Japanese family with autosomal dominant retinitis pigmentosa closely linked to chromosome 19q. *Arch Ophthalmol* 114:318, 1996

Nasr YG, Cherfan GM, Michels RG *et al.*: Goldmann–Favre maculopathy. *Retina* 10:178, 1990

Nishiguchi KM, Sokal I, Yang L *et al.*: A novel mutation (I143NT) in guancylate cyclase-actvating protein 1 (GCAP1) associated with autosomal dominant cone degeneration. *Invest Ophthalmol Vis Sci* 45:3863, 2004

Noble KG: Hereditary pigmented paravenous chorioretinal atrophy. *Am J Ophthalmol* 108:365, 1989

Noble KG, Sherman J: Central pigmentary sheen dystrophy. *Am J Ophthalmol* 108:255, 1989

Novack RL, Foos RY: Drusen of the optic disk in retinitis pigmentosa. *Am J Ophthalmol* 103:44, 1987

O'Gorman S, Flaherty WA, Fishman GA *et al.*: Histopathologic findings in Best's vitelliform macular dystrophy. *Arch Ophthalmol* 106:1261, 1988

Pannarale MR, Grammatico B, Iannaccone A *et al.*: Autosomal dominant retinitis pigmentosa associated with an Arg-135-Trp point mutation of the rhodopsin gene. *Ophthalmology* 103:1443, 1996

Parke DW II: Stickler syndrome: clinical care and molecular genetics. *Am J Ophthalmol* 134:746, 2002

Parminder AH, Murakami A, Inana G *et al.*: Evaluation of the human gene encoding recoverin in patients with retinitis pigmentosa or an allied disease. *Invest Ophthalmol Vis Sci* 38:704, 1997

Patrinely JR, Lewis RA, Font RL: Foveomacular vitelliform dystrophy, adult type: A clinicopathologic study including electron microscopic observations. *Ophthalmology* 92:1712, 1985

Pauleikoff D, Sauer CG, Müller CR *et al.*: Clinical and genetic evidence for autosomal dominant North Carolina macular dystrophy in a German family. *Am J Ophthalmol* 124:412, 1997

Peachey NS, Fishman GA, Kilbride PE *et al.*: A form of congenital stationary night blindness with apparent defect of rod phototransduction. *Invest Ophthalmol Vis Sci* 31:237, 1990

Polk TD, Gass JD, Green WR *et al.*: Familial internal limiting membrane dystrophy: A new sheen retinal dystrophy. *Arch Ophthalmol* 115:878, 1997

Raab MF, Mullen L, Yelchits S *et al.*: A North Carolina macular dystrophy phenotype in a Belizean family maps to the MCDR1 locus. *Am J Ophthalmol* 125:502, 1998

Rabb MF, Tso MOM, Fishman GA: Cone-rod dystrophy: A clinical and histopathologic report. *Ophthalmology* 93:1443, 1986

Richards BW, Brodstein DE, Nussbaum JJ *et al.*: Autosomal dominant crystalline dystrophy. *Ophthalmology* 98:658, 1991

Rodrigues MM, Bardenstein D, Wiggert B *et al.*: Retinitis pigmentosa with segmental massive retinal gliosis: An immunohistochemical, biochemical, and ultrastructural study. *Ophthalmology* 94:180, 1987

Rumelt S, Kraus E, Rehany U: Retinal neovascularization and cystoid macular edema in punctata albescens retinopathy. *Am J Ophthalmol* 114:507, 1992

Runge P, Calver D, Marshall J *et al.*: Histopathology of mitochondrial cytopathy and the Laurence–Moon–Biedl syndrome. *Br J Ophthalmol* 70:782, 1986

Russell-Eggitt IM, Clayton PT, Coffey R *et al.*: Alsröm syndrome: Report of 22 cases and literature review. *Ophthalmology* 105:1274, 1998

Salvador F, García-Arumí J, Corcóstegui B *et al.*: Ophthalmic findings in a patient with cerebellar ataxia, hypogonadotropic hypogonadism, and chorioretinal dystrophy. *Am J Ophthalmol* 120:241, 1995

Sauer CG, Gehrig A, Warneke-Wittstock R *et al.*: Positional cloning of the gene associated with X-linked juvenile retinoschisis. *Nat Genet* 17:164, 1997

Seddon JM, Sharma S, Chong BS *et al.*: Phenotype and genotype correlations in two Best families. *Ophthalmology* 110:1724, 2003

September AV, Vorster AA, Ramesar RS *et al.*: Mutation spectrum and founder chromosomes for the *ABCA4* gene in South African patients with Stargardt disease. *Invest Ophthalmol Vis Sci* 45:1705, 2004

Shroyer NF, Lewis RA, Lupski JR: Analysis of the *ABCR* (*ABCA4*) gene in 4-aminoquinoline retinopathy: Is retinal toxicity by chloroquine and hydroxychloroquine related to Stargardt disease? *Am J Ophthalmol* 131:761, 2001

Shroyer NF, Lewis RA, Yatsenko AN *et al.*: Null missense *ABCR* (*ABCR4*) mutationsin a family with Stargardt disease and retinitis pigmentosa. *Invest Ophthalmol Vis Sci* 42:2757, 2001

Small KW, Puech B, Mullen L *et al.*: North Carolina macular dystrophy phenotype in France maps to the MCDR1 locus. *Am J Ophthalmol* 124:412, 1997

Sneed SR, Sieving PA: Fenestrated sheen macular dystrophy. *Am J Ophthalmol* 112:1, 1991

Souied E, Soubrane G, Benlian P *et al.*: Retinitis punctata albescens associated with the Arg135Trp mutation in the rhodopsin gene. *Am J Ophthalmol* 121:19, 1996

Stefko ST, Zhang K, Gorin MB *et al.*: Clinical spectrum of chromosome 6-linked autosomal dominant drusen and macular degeneration. *Am J Ophthalmol* 130:203, 2000

Steinmetz RL, Garner A, Maguire JI *et al.*: Histopathology of incipient fundus flavimaculatus. *Ophthalmology* 98:953, 1991

Tanna AP, Asrani S, Zeimer R *et al.*: Optical cross-section imaging of the macula with the retinal thickness analyzer in X-linked retinoschisis. *Arch Ophthalmol* 116:1036, 1998

Tantri A, Vrabec TR, Cu-Unjieng *et al.*: X-linked retinoschisis: report of a family with a rare deletion in the XLRS1 gene. *Am J Ophthalmol* 136:547, 2003

To KW, Adamian M, Jakobiec FA *et al.*: Olivopontocerebelar atrophy with retinal degeneration. *Ophthalmology* 100:15, 1993

To KW, Adamian M, Jakobiec FA *et al.*: Clinical and histopathologic findings in clumped pigmentary retinal degeneration. *Arch Ophthalmol* 114:950, 1996

To KW, Adamian M, Jakobiec FA *et al.*: Histopathologic and immunohistochemical study of an autopsy eye with X-linked cone degeneration. *Arch Ophthalmol* 116:100, 1998

To KW, Adamian M, Jakobiec FA *et al.*: Histopathologic and immunohistochemical study of dominant cone dystrophy. *Am J Ophthalmol* 126:140, 1998

To KW, Adamian M, Jakobiec FA *et al.*: Histologic study of retinitis pigmentosa due to a muttion in the RP13 gene (*PRPC8*): comparison with rhodopson Pro23His, Cys110Arg, and Glu18Lys. *Am J Ophthalmol* 137:946, 2004

Toussaint D, Danis P: An ocular pathologic study of Refsum's syndrome. *Am J Ophthalmol* 72:342, 1971

Traboulsi E, O'Neill JF, Maumenee I: Autosomal recessive pericentral pigmentary retinopathy. *Arch Ophthalmol* 106:5321, 1988

Van Lith-Verboeven JJC, Hoyng CB, Van den Helm B *et al.*: The benign concentric annular dystrophy locus maps to 6p12.3-q16. *Invest Ophthalmol Vis Sci* 45:30, 2004

van Soest S, Westerveld A, de Jong PTVM: Retinitis pigmentosa defined from a molecular point of view. *Surv Ophthalmol* 43:321, 1999

Voo I, Blasgow BJ, Flanery J *et al.*: North Carolina macular dystrophy: clinicopathologic correlation. *Am J Ophthalmol* 132:933, 2001

Vrabec TR, Edwards A, Frost A *et al.*: Autosomal dominant Stargardt-like macular dystrophy: identification of a new family with a mutation in the ELOVL4 gene. *Am J Ophthalmol* 136:542, 2003

Vu CD, Brown J J Jr, Körkkö J *et al.*: Posterior chorioretinal atrophy and vitreous phenotype in a family with Stickler syndrome from a mutation in the COL2A1 gene. *Ophthalmology* 110:70, 2003

Weleber RG, Butler NS, Murphey WH *et al.*: X-linked retinitis pigmentosa associated with a 2-base pair insertion in codon 99 of the RP3 gene RPGR. *Arch Ophthalmol* 115:1429, 1997

Weleber RG, Carr RE, Murphey WH *et al.*: Phenotypic variation including retinitis pigmentosa, pattern dystrophy, and fundus flavimaculatus in a single family with a deletion of codon 153 or 154 of the peripheral RDS gene. *Arch Ophthalmol* 111:1531, 1993

Wu G, Pruett RC, Baldiner J *et al.*: Hereditary hemorrhagic macular dystrophy. *Am J Ophthalmol* 111:294, 1991

Yamamoto H, Yakushijin K, Kushara S *et al.*: A novel *RDH5* gene mutation in a patient with fundus albipunctatus presenting with macular atrophy and fading white dots. *Am J Ophthalmol* 136:572, 2003

Yang Z, Lin W, Moshfeghi DM *et al.*: A novel mutation in the RDS/Peripherin gene causes adult-onset foveomacular dystrophy. *Am J Ophthalmol* 135:213, 2003

Yanoff M, Rahn EK, Zimmerman LE: Histopathology of juvenile retinoschisis. *Arch Ophthalmol* 79:49, 1968

Zhang K, Garibaldi DC, Kniazeva M *et al.*: A novel mutation in the ABCR gene in four patients with autosomal recessive Stargardt disease. *Am J Ophthalmol* 128:720, 1999

Zhang K, Garibaldi DC, Li Y *et al.*: Buuterfly-shaped pattern dystrophy. A genetic, clinical, and histologic report. *Arch Ophthalmol* 119:485, 2002

Zhang K, Kniazeva M, Han M, Li W *et al.*: A 5-bp deletion in *ELOVL4* is associated with two related forms of autosomal dominant macular dystrophy. *Nat Gen* 27:89, 2001

Hereditary Secondary Retinal Dystrophies

Aessopos A, Stamatelos G, Savvides P *et al.*: Angioid streaks in homozygous B thalassemia. *Am J Ophthalmol* 108:356, 1989

Aessopos A, Voskaridou E, Kavouklis E *et al.*: Angioid streaks in sickle-thalassemia. *Am J Ophthalmol* 117:589, 1994

Ainsworth JR, Bryce IG, Dudgeon J: Visual loss in infantile osteopetrosis. *J Pediatr Ophthalmol Strabismus* 30:202, 1993

Baker RH, Trautman JC, Younge BR *et al.*: Late juvenile-onset Krabbe's disease. *Ophthalmology* 97:1176, 1990

Bateman JB, Philippart M: Ocular features of the Hagberg–Santavuori syndrome. *Am J Ophthalmol* 102:262, 1986

Bensaoula T, Shibuya H, Katz ML *et al.*: Histopathologic and immunocytochemical analysis of the retina and ocular tissues in Batten disease. *Ophthalmology* 107:1746, 2000

Berard-Badier M, Pellissier J-F, Gambarelli D *et al.*: The retina in Lafora disease: Light and electron microscopy. *Graefes Arch Clin Exp Ophthalmol* 212:285, 1980

Brosnahan DM, Kennedy SM, Converse CA *et al.*: Pathology of hereditary retinal degeneration associated with hypobetalipoproteinemia. *Ophthalmology* 101:38, 1994

Brownstein S, Carpenter S, Polomeno RC *et al.*: Sandhoff's disease (Gm2 gangliosidosis type 2): Histopathology and ultrastructure of the eye. *Arch Ophthalmol* 98:1089, 1980

Chang B, Bronson RT, Hawes NL *et al.*: Retinal degeneration in motor neuron degeneration: A mouse model of ceroid lipofuscinosis. *Invest Ophthalmol Vis Sci* 35:1071, 1994

Cogan DG, Chu FC, Gittinger J *et al.*: Fundal abnormalities of Gaucher's disease. *Arch Ophthalmol* 98:2202, 1980

Dabbs TR, Skjodt K: Prevalence of angioid streaks and other ocular complications of Paget's disease of bone. *Br J Ophthalmol* 74:579, 1990

Dreyer R, Green WR: The pathology of angioid streaks: A study of twenty-one cases. *Trans Pa Acad Ophthalmol Otolaryngol* 31:158, 1978

Duker JS, Belmont J, Bosley TM: Angioid streaks associated with abetalipoproteinemia. *Arch Ophthalmol* 105:1173, 1987

Emery JM, Green WR, Huff DS: Krabbe's disease: Histopathology and ultrastructure of the eye. *Am J Ophthalmol* 74:400, 1972

Erikson A, Wahlberg I: Gaucher disease: Norrbottnian type ocular abnormalities. *Acta Ophthalmol* 63:221, 1985

Font RL, Fine BS: Ocular pathology in Fabry's disease: Histochemical and electron microscopic observations. *Am J Ophthalmol* 73:419, 1972

Gartaganis S, Ismiridis K, Papageorgiou O *et al.*: Ocular abnormalities in patients with B thalassemia. *Am J Ophthalmol* 108:699, 1989

Goebel HH, Lehmann J: An ultrastructural study of the retina in human late infantile neuroaxonal dystrophy. *Retina* 13:50, 1993

Hoshino M, O'Brien TP, McDonnell JM *et al.*: Fucosidosis: Ultrastructural study of the eye in an adult. *Graefes Arch Clin Exp Ophthalmol* 227:162, 1989

Kaback M, Lim-Steele J, Dabholkar D *et al.*: Tay–Sachs disease: Carrier screening, prenatal diagnosis, and the molecular era. *JAMA* 270:2307, 1993

Katz ML, Gao C-L, Prabhakaram M *et al.*: Immunochemical localization of the Batten disease (CLN3) protein in retina. *Invest Ophthalmol Vis Sci* 38:2375, 1997

Katz ML, Rodrigues M: Juvenile ceroid lipofuscinosis: Evidence for methylated lysine in neural storage body protein. *Am J Pathol* 138:323, 1991

Lipson MH, O'Donnell J, Callahan JW et al.: Ocular involvement in Niemann–Pick disease type B. *J Pediatr* 108:582, 1986

Matthews JD, Weiter JJ, Kolodny EH: Macular halos associated with Niemann–Pick disease type B. *Ophthalmology* 93:933, 1986

McGovern MM, Wasserstein MP, Aron A et al.: Ocular manifestations of Neimann–Pick disease. *Ophthalmology* 111:1424, 2004

McLane NJ, Grizzard WS, Kousseff BG et al.: Angioid streaks associated with hereditary spherocytosis. *Am J Ophthalmol* 97:444, 1984

Nagpal KC, Asdourian G, Goldbaum M et al.: Angioid streaks and sickle haemoglobinopathies. *Br J Ophthalmol* 60:31, 1976

Naureckiene S, Sleat DE, Lackland H et al.: Identification of HE1 as the second gene of Niemann–Pick C disease. *Science* 290:2298, 2000

Novak MA, Roth AS, Levine MR: Calcium oxalate retinopathy associated with methoxyflurane abuse. *Retina* 8:230, 1988

Pradham SM, Atchaneeyasakul L-O, Appukuttan B et al.: Electroretinogram in mucolipidosis IV. *Arch Ophthalmol* 120:45, 2002

Rahn EK, Yanoff M, Tucker S: Neuro-ocular considerations in the Pelizaeus–Merzbacher syndrome: A clinicopathologic study. *Am J Ophthalmol* 66:1143, 1968

Ramsey MB, Yanoff M, Fine BS: Ocular histopathology in homocystinuria. *Am J Ophthalmol* 74:377, 1972

Sakamoto T, Maeda K, Sueishi K et al.: Ocular histopathologic findings in a 46-year-old man with primary hyperoxaluria. *Arch Ophthalmol* 109:384, 1991

Schwarz GA, Yanoff M: Lafora bodies, corpora amylacea and Lewy bodies: A morphologic and histochemical study. *Arch Neurobiol (Madr)* 28:801, 1965

Small KW, Letson R, Scheinman J: Ocular findings in primary hyperoxaluria. *Arch Ophthalmol* 108:89, 1990

Small KW, Pollack S, Scheinman J: Optic atrophy in primary oxalosis. *Am J Ophthalmol* 106:96, 1988

Smith JA, Chan C-C, Goldin E et al.: Noninvasive diagnosis and ophthalmic features of mucolipidosis type IV. *Ophthalmology* 109:588, 2002

Traboulsi EI, Maumenee IH: Ophthalmologic findings in mucolipidosis III (pseudo-Hurler polydystrophy). *Am J Ophthalmol* 102:592, 1986

Traboulsi EI, Maumenee IH, Green WR et al.: Olivopontocerebellar atrophy with retinal degeneration: A clinical and ocular histopathologic study. *Arch Ophthalmol* 106:801, 1988

Tsuji S, Choudary PV, Martin BM et al.: A mutation in the human glucocerebrosidase gene in neuronopathic Gaucher's disease. *N Engl J Med* 316:570, 1987

Usui T, Sawaguchi S, Abe H et al.: Late-infantile type galactosialidosis. *Arch Ophthalmol* 109:542, 1991

Wolfsdorf JI, Weinstein DA: Glycogen storage diseases. *Rev Endocr Metab Disord* 4:95, 2003

Wells CG, Johnson RJ, Qingli L et al.: Retinal oxalosis. *Arch Ophthalmol* 107:1638, 1989

Willemsen MAAP, Cruysberg JRM, Rotteveel JJ et al.: Juvenile macular dystrophy associated with deficient activity of fatty aldehyde dehydrogenase in Sjögren–Larsson syndrome. *Am J Ophthalmol* 130:782, 2000

Yanoff M, Schwarz GA: The retinal pathology of Lafora's disease: A form of glycoprotein-acid mucopolysaccharide dystrophy. *Trans Am Acad Ophthalmol Otolaryngol* 69:701, 1965

Systemic Diseases Involving the Retina

See preceding Bibliography under Vascular Disease, Hereditary Primary Retinal Dystrophies, and Hereditary Secondary Retinal Dystrophies.

Tumors

Appiah A, Hirose T: Secondary causes of premacular fibrosis. *Ophthalmology* 96:389, 1989

Apte RS, DiBernardo C, Pearlman JR et al.: Retinal metastasis presenting as a retinal hemorrhage in a patient with adenocarcinoma of the cecum. *Arch Ophthalmol* 123:850, 2005

Bornfeld N, Messmer EP, Theodossiadis G et al.: Giant cell astrocytoma of the retina: Clinicopathologic report of a case not associated with Bourneville's disease. *Retina* 7:183, 1987

Cheng L, Freeman WR, Ozerdem U et al.: Prevalence, correlates, and natural history of epiretinal membranes surrounding idiopathic macular holes. *Ophthalmology* 107:853, 2000

Eagle RC Jr: Carcinomatous retinitis. Presented at the meeting of the Eastern Ophthalmic Pathology Society, Hilton Head, SC, 1989

Farber MG, Smith ME, Gans LA: Astrocytoma of the ciliary body. *Arch Ophthalmol* 105:536, 1987

Fekrat S, Wendel RT, De La Cruz Z et al.: Clinicopathologic correlation of an epiretinal membrane associated with a recurrent macular hole. *Retina* 15:53, 1995

Fine BS, Yanoff M: *Ocular Histology: A Text and Atlas*, 2nd edn. Hagerstown, MD, Harper & Row, 1979:99

Fraser-Bell S, Guzowski M, Rochtchina E et al.: Five-year cumulative incidence and progression of epiretinal membranes: the Blue Mountain Eye Study. *Ophthalmology* 110:34, 2003

Fraser Bell S, Ying-Lai M, Klein R et al.: Prevalence and association of epiretinal membranes in Latinos: the Los Angeles Latino Eye Study. *Invest Ophthalmol Vis Sci* 45:1732, 2004

Guerin CJ, Wolfshagen RW, Elfrig D et al.: Immunocytochemical identification of Müller's glia as a component of human epiretinal membranes. *Invest Ophthalmol Vis Sci* 31:1483, 1990

Inayama Y, Hanashi M, Yazawi T et al.: Masive gliosis of the retina: report of a case investigated by immunohistochemistry and clonal assays. *J Ophthalmol* 140:1176, 2005

Irvine F, O'Donnell N, Kemp E et al.: Retinal vasoproliferative tumors: Surgical management and histological findings. *Arch Ophthalmol* 118:563, 2000

Nork TM, Ghobrial MW, Peyman GA et al.: Massive retinal gliosis: A reactive proliferation of Müller cells. *Arch Ophthalmol* 104:1383, 1986

Robbins SG, Brem RB, Wilson DJ et al.: Immunolocalization of integrins in proliferative retinal membranes. *Invest Ophthalmol Vis Sci* 35:3475, 1994

Sahel JA, Frederick AR, Pesavento R et al.: Idiopathic retinal gliosis mimicking a choroidal melanoma. *Retina* 8:282, 1988

Shields CL, Shields JA, Barrett J et al.: Vasoproliferative tumors of the retina: Classification and clinical manifestations in 103 patients. *Arch Ophthalmol* 113:615, 1995

Sivalingam A, Eagle RC, Duker JS et al.: Visual prognosis correlated with the presence of internal limiting membrane in histopathologic specimens obtained from epiretinal membrane surgery. *Ophthalmology* 97:1549, 1990

Smiddy WE, Michels RG, Green WR: Morphology, pathology, and surgery of idiopathic vitreoretinal macular disorders: A review. *Retina* 10:288, 1990

Spraul CW, Lang GE, Grossniklaus HE et al.: Metastatic adenocarcinoma to the retina in a patient with Muir-Torre syndrome. *Am J Ophthalmol* 120:248, 1995

Yanoff M, Zimmerman LE, Davis R: Massive gliosis of the retina: A continuous spectrum of glial proliferation. *Int Ophthalmol Clin* 11:211, 1971

Retinal Detachment

Bastek JV, Siegel EB, Straatsma BR *et al.*: Chorioretinal juncture: Pigmentary patterns of the peripheral fundus. *Ophthalmology* 89:1455, 1982

Benson WE, Nantawan P, Morse PH: Characteristics and prognosis of retinal detachments with demarcation lines. *Am J Ophthalmol* 84:641, 1977

Boldrey EE: Risk of retinal tears in patients with vitreous floaters. *Am J Ophthalmol* 96:783, 1983

Burton TC: The influence of refractive error and lattice degeneration on the incidence of retinal detachment. *Trans Am Ophthalmol Soc* 87:143, 1989

Byer NE: The natural history of asymptomatic retinal breaks. *Ophthalmology* 89:1033, 1982

Byer NE: Long-term natural history of lattice degeneration of the retina. *Ophthalmology* 96:1396, 1989

Chang C-J, Lai WW, Edward DP *et al.*: Apoptotic photoreceptor cell death after traumatic retinal detachment in humans. *Arch Ophthalmol* 113:880, 1995

Foos RY: Retinal holes. *Am J Ophthalmol* 86:354, 1978

Foos RY, Simons KB: Vitreous in lattice degeneration of retina. *Ophthalmology* 91:452, 1984

Kerkhoff FT, Lamberts QJ, van den Bieson PR *et al.*: Rhegmatogenous retinal detachment and uveitis. *Ophthalmology* 110:427, 2003

Kinyoun JL, Knobloch WH: Idiopathic retinal dialysis. *Retina* 4:9, 1984

Matsuo T: Photoreceptor outer segments in aqueous humor: Key to understanding a new syndrome. *Surv Ophthalmol* 39:211, 1994

Meyer E, Kurz GH: Retinal pits: A study of pathologic findings in two cases. *Arch Ophthalmol* 70:102, 1963

Pastor JC: Proliferative vitreoretinopathy . *Surv Ophthalmol* 43:3, 1998

Powell JO, Bresnick GH, Yanoff M *et al.*: Ocular effects of argon laser radiation: II. Histopathology of chorioretinal lesions. *Am J Ophthalmol* 71:1267, 1971

Robbins SG, Brem RB, Wilson DJ *et al.*: Immunolocalization of integrins in proliferative retinal membranes. *Invest Ophthalmol Vis Sci* 35:3475, 1994

Robinson MR, Streeten BW: The surface morphology of retinal breaks and lattice retinal degeneration: A scanning electron microscopic study. *Ophthalmology* 93:237, 1986

Yanoff M: Formaldehyde-glutaraldehyde fixation. *Am J Ophthalmol* 76:303, 1973

Yanoff M: Prophylactic cryotherapy of retinal breaks. *Ann Ophthalmol* 9:283, 1977

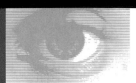

12

Vitreous

NORMAL ANATOMY

I. The transparent vitreous body, or hyaloid (Fig. 12.1), is one of the most delicate connective tissues in the body.
  A. It occupies the posterior or largest compartment of the eye (about 80% of the eye's volume), filling the globe between the internal limiting membrane of the neural retina and the posterior lens capsule.
  B. The structure is composed of a framework of extremely delicate, embryoniclike collagen filaments closely associated with a large quantity of water-binding hyaluronic acid.
II. Embryology
  A. Embryologically, the developing avascular secondary vitreous surrounds and compresses the vascularized primary vitreous into a tube or canal that extends from the optic disc to the back of the lens, forming the hyaloid canal (canal of Cloquet).
  B. The hyaloid vessel, which atrophies and disappears before birth, passes through the canal.
  C. Persisting remnants of the primary vitreous or hyaloid vessel produce congenital anomalies (see later), the most common being retention of tissue fragments on the back of the lens (Mittendorf's dot; Fig. 12.2), retention of tissue on the nasal optic disc (Bergmeister's papilla), and persistent primary vitreous (see p. 747 in Chapter 18).

CONGENITAL ANOMALIES

Persistent Primary Vitreous

I. Remnants of the primitive hyaloid vascular system, either anterior or posterior, may persist, or the entire hyaloid vessel from the optic disc to the back of the lens may remain.

Hyaloid vessel remnants are observed in over 90% of infants of less than 36 weeks' gestation, and in over 95% of infants weighing less than 5 pounds (2.275 kg) at birth.

  A. Anterior remnants (see Fig. 12.2; see also Fig. 9.3)
    1. The lenticular portion of the hyaloid artery may hang free in the vitreous from its lens attachment site.
    2. Mittendorf's dot is an opacity just below and nasal to the lens posterior pole at the lenticular attachment site of the hyaloid artery.
  B. Posterior remnants (Fig. 12.3)
    1. Vascular loops from the optic disc may remain within Cloquet's canal.
    2. Bergmeister's papilla is the glial remnant of the hyaloid system at the optic disc.

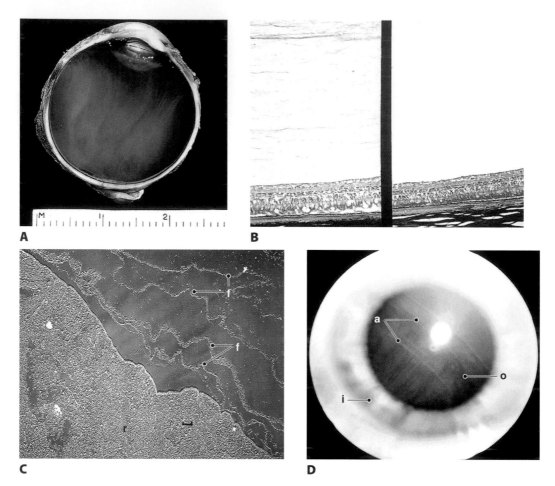

Fig. 12.1 Normal vitreous. **A,** The vitreous compartment is completely filled by the vitreous body. The major components of the vitreous are hyaluronic acid and delicate collagenous filaments. **B,** On the left is a vitreous body stained with colloidal iron so that it appears blue. On the right, the tissue was first treated with hyaluronidase and no staining occurred, indicating that the blue-staining material on the left is hyaluronic acid. **C,** The other major components, the collagenous, delicate vitreous filaments (f), are demonstrated by this electron micrograph of a shadow-cast preparation. The neural retina (r) occupies the diagonal lower left side and the filaments the diagonal upper right side. **D,** A ciliary-body melanoma has elevated the ora serrata region (o) so that it is clearly seen. Note that the attachment site (a) of the vitreous base appears as two white lines, one easily seen just anterior to the ora serrata and the other less easily seen just posterior to the ora serrata. This is the strongest attachment site of the vitreous body. The next strongest attachment site surrounds the optic nerve head, followed by a ring in the clivus of the anatomic fovea centralls (i, iris). (**A,** Armed Forces Institute of Pathology Neg. 57–1284. **B** and **C,** modified from Fine BS, Yanoff M: *Ocular Histology: A Text and Atlas,* 2nd edn. Copyright Elsevier 1979.)

The papilla, which usually occupies the nasal portion of the optic disc, may appear as a solid mass of whitish tissue, as a delicate, ragged strand, or as a well-defined membrane stretching over the disc.

3. Congenital cysts, which are usually pearly gray, wrinkled, and translucent, are the cystic remains of the hyaloid system.

They usually float freely but may be attached to the optic disc or suspended by a pedicle. Some have been shown histologically to consist of gliotic retinal or vascular remnants, whereas others resemble pigment epithelial cells (i.e., choristoma of the primary hyaloid system).

Persistent Hyperplastic Primary Vitreous (Persistent Fetal Vasculature)

I. Anterior (see p. 747 in Chapter 18)
II. Posterior (congenital retinal septum; ablatio falciformis congenita)
   A. Posterior persistent hyperplastic primary vitreous (PHPV; see Fig. 12.3) is most often unilateral and present at birth.
   B. Posterior PHPV consists of vitreous membranes extending from the disc usually toward the equatorial zone, posterior radial retinal fold (usually in the area of the vitreous membrane), disturbances of macular function, and neural retinal detachment.

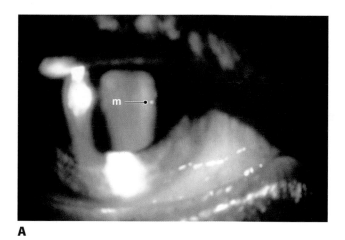

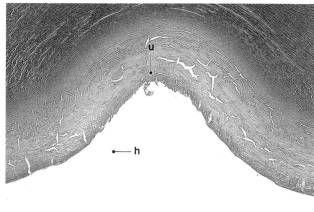

Fig. 12.2 Mittendorf's dot. **A,** Slit-lamp appearance of tiny white Mittendorf's dot (m) at back of lens. **B,** Microscopic appearance of hyaloid vessel (h) as it approaches the posterior capsule (u, posterior umbilication of lens considered to be an artifactitious finding often seen in infants).

Poor vision and strabismus are the most common presenting complaints.

INFLAMMATION

Acute

See Chapter 3.

Chronic

See Chapters 3 and 4.

VITREOUS ADHESIONS

Post Nonsurgical and Surgical Trauma

I. Vitreocorneal adhesions may cause corneal "touch" syndrome (see Fig. 5.5).
   A. Corneal touch syndrome occurs when formed vitreous touches the endothelium of the posterior surface of the cornea, usually after a complicated cataract extraction.
   B. The cornea becomes thickened and edematous in the region of touch.
II. Iridovitreal adhesions may lead to total posterior synechiae (*seclusion of pupil*) with resultant iris bombé, or they may form a membrane across the pupil (*occlusion of pupil*), or both.
III. Cyclovitreal adhesions may lead to a cyclitic membrane and subsequent neural retinal detachment.
IV. Vitreoretinal adhesions may lead to the macular vitreous traction syndrome (cystoid macular edema; Irvine–Gass syndrome; see p. 122 in Chapter 5) or to wrinkling of the internal limiting membrane, namely, "cellophane" retina (see Figs 11.43 to 11.45).

Traction of the vitreous on normal paravascular vitreoretinal attachment sites in an eye with a posterior vitreous detachment can cause neural retinal tears. Neural retinal tears tend to occur in clusters between the equator and the posterior border of the vitreous base.

V. White-without-pressure most likely is related to vitreoretinal adhesions. The areas of white-without-pressure may be migratory.

Postinflammation

See Chapters 3 and 4.

Idiopathic

Idiopathic vitreous adhesions may follow partial vitreoretinal separation (posterior vitreous detachment).

VITREOUS OPACITIES

Hyaloid Vessel Remnants

Muscae volitantes are minute remnants of the hyaloid vascular system or detachments of small folds of poorly differentiated retinal tissue, usually present in the anterior vitreous.

Muscae volitantes also is a historical, obsolete term for acquired vitreous floaters.

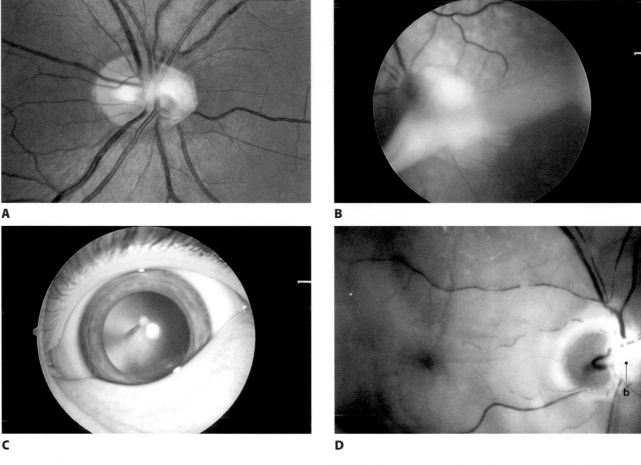

Fig. 12.3 Posterior remnants. Posterior remnants may be mild, as in this Bergmeister's papilla located on the nasal optic disc (**A**), or extreme, as in this posterior hyperplastic vitreous (**B**), which extends from the optic disc to the back of the lens (**C**). **D,** The enucleated eye shows posterior remnants of the hyaloid system over the nasal portion of the optic nerve head (b, Bergmeister's papilla). **E,** Histologic section shows a Bergmeister's papilla (b) in the form of a glial remnant of the hyaloid system.

Acquired Vitreous Strands and Floaters

I. Collapse and condensation of vitreous sheets with aging, especially in myopes, frequently cause the formation of strands and floaters.

II. Separation of the vitreous attachment to the optic disc after posterior vitreoretinal separation may cause a complete or incomplete ringlike floater (vitreous "peephole"; see subsection on vitreous detachment, later).

Inflammatory Cells

I. "Snowball" opacities (microabscesses) may occur with mycotic infections (especially with the mold fungi).

II. Whitish masses ("white balls") may be seen inferiorly with vitreitis (e.g., sarcoidosis).

III. Numerous vitreous opacities, foamy "Whipple" macrophages, may be found in persons with Whipple's disease (Fig. 12.4).

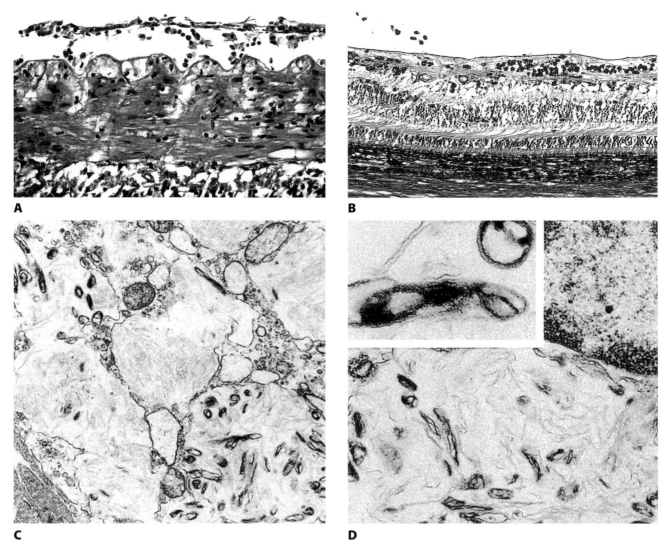

A

B

C

D

Fig. 12.4 Whipple's disease. **A,** Inner retinal layers infiltrated by macrophages that exhibit pale blue cytoplasm and eccentric or paracentral small nuclei. Few macrophages seen along internal limiting membrane (ILM). Epiretinal membrane has caused ILM to wrinkle. **B,** Decreased magnification shows neural retinal nerve fiber layer adjacent to macula containing myriad intensely PAS-positive macrophages. Outer and inner nuclear layers are relatively spared. **C,** Electron microscopy shows macrophage with serpiginous stacks of membranous structures intermixed with degenerating rod-shaped bacteria, both of which are encased in phagocytic vacuoles. **D,** Another macrophage shows almost equal admixture of membranous structures and degenerating bacteria. Inset depicts rod-shaped organism in longitudinal section and in cross-section. (From Font RL *et al.*: *Arch Ophthalmol* 96:1431, 1978. © American Medical Association. All rights reserved.)

A. Whipple's disease is a disorder of men, usually older than 35 years of age.

    1. The detection of the causative agent, *Tropheryma whippelii*, by polymerase chain reaction allows confirmation of the clinical diagnosis.

    2. The Gram-positive bacteria, *Arthrobacter* species, phylogenetically related to *T. whippelii*, may also be causative agents.

B. Arthritis, fever, serous effusions, cough, lymphadenopathy, and malaise may occur for several years preceding the intestinal malabsorption, steatorrhea, and cachexia.

C. Ocular findings, in addition to vitreous opacities, include inflammations and ophthalmoplegia.

D. Foamy macrophages containing periodic acid–Schiff (PAS)–positive cytoplasm may be found in intestinal and rectal mucosa, mesenteric and extra-abdominal lymphatic tissue, heart, lungs, liver, adrenals, spleen, serous membranes, neural retina, and vitreous.

    1. In addition, intracellular and extracellular rod-shaped bacillary bodies and serpiginous membranes are found by electron microscopic examination of macrophages.

    2. It is now assumed that the characteristic macrophages derive their PAS-positivity from ingested rod-shaped bacilli ("Whipple bacteria"—perhaps one of the *Corynebacterium*) and also from

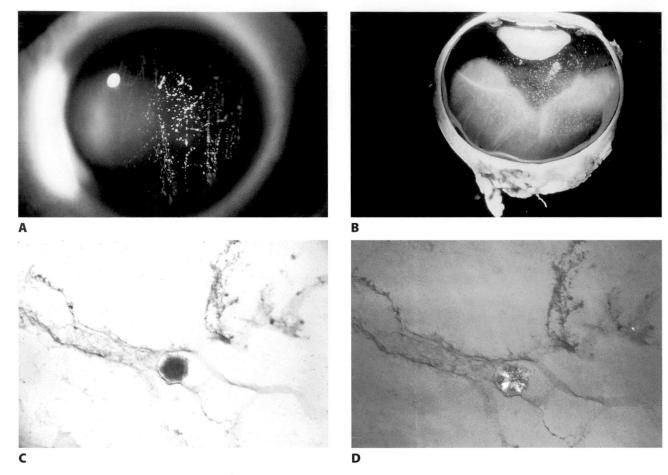

Fig. 12.5 Asteroid hyalosis. **A,** The fundus reflex shows tiny gold-colored balls in the anterior vitreous. **B,** The enucleated globe shows multiple tiny white spherules suspended throughout the vitreous body. Histologic section shows that the spherules stain positively with the acid mucopolysaccharide stain (**C**) and are birefringent to polarized light (**D**).

their residue in autophagic vacuoles of the macrophages.

Red Blood Cells

I. Red blood cells in the vitreous compartment (see Figs 12.11 and 12.12, below) are most often caused by neural retinal tears but may have other causes. Red blood cells may be subvitreal (between vitreous body and internal limiting membrane of the neural retina) or intravitreal (within the vitreous body).

II. Hypoxia of the vitreous body may be demonstrated when blood enters it in a patient who has sickle-cell trait or disease.
   A. Sickling and hemolysis of the erythrocytes increase toward the central vitreous, the most hypoxic area.
   B. On histologic examination of a vitreous specimen or an enucleated globe, occasionally the diagnosis of sickle-cell trait or disease is made in a person not known previously to be so affected.

Iridescent Particles

I. Asteroid hyalosis (Benson's disease; Figs 12.5 and 12.6) consists of complex lipids embedded in an amorphous matrix containing mainly calcium and phosphorus and attached to the vitreous framework.
   A. Diabetes mellitus is a major risk factor; other risk factors include systemic hypertension, atherosclerotic vascular disease, and hyperopia.
   B. Asteroid hyalosis has the following clinical properties:
      1. Asteroid bodies remain attached to collagenous framework and move only when the framework oscillates.

      Asteroid bodies are seen as gold balls when viewed with side illumination (e.g., with the ophthalmoscope) and appear white with direct illumination (e.g., with the slit lamp).
      ---

      2. The condition is usually unilateral and most common in the seventh and eighth decades of life.

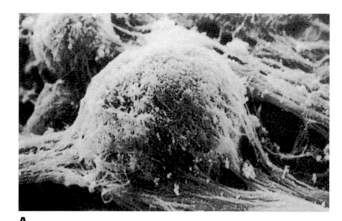

A

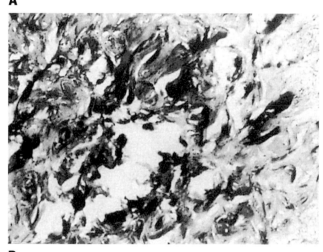

B

Fig. 12.6 Asteroid hyalosis. **A,** Scanning electron micrograph of asteroid bodies intertwined with vitreous collagen. **B,** Center and edge of single asteroid body show core of dense interlacing ribbons surrounded by rim (right side) of delicate strands. (**A,** Courtesy of Dr. RC Eagle, Jr.; **B,** courtesy of Dr. BW Streeten.)

It is infrequently associated with neural retinal detachment.

C. Histologically, asteroid bodies consist of an amorphous matrix that is both PAS-positive and acid mucopolysaccharide-positive and contains birefringent, small crystals when viewed with polarized light.

Electron microscopically, the bodies are composed of finely laminated ribbons of complex lipids, especially phospholipids, lying in a homogeneous background and intertwined with filaments of vitreous framework.

II. Synchysis scintillans (cholesterolosis; see Figs 5.39 and 5.40) consists of degenerative material not attached to the vitreous framework.

When vitreous gains access to the anterior chamber (e.g., in aphakia), a synchysis scintillans of the anterior chamber results.

A. Synchysis scintillans has the following clinical properties:
1. It is golden in color both to retroillumination and to direct view.
2. Usually it is unilateral and most common in men in their fourth or fifth decade.
3. It frequently follows an intravitreal (within vitreous body) hemorrhage.
4. The material settles inferiorly when the eye is immobile.
5. When in the anterior chamber, it disappears (melts) on the application of heat (e.g., as with a sun lamp).
B. Histologically, clefts represent the sites of dissolved-out cholesterol crystals within the vitreous body.

Tumor Cells

I. Retinoblastomas frequently shed their cells into the vitreous body.
II. Primary ocular malignant melanomas and medulloepitheliomas (embryonal type) and metastatic carcinomas, cutaneous melanomas, and lymphomas rarely shed their cells into the vitreous body.

Pigment Dust

I. Pigment dust follows intraocular trauma (nonsurgical or surgical), especially after intracapsular cataract extraction, and is probably derived from the posterior surface of the iris.
II. It also follows intraocular inflammation.

Cysts

I. Congenital (see p. 482 in this chapter)
II. Cysticercus (see p. 92 in Chapter 4)
III. Echinococcus (see p. 92 in Chapter 4)
IV. Embryonal medulloepithelioma (diktyoma), on occasion, may shed cells into the vitreous body, where the cells may then grow as cysts.
V. Retinoblastoma cells not infrequently seed into the vitreous body, where they grow into cysts.

Retinal Fragments

A free-floating operculum is the nonattached or separated neural retinal tissue derived from a neural retinal hole.

Traumatic Avulsion of Vitreous Base

The condition is rare and usually caused by trauma or shrinkage of vitreal fibrous membranes (Fig. 12.7).

Vitreous Detachment

I. Anterior
A. Hyaloideocapsular separation occurs in approximately 0.1% of the population.

B. It has a greater incidence in phakic eyes that contain a neural retinal detachment.

II. Posterior (Figs 12.8 and 12.9)

   A. The condition is present in approximately 65% of people older than 65 years of age and in more than 50% of people between 50 and 65 years of age.

Posterior vitreous detachment often develops in the fellow eye within 2 years of development in the first year.

   B. Partial posterior vitreous detachment is less common than the complete form.

   C. The most common cause of posterior vitreous detachment is senescence; other causes include high myopia, diabetes mellitus, ocular inflammation, and aphakia.

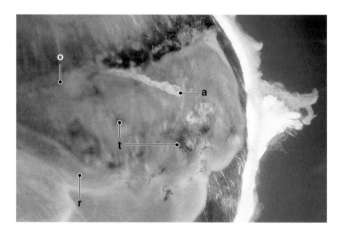

Fig. 12.7 Avulsion of vitreous base. The vitreous base is seen to be partially avulsed (a). The patient had blunt injury to this eye (o, ora serrata; t, traumatic chorloretinal atrophy; r, retina).

D. The most important complication of vitreous detachment, aside from the creation of floaters, is neural retinal tears.

If a neural retinal detachment is to occur, it usually ensues at the time of the vitreous detachment; it is rare as a late event.

E. Syneresis (i.e., one or more areas of central degeneration and liquefaction of the vitreous body) may occur with or without posterior vitreous detachment.

F. Histologically, the vitreous filaments are collapsed anteriorly so as to form a condensed posterior vitreous layer ("membrane").

   The new subvitreal space posteriorly contains a watery fluid but lacks collagenous filaments.

Proteinaceous Deposits

I. Proteinaceous deposits may form diffuse dustlike or cloudlike opacities.

II. They are analogous to plasmoid aqueous and occur chiefly with cyclitis, chorioretinitis, or trauma.

Amyloid

I. Primary familial amyloidosis (AL amyloidosis; Fig. 12.10; see also pp. 238–240 in Chapter 7)

   A. Primary familial amyloidosis has immunoglobulin light-chain amino fragments that are designated as amyloid AL (the same type of amyloid that is found in myeloma-associated amyloid).

   B. Vitreous opacities, frequently in the form of bilateral, sheetlike vitreous veils, are seen along with a retinal perivasculitis.

The nonfamilial form of primary amyloidosis is a rare condition that even more rarely can cause vitreous opacity.

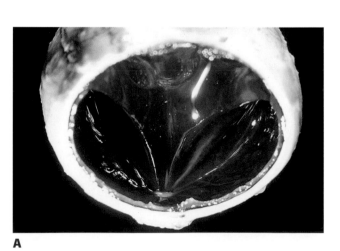

A

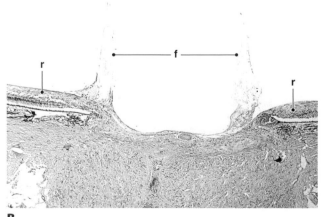

B

Fig. 12.8 Posterior vitreous detachment. **A,** Gross eye shows the vitreous completely detached posteriorly from the neural retina but still attached to the optic nerve head. **B,** Histologic section of eye shown in **A** demonstrates fibrous connection (f) of vitreous to the edges of the optic nerve, but posteriorly detached elsewhere (r, retina).

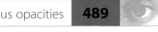

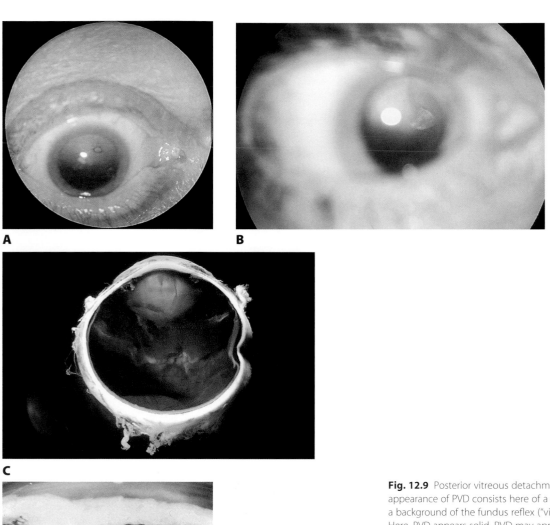

Fig. 12.9 Posterior vitreous detachment (PVD). **A,** Clinical appearance of PVD consists here of a circle viewed against a background of the fundus reflex ("vitreous peephole"). **B,** Here, PVD appears solid. PVD may appear to patient as a circle (doughnut) or, if broken, as J- or C-shaped, or solid, opacity. **C,** Gross specimen shows complete detachment posteriorly of vitreous from neural retina and optic nerve. **D,** Gross specimen of another eye shows the previous attachment site of the vitreous to the optic nerve now floating freely in the central vitreous compartment as a round fibrous band. **E,** Histologic section stained for acid mucopolysaccharide shows the fibrous band.

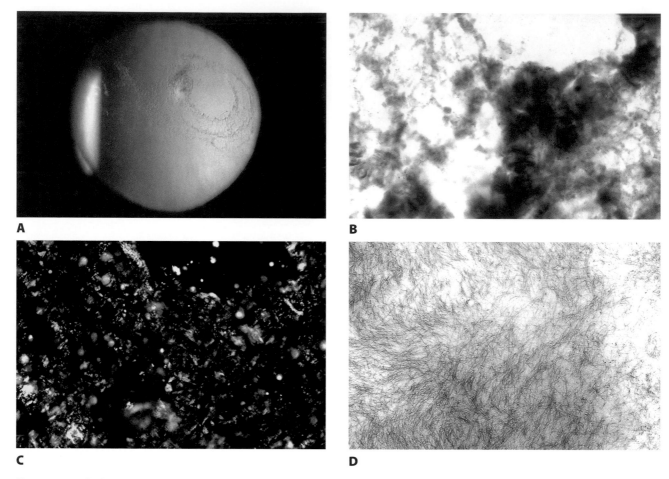

A

B

C

D

Fig. 12.10 Amyloidosis. **A,** Prominent diffuse vitreous opacities present in each eye. Diagnostic vitrectomy was performed. Histologic section of vitreous biopsy shows Congo red-positivity (**B**) and birefingence with polarized light (**C**). **D,** Electron micrograph shows fibrillar material with the individual fibers measuring 7 to 10 nm in diameter and having a faintly banded pattern. (Case presented by Dr. DJ Wilson to the meeting of the Verhoeff Society, 1994.)

C. Amyloid may reach the vitreous directly from affected retinal blood vessels.

D. Ecchymosis of lids, proptosis, ocular palsies, internal ophthalmoplegia, and neuroparalytic keratitis result from amyloid deposition in the lids and orbital connective tissues, muscles, nerves, and ganglia.

E. Glaucoma may be caused by amyloid deposition in the aqueous outflow areas.

F. Systemic amyloid deposition is widespread.

G. Histologically, a pale eosinophilic material is found in the vitreous that binds iodine and Congo red, demonstrates birefringence and dichroism (see later), shows metachromasia with metachromatic dyes such as toluidine blue and crystal violet, shows fluorescence after exposure to thioflavin-T, and has a filamentous ultrastructure.

Birefringence is the change in refractive indices with respect to light polarized in different directions through a substance. *Dichroism* is the property of a substance absorbing light polarized in a certain direction. When light is polarized at right angles to this direction, it is transmitted to a greater extent. In contrast to birefringence, dichroism can be specific for a particular substance. Dichroism can be observed in a microscope with the use of either a polarizer or an analyzer, but not both, because the dichroic substance itself (e.g., amyloid) serves as polarizer or analyzer, depending on the optical arrangement. Amyloid is dichroic only to green light.

---

1. The deposited amyloid filaments found in tissues are portions of immunoglobulin light chains.
2. Filaments of amyloid are difficult to differentiate from normal vitreous filaments.
3. The walls of retinal and choroidal blood vessels may be thickened by the amyloid material.

II. Familial amyloidotic polyneuropathy (FAP)

A. FAP is a hereditary form of systemic amyloidosis that involves vitreous (types I and II) and peripheral nerves.

1. In both FAP types I and II, the responsible protein is mutant transthyretin, designated *amyloid AF*.

In the majority of patients the valin-30 of transthyretin is replaced by methionine.

---

2. Type I FAP includes vitreous amyloidosis and an autonomic and peripheral neuropathy, most often affecting the lower extremities.

FAP has been described in Portuguese, Swedish, and Japanese kindreds.

---

3. Type II FAP includes vitreous amyloidosis and peripheral neuropathy, most often affecting the upper extremities first, along with a cardiomyopathy and sometimes a carpal tunnel syndrome.

FAP was first described in an Indian pedigree with Swiss origins.

---

4. Patients with types III and IV FAP do not acquire vitreous opacities, but do develop peripheral neuropathy, nephropathy, and peptic ulcers.
   a. In type III FAP mutant apolipoprotein A1 is the responsible precursor protein.
   b. In type IV FAP (also called *Meretoja syndrome*), mutant gelsolin is the responsible protein deposited.

Familial Exudative Vitreoretinopathy

I. Familial exudative vitreoretinopathy (FEV) is characterized by organized membranes in all quadrants of the vitreous.
   A. Vitreoretinal traction results from the pull of the membranes.
   B. Snowflakelike opacities are present in the vitreous body.
   C. The vitreous is usually detached posteriorly.
II. Frequently encountered are peripheral neural retinal exudates, localized neural retinal detachment often forming a broad fold temporally from the disc, and peripheral neural retinal neovascularization with recurrent vitreous hemorrhages.

Results of fluorescein angiography suggest a primary abnormality in the peripheral retinal circulation as the cause of the entity.

III. Slowly progressive ocular changes may ultimately lead to a condition that mimics certain aspects of retinopathy of prematurity, Coats' disease, and peripheral uveitis.
IV. FEV is genetically heterogeneous: X-linked; autosomal-dominant (most common); and autosomal-recessive types have been described.
   A. One X-linked and two autosomal-dominant loci have been mapped: *EVR1* on 11q, *EVR2* on Xp, and *EVR3* on 11p.
   B. The defective gene on *EVR1* locus is *FZD4*.

Other autosomal-dominantly inherited retinal disorders include autosomal-dominant vitreoretinochoroidopathy (ADVIRC; see later), autosomal-dominant neovascular inflammatory vitreoretinopathy (ADNIV; see later), autosomal-dominant cystoid macular dystrophy (autosomal-dominant macular edema; see p. 443 in Chapter 11), snowflake degeneration (see p. 440 in Chapter 11), and Wagner's and Stickler's syndromes (see pp. 439 and 440 in Chapter 11). FEV may also have an X-linked recessive inheritance pattern, carried on Xq 21.3 or Xp 11, and perhaps an allelic variant of the Norrie's disease gene.

Autosomal-Dominant Vitreoretinochoroidopathy (ADVIRC, Peripheral Annular Pigmentary Dystrophy of the Retina)

I. ADVIRC clinically shows a stationary or slowly progressive, circumferential (360°), bilateral and symmetric involvement of a coarse, peripheral hyperpigmentation and hypopigmentation of the fundus; a relatively discrete posterior border occurs in the region of the equator.
   A. The retinopathy is associated with fibrillar condensation of the vitreous and superficial and deep, yellowish-white, punctate opacities in the fundus.
   B. Other ocular findings include retinal vascular attenuation, transudation, and neovascularization; cystoid macular edema; choroidal atrophy; and cataract formation.
II. Histologically, disorganization of the peripheral neural retina occurs with focally atrophic retinal pigment epithelium (RPE).
   A. Altered RPE cells surround retinal vessels and line the internal limiting membrane.
   B. The equatorial neural retina shows an unusual multifocal loss of photoreceptors.
   C. An extensive epiretinal membrane consists of condensed vitreous, cellular debris, and layers of Müller cells.

Autosomal-Dominant Neovascular Inflammatory Vitreoretinopathy (ADNIV)

I. ADNIV clinically resembles ADVIRC, except that in the initial stage it shows a characteristic selective reduction of the electroretinogram b-wave amplitude; in addition, the pigmentary changes are less distinctive in ADNIV than in ADVIRC.
II. Cystoid macular edema, vitreous hemorrhage, tractional neural retinal detachment, and neovascular glaucoma can cause a profound loss of vision.

Erosive Vitreoretinopathy

I. Erosive vitreoretinopathy is characterized by pronounced vitreous abnormalities, complicated neural retinal detachments, and a progressive pigmentary retinopathy.
   A. The condition is inherited in an autosomal-dominant pattern. Mutations that cause erosive vitreoretinopathy (and also Wagner's disease) are linked to markers on the long arm of chromosome 5 (5q13–14).
   B. Clinically, nyctalopia, progressive visual field loss, marked vitreous syneresis, progressive atrophy of the

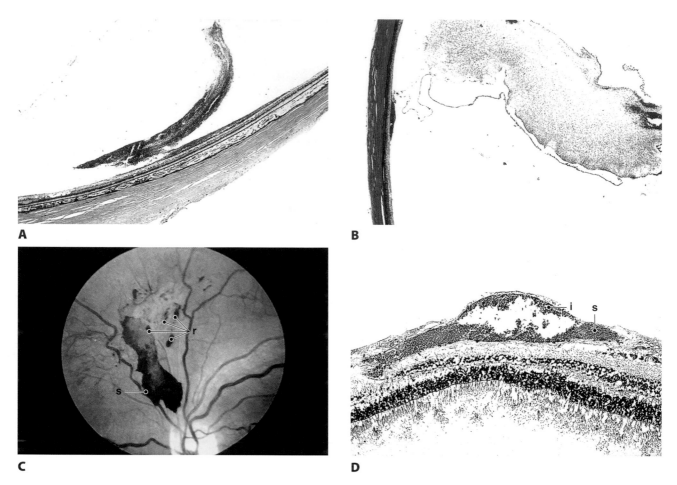

Fig. 12.11 Vitreous hemorrhage. **A,** Histologic section shows blood present between the internal limiting membrane (ILM) of the neural retina, and the posterior "face" of the vitreous (takes weeks to months to clear). **B,** Blood is present in the vitreous body (takes many months to years to clear). **C,** Fundus appearance of hemorrhage completely within the neural retina between the ILM and the nerve fiber layer (intraretinal submembranous hemorrhage) (r, retinal hemorrhage; s, sub-ILM intraretinal hemorrhage). **D,** Histologic section shows blood present between the ILM and the nerve fiber layer completely within the neural retina (intraretinal submembranous hemorrhage) (i, internal surface of retina; s, sub-ILM intraretinal hemorrhage).

RPE, and combined traction–rhegmatogenous neural retinal detachments are seen.

1. Previously normal-appearing RPE seems to thin or erode (hence the term *erosive*) in younger patients, allowing increased visualization of choroidal vessels.
2. Advanced cases show equatorial areas apparently devoid of RPE.
3. Electroretinography demonstrates diffuse rod–cone dysfunction.

> High myopia, epiphyseal dysplasia, orofacial anomalies, and systemic manifestations characteristic of other vitreo-retinopathies are absent.

C. No histologic studies are available.

Knobloch Syndrome

I. Knobloch syndrome is characterized by high myopia, vitreoretinal degeneration, retinal detachment, and a localized defect in the occipital region of the skull.

A. It is inherited as an autosomal recessive
B. A mutation occurs in the *COL1A1* gene, which encodes collagen XVII and its normal product endostatin, an inhibitor of angiogenesis
II. Endostatin is absent from the serum.
III. Persistent hyperplastic primary vitreous may be present (see p. 747 in Chapter 18).

VITREOUS HEMORRHAGE

Definitions

I. Subvitreal hemorrhage (Fig. 12.11)—blood is present between the internal limiting membrane of the neural retina, and the posterior "face" of the vitreous and takes weeks to months to clear. This type of hemorrhage is commonly seen in diabetic patients.
II. Intravitreal hemorrhage (Fig. 12.12; see Fig. 12.11)—blood is present in the vitreous body and takes many months to years to clear.

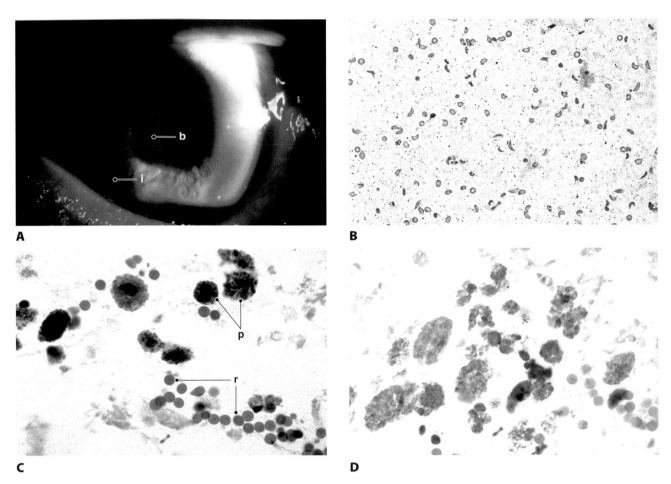

Fig. 12.12 Vitreous hemorrhage. **A,** A hemorrhage is seen in the vitreous body (b, blood in vitreous compartment; i, iris with superior-sector iridectomy). **B,** In this vitrectomy specimen of an intravitreal hemorrhage from a 67-year-old black man, the red blood cells were noted to have a sickle configuration; a diagnosis of sickle-cell trait was made. The diagnosis had not been made previously. **C,** Another vitrectomy specimen shows red blood cells (r) and pigment-containing macrophages (p). **D,** A special stain for iron (Perl's stain) shows that the pigment in some of the macrophages stains positively (blue), signifying hemosiderin; the pigment in other macrophages does not stain, and presumably represents melanin or hemoglobin not yet oxidized to hemosiderin. (**A,** Courtesy of Dr. SH Sinclair; **B–D,** courtesy of Dr. RC Eagle, Jr.)

III. Subhyaloid hemorrhage—this is identical to subvitreal hemorrhage, but use of the term clinically may be confusing.

Sometimes the term *subhyaloid hemorrhage* is used clinically to describe an intraretinal submembranous hemorrhage (i.e., a hemorrhage located mainly between the nerve fiber layer and the internal limiting membrane of the neural retina; see Figs 12.12 and 11.42D).

Causes

I. Causes include blood dyscrasias; choroidal hemorrhage with extension; diabetic retinopathy; Eales' disease; hypertensive retinopathy; juvenile retinoschisis; malignant melanoma; metastatic intraocular tumors; neural retinal neovascularization from any cause; neural retinal tears;

retinal angiomas; retinoblastoma; subneural retinal neovascularization; Terson's syndrome; sickle-cell retinopathy; subarachnoid hemorrhage; trauma; uveitis; and vitreoretinal separation.

II. Terson's syndrome

A. Terson's syndrome consists of hemorrhage into the vitreous compartment associated with intracranial, subarachnoid, or subdural hemorrhage.

Vitreous hemorrhage develops in approximately 16% to 17% of patients in whom spontaneous subarachnoid hemorrhage occurs.

B. Vitreous hemorrhage frequently obscures visualization of the fundus.

1. When visualization of the neural retina is possible, multiple preneural, intraneural (usually subinternal limiting membrane), and subneural retinal hemorrhages are often seen.

2. Other findings include epiretinal membranes, proliferative vitreoretinopathy, pigmentary macular

changes, and perimacular neural retinal folds similar to the folds seen in the battered-baby (shaken-baby) syndrome.

Complications

I. Organization
  A. Membranes may lie on the internal surface of the neural retina (i.e., epiretinal) and cause a cellophane retina or fixed retinal folds (see Figs 11.43 to 11.45).
  B. Many of the delicate epiretinal (on the retinal surface) and preretinal (elevated from the retinal surface) membranes, especially those of the macular and paravascular regions, are believed to form from inward migration and proliferation of the various small glial cells normally present in the nerve fiber and ganglion cell layers.
    1. Other cells, such as RPE cells, fibrocytes, and myofibroblasts, can also be found.
    2. As the membranes shrink or contract, fixed folds of the retina develop (see p. 467 in Chapter 11).
  C. When fibrous RPE or glial membranous proliferations on the internal or external surface of the neural retina are associated with vitreous retraction, a neural retinal detachment and new neural retinal holes may result.
  D. When the membranous process is extensive and associated with a total neural retinal detachment, it is called *proliferative vitreoretinopathy* (PVR); the older terminologies were *massive vitreous retraction* and *massive periretinal proliferation*.
    1. PVR may follow perforating trauma, neural retinal detachment, and surgical manipulation.
    2. Although PVR most often develops posteriorly and equatorially, it may also occur anteriorly, where it results in anterior dragging of the peripheral neural retina.
    3. PVR probably represents a tissue-reparative process and can be thought of as nonvascular granulation tissue.

Some evidence suggests that fibronectin may mediate the initial events in epiretinal membrane formation and that vitronectin may modulate the adhesion mechanisms in established membranes. Transforming growth factor-β_2 levels are increased in eyes that have intravitreal fibrosis associated with PVR, and the levels appear to correlate with the severity of PVR.

  E. Histologically, glial, fibrous, or RPE membranes, or any combination, are seen on the internal, external, or both surfaces of the retina.
    1. T lymphocytes and macrophages may be present in the membranes.
    2. The membrane stroma or matrix is composed primarily of types I, II, and III collagen, accompanied focally by types IV and V collagen, laminin, and heparan sulfate.
II. Hemolytic (ghost cell) glaucoma (see p. 647 in Chapter 16)

BIBLIOGRAPHY

Normal Anatomy

Federman JL, Gouras P, Schubert H *et al.*: Retina and vitreous. In Podos SM, Yanoff M, eds: *Textbook of Ophthalmology*, vol. 9. London, Mosby, 1994:1.8, 1.9, 2.15–2.19

Fine BS, Yanoff M: *Ocular Histology: A Text and Atlas*, 2nd edn. Hagerstown, PA, Harper & Row, 1979:131–145

Yanoff M, Fine BS: *Ocular Pathology: A Color Atlas*, 2nd edn. New York, Gower Medical Publishing, 1992:12.1–12.2

Congenital Anomalies

Flynn WJ, Carlson DW: Pigmented vitreous cyst. *Arch Ophthalmol* 112:1113, 1994

Goldberg MF: Persistent fetal vasculature (PFV): An integrated interpretation of signs and symptoms associated with persistent hyperplastic primary vitreous (PHPV). LIV Edward Jackson Memorial Lecture. *Am J Ophthalmol* 124:587, 1997

Katz B, Wiley CA, Lee VW: Optic nerve hypoplasia and the nevus sebaceous of Jadassohn: A new association. *Ophthalmology* 94:1570, 1987

Lincoff H, Lopez R, Kreissig I *et al.*: Retinoschisis associated with optic nerve pits. *Arch Ophthalmol* 106:61, 1988

Nork TM, Millecchia LL: Treatment and histopathology of a congenital vitreous cyst. *Ophthalmology* 105:825, 1998

Roth AM, Foos RY: Surface structure of the optic nerve head: I. Epipapillary membranes. *Am J Ophthalmol* 74:977, 1972

Rubinstein K: Posterior hyperplastic primary vitreous. *Br J Ophthalmol* 64:105, 1980

Vitreous Adhesions

Fine BS, Yanoff M: *Ocular Histology: A Text and Atlas*, 2nd edn. Hagerstown, PA, Harper & Row, 1979:134

Foos RY, Roth AM: Surface structure of the optic nerve head: 2. Vitreopapillary attachments and posterior vitreous detachment. *Am J Ophthalmol* 76:662, 1973

Nagpal KC, Huamonte F, Constantaras A *et al.*: Migratory white-without-pressure retinal lesions. *Arch Ophthalmol* 94:576, 1976

Robbins SG, Brem RB, Wilson DJ *et al.*: Immunolocalization of integrins in proliferative retinal membranes. *Invest Ophthalmol Vis Sci* 35:3475, 1994

Spencer LM, Foos RY: Paravascular vitreoretinal attachments. *Arch Ophthalmol* 84:557, 1970

Streeten BW: The nature of the ocular zonule. *Trans Am Ophthalmol Soc* 80:823, 1982

Vitreous Opacities

Alkan S, Beals TF, Schnitzer B: Primary diagnosis of Whipple disease manifesting as lymphadenopathy. Use of polymerase chain reaction for detection of *Tropheryma whippelii. Am J Clin Pathol* 116:898. 2001

Bergren RL, Brown GC, Duker JS: Prevalence and association of asteroid hyalosis with systemic disease. *Am J Ophthalmol* 111:289, 1991

Boldrey EE, Egbert P, Gass JDM *et al.*: The histopathology of familial exudative vitreoretinopathy: A report of two cases. *Arch Ophthalmol* 103:238, 1985

Brown DM, Graemiger RA, Hergersberg M *et al.*: Genetic linkage of Wagner's disease and erosive vitreoretinopathy to chromosome 5q13–14. *Arch Ophthalmol* 113:671, 1995

Brown DM, Kimura AE, Weingeist TA *et al.*: Erosive vitreoretinopathy. *Ophthalmology* 101:694, 1994

Chan RY, Yannuzzi LA, Foster CS: Ocular Whipple's disease. Earlier definitive diagnosis. *Ophthalmology* 108:2225, 2001

Cibis GW, Watzke RC, Chua J: Retinal hemorrhages in posterior vitreous detachment. *Am J Ophthalmol* 80:1043, 1975

Ciulla TA, Tolentino F, Morrow JF *et al.*: Vitreous amyloidosis in familial amyloidotic polyneuropathy: Report of a case with the ValsoMet transthyretin mutation. *Surv Ophthalmol* 40:197, 1995

Clement F, Beckford CA, Corral A *et al.*: X-linked familial exudative vitreoretinopathy: Report of one family. *Retina* 15:141, 1995

Duh EJ, Yao Y-G, Dagli M *et al.*: Persistence of fetal vasculature in a patient with Knobloch syndrome. Potential role for endostatin in fetal remodeling of the eye. *Ophthalmology* 111:1885, 2004

Eagle RC Jr, Yanoff M: Cholesterolosis of anterior chamber. *Graefes Arch Klin Ophthalmol* 193:121, 1975

Fine BS, Yanoff M: *Ocular Histology: A Text and Atlas*, 2nd edn. Hagerstown, PA, Harper & Row, 1979:97

Foos RY: Ultrastructural features of posterior vitreous detachment. *Graefes Arch Klin Ophthalmol* 196:103, 1975

Foos RY, Wheeler NC: Vitreoretinal juncture: Synchysis senilis and posterior vitreous detachment. *Ophthalmology* 89:1502, 1982

Gündüz K, Shields JA, Shields CL *et al.*: Cutaneous melanoma metastatic to the vitreous cavity. *Ophthalmology* 105:600, 1998

Han DP, Burke JM, Blaire JR *et al.*: Histopathologic study of autosomal dominant vitreoretinochoroidopathy in a 26-year-old woman. *Arch Ophthalmol* 113:1561, 1995

Hikichi T, Yoshida A: Time course of development of posterior vitreous detachment in the fellow eye after development in the first eye. *Ophthalmology* 111:1705, 2004

Koga T, Ando E, Hirata A *et al.*: Vitreous opacities and outcome of vitreous surgery in patients with familial amyloidotic polyneuropathy. *Am J Ophthalmol* 135:188, 2003

Marano RPC, Vilaró S: The role of fibronectin, laminin, vitronectin and their receptors on cellular adhesion in proliferative vitreoretinopathy. *Invest Ophthalmol Vis Sci* 35:2791, 1994

Miller H, Miller B, Rabinowitz H *et al.*: Asteroid bodies: An ultrastructural study. *Invest Ophthalmol Vis Sci* 24:133, 1983

Moss SE, Klein BEK: Asteroid hyalosis in a population. The Beaver Dam Eye Study. *Am J Ophthalmol* 132:70, 2001

Nishimura JK, Cook BE, Pach JM: Whipple disease presenting as posterior uveitis without prominent gastrointestinal symptoms. *Am J Ophthalmol* 126:130, 1998

Orellana J, O'Malley RE, McPherson AR *et al.*: Pigmented free-floating vitreous cysts in two young adults: Electron microscopic observations. *Ophthalmology* 92:297, 1985

Pena RA, Jerdan JA, Glaser BM: Effects of TGF-β and TGF-β neutralizing antibodies on fibroblast-induced collagen gel contraction: implications for proliferative vitreoretinopathy. *Invest Ophthalmol Vis Sci* 35:2804, 1994

Sandgren O: Ocular amyloidosis with special reference to the hereditary forms with vitreous involvement. *Surv Ophthalmol* 40:1173, 1995

Sandgren D, Holmgren G, Lundgren E *et al.*: Restriction fragment length polymorphism analysis of mutated transthyretin in vitreous amyloidosis. *Arch Ophthalmol* 106:790, 1988

Streeten BW: Vitreous asteroid bodies: Ultrastructural characteristics and composition. *Arch Ophthalmol* 100:969, 1982

Swan N, Skinner M, O'Hara CJ: Bone marrow core biopsy specimens in AL (primary) amyloidosis. *Am J Clin Pathol* 120:610, 2003

Tanner V, Harie D, Tan J *et al.*: Acute posterior vitreous detachment: The predictive value of vitreous pigment and symptomatology. *Br J Ophthalmol* 84:1264, 2000

Toomes C, Bottomley HM, Scott S *et al.*: Spectrum and frequency of FZD4 mutations in familial exudative vitreoretinopathy. *Invest Ophthalmol Vis Sci* 45:2083, 2004

Williams JG, Edward DP, Tessler HH *et al.*: Ocular manifestations of Whipple disease. *Arch Ophthalmol* 116:1232, 1998

Winkler J, Lünsdorf H: Ultrastructure and composition of asteroid bodies. *Invest Ophthalmol Vis Sci* 42:902, 2001

Vitreous Hemorrhage

Butner RW, McPherson AR: Spontaneous vitreous hemorrhage. *Ann Ophthalmol* 14:268, 1982

Forrester JV, Grierson I, Lee WR: The pathology of vitreous hemorrhage: II. Ultrastructure. *Arch Ophthalmol* 97:2368, 1979

Friedman SM, Margo CE: Bilateral subinternal limiting membrane hemorrhage with Terson syndrome. *Am J Ophthalmol* 124:850, 1997

García-Arumí J, Corcostegui B, Tallada N *et al.*: Epiretinal membranes in Terson's syndrome. *Retina* 14:351, 1994

Ogawa T, Kitaoka T, Dake Y *et al.*: Terson syndrome: A case report suggesting the mechanism of vitreous hemorrhage. *Ophthalmology* 108:1654, 2002

Pfausler B, Belcl R, Metzler R *et al.*: Terson's syndrome in spontaneous subarachnoid hemorrhage: A prospective study in 60 consecutive patients. *J Neurosurg* 85:392, 1996

Velikay M, Datlinger P, Wedrich A *et al.*: Retinal detachment with severe proliferative vitreoretinopathy in Terson's syndrome. *Ophthalmology* 101:35, 1994

Yanoff M: Ocular pathology of diabetes. *Am J Ophthalmol* 67:21, 1969

13

Optic Nerve

NORMAL ANATOMY

I. The optic nerve is made up of a number of components (Figs 13.1 and 13.2).
   A. The major component is myelinated nerve fibers or axons (white matter).
      1. The axons of the optic nerve are extensions of the retinal ganglion cells whose unmyelinated axons form much of the nerve fiber layer of the neural retina.
      2. The axons or "nerve fibers" then enter the optic disc by making a sharp turn, where they continue as a series of fascicles or bundles, separated from one another by helical columns of glial cells (astrocytes) and vascular connective tissue septa, to form the optic nerve.
      3. The optic nerve becomes myelinated as it traverses the lamina cribrosa scleralis, doubling its diameter from approximately 1.5 mm at the optic disc to 3 mm as it leaves the scleral canal posteriorly.

   The lamina cribrosa is a series of trabeculae, contiguous with the choroidal (lamina cribrosa choroidalis—glial) and scleral (lamina cribrosa scleralis—vascularized collagen) coats of the eye. The trabeculae form a criss-cross pattern outlining "pores" through which the nerve fiber bundles pass. The myelinated orbital portion of the optic nerve can be considered more a tract of the brain than a true cranial nerve. The optic nerve is continuous at one end with the retina and at the other end with the brain, making it vulnerable to a variety of both ocular and central nervous system (CNS) diseases.

   B. All the CNS meningeal sheaths (dura, arachnoid, and pia) are present and surround the orbital portion of the optic nerve.
      The subarachnoid space of the optic nerve is continuous with that of the intracranial contents.

   An elevation of intracranial pressure, therefore, is directly transmitted to the subarachnoid space surrounding the optic nerve and contained within its dural sheath.

   C. The capillary blood supply to the anterior 2 to 3 mm of the optic nerve (intrachorioscleral portion) is derived exclusively from the ophthalmic artery through two sources.
      1. One source of blood supply, the major supply, consists of peripapillary choroidal branches, which are fed through the choroidal circulation by the short posterior ciliary arteries.
      2. Another source, albeit of much less significance, is the perineural plexus in the most anterior portions of the subarachnoid space surrounding the optic nerve.
   D. The capillary blood supply of the remaining ophthalmic artery vessels enters the nerve from the pial surface in a symmetric, radially distributed pattern.
   E. The central retinal artery first enters the optic nerve approximately 0.8 to 1.5 cm behind the globe.
II. The optic nerve is approximately 30 mm long, longer than the distance from the back of the eye to the optic canal, and so takes a somewhat sinuous course through the posterior orbit.

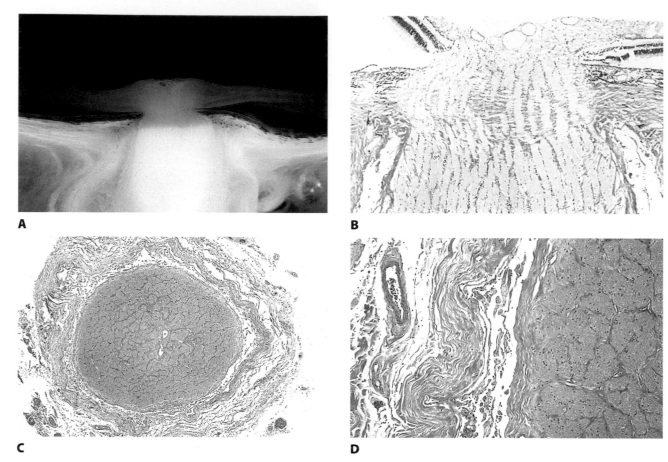

Fig. 13.1 Normal optic nerve. **A** and **B,** Longitudinal sections (gross and microscopic, respectively) of the optic nerve (ON) show the intraocular (in the scleral canal) and retrobulbar portions of the ON. The intraocular portion is divided into three parts or layers: the inner retinal layer anteriorly; the middle choroidal layer where white myelination of the ON begins (**A**); and the outer scleral layer posteriorly. The anterior surface of the retinal layer (the optic disc or ON head) measures approximately 1.5 mm in diameter; as the ON exits the scleral canal posteriorly to form the retrobulbar portion, it measures 3 to 4 mm in diameter; the increased width is mainly due to the addition of myelin (seen as white within the ON in **A**). **C** and **D,** Cross-sections (low and medium magnification, respectively) of the ON show the central parenchyma that contains axons, central retinal artery and vein, other blood vessels, astrocytes, oligodendrocytes, and pial septa. This is surrounded by pia mater, subarachnoid "space," arachnoid mater, subdural "space," and dura. (**A,** Courtesy of Dr. RC Eagle, Jr.; **C** and **D,** courtesy of Dr. MG Farber.)

CONGENITAL DEFECTS AND ANATOMIC VARIATIONS

Aplasia

I. Aplasia of the optic nerve (Fig. 13.3) is rare, especially in eyes without multiple congenital anomalies.

II. Most cases occur as unilateral disorders in otherwise healthy persons, although bilateral cases have been reported.

III. Most probably, the retinal ganglion cells fail to develop properly. Alternatively, the optic nerve aplasia may result from abnormal invagination of the ventral fissure.

IV. Histology

A. The optic nerve, optic nerve head, nerve fibers (axons) in the retinal nerve fiber layer, and retinal vessels are absent.

B. The retinal ganglion cell layer is diminished or absent. When present, the retinal ganglion cells appear undifferentiated, lacking axons or dendrites.

Hypoplasia

I. Although rare, hypoplasia (underdevelopment of the optic nerve) is more common than aplasia (congenital absence of the optic nerve).

A. Hypoplasia of the optic nerve is a major cause of blindness in children.

B. In optic nerve hypoplasia, a small optic disc with central vessels is present.

The term *optic nerve hypoplasia* should be reserved for cases that show hypoplasia as the main or sole anomaly of the nerve (e.g., colobomas of the optic nerve usually show hypoplastic

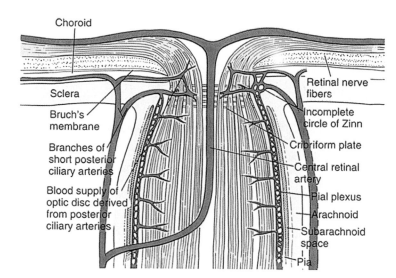

Choroid

Sclera

Bruch's membrane

Branches of short posterior ciliary arteries

Blood supply of optic disc derived from posterior ciliary arteries

Retinal nerve fibers

Incomplete circle of Zinn

Cribriform plate

Central retinal artery

Pial plexus

Arachnoid

Subarachnoid space

Pia

Fig. 13.2 Vascular supply of the anterior optic nerve. Schematic shows that capillaries in laminar region derive from two sources: choroid via short posterior ciliary arteries, and pial plexus. Considerable individual variations occur. (From Hart WM, Jr: In Podos SM, Yanoff M, eds: *Textbook of Ophthalmology*, vol. 6. London, Mosby, 1994:1.14. © Elsevier 1994.)

nerves, but the main event is the coloboma, not the hypoplasia). Also, in those situations where multiple anomalies of the eye or brain or both are present, it is difficult to determine whether the optic nerve is hypoplastic (primary failure of development) or atrophic (secondary degeneration). A hypoplastic or atrophic optic nerve may be found in association with grossly malformed eyes (e.g., microphthalmos) or with deformities of the CNS (e.g., hydrocephalus). Hypoplasia of the optic nerve is also a prominent feature of septo-optic dysplasia *(de Morsier syndrome)*, which consists of optic nerve hypoplasia, absence of the septum pellucidum, and pituitary insufficiency.

II. Optic nerve hypoplasia may be unilateral or bilateral, with or without optic foramina radiographic abnormalities, causes subnormal vision, and shows a decreased number of optic nerve axons.

High-resolution magnetic resonance imaging is an excellent method to detect small optic nerves.

III. Visual acuity is generally markedly decreased.
IV. The cause is failure of the retinal ganglion cells to develop normally.
    A. Because the optic stalk is invaginated by mesoderm, the central retinal artery and vein are present on the disc.
    B. Histologically, the nerve shows partial or complete absence of neurites.

Dysplasia

I. Dysplasia or abnormal development of the optic nerve is usually associated with other optic nerve anomalies such as colobomas and also with gross malformations of the eye.
II. Histologically, a marked disorganization of the nerve occurs, usually accompanied by a partial absence of neurites.

Optic disc dysplasia may be associated with transsphenoidal encephalocele (e.g., when seen with V- or tongue-shaped retinochoroidal anomaly or with the morning-glory syndrome).

Anomalous Shape of Optic Disc and Cup

I. Minor disturbances
   A. Oval discs (vertically, horizontally, or obliquely elongated) are common.
   B. They are congenital and nonprogressive.

A normal disc may appear abnormal when viewed with the direct ophthalmoscope in an eye with a significant degree of astigmatism.

II. Myopia (see p. 504 in this chapter and p. 423 in Chapter 11)
III. Congenital excavation of optic disc (i.e., an exaggeration of physiologic cup)
    A. It almost never extends as far as the edge of the disc (when it does, it usually does so temporally).
        Major retinal blood vessels often pass through the substance of the optic rim.
    B. It is nonprogressive.
    C. Histologically, the optic nerve is normal except for an enlarged physiologic cup in the optic disc. Often the diameter of the choroidal portion of the optic nerve is somewhat larger than normal.
IV. Pseudoneuritis or pseudopapilledema (i.e., the opposite of congenital excavation)
    A. In pseudoneuritis, the nerve fibers and glial tissues are "heaped up."
    B. It is nonprogressive and lacks dilatation of the veins, hemorrhages, or exudates.
    C. Often it is associated with hypermetropia or drusen of the optic nerve head.
    D. Histologically, the optic nerve is normal except for a smaller than usual or absent physiologic cup in the optic disc.

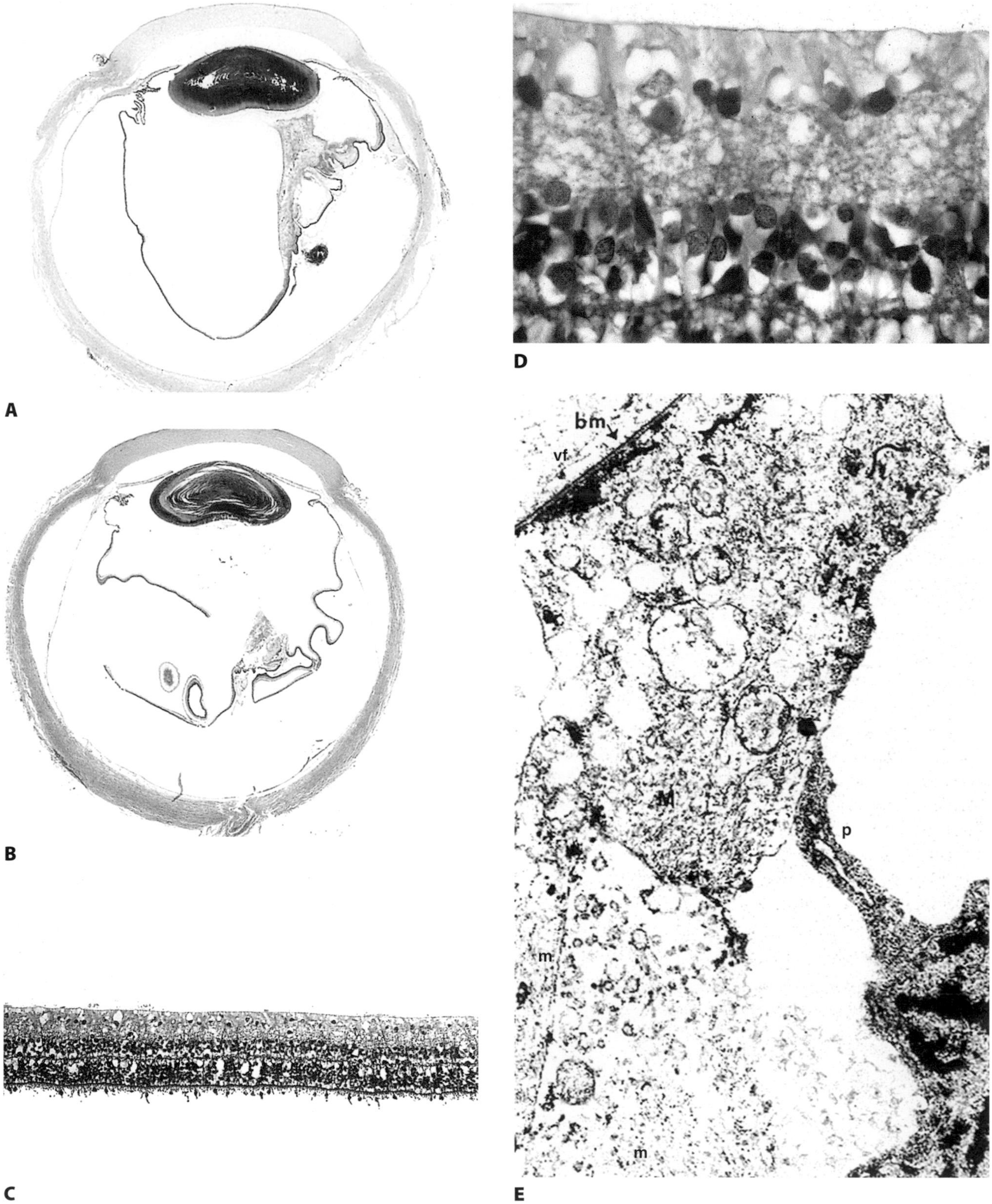

Fig. 13.3 Aplasia of optic nerve. **A** and **B** show both eyes from infant who died at 3 days of age. Step sections of right eye and serial sections of left eye failed to show any posterior attachment of retina. No optic nerve could be identified. **C,** Histologic section of neural retina shows thinned inner layers. **D,** Increased magnification demonstrates immature ganglion cells. **E,** Peripheral retina shows vitreous filaments (vf) present along thin internal limiting membrane of retina (bm). Filamentous Müller cells (m) lie alongside isolated neuronal cell with few, short processes (p), containing dense, nonfilamentous cytoplasm. Latter cell identified as immature ganglion cell. In other sections, external limiting membrane of retina, consisting of series of zonulae adherentes, joining Müller cells and photoreceptor cells in single plane, could be identified. (**B,** trichrome; **A–E,** from Yanoff M *et al.: Arch Ophthalmol* 96:97, 1978, with permission. © American Medical Association. All rights reserved.)

Often, the diameter of the choroidal portion of the optic nerve is smaller than normal and the optic nerve tissue is heaped up on the surface of the optic disc.

Congenital Crescent or Conus

I. A white, semilunar area lies at the margin of the optic disc, usually involving the inferior or inferotemporal margin of the disc. The conus often occurs with an oval disc whose long axis is parallel to the crescent.
II. Vision is usually defective.
III. An associated hypermetropia, often with an associated pit of the optic disc, is frequently seen.
IV. A congenital crescent should not be confused with a myopic crescent. Unlike the former, a myopic crescent is not present at birth, is progressive, has a temporal or annular location about the optic disc, and is associated with other retinal degenerative changes and with myopia.
V. Histologically, retinal pigment epithelium (RPE) and choroid are missing in the area of the conus.

A lack of embryonic development of RPE may be the primary defect.

Congenital (Familial) Optic Atrophies

I. Simple recessive congenital optic atrophy
  A. Simple congenital optic atrophy has an autosomal-recessive inheritance pattern and significant visual disability.
  B. Clinically, its onset is in infancy, is accompanied by a pendular nystagmus, and shows total optic atrophy.
  C. The histology is as described in the section *Optic Atrophy* on p. 514 in this chapter.
II. Behr's syndrome
  A. Behr's syndrome, a heterogeneous group, tends to have an autosomal-recessive inheritance pattern, and its onset is between 1 and 9 years of age.
  B. One form of Behr's syndrome has been reported in Iraqi Jews.
    1. The patients have 3-methylglutaconic aciduria.
    2. The main neurologic signs in these patients, as well as other patients who have Behr's syndrome but presumably no 3-methylglutaconic aciduria, consist of increased tendon reflexes, a positive Babinski sign, progressive spastic paraplegia, dysarthria, head nodding, and horizontal nystagmus.
    3. The optic atrophy tends to be severe, but sometimes only or mostly involving the temporal optic disc.
  C. The histology is as described in the section *Optic Atrophy* on p. 514 in this chapter.
III. Dominant optic atrophy (Kjer)
  A. Dominant optic atrophy is the most common of the inherited optic atrophies; the gene abnormality is in the OPA1 (3q28–3q29), OPA2 9X-linked;X; Xp11.4 to 11.212), OPA3 (autosomal recessive; 19q13.2 to13.3), and *OPA4* autosomal dominant; 18q12.2–121.3).

B. The visual loss in dominant optic atrophy (Kjer type) has an insidious onset in the first 5 or so years of life, with considerable variation in families.

Approximately 58% of affected patients have onset of symptoms before the age of 10 years.

---

  1. Long-term visual prognosis is relatively good, with stable or slow progression of visual loss.
  2. Most patients have blue-yellow dyschromatopsia; the Farnsworth–Munsell test shows the characteristic tritanopia defect.
  3. The optic nerve varies from mild pallor to complete atrophy.

Some nerves are said to have a characteristic focal temporal excavation.

  C. The histology is as described in the section *Optic Atrophy* on p. 514 in this chapter.
IV. Leber's hereditary optic neuropathy (LHON)
  A. LHON, one of the mitochondrial myopathies (see p. 538 in Chapter 14), is inherited through the maternal transmission of one or more mitochondrial DNA (mtDNA) mutations.

The inheritance of these point mutations of mitochondrial DNA is from mothers alone, because the mitochondrial contribution to the embryo comes only from the maternal ovum.

  B. Molecular genetic studies have shown that the condition results from a point mutation in the extranuclear mtDNA.

For example, in the 11778 point mutation, a guanine-to-adenine substitution at nucleotide 11778 of the nicotinamide adenine dinucleotide dehydrogenase subunit 4 gene in mtDNA results in the disease.

---

  1. At least 11 pathogenetic point mutations of mtDNA have been described.
  2. Class I consists of four mutations that are capable of directly causing LHON: in order of decreasing frequency, the point mutations of mtDNA occur at nucleotide positions 11778G–A, 3460G–A, 15257G–G–A, and 14484T–C (previously reported 4160T–C was probably 14484T–C).

Diabetes mellitus, Crohn's disease, and vitamin B_{12} deficiency have also been reported with the 14484 mitochondrial mutation. Secondary mutations such as 13708, 15257, and 15812 may also occur.

---

  3. Class II contains five mutations and carries a much lower risk of blindness, but the mutations have an enhancing or predisposing effect when present with each other or with class I mutations.

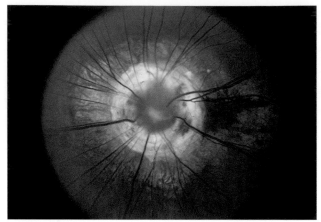

A

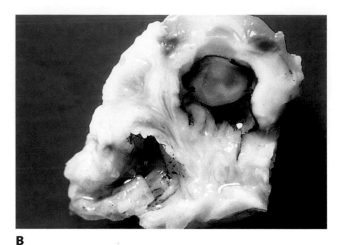

B

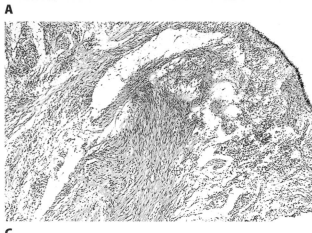

C

Fig. 13.4 Coloboma of optic nerve. **A,** The enlarged, deeply excavated optic disc resembles a morning-glory flower, hence the name *morning-glory syndrome*, another form of optic nerve coloboma. **B,** Another patient had bilateral microphthalmos with cyst secondary to 18 chromosome deletion defect. **C,** Histologic section shows smooth muscle, like that found in contractile peripapillary staphyloma, near a coloboma of optic nerve (see also Fig. 2.10). (**B** and **C,** From Yanoff M *et al.: Am J Ophthalmol* 70:391. © Elsevier 1970.)

4. Class I/II contains two mutations that have an intermediate effect between classes I and II.
5. LHON mainly affects men in European families, but only slightly more men than women in Japanese families.

> An unusual type of epidemic neuropathy in Cuba that resembles LHON, but is not associated with the primary and most common DNA mutations associated with LHON, has been described.

Presumably a gene (or genes) on the X chromosome (tentatively localized to the subregion p11.3) influences the expression of LHON mutations, and an ethnic variant exists in Europeans that predisposes to disease.

C. LHON is characterized by a subacute, sequential, bilateral, central loss of vision mainly in young men (usually between the ages of 18 and 30 years).
   1. The acute neuropathy is characterized by circumpapillary, telangiectatic neuropathy; swelling of the nerve fiber layer around the optic disc (pseudopapilledema); and absence of disc leakage on fluorescein angiography.

2. Color vision is affected early.
3. The acute neuropathy is followed by nerve fiber loss mainly in the papillomacular bundle, optic atrophy, and mostly irreversible visual loss.

> A transient worsening of visual function with exercise or warming (*Uhthoff's symptom*) is not unusual.

4. The optic nerve and inner retinal atrophy in LHON may be a result of metabolic mitochondrial dysfunction that leads to intramitochondrial calcification.

D. The histology is as described in the section *Optic Atrophy* on p. 514 in this chapter.

Coloboma

I. A coloboma (Figs 13.4 and 13.5) may involve the optic disc alone or may be part of a complete coloboma involving the entire embryonic fissure.
   A. Its clinical appearance may vary from a deep physiologic cup to a large hole associated with a retrobulbar cyst.
   B. The surrounding retina may be involved.

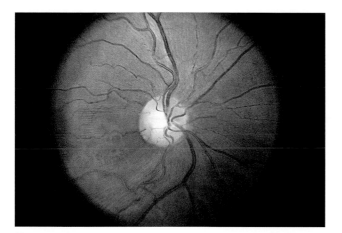

A

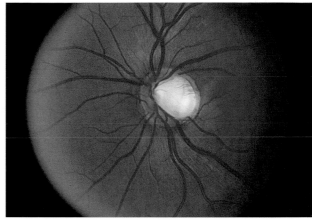

B

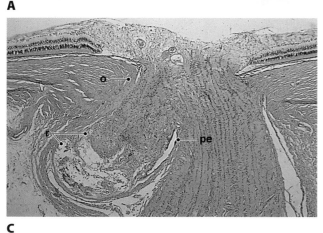

C

Fig. 13.5 Optic pit. Right (**A**) and left (**B**) eyes from same patient. Left eye shows large pit (another form of optic nerve coloboma) in the inferior temporal optic nerve head. **C,** Histologic section of another case shows herniation of retinal tissue through an enlarged scleral opening along one side of the optic nerve (o, area of optic pit; pe, pigment epithelium; r, primitive retinal tissue). (**C,** Courtesy of Dr. JB Crawford, from Irvine AR *et al.: Retina* 6:146, 1986, with permission.)

II. It is usually unilateral, and the cause is either a failure in fusion of the proximal end of the embryonic fissure or aplasia of the primitive Bergmeister's papilla.

III. A coloboma of the optic disc may be associated with other ocular anomalies such as congenital nonattachment of the retina, coloboma of the neural retina and choroid, and persistent hyaloid artery.

A coloboma of the optic nerve (cavitary optic disc anomaly) may be inherited as an autosomal-dominant trait. It then is usually bilateral and shows evidence of a serous detachment of the macular or extramacular neural retina. The types of anomalies in an individual family range to all possible combinations of coloboma of the optic disc, including optic nerve pit. Some family members show progressive optic nerve cupping with increasing age. Mutations in the *PAX2* gene may occur in patients who have optic nerve colobomas and renal abnormalities.

IV. Vision may be normal but is usually defective.

V. Histologically, the coloboma appears as a large defect at the side of the nerve usually involving the neural retina, choroid, and sclera.

    A. Fibrous tissue lines the defect, which often contains hypoplastic or gliotic retina. The gliosis may be so massive as to simulate a neoplasm.

    B. The wall of the defect may contain adipose tissue and even smooth-muscle cells.

A *contractile peripapillary staphyloma* may result from the presence of smooth-muscle cells.

    C. The coloboma may protrude into the retrobulbar tissue and cause microphthalmos with cyst (see Fig. 13.4B and C and p. 531 in Chapter 14).

VI. An optic nerve pit (see Fig. 13.5) is a form of coloboma of the optic nerve that shows a small, circular or triangular depression approximately one-eighth to one-half the diameter of the optic disc, usually located in the inferotemporal quadrant of the disc.

    A. It tends to be unilateral, and more than one may be present.

Bilateral optic pits have been reported in monozygotic siblings.

    B. The optic disc is usually of greater size than the one in the uninvolved fellow eye.

Less frequently, a centrally placed pit of the optic disc may occur. The presenting symptom may be decreased vision or a defect in the visual field that usually remains unchanged. Central serous choroidopathy (retinopathy) does not occur with a central pit.

Rarely, an autosomal-dominant inheritance pattern is present.

C. In approximately one-third to one-half of cases, the optic pit may be associated with macular changes such as serous detachment of the macula, hemorrhages, pigmentary changes, cysts, and holes.

Serous detachment of the macula is probably the basic lesion that causes the other macular changes.

An alternative theory is that a macular detachment develops secondarily to a pre-existing schisis-like lesion consisting of severe outer neural retinal edema. Fluid may enter the retina directly from the optic pit, rather than entering the neural retina from the subneural retinal space.

a. The condition usually occurs in people between 20 and 40 years of age and carries a poor visual prognosis.

b. There is no angiographic evidence of leakage of fluorescein dye into the area of the detached retina.

c. Subretinal fluid probably consists of vitreous fluid leaked into the area through the pit or, less likely, cerebrospinal fluid leaked around the pit into the subneural retinal space.

One reported attempt at intrathecal injection of fluorescein failed to show fluorescein leakage into the subretinal space in a case of optic nerve pit with a serous detachment of the macula. Only a minute amount of fluorescein, however, was injected. A second attempt used radioisotope cisternography in a patient who had serous detachment of the macula associated with a coloboma of the optic nerve; radioactivity of the subretinal fluid was not demonstrated. Rarely, peripapillary subretinal neovascularization may occur.

D. The optic pit is probably caused by an anomalous development of the primordial optic nerve papilla and failure of complete resolution of peripapillary neuroectodermal folds, which are part of the normal development of the optic nerve head.

Pitlike localized cupping of the optic nerve (acquired pit of the optic nerve) can occur in glaucoma, especially in normotensive ("low-tension") glaucoma.

E. Histologically, the pit is an outpouching of neurectodermal tissue surrounded by a connective tissue capsule. The pit passes posteriorly through a defect in the lamina cribrosa and protrudes into the subarachnoid space.

VII. The *morning-glory syndrome* (see Fig. 13.4A) is a form of coloboma of the optic nerve that shows an enlarged, deeply excavated optic disc, resembling the morning-glory flower.

A. Although the condition is usually unilateral, rare bilateral cases have been reported.

B. Girls are affected twice as often as boys.

C. The visual acuity is usually poor.

D. The tissue that surrounds the funnel-shaped staphylomatous excavation involving the nerve proper and peripapillary retina often appears elevated.

E. The demarcation of the elevated peripapillary tissue and normal surrounding retina is indistinct.

F. The retinal vessels seem to originate from deep within the excavation, travel along the peripheral optic disc and peripapillary neural retinal tissue, and exit radially.

G. Glial tissue may obscure the anomalous cup, and surrounding retinal pigment epithelial alterations may occur.

H. Neural retinal detachment, retinal vascular anomalies, and displacement (ectopia) of the macula may be seen.

Systemic abnormalities such as transsphenoidal encephalocele, agenesis of the corpus callosum, midline CNS anomalies, endocrine dysfunction, cleft lip and palate, and renal anomalies have been reported.

I. Histologically, the optic disc is displaced deeply in the posterior, staphylomatous, colobomatous defect.

VIII. Choristoma

A. Rarely, choristomatous elements can be found in the optic nerve in the absence of a coloboma.

B. Because of the absence of a coloboma, these cases are usually mistaken for an optic nerve glioma (ONG).

C. Histologically, choristomatous elements such as adipose tissue and smooth muscle replace most of the parenchyma of the optic nerve.

Myopia

I. Even before the onset of juvenile myopia, children of myopic parents have longer-than-normal eyes (Fig. 13.6; see p. 423 in Chapter 11).

II. The optic disc in myopia is oblique, with exaggeration of the normally raised nasal and flattened temporal edges. A surrounding white scleral crescent is usually present temporally.

III. The optic nerve head is ovoid, with a long vertical axis.

IV. Histologically, the optic nerve passes obliquely through the scleral canal.

A. Temporal side of optic disc

1. The RPE and Bruch's membrane do not extend to the temporal margin of the optic disc.

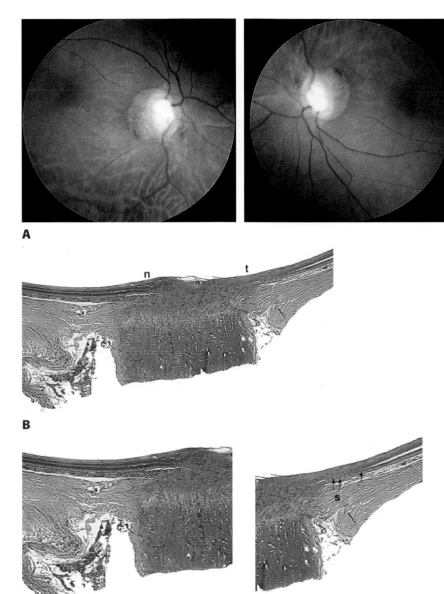

Fig. 13.6 Myopia. **A,** Typical myopic discs show bilateral temporal crescent. **B,** Histologic section shows oblique, myopic optic disc with exaggeration of normally raised nasal (n) and flattened temporal (t) edges. **C,** Increased detail of nasal side of disc shows overlapping tissue [i.e., sensory retina, retinal pigment epithelium (RPE), Bruch's membrane, and choroid] extending over nasal aspect of scleral opening of optic nerve. **D,** Temporal side of disc shows RPE and Bruch's membrane (*single arrow*) stopping short of disc. Choroid (*double arrows*) also stops short of disc, allowing sclera (s) to be seen through transparent sensory retina as white scleral crescent.

2. The choroid extends farther toward the temporal margin of the disc than do the RPE and Bruch's membrane.

   > The sclera exposed just temporal to the optic disc margin is seen through the transparent neural retina as a white crescent.

B. Nasal side of disc

   Overlapping tissue (i.e., neural retina, RPE, Bruch's membrane, and choroid) may extend as far as halfway over the nasal half of the scleral opening.

OPTIC DISC EDEMA

General Information (Fig. 13.7; see Fig. 13.22)

I. Usually, visual acuity is not affected.

II. Because the term *papilledema* is widely interpreted as a swollen optic nerve head secondary to raised intracranial pressure, the term *optic disc edema*, which is the generic term, is preferred for all noninflammatory causes of a swollen optic nerve head.

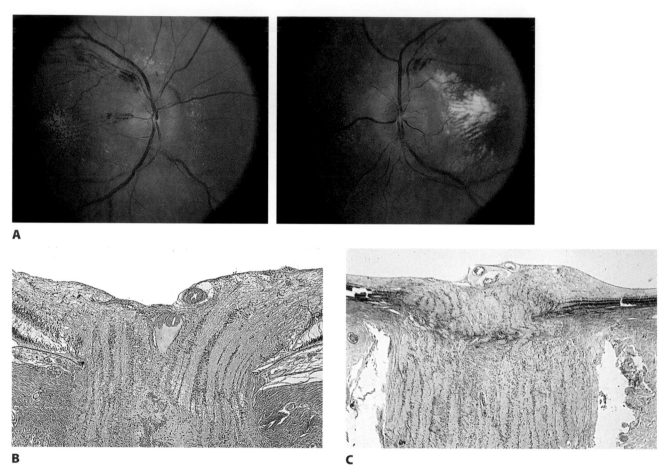

Fig. 13.7 Optic disc edema. **A,** Patient has bilateral optic disc edema secondary to grade IV malignant hypertension. **B,** Histologic section shows optic disc edema secondary to ocular hypertension caused by phacolytic glaucoma. **C,** Optic disc edema secondary to ocular hypotony caused by a ruptured globe. Optic disc edema can be caused by increased intracranial pressure (**A**) or increased (**B**) or decreased (**C**) intraocular pressure. The main findings in **B** and **C** consist of increased mass of anterior optic nerve caused by axonal swelling, optic nerve head tissue edema and vascular congestion, and lateral displacement of photoreceptors from the end of Bruch's membrane, which terminates in a ring at the optic nerve.

Fluorescein studies of optic disc edema show late fluorescence.

III. The term *papillitis* is used for a swollen optic nerve head secondary to inflammation.

Causes

I. Relative or absolute increase in venous pressure at the lamina cribrosa or posterior to it, such as occurs in acute glaucoma, optic nerve tumors, orbital tumors, brain tumors, subarachnoid hemorrhage, meningitis, encephalitis, malignant hypertension, and from drugs (e.g., tetracycline)

II. Relative increase in venous pressure at the lamina cribrosa or anterior to it, such as occurs in accidental penetrating wounds, intraocular surgery, uveitis, central retinal vein thrombosis, and ocular hypotony from any cause (acute or chronic)

III. Local phenomena (e.g., the Irvine–Gass syndrome, iron-deficiency anemia, gastrointestinal hemorrhage, papillitis, juxtapapillary choroiditis, mucopolysaccharidoses, and perhaps from oral contraceptives)

IV. Axoplasmic transport (flow)

A. Orthograde axoplasmic transport occurs at various rates, including a rapid component (200 to 1000 mm/day) and a slow component (0.5 to 3 mm/day). Retrograde axoplasmic transport also occurs.

B. Blockage of optic nerve axoplasmic flow at the level of the lamina choroidalis and lamina scleralis occurs through increased intracranial pressure, ocular hypotony, or increased intraocular pressure and results in increased mass or bulk of the optic nerve head.

Pseudopapilledema

Optic disc edema may be simulated by hypermetropic optic disc, drusen of optic nerve head, congenital developmental abnormalities, optic neuritis and perineuritis, and myelinated (medullated) nerve fibers.

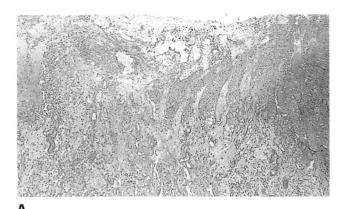

A

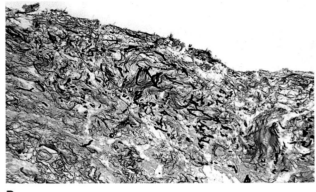

B

Fig. 13.8 Optic neuritis presumably caused by orbital aspergillosis. **A,** Acid-fast stain negative for acid-fast organisms. Optic nerve is undergoing necrosis with macrophages phagocytosing disintegrating myelin. **B,** Grocott's stain shows hyphae compatible with *Aspergillus* fungi, mainly in anterior optic nerve.

Histology of Optic Disc Edema

I. Acute (see Fig. 13.7)
   A. Edema and vascular congestion of the nerve head result in increased tissue volume.
     1. Hemorrhages may be seen in the optic nerve or in the retinal nerve fiber layer.
     2. The increased tissue mass causes the physiologic cup to narrow.

> Axonal swelling, caused by blockage of axoplasmic flow, rather than vascular alterations, appears to be the major factor in overall increase in tissue volume of the optic nerve head.

   B. The aforementioned changes result in a displacement of the neural retina away from the edge of the optic disc.
     1. The outer layers of the neural retina may buckle (retinal and choroidal folds are seen clinically).
     2. The rods and cones are displaced away from the end of Bruch's membrane.

> The lateral displacement of the rods and cones results in enlargement of the blind spot. Sometimes the pigment epithelial cells are also pushed laterally so that the peripapillary RPE is flattened and cells farther away are "squeezed" together.

     3. There may be a peripapillary neural retinal detachment, and this can add to the density of the peripapillary scotoma.
II. Chronic
   A. Degeneration of nerve fibers may occur.
   B. Gliosis and optic atrophy are most likely to occur with long-standing or chronic optic disc edema rather than with short-term or acute optic disc edema.

> Optic disc edema secondary to increased intraocular pressure (e.g., acute closed-angle glaucoma) may cause necrosis of optic nerve fibers. Optic atrophy and even cavernous optic atrophy may result. The fibers in the optic nerve are more susceptible to injury by high intraocular pressure than are the retinal ganglion cells and nerve fiber layer.

OPTIC NEURITIS

In general, visual acuity is severely affected.

Causes

   I. Secondary to ocular disease (e.g., acute corneal ulcer; anterior or posterior uveitis; endophthalmitis or panophthalmitis; and retinochoroiditis; see Fig. 4.26)
   II. Secondary to orbital disease [Fig. 13.8; e.g., as bilateral idiopathic inflammation of the optic nerve sheaths, cellulitis (may be primary, but more commonly secondary to sinusitis), thrombophlebitis, arteritis, and midline granuloma syndrome]
   III. Secondary to intracranial disease (e.g., meningitis, encephalitis, and meningoencephalitis)
   IV. Secondary to spread of distant infection (e.g., acquired immune deficiency syndrome, syphilis, tuberculosis, coccidioidomycosis, and bacterial endocarditis)
   V. Secondary to vascular disease [Figs 13.9 and 13.10; e.g., temporal arteritis, periarteritis nodosa, pulseless (Takayasu's) disease, and arteriosclerosis]
     A. Temporal (cranial, giant cell) arteritis (see Figs 13.9 and 13.10)
       1. Temporal arteritis (ischemic arteritic optic neuropathy) is most commonly found in middle-aged or elderly women.

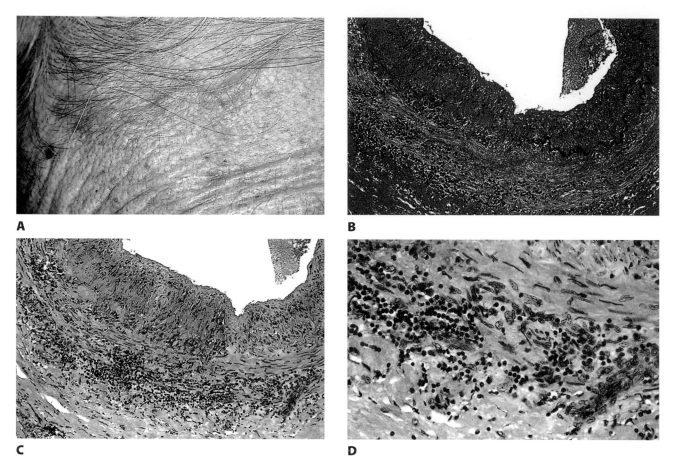

Fig. 13.9 Atypical temporal arteritis. **A,** Patient had an enlarged temporal artery and decreased vision. Temporal artery biopsy was performed. **B,** Histologic section, stained for elastic tissue, shows a vasculitis, involving all coats, and fragmentation of the internal elastic lamina. **C** and **D,** Increased magnification, however, failed to show any giant cells or granulomatous inflammation. The case was signed out as chronic nongranulomatous (nongiant cell) temporal arteritis.

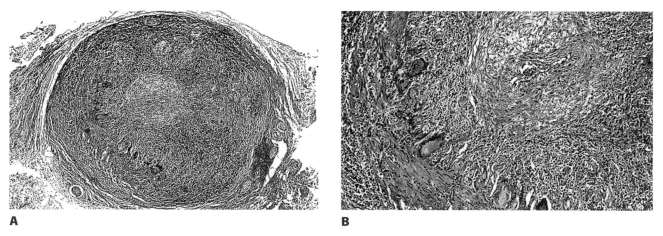

Fig. 13.10 Typical temporal arteritis. **A,** Histologic section shows a vasculitis involving all coats of the temporal artery. **B,** Increased magnification shows the typical giant cell granulomatous inflammation. (Courtesy of Dr. MM Rodrigues.)

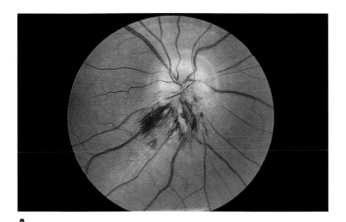

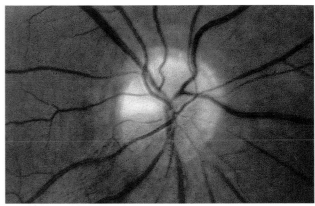

A

B

Fig. 13.11 Anterior ischemic optic neuropathy (ANION). The clinical appearance of ANION can be confused with multiple sclerosis papillitis. **A** and **B,** ANION acutely with optic disc edema and hemorrhages (**A**) and 1 year later with superior temporal sector optic atrophy (**B**).

2. It is often associated with malaise, weight loss, fever, headaches, scalp pain, neck pain, intermittent jaw claudication, scalp necrosis, and visual loss.

   Jaw claudication is the most reliable clinical sign, followed by neck pain.

3. The superficial temporal artery may be red, tender, firm, enlarged, and pulseless, or it may be normal.

   The erythrocyte sedimentation rate (ESR) becomes elevated (usually above 44 mm/hour), often to a high degree.

   C-reactive protein above 2.45 mg/dl and an ESR of 47 mm/hour or more is highly specific (97%) for temporal arteritis.

4. The aorta and its larger branches, including coronary arteries, may be involved in up to 10% to 15% of cases.

5. Marked impairment of visual acuity, often with involvement of the second eye within days or weeks of involvement of the first eye, is the most frequent ocular problem, but ptosis and muscle palsies may also occur.
   a. Approximately 14% to 27% of patients have permanent visual loss.
   b. Regional choroidal nonperfusion, presumably secondary to arteritis of a ciliary artery, may cause a reversible (with steroid therapy) visual loss.

   Choroidal ischemia may be the first sign of temporal arteritis in elderly patients who have loss of vision.

6. Although most teaching is that a temporal artery biopsy should be performed before steroid therapy is instituted, some authorities suggest that it can be performed within 48 hours or even more, after treatment with steroid therapy has begun.

   Temporal artery biopsy may be positive even after up to 1 month of steroid therapy for presumed temporal arteritis.

7. Histologically, a granulomatous reaction centering about a fragmented internal elastic lamina and spreading into the media and adventitia of the temporal artery is characteristic.
   a. Giant cells are frequently present (see Fig. 13.10) but may be absent (see Fig. 13.9).
   b. Rarely, a chronic nongranulomatous reaction with lymphocytes and plasma cells without epithelioid or giant cells is seen (see Fig. 13.9).
   c. The inflammatory reaction tends to be spotty, so that microscopic sections cut at many levels may have to be done; thus, a positive finding is more significant than a negative one.

   It is unclear whether the pathogenesis involves humoral immunity (direct immunofluorescence demonstrates immunoglobulin) or cell-mediated immunity (almost all lymphocytes in the inflammation are T lymphocytes and often surrounding macrophages express human leukocyte antigen-DR). A significant association exists between varicella-zoster virus (VZV) DNA in temporal artery biopsies from patients who have temporal arteritis as compared to patients who do not have the condition. VZV may play a role in the pathogenesis of some cases of temporal arteritis.

B. Anterior ischemic optic neuropathy (ANION; Fig. 13.11)
   1. ANION (nonarteritic) occurs primarily in 55- to 70-year-old people who are usually otherwise well, except that approximately half have mild hypertension.

Cigarette smoking is an important risk factor in the development of ANION. Also, ANION has been reported as a complication secondary to treatment with interferon-alfa.

2. Extracranial carotid occlusive disease is not significantly associated, and long-term follow-up shows no increased incidence of stroke.

In the presence of Hollenhorst plaques, however, long-term follow-up shows increased incidence of stroke.

3. Clinically, a sudden or rapidly progressive monocular visual acuity loss is associated with pallid optic disc edema, followed by a stable visual field defect of variable degree.

The most common visual field defect is altitudinal, with a 3:1 preference for the inferior half of the field. The fixational area is spared at least as often as it is involved.

4. The second eye is involved in about 15% of patients over a 5-year period.

No form of therapy has proved efficacious. Old optic atrophy coupled with fresh contralateral disc infarction may be confused with the Foster–Kennedy syndrome.

5. The ESR is usually below 44 mm/hour, unlike the elevated ESR in temporal arteritis.
6. The pathophysiology and the anatomic background of ANION are not well understood. Histologic findings are consistent with optic disc edema of a noninflammatory type.

In some cases, the optic nerve infarction is caused by embolic occlusion of small arteries supplying the anterior portion of the optic nerve.

7. A condition that has numerous similarities to ANION (abrupt onset, absence of ocular pain, altitudinal field loss, and lack of subsequent improvement) is called *neuroretinitis* (previously called *Leber's stellate maculopathy*).
   a. Neuroretinitis differs from ANION in involving a relatively young group (average age 27 years), the tendency to recur, and macular star formation (more common than in ANION).
   b. Neuroretinitis differs from "garden-variety" optic neuritis in the absence of ocular pain, tendency to spare fixation, lack of visual recovery, macular star formation, and no increased risk for development of multiple sclerosis (MS).

VI. Secondary to demyelinating disease
   A. MS (Fig. 13.12; see Fig. 13.11)
      1. Retrobulbar neuritis
         a. Retrobulbar neuritis has an acute onset in one eye with sudden loss of vision, usually preceded by orbital pain (especially with ocular movement).
         b. Vision tends to recover in a few weeks to months.

With loss of vision, a central scotoma can be demonstrated on central visual field examination. Frequently, after the first eye has recovered, the second eye is involved. In MS, lesion progression is associated with large numbers of helper (inducer) T cells in the adjacent normal white matter, whereas suppressor-cytotoxic T cells are limited to the lesion margin. Demyelination seems to depend on the presence of macrophages. Evidence implicates cell-mediated immunity as the cause of MS.

         c. The ophthalmoscopic appearance may be normal, or papillitis may simulate optic disc edema.
         d. Associated sheathing of retinal veins is seen in 10% to 20% of patients.
         e. The risk development of MS after an uncomplicated optic neuritis is 3.5 times greater in women than in men.

In one study, 13% to 15% of patients who had MS presented with optic neuritis, and 27% to 37% of patients who had MS showed evidence of optic neuritis during the course of the disease. MS develops in approximately 17% to 38% of patients who have optic neuritis; younger patients have a higher incidence.

      2. Ocular muscle palsies may occur (conjugate movements may be involved) along with nystagmus, frequently of the cerebellar type. Internuclear ophthalmoplegia may also occur.

Variable, uncharacteristic pupillary changes may also be noted.

      3. A link may exist between pars planitis and MS, especially when retinal periphlebitis is present at the time of diagnosis of pars planitis (MS develops in perhaps 15% of patients with pars planitis followed for at least 8 years).

Other ocular inflammations associated with MS to a lesser extent include periphlebitis, granulomatous uveitis (especially anteriorly), and neuroretinitis.

   B. Neuromyelitis optica (encephalomyelitis optica; Devic's disease) consists of bilateral optic atrophy and paraplegia.
      1. Bilateral optic atrophy
         a. The loss of vision is acute in onset and rapid in progression, even to complete blindness.

Unlike in MS, pain precedes loss of vision in very few cases. The loss of vision precedes onset of paraplegia in approximately 80% of cases.

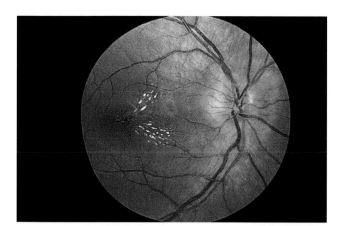

A

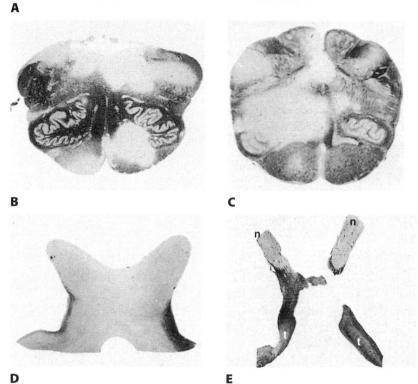

B

C

D

E

Fig. 13.12 Multiple sclerosis. **A,** Patient presented acutely with papillitis. Multiple sclerosis was subsequently diagnosed. **B** and **C,** Large astrocytic plaques present in different areas of brainstem of another patient. Note irregular distribution of plaques at different levels. **D,** Almost total demyelination of chiasm. **E,** Another case shows demyelination of optic nerves (n) but preservation of myelin in optic tracts (t). (**B–E,** Kluver–Barerra stain; courtesy of Dr. LB Rorke.)

b. The ophthalmoscopic appearance may be normal, or a papillitis may simulate optic disc edema.
c. Bilaterality of optic atrophy along with paraplegia is characteristic.
2. Extraocular muscle palsies and nystagmus may be seen infrequently.

Pupillary changes are not characteristic.

3. Paraplegia usually follows loss of visual acuity in days to weeks, but may follow in months or, rarely, in years.
C. Diffuse cerebral sclerosis primarily involves white matter of the CNS and includes Schilder's disease (Fig. 13.13), Krabbe's disease, Pelizaeus–Merzbacher syndrome, adrenoleukodystrophy, and metachromatic leukodystrophy.

A number of childhood diseases [e.g., neonatal and X-linked (childhood) adrenoleukodystrophy, infantile Refsum's disease, and primary hyperoxaluria type 1] may be attributed to the malfunction of the subcellular organelle peroxisome.

VII. Secondary to nutritional or toxic or metabolic disease [e.g., starvation (nutritional); tobacco–alcohol toxicity; methyl alcohol; diabetes mellitus; hyperthyroidism; amiodarone; disulfiram; iodochlorohydroxyquinoline; ethambutol; and chloramphenicol]
VIII. Secondary to hereditary conditions (see p. 514 in this chapter)

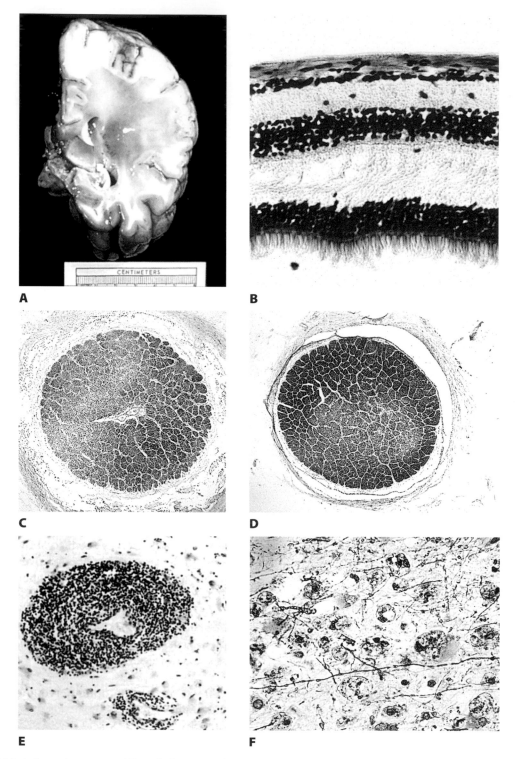

Fig. 13.13 Schilder's disease in an 8-year-old boy. **A,** Gross coronal section shows giant plaque in occipital lobe. **B,** The macular neural retina shows a thinning of the nerve fiber layer and a loss of ganglion cells (descending atrophy). **C,** Left optic nerve near globe shows descending optic atrophy involving mainly upper left periphery of nerve. **D,** Optic nerve near chiasm shows descending optic atrophy involving mainly central nerve. **E,** Perivascular cuffing of predominantly lymphocytes present in occipital area of brain. **F,** Surrounding brain shows loss of myelin, preservation of some axons, and a reactive gliosis with proliferating astrocytes.

IX. Secondary to idiopathic or unknown causes
X. Secondary to radiation (e.g., after radiation therapy for pituitary adenoma, a delayed necrosis of the perisellar optic nerves and chiasm may occur)

Histology of Optic Neuritis

I. General information
   A. *Optic neuritis, retrobulbar neuritis, papillitis,* and *neuro-retinitis* are clinical terms and do not connote specific causes. Actually, many causes exist (e.g., inflammatory, vascular, and degenerative).

   The suffix *-itis*, therefore, as generally used here, is not necessarily synonymous with *inflammation.*

   B. Topographic histologic classification of optic neuritis
      1. Perineuritis: leptomeningeal involvement (e.g., extension of intracranial meningitis, of orbital inflammation, or from intraocular inflammations)
      2. Periaxial neuritis: leptomeningeal involvement spreads to the optic nerve parenchyma, usually in its periphery
      3. Axial neuritis: inner or central portions of the optic nerve involved (e.g., MS, toxic factors, malnutrition, and vascular factors)
      4. Transverse neuritis: total cross-sectional destruction of a variable length of optic nerve (e.g., Devic's disease)
II. Specific types of tissue reaction
   A. Inflammatory disease: the types of inflammatory disease of the optic nerve depend on the cause (see Figs 13.8 and 13.13; see also Fig. 4.26; section on *Inflammation* in Chapter 1; and Chapters 3 and 4).
   B. Vascular disease: the clinicopathologic picture depends on the type of vascular disease involving the optic nerve.
      1. Temporal (cranial) arteritis: a granulomatous arteritis (usually has giant cells) with necrosis of the arterial wall and a splitting and destruction of the inner elastic lamina (see Figs 13.9 and 13.10)
      2. Nonarteritic (ischemic) optic neuropathy (see Fig. 13.11)
      3. Periarteritis nodosa: a fibrinoid necrosis of muscular arteries and arterioles with acute and chronic non-granulomatous intra-arterial wall inflammatory reaction
      4. Pulseless disease and arteriosclerosis: coagulative or ischemic type of necrosis
   C. Demyelinating diseases
      1. Demyelinating stage (see Figs 13.11 to 13.13)
         a. Early breakdown of myelin sheaths occurs.
         b. Macrophages phagocytose the disintegrated myelin.
         c. The "fat-laden" phagocytes then move to perivascular locations.
         d. A perivascular "cuffing" or exudation of fluid, lymphocytes, and plasma cells around blood vessels frequently is seen in areas remote from the acute reaction.
      2. Healing stage (see Fig. 13.13B)
         a. Astrocytic response occurs in areas of demyelination.
         b. Ultimately, the area of involvement shows gliosis.
   D. Nutritional or toxic or metabolic diseases
      1. Little is known of the acute reaction.
      2. These conditions may cause considerable destruction of optic nerve parenchyma with resultant secondary optic atrophy.

OPTIC ATROPHY*

Causes

I. Ascending optic atrophy
   A. The primary lesion is in the neural retina or optic disc, e.g., glaucoma* (see Figs 16.32 and 16.33); retinochoroiditis†; retinitis pigmentosa†; traumatic or secondary retinitis pigmentosa†; central retinal artery occlusion* (see Fig. 11.10); chronic optic disc edema†; toxic or nutritional causes (e.g., chloroquine*), and Alzheimer's disease (AD).*
      1. AD
         a. AD primarily causes over 50% of all dementia in the United States, affecting approximately 8% of the population 65 years of age or older.
         b. Patients may present with visual signs and symptoms, e.g., difficulties with reading and writing, problems with navigation, and difficulty recognizing familiar objects.
         c. The apolipoprotein E gene and a putative AD gene(s) on chromosome 10q are two known risk factors for late-onset AD.

         The rare, early-onset autosomal-dominant form of AD results from mutations in at least three different genes: amyloid precursor protein gene on chromosome 21; presenilin-1 gene on chromosome 14; and presenilin-2 gene on 14 chromosome 1.

         ---

         d. The diagnosis of AD depends on antemortem evidence of dementia and postmortem findings of neuritic plaques, neurofibrillary tangles, and neuronal cell loss primarily in subcortical brain areas, such as hippocampus, amygdala, and locus ceruleus.

         Although a few individual patients who have AD may exhibit a marked hypersensitivity in their pupillary

---

*Usually very little, if any, gliotic reaction on surface of optic disc, hence "white" or primary optic atrophy.
†Usually gliotic reaction on surface of optic disc, hence "dirty" or secondary optic atrophy.

response (i.e., rapid pupillary dilatation) to the topically administered cholinergic antagonist tropicamide, in most patients with AD the pupillary response is no different than in control subjects.

    e. Histologically, the optic nerves seem to show preferential loss of the large-caliber fibers derived from the largest class of neural retinal ganglion cells (M cells).

> The M-cell system mediates specific visual functions, and selective involvement in AD leads to clinically measurable neuro-ophthalmic and psychophysical impairments.

  B. The secondary effects are on the optic nerve and white tracts in the brain.

  II. Descending optic atrophy

    A. The primary lesion is in the brain or optic nerve [e.g., tabes dorsalis*; Creutzfeldt–Jakob disease*; hydrocephalus*; meningioma* (see Figs 13.18 and 13.19); ONG*; traumatic transection of the optic nerve*]; toxic or nutritional causes (e.g., methyl alcohol*); and genetically determined disorders* [e.g., Schilder's disease (see Fig. 13.13), Pelizaeus–Merzbacher syndrome, adrenoleukodystrophy, and Krabbe's disease].

    B. The secondary effects are on the optic disc and neural retina.

  III. Inherited optic atrophy

    A. Familial optic atrophies (Table 13.1; and see subsection *Congenital (Familial) Optic Atrophies* on p. 501 in this chapter)

    B. Glucose-6-phosphate dehydrogenase (G-6-PD) Worcester

      1. G-6-PD Worcester is a variant of G-6-PD deficiency with congenital, nonspherocytic hemolytic anemia, absent erythrocyte G-6-PD activity, and optic atrophy.

      2. It is inherited as a sex-linked recessive trait.

    C. Friedreich's ataxia

Histology of Optic Atrophy

  I. Shrinkage or loss of parenchyma and loss of both myelin and axis cylinders are seen (Figs 13.14 and 13.15; see Fig. 13.13).

    A. Shrinkage results in widening of the subarachnoid and subdural spaces and redundancy of the dura.

    B. Pial septa widen to occupy the space made by the loss of parenchyma.

    C. The normal spongy texture of the optic nerve is lost.

  II. Optic nerve gliosis and proliferation of astrocytes are prominent.

  III. The physiologic cup widens or deepens and results in a baring of the lamina cribrosa.

  IV. Secondary changes

    A. Glial proliferation on the surface of the disc results in a "secondary" optic atrophy.

see footnote on p. 513.

  B. Hyaluronic acid accumulates in the anterior portion of the optic nerve [i.e., cavernous (Schnabel's) optic atrophy; see Fig. 16.33] after long-standing glaucoma (see p. 659 in Chapter 16).

INJURIES

See Chapter 5.

TUMORS

Primary

  I. "Glioma" (more properly called *juvenile pilocytic astrocytoma*) of optic nerve (Figs 13.16 and 13.17)

    A. The prevalence is slightly greater in girls than in boys.

      1. The median age at onset is approximately 5 years, with over 80% of patients younger than 15 years of age; 71% of the tumors occur during the first decade of life.

      2. Gliomas of the optic pathways account for 2% to 5% of intracranial tumors in children.

      3. The tumor is quite rare after the second decade of life (approximately two-thirds are diagnosed in the first 5 years of life).

    B. Proptosis, predominantly temporal, is the most common presenting sign; loss of vision is the next most common sign.

      1. When intracranial involvement occurs, the presenting signs may be nystagmus, headache, vomiting, and convulsions.

      2. Occasionally, the presenting sign clinically may be a central retinal vein occlusion; more commonly, however, it occurs as a late phenomenon.

    C. Neurofibromatosis [NF: mainly NF type 1 (NF-1)] is present in approximately 25% of patients who have ONG; conversely, approximately 15% of patients who have NF have ONG.

> Although a rare case of ONG may occur in NF-2, most occur in NF-1. Gliomas in patients who have NF-1 appear to be more indolent than in patients who do not have NF-1, and tend to occur at a later age (average 7.1 years) than in patients without NF-1.

    D. Optic disc edema followed by optic atrophy is a frequent clinical finding.

    E. The ONG is most often located in the orbital portion of the optic nerve alone, with combined involvement of both orbital and intracranial portions next most common (Table 13.2).

    F. If the ONG is limited to the orbital or intracranial portion of the optic nerve, the optic foramen may still be enlarged.

TABLE 13.1 Optic Atrophies

	CONGENITAL		JUVENILE			
	Dominant	**Recessive**	**Dominant**	**Recessive**	**Leber's**	**Behr's**
Inheritance	Dominant	Recessive	Dominant locus on chromosome 2	Recessive	X-linked	Recessive
Systemic signs and symptoms	—	—	—	Diabetes, decreased hearing	Headache, vertigo, nervousness, palpitations	Increased tendon reflexes, + Babinski, ataxia, + Romberg, muscular rigidity, mental debility
Onset	Congenital or neonatal	Congenital or neonatal	Insidious onset, 2–6 years of age	Insidious onset, 6–12 years of age	Acute onset, 16–30 years of age	1–9 years of age
Nystagmus	Yes	Yes	No	No	No	Possibly
Vision	20/100 to hand movements	Marked loss	20/20 to 3/400	May be hand movements or light perception	Usually 10/200	Usually 10/200
Fields	Constricted peripheral; no characteristic scotoma	—	Central scotoma; possibly bitemporal defect; blue inside red	—	Central scotoma, peripheral fields normal	Central scotoma, peripheral fields normal
Fundi	Marked atrophy of entire disc; narrow arteries	Total atrophy	Temporal atrophy	Total atrophy	Hyperemia or optic disc edema at onset; white disc develops after neuritis; arteries are narrow	Temporal atrophy
Color testing	May be reduced	—	Possible blue–green defect	—	Red–green defect	—
Electroretinogram	—	—	Normal	Normal	Normal	Normal
Visually evoked cortical potential	—	—	Possibly diminished	—	—	—
Dark adaptation	—	—	Possibly diminished	Normal	Diminished	Normal
Clinical course	May progress slowly; usually in school for blind	—	Atrophy is stationary or may progress	—	Acute course may progress, or regress to normal or near-normal vision	Evolution of neurologic symptoms for years; then stabilization
Pathology	—	—	Optochiasmatic arachnoiditis seen at surgery	—	Atrophy of retinal ganglion cells, especially foveal, demyelination in optic nerve and temporal lobe	Degeneration of second retinal neuron

Secondary meningeal hyperplasia may travel proximally (or distally) and is responsible for the enlargement of the optic foramen. An enlarged optic foramen, therefore, is not necessarily proof of intracranial extension of an orbital ONG. Conversely, the optic foramen may be normal in the face of intracranial or chiasmal ONG.

G. The mortality rate is significant.
1. If the astrocytoma is limited to the orbital portion of the optic nerve, the prognosis is excellent. Surgical removal, even when incomplete, usually cures.
2. With involvement of the intracranial optic nerve, the prognosis is guarded.

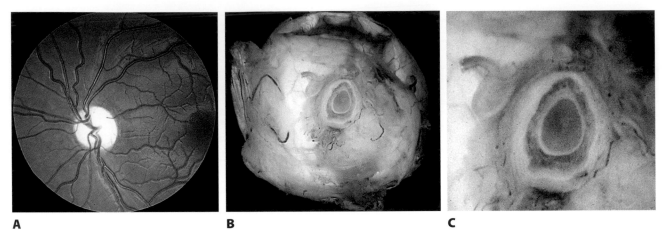

Fig. 13.14 Optic atrophy. **A,** Optic atrophy in child secondary to increased intracranial pressure. **B,** Gross appearance of optic atrophy (shown at increased magnification in **C**). Note small nerve, widened subarachnoid space, and redundant dura.

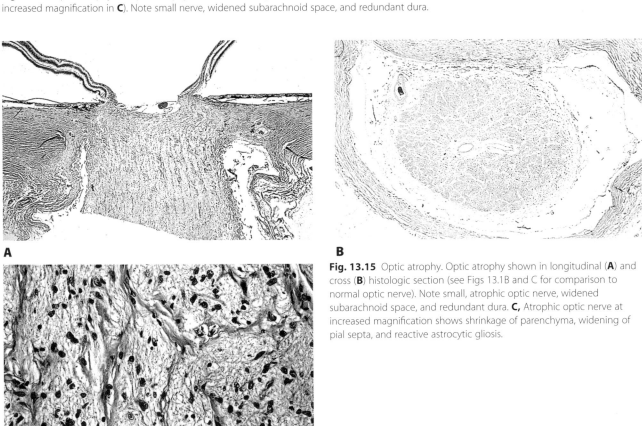

Fig. 13.15 Optic atrophy. Optic atrophy shown in longitudinal (**A**) and cross (**B**) histologic section (see Figs 13.1B and C for comparison to normal optic nerve). Note small, atrophic optic nerve, widened subarachnoid space, and redundant dura. **C,** Atrophic optic nerve at increased magnification shows shrinkage of parenchyma, widening of pial septa, and reactive astrocytic gliosis.

H. Histology
 1. Three main patterns may all be present in different parts of the same tumor:
  a. Transitional area: the tumor merges into the normal optic nerve and is difficult to differentiate from reactive gliosis.
   1). Glial nuclei are more numerous and less orderly than in the normal nerve.
   2). The increase in the number and size of glial cells results in enlarged nerve bundles.
   3). The area has a finely reticulated appearance.
  b. Coarsely reticulated and myxomatous area: microcystoid spaces in the tumor are probably secondary to tumor necrosis. The spaces contain acid mucopolysaccharides that are partially sensitive to hyaluronidase.

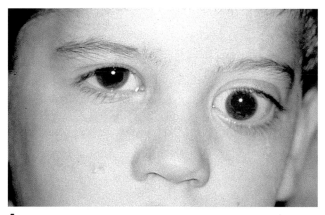

A

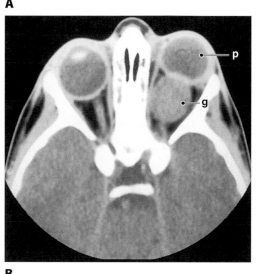

B

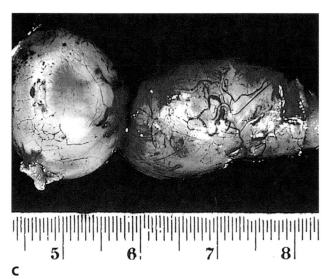

C

Fig. 13.16 Optic nerve "glioma." **A,** The patient has proptosis of the left eye caused by a glioma of the optic nerve. Most of the time the proptosis is in a downward and outward direction. **B,** Computed tomography scan of this case shows the glioma (g) enlarging the retrobulbar optic nerve (p, proptotic eye). **C,** This gross specimen from another case shows the optic nerve thickened by tumor, starting just behind the globe. (**A** and **B,** Case presented by Dr. JA Shields to the meeting of Armed Forces Institute of Pathology Alumni, 1987; **C,** courtesy of Dr. WC Frayer.)

c. Astrocytic areas: the areas resemble juvenile astrocytomas of the cerebellum and probably are the same type of tumor.
  1). The cellular areas show spindle cell formation.
  2). Rosenthal fibers, which are cytoplasmic, eosinophilic structures in astrocytes, may be prominent.

> Although Rosenthal fibers are characteristically found in ONG, they are not pathognomonic. The fibers may be found in astrocytes in a number of inflammatory (e.g., *Alexander's disease*) and other neoplastic processes involving the CNS. Rosenthal fibers are collections of ubiquitinated intermediate filaments (i.e., ubiquitinated glial fibrillary acidic protein).

2. Neoplastic astrocytes stain positively for glial fibrillary acidic protein, HNK-1 (type 1 astrocyte pre-cursor marker), S-100, and vimentin, suggesting origin from type 1 astrocytes.

3. Secondary effects

> Rarely, synaptophysin-positive neuronal cells may be present. The appropriate name then is *ganglioglioma*, which probably has the same prognosis as ONG.

  a. Infiltration by the ONG through the pia with resultant arachnoid hyperplasia is seen.

> Secondary or reactive arachnoid (meningothelial) hyperplasia may extend well beyond the limits of the ONG. The hyperplasia may mimic a meningioma of the optic nerve sheath.

  b. The tumor itself may enlarge the optic foramen (as may proliferating meningothelial cells).
  c. The ONG may cause edema or atrophy of the optic nerve.

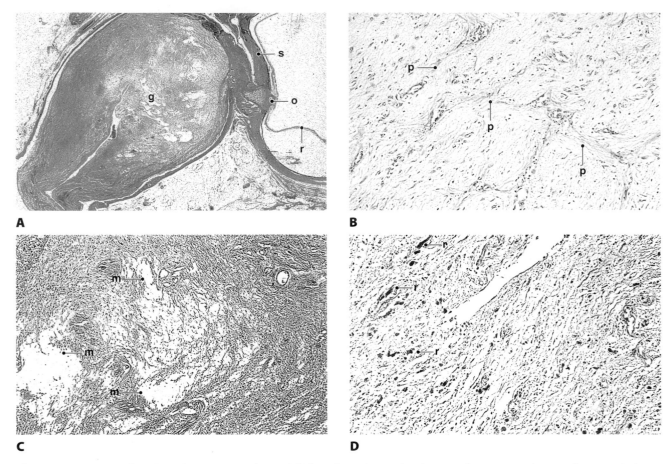

Fig. 13.17 Optic nerve "glioma." **A,** A large tumor involves and thickens the optic nerve (s, sclera; o, optic nerve; g, optic nerve glioma; r, retina).
B, Increased magnification shows enlarged neural bundles between the spread-out pial septa. The neural bundles contain expanded, disordered glial cells and a few axons (p, pial septa separating tumor). **C,** An area of necrosis in the tumor shows myxomatous microcystoid and macrocystoid spaces (m). **D,** Many astrocytes contain intracytoplasmic eosinophilic structures, called *Rosenthal fibers* (r).

TABLE 13.2 Juvenile Pilocytic Astrocytoma of the Optic Nerve: Location of Astrocytoma

Location	Number	Percent
Orbital	27	47
Intracranial and orbital	15	26
Intracranial	6	10
Intracranial and chiasm	7	12
Chiasm	3	5
Total	58	100

(Adapted from Yanoff M et al.: Juvenile pilocytic astrocytoma ["glioma"]. In Jakobiec FA, ed: Ocular and Adnexal Tumors. Birmingham, Aesculapius, 1978:685.)

    d. The ONG may infiltrate the optic nerve head.
    e. The tumor may compress or occlude the central retinal vein.
  II. Other astrocytic neoplasms
    A. Oligodendrocytomas are rare.

> More often, but still quite rarely, small collections of oligodendrocytes may be seen in ONGs that are made up predominantly of astrocytes.

    B. Rarely, malignant astrocytic neoplasms may involve the optic nerve primarily, most commonly in adults.
        Histologically, the neoplasms are marked by areas of anaplasia and classed as low-grade astrocytomas, anaplastic astrocytomas, and glioblastoma multiforme.
      1. Necrosis is the sine qua non of glioblastoma multiforme.
      2. DNA analysis, combined with histologic grading, improves prognosis designation.
 III. Meningioma (Figs 13.18 and 13.19)
    A. Primary meningioma of the intraorbital meninges of the optic nerve is more common in women than in men (5:1).

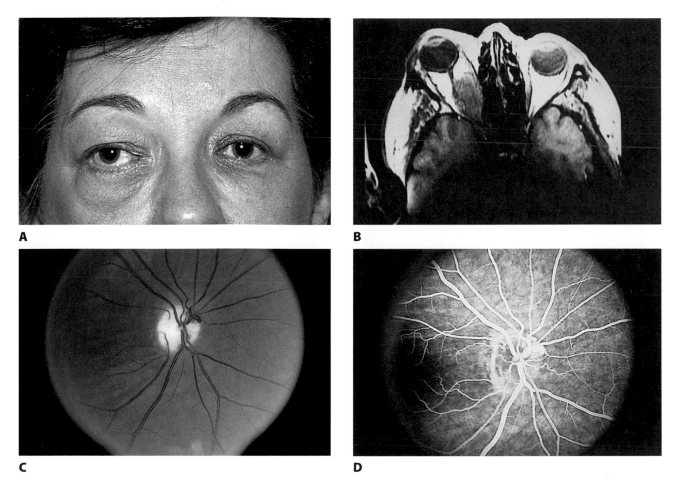

Fig. 13.18 Meningioma of optic nerve in 50-year-old woman. **A,** Clinical appearance of right exophthalmos and extropia. **B,** Magnetic resonance imaging appearance after biopsy. Tumor still present nasally in right orbit. **C,** Chorioretinal striae and optociliary shunt vessel present on atrophic right optic nerve head. **D,** Fluorescein angiography shows shunt vessel diverting retinal venous blood around obstructed optic nerve toward choroid. Biopsy showed a proliferation of meningothelial cells (see Fig. 13.19C).

B. The average age at onset is 32 years (range, 3.5 to 73 years), with the median 38 years.

Approximately 40% of the tumors occur in patients younger than 20 years of age and 25% in patients younger than 10 years.

C. The main clinical presentations are loss of vision and progressive exophthalmos.

D. Optociliary (opticociliary) shunt vessels may be seen in approximately 25% of cases.

Optociliary shunt vessels may also be found in association with central retinal vein occlusion or as a congenital anomaly. The vessels have also been reported with optic nerve juvenile pilocytic astrocytomas (gliomas), arachnoid and optic nerve cysts, optic nerve colobomas and drusen, and with chronic atrophic optic disc edema. Primary intracranial meningioma may extend into the orbit secondarily and even involve the optic nerve. Also, theoretically, a meningioma may arise primarily in the orbit from ectopic meningeal tissue.

E. There may be associated neurofibromatosis (mainly NF-2) in 16% of patients.

F. The prognosis for life depends somewhat on age at onset.

With onset in childhood, the meningiomas tend to be much more aggressive and to have a much worse prognosis than with onset at an older age. In one series, 2 of 8 patients younger than 20 years of age were alive without recurrence (follow-up less than 2 years), 4 had recurrent tumor (1 with intracranial extension and 3 without), and 1 died during an attempt to excise the recurrent tumor. In the same series, 10 of 13 patients older than 20 years of age were alive and well without recurrent tumor (follow-up, 3 to 21 years), and 3 patients had died (1 an operative death). Adult patients who have primary optic nerve sheath meningiomas but do not have NF, followed over time after their diagnosis, tend to have a relatively stable course and some may even show slight improvement.

G. Histologically, the tumors have a meningotheliomatous or a mixed-type pattern.

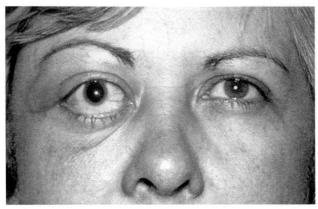

A

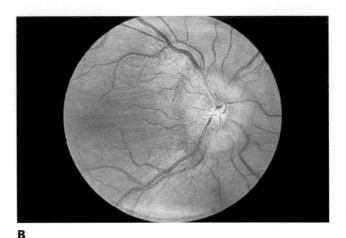

B

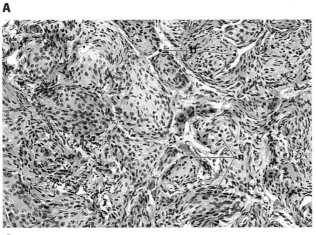

C

Fig. 13.19 Meningioma of optic nerve. **A,** A meningioma of the orbital portion of the optic nerve has caused proptosis of the right eye. **B,** Fundus examination shows optic disc edema of long-term duration. **C,** A biopsy of another case (see Fig. 13.18) shows a proliferation of meningothelial cells. As is often the case, no psammoma bodies are present (b, blood vessels; n, nests of meningothelial cells). (**A** and **B,** Courtesy of Dr. WC Frayer.)

1. Fibroblastic and angiomatous types of meningiomas rarely occur primarily in the orbit.

   "Angioblastic type" of meningioma, once thought to be of meningeal origin, is now generally accepted to be a hemangiopericytoma of the CNS. However, a case of primary orbital angiomatous meningioma, not arising from the optic nerve, has been reported.

   ---

2. Frequently, meningiomas extend extradurally to invade the orbital tissue.
3. Uncommonly, they invade the optic nerve and sclera and may even invade into the choroid and retina.

   Malignant meningioma may be diagnosed if the tumor shows either, or both, unequivocal anaplasia or invasion of brain parenchyma (<10% of intracranial meningiomas are malignant).

IV. Melanocytoma (see p. 721 in Chapter 17)
V. Hemangioma is usually associated with the phakomatoses (see p. 30 in Chapter 2).

Hemangiomas, usually cavernous, rarely capillary, infrequently may occur as a primary optic nerve tumor unassociated with the phakomatoses.

VI. Medulloepithelioma may rarely arise from the distal end of the optic nerve (see p. 686 in Chapter 17).
VII. Giant drusen of the anterior portion of the optic nerve are astrocytic hamartomas usually associated with tuberous sclerosis (see pp. 34–35 in Chapter 2).
VIII. Ordinary drusen of the anterior portion of the optic nerve (Fig. 13.20)
   A. Ordinary optic disc drusen occur in 3.4 to 24 per 1000 population and are bilateral in about 75%.

      The drusen tend to increase in size with age because of increased calcium deposition.
   B. These may present as pseudopapilledema.

      Ordinary drusen of the optic nerve may occur in retinitis pigmentosa or pseudoxanthoma elasticum.

Drusen of the optic nerve occur 20 to 50 times more often in pseudoxanthoma elasticum than in the general, healthy population.

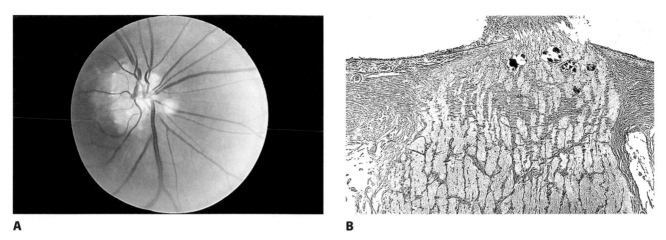

A   **B**

Fig. 13.20 Ordinary drusen of optic nerve. **A,** Clinical appearance of buried drusen of optic nerve head. **B,** Dark, basophilic, calcareous, laminated acellular bodies of different sizes and shapes are located in the substance of the optic disc anterior to the scleral lamina cribrosa. These bodies stain periodic acid–Schiff and acid mucopolysaccharide-positive.

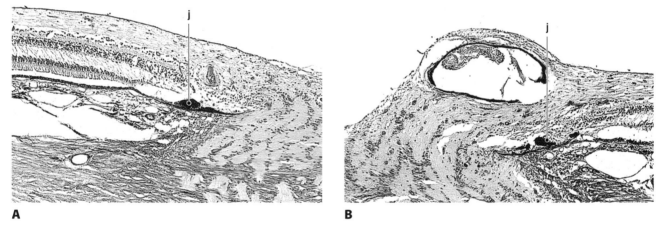

A   **B**

Fig. 13.21 Drusen of the adjacent retinal pigment epithelium (RPE) in same eye. Periodic acid–Schiff-positive drusen (j) of the RPE are seen at the end of Bruch's membrane adjacent to the lateral aspect of the retinal layer of the optic nerve head (**A** and **B**).

C. Although field defects are common (87% in one series), very rarely does a patient lose central vision.
D. Hemorrhage of the optic disc is a rare complication.
   1. The hemorrhage may extend into the vitreous or under the surrounding retina.
   2. Peripapillary subretinal neovascularization may occur.
E. Histologically, basophilic, calcareous, laminated acellular bodies of different sizes and shapes are located in the substance of the optic disc anterior to the scleral lamina cribrosa.

Drusen seem to start intracellularly, but then enlarge and become extracellular. Alterations in axoplasmic transport (flow) may play a role in the formation of these drusen.

IX. Drusen of the adjacent RPE may protrude into the lateral aspect of the retinal layer of the optic nerve head.

Although drusen of the RPE and of the optic nerve have the same name, they are quite different. RPE drusen are basement membrane secretions of the RPE (Fig. 13.21), whereas optic nerve drusen are structurally as described previously and may be degenerative products of optic nerve glial cells, presumably astrocytes anterior to the scleral lamina cribrosa.

X. Corpora amylacea—these are intracellular, basophilic, periodic acid–Schiff-positive structures often observed in the white matter of the brain, including optic nerve and neural retina (mainly nerve fiber layer).
A. The structures are composed of a glycoprotein–acid mucopolysaccharide complex produced within neuronal axons, and probably represent products of axonal degeneration.
B. They have no clinical significance and are considered an aging phenomenon.

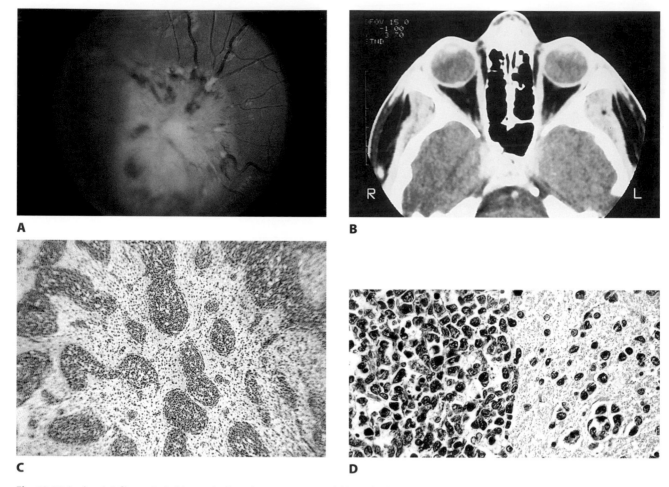

Fig. 13.22 Leukemic infiltrate. **A,** Striking optic disc edema in a 16-year-old boy who had acute lymphoblastic leukemia. **B,** Computed tomography shows bilateral optic disc infiltrate. **C,** Histologic section of another case shows markedly thickened optic nerve pial septa. **D,** Increased magnification shows pial septa thickened by blastic leukemic cells.

Corpora amylacea in the retinal ganglion cell layer may decrease in number with advancing glaucoma.

XI. Corpora arenacea (psammoma bodies)
   A. These are laminated, basophilic bodies produced by the arachnoid meningothelial cells.
   B. They are of no clinical significance and are an aging phenomenon.

Morphologically identical structures, psammoma bodies, may be found in meningiomas and in a variety of papillary carcinomas.

XII. Cysts of the optic nerve may be congenital, arise de novo, or occur secondary to conditions such as optic nerve juvenile pilocytic astrocytomas (gliomas), NF, empty sella syndrome, or hemangioma of leptomeningeal origin.

Optociliary veins (shunt vessels) may be found in the presence of optic nerve cysts.

XIII. Choristoma
XIV. Buscaiano bodies resemble corpora amylacea but are fixation artifacts.

Secondary

   I. Retinoblastoma
  II. Malignant melanoma of choroid
 III. Pseudotumor of RPE
  IV. Intracranial meningioma
   V. Metastatic carcinoma
      A. Metastatic to parenchyma
      B. Metastatic to meninges
  VI. Glioblastoma multiforme of brain
 VII. Lymphoma or leukemia (Fig. 13.22)
VIII. Macroscopically, artifacts may simulate secondary (or primary) optic nerve tumors (e.g., myelin).

BIBLIOGRAPHY

Normal Anatomy

Fine BS, Yanoff M: *Ocular Histology: A Text and Atlas*, 2nd edn. Hagerstown, PA, Harper & Row, 1979:273–286

Hart MH Jr: Clinical perimetry and topographic diagnosis in diseases of the afferent visual system. In Podos SM, Yanoff M, eds: *Textbook of Ophthalmology*, vol. 6. London, Mosby, 1994:1.12–1.16

Hupp SL, Kline KB: Magnetic resonance imaging of the optic chiasm. *Surv Ophthalmol* 36:207, 1991

Onda E, Cioffi GA, Bacon DR et al.: Microvasculature of the human optic nerve. *Am J Ophthalmol* 120:92, 1995

Yanoff M, Fine BS: *Ocular Pathology: A Color Atlas*, 2nd edn. New York, Gower Medical Publishing, 1994:9.1–9.3

Congenital Defects and Anatomic Variations

Akiba J, Kakehashi A, Hikichi T et al.: Vitreous findings in cases of optic nerve pits and serous macular detachment. *Am J Ophthalmol* 116:38, 1993

Brodsky MC: Congenital optic disk anomalies. *Surv Ophthalmol* 39:89, 1994

Brodsky MC, Glasier CM, Pollock SC et al.: Optic nerve hypoplasia. *Arch Ophthalmol* 108:1562, 1990

Brodsky MC, Hoyt WF, Hoyt CS et al.: Atypical retinochoroidal coloboma in patients with dysplastic optic discs and transsphenoidal encephalocele: Report of five cases. *Arch Ophthal*mol 113:624, 1995

Curtin BJ, Iwamoto T, Renaldo DP: Normal and staphylomatous sclera of high myopia: An electron microscopic study. *Arch Ophthalmol* 97:912, 1979

Eliott D, Traboulsi EI, Maumenee IH: Visual prognosis in autosomal dominant optic atrophy. *Am J Ophthalmol* 115:360, 1993

Eustis HS, Sanders MR, Zimmerman T: Morning glory syndrome in children. *Arch Ophthalmol* 112:204, 1994

Fournier AV, Damji KF, Epstein DL et al.: Disc elevation in dominant optic atrophy: Differentiation from normal tension glaucoma. *Ophthalmology* 108:1595, 2002

Guy J, QiIX, Pallotti F et al.: Rescue of a mitochondrial deficiency causing Leber hereditary optic neuropathy. *Ann Neurol* 52:534, 2002

Harding AE, Sweeney MG, Govan GG et al.: Pedigree analysis in Leber hereditary optic neuropathy families with a pathogenic mtDNA mutation. *Am J Hum Genet* 57:77, 1995

Irvine AR, Crawford JB, Sullivan JH: The pathogenesis of retinal detachment with morning glory disc and optic pit. *Retina* 6:146, 1986

Javitt JC, Spaeth GL, Katz LJ et al.: Acquired pits of the optic nerve. *Ophthalmology* 97:1038, 1990

Johns DR, Heher KL, Miller NR et al.: Leber's hereditary optic neuropathy. *Arch Ophthalmol* 111:495, 1993

Johns DR, Smith KH, Savino PJ et al.: Leber's hereditary optic neuropathy. *Ophthalmology* 100:981, 1993

Jonas JB, Freisler KA: Bilateral congenital optic nerve head pits in monozygotic twins. *Am J Ophthalmol* 124:844, 1997

Kalina RE, Conrad WC: Intrathecal fluorescein for serous macular detachment (letter). *Arch Ophthalmol* 94:1421, 1976

Keller-Wood H, Robertson N, Govan GG et al.: Leber's hereditary optic neuropathy mitochondrial DNA mutations in multiple sclerosis. *Ann Neurol* 36:109, 1994

Kerrison JB, Arnold VJ, Feraz Sallum JM et al.: Genetic heterogeneity of dominant optic atrophy, Kjer type: Identification of a second locus on chromosome 18q12.2–12.3. *Arch Ophthalmol* 117:803, 1999

Kerrison JB, Howell N, Miller NR et al.: Leber hereditary optic neuropathy: Electron microscopy and molecular genetic analysis of a case. *Ophthalmology* 102:1509, 1995

Kim SH, Choi MY, Yu YS et al.: Peripapillary staphyloma: clinical features and visual outcome in 19 cases, *Arch Ophthalmol* 123:1371, 2005

Larsson N-G: Leber hereditary optic neuropathy: a nuclear solution of a mitochondrial problem. *Ann Neurol* 52:529, 2002

Latkany P, Ciulla TA, Cacchillo PF et al.: Mitochondrial maculopathy: Geographic atrophy of the macula in the MELAS associated A to G 3243 mitochondrial DNA point mutation. *Am J Ophthalmol* 128:112, 1999

Lott MT, Voljavec AS, Wallace DC: Variable genotype of Leber's hereditary optic neuropathy patients. *Am J Ophthalmol* 109:625, 1990

Mashima Y, Hiida Y, Saga M et al.: Risk of false-positive molecular genetic diagnosis of Leber's hereditary optic neuropathy. *Am J Ophthalmol* 119:245, 1995

Moore M, Salles D, Jampol LM: Progressive optic nerve cupping and neural rim decrease in a patient with autosomal dominant optic nerve colobomas. *Am J Ophthalmol* 129:517, 2000

Morris MA: Mitochondrial DNA mutations and disease: It's the quantity that counts. *Neuroophthalmology* 13:243, 1993

Newman NJ: Hereditary optic neuropathies: from the mitochondria to the optic nerve. *Am J Ophthalmol* 140:517, 2005

Newman NJ, Lott MT, Wallace DC: The clinical characteristics of pedigrees of Leber's hereditary optic neuropathy with the 11778 mutation. *Am J Ophthalmol* 111:750, 1991

Newman NJ, Wallace DC: Mitochondria and Leber's hereditary optic neuropathy. *Am J Ophthalmol* 109:726, 1990

Newman NJ, Torroni A, Brown MD et al.: Epidemic neuropathy in Cuba not associated with mitochondrial DNA mutations found in Leber's hereditary neuropathy patients. *Am J Ophthalmol* 118:158, 1994

Nikoskelainen E, Huoponen K, Juvonen V et al.: Ophthalmic findings in Leber hereditary optic neuropathy, with special reference to mtDNA mutations. *Ophthalmology* 103:504, 1996

Oostra RJ, Bolhuis PA, Wijburg FA et al.: Leber's hereditary optic neuropathy: Correlations between mitochondrial genotype and visual outcome. *J Med Genet* 31:280, 1994

Payune M, YangZ, Katz BJ et al.: Dominant optic atrophy, sensorineural hearing loss, ptosis, and ophthalmoplegia: a syndrome caused by a missense mutation in *OPA1*. *Am J Ophthalmol* 138:749, 2004

Ravine D, Ragge NK, Stephens D et al.: Dominant coloboma-microphthalmos syndrome associated with sensorineural hearing loss, hematuria, and cleft-lip/palate (abstract). *Am J Hum Genet* 59S:A558, 1996

Riordan-Eva P, Sanders MD, Govan GG et al.: The clinical features of Leber's hereditary optic neuropathy defined by the presence of a pathogenic mitochondrial DNA mutation. *Brain* 118:319, 1995

Rutledge BK, Puliafito CA, Duker JS et al.: Optical coherence tomography of macular lesions associated with optic nerve head pits. *Ophthalmology* 103:1047, 1996

Saddun AA, Carelli V, Saomao SR et al.: A very large Brazilian pedigree with 11778 Leber's hereditary optic neuropathy. *Am Ophthalmol Soc* 100:169, 2003

Saddun AA, De Negri AM, Carelli V et al.: Ophthalmologic finding in a large pedigree of 11778/Haplogroup J Leber hereditary optic neuropathy. *Am J Ophthalmol* 137:271, 2004

Saddun AA, Kashima Y, Wurdeman AE et al.: Morphological findings in the visual system in a case of Leber's hereditary optic neuropathy. *Clin Neurosci* 2:165, 1994

Schimmenti LA, Cunliffe HE, McNoe LA: Further delineation of renal-coloboma syndrome in patients with extreme variability of phenotype and identical PAX2 mutations. *Am J Hum Genet* 60:869, 1997

Scott IU, Warman R, Altman N: Bilateral aplasia of the optic nerves, chiasm, and tracts in an otherwise healthy infant. *Am J Ophthalmol* 124:409, 1997

Sheffer RN, Zlotogora J, Elpeleg ON et al.: Behr's syndrome and 3-methylglutaconic aciduria. *Am J Ophthalmol* 114:494, 1992

Slusher MM, Weaver G, Greven C et al.: The spectrum of cavitary optic disc anomalies in a family. *Ophthalmology* 96:342, 1989

Sobol WM, Blodi CF, Folk JC et al.: Long-term visual outcome in patients with optic nerve pit and serous retinal detachment of the macula. *Ophthalmology* 97:1539, 1990

Sperduto RD, Seigel D, Roberts J et al.: Prevalence of myopia in the United States. *Arch Ophthalmol* 101:405, 1983

Spruijt L, Kolbach DN, de Coo RF et al.: Influence of mutation type on clinical expression of Leber hereditary optic neuropathy. *Am J Ophthalmol* 141:676, 2006

Stefko ST, Campochiaro P, Wang P et al.: Dominant inheritance of optic pits. *Am J Ophthalmol* 124:112, 1997

Stone EM, Coppinger JM, Kardon RH et al.: Mae III positively detects the mitochondrial mutation associated with type 1 Leber's hereditary optic neuropathy. *Arch Ophthalmol* 108:1417, 1990

Votruba M, Fitzke FW, Holder GE et al.: Clinical features in affected individuals from 21 pedigrees with dominant optic atrophy. *Arch Ophthalmol* 116:351, 1998

Willis R, Zimmerman LE, O'Grady R et al.: Heterotopic adipose tissue and smooth muscle in the optic disc. *Arch Ophthalmol* 88:139, 1972

Yanoff M, Rorke LB: Ocular and central nervous system findings in tetraploid–diploid mosaicism. *Am J Ophthalmol* 75:1036, 1973

Yanoff M, Rorke LB, Allman MI: Bilateral optic system aplasia with relatively normal eyes. *Arch Ophthalmol* 96:97, 1978

Yanoff M, Rorke LB, Niederer BS: Ocular and cerebral abnormalities in chromosome 18 deletion defect. *Am J Ophthalmol* 70:391, 1970

Zadnik K, Satariano WA, Mutti DO et al.: The effect of parental history of myopia on children's eye size. *JAMA* 271:1323, 1994

Zimmerman LE, Arkfeld DL, Schenken JB et al.: A rare choristoma of the optic nerve and chiasm. *Arch Ophthalmol* 101:766, 1983

Optic Disc Edema

Cartlidge NEF, Ng RCY, Tilley PJB: Dilemma of the swollen optic disc: a fluorescein retinal angiography study. *Br J Ophthalmol* 61:385, 1977

Collins ML, Traboulsi EI, Maumenee IH: Optic nerve head swelling and optic atrophy in the systemic mucopolysaccharidoses. *Ophthalmology* 97:1445, 1990

Green GJ, Lessell S, Loewenstein JI: Ischemic optic neuropathy in chronic papilledema. *Arch Ophthalmol* 98:502, 1980

Hayreh SS: Optic disc edema in raised intracranial pressure: V. Pathogenesis. *Arch Ophthalmol* 95:1553, 1977

Hayreh SS: Fluids in the anterior part of the optic nerve in health and disease. *Surv Ophthalmol* 23:1, 1978

Laibovitz RA: Presumed phlebitis of the optic disc. *Ophthalmology* 86:313, 1979

Lazaro EJ, Cinotti AA, Eichler PN et al.: Amaurosis due to massive gastrointestinal hemorrhage. *Am J Gastroenterol* 55:50, 1971

Morris AT, Sanders MD: Macular changes resulting from papilloedema. *Br J Ophthalmol* 64:211, 1980

Radius RL, Anderson DR: Fast axonal transport in early experimental disc edema. *Invest Ophthalmol* 19:158, 1980

Rosenberg MA, Savino PJ, Glaser JS: A clinical analysis of pseudopapilledema: I. Population, laterality, acuity, refractive error, ophthalmoscopic characteristics and coincident disease. *Arch Ophthalmol* 97:65, 1979

Savino PJ, Glaser JS, Rosenberg MA: A clinical analysis of pseudopapilledema: II. Visual field defects. *Arch Ophthalmol* 97:71, 1979

Sher NA, Wirtschafter J, Shapiro SK et al.: Unilateral papilledema in "benign" intracranial hypertension (pseudotumor cerebri). *JAMA* 250:2346, 1983

Trujillo MH, Desenne JJ, Pinto HB: Reversible papilledema in iron deficiency anemia: Two cases with normal spinal fluid pressure. *Ann Ophthalmol* 4:378, 1972

Tso MOM, Fine BS: Electron microscopic study of human papilledema. *Am J Ophthalmol* 82:424, 1976

Tytell M, Black MM, Garner JA et al.: Axonal transport: each major rate component reflects the movement of distinct macromolecular complexes. *Science* 214:179, 1981

Optic Neuritis

Achkar AA, Lie JT, Hunder GG et al.: How does previous corticosteroid treatment affect the biopsy findings in giant cell (temporal) arteritis? *Ann Intern Med* 120:987, 1994

Aiello PD, Trautmann JC, McPhee TJ et al.: Visual prognosis in giant cell arteritis. *Ophthalmology* 100:550, 1993

Arnold AC, Hepler RS: Fluorescein angiography in acute nonarteritic anterior ischemic optic neuropathy. *Am J Ophthalmol* 117:222, 1994

Arnold AC, Pepose JS, Hepler RS et al.: Retinal periphlebitis and retinitis in multiple sclerosis: I. Pathologic characteristics. *Ophthalmology* 91:255, 1984

Baumbach GL, Cancilla PA, Martin-Amat G et al.: Methyl alcohol poisoning: IV. Alterations of the morphological findings of the retina and optic nerve. *Arch Ophthalmol* 95:1859, 1977

Beck RW, Cleary PA, Trobe JD et al.: The effect of corticosteroids for acute optic neuritis on the subsequent development of multiple sclerosis. *N Engl J Med* 329:1764, 1993

Beri M, Klugman MR, Kohler JA et al.: Anterior ischemic optic neuropathy: VII. Incidence of bilaterality and various influencing factors. *Ophthalmology* 94:1020, 1987

Birch MK, Barbosa S, Blumhardt LD et al.: Retinal venous sheathing and the blood–retinal barrier in multiple sclerosis. *Arch Ophthalmol* 114:34, 1996

Brownstein S, Jannotta FS: Sarcoid granulomas of the retina and optic nerve. *Can J Ophthalmol* 9:372, 1974

Chung SM, Gay CA, McCrary JA: Nonarteritic ischemic optic neuropathy. *Ophthalmology* 101:779, 1994

Corcoran GM, Prayson RA, Herzog KM: The significance of perivascular inflammation in the absence of arteritis in temporal artery biopsy specimens. *Am J Clin Pathol* 115:342, 2001

Currie JN, Lessell S, Lessell IM et al.: Optic neuropathy in chronic lymphatic leukemia. *Arch Ophthalmol* 106:654, 1988

Danesh-Meyer H, Savino PJ, Gamble GG: Poor prognosis of visual outcome after visual loss from giant cell arteritis. *Ophthalmology* 112:1098, 2005

Dudenhoefer EJ, Cornblath WT, Schatz MP: Scalp necrosis with giant cell arteritis. *Ophthalmology* 105:1875, 1998

Folz SJ, Trobe JD: The peroxisome and the eye. *Surv Ophthalmol* 35:353, 1991

Frohman EM, Frohman TC, Zee DS et al.: The neuro-ophthalmology of multiple sclerosis. *Lancet Neurol* 4:111, 2005

Glasgow BJ, Brown HH, Hannah JB et al.: Ocular pathologic findings in neonatal adrenoleukodystrophy. *Ophthalmology* 94:1054, 1987

Guyer DR, Miller NR, Auer CL et al.: The risk of cerebrovascular and cardiovascular disease in patients with anterior ischemic optic neuropathy. *Arch Ophthalmol* 103:1136, 1985

Hayreh SS: Anterior ischemic optic neuropathy: I. Terminology and pathogenesis. II. Fundus on ophthalmoscopy and fluorescein angiography. III. Treatment, prophylaxis and differential diagnosis. *Br J Ophthalmol* 58:955, 964, 981, 1974

Hayreh SS: Anterior ischemic optic neuropathy: IV. Occurrence after cataract extraction. *Arch Ophthalmol* 98:1410, 1980

Hayreh SS: Anterior ischemic optic neuropathy: V. Optic disc edema: an early sign. *Arch Ophthalmol* 99:1030, 1981

Hayreh MS, Hayreh SS, Baumbach GL *et al.*: Methyl alcohol poisoning: III. Ocular toxicity. *Arch Ophthalmol* 95:1851, 1977

Hayreh SS, Podhajsky PA, Zimmerman B: Occult giant cell arteritis: Ocular manifestations. *Am J Ophthalmol* 125:521, 1996

Hedges III TR, Gieger GL, Albert DM: The clinical value of negative temporal artery biopsy specimens. *Arch Ophthalmol* 101:1251, 1983

Henkind P, Charles NC, Pearson J: Histopathology of ischemic optic neuropathy. *Am J Ophthalmol* 69:78, 1970

Hwang J-M, Girkin CA, Perry JD *et al.*: Bilateral ocular ischemic syndrome secondary to giant cell arteritis progressing despite corticosteroid treatment. *Am J Ophthalmol* 127:102, 1999

Hupp SL, Nelson GA, Zimmerman LE: Generalized giant-cell arteritis with coronary artery involvement and myocardial infarction. *Arch Ophthalmol* 108:1385, 1990

Galor A, Lee MS: Slowly progressive vision loss in giant cell arteritis, Arch Ophthalmol 124:416, 2006

Katz PR, Karuza J, Gutman SI *et al.*: A comparison between erythrocyte sedimentation rate (ESR) and selected acute-phase proteins in the elderly. *Am J Clin Pathol* 94:637, 1990

Lim JI, Tessler HH, Goodwin JA: Anterior granulomatous uveitis in patients with multiple sclerosis. *Ophthalmology* 98:142, 1991

Liu GT, Glaser JS, Schatz NJ *et al.*: Visual morbidity in giant cell arteritis: Clinical characteristics and prognosis for vision. *Ophthalmology* 101:1779, 1994

Macaluso DC, Shults WT, Fraunfelder FT: Features of amiodarone-induced optic neuropathy. *Am J Ophthalmol* 127:610, 1999

Malinowski SM, Pulido JS, Folk JC: Long-term visual outcome and complications associated with pars planitis. *Ophthalmology* 100:818, 1993

Margo CE, Levy MH, Beck RW: Bilateral idiopathic inflammation of the optic nerve sheaths. *Ophthalmology* 96:200, 1989

Martin-Amat G, Tephly TR, McMartin KE *et al.*: Methyl alcohol poisoning: II. Development of a model for ocular toxicity in methyl alcohol poisoning using the rhesus monkey. *Arch Ophthalmol* 95:1847, 1977

McDonnell PJ: Ocular manifestations of temporal arteritis. *Curr Opin Ophthalmol* 1:158, 1990

Mitchell BM, Font RL: Detection of varicella virus DNA in some patients with giant cell arteritis. *Invest Ophthalmol Vis Sci* 42:2572, 2001

Newman NJ, Scherer R, Langenberg P *et al.*: The fellow eye in NAION: report from the ischemic optic neuropathy decompression trial follow-up study. *Am J Ophthalmol* 134:317, 2002

Niederkohr RD, Levin LA: Management of the patient with temporal arteritis: a decision-analytic approach. *Ophthalmology* 112:744, 2005

Patel SS, Rutzen AR, Marx JL *et al.*: Cytomegalic papillitis in patients with acquired immune deficiency syndrome. *Ophthalmology* 103:1476, 1996

Purvin VA: Anterior ischemic optic atrophy secondary interferon alpha. *Arch Ophthalmol* 113:1041, 1995

Purvin VA, Chioran G: Recurrent neuroretinitis. *Arch Ophthalmol* 112:365, 1994

Quillen DA, Cantore WA, Schwartz SR *et al.*: Choroidal nonperfusion in giant cell arteritis. *Am J Ophthalmol* 116:171, 1993

Ray-Chaudhuri N, Kiné DA, Tijani SO *et al.*: Effect of prior steroid treatment on temporal artery biopsy findings in giant cell arteritis. *Br J Ophthalmol* 86:530, 2002

Rizzo JF, Lessell S: Tobacco amblyopia. *Am J Ophthalmol* 116:84, 1993

Sack GH, Morrell JC: Visual pigment gene changes in adrenoleukodystrophy. *Invest Ophthalmol Vis Sci* 34:2634, 1993

Schmidt D, Löffler KU: Temporal arteritis: Comparison of histologic and clinical findings. *Acta Ophthalmol* 72:319, 1994

De Seze J, Stojkovic T, Ferriby D *et al.*: Devic's neuromyelitis optica: clinical, laboratory, MRI and outcome profile. *J Neurol Sci* 197:57, 2002

Slavin ML, Barondes MJ: Visual loss caused by choroidal ischemia preceding anterior ischemic optic neuropathy in giant cell arteritis. *Am J Ophthalmol* 117:81, 1994

Sørensen TL, Frederiksen JL, Brøonnum-Hansen H *et al.*: Optic neuritis as onset manifestation of multiple sclerosis: a nationwide, long-term survey. *Neurology* 53:473, 1999

To KW, Enzer YR, Tsiaras WG: Temporal artery biopsy after one month of corticosteroid therapy. *Am J Ophthalmol* 117:265, 1994

Warwar RE, Bullock JD, Shields JA *et al.*: Coexistence of three tumors of neural crest origin: Neurofibroma, meningioma, and uveal melanoma. *Arch Ophthalmol* 116:1241, 1978

Wells KK, Folberg R, Goeken JA *et al.*: Temporal artery biopsies. *Ophthalmology* 96:1058, 1989

Williams KE, Johnson LN: Neuroretinitis in patints with multiple sclerosis. *Ophthalmology* 111:335, 2004

Wingerchuk DM, Hoganncamp WF, O'Brian PC *et al.*: The clinical course of neuromyelitis optica (Devic syndrome). *Neurology* 53:1107, 1999

Optic Atrophy

Bertram L, Blacker D, Mullin K *et al.*: Evidence for genetic linkage of Alzheimer's disease to chromosome 10q. *Science* 290:2302, 2000

Brinton GS, Norton EWD, Zahn JR *et al.*: Ocular quinine toxicity. *Am J Ophthalmol* 90:403, 1980

Downes SM, Black GCM, Hyman N *et al.*: Visual loss due to progressive multifoval leukoencephalopathy in a congenital immunodeficiency disorder. *Arch Ophthalmol* 119:1377, 2001

Ertekin-Taner N, Graff-Radford N, Youkin LH: Linkage of plasma Aβ42 to a quantitative locus on chromosome 10 in late-onset Alzheimer's disease pedigrees. *Science* 290:2303, 2000

Hinton DR, Sadun AA, Blanks JC *et al.*: Optic-nerve degeneration in Alzheimer's disease. *N Engl J Med* 315:485, 1986

Johnston RL, Seller MJ, Behnam JT *et al.*: Dominant optic atrophy: Refining the clinical diagnostic criteria in light of genetic linkage studies. *Ophthalmology* 106:1233, 1999

Kollarits CR, Pinheiro ML, Swann ER *et al.*: The autosomal dominant syndrome of progressive optic atrophy and congenital deafness. *Am J Ophthalmol* 87:789, 1979

Lee AG, Martin CO: Neuro-ophthalmic findings in the visual variant of Alzheimer's disease. *Ophthalmology* 111:376, 2004

Lesser RL, Albert DM, Bobowick AR *et al.*: Creutzfeldt–Jakob disease and optic atrophy. *Am J Ophthalmol* 87:317, 1979

Loupe DN, Newman NJ, Green RC *et al.*: Pupillary response to tropicamide in patients with Alzheimer disease. *Ophthalmology* 103:495, 1996

Merz B: Eye disease linked to mitochondrial defect. *JAMA* 260:894, 1988

Myers A, Holmans P, Marshall H *et al.*: Susceptibility locus for Alzheimer's disease on chromosome 10. *Science* 290:2304, 2000

Ormerod LD, Rhodes RH, Gross SA *et al.*: Ophthalmologic manifestations of acquired immune deficiency syndrome-associated progressive multifocal leukoencephalopathy. *Ophthalmology* 103:899, 1996

Rahn EK, Yanoff M, Tucker S: Neuro-ocular considerations in the Pelizaeus–Merzbacher syndrome: A clinicopathologic study. *Am J Ophthalmol* 66:1143, 1968

Roth AM, Keltner JL, Ellis WG *et al.*: Virus-simulating structures in the optic nerve head in Creutzfeldt–Jakob disease. *Am J Ophthalmol* 87:827, 1979

Sadun AA, Bassi CJ: Optic nerve damage in Alzheimer's disease. *Ophthalmology* 97:9, 1990

Scinto LFM, Daffner KR, Dressler D *et al.*: A potential noninvasive neurobiological test for Alzheimer's disease. *Science* 266:1051, 1994

Tumors

Auw-Haedrich C, Staubach F, Witschel H: Optic disk drusen. *Surv Ophthalmol* 47:515, 2000

Alvord EC Jr, Lofton S: Gliomas of the optic nerve or chiasm: Outcome by patients' age, tumor site, and treatment. *J Neurosurg* 68:85, 1988

Beck RW, Corbett JJ, Thompson HS *et al.*: Decreased visual acuity from optic disc drusen. *Arch Ophthalmol* 103:1155, 1985

Bergin DJ, Johnson TE, Spencer WH *et al.*: Ganglioma of the optic nerve. *Am J Ophthalmol* 95:146, 1988

Bosch MM, Wichmann WW, Boltshauser E *et al.*: Optic nerve sheath meningiomas in patients with neurofibromatosis type 2. *Arch Ophthalmol* 124:379, 2006

Christmas NJ, Mead MD, Richardson EP *et al.*: Secondary optic nerve tumors. *Surv Ophthalmol* 36:196, 1991

Cibis GW, Whittaker CK, Wood WE: Intraocular extension of optic nerve meningioma in a case of neurofibromatosis. *Arch Ophthalmol* 103:404, 1985

Cogan DG, Kuwabara T: Myelin artifacts. *Am J Ophthalmol* 64:622, 1967

Coleman K, Ross MH, McCabe M *et al.*: Disk drusen and angioid streaks in pseudoxanthoma elasticum. *Am J Ophthalmol* 112:166, 1991

Dossetor FM, Landau K, Hoyt WF: Optic disk glioma in neurofibromatosis type 2. *Am J Ophthalmol* 602, 1989

Dutton JJ: Optic nerve sheath meningiomas. *Surv Ophthalmol* 37:167, 1992

Dutton JJ: Gliomas of the anterior visual pathway (review). *Surv Ophthalmol* 38:427, 1994

Egan RA, Lessell S: A contribution to the natural history of optic nerve sheath meningiomas. *Arch Ophthalmol* 120:1505, 2002

Elahi E, Meltzer MA, Friedman AH *et al.*: Primary orbital angiomatous meningioma. *Arch Ophthalmol* 121:124, 2003

Fine BS, Yanoff M: *Ocular Histology: A Text and Atlas*, 2nd edn. Hagerstown, PA, Harper & Row, 1979:103

Gallie BL, Graham JE, Hunter WS: Optic nerve head metastasis. *Arch Ophthalmol* 93:983, 1975

Garrity JA, Trautmann JC, Bartley GB *et al.*: Optic nerve sheath meningoceles. *Ophthalmology* 97:1519, 1990

Guigis MF, White FV, Dunbar JA *et al.*: Optic nerve teratoma and odontogenic dermoid cyst in a neonate with persistent fetal vasculature. *Arch Ophthalmol* 120:1582, 2002

Imes RK, Schatz H, Hoyt WF *et al.*: Evolution of optociliary veins in optic nerve sheath meningioma. *Arch Ophthalmol* 103:59, 1985

Janss AJ, Grundy R, Cnaan A *et al.*: Optic pathway and hypothalamic/chiasmatic gliomas in children younger than 5 years with a 6-year follow-up. *Br J Cancer* 75:1051, 1995

Karp LA, Zimmerman LE, Borit A *et al.*: Primary intraorbital meningiomas. *Arch Ophthalmol* 91:24, 1974

Kazim M, Kennerdell JS, Maroon J *et al.*: Choristoma of the optic nerve and chiasm. *Arch Ophthalmol* 110:236, 1992

Kiss R, Dewitte O, Decaestecker C *et al.*: The combined determination of proliferative activity and cell density in the prognosis of adult patients with supratentorial high-grade astrocytic tumors. *Am J Clin Pathol* 107:321, 1997

Kubota T, Naumann GOH: Reduction in number of corpora amylacea with advancing histological changes of glaucoma. *Graefes Arch Clin Exp Ophthalmol* 231:249, 1993

Kubota T, Holbach LM, Naumann GOH: Corpora amylacea in glaucomatous and non-glaucomatous optic nerve and retina. *Graefes Arch Clin Exp Ophthalmol* 231:7, 1993

Kuenzle C, Weissert M, Roulet E *et al.*: Follow-up of optic pathway gliomas in children with neurofibromatosis type 1. *Neuropediatrics* 25:295, 1994

Lindblom B, Truwit CL, Hoyt WF: Optic nerve sheath meningioma. *Ophthalmology* 99:560, 1992

Listernick R, Charrow J, Greenwald MJ: Emergence of optic pathway gliomas in children with neurofibromatosis type 1 after normal neuroimaging results. *J Pediatr* 121:584, 1992

Loeffler KU, Edward DP, Tso MOM: Tau-2 immunoreactivity of corpora amylacea in the human retina and optic nerve. *Invest Ophthalmol Vis Sci* 34:2600, 1993

Malecha MA, Haik BG, Morris WR: Capillary hemangioma of the optic nerve head and juxtapapillary retina. *Arch Ophthalmol* 118:289, 2000

Martidis A, Yee RD, Azzarelli B *et al.*: Neuro-ophthalmic, radiographic, and pathologic manifestations of Alexander disease. *Arch Ophthalmol* 117:265, 1999

McCartney ACE: Lineage and ubiquination in optic nerve gliomas. Presented at the joint meeting of Verhoeff and European Ophthalmic Pathology Societies, May 1991

Newman NJ, Grossniklaus HE, Wojno TH: Breast carcinoma metastatic to the optic nerve. *Arch Ophthalmol* 114:102, 1996

Novack RL, Foos RY: Drusen of the optic disk in retinitis pigmentosa. *Am J Ophthalmol* 103:44, 1987

Radley MG, di Sant'Agnese PA, Eskin TA: Epithelial differentiation in meningiomas. *Am J Clin Pathol* 92:266, 1989

Roh S, Mawn L, Hedges TR III: Juvenile pilocytic astrocytoma masquerading as amblyopia. *Am J Ophthalmol* 123:692, 1997

Saeed P, Rootman J, Nugent RA *et al.*: Optic nerve sheath meningiomas. *Ophthalmology* 110:2019, 2003

Schwarz GA, Yanoff M: Lafora bodies, corpora amylacea, and Lewy bodies: A morphologic and histochemical study. *Arch Neurobiol (Madr)* 28:803, 1965

Sedun F, Hinton DR, Sedun AA: Rapid growth of an optic nerve ganglioglioma in a patient with neurofibromatosis 1. *Ophthalmology* 103:794, 1996

Shields JA, Shields CL, Singh AD: Metastatic neoplasms in the optic disc: The Bjerrum lecture: Part 2. *Arch Ophthalmol* 118:217, 2000

Spoor TC, Kennerdell JS, Martinez AJ *et al.*: Malignant gliomas of the optic nerve pathways. *Am J Ophthalmol* 89:284, 1980

Strominger MB, Schatz NJ, Glaser JS: Lymphomatous optic neuropathy. *Am J Ophthalmol* 116:774, 1993

Taphoorn MJB, De Vries-Knoppert WAEJ, Ponsen H *et al.*: Malignant optic glioma in adults. *J Neurosurg* 70:277, 1989

Thiagalingam S, Flaherty M, Billson F *et al.*: Neurofibromatosis type 1 and optic pathway gliomas: follow-up of 54 patients. *Ophthalmology* 111:568, 2004

Wallace RT, Shields JA, Shields CL *et al.*: Leukemic infiltration of the optic nerve. *Arch Ophthalmol* 109:1027, 1991

Wineck RR, Scheithauer BW, Wick MR: Meningioma, meningeal hemangiopericytoma (angioblastic hemangiopericytoma), peripheral hemangiopericytoma, and acoustic schwannoma: A comparative immunohistochemical study. *Am J Surg Pathol* 13:251, 1989

Woodford B, Tso MOM: An ultrastructural study of the corpora amylacea of the optic nerve head and retina. *Am J Ophthalmol* 90:492, 1980

Wright JE, McNab AA, MacDonald WI: Primary optic nerve sheath meningioma. *Br J Ophthalmol* 73:960, 1989

Wulc AE, Bergin DJ, Barnes D *et al.*: Orbital optic nerve glioma in adult life. *Arch Ophthalmol* 107:1013, 1989

Yanoff M, Davis R, Zimmerman LE: Juvenile pilocytic astrocytoma ("glioma") of optic nerve: Clinicopathologic study of 63 cases. In Jakobiec FA, ed: *Ocular and Adnexal Tumors*. Birmingham, AL, Aesculapius, 1978:685

Zimmerman LE, Fine BS: Myelin artifacts in the optic disc and retina. *Arch Ophthalmol* 74:394, 1965

Zimmerman CF, Schatz NJ, Glaser JS: Magnetic resonance imaging of optic nerve meningiomas. *Ophthalmology* 97:585, 1990

Zimmerman LE, Arkfeld DL, Schenken JB *et al.*: A rare choristoma of the optic nerve and chiasm. *Arch Ophthalmol* 101:766, 1983

Zimmerman RA, Bilaniuk LT, Yanoff M *et al.*: Orbital magnetic resonance imaging. *Am J Ophthalmol* 100:312, 1985

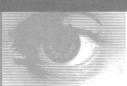

14

Orbit

NORMAL ANATOMY

I. The orbital volume is approximately 30 ml, and the orbital depth (anterior to posterior) is approximately 4.5 cm (Figs 14.1 to 14.5).

A. The medial orbital wall is quite thin (<0.5 mm) and transparent.

B. The roof of the orbit, composed mainly of the orbital plate of the frontal bone, is thinnest anteriorly, where it is adjacent to the frontal sinus, and separates the orbit from the frontal lobes of the brain.

C. The orbital floor is composed of the orbital plates of the maxilla and zygomatic bones and a small contribution from the palatine bone posteriorly.

D. The floor is also thin, 0.5 to 1 mm, and thus is easily fractured, especially medial to the infraorbital canal.

E. Conversely, the lateral orbital wall is thick, composed anteriorly by the zygomatic bone and posteriorly by the greater wing of the sphenoid.

II. In addition to the bony walls, the eye, and the optic nerve, the orbit contains many soft-tissue structures such as fat, muscle (striated and nonstriated), cartilage, bone, fibrous tissue, nerves, and blood vessels.

A. Other than the epithelia within the eyeball, the lacrimal gland is the only epithelial structure in the orbit.

B. All orbital structures may be involved in disease processes.

C. Orbital disease, whatever its cause, tends to increase the bulk of the orbit, so the main presenting sign is exophthalmos.

EXOPHTHALMOS

I. The main clinical manifestation of orbital disease is exophthalmos (ocular proptosis), the extent and direction of which depend on a number of factors*: (1) size of lesion; (2) character of lesion (expansile versus infiltrative growth, rapid versus slow growth); (3) location of the lesion in the orbit (small lesion in muscle cone causes more exophthalmos than lesion of same size outside the muscle cone; lesions anterior to septum orbitale do not produce exophthalmos unless they also grow posteriorly); and (4) lesion's effect on the extraocular muscles (complete paralysis of all muscles by itself can cause 2 mm of exophthalmos)

II. Exophthalmos may be simulated by many conditions: lid retraction due to any cause (most commonly Graves' disease); unilateral enlargement of the globe; high myopia; buphthalmos; sagging lower lid; relaxation of the rectus muscle(s); enophthalmos or microphthalmos of the oppo-

*Exophthalmos *refers specifically to protrusion of the eyes, whereas* proptosis *refers to protrusion of any part of the body.*

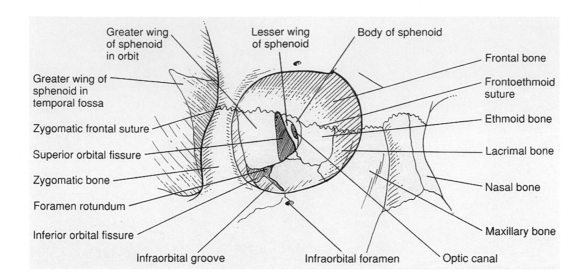

Fig. 14.1 Normal orbit. Composite illustration of the seven bones of the orbit. (From Levine MR, Larson DW: In Podos SM, Yanoff M, eds: *Textbook of Ophthalmology,* vol. 4. © Elsevier 1993; adapted from Zide B, Jelks G: *Surgical Anatomy of the Orbit.* New York, Raven Press, 1985.)

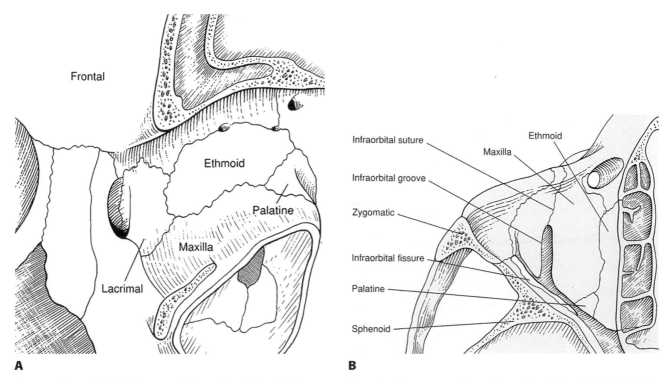

Fig. 14.2 Normal orbit. **A,** Anatomy of the medial orbital wall. **B,** Anatomy of the orbital floor as viewed from above. (From Wojno TH: In Podos SM, Yanoff M, eds: *Textbook of Ophthalmology,* vol. 4. New York, Gower Medical Publishing, 1993:9.1–9.4. © Elsevier 1993.)

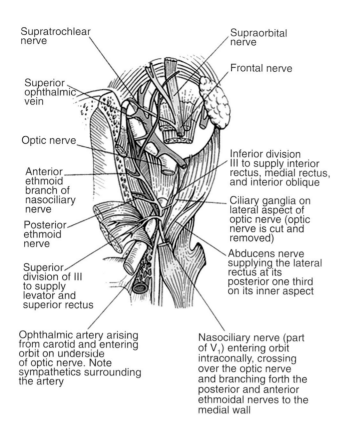

Supratrochlear nerve

Supraorbital nerve

Frontal nerve

Superior ophthalmic vein

Optic nerve

Inferior division III to supply interior rectus, medial rectus, and interior oblique

Anterior ethmoid branch of nasociliary nerve

Posterior ethmoid nerve

Ciliary ganglia on lateral aspect of optic nerve (optic nerve is cut and removed)

Abducens nerve supplying the lateral rectus at its posterior one third on its inner aspect

Superior division of III to supply levator and superior rectus

Ophthalmic artery arising from carotid and entering orbit on underside of optic nerve. Note sympathetics surrounding the artery

Nasociliary nerve (part of V₁) entering orbit intraconally, crossing over the optic nerve and branching forth the posterior and anterior ethmoidal nerves to the medial wall

Fig. 14.3 Normal orbit. Right orbital structures and their basic relationships as seen from above. (From Levine MR, Larson DW: In Podos SM, Yanoff M, eds: *Textbook of Ophthalmology*, vol. 4. New York, Gower Medical Publishing, 1993:10.4–10.13. © Elsevier 1993.)

site eye; asymmetry of the bony orbits; and shallow orbits

III. The most common causes of exophthalmos are: thyroid disease (most common for both unilateral and bilateral exophthalmos); hemangioma; inflammatory pseudotumors; and benign and malignant lymphoid tumors (all others are relatively rare)

Although dermoids are one of the most common orbital tumors, if not the most common, they rarely cause exophthalmos because of their position, which is usually anterior to the septum orbitale.

DEVELOPMENTAL ABNORMALITIES

Developmental Abnormalities of Bony Orbit

Developmental abnormalities are usually associated with abnormalities of the cranial and facial bones such as tower skull or hypertelorism.

Microphthalmos with Cyst

I. Microphthalmos with cyst (see Fig. 2.10) is usually a unilateral condition, but may be bilateral.

II. The cyst may be so large as to obscure the microphthalmic eye.

III. Proliferated neuroectodermal tissue (i.e., pseudogliomatous hyperplasia) may simulate an orbital neoplasm.

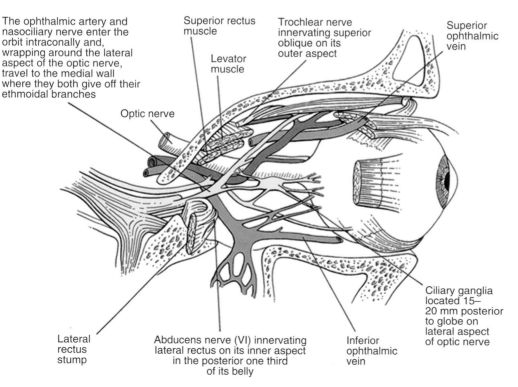

The ophthalmic artery and nasociliary nerve enter the orbit intraconally and, wrapping around the lateral aspect of the optic nerve, travel to the medial wall where they both give off their ethmoidal branches

Superior rectus muscle

Trochlear nerve innervating superior oblique on its outer aspect

Superior ophthalmic vein

Levator muscle

Optic nerve

Lateral rectus stump

Abducens nerve (VI) innervating lateral rectus on its inner aspect in the posterior one third of its belly

Inferior ophthalmic vein

Ciliary ganglia located 15–20 mm posterior to globe on lateral aspect of optic nerve

Fig. 14.4 Normal orbit—side view. Retrobulbar contents of orbit. (From Levine MR, Larson DW: In Podos SM, Yanoff M, eds: *Textbook of Ophthalmology*, vol. 4. New York, Gower Medical Publishing, 1993:10.4–10.13. © Elsevier 1993.)

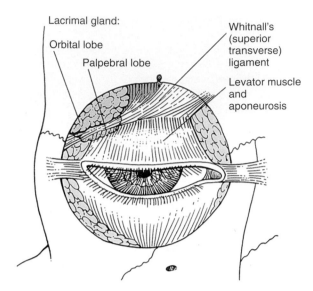

Fig. 14.5 Normal orbit—front view. Lacrimal gland and surrounding structures. (From Buffam FV: In Podos SM, Yanoff M, eds: *Textbook of Ophthalmology*, vol. 4. New York, Gower Medical Publishing, 1993:7.1–7.6. © Elsevier 1993.)

IV. The condition is caused by incomplete closure of the fetal cleft.

Although microphthalmos with cyst usually has no known cause, it may be associated with the 13q deletion or chromosome 18 deletion defect (partial 18 monosomy). A congenital cystic eye may also be associated with contralateral persistent hyperplastic vitreous and cerebrocutaneous abnormalities, called cranial ectodermopathy.

V. Histologically, the eye may range from relative normality to complete disorder, and may contain structures such as ectopic smooth muscle and cartilage.

The cyst may be lined by gliotic retina or it may be filled with proliferated glial tissue that can reach massive amounts (massive gliosis) and simulate a glial neoplasm.

Cephaloceles

I. Cephaloceles are caused by a developmental malformation in which brain tissue or meninges, or both, are present in the orbit.
   A. Meningocele—only meninges are present
   B. Encephalocele—only brain tissue is present; hydroencephalocele—considerable fluid is present in the cyst
   C. Meningoencephalocele—meninges and brain tissue are present
   D. All of the preceding may communicate with the brain. Although the initial communication usually closes, it may rarely remain open.

II. Most cephaloceles are developmental displacements of brain tissue, and are generally referred to as *ectopic* brain tissue.

III. Histologically, most cephaloceles show a structure similar to that of the optic nerve (i.e., white matter separated by pial septa).

Congenital Alacrima

I. Hereditary congenital alacrima is part of a systemic disturbance such as the Riley–Day syndrome or anhidrotic ectodermal dysplasia.

II. An isolated case of congenital alacrima, presumably caused by hypoplasia of the lacrimal gland, has been reported.

ORBITAL INFLAMMATION

Acute

I. Nonsuppurative (see section *Nonsuppurative, Chronic Nongranulomatous Uveitis and Endophthalmitis* in Chapter 3) —orbital cellulitis is most commonly caused by extension of an inflammation from the paranasal sinuses (Fig. 14.6).

II. Suppurative (see section *Suppurative Endophthalmitis and Panophthalmitis* in Chapter 3)
   A. Purulent infection (e.g., with *Staphylococcus*) occurs commonly after trauma.

A rare causative agent of posttraumatic acute orbital inflammation is atypical mycobacteria.

   B. Phycomycosis (mucormycosis) is a devastating cause of suppurative orbital inflammation (Fig. 14.7; see p. 86 in Chapter 4.)
      1. It is usually associated with other disease, especially when acidosis is present (e.g., diabetes mellitus, renal disease, and malignancies).
      2. Thrombotic complications may dominate the clinical picture.

Chronic

I. Nongranulomatous
   A. Chronic nongranulomatous inflammation is the most common inflammatory lesion of the orbit and is of unknown cause (see pp. 571–573 in this chapter).
   B. A rare cause is the benign lymphoepithelial lesion of Godwin*; Fig. 14.8.

---

*Mikulicz's disease *is the old name for* benign lymphoepithelial lesion. Mikulicz's syndrome *is a confusing term that has been used to describe secondary diseases of the lacrimal or salivary glands, as may occur in tuberculosis, metastatic cancer, malignant lymphomas, and leukemia. Because what Mikulicz originally described is uncertain, the terms* Mikulicz's disease *and* Mikulicz's syndrome *should be completely avoided. This will eliminate much confusion that now exists in the literature and in clinical terminology.*

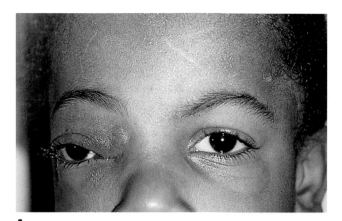

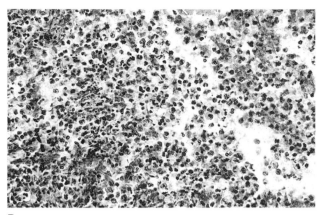

B

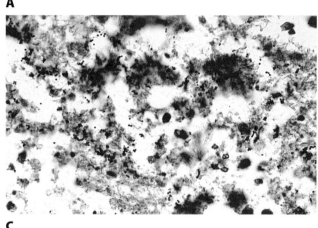

C

Fig. 14.6 Orbital cellulitis secondary to acute ethmoiditis. **A,** Acute purulent inflammatory infiltrate present around right eye in child. **B,** Similar purulent reaction, consisting mainly of neutrophils, is seen in tissue removed from another child. **C,** Special stain shows many Gram-positive cocci.

1. It is characterized by painless unilateral or bilateral enlargement of the salivary or, rarely, the lacrimal glands.
2. It may be part of Sjögren's syndrome (see later).
3. Rarely, it may become malignant.
4. Histologically, two features characterize benign lymphoepithelial lesion: (a) replacement of the glandular parenchyma by a benign lymphoid infiltrate and general preservation of the lobular architecture of the lacrimal gland; and (b) epimyoepithelial islands of proliferation in the glandular ducts.

C. Sjögren's syndrome (see Fig. 14.8)
1. Sjögren's syndrome is defined as a chronic autoimmune disorder characterized by lymphoid inflammatory infiltration of the lacrimal and salivary glands, destroying acinar tissue.

> Autoantibodies to the ribonucleoprotein (RNP) particles SS-A (also called Ro RNA particle) and SS-B (also called La snRNA) are produced systemically. The immune response to 120-kD α-fodrin may be important in the initial development of Sjögren's syndrome.

2. The tissue destruction results in the symptoms of keratoconjunctivitis sicca and xerostomia.

> The tissue destruction in the lacrimal gland may be related to elaboration of granzyme A and perforin. Rarely, the infiltrate can extend outside the lacrimal gland into the orbit.

3. Indirect support exists for a putative role of the Epstein–Barr virus (see p. 63 in Chapter 3) in the pathogenesis of the disease.

D. Inflammatory pseudotumor (see pp. 571–573 in this chapter)

II. Granulomatous
A. Granulomatous inflammations rarely involve the orbit.
B. Causes include tuberculosis, sarcoidosis, syphilis, fungi, parasites (trichinosis, schistosomiasis, and so forth), Crohn's disease, cat-scratch disease, midline lethal granuloma syndrome (polymorphic reticulosis), and giant cell polymyositis (giant cell granulomatous necrotizing myositis).

> *Tolosa–Hunt syndrome* is a benign granulomatous orbital inflammation of unknown cause that presents as a painful ophthalmoplegia. Symptoms usually disappear after steroid therapy.

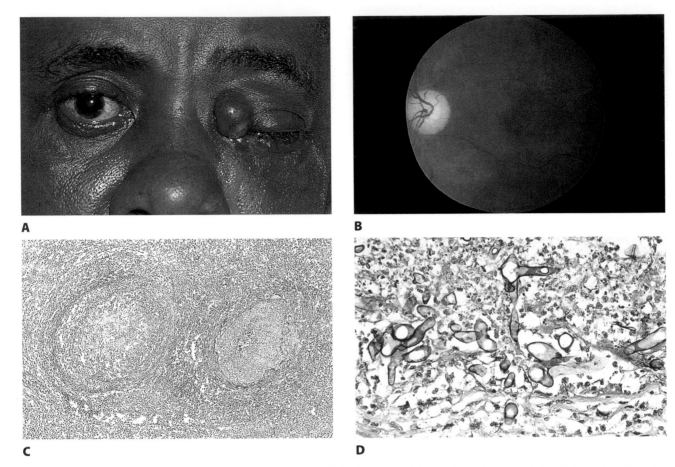

Fig. 14.7 Orbital phycomycosis. **A,** Diabetic man had phycomycosis of left orbit, causing left central retinal artery occlusion. **B,** Systemic antifungal therapy arrested condition. **C,** Orbital tissue obtained from another patient who died from phycomycosis shows two large thrombosed orbital vessels surrounded by acute suppurative inflammation. Even under this low magnification, large, hematoxylinophilic, nonseptate fungal hyphae (round bodies) can be seen in the wall of the smaller vessel (artery) on the right. **D,** Increased magnification of another case stained with periodic acid–Schiff clearly shows the organisms. (**A** and **B,** Courtesy of Dr. LA Karp; **C,** courtesy of Dr. H Ring.)

C. Cholesterol granuloma
1. Cholesterol granuloma has also been called *cholesteatoma, lipid granuloma of the frontal bone, xanthomatosis of the orbit, hematoma,* and *chronic hematic cyst.*

> Some authors incorrectly use the term *cholesteatoma* interchangeably with *epidermoid cyst.* The term *epidermoid cyst* should not be used, or should be restricted to postinflammatory tumors that contain squamous epithelium and keratin debris; cholesterol granuloma is never associated with any epithelial elements.

2. Cholesterol granuloma of the orbital bones is a rare extraperiosteal condition that usually involves the frontal bone above the lacrimal fossa.

3. The cause seems to be a hemorrhage into the diploë of the bone, probably secondary to trauma, but perhaps, secondary to an anomaly in the diploë that could initiate a hemorrhage.
4. Histologically, a granulomatous reaction surrounds cholesterol crystals and altered blood.
D. Inflammatory pseudotumor (see pp. 571–573 in this chapter)

INJURIES

Penetrating Wounds

I. Direct effect on whatever tissue may be wounded by the injury

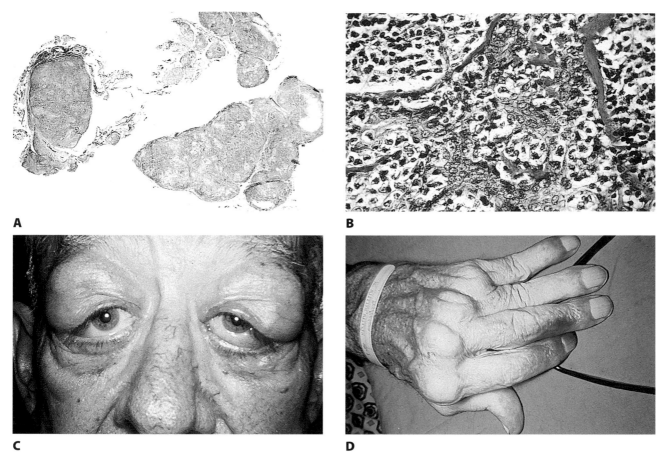

Fig. 14.8 Benign lymphoepithelial lesion (of Godwin) and Sjögren's syndrome. Benign lymphoepithelial lesion is characterized by: (1) the glandular parenchyma being replaced by benign lymphoid infiltrate (**A**); (2) general preservation of the glandular lobular architecture (**A**); and (3) epimyoepithelial islands of proliferation within glandular ducts (**B**). Note thickened ductal basement membrane. **C,** Patient who has Sjögren's syndrome shows bilateral lacrimal gland enlargement caused by Godwin's lesion and also rheumatoid arthritis (**D**). (**A** and **B,** From Font RL *et al.: Am J Clin Pathol* 48:365, 1968, with permission; **C** and **D,** modified from Meyer D *et al.: Am J Ophthalmol* 71:516. © Elsevier 1971.)

II. Complications (indirect effect)

  A. Infection

    1. Organisms may be introduced at the time of injury.

      a. Bacteria cause an acute purulent inflammation.

      b. Fungi cause a delayed, chronic, granulomatous inflammation.

  B. Inflammation

    1. The inflammation may be secondary to toxic products of tissue destruction.

    2. Orbital thrombophlebitis may result.

    3. A retained intraorbital foreign body may induce inflammation.

      a. Frequently, cilia and pieces of skin, bone, wood, and so forth may be introduced into the orbit at the time of injury and cause a foreign-body granulomatous inflammatory reaction.

      b. Fungi may enter as a coincidental saprophyte along with the penetrating foreign body, which usually causes a granulomatous inflammatory reaction or even superimposed infection if the organism proliferates.

  C. Orbital inflammation may lead to other complications such as cavernous sinus thrombosis, central retinal vein thrombosis, glaucoma, and proptosis.

Nonpenetrating Wounds

The effects of nonpenetrating wounds are those secondary to contusion and concussion, mainly hemorrhage, secondary muscle palsies, and infraorbital nerve involvement.

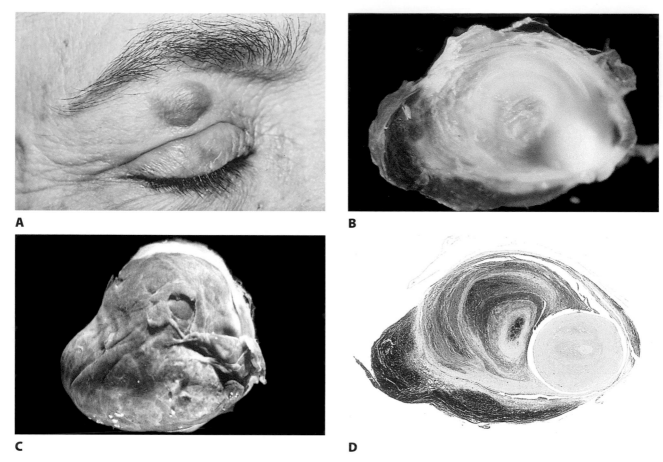

Fig. 14.9 Orbital varix. **A,** Clinical appearance of varix before removal. Gross appearance of skin (**B**) and internal (**C**) side of removed varix. **D,** Trichrome stains show microscopic appearance of clotted vein.

VASCULAR DISEASE

Primary

  I. Primary orbital vascular disease is rare
  II. Causes include varices, arteriovenular aneurysm, thrombophlebitis, and cavernous sinus thrombosis

> Orbital varix, also called *distensible venous malformation* (Fig. 14.9), may occur anterior to the septum orbitale and not cause exophthalmos, or it may occur posterior to the septum orbitale, causing exophthalmos. The exophthalmos may be acute if the varix undergoes thrombosis.

Part of Systemic Disease

  I. Collagen diseases (see pp. 182–184 in Chapter 6, and p. 540 in this chapter)
  II. Midline lethal granuloma syndrome (*natural killer (NK)/T-cell lymphoma*, polymorphic or malignant reticulosis; see section later this chapter and p. 184 in Chapter 6)
  III. Allergic granulomatosis (vasculitis; see p. 184 in Chapter 6)
  IV. Temporal (cranial) arteritis (see p. 507 in Chapter 13)

OCULAR MUSCLE INVOLVEMENT IN SYSTEMIC DISEASE

Graves' Disease (Fig. 14.10)

  I. Classification of eye changes of Graves' disease (Table 14.1)
  II. Mild form ("thyrotoxic" exophthalmos)
    A. The mild form of Graves' ophthalmopathy has its onset in early adult life, with women predominantly affected (approximately 2:1).

> Smokers have an increased risk for development of both Graves' disease and thyroid ophthalmopathy. Temporally, the diagnosis of Graves' ophthalmopathy tends to follow the diagnosis of hyperthyroidism. Treatment of hyperthyroidism with iodine-131 does not seem to alter the course of Graves' ophthalmopathy.

    B. It may present initially with unilateral involvement, but usually becomes bilateral.
    C. Clinically and chemically, the patient is hyperthyroid.
    D. Lid retraction may simulate exophthalmos.

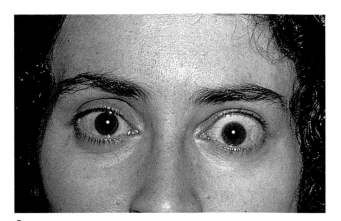

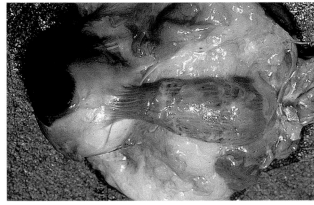

A

B

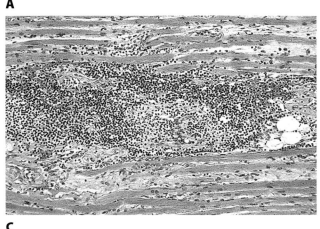

C

Fig. 14.10 Graves' disease. **A,** In Graves' disease, exophthalmos often looks more pronounced than it actually is because of the extreme lid retraction that may occur. This patient, for instance, had minimal proptosis of the left eye but marked lid retraction. **B,** The orbital contents obtained postmortem from a patient with Graves' disease. Note the enormously thickened extraocular muscle. **C,** A histologic section shows both fluid and inflammatory cells separating the muscle bundles. The inflammatory cells are predominantly lymphocytes, plus plasma cells. (**A,** Courtesy of Dr. HG Scheie; **B** and **C,** courtesy of Dr. RC Eagle, Jr., case in **B** and **C** reported in Hufnagel TJ *et al.: Ophthalmology* 91:1411. © Elsevier 1984.)

TABLE 14.1 Eye Changes in Graves' Disease	
Class	**Ocular Symptoms and Signs**
0	No signs or symptoms
1	Only signs, no symptoms
2	Soft-tissue involvement with symptoms and signs
3	Proptosis of the eyes
4	Extraocular muscle involvement
5	Corneal involvement
6	Sight loss with optic nerve involvement

(Modified from Werner SC: Am J Ophthalmol 68:646, 1969.)

Lid retraction is the most common clinical sign of Graves' ophthalmopathy.

   E. Occasionally exophthalmos is present.

   F. Prognosis for vision is good.

III. Severe form ("thyrotropic" or "malignant" exophthalmos; thyroid ophthalmopathy; thyroid orbitopathy)

A. The severe form is an autoimmune disease that affects people in middle age (average age, 50 years).

   1. The disease is characterized by an increased percentage of suppressor/cytotoxic T lymphocytes.

   2. Circulating T cells are directed against thyroid follicular cell antigens.

B. The severe form is most common in men, especially those older than 50 years of age. The disease is usually bilateral and asymmetric.

C. Clinically and chemically, the patient may be hyperthyroid, hypothyroid, or euthyroid.

The term *euthyroid Graves' disease* describes ocular manifestations of Graves' disease in patients who are "euthyroid," and have no past history suggesting hyperthyroidism. The eye signs are frequently asymmetric. The patients may have a family history of thyroid disease or pernicious anemia. All of the euthyroid patients, however, do show some mild thyroid abnormality (e.g., thyroid autoantibodies, negative thyrotropin-releasing hormone test, negative triiodothyronine suppression test, goiter).

D. Exophthalmos is severe, and frequently associated with pretibial myxedema. Chemosis, dilated vessels (especially over the rectus muscles), and limitation of ocular motility often accompany the exophthalmos.

Orbital accumulation of glycosaminoglycans and increased adipogenesis may play an important role in the development of Graves' ophthalmopathy.

E. Prognosis for vision is poor.
F. Histologically, the orbital tissue is characterized predominantly by extraocular and periorbital muscle involvement by edema, lymphocytic infiltration (mainly CD4+ and CD8+ T cells along with some focal aggregates of B cells, plasma cells, and mast cells), endomysial fibrosis, and mucopolysaccharide deposition.
   1. Positive staining occurs in extraocular and periorbital muscle for immunoglobulin A1 (IgA1) and IgE antibodies, and C3bi (the terminal attack complex) complement component.

The inferior rectus muscle is most prone to fibrosis. If the patient is looking up during tonometry, abnormally high readings may be obtained. It is important, therefore, that the patient be looking straight ahead during applanation tonometry.

Myasthenia Gravis

I. Myasthenia gravis is an autoimmune disorder (defect on chromosome 19q13.3) that involves the extraocular muscles, especially the levator palpebrae superioris. A reduction in available acetylcholine receptors occurs at the neuromuscular junctions of skeletal muscles.
II. The most common clinical manifestation is ptosis of the eyelid.

As a rough test, the ptosis can often be aggravated by having the patient raise and lower the eyes 10 to 30 times in rapid succession. The normal patient can do this easily with no ptosis afterward.

III. Histologically, the ocular muscles are edematous and infiltrated by lymphocytes.

Myotonic Dystrophy (Myotonia Dystrophica; Steinert's Disease)

I. Myotonic dystrophy, an autosomal-dominant condition, is characterized by myotonia (i.e., failure to relax a contracted muscle voluntarily).

Myotonic dystrophy, like Huntington's disease, is caused by an expansion of a repeated sequence of three nucleotides. In myotonic dystrophy the expansion occurs in the 3' untranslated region of the *DM* gene. Perhaps disrupted activity of a CUG-binding protein induced by repeats in RNA prevents the protein from doing its normal job of splicing a certain family of genes.

A. Its onset is between 20 and 30 years of age, with patients rarely living beyond 40 or 50 years.
B. Frontal baldness and endocrinopathy, especially testicular atrophy, are common.

II. Ocular findings
   A. Cataracts showing iridescent dots in the anterior and posterior cortex, and a stellate grouping of opacities at the posterior pole of the lens along the posterior suture lines
   B. Foveal dystrophy that hardly affects vision
   C. Pigmentary retinopathy
   D. Ocular hypotension
III. Histologically, selective atrophy of muscle fibers is seen.

Myotonia Congenita (Thomsen's Disease)

I. Myotonia congenita, an autosomal-dominant or recessive condition, is characterized by myotonia
   A. Its onset is early in life and may involve muscles of the face and eyelids.
   B. It does not cause death and rarely causes severe disability.
II. Histologically, the muscles are not atrophic; individual muscle fibers may be larger than normal with an increase in sarcolemmal nuclei

Mitochondrial Myopathies

I. Mitochondrial myopathies (cytopathies) are rare multisystem diseases that mainly affect the central nervous and musculoskeletal systems.
   Abnormal mitochondria are found in the periphery of skeletal muscle fibers, which have a characteristic "ragged-red" appearance when stained with the modified trichrome stain.
II. Four of these entities are of major ophthalmic importance: Leber's hereditary optic atrophy, chronic progressive external ophthalmoplegia (CPEO), Kearns–Sayre syndrome, and the syndrome of mitochondrial encephalomyopathy, lactic acidosis, and strokelike episodes (MELAS).

The inheritance of these point mutations of mitochondrial DNA is from mothers alone because the mitochondrial contribution to the embryo comes only from the maternal ovum.

A. Leber's hereditary optic atrophy (see p. 501 in Chapter 13)
B. CPEO
   1. CPEO, one of the mitochondrial myopathies, is a slowly progressive, bilaterally symmetric, ocular muscle dystrophy that starts in late childhood or adulthood.
   2. CPEO is inherited through the maternal transmission of one or more mitochondrial large-deletion DNA mutations.
   3. Ptosis, external ophthalmoplegia, and often a pigmentary retinopathy can be seen.
   4. Histology of muscle fibers
      a. Atrophy, large variation in diameter, and granular and vacuolar degeneration

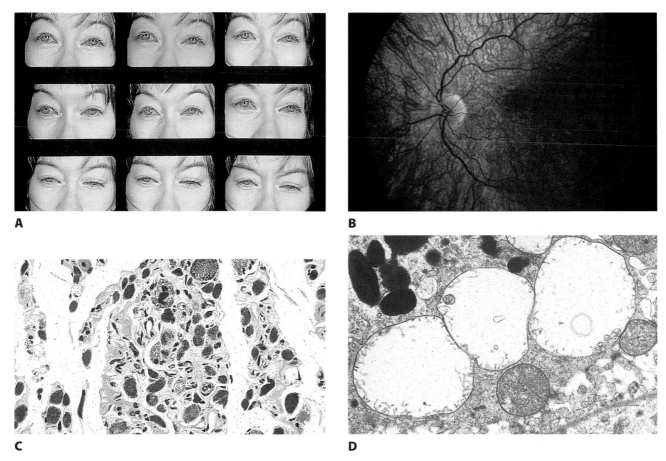

Fig. 14.11 Mitochondrial encephalomyopathy, lactic acidosis, and strokelike episodes (MELAS) syndrome. **A,** Complete external ophthalmoplegia present in 20-year-old woman. **B,** Fundus shows a fine, dustlike, "salt-and-pepper" appearance. **C,** Microscopic section of degenerated extraocular muscles stained with trichrome shows "ragged-red" fibers. **D,** Cytoplasm of retinal pigment epithelial cells packed with many ballooned, structurally abnormal ("giant") mitochondria. (Case presented by Dr. R Folberg to the meeting of the Verhoeff Society, 1993 and reported by Rummelt V *et al.: Ophthalmology* 100:1757. © Elsevier 1993.)

b. Absence of glycogen, cross-striations, myofibrillar structure, and succinic dehydrogenase
c. Fibrous and fatty replacement of tissue
d. Preservation of myelinated nerve fibers and myoneural junctions

---

Mitochondria of selective muscle fibers appear abnormal in size, shape, number, and internal structure, whereas others seem normal, resembling the changes found in Leber's hereditary optic atrophy. Because the modified trichrome stain colors the abnormal muscle fibers red, the fibers have been called *ragged-red fibers.*

C. Kearns–Sayre syndrome
1. Kearns–Sayre syndrome consists of the triad of external ophthalmoplegia, pigmentary retinopathy, and heart block. Other findings include mental retardation, hearing loss, endocrinopathy, and cerebellar ataxia.
2. Kearns–Sayre syndrome is inherited through the maternal transmission of one or more mitochondrial large-deletion DNA mutations.

3. Histologically, along with the characteristic ragged-red appearance seen under light microscopy with the modified trichrome stain, electron microscopy shows well-preserved, swollen mitochondria containing circular cristae or granular deposits.
D. MELAS (Fig. 14.11)
1. MELAS usually has an abrupt onset before the age of 15 years with symptoms of visual loss, hemiparesis or hemianopia, strokelike episodes, headaches, and convulsions.
2. Patients have short stature and increased serum and cerebrospinal fluid lactate levels.
3. MELAS is inherited through the maternal transmission of one or more mitochondrial point DNA mutations (nucleotide positions 3243 and 3271).
4. Ocular findings include external ophthalmoplegia, atypical pigmentary retinopathy, and nuclear cataract.
5. Histologically, along with the characteristic ragged-red appearance seen under light microscopy with the modified trichrome stain, electron microscopy

shows an increased number of mitochondria containing abnormal cristae.

a. The eyes show abnormalities of the macular photoreceptor–retinal pigment epithelium (RPE)–choriocapillaris complex, namely, absent or degenerated outer segments and hyperpigmented and hypopigmented RPE.

1). The cytoplasm of RPE cells show ballooned, structurally abnormal ("giant") mitochondria.

2). The photoreceptor inner segments demonstrate markedly altered mitochondria (increased number, loss of cristae, circular cristae, ballooned mitochondria, and paracrystalline inclusions).

b. Abnormal mitochondria are also found in choriocapillaris endothelial cells and smooth-muscle cells of choroidal and retinal blood vessel walls.

Dermatomyositis

I. Dermatomyositis is a collagen disease of unknown cause with a poor prognosis; death is a frequent outcome.

II. Men predominate and may acquire the disease in childhood.

III. Conjunctivitis, iritis, ptosis, paralysis of external ocular muscles, horizontal nystagmus, and exophthalmos may be present.

Erythematous, edematous patches of skin are frequently seen. A predilection for the face and periorbital region exists, where a violaceous heliotrope may occur around the eyes, on the lids, and on the cheeks.

IV. A retinitis may be seen with superficial whitish exudates in the macula, and round and flame-shaped hemorrhages.

V. Histologically, lymphocytes are present in the muscles (myositis) and in the walls of blood vessels (vasculitis), giving a picture of a nonspecific chronic nongranulomatous inflammation.

NEOPLASMS AND OTHER TUMORS*

See Table 14.2 for classification of neoplasms and other tumors.

Primary Orbital Tumors

Orbital tumors in the senior adult population are malignant in 63% of cases, malignant lymphoma being the most common.

In the following text, a dagger (†) after the name of the tumor denotes that the tumor is common, important, or both; a double dagger (‡) denotes that the tumor is uncommon, unimportant, or both.

I. Choristomas—these are congenital tumors not normally present at the involved site.

A. Epidermoid cyst†

1. An epidermoid cyst is composed of epidermis (i.e., stratified squamous epithelium with no epidermal appendages in the wall of the cyst) and contains desquamated keratin in the cyst, which appears as a cheesy material.

a. An epidermoid cyst tends to occur in the superotemporal aspect of the orbit, often anterior to the septum orbitale.

Rarely, an epidermoid cyst may originate in the diploic space of the orbital bone, called an *intradiploic* epidermoid cyst. Also rarely, squamous cell carcinoma may develop in an epidermoid or dermoid cyst.

---

b. A much rarer type of congenital epithelial cyst is called *primary nonkeratinized epithelial cyst* ("conjunctival cyst"; see Fig. 14.12D and E). It is usually found in the superonasal aspect of the orbit, is lined by nonkeratinizing epithelium that resembles conjunctival epithelium, contains no adnexal structures in its wall, and is filled with clear fluid.

2. Histologically, a congenital epidermoid cyst and an acquired (usually secondary to trauma) epithelial inclusion cyst appear identical.

Rarely, an epithelial conjunctival inclusion cyst may occur in an orbit after enucleation.

B. Dermoid cyst† (Fig. 14.12)

1. A dermoid cyst is probably a result of the sequestration of surface ectoderm pinched off at bony suture lines or along lines of embryonic closure.

a. It is most often found in the superotemporal quadrant of the orbit (rarely, a dermoid may occur in the lateral rectus muscle).

b. A dermoid may have a pedicle attached to the periorbita and may produce bony changes detectable on radiography.

c. A much rarer type, which is lined by nonkeratinizing epithelium (resembling conjunctival epithelium), contains adnexal structures in its wall, and is filled with clear fluid, is called *primary nonkeratinized epidermoid cyst* ("conjunctival cyst").

Primary nonkeratinized epidermoid cysts probably represent developmental sequestrations of forniceal or caruncular conjunctival epithelium. They are found in the superonasal quadrant (see Fig. 14.12D and E) and are not associated with an osseous defect. They constitute approximately 75% of the superonasal dermoids, the other 25% being the typical dermoids lined by keratinizing squamous epithelium.

TABLE 14.2 Classification of Neoplasms and Other Tumors

PRIMARY ORBITAL TUMORS

Choristomas

Epidermoid cyst†
Dermoid cyst† (see Figs 14.12 and 14.13)
Teratoma‡ (see Fig. 14.14)
Ectopic lacrimal gland‡ (see Fig. 14.15)

Hamartomas

Phakomatoses† (see Chapter 2)
Hemangioma
    Capillary hemangioma† (see Figs 14.16 and 14.17)
    Cavernous hemangioma† (see Fig. 14.18)
    Arteriovenous communication‡ (see Chapter 2)
    Telangiectasia‡ (see Chapter 2)
Lymphangioma† (see Fig. 14.19)

Mesenchymal Tumors

Vascular
    Hemangiopericytoma‡
    Glomus tumor‡ (see Fig. 14.20)
    Hemangiosarcoma‡
    Kaposi's sarcoma‡ (see Fig. 14.21)
Fatty
    Lipoma† (see Fig. 14.22)
    Liposarcoma‡ (see Fig. 14.23)
Fibrous
    Reactive fibrous proliferations
        Nodular fasciitis†
        Juvenile fibromatosis‡
    Neoplastic fibrous proliferations
        Fibrous histiocytoma† (see Fig. 14.24)
        Fibroma‡ and fibrosarcoma‡ (see Fig. 14.25)
        Solitary fibrous tumor‡
        Giant cell angiofibroma‡
Muscle
    Leiomyoma (see Fig. 14.26)‡ and leiomyosarcoma‡
    Mesectodermal leiomyosarcoma‡ (see Chapter 9)
    Rhabdomyoma‡
    Rhabdomyosarcoma† (see Figs 14.27 and 14.28; see also Fig. 17.26)
Cartilage
    Chondroma‡ and chondrosarcoma‡
Bone
    Aneurysmal bone cyst‡
    Fibrous dysplasia† (see Fig. 14.29)
    Giant cell tumor‡
    Juvenile fibromatosis‡
Leontiasis ossea‡

Osteitis fibrosa cystica†

Osteopetrosis‡
Paget's disease†
Osteoma‡ and osteogenic sarcoma (osteosarcoma)‡

Neural Tumors

Amputation neuroma‡
Neurofibroma† (see Chapter 2)
Neurilemmoma† (see Figs 14.30 and 14.31)
Juvenile pilocystic astrocytoma† (see Chapter 13)
Peripheral primitive neuroectodermal tumors (PNETs)‡ (see Fig. 14.32)

Miscellaneous Tumors

Meningioma† (see Chapter 13)
Nonchromaffin paraganglioma‡
Granular cell tumor‡ (see Fig. 14.33)
Alveolar soft-part sarcoma‡ (see Fig. 14.34)
Malignant melanoma‡ (see Chapter 17)
Endodermal sinus tumor‡

Epithelial Cysts and Neoplasms of Lacrimal Gland

Lacrimal ductal cysts†
Benign mixed tumor† (see Fig. 14.35)
Malignant mixed tumor† (see Fig. 14.36)
Adenoid cystic carcinoma† (see Fig. 14.37)
Other types of carcinoma‡ (see Fig. 14.38)

Reticuloendothelial System, Lymphatic System, and Myeloid System

Reticuloendothelial system
    Langerhans' granulomatoses (histiocytosis X)†
        Eosinophilic granuloma† (see Fig. 14.39)
        Hand–Schüller–Christian disease†
        Letterer–Siwe disease‡ (see Fig. 14.40)
        Juvenile xanthogranuloma† (see Chapter 9)
        Sinus histiocytosis‡ (see Fig. 14.41)
    Inflammatory pseudotumor† (see Fig. 14.42)
    Malignant lymphoma† (see Figs. 14.43–14.46)
    Leukemia† (see Fig. 14.47)
    Multiple myeloma‡ (see Fig. 14.48)
    Monoclonal and polyclonal gammopathies‡

SECONDARY ORBITAL TUMORS

Direct Extension† (see Fig. 14.49)

Metastatic†

†*The tumor is common, important, or both.*
‡*The tumor is uncommon, unimportant, or both.*

  2. Histologically, a dermoid cyst, derived from ectoderm, is composed of a wall surrounding a cavity.
      a. The wall is lined by keratinizing, stratified squamous epithelium and contains epidermal appendages (e.g., hair follicles, sebaceous glands, sweat glands).

Rupture of a dermoid cyst can cause a chronic granulomatous inflammatory reaction (Fig. 14.13). Rarely, squamous cell carcinoma may develop in an epidermoid or dermoid cyst.

      b. The cavity contains desquamated keratin, hair shafts, and debris.

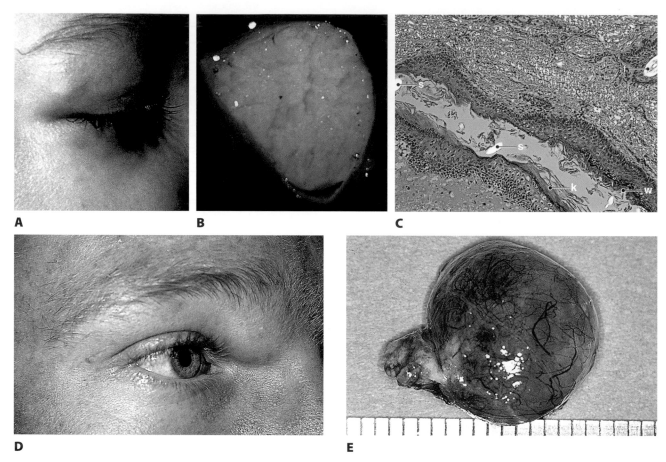

Fig. 14.12 Dermoid cyst. **A,** A dermoid tumor is present in its most common location: the superior temporal portion of the orbit. **B,** Gross examination of the cut surface of the tumor shows a cyst filled with "cheesy" material. **C,** A histologic section, viewed using polarized light, shows a cyst lined by stratified squamous epithelium. Hair follicles (which contain birefringent hair shafts) and other epidermal appendages are contained in the wall of the cyst. The cyst itself contains keratin debris (k) and hair shafts (s) which are birefringent in the polarized light (f, hair follicle; w, wall of cyst). **D** and **E,** A much rarer type, found in the superonasal quadrant, containing clear fluid, and lined by nonkeratinizing epithelium, is called *primary nonkeratinized epidermoid cyst* ("conjunctival cyst"). The cyst in **D** and **E** contained adnexal structures in its wall. (**A,** Courtesy of Dr. JA Katowitz.)

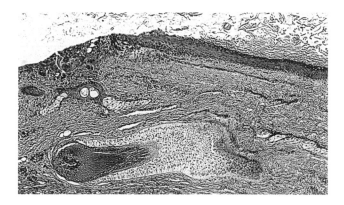

Fig. 14.13 Dermoid cyst. Rupture of the dermoid cyst has caused a chronic granulomatous inflammatory reaction.

C. Teratoma‡ (Fig. 14.14)

1. An orbital teratoma is an embryonic tumor composed of all three embryonic germinal cell layers (ectoderm, endoderm, and mesoderm).

A rare teratoma has been reported in an intraocular location. A teratoma can also have both an orbital and an extraorbital (limited intracranial extension) or periorbital (beneath the skin and scalp) location.

---

2. It characteristically causes massive exophthalmos at birth and may contain structures such as stratified squamous epithelium, colonic mucosa, and central nervous system tissue.

3. It has malignant potential and may also involve the eye.

D. Cholesterol granuloma and cholesteatoma (see p. 534 in this chapter)

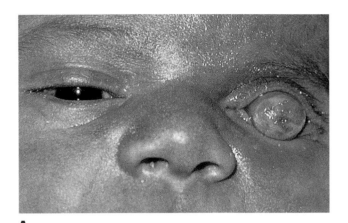

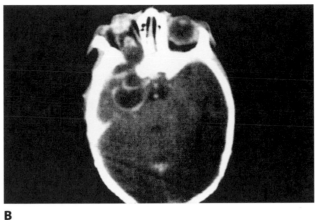

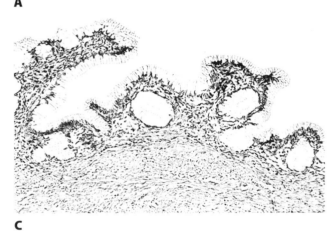

Fig. 14.14 Teratoma. **A,** Child presented with a cystic eyeball protruding between the left eyelids. **B,** Computed tomography scan shows cystic structures extending back into brain. **C,** Removal of left orbital cystic contents showed a large teratoma, which was behind an atrophic eyeball. The teratoma contained many choristomatous structures, including intestinal tract lined by colonic mucosa. (**A** and **B,** Courtesy of Dr. JA Katowitz.)

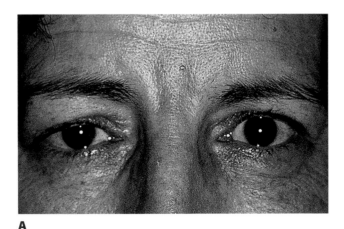

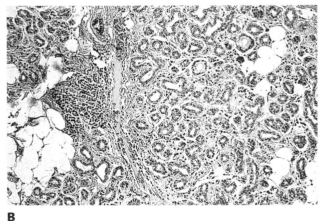

Fig. 14.15 Ectopic lacrimal gland. **A,** Proptosis of left eye. **B,** Biopsy of retrobulbar mass, which was not connected to the lacrimal gland, shows glandular tissue that resembles lacrimal gland, with foci of chronic nongranulomatous inflammation. (**A,** Courtesy of Dr. HG Scheie.)

E. Ectopic lacrimal gland‡ (Fig. 14.15)
   1. Ectopic lacrimal gland consists of lacrimal gland tissue found anywhere except in the lacrimal fossa.
   2. It may be associated with other choristomatous tissues such as muscle, nerve, cartilage, or various dermal appendages, or it may occur alone.

   3. It usually causes symptoms only when inflamed; the origin of the inflammation is unknown.
   4. Histologically, it is composed of relatively normal-looking lacrimal gland tissue with a mild inflammatory infiltrate of lymphocytes and plasma cells.
II. Hamartomas—these are congenital tumors normally found at the involved site.

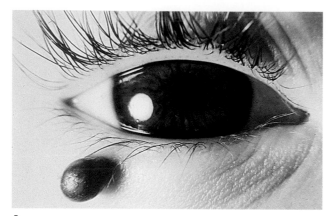

A

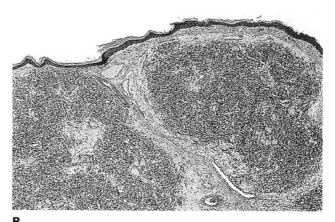

B

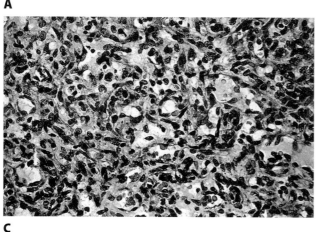

C

Fig. 14.16 Capillary hemangioma. **A,** Clinical appearance of tumor. **B,** Tumor composed of blood vessels of predominantly capillary size. **C,** High magnification shows capillaries and endothelial cells.

A. Phakomatoses (see Chapter 2)
B. Hemangioma
1. Capillary hemangioma ("cherry" hemangioma)† (Fig. 14.16)
   a. A capillary hemangioma, the most common periocular vascular tumor in infancy and childhood, is usually solitary, bright red, and smooth.

   Another form occurs in middle-aged or older people, often those with cardiovascular problems.

   ---

   b. Usually, a capillary hemangioma begins before 2 months of age, reaches maximum size by 6 to 12 months, and then tends to regress (involute) spontaneously by 4 to 7 years. Although it usually regresses, it can cause deprivation or anisometropic amblyopia, strabismus, and other problems before regression is attained.
   c. A form of capillary hemangioma is found in angiomatosis retinae (see p. 29 in Chapter 2).
   d. A variant of capillary hemangioma, often called *hemangioendothelioma* (Fig. 14.17), is observed at birth (20%), infancy, or early childhood. Typically, it appears suddenly, grows rapidly, and is characterized by relatively solid cords of round, multilayered endothelial cells with little or no evidence of lumen.

   The tumor has also been called *benign hemangioendothelioma* and *strawberry, infantile,* and *juvenile hemangioma*. The lesion, although benign, may arise in a number of areas simultaneously and thereby simulate invasion and malignancy. The tumor almost always regresses spontaneously. Histologically, it consists mainly of plump endothelial cells, some of which form a capillary lumen.

   ---

   e. Histologically, the capillary hemangioma is composed primarily of capillaries lined by plump endothelial cells.
2. Cavernous hemangioma† (orbital cavernoma) (Fig. 14.18)
   a. Cavernous hemangioma is the *most common* primary orbital tumor producing exophthalmos.
   b. It may press on the coats of the eye and cause chorioretinal striae.
   c. It is a well-encapsulated tumor, usually within the muscle cone, and can often be shelled out easily with little or no bleeding.

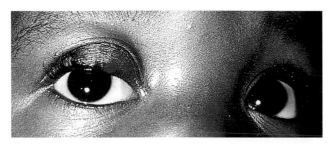

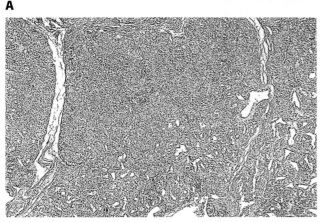

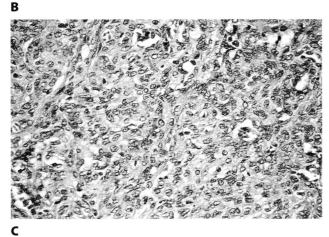

Fig. 14.17 Hemangioendothelioma variant of capillary hemangioma. **A,** Child shows diffuse thickening of right upper lid. **B,** Biopsy shows tumor composed primarily of endothelial cells and occasional capillaries. **C,** High magnification shows endothelial cells. (**A,** Courtesy of Dr. RE Shannon.)

Rarely, the tumor may arise in the orbital bones. Even more rarely, the tumor may be associated with the *blue rubber bleb nevus syndrome* (multiple cutaneous and visceral bluish-red, rubbery hemangiomas; may be autosomal dominant but most cases are sporadic). If bilateral orbital hemangiomas are present, they may be part of the *blue rubber bleb nevus syndrome* or *Maffuci's syndrome* (nonhereditary disease characterized by hemangiomas and enchondromas).

   d. No feeder vessels are demonstrated by dye study techniques.

Rarely, a cavernous hemangioma may bleed and give rise to a *hematic cyst*. The cyst contains birefringent crystals and altered blood that seem to initiate a granulomatous inflammation (similar to a cholesterol granuloma—see p. 534 in this chapter). Other causes of hematic cyst include blunt trauma, spontaneous orbital hemorrhage, blood dyscrasias, vascular disease, and lymphangioma.

   e. Histologically, it is composed of large, blood-filled spaces, lined by endothelium and separated by fibrous septa ranging from quite thin to fairly thick.

The endothelial cells of hemangiomas give a strong reaction for factor VIII-related antigen (FVIII-RAG).

3. Arteriovenous communication‡
   a. Arteriovenous communication (arteriovenous or varix aneurysm; tumor cirsoides; angiomatous malformation; cirsoid, serpentine, plexiform, racemose, or cavernous angioma) is a rare malformation or developmental anomaly between the arterial and venous systems.
   b. It occurs in arteriovenous communication of retina and brain or as an incidental finding.
   c. Histologically, it is composed of mature blood vessels that may be hypertrophied.

      The malformation seems to be a mature artery (albeit hypertrophied) that is becoming a mature vein (also often hypertrophied) without passing through a vascular (i.e., capillary) bed.

4. Telangiectasia‡
   a. Telangiectasia of the orbit is rare.
   b. Telangiectasia is found in meningocutaneous angiomatosis (see pp. 30–31 in Chapter 2), ataxia–telangiectasia (see p. 36 in Chapter 2), and Osler–Rendu–Weber disease (see p. 225 in Chapter 7).
   c. Histologically, it is composed of dilated and tortuous capillaries.

C. Lymphangioma† (Fig. 14.19)

Often lymphangiomas contain both venous and lymphatic components, hence, another term for the lesions is *combined venous lymphatic malformations*. The lesions may be associated with noncontiguous intracranial vascular anomalies.

1. Frequently, the clinical onset of lymphangioma is in children younger than 10 years of age.
2. It may diffusely involve the orbit, conjunctiva, and lids, and tends to be invasive and slow-growing.
   a. Clinically at presentation, proptosis occurs in 85% of cases, blepharoptosis in 73%, and restriction of eye movements in 46%.
   b. Although retinal folds may be seen, compressive optic neuropathy is rare.

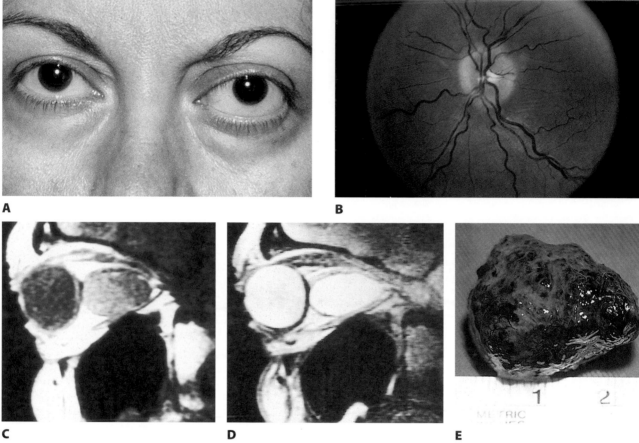

A, **B,** **C,** **D,** **E,**

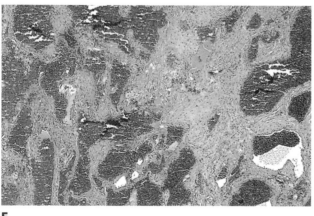

F,

Fig. 14.18 Cavernous hemangioma. **A,** Clinical appearance of left exophthalmos. **B,** Pressure of tumor on optic nerve has caused optic disc edema. **C,** Magnetic resonance imaging shows optic nerve stretched over tumor in T1-weighted image. **D,** Tumor "lights up" in T2-weighted image, characteristic of a hemangioma. **E,** Gross appearance of surgically removed hemangioma. **F,** Histologic section shows large, blood-filled spaces of tumor lined by endothelium and separated by fibrous septa of different thicknesses. (Case presented by Dr. WC Frayer to the meeting of the Verhoeff Society, 1989.)

3. The tumor probably regresses somewhat in time, but easily becomes infected.
4. Histologically, it is composed of lymph-filled spaces of different sizes, lined by endothelium and separated by thin, delicate walls.

    Hemorrhage in the lesion produces a "chocolate cyst."

III. Mesenchymal tumors
  A. Vascular
    1. Hemangiomas and lymphangioma (see earlier under discussion of hamartomas)
    2. Hemangiopericytoma‡

a. This rare orbital tumor is most common in the fourth decade.

Rarely, a hemangiopericytoma can involve the epibulbar region anteriorly.

b. It may be malignant in 12% to 57% of cases (varies according to authors' series).

It seems that the longer the follow-up, the greater the mortality rate from the tumor.

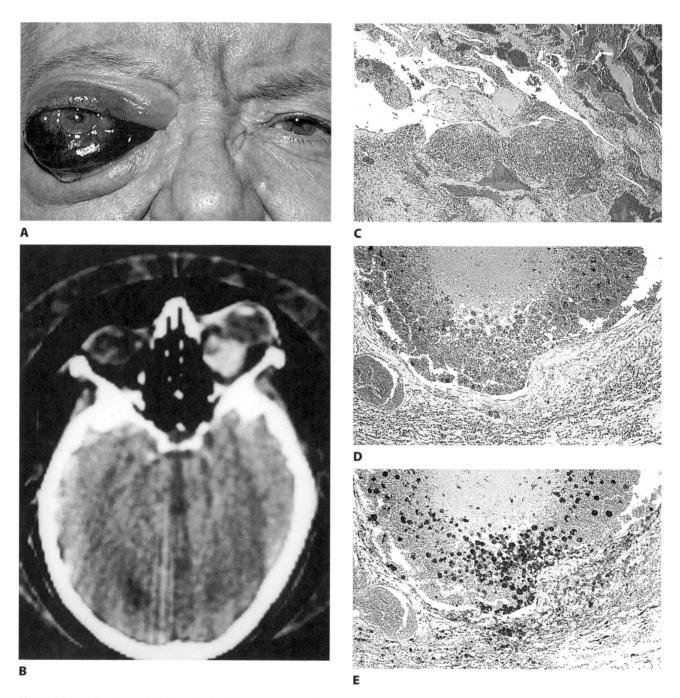

Fig. 14.19 Lymphangioma. **A,** Patient developed acute proptosis of right eye. **B,** Computed tomographic appearance of retrobulbar tumor. **C,** Histologic section of surgically removed specimen shows tumor composed of lymph-filled spaces of varying sizes (some of the spaces contain blood). Note lymphoid collections in walls of tumor. **D,** Other areas show older blood (hemosiderin) in the lumen and septum that stains positively with Perl's stain for iron (blue color in **E**). Presumably, a hemorrhage into the lymphangioma caused the acute exophthalmos.

c. The clinical course cannot always be predicted from the histologic appearance, especially when the cytology "appears" benign.

d. The tumor probably arises from pericytes.

"Angioblastic type" of meningioma, once thought to be of meningeal origin, is now generally accepted to be a hemangiopericytoma of the central nervous system.

e. Histologically, an increased number of thin-walled vascular channels are separated by tumor cells in a network of extracellular material.

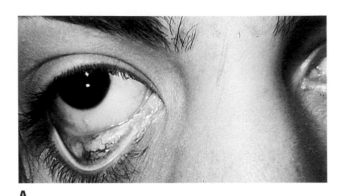

A

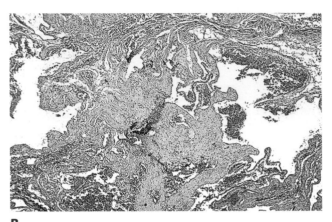

B

Fig. 14.20 Glomus tumor. **A,** A bluish tumor is present in the right lower lid. **B,** Histologic section shows vascular spaces lined by a single layer of endothelial cells and surrounded by layers of glomus cells. (Presented by Dr. NC Charles to the meeting of the Eastern Ophthalmic Pathology Society, 1975 and reported in Charles NC: *Arch Ophthalmol* 94:1283, 1976. © American Medical Association. All rights reserved.)

1). Perivascular massing of pericytes is present.
2). Silver-stained material reveals reticulin characteristically segregating cells into groups.
3). Cell morphology is uniform.

> The tumor is more likely to be malignant if the following occur: increased mitotic activity (>4 mitotic figures per 400 field), necrotic foci, pleomorphism, S-phase greater than 9, and a proliferative index greater than 11 (the last two determined by cell cycle analysis). Hemangiopericytoma resembles the vascular form of fibrous histiocytoma (FH; see pp. 551 in this chapter).

4). Focal staining for vimentin, CD34, and factor XIIIa occurs

3. Glomus tumor (glomangioma‡; Fig. 14.20)
   a. The glomus cell is probably a specialized smooth-muscle cell.
   b. A tumor composed of glomus cells, a very rare tumor, occurs in two forms: a solitary form and a familial form that shows multiple tumors involving face, palate, eyelid, and anterior orbit.
   c. Histologically, small vessels lined by a single layer of endothelial cells are surrounded by one or more layers of glomus cells.
      1). The cells are round and have small, round nuclei and clear cytoplasm.
      2). Immunohistochemically, the cells are positive for muscle-specific actin and vimentin, and are negative for factor VIII and other endothelial markers.

4. Hemangiosarcoma‡ (angiosarcoma, malignant hemangioendothelioma)
   a. This is a rare orbital tumor.

> *Intravascular papillary endothelial hyperplasia,* a benign lesion, has been confused with hemangiosar-

coma. Another benign lesion, probably a reactive or immunologic inflammatory process, angiolymphoid hyperplasia with eosinophilia (*Kimura's disease*; see p. 572 in this chapter), has also been mistaken for hemangiosarcoma.

   b. Histologically, it is composed of intercommunicating channels or irregular vascular spaces lined by atypical endothelial cells confined in a thin reticulin network.
      1). The endothelial cells may form a single layer, proliferate in focal areas, or produce papillary projections.

> The endothelial cells stain positively for FVIII-RAG and *Ulex europaeus* agglutinin I.

      2). Marked histologic variation is seen in the tumor, and from tumor to tumor.

5. Kaposi's sarcoma (KS‡; Fig. 14.21)
   a. KS, previously a disease of elderly men of Mediterranean or Eastern European Jewish ancestry, young black African men, or chemotherapy-immunosuppressed patients, now is associated with acquired immunodeficiency syndrome (AIDS) in almost all cases.

> Approximately 20% of patients who have AIDS also have KS (second only to *Pneumocystis carinii* infection as a presenting manifestation). In addition to AIDS, an association exists between KS and other cancers such as malignant lymphoma (especially Hodgkin's disease), leukemia, or a primary carcinoma with a separate histogenesis.

   b. KS is a multicentric vascular neoplasm that affects skin, mucous membranes, internal organs, and lymph nodes.

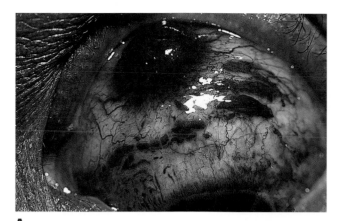

A

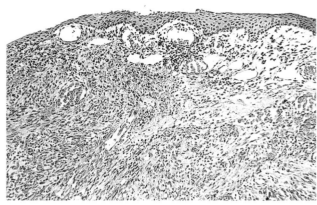

B

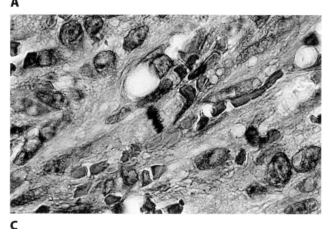

C

Fig. 14.21 Kaposi's sarcoma. **A,** A patient who was subsequently found to have the acquired immunodeficiency syndrome presented with a conjunctival tumor. **B,** Biopsy shows neoplastic cells that contain spindle-shaped nuclei and conspicuous nucleoli that are forming bundles or are lining vascular clefts. **C,** A mitotic figure is seen. (Case reported by Bedrick JJ *et al.: Arch Ophthalmol* 99:1607, 1981. © American Medical Association. All rights reserved.)

New herpesvirus-like DNA sequences (KSHV) have been found in classic, endemic, and AIDS-associated KS. KSHV is also associated with lesions other than KS in non-AIDS-immunosuppressed patients, and may be involved in the pathogenesis of the various forms of proliferative skin lesions in organ transplant recipients. The human herpesvirus 8 (HHV-8) is the infectious agent responsible for KS in patients with and without human immunodeficiency virus infection. The latent nuclear antigen-1 (LNA-1) of HHV-8 is a nuclear antigen expressed in all cells latently infected by the virus.

    c. Characteristically, it originates as a bluish-red skin macule, often on the lower extremities, that multiplies, coalesces, and eventually spreads to internal viscera.

    d. Approximately 22% of patients with AIDS have involvement of the lids and conjunctiva, often as multifocal tumors.

KS may present in the bulbar conjunctiva as the initial clinical manifestation of AIDS.

    e. Histologically, it is composed of many foci of capillary clusters in a stroma of malignant spindle cells.

KSHV is a reliable marker (by polymerase chain reaction) to distinguish KS, particularly at its early stage, from other vascular lesions.

1). Type I consists of a flat lesion with thin, dilated vascular channels lined by flat endothelial cells with lumen-containing erythrocytes.
2). Type II consists of a flat lesion with plump, fusiform endothelial cells, often containing hyperchromic nuclei, and foci of immature spindle cells and occasionally slit vessels.
3). Type III consists of a nodular (>3 mm in height) lesion with large aggregates of densely packed spindle cells containing hyperchromic nuclei, occasional mitotic figures, and abundant slit vessels, often with erythrocytes in between.

Commonly, the tumor is admixed with lymphocytes, hence the term *malignant granulation tissue*. The endothelial cells lining well-formed tumor blood vessels give a strong reaction with immunohistochemical staining for FVIII-RAG when the peroxidase–antiperoxidase technique is used. The proliferating spindle cells that form the capillary clusters ("vascular slits"), however, give a negative reaction.

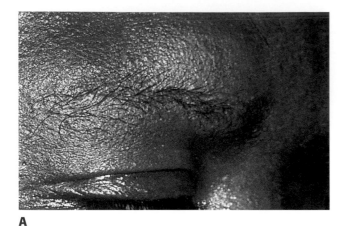

A

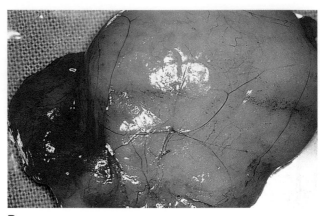

B

Fig. 14.22 Lipoma. **A,** Clinical appearance of lipoma of right brow. **B,** Gross specimen of another case in a 14-year-old girl has "fatty" appearance. **C,** Microscopic section shows that the tumor is composed of lobules of mature fat separated from each other by delicate fibrovascular septa. (**A,** Courtesy of Dr. WR Green; **B** and **C,** presented by Dr. CJ Lee, Jr. to the meeting of the Eastern Ophthalmic Pathology Society, 1989.)

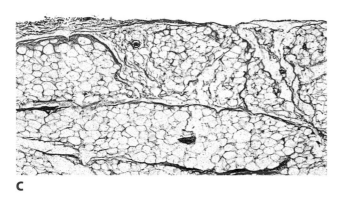

C

B. Fatty
  1. Lipoma† (Fig. 14.22)
     a. It is easier to determine clinically than histologically whether a tumor is a primary orbital lipoma or herniated orbital fat.

     Variants of benign lipoma include angiolipoma, angiomyolipoma, spindle cell lipoma, pleomorphic lipoma, benign lipoblastoma, and hibernoma (multivacuolar brown fat cells).

     ---

     b. Histologically, a lipoma is composed of groups of mature, univacuolar, white, fat cells separated from other groups by delicate fibrovascular septa.
        1). Coarser septa divide the tumor into lobules.
        2). A true lipoma usually has a thin, fibrous capsule.
  2. Liposarcoma‡ (Fig. 14.23)
     a. This extremely rare orbital tumor may be primary, or secondary to radiation therapy.
     b. Histologically, liposarcomas tend to be well differentiated or myxoid.
        1). The tumors are composed of univacuolar signet-ring lipoblasts.
        2). Scattered, bizarre, hyperchromatic cells without prominent lipidization may also be present.

C. Fibrous–histiocytic–reactive
  1. Nodular fasciitis†
     a. This is a benign proliferation of connective tissue.

     The tumor is also called subcutaneous pseudosarcomatous fibromatosis, pseudosarcomatous fasciitis, and nodular fibrositis.

     ---

     b. Clinically, it presents as a rapidly growing mass.
     c. Histologically, it is composed of nodular proliferations of plump, stellate, or spindle-shaped fibroblasts arranged in parallel bundles or haphazardly (the cells resemble tissue culture fibroblasts).
        1). A variable amount of intercellular myxoid ground substance is present.
        2). Abundant reticulin fibers and moderate numbers of collagen fibers can be demonstrated.
        3). Proliferation of slitlike vascular spaces or well-formed capillaries is characteristic.
  2. Juvenile fibromatosis‡ (psammomatoid ossifying fibroma)
     a. This is usually seen in children.

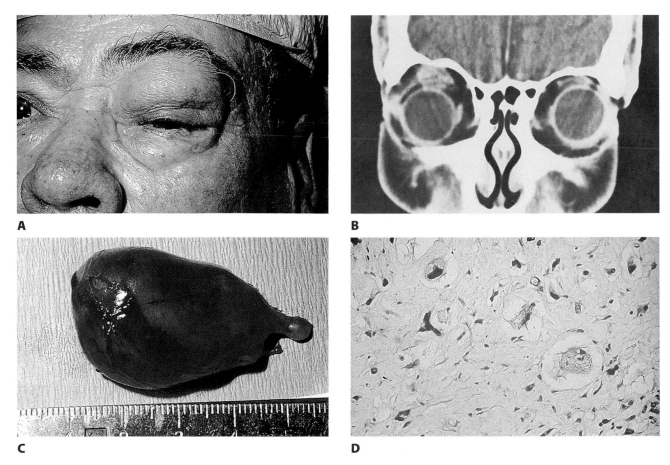

Fig. 14.23 Liposarcoma. **A,** A 78-year-old man has swelling and ptosis of the left upper lid. **B,** Computed tomography scan shows a mass superior to the globe. **C,** Appearance of gross specimen. **D,** Microscopic section shows bizarre lipoblasts. (Presented by Dr. CJ Lee, Jr. to the AOA–Armed Forces Institute of Pathology Alumni meeting, 1989.)

The group of tumors includes keloids, desmoids, fibromatoses of palmar and plantar fascias and of sternomastoid muscle, radiation fibromatosis, and congenital progressive polyfibromatosis.

    b. It may recur after excision and is frequently mistaken for fibrosarcoma.
    c. Histologically, it is composed of fibrous tissue interlacing with numerous mature capillaries.

A rare tumor in infants contains both fibroblastic and smooth-muscle elements and is called *infantile myofibromatosis.*

D. Fibrous–histiocytic–neoplastic
    1. Fibrous histiocytoma (FH)† (xanthoma; Fig. 14.24)

Xanthoma consists of an intracellular accumulation of fat, as opposed to a *lipogranuloma*, which is composed of an extracellular accumulation of fat.

    a. FH is the most common primary mesenchymal orbital tumor of adults.

In the past, FH has been misdiagnosed as hemangiopericytoma, sclerosing hemangioma, dermatofibrosarcoma protuberans (DFSP), and even neurofibroma. When associated with multinucleated giant cells and lipid-filled histiocytes, FH has been misdiagnosed as synovial giant cell tumor and villonodular synovitis.

    b. FH may involve ocular structures such as orbit (most commonly), lids, conjunctiva, and corneoscleral limbus.
    c. Although its cell of origin has been thought to be the histiocyte or the fibroblast, it is most probably a primitive mesenchymal cell that shows divergent lines of differentiation, expressing fibroblastic, histiocytic, and even myofibroblastic phenotypes.
    d. A variant of FH that forms no fibers at all and is entirely composed of histiocytes is called a *histiocytoma.*
    e. FH has a malignant potential.

Malignant FH (MFH), is considered to be a sarcoma having an undifferentiated mesenchymal cell origin

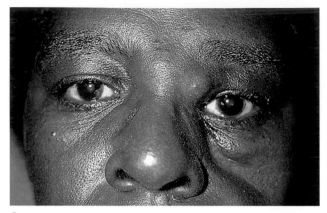

A

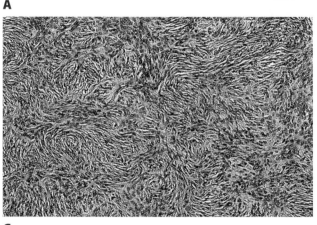

C

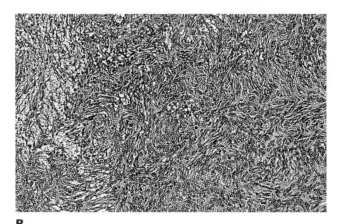

B

Fig. 14.24 Fibrous histiocytoma. **A,** This is the fourth recurrence of an orbital tumor that had first been excised 10 years previously. The histology of the primary lesion and of the four recurrences appears identical. **B,** A histologic section shows the diphasic pattern consisting of a histiocytic component (h) (mainly on far left) and a fibrous component (f). **C,** Increased magnification shows that the fibrous component forms a storiform or matted pattern. Controversy exists as to whether the tumor arises from histiocytes or fibroblasts (most of the evidence points toward a primitive mesenchymal cell origin). (Case reported by Jones WD III *et al.: Br J Plast Surg* 32:46, 1979. Copyright 1979 with permission from Elsevier.)

that differentiates along a broad fibroblastic and histiocytic (fibrohistiocytic) spectrum and usually has a predominant "fibroblastic" component.

   f. Histologically, FH shows a characteristic, diphasic pattern with mainly "storiform" (matted) areas composed of fibrous spindle cells along with scattered areas showing single or grouped foamy histiocytes.
      1). FH can be richly vascularized and then easily confused with hemangiopericytoma.
      2). MFH shows a mixture of storiform and pleomorphic features.

> MFH may be difficult to differentiate from other pleomorphic soft-tissue tumors such as pleomorphic liposarcoma, pleomorphic rhabdomyosarcoma, malignant schwannoma, leiomyosarcoma, and *epithelioid sarcoma*—a very rare orbital malignancy presumably of tendon sheath origin, having both epithelial and mesenchymal features. KP-1 (CD68), a recently described monoclonal antibody to a cytoplasmic epitope present on tissue histiocytes and macrophages, may have specific marker properties to help identify MFH. Vimentin also is usually positive. Finally, molecular assays for spe-

cific gene fusion provide a genetic approach to the differential diagnosis of soft-tissue sarcomas.

   2. Atypical fibroxanthoma (AFX)‡
      a. AFX usually occurs in the sun-damaged skin of the head and neck in the elderly.
      b. Histologically, spindle cells and pleomorphic polyhedral cells occur with many giant cells and mitotic figures.
         1). Despite its anaplastic appearance, AFX is regarded as a low-grade malignant tumor, usually acts benign, but rarely may metastasize.
         2). Immunohistochemically, AFX and Dermatofibrosarcoma (DFSP) (see later) stain nearly identically: negative for cytokeratin, desmin, S-100 protein, and melanoma antibodies HMB-45 and HMB-50; strongly positive for vimentin and NKI/C3, and variable positivity for muscle-specific actin (HHF-35).

> Although AFX and DFSP can be confused with spindle cell, squamous cell carcinoma and desmoplastic malignant melanoma, the absence of cytokeratin, HMB-45, and HMB-50 staining easily distinguishes AFX and DFSP from the others.

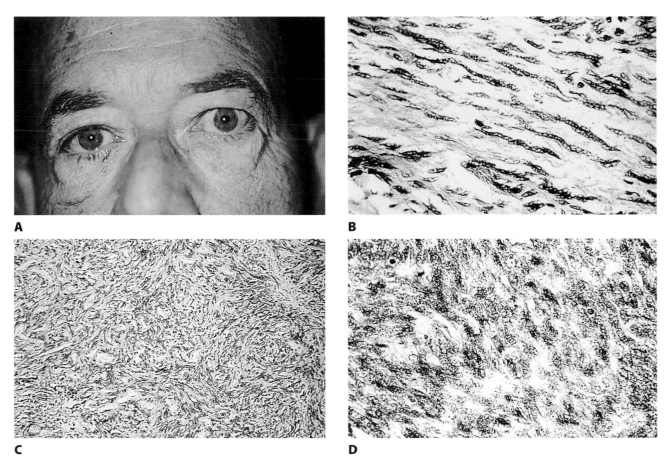

Fig. 14.25 Fibrosarcoma. **A,** A 60-year-old man presented with exophthalmos of left eye. **B,** Histologic section of removed orbital tumor shows well-differentiated fibrosarcoma with "herringbone" pattern and bland spindle nuclei. **C,** Recurrent tumor excised 3 years later by exenteration is much more cellular and less well differentiated than primary (shown with increased magnification in **D**). At time of death 9 years later from a heart condition, two small tumors had developed (presumably recurrences), one at temple over removed eye and other on cheek on same side. (From Yanoff M, Scheie HG: *Cancer* 19:1711, 1966. © American Cancer Society. Reproduced by permission of Wiley-Liss, Inc., a subsidiary of John Wiley & Sons, Inc.)

3. Dermatofibrosarcoma (DFSP)‡
    a. DFSP usually occurs in young or middle-aged persons as large cutaneous nodules.
    b. Histologically, DFSP is composed of relatively uniform spindle cells with a conspicuous storiform pattern (similar to FH except for the lack of a histiocytic component).
        1). DFSP is regarded as a low-grade malignant tumor, usually acts benign, but extremely rarely may metastasize.
        2). Immunohistochemically, DFSP and AFX (see earlier) stain nearly identically.
4. Fibroma‡ and fibrosarcoma‡
    a. True orbital fibroma is rare.

An even rarer tumor is the *elastofibroma*, which consists of a fibrous proliferation of abundant elastinophilic polymorphic structures.

Histologically, orbital fibroma is composed of scattered spindle-shaped cells, sometimes showing a herringbone pattern, but lacking atypia and mitotic figures.

b. Fibrosarcoma (Fig. 14.25) is a very rare, slow-growing, orbital tumor.

Histologically, fibrosarcoma is composed of interlacing bundles of spindle-shaped cells forming a herringbone pattern, often with atypical cells and mitotic figures.

5. Solitary fibrous tumor‡
    a. Solitary fibrous tumor is a rare tumor of mesenchymal origin that most often involves the pleura; rarely, the orbit is involved.

The tumor may arise from mesenchymal cells that show fibroblastic differentiation.

---

b. Although usually benign, it can recur locally and rarely metastasizes.
c. Histologically, usually strong CD34- and vimentin-positive spindle cells with elongated, wavy nuclei and inconspicuous nucleoli in hypocellular collagen-rich areas form a characteristic "patternless pattern."

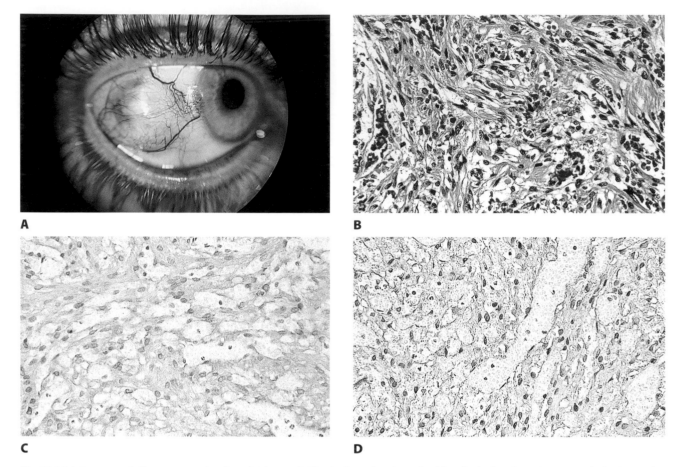

Fig. 14.26 Leiomyoma. **A,** Tumor present in sclera of right eye. **B,** Histologic section shows fascicles of spindle cells against a vascular background. Spindle cells are positive for muscle-specific actin (**C**) and smooth-muscle actin (**D**). (Presented by Dr. CL Shields to the meeting of the Eastern Ophthalmic Pathology Society, 1989; case reported in Shields CL *et al.:* Ophthalmology 98:84. © Elsevier 1991.)

Solitary fibrous tumor resembles giant cell angiofibroma but lacks multinucleated giant cells and pseudovascular spaces

---

6. Fibrous hamartoma of infancy‡
   a. Benign solitary tumor (0.5 to 4.0 cm) present at birth or at a very young age
   b. Male to female ratio 2:1
   c. Growth slows with age without malignant transformation
   d. Histologically it consists of well-defined bundles of dense fibrocollagenous tissue, immature and primitive mesenchyme arranged in nests, concentric whorls or bands, and mature adipose tissue intimately admixed with the other components.
7. Giant cell angiofibroma‡
   a. Giant cell angiofibroma, probably a benign tumor, occurs mainly in men from the third to the eighth decades.
   b. Although most occur in the orbit, they can also occur in the lids and, rarely, conjunctiva.
   c. Histologically the tumors are richly vascularized and contain a patternless proliferation of spindle

cells, numerous multinucleated giant cells, and some pseudovascular spaces, all embedded in variably collagenized stroma.
1). Myxoid stromal deposition may be present.
2). The spindle cells and multinucleated giant cells stain intensely positive with CD34 and vimentin.

Solitary fibrous tumor, which resembles giant cell angiofibroma, lacks multinucleated giant cells and pseudovascular spaces. Stains for KP1 (CD68) are negative, unlike in FH, where they are positive.

E. Muscle
1. Leiomyoma‡ and leiomyosarcoma‡ are very rare orbital tumors.

An even rarer tumor, composed of myofibroblasts surrounding a hemangiopericytoma-like stroma, is *infantile myofibromatosis.*

Histologically, leiomyoma (Fig. 14.26) consists of interlacing fascicles of smooth-muscle cells.

1). Immunohistochemistry shows strong positivity for the sensitive marker muscle-specific actin and focal positivity for desmin.

2). Electron microscopy shows the characteristic findings for smooth muscle, namely cytoplasmic filaments associated with dense bodies, plasmalemmal densities, and pinocytotic vesicles, and investing thin basement membrane.

3). Leiomyosarcoma, in addition, shows atypical nuclei and mitotic figures.

2. Mesectodermal leiomyoma‡ (see p. 350 in Chapter 9) and leiomyosarcoma‡ are very rare orbital tumors whose origin seems to be from tissue derived from neural crest.

Histologically, mesectodermal leiomyoma resembles ganglionic, astrocytic, and peripheral nerve tumors.

Electron microscopy, however, demonstrates the smooth-muscle origin of the tumor.

Mesectodermal leiomyoma also occurs in the ciliary body. The tumor has some similarities to a malignant schwannoma or rhabdomyosarcoma by light microscopy. Electron microscopy aids in identifying the smooth-muscle nature of the tumor. Finally, molecular assays for specific gene fusion provide a genetic approach to the differential diagnosis of soft-tissue sarcomas.

3. Malignant rhabdoid tumor‡
   a. Malignant rhabdoid tumor is a rare, highly aggressive renal tumor of infants.
      1). The tumor rarely involves extrarenal sites in children and adults, and even more rarely involves the orbit.
      2). Although its name, *malignant rhabdoid tumor*, implies a muscle origin, more likely the tumor arises from epithelium.
   b. Histologically, the tumor is composed of dyscohesive, globoid, and eosinophilic cells, often containing cytoplasmic inclusions.
      1). Immunohistochemically, the inclusions consist of whorls of vimentin-positive (intermediate) filaments, and the cells express epithelial membrane antigen and cytokeratin positivity (evidence of epithelial origin).
      2). Electron microscopy shows intercellular junctions and interrupted segments of thin basement membrane material, further evidence of epithelial origin.
4. Rhabdomyoma‡ is a very rare, benign orbital tumor.

Histologically, well-differentiated rhabdomyoblasts are present.
5. Rhabdomyosarcoma†
   a. Rhabdomyosarcoma is the most common malignant mesenchymal orbital neoplasm, and is the most common primary malignant orbital tumor in children.

b. Although found in many parts of the body, rhabdomyosarcoma has a predilection for the orbit.

It can rarely occur in the eyelid, conjunctiva, and uveal tract.

c. The average age of onset is approximately 6 years, with most children younger than 10 years of age; it is extremely rare after 25 years of age.
d. The tumor is characterized clinically by a very rapid onset, often simulating an orbital cellulitis.
e. Three types exist: embryonal, differentiated, and alveolar.
f. Embryonal type (Fig. 14.27)—most common type.

An undifferentiated tumor that resembles rhabdomyosarcoma, but without demonstrable rhabdomyoblasts, should be classified as *embryonal sarcoma*. Many of the metastases, however, show rhabdomyoblasts with cross-striations; then the classification embryonal rhabdomyosarcoma (or alveolar rhabdomyosarcoma, according to pattern) is appropriate.

1). When it arises in the submucosa of the conjunctiva, it is identical to the vaginal submucosal tumor of infancy, *sarcoma botryoides*.
2). Histologically, it is composed of malignant embryonal cells, rhabdomyoblasts, in a loose syncytial arrangement of fascicles of spindle cells running in a haphazard arrangement, usually showing frequent mitotic figures.
   a). The cells are round, oval, elongate, or stellate, with nuclei rich in chromatin and cytoplasm rich in glycogen.
   b). A ribbon of eosinophilic cytoplasm may be seen around the nucleus.

Usually, only undifferentiated embryonal cells with large hyperchromic nuclei and a scant amount of cytoplasm are present. In some areas, however, cells with a ribbon of pink cytoplasm can be seen. Cross-striations are most likely to be found in these latter areas.

   c). Cross-striations may sometimes be present in the metastases even though they were not found in the primary tumor.
   d). Immunohistochemistry shows positivity for vimentin, myosin, myoglobin, muscle-specific actin, and desmin.

Insulin-like growth factor-2, which acts as an autocrine growth and motility factor, may be operating in rhabdomyosarcomas. The expres-

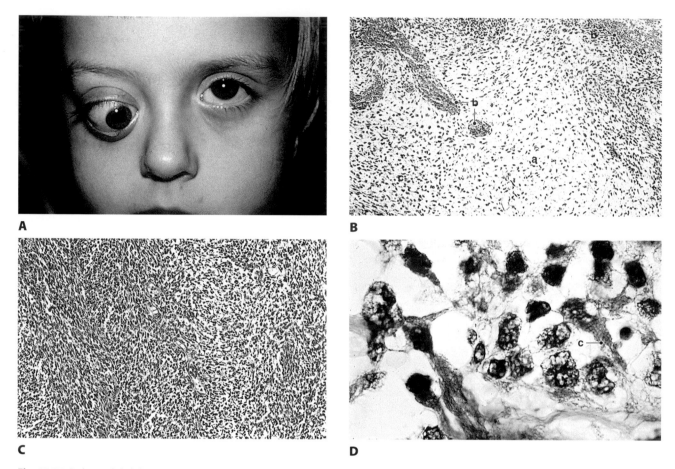

Fig. 14.27 Embryonal rhabdomyosarcoma. **A,** The patient has a unilateral right ocular proptosis of very recent onset. Often, rhabdomyosarcoma presents rapidly, causes lid redness, and is mistaken for orbital inflammation. **B,** A histologic section shows a marked embryonic cellular pattern, hence the term *embryonal rhabdomyosarcoma* (a, relatively acellular area; b, blood vessels; c, relatively cellular area). **C,** Increased magnification of a cellular area shows the primitive nature of the rhabdomyoblasts; these tend to cluster in groups, separated by relatively acellular areas. **D,** A trichrome stain shows characteristic cross-striations (c) in the cytoplasm of some of the rhabdomyoblasts. Cross-striations, although not abundant in embryonal rhabdomyosarcoma, can be seen in sections stained with hematoxylin and eosin but are easier to see with special stains.

sion of the myogenic determination gene *MyoD*, a member of the helix–loop–helix family of transcription factors, is the most sensitive marker for rhabdomyosarcoma. Rhabdomyosarcomas seem to be deficient in a factor required for *MyoD* activity.

e). Electron microscopy shows, in better-differentiated tumors, the characteristic findings for striated muscle (formed sarcomeres containing interdigitated thick myosin and thin actin filaments outlined by transverse Z-bands), but in primitive cases may show only focal myofilamentary differentiation.

g. Differentiated type
1). The differentiated form of rhabdomyosarcoma is the least common type, but seems to have the best prognosis.
2). Cross-striations are easily found in the differentiated type.

The adult pleomorphic form of rhabdomyosarcoma rarely, if ever, involves the orbit.

h. Alveolar type (Fig. 14.28)
1). The alveolar form of rhabdomyosarcoma seems to have the worst prognosis.
a). The diagnosis of alveolar rhabdomyosarcoma depends heavily on the presence of rearrangement of the *FKHR* (forkhead) gene located on chromosome 13q14.
b). The tumor is characterized by a tumor-specific translocation, t(2;13)(q35;q14) and t(1;3)(p36;q14)
c). Molecular confirmation of alveolar rhabdomyosarcoma is important in the treatment of this tumor
2). The individual cell type is similar to that seen in the embryonal type, but the tumor has a distinct alveolar pattern.

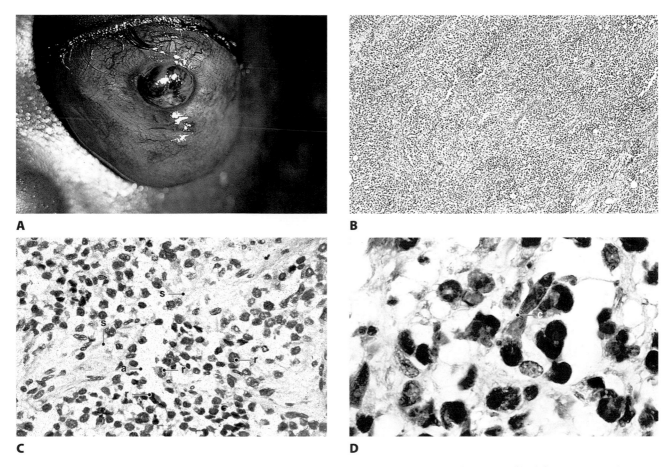

Fig. 14.28 Alveolar rhabdomyosarcoma. **A,** This 21-year-old man presented with marked chemosis and proptosis of his left eye. **B,** A reticulin stain shows delicate septa, which give the tumor an alveolated appearance (hence the term *alveolar rhabdomyosarcoma*). **C,** Increased magnification shows that the cytoplasm of the rhabdomyoblasts makes up part of the septa (s, septa made up of cytoplasm of rhabdomyoblasts; a, "alveolus"; r, rhabdomyoblast nuclei). **D,** A trichrome stain shows typical cross-striations (c). Cross-striations are least abundant and hardest to find in alveolar rhabdomyosarcoma. In the third type of rhabdomyosarcoma (differentiated), unlike in embryonal and alveolar types, most of the cells are differentiated, and cross-striations are easy to find.

3). Some rhabdomyoblastic cell processes fuse to form the walls of the alveoli, whereas other rhabdomyoblasts lie free in the alveolar lumen.

4). It is the most difficult tumor in which to find cross-striations.

Molecular assays for specific gene fusion provide a genetic approach to the differential diagnosis of soft-tissue sarcomas.

I. Prognosis

1). If the tumor is confined to the orbit, the survival rate is 90% with a combination of chemotherapy and radiation.

2). If there is bone destruction and extension beyond the orbit exist, the survival rate decreases to 65%.

3). Most deaths occur within the first 3 years, so that a 5-year cure probably is a valid one.

4). DNA content is an important variable in predicting prognosis. DNA hyperdiploid and tetradiploid rhabdomyosarcomas have a favorable prognosis, whereas DNA diploid and polyploid tumors have a poor prognosis.

F. Cartilage—chondroma‡ and chondrosarcoma‡

1. Chondroma and chondrosarcoma are extremely rare orbital tumors.

2. Chondrosarcoma may be congenital or may arise primarily without antecedent cause, but most frequently it follows radiation for retinoblastoma or pre-existing Paget's disease.

Enchondroma, a tumor that originates from misplaced islands of cartilage in the intramedullary canal of bone, is extremely rare.

G. Bone

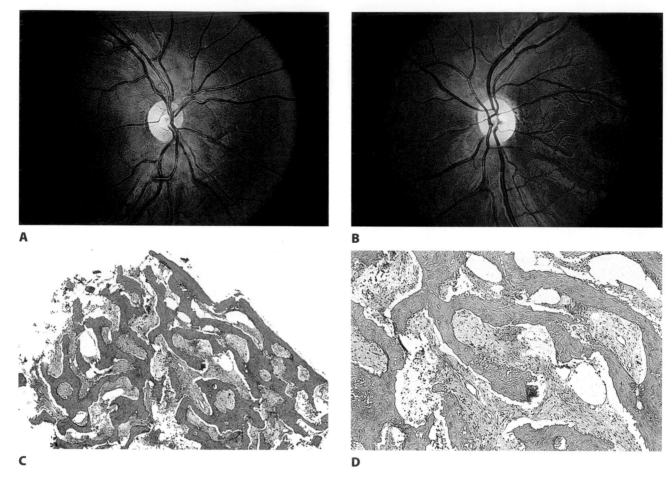

Fig. 14.29 Fibrous dysplasia. **A** (fundus OD) and **B** (fundus OS): A 13-year-old girl had a vision of 20/20 OD and 20/30 OS, a left afferent pupillary defect, and mild optic nerve pallor OS. **C,** Histologic section of sphenoid bone shows highly characteristic bone structure composed of moderately cellular and loosely textured fibrous connective tissue, enclosing poorly formed bone spicules, demonstrating both formative and resorptive changes, shown with increased magnification in **D.**

Nonneoplastic and neoplastic diseases of bone usually cause exophthalmos by decreasing orbital volume.

a. Aneurysmal bone cyst‡
b. Fibrous dysplasia† (Fig. 14.29)
c. Giant cell tumor‡
d. Giant cell reparative granuloma‡
e. Juvenile fibromatosis‡ (psammomatoid ossifying fibroma)
f. Cholesterol granuloma‡ and cholesteatoma‡ (see p. 534 in this chapter)
g. Leontiasis ossea‡
h. Osteitis fibrosa cystica (brown tumor)†
i. Osteopetrosis‡
j. Paget's disease†
k. Osteoma‡, osteoblastoma‡, and osteogenic sarcoma (osteosarcoma)‡
l. Benign osteoblastoma‡
1). All are extremely rare orbital tumors.

Osteomas may occur in Gardner's syndrome, an autosomal-dominant disorder characterized by intestinal polyposis, various skin and soft-tissue tumors, retinal pigment epithelial hypertrophy, and osteomas.

2). Osteogenic sarcoma (osteosarcoma)‡ may rarely be primary, may be associated with Paget's disease of bone, or may follow radiation for retinoblastomas.
m. Ameloblastoma‡
IV. Neural tumors
A. Amputation neuroma‡
1. An amputation neuroma is rare in the orbit.
2. Histologically, it is composed of a haphazard entanglement of regenerated nerve fibers from the cut end of the peripheral ciliary nerve(s).
B. Neurofibromas† (see Figs 2.3 to 2.5)
C. Neurilemmoma (schwannoma†; Figs 14.30 and 14.31)
1. A neurilemmoma is a rare orbital tumor composed of neoplastic Schwann cells.

Even more rarely, the tumor may occur in the uveal tract or in the conjunctiva.

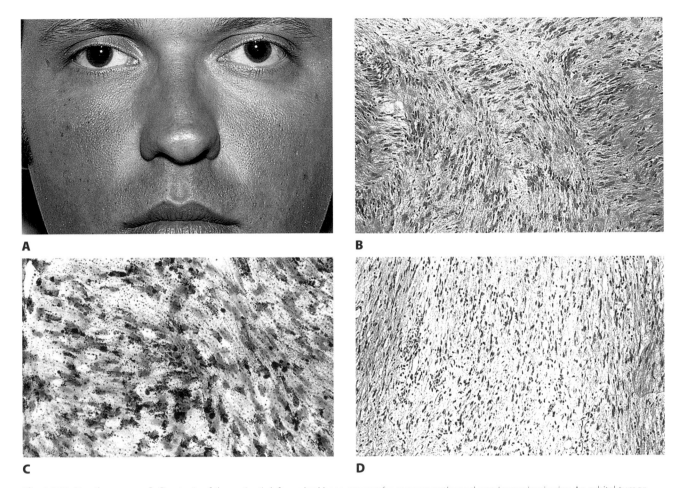

Fig. 14.30 Neurilemmoma. **A,** Proptosis of the patient's left eye had been present for many months and was increasing in size. An orbital tumor was removed. **B,** A histologic section shows ribbons of spindle Schwann cell nuclei, which show a tendency toward palisading. Areas of relative acellularity, mimicking tactile corpuscles, are called *Verocay bodies*. This pattern is called the *Antoni type A* pattern. **C,** Oil red-O stain shows that the cytoplasm of the tumor cells is clearly lipid-positive. **D,** In this area of necrosis, inflammatory cells and microcystoid degeneration are present, a pattern called the *Antoni type B* pattern.

2. Histologically, nuclei of spindle-shaped Schwann cells show a tendency toward palisading.
    a. When the texture is compact and composed of interwoven bundles of long bipolar spindle cells, often with ribbons of palisading cells alternating with relatively acellular areas, the *Antoni type A* pattern is present.
        1). Areas of the tumor may mimic tactile corpuscles and are called *Verocay* bodies.
        2). The tumor may have a haphazard arrangement, a loose texture, and mucinous and microcystoid areas of necrosis; this type of degenerative pattern is called the *Antoni type B* pattern.
    b. The tumor is usually encapsulated in the perineurium of the originating nerve.
    c. Immunohistochemistry shows positivity for human nerve growth factor (NGF), laminin, the major glycoprotein of basement membranes, HMB-45, and S-100 protein.

Immunohistochemistry may be quite helpful in differentiating the very rare melanotic neurilemmoma from a malignant melanoma, especially if the former arises in the choroid. A rare histologic variant of neurilemmoma, called *ancient schwannoma*, shows distinctive areas of hypercellularity and hyperchromic nuclei suggesting fibrosarcoma, as well as hypocellular areas containing considerable fibrosis; the clinical course, however, tends to be benign.

    d. Electron microscopy may show Luse bodies (see Fig. 14.31C; i.e., aggregates of long-spaced collagen).
3. Malignant peripheral nerve sheath tumor (malignant schwannoma, malignant neurilemmoma, neurofibrosarcoma, perineural fibrosarcoma, neurogenic sarcoma)‡ is extremely rare, but when present is associated with neurofibromatosis in 50% of cases.
    S-100 protein and NGF positivity and electron microscopic evidence of basement membrane mate-

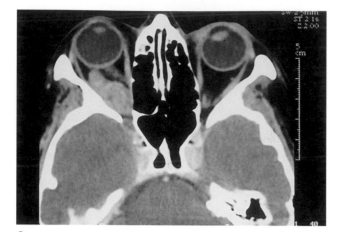

A

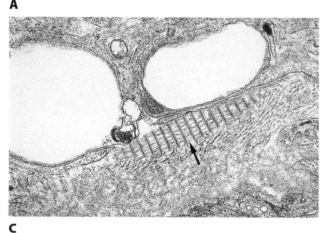

C

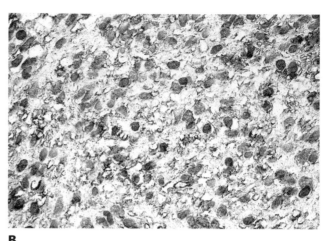

B

Fig. 14.31 Neurilemmoma. **A,** A 61-year-old patient had decreased vision in the right eye for 8 months. The computed tomography scan shows a right orbital mass. **B,** Histologic section was characteristic of neurilemmoma and, as seen in this figure, is positive for S-100 protein. **C,** Electron microscopy shows a Luse body (i.e., an aggregate of long-spaced collagen), often found in neurilemmomas. (Case presented by Dr. HE Grossniklaus to the meeting of the Verhoeff Society, 1994.)

rial and mesaxon or pseudomesaxon formation help to identify these often poorly differentiated tumors.

> Mutations in the *p53* tumor suppressor gene, located on the short arm of chromosome 17 at position 17p13.1, represent the most frequent genetic alteration detected in human solid malignancies. In approximately half of all cancer cases, *p53* is inactivated by mutations and other genomic alterations, and in many of the remaining cases, *p53* is functionally inactivated by the binding of the cellular MDM2 oncoprotein, a cellular inhibitor of the *p53* tumor suppressor. The *p53* gene encodes a 53-kD nucleophosphoprotein that binds DNA and negatively regulates cell division, preventing progression from G1 to S phase. Approximately 25% of adult sarcomas of different types are associated with *p53* abnormalities. It also appears to be a marker of tumor progression (i.e., a direct correlation seems to exist between mutations at the *p53* locus and increasing histologic grade). This correlation may be especially applicable to malignant peripheral nerve sheath tumors.

  4. Juvenile pilocytic astrocytoma (glioma) of optic nerve† (see pp. 514–518 in Chapter 13)
D. Peripheral primitive neuroectodermal tumors (PNETs‡; Fig. 14.32)
  1. PNETs are a group of soft-tissue tumors of presumed neural crest origin arising outside the central and sympathetic nervous system.

  a. PNETs include adult neuroblastoma, neuroepithelioma, primitive neuroectodermal tumor of bone, and malignant small cell tumors of the thoracopulmonary region (Askin's tumor).
  b. All share in a chromosomal aberration translocation (11;22)(q24]2).

> *Ewing's sarcoma* also has the same genetic abnormality and may represent the opposite end of the same spectrum. However, despite their genetic and antigenic similarity, most authors recognize PNET and extraosseous Ewing's sarcoma as separate entities, a distinction based primarily on the more neural differentiation of PNET and its graver prognosis.

  c. Histologically, scattered nests of small tumor cells containing an even chromatin pattern, similar to Ewing's sarcoma cells, are set in a highly desmoplastic stroma.

> *Ewing's sarcoma* stains positively for periodic acid–Schiff (PAS) stain, vimentin, and especially terminal deoxynucleotidyl transferase and MIC-2 (CD99), a cell surface glycoprotein encoded by genes on chromosomes X and Y. The histologic differentiation includes other small cell tumors such as lymphomas, rhabdo-

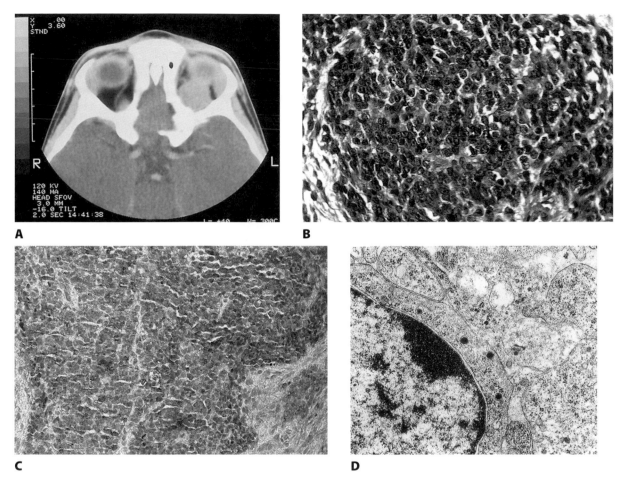

Fig. 14.32 Peripheral primitive neuroectodermal tumor. **A,** Computed tomogram in a 4-year-old child shows a large, homogeneous orbital mass behind the left eye. **B,** Biopsy shows small tumor cells containing an even chromatin pattern. **C,** The tumor cells stain positively for neuron-specific enolase. **D,** Electron microscopy demonstrates cytoplasmic neurosecretory granules.

myosarcoma, neuroblastoma, PNET, nephroblastoma, small cell variant of osteosarcoma, and carcinomas with various degrees of neuroendocrine differentiation.

---

    d. Immunohistochemically, the cells are positive for low-molecular-weight cytokeratin, epithelial membrane antigen, and neuron-specific enolase.

    e. Electron microscopically, cytoplasmic processes, cytoplasmic glycogen, cytoplasmic filaments, and occasional neurosecretory granules are seen.

  2. Adult neuroblastoma (one of the PNETs)

    a. Adult neuroblastoma most rarely involves the orbit as a primary tumor.

    b. The two-mutation model of tumorigenesis applies to neuroblastoma as well as to retinoblastoma.

    c. More commonly, it is a childhood metastatic disease (see p. 483 in this chapter).

V. Miscellaneous tumors

  A. Meningioma† (see p. 518 in Chapter 13)

  B. Nonchromaffin paraganglioma (carotid body tumor)‡

    1. Nonchromaffin paraganglioma is a rare, benign orbital tumor probably of neurogenic origin.

It occurs chiefly outside the orbit at the bifurcation of the common carotid artery.

---

    2. Histologically, it is composed of clusters of relatively clear (epithelioid) or dark (chief) cells surrounded by a vascularized connective tissue stroma.

    a. Typically, silver stains show that reticulin separates or surrounds tumor cell clusters but does not surround individual cells.

    b. By electron microscopy, two cellular elements are present.

     1). Central chief cells containing membrane-bound neurosecretory granules in great abundance

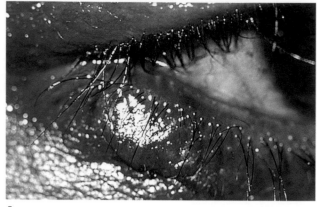

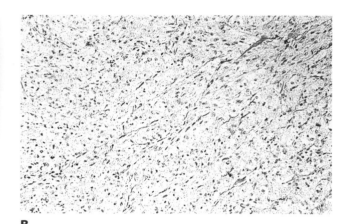

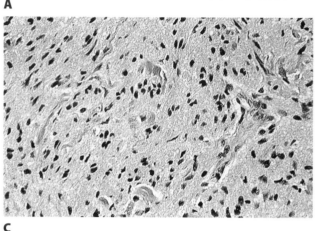

Fig. 14.33 Granular cell tumor. **A,** A 48-year-old woman had a hard tumor of the right lower lid. **B,** Histologic section shows solid groups and cords of cells. **C,** Increased magnification of small nuclei and granular eosinophilic cytoplasm of round and polygonal cells.

2). Fibroblast-like sustentacular cells at the periphery of cell clusters

C. Granular cell tumor (granular cell myoblastoma‡; Fig. 14.33)

1. Granular cell tumor is a rare, benign orbital tumor.

> The histogenesis of the tumor is uncertain, and skeletal muscle, fibroblasts, undifferentiated mesenchymal cells, histiocytes, and neural or Schwann cells have all been proposed as cells of origin. Most of the evidence would suggest that the Schwann cell is the cell of origin. Rarely, the tumor can occur in the epibulbar region or in the ciliary body.

2. Histologically, it is composed of round to polygonal cells in solid groups and cords and occasionally in alveolated collections.

   a. The cells are frequently contiguous to adjacent skeletal muscle.

   b. The nuclei are round and relatively small in relation to the voluminous, finely granular, eosinophilic cytoplasm, which is PAS-positive and diastase-resistant.

   c. Silver stains frequently show reticulin surrounding individual cells.

d. Electron microscopy reveals oval and round membrane-bound cytoplasmic bodies.

D. Alveolar soft-part sarcoma‡ (Fig. 14.34)

1. An alveolar soft-part sarcoma is a rare, malignant orbital tumor.

> Another entity, *malignant mesenchymoma*, a very rare orbital tumor, was thought to be a subtype of alveolar soft-part sarcoma, but probably represents a separate enty, although this is controversial. The tumor, which usually affects patients older than 60 years, is composed of two or three distinct malignant components, e.g., rhabdomyosarcoma, chondrosarcoma, and osteogenic sarcoma.

2. Histologically, it is composed of alveolated groups of round and polygonal cells circumscribed by bands of connective tissue, some of which contain delicate vascular channels in a distinct organoid pattern.

   a. Cytoplasm of tumor cells contains scattered eosinophilic and PAS-positive, diastase-resistant, crystalline granules as well as larger refractile bodies.

   b. Immunohistochemistry shows positive staining with desmin, myoglobin, muscle actin, S-100

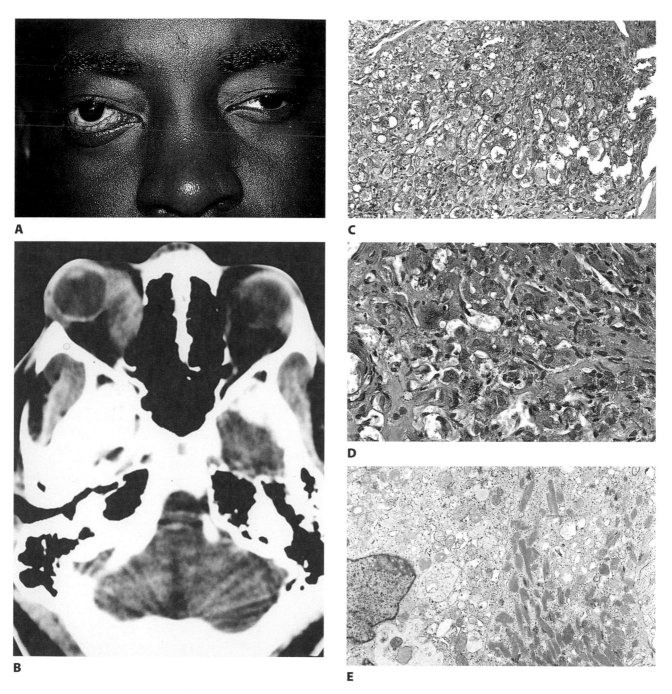

Fig. 14.34 Alveolar soft-part sarcoma. **A,** Clinical appearance of right exophthalmos. **B,** Computed tomography scan shows tumor in nasal orbit. **C,** Histologic section stained with periodic acid–Schiff (PAS) shows alveolated groups of round and polygonal cells circumscribed by bands of connective tissue. **D,** Increased magnification demonstrates PAS-positive, diastase-resistant crystalline granules and larger refractile bodies. **E,** Electron microscopy reveals intracytoplasmic crystalline inclusions exhibiting a variety of geometric configurations. (Case presented by Dr. VT Curtin to the meeting of the Eastern Ophthalmic Pathology Society, 1990.)

protein, and NKI/C3 (melanoma marker), but negative staining with HMB-45 (melanoma-specific marker), vimentin, and synaptophysin (neuroendocrine marker), suggesting a muscle cell origin rather than nerve cell or paraganglionic origin.

c. Electron microscopy reveals intracytoplasmic crystalline inclusions that exhibit a variety of geometric configurations.

The cytoplasmic crystalloids are similar to the rods observed in benign rhabdomyoma cells. The tumor, therefore, has been thought by some to be a unique type of rhabdomyosarcoma instead of being of neural derivation.

E. Malignant melanoma‡ (see p. 722 in Chapter 17)
F. Endodermal sinus tumor (parietal yolk sac carcinoma)‡
   1. Always malignant, endodermal sinus tumor usually arises in the gonads but rarely can arise primarily from ectopic, extraembryonic germ cells in the orbit.
   2. Histologically, the tumor is composed of a meshwork of spaces and cords lined by flat to cuboidal primitive epithelium, scant myxomatous stroma, and frequent mitotic figures.

The tumors may contain Schiller–Duval bodies (i.e., pseudopapillary formations that contain a central vascular core that resembles a glomerulus).

G. Myxoma‡
   1. Myxoma may arise in orbital bones as a benign solitary lesion, or be part of Carney's syndrome (see p. 244 in Chapter 7).
   2. Histologically, stellate spindle cells, some of which contain PAS-positive, diastase-resistant intracytoplasmic inclusions, are present within a myxoid stroma.
V. Epithelial cysts and neoplasms of lacrimal gland
   A. Lacrimal ductal cysts (dacryops)†
      1. Cysts (dacryops) can occur in any location where lacrimal gland is present and account for 6% of all epithelial lesions of the lacrimal gland.
         a. Palpebral lobe cysts
         b. Orbital lobe cysts
         c. Cysts of the accessory lacrimal glands of Krause and Wolfring
         d. Cysts of ectopic lacrimal gland
      2. Histologically, the cyst is lined by a double layer of epithelium.
   B. Localized amyloidosis of the lacrimal gland‡
      1. Localized amyloidosis of the lacrimal gland can occur unilaterally or bilaterally.
      2. Characteristic amyloid (see p. 238 in Chapter 7) is found by light and electron microscopy and by immunohistochemistry (monoclonal lambda light chains).
   C. General information on neoplasms
      1. Characteristically, lacrimal gland tumors cause a "down and in" type of proptosis.
      2. The lacrimal gland is composed exclusively of serous cells, entirely lacking mucinous cells. Myoepithelial cells surround the secretory cells of the acini.
      3. Although "classic teaching" states that epithelial and nonepithelial lacrimal gland lesions occur with equal frequency, recent studies have shown that approximately 25% of lacrimal gland tumors are epithelial, and the remaining 75% are nonepithelial

(mainly lymphoid tumors or inflammatory pseudotumors).

The lymphoid tumors and pseudotumors are identical to those occurring elsewhere in the orbit (see pp. 571–581 in this chapter).

---

   4. Pleomorphic adenoma (benign mixed tumor) is the most common benign neoplasm of the salivary glands and of the lacrimal gland.
   5. Mucoepidermoid carcinoma, the most common carcinoma of the salivary gland, is uncommon in the lacrimal gland.

Mucoepidermoid carcinoma can also arise from the conjunctiva and the caruncle.

---

   6. Simplified classification of tumors of the lacrimal gland
      a. Lymphoid tumors and inflammatory pseudotumors: 75% (most benign)
      b. Epithelial and cystic lesions: 25%
         1). Benign epithelial lesions: approximately 78% (approximately two-thirds pleomorphic adenomas and one-third dacryops)
         2). Malignant epithelial tumors (carcinomas): approximately 22% (slightly greater numbers of adenoid cystic carcinoma than malignant mixed tumor, along with a rare adenocarcinoma, mucinous carcinoma, mucoepidermoid carcinoma, or undifferentiated carcinoma)

Aside from malignant lacrimal gland tumors, the only other malignant epithelial tumor that may occur primarily in the orbit is the carcinoid tumor.

---

   7. Prognosis
      a. Pleomorphic adenomas: the mortality rate is well under 10%, with the deaths due mainly to multiple recurrences and intracranial extension.
      b. All malignant tumors: the mortality rate is 50% or more.
D. Pleomorphic adenoma (benign mixed tumor)†; Fig. 14.35)
   1. Pleomorphic adenoma occurs in young adults, with a median age of 35 years.
   2. Males predominate 2:1.
   3. It is a locally invasive tumor and may infiltrate its own pseudocapsule to involve adjacent periosteum.
      a. Acute pain and progression are rare.
      b. With incomplete removal, the tumor may recur in the soft tissues or the bony wall.
      c. If removed in piecemeal fashion, multiple recurrences may occur.
   4. Histologically, the tumor shows marked structural variation from patient to patient and within the same tumor.

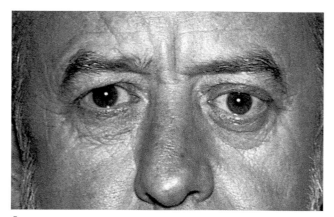

A

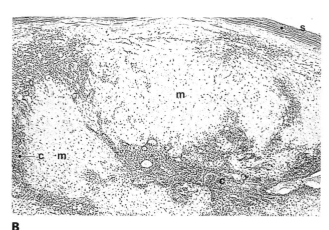

B

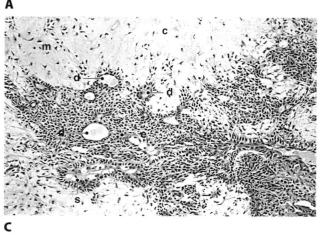

C

Fig. 14.35 Benign mixed tumor. **A,** The patient had proptosis of the left eye for a long time. It had gradually increased in severity. **B,** A histologic section shows the characteristic diphasic pattern, consisting of a pale background that has a myxomatous stroma and a relatively amorphous appearance, contiguous with quite cellular areas that contain mainly epithelial cells (s, surface of tumor; m, myxomatous stroma; c, cellular epithelial areas). **C,** Increased magnification shows the characteristic epithelial ductal structures lined by two layers of epithelium. The outer layer often undergoes myxoid and even cartilaginous metaplasia, whereas the inner layer may secrete mucus or may undergo squamous metaplasia, both of which are present here (c, area resembling cartilage; m, mesenchymal component; d, ducts filled with mucin; e, epithelial component; s, squamous metaplasia).

a. Almost all, at least in some areas, have tubular structures arranged in an irregularly anastomosing pattern, lying in a myxoid stroma.

> The juxtaposition of highly cellular epithelial areas with the relatively acellular myxomatous areas gives the tumor its characteristic diphasic pattern. The stroma is rich in a hyaluronidase-resistant acid mucopolysaccharide.

b. A double layer of epithelium lines the tubes or ducts.
  1). The inner layer of epithelium may secrete mucus or undergo squamous metaplasia.
  2). The outer layer of epithelium may undergo metaplasia to form a myxoid, fibrous, or cartilaginous stroma.
c. Pressure of the tumor on surrounding tissue forms a pseudocapsule; the tumor almost always infiltrates its pseudocapsule in some area.
d. Positive immunohistologic staining with cytokeratin, muscle-specific actin, and glial fibrillary acidic protein, in both benign and malignant mixed tumors, suggests that ductal epithelium develops into the epithelial component and some cells in the stroma, and myoepithelium develops into some cells in the stroma.

E. Other types of benign tumors (all are rare)
  1. Hemangioma‡
  2. Warthin's tumor‡
F. Malignant mixed tumor† (Fig. 14.36)
  1. Malignant mixed tumor occurs in an older age group than pleomorphic adenoma, with a median age of 51 years.
  2. No sex predilection exists.
  3. It arises from a pleomorphic adenoma.
  4. Histologically, areas resembling a pleomorphic adenoma are seen along with adenocarcinomatous areas.
G. Adenoid cystic carcinoma† (malignant cylindroma; Fig. 14.37)
  1. The tumor occurs in young adults, with a median age of approximately 38 years.

> Rarely, the tumor occurs in young people (6.5 to 18 years of age) and seems to have a more favorable prognosis in this young group.

  2. No sex predilection exists.
  3. The tumor soon invades perineural lymphatics and has an extremely poor prognosis.
  4. Acute pain and progression are common.

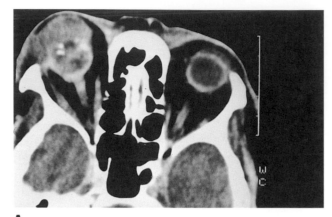

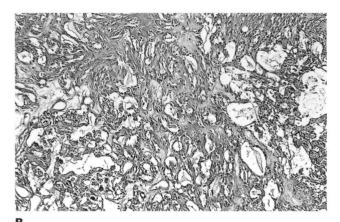

A

B

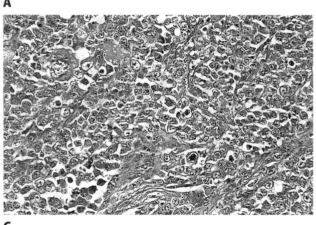

C

Fig. 14.36 Malignant mixed tumor. **A,** Computed tomography shows large anterior orbital tumor arising from lacrimal gland. **B,** Histologic section shows areas resembling benign mixed tumor. **C,** High magnification of another area shows sheets of malignant epithelial cells. (Case presented by Dr. HE Grossniklaus to the meeting of the Eastern Ophthalmic Pathology Society, 1989.)

Rarely, the tumor can occur in the nasal orbit, presumably from ectopic lacrimal gland.

5. Histologically, under lower power it has a characteristic "Swiss-cheese" pattern.
   a. Aggregates or islands of poorly differentiated, small, tightly packed epithelial cells are sharply outlined against the surrounding typical, hyaline-like stroma.
      1). Aggregates may be very small, moderate, or quite large, but are always sharply outlined.
      2). Aggregates contain mucin-filled cystic spaces of different sizes, hence the Swiss-cheese pattern.
   Hyaline stroma surrounding the nests of neoplastic cells is an important finding in differentiating adenoid cystic carcinoma from similarly appearing basal cell or adnexal cell carcinomas. Instead of a hyaline, relatively acellular stroma, the basal cell and adnexal cell carcinomas have a highly cellular, sarcomatous-like, "desmoplastic" stroma surrounding the nests of neoplastic cells.
   b. Some tumors have solid sheets or nests of basaloid cells in addition to the typical cribriform or Swiss-cheese pattern.

Patients who have a basaloid pattern in their tumor have a 5-year survival rate of 21%, compared with a 71% survival rate when no basaloid pattern is present. "Bad" prognostic signs include a basaloid (solid) pattern, presence of tumor at resection margins, and presence of abnormal S-phase (proliferative) fraction. A basaloid pattern in an adenoid cystic carcinoma must be differentiated from the entity basal cell adenocarcinoma (see later), which has a lower degree of malignancy and a more favorable prognosis than adenoid cystic carcinoma.

H. Other types of carcinomas (all are rare)‡
   1. Mucoepidermoid carcinoma, adenocarcinoma (including the less malignant subtypes salivary duct carcinoma, epithelial–myoepithelial carcinoma, and polymorphous low-grade adenocarcinoma), mucinous carcinoma, undifferentiated carcinoma, myoepithelioma (spindle cell variety), lymphoepithelial carcinoma, primary cystadenocarcinoma, and carcinoid tumor occur.
   2. Median age group is approximately 53 years, with a 3 : 1 male predominance.
   3. All have a very poor prognosis.
   4. Mucoepidermoid carcinoma (Fig. 14.38) is the most common primary carcinoma of the major salivary glands, but is rare in the lacrimal gland. The

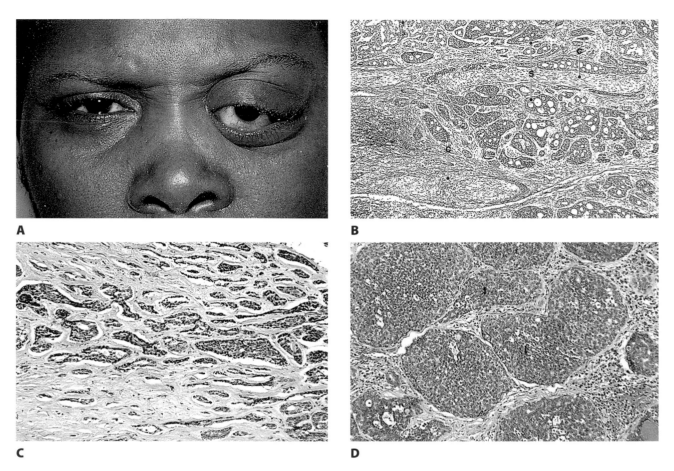

A

B

C

D

Fig. 14.37 Adenoid cystic carcinoma. **A,** The patient had a rapidly progressing proptosis of the left eye. **B,** A histologic section shows the characteristic "Swiss-cheese" pattern (s) of adenoid cystic carcinoma. The Swiss-cheese pattern is also present in the perineural sheath around a ciliary nerve (c). Adenoid cystic carcinoma is noted for its rapid invasion of ciliary nerves. **C,** The tumor may superficially resemble a basal cell carcinoma, but it tends to have a relatively acellular hyalin-like stroma between the islands of poorly differentiated, tightly packed, small, dark, epithelial cells. A basal cell carcinoma tends to have a very cellular desmoplastic stroma between the nests of malignant basal cells. **D,** In this area, a more solid pattern (basaloid pattern) is seen [l, lobules of solid (basaloid) tumor]. This type of pattern is present in approximately 50% of tumors. If no basaloid pattern is present, the 5-year survival rate is 71%; with a basaloid pattern, the 5-year survival rate is 21%.

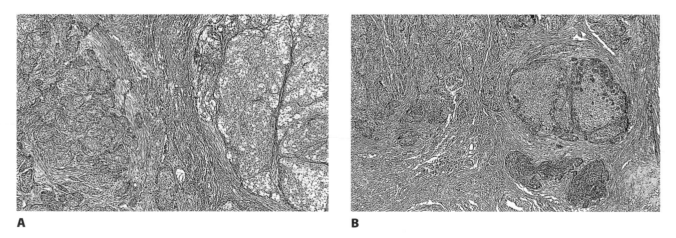

A

B

Fig. 14.38 Mucoepidermoid carcinoma. **A,** Both epidermal cells (mainly on left) and clear cells (mainly on right) are present. **B,** Clear cells stain positively with mucicarmine. (Case courtesy of Dr. LE Zimmerman and reported by Byers RM *et al.: Am J Ophthalmol* 79:53. © Elsevier 1975.)

tumor contains both epidermoid (squamous) and mucin-producing cells.

5. Myoepitheliomas can occur in a spindle form or clear cell form; the latter needs to be differentiated from clear cell variants of oncocytoma, mucoepidermoid carcinoma, carcinoid tumor, and others.

6. Acinic cell carcinoma is rare in the parotid gland (2% to 4% of tumors), and even rarer in the lacrimal gland.

7. Basal cell adenocarcinoma, a very rare neoplasm of the lacrimal gland, has a similar appearance to those adenoid cystic carcinomas that have a large basaloid component, but is less malignant and has a more favorable prognosis than the latter.

VI. Reticuloendothelial system
   A. Langerhans' cell histiocytosis (LCH; Langerhans' granulomatosis, histiocytosis X)†
      1. LCH occurs primarily in children, adolescents, and young adults.
         a. Bone is involved in approximately 80% of cases; other common sites include skin, liver, lymph nodes, spleen, bone marrow, lungs, eyes, and ears.
         b. LCH is characterized by a proliferation of Langerhans' cells in an inflammatory background, often containing many eosinophils.
            1). Langerhans' cells, found primarily in skin and mucosa (including conjunctiva), bear human leukocyte antigen-DR antigens, leukocyte common antigen (CD45-positive in frozen sections but negative in paraffin sections), and express CD1 and S-100 protein.

Langerhans' cells act as antigen-presenting cells, having lost most of their phagocytic function.

---

            2). Langerhans' cells are large cells with abundant, ill-defined cytoplasm, and contain typical oval or indented nuclei, some of which are shaped like coffee beans with long, central, longitudinal grooves.
            3). Immunohistochemically, Langerhans' cells stain positively for vimentin, S-100 protein, CD1a, LN-2, LN-3, CD4, CD11c, CD14, CD15, HAM 56, CD68 (KP1), and peanut agglutinin, and negative for factor VIII, and CD30.

The histopathologic diagnosis of LCH is made if two or more of the following features are found: positive staining for adenosine triphosphatase, S-100 protein, α-mannosidase, or peanut lectin binding.

---

            4). Electron microscopically, the characteristic, rod-shaped granules, called *Birbeck granules*, contain a central dense core (imparting a grooved appearance) and a thick outer sheath.

Birbeck granules have an expanded, rounded end, resembling a tennis racket.

      2. LCH, previously called *histiocytosis X* and then *Langerhans' granulomatosis*, consists of the interrelated clinicopathologic entities of eosinophilic granuloma of bone, Hand–Schüller–Christian disease, and Letterer–Siwe disease.
      3. Eosinophilic granuloma of bone (solitary†; Fig. 14.39)
         a. An eosinophilic granuloma is a relatively benign tumor that usually involves a single bone, often the outer part of the upper orbital rim, in a destructive process.

Rarely, orbital eosinophilic granuloma can be bilateral.

---

         b. Histologically, the tumor is composed of Langerhans' cells admixed with eosinophils; Langerhans' cells are essential for the diagnosis (see earlier for immunohistochemistry and electron microscopy under discussion of LCH).
      4. Hand–Schüller–Christian disease (multifocal eosinophilic granuloma)†
         a. Characteristic triad: bony lesions in the skull, exophthalmos, and diabetes insipidus
         b. The disease may be fatal.
         c. Histologically, Langerhans' cells infiltrate the orbit (see earlier for immunohistochemistry and electron microscopy under discussion of LCH).
      5. Letterer–Siwe disease (diffuse histiocytosis‡; Fig. 14.40)
         a. Letterer–Siwe disease affects infants and very young children.
         b. It is a rapidly progressive disease that is almost always fatal. The disease rarely involves the orbit.
         c. Histologically, Langerhans' cells infiltrate the involved tissues (see earlier for immunohistochemistry and electron microscopy under discussion of LCH).

When the uveal tract is involved in the disease, which is rare, the process is usually restricted to the choroid.

   B. Juvenile xanthogranuloma (nevoxanthoendothelioma†; see p. 343 in Chapter 9)
      The histiocytes in juvenile xanthogranuloma do not contain Birbeck granules, are negative for S-100 protein, and should not be included in LCH.
   C. Reactive histiocytic disorders
      1. Reactive histiocytic disorders are a group of diseases characterized by a systemic or localized proliferation of benign histiocytes and include sinus histiocytosis, X-linked lymphoproliferative syndrome, virus-associated hemophagocytic syndrome, and familial erythrophagocytic lymphohistiocytosis.

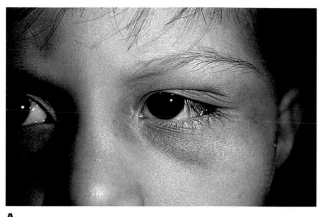

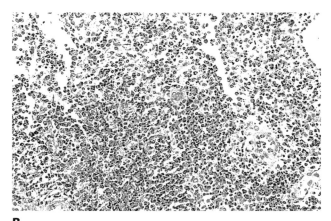

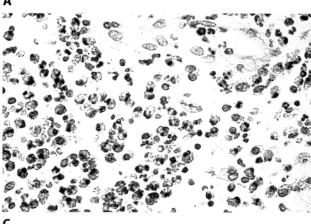

A

B

Fig. 14.39 Eosinophilic granuloma. **A,** A 4-year-old boy presented clinically with rapid onset of erythema and swelling over lateral edge of left orbit. Osteomyelitis versus rhabdomyosarcoma diagnosed clinically; area explored surgically. **B,** Histologic section shows large histiocytes (abnormal Langerhans' cells) and numerous eosinophils characteristic of a solitary eosinophilic granuloma, seen with increased magnification in **C.** (**A,** Courtesy of Dr. DB Schaffer.)

C

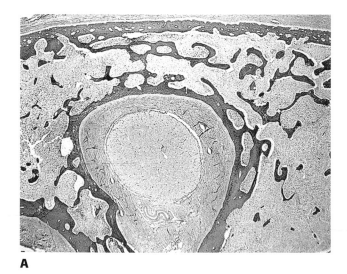

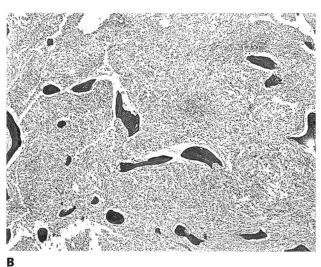

A

B

Fig. 14.40 Letterer–Siwe disease (diffuse histiocytosis). At autopsy, some lesions showed transition to Hand–Schüller–Christian disease (multifocal eosinophilic granuloma). **A,** Bone around optic nerve (large, central, circular area) and optic canal replaced massively by histiocytes (abnormal Langerhans' cells). **B,** Increased magnification of orbital bone to show histiocytes. (Courtesy of Dr. LE Zimmerman; case illustrated by Hogan MJ, Zimmerman LE, eds: Ophthalmic Pathology: An Atlas and Textbook. © Elsevier 1962.)

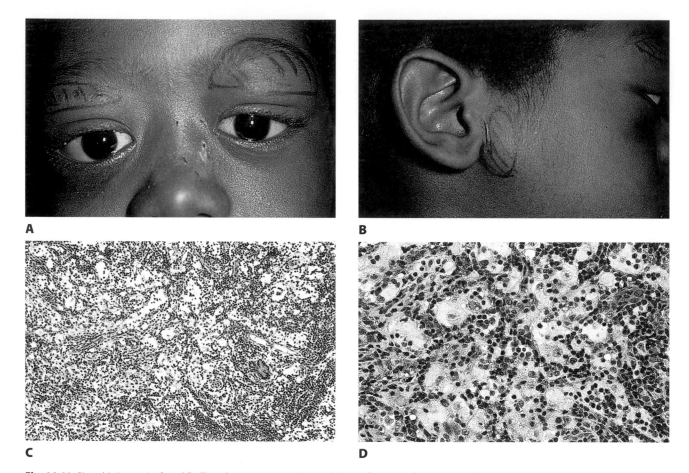

Fig. 14.41 Sinus histiocytosis. **A** and **B**, Clinical appearance in 3-year-old boy of tumors of both upper lids and preauricular area. **C**, Histologic section shows diffuse infiltration of lymphocytes, plasma cells, and histiocyte-like cells. **D**, "Histiocytes" prominent and characterized by large, pale, vesicular nuclei. Note abundant foamy cytoplasm and that some histiocyte-like cells contain plasma cells or lymphocytes in their cytoplasm. (Courtesy of Dr. ME Smith; case reported by Pickering L, Phelan E: *J Pediatr* 86:745. © Elsevier 1975.)

2. Sinus histiocytosis (Rosai–Dorfman disease‡; Fig. 14.41)
    a. Sinus histiocytosis is a benign disease, tends to run a protracted course, and mainly affects children and young adults.
       1). The main clinical finding is cervical lymphadenopathy.
       2). Low-grade fever, anemia, leukocytosis, and elevated IgG levels occur.
    b. Ocular findings include orbital (proptosis that may lead to exposure keratitis) and lid involvement, rarely epibulbar involvement, corneal ulceration, bilateral retinal detachment, lacrimal sac and duct involvement, endophthalmitis, and even loss of the eye.
    c. Histologically, a proliferation of large, bland, histiocyte-like cells intermixed with lymphocytes and plasma cells is noted.
       1). Lymphocytes (mainly), plasma cells, and occasionally other hematopoietic cells (leukophagocytosis, sometimes striking) or erythrocytes (erythrophagocytosis) may be seen in the cytoplasm of the "histiocytes."

       2). The histiocyte-like cells share some properties of histiocytes (express monocyte–macrophage markers α_1-antitrypsin, α_1-chymotrypsin, lysozyme, Mac 386) and some of interdigitating reticulum cells and Langerhans' cells (express the dendritic cell-associated marker S-100 protein, but not CD1).

       Reticulohistiocytoma (reticulohistiocytic granuloma), a rare, benign histiocytic lesion that occurs as an isolated nodule or part of a systemic disorder, may be confused with sinus histiocytosis, as well as with LCH, juvenile xanthogranuloma, ganglioneuroma, and amelanotic melanoma.

       ---

3. X-linked lymphoproliferative syndrome (see p. 64 in Chapter 3)
4. Virus-associated hemophagocytic syndrome and familial erythrophagocytic lymphohistiocytosis rarely have ocular manifestations.
D. Lymphomatoid granulomatosis
    1. Lymphomatoid granulomatosis behaves like a malignant lymphoma.

TABLE 14.3 Diagnostic Criteria for Extranodal Lymphomas

HISTOLOGIC CRITERIA
Features Strongly Associated with Lymphoma

Relatively monomorphic lymphoid infiltrate
Cytologic atypia
Infiltrative growth with effacement of architecture
Dutcher bodies

Features Suggestive of Lymphoma

Lymphoepithelial lesions

Reactive Features Often Associated with Low-Grade Extranodal Lymphomas

Reactive follicular centers; mantle zones often irregular or absent
Plasma cells

IMMUNOPHENOTYPIC CRITERIA

Monoclonal immunoglobin (light-chain restriction)*
Aberrant expression of T- or B-cell-associated antigens
Marked predominance of B cells

MOLECULAR GENOTYPIC CRITERIA

Clonal rearrangement of immunoglobin or T-cell receptor genes*
Rearrangement of lymphoma-associated oncogenes, such as *bcl-1*, *bcl-2*, or *c-myc*

Light-chain restriction and clonal immunoglobin and T-cell receptor gene rearrangements have been reported in some benign lymphoid proliferations.
(From Salhany KE, Pietra GC: *Am J Clin Pathol* 99:472, 1993.)

2. Lymphomatoid granulomatosis is an uncommon, often fatal, lymphoreticular disease that primarily involves the lungs, skin, and central nervous system.
3. Ocular findings are usually lid lesions, but also reported are uveitis, scleritis and episcleritis, central retinal artery occlusion, and peripheral vasculitis.
4. Histologically, an angiocentric pattern of polymorphic cellular infiltrate (atypical mononuclear cells, plasma and plasmacytoid cells, epithelioid cells, inflammatory giant cells) is seen invading blood vessels (necrotizing vasculitis)

VII. Inflammatory pseudotumor†—any nonneoplastic, space-occupying orbital lesion that presents clinically as a neoplasm (Table 14.3)

Rarely, the tumors can extend beyond the orbit, intracranially or into the sinuses.

A. The signs and symptoms include pain, proptosis, chemosis, lid swelling, and ductional (motility) defects.

Similar findings occur in carotid–cavernous fistula, infectious cellulitis, metastatic neoplasm, cavernous sinus thrombosis, and Graves' ophthalmopathy.

B. On the basis of combined histologic and immunologic information, these tumors show unequivocal chronic inflammation, either granulomatous or nongranulomatous.
C. Chronic granulomatous
  1. Foreign body
  2. Ruptured dermoid
  3. Fat necrosis or lipogranuloma
  4. Sarcoidosis
  5. Tuberculosis
  6. Many others (see Chapter 4)
D. Chronic nongranulomatous
  1. Inflammatory—localized (Fig. 14.42)
    a. Most inflammatory pseudotumors are idiopathic (also called idiopathic orbital inflammation), are usually unilateral but often are bilateral, have an equal sex incidence, and mostly occur in the fourth, fifth, and sixth decades.
    b. The histologic presentation may be quite varied.
      1). Inflammatory pseudotumor is probably an abnormal response pattern with multiple causes, involving predominantly a fibrohistiocytic cell [vimentin and CD68 (KP-1)-positive].
      2). The hallmark is the following histologic tetrad:
        a). Cellular polymorphism (i.e., different types of inflammatory cells, including lymphocytes, non-Dutcher body-containing plasma cells, histiocytes, and eosinophils).
        b). Lymphoid follicles with germinal centers.

Mitotic figures are normally found in the germinal centers of lymphoid follicles. Although lymphoid follicles are highly suggestive of inflammatory pseudotumors, they may occur in small B-cell lymphomas [e.g., mucosal-associated lymphoid tissue (MALT) lymphomas].

        c). Absence of atypia.

Absence of atypia, however, can also occur in small B-cell lymphomas.

        d). Ancillary evidence of inflammation (e.g., plasmacytoid cells, Russell bodies, and proliferation of capillaries with swollen, enlarged endothelial cells)
      3). The response can be cellular, or predominantly collagen and relatively acellular.
      4). The response can also involve mainly ocular muscles (myositis), the lacrimal gland (dacryoadenitis), or the orbital vessels (vasculitis), or result from changes in a pre-existing hemangioma with hemorrhage, organization, and inflammation.

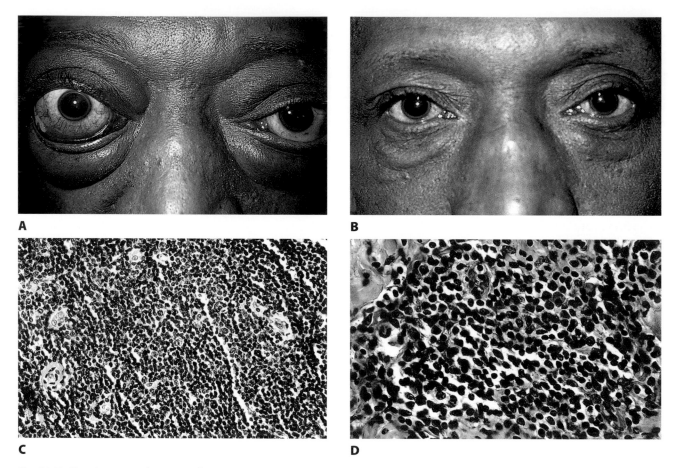

Fig. 14.42 Chronic nongranulomatous inflammatory pseudotumor. **A**, A 45-year-old man had bilateral exophthalmos, much worse OD. After orbital biopsy, the patient was given a short course of systemic steroid therapy and bilateral orbital X-ray therapy. **B**, Six years later. **C**, Biopsy shows endothelial cell proliferation, plasma cells, and lymphocytes, shown with increased magnification in **D**. Concurrently, presumed nonrelated, chronic lymphatic leukemia was detected in peripheral blood smear and verified on bone marrow examination, and immunoglobulin M paraprotein discovered on serum immunoelectrophoresis; both continued when patient last seen 11 years after the initial onset of bilateral exophthalmos.

c. Idiopathic sclerosing inflammation of the orbit
   1). Idiopathic sclerosing inflammation is a clinicopathologic entity, similar to retroperitoneal fibrosis, characterized by primary, chronic, and immunologically mediated fibrosis, poor response to steroid therapy or radiation therapy, and frequent visual disability.
   2). Histologically, the fibrosis appears consistently and early.
2. Inflammatory—part of systemic disease
   a. Graves' ophthalmopathy
   b. Sjögren's syndrome
   c. Abnormalities of IgA, IgG, or IgM serum fractions (polyclonal), and may be associated with inflammation and PAS-positive inclusions called *Dutcher bodies* (see Fig. 14.43D).

Dutcher bodies appear as intranuclear inclusion bodies but are cytoplasmic invaginations of immunoglobulin into the nucleus. Usually, if Dutcher bodies are found, the lymphoma is malignant.

---

d. Kimura's disease (angiolymphoid hyperplasia with eosinophilia)‡
   1). Kimura's disease is characterized by single or multiple painless, subcutaneous tumors of the head and neck in young Asian males; the orbit is rarely involved.
   2). Increased serum IgE levels and peripheral blood eosinophilia are common.
   3). Histologically, vascular hyperplasia with plump endothelial cells is accompanied by varying degrees of mixed cellular infiltrate, usually a significant number of eosinophils in a background of lymphoid cells.

Kimura's disease and epithelioid hemangioma, also called *angiolymphoid hyperplasia with eosinophilia* (see later) are two different distinct clinicopathologic entities. Kimura's disease occurs almost exclusively in Asian men and shows florid lymphoid infiltrates with formation of prominent lymphoid follicles, germinal center necrosis and vasculariza-

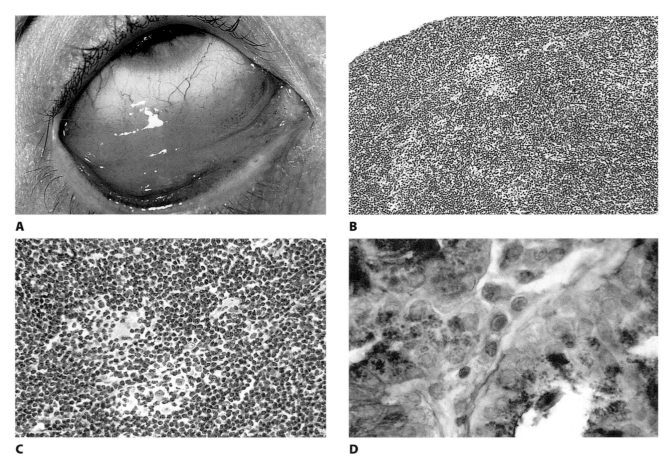

Fig. 14.43 Reactive lymphoid hyperplasia. **A,** The patient noted a fullness of the lower right lid. Large, thickened, redundant folds of conjunctiva in the inferior cul de sac are seen. The characteristic "fish flesh" appearance of the lesion suggests the clinical differential diagnosis of a lymphoid or leukemic infiltrate or amyloidosis. **B,** A histologic section shows a lymphoid infiltrate. **C,** Increased magnification shows that the lymphocyes are mature, quite small, and uniform; occasional plasma cells and large monocytoid lymphocytes are seen. The uniformity of the lymphocytes makes it difficult to differentiate this benign lesion from a well-differentiated lymphosarcoma. The very mature appearance of the cells and the absence of atypical cells, along with the presence of plasma cells, suggests the diagnosis of a benign lesion. In such cases, testing using monoclonal antibodies may be helpful. If the population is of mixed B and T cells, the chances are that the tumor is benign. If it is predominantly of one cell type or the other, usually B-cell, it is probably malignant and may represent mucosal-associated lymphoid tissue (MALT) of the conjunctiva. **D,** Dutcher bodies (periodic acid–Schiff-positive, eosinophilic, intranuclear inclusions) are a sign of malignancy.

tion, marked eosinophilia with or without abscess formation, proliferation of cuboidal endothelium-lined venules, and focal fibrosis. Epithelioid hemangioma occurs in all races, has smaller lesions, and is characterized by exuberant proliferation of "epithelioid" endothelium-lined vessels with irregular nuclei and cytoplasmic vacuoles, supported in a fibromyxoid stroma containing infiltrates of small lymphocytes and eosinophils.

e. Epithelioid hemangioma (angiolymphoid hyperphilia)‡
1). Epithelioid hemangioma is a benign vascular tumor typically occurring in middle-aged women.
2). A small proportion of patients have regional lymphadenopathy and peripheral blood eosinophilia.

3). Histologically, the lesions are mainly vascular and show characteristic plump endothelial cells that contain abundant eosinophilic cytoplasm and have scalloped borders, simulating epithelial cells (plump epithelioid cells), lining blood vessels and protruding into the lumina.

VIII. Malignant lymphoma† (Figs 14.43 to 14.46; see Tables 14.3 and 14.4)
A. Among extraconal orbital tumors, 22% are reactive lymphoid hyperplasia and 20% are malignant lymphoma.

In one study, 20% of orbital lymphoid lesions were idiopathic chronic inflammation, 40% were lymphoid hyperplasias, and 40% were lymphomas. The relative percentage of B cells in the various lesions was inflammation, 35%; hyperplasia, 65.9%; and lymphoma, 87.3%. If one considers ophthalmic and intraocular

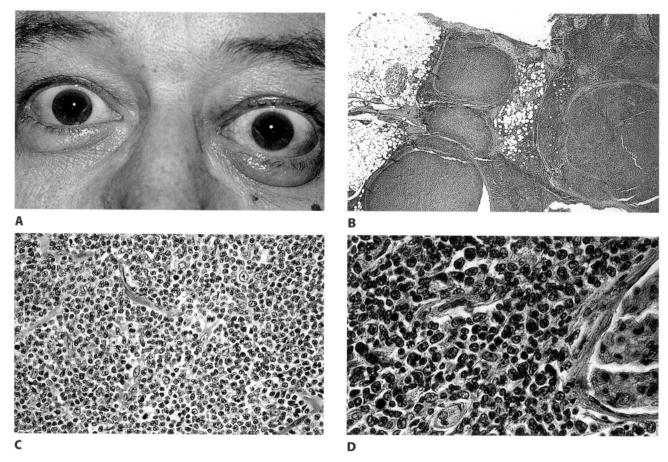

Fig. 14.44 Non-Hodkin's lymphoma—B-cell. **A**, Clinical appearance of left exophthlmos. **B**, Histologic section shows extensive nodular lymphoid infiltrate of orbital tissue. **C**, Increased magnification shows monotonous uniform lymphocytic infiltrate and many mitotic figures. **D**, Same nodular lymphomatous infiltrate replaces kidney parenchyma; glomerulus present toward right. (From Yanoff M, Scheie HG: *Surv Ophthalmol* 12:133. © Elsevier 1967.)

non-Hodgkin's lymphoma, 42% are intraorbital and 35% are conjunctival. There may be a high incidence of orbital malignant lymphoma among Japanese patients. About 3% of patients who have chronic lymphocytic leukemia develop non-Hodgkin's syndrome (usually large B-cell lymphoma); this sequence of malignancies is called *Richter's syndrome*. In general, ocular involvement with chronic lymphocytic leukemia is rare.

1. Orbital lymphomatoid lesions usually present as a palpable mass with proptosis, diplopia, and conjunctival ("salmon-pink") swelling. Uncommon presentations include ptosis.

B. Reactive lymphoid or plasma cell hyperplasia (see Fig. 14.43)
1. Although previously classified as inflammatory pseudotumors, these tumors are in the "gray zone" and are very difficult to differentiate histologically from malignant lymphomas (or plasmacytomas), and probably many, if not most represent small B-cell lymphomas.

They probably represent approximately 11% of the cases of lymphoproliferative lesions of the ocular adnexa.

2. "True" reactive lymphoid hyperplasia usually consists of a virtually pure lymphoproliferative lesion of small lymphocytes that, by immunophenotyping and immunogenotyping, shows a polyclonal T- and B-cell infiltrate and an absence of Dutcher bodies; mitoses, if present, are restricted to germinal centers where macrophages contain scattered debris (tingible bodies).
   a. Reactive lymphoid follicles reminiscent of normal lymphoid architecture are usually seen within the infiltrate.
   b. No polymorphism or ancillary evidence of inflammation occurs.
   c. The tumors lack anaplasia.

C. Non-Hodgkin's lymphoma—B-cell
1. The following diagnostic criteria point to malignant extranodal B-cell lymphoma:
   a. The absence of the following histologic tetrad:

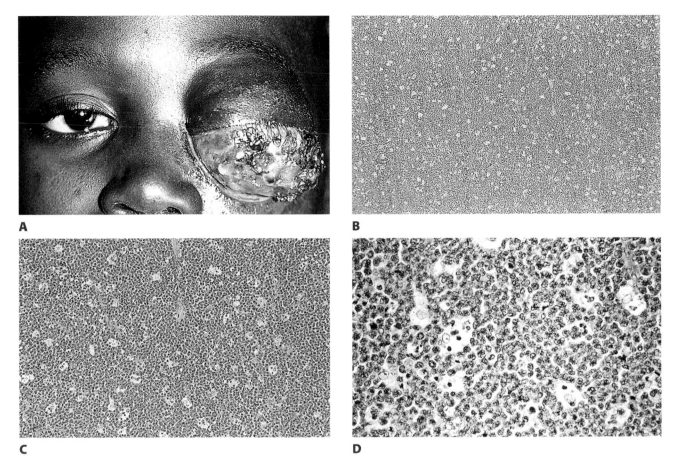

Fig. 14.45 Burkitt's (undifferentiated) lymphoma. **A**, African boy (Zaire) has massive left orbital infiltrate. **B** and **C**, Histiocytes, which often display phagocytosis, scattered among lymphoid tumor cells, giving characteristic "starry-sky" appearance. **D**, Undifferentiated, anaplastic, large lymphoid cells contain ovoid vesicular basophilic nuclei and prominent nucleoli. Histiocytes contain abundant, almost clear cytoplasm and phagocytosed cellular debris. (**A**, Courtesy of Dr. RE Shannon.)

1). Cellular polymorphism (i.e., different types of inflammatory cells, including lymphocytes, non-Dutcher body-containing plasma cells, histiocytes, and eosinophils)

2). Lymphoid follicles with germinal centers.

Mitotic figures are normally found in the germinal centers of lymphoid follicles. Although lymphoid follicles are highly suggestive of inflammatory pseudotumors, they may occur in small B-cell lymphomas (e.g., MALT lymphomas).

---

3). Absence of atypia.

Absence of atypia, however, can also occur in small B-cell lymphomas.

---

4). Ancillary evidence of inflammation (e.g., plasmacytoid cells, Russell bodies, and proliferation of capillaries with swollen, enlarged endothelial cells)

b. Formation of a mass, tissue architectural effacement, cellular monomorphism, cytologic atypia, presence of proliferative centers, and plasma cells containing Dutcher bodies are all features of low-grade B-cell lymphomas.

c. Immunoglobulin light-chain restriction or an aberrant B-cell phenotype are immunologic features that, if demonstrated, help to support a malignant diagnosis.

1). A ratio of κ/λ immunoglobulin light-chain-expressing B lymphocytes in excess of 5:1 or less than 0.5:1 indicates a monoclonal κ or λ B-cell population.

2). In general, CD5+ B-cell proliferative disorders are considered to be malignant.

1. Immunoglobulin light-chain restriction is accepted as a marker of clonality in identifying B-cell lymphomas.

Abnormal chromosome translocations are important mechanisms in the pathogenesis of non-Hodgkin's lymphoma, especially translocations involving the region of the immunoglobulin heavy-chain gene on band 14q32.

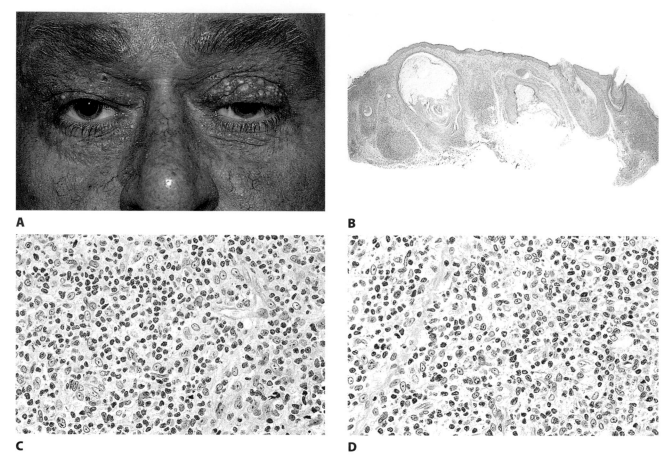

Fig. 14.46 Mycosis fungoides. **A**, Clinical appearance of skin lesions in patient who had known mycosis fungoides. **B**, Histologic section of skin biopsy shows an extensive perifollicular infiltrate, including a population of lymphocytes with hyperchromic convoluted nuclei (cerebriform nuclei) with scanty cytoplasm, shown with increased magnification in **C** and **D**. Pautrier microabscesses (small intradermal groups of tightly packed mononuclear cells) who are not present. Immunologic characterization demonstrated predominantly T cells with a slight preponderance of helper (CD4) over suppressor (CD8) forms. A diagnosis of cutaneous T-cell lymphoma was made. (Case courtesy of Dr. H Levy.)

2. Small B-cell lymphomas can be classified in many ways.
   a. Kiel classification of nodal, low-grade B-cell lymphomas composed of small B cells with a minority of blast cells: chronic lymphocytic leukemia, centrocytic (mantle cell) lymphoma, centroblastic/centrocytic lymphoma, MALT or bronchial-associated lymphoid tissue, lymphoma/immunocytoma/monocytoid B-cell lymphoma, and unclassified. In the World Health Organization classification, system MALT lymphomas are classified as extranodal marginal-zone lymphomas.
      1). Primary orbital lymphomas have a favorable prognosis.
      2). A high percentage of them have clinical, pathologic, and biologic MALT characteristics.
         a). Clinically, MALT tumors arise in extranodal sites from postgerminal center memory B cells, mainly mucosal.
      b). Nongastric marginal-zone B-cell lymphomas present in a single site in 90% of cases. The most frequent such locations are: skin (26%), salivary glands (18%), orbit (14%), Waldeyer's ring (13%), and 39% and 28% have nodal involvement and bone marrow involvement, respectively.
      c). Pathologically, the tumors recapitulate Peyer's patches (i.e., reactive follicles), marginal-zone or monocytoid B cells, plasma cells, occasional Dutcher bodies, scattered transformed blasts (entoblasts and immunoblasts), and sometimes epithelial lesions in the form of lymphoepithelium.

The tumor cells are CD5⁻, CD10⁻, cyclin D1⁻, CD23 and CD43-variable, and proliferating cell nuclear antigen (PCNA) KI 67⁺.

TABLE 14.4 Morphological, Immunophenotypic, Molecular-Biological and Clinical Characteristics of the 5 Lymphoma Subtypes Presented

Lymphoma Subtype	Morphology	Tumor Cell Immune Profile	Molecular Biological Changes*	Cell of Origin	Clinical Characteristics
EMZL	• Expansive growth in the marginal zone between reactive secondary follicles • Heterogeneous cell population: centrocyte-like cells, monocytoid B-cells, plasmacytoid cells, occasional blasts • Possibly "Follicular Colonization" • Possibly "Lymphoepithelial lesions" • Often multifocal growth	• CD79a+, CD20+, CD43+ (usually), BCL-2± • IgM+, IgD− • CD10−, CD23−, CD5−, cyclin D1− • Presence of FDC's in reactive secondary follicles • Monotypic cytoplasmic Ig in 10%	• Clonal Ig-H and Ig-L rearrangements • Mutations in V-region of IgH-gene • t(11;18)(q21;q21) in ca. 50% • Trisomy 3 in ca. 50%	• "Memory" B-cell	• 8% of all NHL • Peak age, 65 years • Females > Males • Rare involvement of BM or spleen at time of diagnosis • Possible concurrent or subsequent involvement of other extranodal sites • Tendency to recur
DLBCL	• Diffuse growth pattern • Centroblastic: large centroblast-like tumor cells with variable content of immunoblasts • Immunoblastic: >90% immunoblastic tumor cells • Anaplastic: polymorphic often bizarre tumor cells • T-cell rich: only 10% tumor cells with 90% T-cell infiltrate and macrophages	• CD79a+, CD20a+, • BCL-6+ (ca. 70% of cases) • CD10+ (ca. 25–50%) • IgM > IgG > IgA in 50%–75% of cases • CD30+ in lymphoma with anaplastic morphology • Rarely CD5+ or CD23+ • No FDC-MW • Ki-67 nearly always >40%	• Clonal Ig-H and Ig-L rearrangements** • Numerous mutations in V-Region of IgH-Gene • Bcl-6 gene rearrangements in up to 40% of cases • Bcl-2 gene rearrangements in 20–30% of cases • C-myc gene rearrangements extremely rare • REL gene amplification in 20% mainly extranodal lymphoma • P53-Gene mutations only in secondary lymphoma arising from a FL	• Mature germinal center-B-cell or post-germinal center-B-cell (memory) B-cell	• 40% extranodal (gastrointestinal tract > skin > soft tissue > central nervous system) • 60% nodal • Average age: 60–70 years • Rapidly growing solitary nodal or extranodal tumor • Aggressive clinical course
FL	• Usually follicular growth pattern with occasional diffuse areas; rarely purely diffuse • Mixture of centrocytes and centroblasts with dominance of former • Obvious reduction in growth fraction in neoplastic GCs • Monomorphic GCs with loss of zonation • Minimal or no apoptosis in GC • Usually no macrophages with tingible bodies • Thin or even absence of the follicle mantle • Rarely pure diffuse growth pattern	• CD20+, CD10+, BCL-2+ (90%), BCL-6+, IgM+ (50%), IgG (50%) • CD43- (95%), CD23-, CD5- • Dense follicular FDC MW • Obvious reduction in growth fraction in neoplastic GCs versus reactive GCs, particularly in BCL-2+ cases • Often CD10+ and BCL-6+ B-cells in the interfollicular region • Dense well-defined FDC meshworks in neoplastic germinal centers (demonstrated with CD 21)	• Clonal Ig-H and Ig-L rearrangements** • Numerous mutations in V-region of IgH-Gene with "ongoing" mutations (intraclonal diversity) • t(14;18) in 90%, resulting in the expression of BCL-2 in neoplastic germinal centers • Mutations of p 53 gene and c-myc-rearrangement in high-grade transformed cases	• Germinal center-B-cell	• 40% of all NHL in the USA, 2C–30% in Europe • Fifth and sixth decades of life (mean age, 59 years), unusual before 20 years of age • M:F = 1:1 • Lymph nodes mainly infiltrated, but also spleen, bone marrow and skin • Often advanced disease (Stage III/IV) at the time of diagnosis • 5-year survival rate: 75% Transformation to DLBCL in 30% of cases

TABLE 14.4 *Continued*

Lymphoma Subtype	Morphology	Tumor Cell Immune Profile	Molecular Biological Changes*	Cell of Origin	Clinical Characteristics
Classical BL	• Diffuse monotonous infiltration pattern • Medium-sized tumor cells, round nuclei, clumped chromatin, basophilic cytoplasm • Extremely high proliferation rate with numerous mitoses and apoptotic bodies • Starry sky pattern due to admixed histiocytes	• CD79a+, CD20+, CD10+, BCL-6+, IgM+ • CD21+ (endemic form) • CD5–, CD23–, TdT–, BCL-2– • Ki-67 = 100%	• Clonal IgH-rearrangements with somatic mutations • Translocation of MYC: t(8;14), t(2;8) or t(8;22) • Inactivation of TP53 due to mutations (30%) • EBV genomes can be demonstrated in tumor cells in nearly all endemic cases, 25–40% immunodeficient cases and <30% in sporadic cases	• Germinal center-B-cell	• Endemic form: children > adults (ages 4–7 years), M : F = 2 : 1, mandible maxilla and orbital bones • Sporadic form: children > adults, 1–2% of all NHL in USA, M : F = 2 or 3 : 1, distal ileum, cecum and mesenteric lymph nodes • Immunodeficiency associated BL: adults > children, HIV-infection, predominantly lymph nodes • Often bulky tumor disease due to rapid proliferation rate of tumors • Prognosis dependant on Stage, particularly bone marrow involvement
Classical HL	• Tumor cells: typical HRS-cells • Architecture: mainly diffuse or an interfollicular infiltrate composed of eosinophils neutorphils, lymphocytes, plasmacells and macrophages	• CD30+, CD15+, • EBV+ (40–50%) • EMA 5%+ • CD20–/+, CD79–/+ • CD45–, J-chain–	• Clonal IgH-rearrangements with numerous somatic mutations without "ongoing" mutations	• Germinal center-B-cell	• Mainly 30–40 years • M : F—3 : 1 • Lymph node enlargement, particularly cervical, axillary and inguinal • Extranodal involvement mainly in mediastinum, spleen, less often lung, liver and bone marrow • B-symptoms in 35% of cases • Prognosis dependant on Stage of disease at diagnosis • 5 year survival: 85–90%

*These results arise from investigations of Non-Hodgkin lymphomas in other locations.

**Rearrangements demonstrable only in 50–70% of cases due to presence of somatic mutations.

EMZL = Extranodal marginal zone B-cell lymphoma; DLBCL = Diffuse large cell B-cell lymphoma+; FL = Follicular lymphoma; BL = Burkitt lymphoma; HL = Hodgkin's lymphoma; NHL = Non-Hodgkin's lymphoma; FDC-MW = follicular dendritic cell meshworks; Ig-L = Immunoglobulin Light chain; Ig-H = Immunoglobin Heavy chain; EBV = Epstein-Barr Virus.

(From Coupland SE, Hummel M, Stein H: Ocular adnexal lymphomas: five case presentations and a review of the literature. Surv Ophthalmol 47:470, 2002, with permission from Elsevier.)

d). Biologically, the tumor cells are B cells, proliferate in mucosal and other extranodal sites, and usually show reactive germinal centers, often interacting with epithelium.

1). Chronic antigenic stimulation, particularly in the setting of chronic infection, may contribute to the development of these lesions.

e). Rarely, MALT tumors can present as a scleritis.

f). These lesions are radiosensitive, with orbital lesions and ocular adnexal lesions demonstrating a high rate of complete response to radiotherapy.

g). Somatostatin receptor scintigraphy may be helpful in the staging and noninvasive therapy-monitoring in extragastric MALT-type lymphoma irrespective of the site of presentation.

b. Modified Rappaport and the working formulation classification of diffuse B-cell lymphomas composed of small to medium-sized B cells: well-differentiated lymphocytic lymphoma (without bone marrow involvement) or well-differentiated lymphocytic leukemia (with bone marrow involvement), intermediate lymphocytic lymphoma, and poorly differentiated lymphocytic lymphoma (small cleaved-cell lymphoma)

c. Others classify small B-cell lymphomas in different ways [e.g., Pangalis: small lymphocytic (well-differentiated) non-Hodgkin's lymphoma, lymphoplasmacytic lymphoma (Waldenström's macroglobulinemia), and chronic lymphocytic leukemia].

d. Obviously, the perfect classification does not yet exist, but the World Health Organization has completed a "consensus" classification of hematologic malignant lymphomas, which is a modification of the Revised European American Lymphoma (REAL) classification.

The use of *in vitro* immunologic and immunohistochemical techniques can aid in the diagnosis of orbital lymphoreticular neoplasms by demonstrating immunologic markers. Most lymphoid malignancies in adults have been shown to be B-cell (e.g., CD19[+], CD20[+], and CD22[+]). For example, non-Hodgkin's lymphoma of the central nervous system (reticulum cell sarcoma) is composed of B cells at least 70% of the time, T cells (e.g., CD2[+], CD3[+], CD4[+], CD5[+], and CD7[+]) approximately 20% of the time, and histiocytes (e.g., CD1[+], CD4[+], CD11b[+] and CD11c[+], CD14[+], CD15[+], and CD45[+]) less than 10%. The most common acute lymphoblastic leukemia in children does not have demonstrable immunologic markers (null cell). More than 90% of T-cell lymphomas, mantle cell lymphomas (MCLs), B-cell small lymphocytic lymphomas, and Burkitt's lymphomas are positive for CD43.

---

e. According to Bertoni and Zucca, at least three different, apparently site-specific, chromosomal translocations, all affecting the NF-kappaB pathway, have been implicated in the development and progression of MALT lymphoma. The most common is said to be the translocation t(11;18)(q21;q21), which is present in more than one-third of cases, but is rare in the conjunctiva and orbit. Among MALT lymphomas screened by Streubel and colleagues for translocations t(11;18)(q21;q21), t(14;18)(q32;q21), and t(1;14)(p22;q32), and trisomies 3 and 18, these translocations occurred mutually exclusively and were detected overall in 13.5%, 10.8%, and 1.6% of cases respectively; trisomy 3 and/or 18 occurred in 42.1%. t(14;18)(q32;q21) was most commonly found in lesions of the ocular adnexa/orbit, skin, and salivary glands, and trisomies 3 and 18 each occurred most frequently in intestinal and salivary gland MALT lymphomas. Another study of orbital MALT lymphoma found aneuploidy in six of 10 cases studied, and gains were more frequent than losses. Duplications of chromosome 3 (common region at 3q24-qter), which is said to be expected in marginal-zone lymphoma, and chromosome 6 (common region at 6p21.1–21.3), which is said to be typical of an orbital location, were the most frequently detected.

3. Other B-cell lymphomas (mixed small and large cell, large cell, large cell–immunoblastic, angioimmunoblastic lymphadenopathy). Spontaneous regression of a large B-cell-type lymphoma of the conjunctiva and orbit has been reported.

a. Burkitt's lymphoma (see Fig. 14.45)

1). Burkitt's lymphoma (a diffuse, poorly differentiated, large B-cell lymphoma) is the most common malignant tumor among children in tropical Africa (it is the most common orbital tumor in Uganda, regardless of age); its distribution, however, is worldwide. It is one of the fastest-growing malignancies in the pediatric population in the United States.

a). It can be subdivided into African (endemic), sporadic, and human immunodeficiency-associated subtypes.

Burkitt's lymphoma and diffuse large B-cell lymphoma constitute the majority of nonlymphoblastic lymphomas in the pediatric population.

---

2). The tumor has a predilection for the face and jaws, and may be induced by an insect-vectored agent.

The incidence of Burkitt's lymphoma is markedly increased when associated with infection with the malarial organism *Plasmodium falciparum*.

3). The c-*myc* oncogene is rearranged in Burkitt's lymphoma so that one of the immunoglobulin genes is brought in proximity to c-*myc* and disrupts its normal regulation.

Considerable evidence has been accumulated associating a herpesvirus, the Epstein–Barr virus (see p. 63 in Chapter 3), with Burkitt's lymphoma, probably by its role in the development of the point mutations in the c-*myc* area.

---

4). The prognosis for life is poor.
5). Histologically, the tumor shows tightly packed, undifferentiated, large B-type lymphoid cells and scattered large histiocytes that contain abundant, almost clear cytoplasm and phagocytosed cellular debris.

Burkitt's lymphoma and diffuse large B-cell lymphoma have distinctive immunohistochemical profiles. Staining for c-*myc*, MIB-1, and *bcl-2* may be useful in morphologically difficult cases.

---

b. Mantle cell lymphoma (MCL)
   1). MCL represent about 6 to 7% of all non-Hodgkin's lymphomas.
   2). It is a disease mainly of the elderly and has a male preponderance.
   3). Immunohistochemical staining is generally positive for CD20 and cyclin-D1; CD5 is positive in about 70% of cases, and p53 is negative in most cases.
   4). MCL presenting in the ocular adnexal region is associated with advanced-stage disease and short progression-free survival, but an overall survival similar to MCL at other sites.
c. Cutaneous precursor B-cell lymphoblastic lymphoma is rare but has presented with orbital bone involvement.
   1). Immunohistochemical staining was positive for CD79a and CD43 in all six cases in one report. Cell marker studies by flow cytometry are positive for CD10 and CD19.
4. The majority of extranodal non-Hodgkin's lymphomas, including those that involve the orbit, are of the B-cell variety (conversely, most that involve the skin are T-cell).
5. A morphologic progression of low-grade, small B-cell lymphoma to diffuse, large-cell lymphoma is well recognized.
D. Non-Hodgkin's lymphoma—T-cell‡
1. No single immunologic clonal marker has been identified for malignant T-cell disorders.
   a. Molecular hybridization studies have shown that rearrangements of the T-cell receptor β-chain gene provide a practical means of identifying clonal T-cell proliferations.

b. Although antibodies such as CD3 and CD4 (OPD4) are very specific for T-cell neoplasms, they may recognize only 60% to 70% of T-cell lymphomas. Other antibodies used to identify T-cell processes, such as CD43 (L60, Leu-22, MT-1), CD45RA (MT-2), CD45RO (UCHL-1), and CD5, suffer from a lack of specificity.

Primary localized skin lymphomas that have a predominance of anaplastic Reed–Sternberg-like cells and CD30 positivity appear to have a better prognosis than many other large cell cutaneous lymphomas. More than 90% of T-cell lymphomas, MCLs, B-cell small lymphocytic lymphomas, and Burkitt's lymphomas are positive for CD43.

---

2. Non-Hodgkin's T-cell lymphomas can be divided into three groups:
   a. Those derived from prethymic and thymic T cells (lymphoblastic lymphoma/leukemia)

Lymphoblastic lymphoma/leukemia (T-cell leukemia/ lymphoma) has an association with a retrovirus, the human T-lymphotropic virus type I (HTLV-I). It has presented with bilateral orbital tumors.

---

b. Those derived from postthymic or peripheral T cells (called *peripheral T-cell lymphomas*) and composed of a morphologically and immunologically heterogeneous group of lymphoproliferative disorders (T-cell chronic lymphocytic leukemia, T-prolymphocytic leukemia, monomorphous T-cell lymphoma, immunoblastic T-cell lymphoma)

Immunohistochemistry has shown that the following appear to be abnormal or neoplastic T-cell lymphoproliferative disorders: benign lymphocytic vasculitis, lymphomatoid granulomatosis, midline malignant reticulosis, angiocentric lymphoma, and many cases of angioimmunoblastic lymphadenopathy. NK/T-cell malignancies are uncommon and were previously known as polymorphic reticulosis or angiocentric T-cell lymphomas. The World Health Organization further divides these lesions into NK/T-cell lymphoma (nasal and extranasal) type and aggressive NK-cell leukemia.

---

c. Mycosis fungoides and Sézary's syndrome are special forms of cutaneous T-cell lymphomas that have a relatively protracted course (see Fig. 14.46).
   1). The neoplastic T cells most typically express a CD3⁺, CD4⁺, CD8⁻, CD7⁻ surface phenotype, although exceptions may occur.

The proliferating small lymphocytes show cerebriform nuclei.

2). The percentage of CDR⁺, CD7⁻ cells is elevated in the peripheral blood of patients who have Sézary's syndrome.

3). Although mycosis fungoides rarely involves the orbit, it does so more commonly than the other T-cell lymphomas.

Very rarely, mycosis fungoides can involve the vitreous.

---

4). Altered forms of the retrovirus HTLV-I and HTLV-II have been incriminated in the causation of some cases of mycosis fungoides and Sézary's syndrome.

E. Hodgkin's disease‡

1. Hodgkin's disease very rarely presents initially with orbital involvement, and orbital involvement is rare in any stage of the disease.

2. Hodgkin's disease may be a direct consequence of a *bcl-2* translocation through additional genomic events to be clarified in the future.

The *bcl-2* oncogene acts mainly on the pathways of *apoptosis* (programmed death) and plays a crucial role in the control of cellular growth of lymphoid and nonlymphoid cells. Two other types of oncogenes are recognized: oncogenes such as *myc*, *ras*, and *abl* act as growth and proliferative regulatory genes; and oncogenes such as *Rb* and *p53* inhibit growth and proliferation.

---

3. Differentiation of Hodgkin's disease from non-Hodgkin's lymphoma is based on finding Reed–Sternberg cells in the former. Also helpful is the presence of markers for the Reed–Sternberg cells [e.g., CD30 (Ki-1), and CD15], and the absence of CD45.

In the absence of any Reed–Sternberg cells and the presence of CD30 positivity, the diagnosis of anaplastic Ki-1⁺ (CD30) large cell lymphoma should be considered. Four types of Ki-1⁺ large cell lymphoma may exist: common, Hodgkin's-related, giant cell-rich, and lymphohistiocytic. The tumor cells stain intensely positive with CD30. Approximately 70% of cases are of T-cell type, 15% are of B-cell type, 5% are mixed B- and T-cell types, and 10% are null type.

---

4. Epstein–Barr virus is found in a high percentage of cases of Hodgkin's disease (see p. 63 in Chapter 3)

5. The origin of the neoplastic cells in Hodgkin's disease remains an enigma in spite of the advances in immunology, cytogenetics, and molecular biology.

IX. Leukemia† (Fig. 14.47; see p. 353 in Chapter 9)

A. Orbital leukemic infiltrates most commonly occur late in the disease.

B. Occasionally, acute leukemia, usually granulocytic (myeloid or myelogenous) or stem cell, may present

initially with exophthalmos. Acute angle closure glaucoma has accompanied bilateral orbital infiltration with acute myeloid leukemia. Ultrasonography revealed uveoscleral thickening and anterior rotation of the ciliary body.

Rarely, the first sign of granulocytic leukemia relapse is ocular adnexal involvement. Occasionally, granulocytic sarcoma of the orbit has been reported as an isolated lesion.

---

1. The initial blood count may be normal or low with no circulating leukemic cells.

2. The bone marrow initially may be normal or hypocellular.

3. Exophthalmos is caused by an infiltrate of leukemic cells, called *myeloid (granulocytic) sarcoma*.

Because the pigment myeloperoxidase is sometimes present, the tumors appear greenish; hence the term *chloroma*.

The World Health Organization recommends the term *myeloid sarcoma* for a localized extramedullary tumor composed of immature myeloid cells; other terms are *chloroma* and *granulocytic sarcoma*.

---

4. Approximately two-thirds of patients who have myeloid leukemia present with some blurring of vision and accompanying fundus changes.

C. Histologically, leukemic cells infiltrate the orbit (see p. 353 in Chapter 9).

1. Auer rods (splinter-shaped, azurophilic, cytoplasmic crystalline inclusions) may be found in the blast cells of acute myeloid leukemia (see Fig. 14.47D).

2. The myeloid nature of the tumor is identified by chloroacetate esterase staining of the neoplastic cells.

The cells are CD43, CD45, Leder, and antilysozyme positive.

X. Monoclonal and polyclonal gammopathies‡

A. Monoclonal (single species of antibody) and polyclonal (multiple species of antibodies) macroglobulinemia may be seen in a variety of lymphoproliferative disorders such as nodular lymphoid hyperplasia, immunoblastic lymphadenopathy, nodular malignant lymphoma, and the plasma cell dyscrasias multiple myeloma, Waldenström's macroglobulinemia, and the rare entities such as light-chain deposition disease and heavy-chain disease.

1. Monoclonal gammopathies are immunoglobulin products of single clones of plasma cells and B lymphocytes; polyclonal gammopathies are produced by more than one clone.

2. Most monoclonal gammopathies do not evolve into a malignant condition (all polyclonal gammopathies do not so evolve) and are termed *monoclonal gammopathies of undetermined significance*.

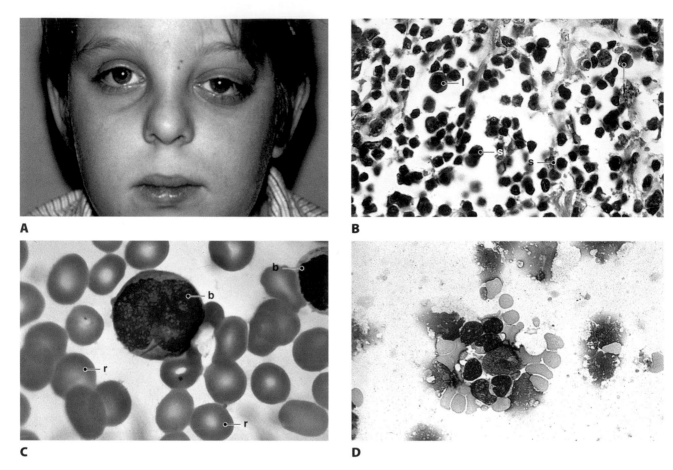

Fig. 14.47 Leukemia. **A**, A 9-year-old boy who presented with a left, painless exophthalmos died approximately 2 years after diagnosis. Initially, the work-up, including a complete blood count, showed normal results. Orbital biopsy was performed. **B**, Histologic section shows a diffuse cellular infiltratae of primitive granulocytic leukemic cells (l, large blast cells; s, small blast cells). **C**, Bone marrow smear shows blast cells (b, blast cells; r, red blood cells). Acute granulocytic leukemia diagnosed. **D**, A touch preparation of another case of granulocyte sarcoma shows Auer rods. (Case in **A–C** reported by Brooks HW *et al.: Arch Otolaryngol* 100:304, 1974; **D**, courtesy of Dr. RC Eagle, Jr., who presented case to the meeting of the Verhoeff Society, 1994.)

B. Multiple myeloma‡ (Fig. 14.48)
1. Multiple myeloma shows evidence of bone marrow plasmacytosis, monoclonal gammopathy in serum or urine (Bence Jones protein), and lytic bone lesions.
2. Direct orbital infiltration by myeloma cells, mimicking a primary orbital tumor, is uncommon.
   a. The orbital involvement, however, may be the initial manifestation of the systemic disease.
   b. Solitary orbital extramedullary plasmocytoma is a rare tumor; fewer than 15 cases have been described.

Some cases show necrobiotic xanthogranuloma of the eyelid. The eyelids may also show characteristic hemorrhagic lesions (see Fig. 7.13).

C. Waldenström's macroglobulinemia‡
1. Waldenström's macroglobulinemia is a small B-cell lymphocytic lymphoma that produces monoclonal

IgM, a pentameric immunoglobulin of high molecular weight.
2. Clinical symptoms are mainly related to anemia, bleeding, or symptoms of hyperviscosity.

A progressive macroglobulinemia-associated retinopathy may develop with associated antibodies against the connecting cilia of the photoreceptors.

D. *In vitro* immunologic and immunohistochemical techniques can aid in the diagnosis of plasma cell infiltrates.
E. Corneal, and even iris, crystals can be found in some patients who have monoclonal gammopathy.
F. Intranuclear and intracytoplasmic inclusions may be found in plasma cells and lymphocytes.
1. Intranuclear inclusions (Dutcher bodies; see Fig. 14.43D) are PAS-positive collections of monoclonal macroglobulins.

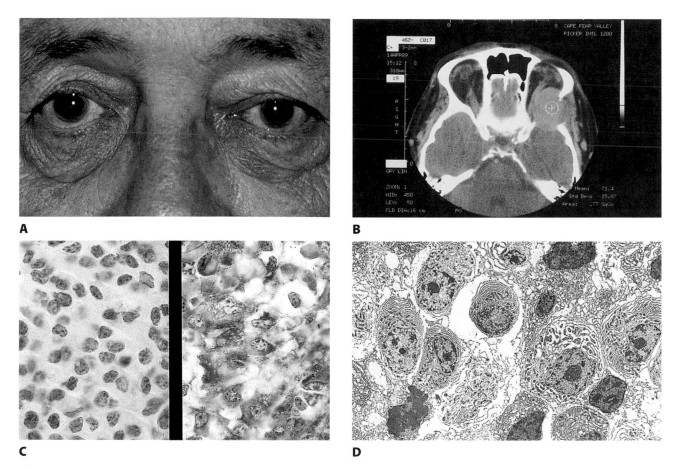

Fig. 14.48 Multiple myeloma. **A**, Left exophthalmos present. **B**, Computed tomography scan shows mass (+) in orbital region. **C**, Immunoperoxidase-stained sections show many plasma cells with negative staining for λ light chains on left panel and positive staining for κ light chains on right. **D**, Electron microscopy shows abnormal plasma cells. (Case presented by Dr. MW Scroggs to the meeting of the Eastern Ophthalmic Pathology Society, 1989.)

Actually, the inclusions are cytoplasmic invaginations into the nucleus. In some cases, the inclusions show no PAS positivity.

---

2. Intracytoplasmic inclusions (Russell bodies; see Fig. 1.13, and p. 12 in Chapter 1) are PAS-positive collections of monoclonal or polyclonal macroglobulins.

Secondary Orbital Tumors

I. Direct extension†
  A. Intraocular neoplasms, especially malignant melanoma and retinoblastoma
  B. Eyelid neoplasms, especially basal cell carcinoma, squamous cell carcinoma, malignant melanoma, and sebaceous gland carcinoma
  C. Conjunctival neoplasms, especially squamous cell carcinoma and malignant melanoma

  D. Paranasal sinus cysts (mucoceles; Fig. 14.49) and neoplasms, especially squamous cell carcinoma, adenoid cystic carcinoma (malignant cylindroma), and mucoepidermoid carcinoma
  E. Intracranial, especially meningioma
II. Metastatic†
  A. Neuroblastoma in children usually occurs as a late manifestation of the disease. Frequently, the orbital metastases are heralded by the onset of lower-lid ecchymosis (Fig. 14.50).
  B. Lung carcinoma in adult men
  C. Breast and lung carcinoma in adult women

In the past, breast carcinoma was much more common in women than lung carcinoma. With increased smoking by women, however, lung carcinoma has become much more common. Lung carcinoma tends to metastasize early, whereas breast metastases tend to be a late manifestation.

  D. All other sites of primary neoplasms are rare.

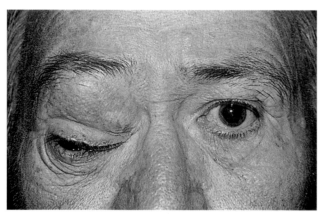

A

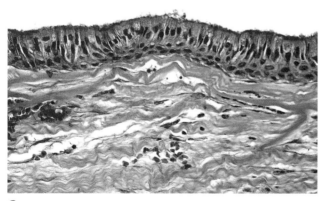

C

Fig. 14.49 Orbital mucocele. **A**, A 66-year-old man had left exophthalmos for 6 months and a 40-year history of sinusitis and a number of facial injuries. **B**, Histologic section of the surgically removed mucocele shows that the lumen is lined by respiratory-type, pseudostratified, ciliated columnar epithelium (shown with increased magnification in **C**) and contains scattered round inflammatory cells in its wall. (Courtesy of Dr. WR Green.)

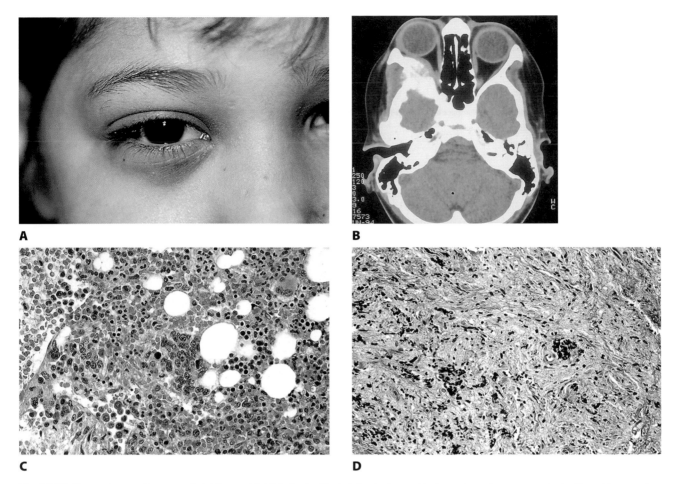

Fig. 14.50 Metastatic neuroblastoma. **A**, A 12-year-old child who had had abdominal neuroblastoma at age 4 years presented with sudden-onset ecchymosis of right lower lid. **B**, Computed tomography scan shows mass in right temporal fossa and erosion into sphenoid sinus and orbit. Histologic appearance similar to retinoblastoma in bone marrow (**C**) and orbit (**D**). (Case presented by Dr. E Torczynski at the meeting of the Eastern Opthalmic Society, 1994.)

BIBLIOGRAPHY

Normal Anatomy

Buffam FV: Lacrimal disease. In Podos SM, Yanoff M, eds: *Textbook of Ophthalmology*, vol. 4. New York, Gower Medical Publishing, 1993:7.1–7.6

Dutton JJ: Clinical anatomy of the orbit. In Ynaoff M, Duker JS, eds. *Ophthalmology*, 2nd edn. St. Louis, Mosby, 2004:641–648

Levine MR, Larson DW: Orbital tumors. In Podos SM, Yanoff M, eds: *Textbook of Ophthalmology*, vol. 4. New York, Gower Medical Publishing, 1993:10.4–10.13

Obata H, Yamamoto S, Horiuchi H *et al.*: Histopathologic study of human lacrimal gland: Statistical analysis with special reference to aging. *Ophthalmology* 102:678, 1995

Wojno TH: Orbital trauma and fractures. In Podos SM, Yanoff M, eds: *Textbook of Ophthalmology*, vol. 4. New York, Gower Medical Publishing, 1993:9.1–9.4

Exophthalmos

Char DH, Sobel D, Kelly WM *et al.*: Magnetic resonance scanning in orbital tumor diagnosis. *Ophthalmology* 92:1305, 1985

Hyman RA, Edwards JH: MR imaging versus CT in the evaluation of orbital lesions. *Geriatr Ophthalmol* 1:15, 1985

Kodsi SR, Shetlar DJ, Campbell RJ *et al.*: A review of 340 orbital tumors in children during a 60-year period. *Am J Ophthalmol* 117:177, 1994

Shields JA, Bakewell B, Augsburger JJ *et al.*: Classification and incidence of space-occupying lesions of the orbit: A survey of 645 biopsies. *Arch Ophthalmol* 102:1606, 1984

Zimmerman RA, Bilaniuk LT, Yanoff M *et al.*: Orbital magnetic resonance imaging. *Am J Ophthalmol* 100:312, 1985

Developmental Abnormalities

Hoepner J, Yanoff M: Craniosynostosis and syndactylism (Apert's syndrome) associated with a trisomy 21 mosaic. *J Pediatr Ophthalmol* 8:107, 1971

Kivelä T, Tarkkanen A: Orbital germ cell tumors revisited: A clinico-pathological approach to classification. *Surv Ophthalmol* 38:541, 1994

Pasquale LR, Romayananda N, Kubacki J et al.: Congenital cystic eye with multiple ocular and intracranial anomalies. *Arch Ophthalmol* 109:985, 1991

Pokorny KS, Hyman BM, Jakobiec FA et al.: Epibulbar choristomas containing lacrimal tissue: Clinical distinction from dermoids and histologic evidence of an origin from the palpebral lobe. *Ophthalmology* 94:1249, 1987

Shields JA, Shields CL: Orbital cysts of childhood—classification, clinical features, and management. *Surv Ophthalmol* 49:281, 2004

Wilkins RB, Hoffmann RJ, Byrd WA et al.: Heterotopic brain tissue in the orbit. *Arch Ophthalmol* 105:390, 1987

Yanoff M, Rorke LB, Niederer BS: Ocular and cerebral abnormalities in 18 chromosome deletion defect. *Am J Ophthalmol* 70:391, 1970

Orbital Inflammation

Duker JS, Brown GC, Brooks L: Retinal vasculitis in Crohn's disease. *Am J Ophthalmol* 103:664, 1987

Fairley C, Sullivan TJ, Bartley P et al.: Survival after rhino-orbital-cerebral mucormycosis in an immunocompetent patient. *Ophthalmology* 107:555, 2000

Font RL, Yanoff M, Zimmerman LE: Benign lymphoepithelial lesion of the lacrimal gland and its relationship to Sjögren's syndrome. *Am J Clin Pathol* 48:365, 1967

Gravanis MB, Giansanti DMD: Malignant histopathologic counterpart of the benign lymphoepithelial lesion. *Cancer* 26:1332, 1970

Haneji N, Nakamura T, Takio K et al.: Identification of α-fodrin as a candidate antigen in primary Sjögren's syndrome. *Science* 276:604, 1997

Hunt WE: Tolosa–Hunt syndrome: One cause of painful ophthalmoplegia. *J Neurosurg* 44:544, 1976

Jones DT, Monroy D, Ji Z et al.: Sjögren's syndrome: Cytokine and Epstein–Barr viral gene expression within the conjunctival epithelium. *Invest Ophthalmol Vis Sci* 35:3493, 1994

Kattah JC, Zimmerman LE, Kolsky MP et al.: Bilateral orbital involvement in fatal giant cell polymyositis. *Ophthalmology* 978:520, 1990

Klapper SR, Patrinely JR, Kaplan SL et al.: Atypical mycobacterial infection of the orbit. *Ophthalmology* 102:1536, 1995

McNab AA, Wright JE: Orbitofrontal cholesterol granuloma. *Ophthalmology* 97:28, 1990

Meyer D, Yanoff M, Hanno H: Differential diagnosis in Mikulicz's syndrome, Mikulicz's disease and similar disease entities. *Am J Ophthalmol* 71:516, 1971

Parken B, Chew JB, White VA et al.: Lymphocytic infiltration and enlargement of the lacrimal glands: a new subtype of primary Sjögren's syndrome? *Ophthalmology* 112:2040, 2005

Streeten BW, Rabuzzi DD, Jones DB: Sporotrichosis of the orbital margin. *Am J Ophthalmol* 77:750, 1974

Tsubota K, Fujita H, Tsuzaka K et al.: Mikulicz's disease and Sjögren's syndrome. *Invest Ophthalmol Vis Sci* 41:1666, 2000

Tsubota K, Saito I, Miyasaka N: Granzyme A and perforin expressed in the lacrimal glands of patients with Sjögren's syndrome. *Am J Ophthalmol* 117:120, 1994

Injuries

See Chapter 5 for bibliography.

Vascular Disease

See bibliography under appropriate sections.

Foroozan R, Shields CL, Shields JA et al.: Congenital orbital varices causing extreme neonatal proptosis. *Am J Ophthalmol* 129:693, 2000

Lacey B, Rootman J, Vangveeravong S et al.: Distensible venous malformations of the orbit. *Ophthalmology* 106:1197, 1999

Wright JF, Sullivan TJ, Garner A et al.: Orbital venous abnormalities. *Ophthalmology* 104:905, 1997

Ocular Muscle Involvement in Systemic Disease

Bahn RS, Dutton CM, Heufelder AE et al.: A genomic point mutation in the extracellular domain of the thyrotropin receptor in patients with Graves' ophthalmopathy. *J Clin Endocrinol Metab* 78:256, 1994

Bartalena L, Marcocci C, Bogazzi F et al.: Relation between therapy for hyperthyroidism and the course of Graves' ophthalmopathy. *N Engl J Med* 338:73, 1998

Bartley GB, Gorman CA: Diagnostic criteria for Graves' disease. *Am J Ophthalmol* 119:792, 1995

Bartley GB, Fatourechi V, Kadrmas EF et al.: Clinical features of Graves' ophthalmopathy in an incidence cohort. *Am J Ophthalmol* 121:284, 1996

Bartley GB, Fatourechi V, Kadrmas EF et al.: The chronology of Graves' ophthalmopathy in an incidence cohort. *Am J Ophthalmol* 121:426, 1996

Bartley GB, Fatourechi V, Kadrmas EF et al.: Long-term follow-up of Graves' ophthalmopathy in an incidence cohort. *Ophthalmology* 103:958, 1996

Carta A, D'Adda T, Carrara F et al.: Ultrastructural analysis of external muscle in chronic progressive external ophthalmoplegia. *Arch Ophthalmol* 118:1441, 2000

Chang TS, Johns DR, Walker D et al.: Ocular clinicopathologic study of the mitochondrial encephalomyopathy overlap syndromes. *Arch Ophthalmol* 111:1254, 1993

Crisp M, Starkey KJ, Lane C et al.: Adipogenesis in thyroid eye disease. *Invest Ophthalmol Vis Sci* 41:3249, 2000

De Carli M, D'Elios MM, Mariotti S et al.: Cytolytic T cells with Th1-like cytokine profile predominate in retroorbital lymphocytic infiltrates of Grave's ophthalmology. *J Clin Endocrinol Metab* 77:1120, 1993

Drachman DB: Myasthenia gravis. *N Engl J Med* 330:1797, 1994

Eshaghian J, March WF, Goossens W et al.: Ultrastructure of cataract in myotonic dystrophy. *Invest Ophthalmol Vis Sci* 17:289, 1978

Folberg R, Rummelt V, Ionasescu V: MELAS syndrome. Presented at the meeting of the Verhoeff Society, 1993

Herzberg NH, van Schooneveld MJ, Bleeker-Wagemakers EM et al.: Kearns–Sayre syndrome with a phenocopy of choroideremia instead of pigmentary retinopathy. *Neurology* 43:218, 1993

Jaume JC, Portolano S, Prummel MF et al.: Molecular cloning and characterization of genes for antibodies generated by orbital tissue-infiltrating B-cells in Graves' ophthalmopathy. *J Clin Endocrinol Metab* 78:348, 1994

Leib ML, Odel JG, Cooney MJ: Orbital polymyositis and giant cell myocarditis. *Ophthalmology* 101:950, 1994

Nunery WR, Martin RT, Heinz GW et al.: The association of cigarette smoking with clinical subtypes of ophthalmic Graves' disease. *Ophthalmic Plast Reconstr Surg* 9:77, 1993

Ohtsuka K, Hashimoto M: [1]H-magnetic resonance spectroscopy of retrobulbar tissue in Graves ophthalmopathy. *Am J Ophthalmol* 128:715, 1999

Philips AV, Timchenko LT, Cooper TA: Disruption of splicing regulated by a CUG-binding protein in myotonic dystrophy. *Science* 280:737, 1998

Rosen CE, Parisi F, Raikow RB *et al.*: Immunohistochemical evidence for C3bi involvement in Graves' ophthalmopathy. *Ophthalmology* 99:1325, 1992

Rosen CE, Raikow RB, Burde RM *et al.*: Immunohistochemical evidence for IgA₁ involvement in Graves' ophthalmopathy. *Ophthalmology* 99:146, 1992

Rummelt V, Folberg R, Ionasescu V *et al.*: Ocular pathology of MELAS syndrome with mitochondrial DNA nucleotide 3243 point mutation. *Ophthalmology* 100:1757, 1993

Small RG: Enlargement of levator palpebrae superioris muscle fibers in Graves' ophthalmopathy. *Ophthalmology* 96:424, 1989

Sue CM, Mitchell P, Crimmins DS *et al.*: Pigmentary retinopathy associated with the mitochondrial DNA 3243 mutation. *Neurology* 49:1013, 1997

Van Dyk HJL: Orbital Graves' disease: A modification of the "no specs" classification. *Ophthalmology* 88:479, 1981

Weinberg DA, Lesser RL, Vollmer TL: Myasthenia gravis: A protein disorder. . *Surv Ophthalmol* 39:169, 1994

Yanoff M: Pretibial myxedema: A case report. *Med Ann DC* 34:319, 1965

Tumors: Choristoma

Boynton JR, Searl SS, Ferry AP *et al.*: Primary nonkeratinized epithelial ("conjunctival") orbital cysts. *Arch Ophthalmol* 110:1238, 1992

Eijpe AA, Koornneef L, Verbeeten B *et al.*: Intradiploic epidermoid cysts of the bony orbit. *Ophthalmology* 98:1737, 1991

Goldstein MH, Soparkar CNS, Kersten RC *et al.*: Conjunctival cysts of the orbit. *Ophthalmology* 105:2056, 1998

Holds JB, Anderson RL, Mamalis N *et al.*: Invasive squamous cell carcinoma arising from asymptomatic choristomatous cysts of the orbit. *Ophthalmology* 100:1244, 1993

Howard GR, Nerad JLA, Bonavolonta G *et al.*: Orbital dermoid cysts located within the lateral rectus muscle. *Ophthalmology* 101:767, 1994

Meyer DR, Lessner AM, Yeatts P *et al.*: Primary temporal fossa dermoid cyst: Characterization and surgical management. *Ophthalmology* 106:342, 1999

Pokorny KS, Hyman BM, Jakobiec FA *et al.*: Epibulbar choristomas containing lacrimal tissue: Clinical distinction from dermoids and histologic evidence of an origin from the palpebral lobe. *Ophthalmology* 94:1249, 1987

Prause JU, Børgesen SE, Carstensen H *et al.*: Cranio-orbital teratoma. *Acta Ophthalmol Scand Suppl* 219:53, 1996

Rush A, Leone CR Jr: Ectopic lacrimal gland cyst of the orbit. *Am J Ophthalmol* 92:198, 1981

Shields JA, Shields CL: Orbital cysts of childhood—classification, clinical features, and management. *Surv Ophthalmol* 49:281, 2004

Tumors: Hamartomas

Bowen JH, Christensen FH, Klintworth GK *et al.*: A clinicopathologic study of a cartilaginous hamartoma of the orbit: A rare cause of proptosis. *Ophthalmology* 88:1356, 1981

Burnstine MA, Frueh BR, Elner VM: Angiosarcoma metastatic to the orbit. *Arch Ophthalmol* 114:93, 1996

Canavan YM, Logan WC: Benign hemangioendothelioma of the lacrimal gland fossa. *Arch Ophthalmol* 97:1112, 1979

Chang EL, Rubin PAD: Bilateral multifocal hemangilas of the orbit in the blue rubber bleb nevus syndrome. *Ophthalmology* 109:258, 2002

Ferry AP, Kaltreider SA: Cavernous hemangioma of the lacrimal sac. *Am J Ophthalmol* 110:316, 1990

Geyer O, Neudorfer M, Stolevitch C *et al.*: Giant cavernous hemangioma of the face. *Arch Ophthalmol* 112:123, 1994

Haik BG, Karcioglu ZA, Gordon RA *et al.*: Capillary hemangioma (infantile periocular hemangioma). *Surv Ophthalmol* 38:399, 1994

Harris GJ, Sakol PJ, Bonavolonta G *et al.*: An analysis of thirty cases of orbital lymphangioma. *Ophthalmology* 97:1583, 1990

Henderson JW, Farrow GM, Garrity JA: Clinical course of an incompletely removed cavernous hemangioma of the orbit. *Ophthalmology* 97:625, 1990

Imayama S, Murakamai Y, Hashimoto H *et al.*: Spindle cell hemangioendothelioma exhibits the ultrastructural features of reactive vascular proliferation rather than of angiosarcoma. *Am J Clin Pathol* 97:279, 1992

Katz SE, Rootman J, Vangveeravong S *et al.*: Combined venous lymphatic malformations of the orbit (so-called lymphangiomas): Association with noncontiguous intracranial vascular anomalies. *Arch Ophthalmol* 105:176, 1998

Kazim M, Kennerdell JS, Rothfus W *et al.*: Orbital lymphangioma. *Ophthalmology* 99:1588, 1993

Neufeld M, Pe'er J, Rosenman E *et al.*: Intraorbital glomus cell tumor. *Am J Ophthalmol* 117:539, 1994

Relf SJ, Bartley GB, Unni KK: Primary orbital intraosseous hemangioma. *Ophthalmology* 98:541, 1991

Reeves SW, Miele DL, Woodward JA *et al.*: Retinal folds as initial manifestation of orbital lymphangioma. *Arch Ophthalmol* 123:1756, 2005

Scheuerle AF, Steiner HH, Kolling G *et al.*: Treatment and long-term outcome of patients with orbital cavernomas. *Am J Ophthalmol* 138:237, 2004

Tunç M, Sadri E, Char DH: Orbital lymphangioma: An analysis of 26 patients. *Br J Ophthalmol* 83:76, 1999

Tumors: Mesenchymal–Vascular

Alles JU, Bosslet K: Immunocytochemistry of angiosarcomas: A study of 19 cases with special emphasis on the applicability of endothelial cell specific markers to routinely prepared tissues. *Am J Clin Pathol* 89:463, 1988

Cheuk W, Wong KOY, Wong CSC *et al.*: Immunostaining for human herpesvirus 8 latent nuclear antigen—1 helps distinguish Kaposi sarcoma from its mimickers. *Am J Clin Pathol* 121:335, 2004

Chow LTC, Yuen RWS, Tsui WMS *et al.*: Cytologic features of Kimura's disease in fine-needle aspirates: A study of eight cases. *Am J Clin Pathol* 102:316, 1994

Fajardo LF: The complexity of endothelial cells. *Am J Clin Pathol* 92:241, 1989

Fetsch JF, Weiss SW: Observations concerning the pathogenesis of epithelioid hemangioma (angiolymphoid hyperplasia). *Mod Pathol* 4:449, 1991

Finn WG, Goolsby CL, Rao MS: DNA flow cytometric analysis of hemangiopericytoma. *Am J Clin Pathol* 101:181, 1994

Ghabrial R, Quivey JM, Dunn JP *et al.*: Radiation therapy of acquired immunodeficiency syndrome-related Kaposi's sarcoma of the eyelids and conjunctiva. *Arch Ophthalmol* 110:1423, 1992

Jin Y-T, Tsai S-T, Yan J-J *et al.*: Detection of Kaposi's sarcoma-associated herpesvirus-like DNA sequence in vascular lesions: A reliable diagnostic marker for Kaposi's sarcoma. *Am J Clin Pathol* 105:360, 1996

Karcioglu ZA, Nasr A, Haik BG: Orbital hemangiopericytoma: Clinical and morphologic features. *Am J Ophthalmol* 124:661, 1997

Kledal TN, Rosenkilde MM, Coulin F *et al.*: A broad spectrum chemokine antagonist encoded by Kaposi's sarcoma-associated herpesvirus. *Science* 277:1656, 1997

Kurumety UR, Lustbader JM: Kaposi's sarcoma of the bulbar conjunctiva as an initial clinical manifestation of acquired immunodeficiency syndrome. *Arch Ophthalmol* 113:978, 1995

Lee JT, Pettit TH, Glascow BJ: Epibulbar hemangiopericytoma. *Am J Ophthalmol* 124:546, 1997

McEachren TM, Brownstein S, Jordan DR *et al.*: Epithelioid hemangioma of the orbit. *Ophthalmology* 107:806, 2000

Rettig MB, Ma RJ, Vescio RA *et al.*: Kaposi's sarcoma-associated herpesvirus infection of bone marrow dendritic cells from multiple myeloma patients. *Science* 276:1851, 1997

Saxe SJ, Grossniklaus HE, Wojno TH *et al.*: Glomus cell tumor of the eyelid. *Ophthalmology* 100:139, 1993

Sekundo W, Roggenkämper P, Tschubel K *et al.*: Hemangio pericytoma of the inner canthus. *Am J Ophthalmol* 121:445, 1996

Tumors: Mesenchymal–Fatty

Brown HH, Kersten RC, Kulwin DR: Lipomatous hamartoma of the orbit. *Arch Ophthalmol* 109:240, 1991

Daniel CS, Beaconsfield M, Rose GF *et al.*: Pleomorphic lipoma of the orbit: a case series and review of the literature. *Ophthalmology* 110:101, 2003

Feinfield RE, Hesse RJ, Scharfenberg JC: Orbital angiolipoma. *Arch Ophthalmol* 106:1093, 1988

Gibis Z, Miettinen M, Limon J *et al.*: Cytogenetic and immunohistochemical profile of myxoid liposarcoma. *Am J Clin Pathol* 103:20, 1995

Sabb PC, Syed NA, Sires BS *et al.*: Primary orbital myxoid liposarcoma presenting as orbital pain. *Arch Ophthalmol* 114:353, 1996

Small ML, Green WR, Johnson LC: Lipoma of the frontal bone. *Arch Ophthalmol* 97:129, 1979

Yoganathan P, Meyer DR, Farber MG: Bilateral lacrimal gland involvement with Kimura disease in an African American male. *Arch Ophthalmol* 122:917, 2004

Tumors: Mesenchymal–Fibrous–Histiocytic

Allaire GS, Corriveau C, Teboul N: Malignant fibrous histiocytoma of the conjunctiva. *Arch Ophthalmol* 117:685, 1999

deBacker CM, Bodker F, Putterman AM *et al.*: Solitary fibrous tumor of the orbit. *Am J Ophthalmol* 121:447, 1996

Barr FG, Chatten J, D'Cruz *et al.*: Molecular assays for chromosomal translocations in the diagnosis of pediatric soft tissue sarcomas. *JAMA* 273:553, 1995

Bernardini FP, de Concilius C, Schneider S *et al.*: Solitary fibrous tumor of the orbit: is it rare? Report of a case series and review of the literature. *Ophthalmology* 110:1442, 2003

Boynton JR, Markowitch W, Searl SS: Atypical fibroxanthoma of the eyelid. *Ophthalmology* 96:1480, 1989

Conway RM, Holbach LM, Naumann GOH *et al.*: Benign fibrous histiocytoma of the corneoscleral limbus: unique clinicopathologic features. *Arch Ophthalmol* 121:1776, 2003

Dei Tos AP, Seregard S, Calonje E *et al.*: Giant cell angiofibroma: A distinctive orbital tumor in adults. *Am J Surg Pathol* 19:1286, 1995

Dickey GE, Sotelo-Avila C: Fibrous hamartoma of infancy: current review. *Pediatr Dev Pathol* 2:236, 1999

Dorfman DM, To K, Dickerson GR *et al.*: Solitary fibrous tumor of the orbit. *Am J Surg Pathol* 18:281, 1994

Ferry AP, Sherman SE: Nodular fasciitis of the conjunctiva apparently originating in the fascia bulbi (Tenon's capsule). *Am J Ophthalmol* 78:514, 1974

Font RL, Hidayat AA: Fibrous histiocytoma of the orbit: A clinicopathologic study of 150 cases. *Hum Pathol* 13:199, 1982

Gold JS, Antonescu CR, Hajdu C *et al.*: Clinicopathologic correlates of solitary fibrous tumors. *Cancer* 94:1057, 2002

Hartstein ME, Grove AS Jr, Woog JJ *et al.*: The multidisciplinary management of psammomatoid ossifying fibroma of the orbit. *Ophthalmology* 105:591, 1998

Hasegawa T, Hirose T, Seki K *et al.*: Solitary fibrous tumor of the soft tissue. An immunohistochemical and ultrastructural study. *Am J Clin Pathol* 106:325, 1996

Hayashi N, Borodic G, Karesh JW *et al.*: Giant cell angiofibroma of the orbit and eyelid. *Ophthalmology* 106:1223, 1999

Heathcote JG: Solitary fibrous tumor of the orbit. *Can J Ophthalmol* 32:432, 1997

Ing EB, Kennerdell JS, Olsen PR *et al.*: Solitary fibrous tumor of the orbit. *Ophthalmic Plast Reconstr Surg* 14:57, 1997

Jakobiec FA: Solitary fibrous tumor. Presented at the meeting of the Verhoeff Society, 1994

Jakobiec FA, Klapper D, Maher E *et al.*: Infantile subconjunctival and anterior orbital fibrous histiocytoma: Ultrastructural and immunohistochemical studies. *Ophthalmology* 95:516, 1988

Jakobiec FA, Sacks E, Lisman RL *et al.*: Epibulbar fibroma of the conjunctival substantia propria. *Arch Ophthalmol* 106:661, 1988

John T, Yanoff M, Scheie HG: Eyelid fibrous histiocytoma: *Ophthalmology* 88:1193, 1981

Jones WD III, Yanoff M, Katowitz JA: Recurrent facial fibrous histiocytoma. *Br J Plast Surg* 32:46, 1979

Krishnakumar S, Subramanian N, Mohan ER *et al.*: Solitary fibrous tumor of the orbit: a clinicopathologic study of six cases with review of the literature. *Surv Ophthalmol* 48:544, 2003

Lakshminarayanan R, Konia T, Welborn J: Fibrous hamartoma of infancy. *Arch Pathol Lab Med* 129:520, 2005

Linder JS, Harris GJ, Segura AD: Periorbital infantile myofibromatosis. *Arch Ophthalmol* 114:219, 1996

Ma CK, Zarbo RJ, Gown AM: Immunohistochemical characterization of atypical fibroxanthoma and dermatofibrosarcoma protuberans. *Am J Clin Pathol* 97:478, 1992

Martin AJ, Summersgill BM, Fisher C *et al.*: Chromosomal imbalances in meningeal solitary fibrous tumors. *Cancer Genet Cytogenet* 135:160, 2002

Rice CD, Gross DJ, Dinehart SM *et al.*: Atypical fibroxanthoma of the eyelid and cheek. *Arch Ophthalmol* 109:922, 1991

Scott IU, Tanenbaum M, Rubin D *et al.*: Solitary fibrous tumor of the lacrimal gland fossa. *Ophthalmology* 103:1613, 1996

Song A, Syed N, Kirby PA *et al.*: Giant cell angiofibroma of the ocular adnexae. *Arch Ophthalmol* 123:1438, 2005

Weiner JM, Hidayat AA: Juvenile fibrosarcoma of the orbit and eyelid. *Arch Ophthalmol* 101:253, 1983

Westfall AC, Mansoor A, Sullivan SS *et al.*: Orbital and periorbital myofibromas in childhood: two case reports. *Ophthalmology* 110:2000, 2003

Westra WH, Gerald WL, Rosai J: Solitary fibrous tumor of the orbit: consistent CD34 immunoreactivity and occurrence in the orbit. *Am J Surg Pathol* 18:992, 1994

White VA, Heathcote G, Hurwitz JJ *et al.*: Epithelioid sarcoma of the orbit. *Ophthalmology* 101:1689, 1994

Wiley EL, Stewart D, Brown M *et al.*: Fibrous histiocytoma of the parotid gland. *Am J Clin Pathol* 97:512, 1992

Yanoff M, Scheie HG: Fibrosarcoma of the orbit: Report of two cases. *Cancer* 19:1711, 1966

Tumors: Mesenchymal–Muscle

Azumi N, Ben-Ezra J, Battifora H: Immunophenotypic diagnosis of leiomyosarcomas and rhabdomyosarcomas with monoclonal antibodies to muscle-specific actin and desmin in formalin-fixed tissue. *Mod Pathol* 1:469, 1988

Barr FG, Chatten J, D'Cruz *et al.*: Molecular assays for chromosomal translocations in the diagnosis of pediatric soft tissue sarcomas. *JAMA* 273:553, 1995

Van den Broek PP, de Faber J-THN, Kliffen M *et al.*: Anterior orbital leiomyoma. Possible pulley smooth muscle tissue tumor. *Arch Ophthalmol* 123:1614, 2005

Duffy MT, Harris M, Hornblass A: Infantile myofibromatosis of orbital bone: A case report with computed tomography, magnetic resonance imaging, and histologic findings. *Ophthalmology* 104:1471, 1997

Frayer WC, Enterline HT: Embryonal rhabdomyosarcoma of the orbit in children and young adults. *Arch Ophthalmol* 62:203, 1959

Gündüz K, Shields JA, Eagle RC Jı *et al.*: Malignant rhabdoid tumor of the orbit. *Arch Ophthalmol* 116:243, 1998

Hill DA, O'Sullivan MJ, Zhu X *et al.*: Practical application of molecular genetic testing as an aid to the surgical patthologic diagnosis of sarcomas: a prospective study. *Am J Surg Pathol* 26:965, 2002

Hou LC, Murphy MA, Tung GA: Primary orbital leiomyosarcoma: a case report with MRI findings. *Am J Ophthalmol* 135:408, 2003

Karcioglu ZA, Hadjistilianou D, Rozans M *et al.*: Orbital rhabdomyosarcoma. *Cancer Control* 11:328, 2004

Miguel-Fraile PS, Carrillo-Gijón R, Rodriguez-Peralto JL *et al.*: Prognostic significance of DNA ploidy and proliferative index (MIB-1 index) in childhood rhadomyosarcomas. *Am J Clin Pathol* 121:358, 2004

Parthaam DM, Weeks DA, Beckwith JB: The clinicopathologic spectrum of putative extrarenal rhabdoid tumors: An analysis of 42 cases studied with immunohistochemistry or electron microscopy. *Am J Surg Pathol* 18:1010, 1994

Porterfield JF, Zimmerman LE: Orbital rhabdomyosarcoma: A clinicopathologic study of 55 cases. *Virchows Arch Pathol Anat* 335:329, 1962

Shields CL, Shields JA: Rhabdomyosarcoma: review for the ophthalmologist. *Surv Ophthalmol* 48:39, 2003

Taylor SF, Yen KG, Patel BCK: Primary conjunctival rhabdomyosarcoma. *Arch Ophthalmol* 120:668, 2002

Xia SJ, Pressey JG, Barr FG: Molecular pathogenesis of rhabdomyosarcoma. *Cancer Biol Ther* 1:2:97, 2002

Tumors: Mesenchymal–Cartilage

Jacobs JL, Merriam JC, Chadburn A *et al.*: Mesenchymal chondrosarcoma of the orbit: Report of three new cases and review of the literature. *Cancer* 73:399, 1994

Pasternak S, O'Connell JX, Verchere C *et al.*: Enchondroma of the orbit. *Am J Ophthalmol* 122:444, 1996

Tuncer S, Kebudi R, Peksayar G *et al.*: Congenital mesenchymal chondrosarcoma of the orbit: case report and review of the literature. *Ophthalmology* 111:1016, 2004

Tumors: Mesenchymal–Bone

Dailey R, Gilliland G, McCoy GB: Orbital aneurysmal bone cyst in a patient with renal cell carcinoma. *Am J Ophthalmol* 117:643, 1994

Katz BJ, Nerad JA: Ophthalmic manifestations of fibrous dysplasia: A disease of children and adults. *Ophthalmology* 105:2207, 1998

Leone CR, Lawton AW, Leone RT: Benign osteoblastoma of the orbit. *Ophthalmology* 95:1554, 1988

Mercado GV, Shields CL, Gunduz K *et al.*: Giant cell reparative granuloma of the orbit. *Am J Ophthalmol* 127:485, 1999

Mooy CM, Naus NC, de Klein A *et al.*: Orbital chondrosarcoma developing in a patient with Paget's disease. *Am J Ophthalmol* 127:619, 1999

Parmar DN, Luthert PH, Cree IA *et al.*: Two unusual osteogenic orbital tumors: presumed parosteal osteosarcoma. *Ophthalmology* 108:1452, 2001

Parrish CM, O'Day DM: Brown tumor of the orbit: Case report and review of the literature. *Arch Ophthalmol* 104:1199, 1986

Sires BS, Benda PM, Stanley RB Jr *et al.*: Orbital osteoid osteoma. *Arch Ophthalmol* 117:414, 1999

Trevisani MG, Fry CL, Hesse RJ *et al.*: A rare case of orbital osteogenic sarcoma. *Arch Ophthalmol* 114:494, 1996

Weiss JS, Bressler SB, Jacobs EF *et al.*: Maxillary ameloblastoma with orbital invasion: A clinicopathologic study. *Ophthalmology* 92:710, 1985

Tumors: Neural

Allman MI, Frayer WC, Hedges TR Jr: Orbital neurilemoma. *Ann Ophthalmol* 9:1409, 1977

Andreoli CA, Hatton M, Semple JP *et al.*: Perilimbal conjunctival schwannoma. *Arch Ophthalmol* 122:388, 2004

Arora R, Sarkar C, Betharia SM: Primary orbital primitive neuroectodermal tumor with immunohistochemical and electron microscopic confirmation. *Orbit* 12:7, 1993

Brannan PA, Schneider S, Grosniklaus HE *et al.*: Malignant mesenchymoma of the orbit. Case report and review of the literature. *Ophthalmology* 110:314, 2003

Briscoe D, Mahmood S, O'Donovan DG *et al.*: Malignant peripheral nerve sheath tumor in the orbit of a child with acute proptosis. *Arch Ophthalmol* 120:653, 2002

Bullock JD, Goldberg SH, Rakes S *et al.*: Primary orbital neuroblastoma. *Arch Ophthalmol* 107:1031, 1989

Chan C-C, Pack S, Pak E *et al.*: Translocation of chromosome 11 and 22 in choroidal metastatic Ewing sarcoma detected by fluorescent in situ hybridization. *Am J Ophthalmol* 127:226, 1999

Charles NC, Fox DM, Avendaño JA *et al.*: Conjunctival neurilemoma. *Arch Ophthalmol* 115:547, 1997

Choi RY, Lucarelli MJ, Imesch PD *et al.*: Primary orbital Ewing sarcoma in a middle-aged woman. *Arch Ophthalmol* 117:535, 1999

Cibis GW, Freeman WI, Pang V *et al.*: Bilateral choroidal neonatal neuroblastoma. *Am J Ophthalmol* 109:445, 1990

Coira BM, Sachdev R, Moscovic E: Skeletal muscle markers in alveolar soft part sarcoma. *Am J Clin Pathol* 94:790, 1990

Furman J, Murphy WM, Jelsma PF *et al.*: Primary primitive neuroectodermal tumor of the kidney: Case report and review of the literature. *Am J Clin Pathol* 106:339, 1996

Halling KC, Scheithauer BW, Halling AC *et al.*: p53 expression in neurofibroma and malignant peripheral nerve sheath tumors: An immunohistochemical study of sporadic and ND-1 associated tumors. *Am J Clin Pathol* 106:282, 1996

Hill DA, Pfeifer JD, Marley EF *et al.*: WT1 staining reliably differentiates desmoplastic small round cell tumor from Ewing sarcoma/primitive neuroectodermal tumor: an immunohistochemical and molecular diagnostic study. *Am J Clin Pathol* 114:345, 2000

Khwang SI, Lucarelli MJ, Lemke BN *et al.*: Ancient schwannoma of the orbit. *Arch Ophthalmol* 117:262, 1999

Kussie PH, Gorina S, Marechal V *et al.*: Structure of the MDM2 oncoprotein bound to the p53 tumor suppressor transactivation domain. *Science* 274:948, 1996

Le Marc'hadour F, Romanet JP, Péoc'h M *et al.*: Schwannoma of the bulbar conjunctiva. *Arch Ophthalmol* 114:1258, 1996

Li T, Goldberg RA, Becker B *et al.*: Primary orbital extraskeletal Ewing sarcoma. *Arch Ophthalmol* 121:1049, 2003

Lucas DR, Bentley G, Dan ME *et al.*: Ewing sarcoma vs. lymphoblastic lymphoma: A comparative immunohistochemical study. *Am J Clin Pathol* 115:11, 2001

Messmer EP, Camara J, Boniuk M *et al.*: Amputation neuroma of the orbit: Report of two cases and review of the literature. *Ophthalmology* 91:1420, 1984

Pineda R II, Urban RC, Bellows AR *et al.*: Ciliary body neurilemoma. *Ophthalmology* 102:918, 1995

Renshaw AA, Perez-Atayde AR, Fletcher JA *et al.*: Cytology of typical and atypical Ewing's sarcoma/PNET. *Science* 274:948, 1996

Shields JA, Font RL, Eagle RC *et al.*: Melanotic schwannoma of the choroid. *Ophthalmology* 101:843, 1994

Singh AD, Husson M, Shields CL *et al.*: Primitive neuroectodermal tumor of the orbit. *Arch Ophthalmol* 112:217, 1994

Warwar RE, Bullock JD, Shields JA *et al.*: Coexistence of 3 tumors of neural crest origin: Neurofibroma, meningioma, and uveal melanoma. *Arch Ophthalmol* 116:1241, 1997

Weiss SW: p53 gene alterations in benign and malignant nerve sheath tumors. *Am J Clin Pathol* 106:271, 1996

Tumors: Miscellaneous

Archer KF, Hurwitz JJ, Balogh JM *et al.*: Orbital nonchromaffin paraganglioma. *Ophthalmology* 96:1659, 1989

Candy EJ, Miller NR, Carson BS: Myxoma of bone involving the orbit. *Arch Ophthalmol* 109:919, 1991

Charles NC, Fox DM, Glasberg SS *et al.*: Epibulbar granular cell tumor: Report of a case and review of the literature. *Ophthalmology* 104:1454, 1997

Hashimoto M, Ohtsuka K, Suzuki T *et al.*: Orbital granular cell tumor developing in the inferior oblique muscle. *Am J Ophthalmol* 124:405, 1997

Jordan DR, MacDonald H, Noel L *et al.*: Alveolar soft-part sarcoma of the orbit. *Ophthalmic Surg* 26:269, 1995

Margo CE, Folberg R, Zimmerman LE *et al.*: Endodermal sinus tumor (yolk sac tumor) of the orbit. *Ophthalmology* 90:1426, 1983

Sabet SJ, Tarbet KJ, Lemke BN *et al.*: Granular cell tumor of the lacrimal sac and nasolacrimal duct. No invasive behavior with incomplete resection. *Ophthalmology* 107:1992, 2000

Vogel MH: Granular cell myoblastoma of the ciliary body. Presented at the combined Meeting of the Verhoeff Society and the European Ophthalmic Pathology Society, Houston, TX, April, 1996

Tumors: Epithelial of Lacrimal Gland

Alyahya GA, Stenman G, Persson F *et al.*: Pleomorphic adenoma arising in an accessory lacrimal gland of Wolfring. *Ophthalmology* 113:879, 2006

Bonavolontà G, Tranfa F, Staibano S *et al.*: Warthin tumor of the lacrimal sac. *Am J Ophthalmol* 124:857, 1997

Bullock JD, Fleishman JA, Rosset JS: Lacrimal ductal cysts. *Ophthalmology* 93:1355, 1986

Conlon MR, Chapman WB, Burt WL *et al.*: Primary localized amyloidosis of the lacrimal glands. *Ophthalmology* 98:1556, 1991

Devoto MH, Croxatto O: Primary cystadenocarcinoma of the lacrimal gland. *Ophthalmology* 110:2006, 2003

Font RL, Patipa M, Rosenbaum PS *et al.*: Correlation of computed tomographic and histopathologic features in malignant transformation of benign mixed tumor of lacrimal gland. *Surv Ophthalmol* 34:449, 1990

Font RL, Smith SL, Bryan RG: Malignant epithelial tumors of the lacrimal gland: A clinicopathologic study of 21 cases. *Arch Ophthalmol* 116:589, 1998

Grossniklaus HE, Abbuhl MF, McLean IW: Immunohistologic properties of benign and malignant mixed tumor of the lacrimal gland. *Am J Ophthalmol* 110:540, 1990

Grossniklaus HE, Wojno TH, Wilson MW *et al.*: Myoepithelioma of the lacrimal gland. *Arch Ophthalmol* 115:1588, 1997

Harris NL: Lymphoid proliferations of the salivary glands. *Am J Clin Pathol* 111(Suppl. 1):S94, 1999

Heathcote JG, Hurwitz JJ, Dardick I: A spindle-cell myoepithelioma of the lacrimal gland. *Arch Ophthalmol* 108:1135, 1990

Khalil M, Arthurs B: Basal cell adenocarcinoma of the lacrimal gland. *Ophthalmology* 107:164, 2000

Levin LA, Popham J, To K *et al.*: Mucoepidermoid carcinoma of the lacrimal gland. *Ophthalmology* 98:1551, 1991

Milman T, Shields JA, Husson M *et al.*: Primary ductal adenocarcinoma of the lacrimal gland. *Ophthalmology* 112:2052S, 2005

Ostrowski ML, Font RL, Halpern J *et al.*: Clear cell epithelial-myoepithelial carcinoma arising in pleomorphic adenoma of the lacrimal gland. *Ophthalmology* 101:925, 1994

Rao NA, Kaiser E, Quiros PA *et al.*: Lymphoepithelial carcinoma of the lacrimal gland. *Arch Ophthalmol* 120:1745S, 2002

Rodman RC, Frueh BR, Elner VM: Mucoepidermoid carcinoma of the caruncle. *Am J Ophthalmol* 123:564, 1997

Rosenberg PS, Mahadevia PS, Goodman LA *et al.*: Acinic cell carcinoma of the lacrimal gland. *Arch Ophthalmol* 113:781, 1995

Selva D, Davis GJ, Dodd T *et al.*: Polymorphous low-grade adenocarcinoma of the lacrimal gland. *Arch Ophthalmol* 122:915, 2004

Shields CL, Shields JA, Eagle RC *et al.*: Adenoid cystic carcinoma in the nasal orbit. *Am J Ophthalmol* 123:398, 1997

Shields CL, Shields JA, Eagle RC *et al.*: Adenoid cystic carcinoma of the lacrimal gland simulating a dermoid cyst in a 9-year-old boy. *Arch Ophthalmol* 116:1673, 1998

Tellado MV, McClean IW, Specht CS *et al.*: Adenoid cystic carcinomas of the lacrimal gland in childhood and adolescence. *Ophthalmology* 104:1622, 1997

Vangveeravong S, Katz SE, Rootman J *et al.*: Tumors arising in the palpebral lobe of the lacrimal gland. *Ophthalmology* 103:1606, 1996

Zimmerman LE, Stangl R, Riddle PJ: Primary carcinoid tumor of the orbit: A clinicopathologic study with histochemical and electron microscopic observations. *Arch Ophthalmol* 101:1395, 1983

Tumors: Reticuloendothelial System

Allaire GS, Hidayat AA, Zimmerman LE *et al.*: Reticulohistiocytoma of the limbus and cornea. *Ophthalmology* 97:1018, 1990

Ben-Ezra JM, Koo CH: Langerhans' cell histiocytosis and malignancies of the M-Pire system. *Am J Clin Pathol* 99:464, 1993

Chikama T-I, Yoshino H, Nishida T *et al.*: Langerhans cell histiocytosis localized to the eyelid. *Arch Ophthalmol* 116:1375, 1998

Demirci H, Shields CL, Shields JA *et al.*: Bilateral sequential orbital involvement by eosinophilic granuloma. *Arch Ophthalmol* 120:978, 2002

DeStafeno JJ, Carlson A, Myer DR: Solitary spindle-cell xanthogranuloma of the eye lid. *Ophthalmology* 109:258, 2002

Font RL, Rosenbaum PS, Smith JL: Lymphomatoid granulomatosis of eyelid and brow with progression to lymphoma. *J Am Acad Dermatol* 23:334, 1990

Harbour JW, Char DH, Ljung BM *et al.*: Langerhans cell histiocytosis diagnosed by fine needle biopsy. *Arch Ophthalmol* 115:1212, 1997

Hogan MJ, Zimmerman LE, eds: *Ophthalmic Pathology: An Atlas and Textbook*. Philadelphia, WB Saunders, 1962:778

Ireland KC, Hutchinson AK, Grossniklaus HE: Sinus histiocytosis presenting as bilateral epibulbar masses. *Am J Ophthalmol* 127:360, 1999

Jordan DR, McDonald H, Noel L *et al.*: Eosinophilic granuloma. *Arch Ophthalmol* 111:134, 1993

Kramer TR, Noecker RJ, Miller JM *et al.*: Langerhans cell histiocytosis with ocular involvement. *Am J Ophthalmol* 124:814, 1997

Lee-Wang M, Oryschak A, Attariwala G et al.: Rosai–Dorfman disease presenting as bilateral lacrimal gland enlargement. *Am J Ophthalmol* 131:677, 2001

Malone M: The histiocytosis of childhood. *Histopathology* 19:105, 1991

Meyer CT, Sel S, Hörle S et al.: Rosai–Dorfman disease with bilateral retinal detachment. *Arch Ophthalmol* 121:733, 2003

Miller ML, Sassani JW, Sexton FM: Diffuse histiocytosis X involving the eyelid of a 65-year-old woman. *Am J Ophthalmol* 113:458, 1992

Mittleman D, Apple DJ, Goldberg MF: Ocular involvement in Letterer–Siwe disease. *Am J Ophthalmol* 75:261, 1973

Trocme SD, Baker RH, Bartley GB et al.: Extracellular deposition of eosinophil major basic protein in orbital histiocytosis X. *Ophthalmology* 98:353, 1991

Tsai JH, Galaydh F, Ching SST: Anterior uveitis and iris nodules that are associated with Langerhans cell histiocytosis. *J Ophthalmol* 140:1143, 2005

Woda BA, Sullivan JL: Reactive histiocytic disorders. *Am J Clin Pathol* 99:459, 1993

Tumors: Inflammatory Pseudotumor

Ahn Yuen SJ, Rubin PAD: Idiopathic orbital inflammation. Distribution, clinical features, and treatment outcome. *Arch Ophthalmol* 121:491, 2003

Cockerham GC, Hidayat AA, Bijwaard KE et al.: Re-evaluation of "reactive lymphoid hyperplasia of the uvea": An immunohistochemical and molecular analysis of ten cases. *Ophthalmology* 107:151, 2000

Coupland SE, Krause L, Delecluse H-J et al.: Lymphoproliferative lesions of the ocular adnexa: Analysis of 112 cases. *Ophthalmology* 105:1430, 1998

Feinberg AS, Spraul CW, Holden JT et al.: Conjunctival lymphocytic infiltrate associated with Epstein–Barr virus. *Ophthalmology* 107:159, 2000

Jakobiec FA, Neri A, Knowles DM: Genotypic monoclonality in immunophenotypically polyclonal orbital lymphoid tumors: A model of tumor progression in the lymphoid system. *Ophthalmology* 94:980, 1987

Krishnan J, Danon AD, Frizzera G: Reactive lymphadenopathies and atypical lymphoproliferative disorders. *Am J Clin Pathol* 99:385, 1993

Mahr MA, Salomao DR, Garrity JA: Inflammatory pseudotumor with extension beyond the orbit. *Am J Ophthalmol* 138:396, 2004

Mombaerts I, Goldschmeding R, Schlingemann R et al.: What is orbital pseudotumor? *Surv Ophthalmol* 41:66, 1996

Pettinato G, Manivel C, De Rose N et al.: Inflammatory myofibroblastic tumor (plasma cell granuloma). *Am J Clin Pathol* 94:538, 1990

Rootman J, McCarthy M, White V et al.: Idiopathic sclerosing inflammation of the orbit. *Ophthalmology* 101:570, 1994

Sheren SB, Custer PL, Smith ME: Angiolymphoid hyperplasia with eosinophilia of the orbit associated with obstructive airway disease. *Am J Ophthalmol* 108:167, 1989

Sigudardoottir M, Sigurdsson H, Björk Bakardottir R et al.: Lymphoid tumors of the ocular adnexa: a morphologic and genotypic study of 15 cases. *Acta Ophthalmol Scand* 81:299, 2003

Yanoff M, Nix R, Arvan D: Bilateral lacrimal gland enlargement associated with a diffuse gamma globulin elevation: A case report. *Ophthalmol Res* 1:245, 1970

Tumors: Malignant Lymphoma

Akpek EK, Polcharoen W, Ferry JA et al.: Conjunctival lymphoma masquerading as chronic conjunctivitis. *Ophthalmology* 106:757, 1999

Al-Hazzaa SAF, Green WR, Mann RB: Uveal involvement in systemic angiotropic large cell lymphoma. *Ophthalmology* 100:961, 1993

Antle CM, White VA, Horsman DE et al.: Large cell orbital lymphoma in a patient with acquired immune deficiency syndrome. *Ophthalmology* 97:1494, 1990

Arcaini L, Burcheri S, Rossi A et al.: Nongastric marginal-zone B-cell MALT lymphoma: prognostic value of disease dissemination. *Oncologist* 11:285, 2006

Au Eong KG, Choo CT: Burkitt lymphoma manifesting as acute proptosis. *Am J Ophthalmol* 123:856, 1997

Bairey O, Kremer I, Radkowsky E et al.: Orbital and adnexal involvement in systemic non-Hodgkin's lymphoma. *Cancer* 73:2395, 1994

Banthia V, Jen A, Kacker A. Sporadic Burkitt's lymphoma of the head and neck in the pediatric population. *Int J Pediatr Otorhinolaryngol* 67:59, 2003

Banks PM, Isaacson PG: MALT lymphomas in 1997. *Am J Clin Pathol* 111(Suppl. 1):S75, 1999

Barcos M: Mycosis fungoides. *Am J Clin Pathol* 99:452, 1993

Bardenstein DS. Ocular adnexal lymphoma: classification, clinical disease, and molecular biology. *Ophthalmol Clin North Am* 18:187, 2005

Ben-Ezra JM, Kornstein MJ: Antibody NCL-CD5 fails to detect neoplastic CD5+ cells in paraffin sections. *Am J Clin Pathol* 106:370, 1996

Bertoni F, Zucca E. Delving deeper into MALT lymphoma biology. *J Clin Invest* 116:22, 2006

Buchan J, McKibbin M, Burton T. The prevalence of ocular disease in chronic lymphocytic leukaemia. *Eye* 17:27, 2003

Burke JS: Are there site-specific differences among the MALT lymphomas: Morphologic, clinical? *Am J Clin Pathol* 111(Suppl. 1):S133, 1999

Burke JS: Extranodal hematopoietic/lymphoid disorders. *Am J Clin Pathol* 111(Suppl. 1):S40, 1999

Carbone A, Gloghini A, Volpe R et al.: Follicular lymphoma of compartmentalized small cleaved center cells and mantle zone lymphocytes. *Am J Clin Pathol* 98:437, 1992

Chan JKC, Banks PM, Cleary ML et al.: A revised European-American classification of lymphoid neoplasms proposed by the International Lymphoma Study Group. *Am J Clin Pathol* 103:543, 1995

Chang YC, Chang CH, Liu YT et al.: Spontaneous regression of a large-cell lymphoma in the conjunctiva and orbit. *Ophthalm Plast Reconstr Surg* 20:461, 2004

Chi-chu S, Wong K-F, Siu LL et al.: Large cell transformation of Sézary syndrome: A conventional and molecular cytogenetic study. *Am J Clin Pathol* 113:792, 2000

Chott A, Vesely M, Simonitsch I et al.: Classification of intestinal T-cell neoplasms and their differential diagnosis. *Am J Clin Pathol* 111(Suppl. 1):S68, 1999

Clarke B, Legodi E, Chrystal V et al.: Systemic anaplastic large cell lymphoma presenting with conjunctival involvement. *Arch Ophthalmol* 121:569, 2003

Cockerham GC, Hidayat AA, Bijwaard KE et al.: Re-evaluation of "reactive lymphoid hyperplasia of the uvea": An immunohistochemical and molecular analysis of ten cases. *Ophthalmology* 107:151, 2000

Coffee R, Lazarchick J, Chévez-Barrios P et al.: Rapid diagnosis of orbital mantle cell lymphoma utilizing in situ hybridization technology. *Am J Ophthalmol* 140:554, 2005

Cook BE Jr, Bartley GB, Pittelkow MR: Ophthalmic abnormalities in patients with cutaneous T-cell lymphoma. *Ophthalmology* 106:1339, 1999

Corbally N, Grogan L, Keane MM et al.: Bcl-2 rearrangement in Hodgkin's disease and reactive lymph nodes. *Am J Clin Pathol* 101:756, 1994

Coupland SE, Krause L, Delecluse H-J *et al.*: Lymphoproliferative lesions of the ocular adnexa: Analysis of 112 cases. *Ophthalmology* 105:1430, 1998

Demirci H, Shields CL, Shields JA *et al.*: Orbital tumors in the older population. *Ophthalmology* 109:243, 2002

Edelstein C, Shields JA, Shields CL *et al.*: Non-African Burkitt lymphoma presenting with oral thrush and an orbital mass in a child. *Am J Ophthalmol* 124:859, 1997

Elghetany MT, Kurec AS, Schuehler K *et al.*: Immunophenotyping of non-Hodgkin's lymphomas in paraffin-embedded tissue sections. *Am J Clin Pathol* 95:517, 1991

Feinberg AS, Spraul CW, Holden JT *et al.*: Conjunctival lymphocytic infiltrate associated with Epstein–Barr virus. *Ophthalmology* 107:159, 2000

Fernandez-Suntay JP, Gragoudas ES, Ferry JA *et al.*: High-grade uveal B-cell lymphoma as the initial feature in Richter syndrome. *Arch Ophthalmol* 120:1383, 2002

Frizzera G, Wu CD, Inghirami G: The usefulness of immunophenotypic and genotypic studies in the diagnosis and classification of hematopoietic and lymphoid neoplasms. *Am J Clin Pathol* 111(Suppl. 1):S13, 1999

Frost M, Newell J, Lones MA *et al.*: Comparative immunohistochemical analysis of pediatric Burkitt lymphoma and diffuse large B-cell lymphoma. *Am J Clin Pathol* 121:384, 2004

Galindo LM, Garcia FU, Hanau CA *et al.*: Fine-needle aspiration biopsy in the evaluation of lymphadenopathy associated with cutaneous T-cell lymphoma (mycosis fungoides/Sézary syndrome). *Am J Clin Pathol* 113:865, 2000

Gilles FJ, O'Brian SM, Keating MJ: Chronic lymphocytic leukemia in (Richter's) transformation. *Semin Oncol* 25:117, 1998

Gordon KB, Rugo HS, Duncan JL *et al.*: Ocular manifestations of leukemia: leukemic infiltration vs infectious process. *Ophthalmology* 108:2293, 2001

Groom D, Wong D, Brynes RK *et al.*: Auer rod-like inclusions in circulating lymphoma cells. *Am J Clin Pathol* 96:111, 1991

Hara Y, Nakamura N, Kuze T *et al.*: Immunoglobulin heavy chain gene analysis of ocular adnexal extranodal marginal zone B-cell lymphoma. *Invest Ophthalmol Vis Sci* 42:2450, 2001

Harris NL: Lymphoid proliferations of the salivary glands. *Am J Clin Pathol* 111(Suppl. 1):S94, 1999

Harris NL, Isaacson PG: What are the criteria for distinguishing MALT from non-MALT lymphoma at extranodal sites? *Am J Clin Pathol* 111(Suppl. 1):S126, 1999

Hasegawa M, Kojima M, Shioya M *et al.*: Treatment results of radiotherapy for malignant lymphoma of the orbit and histopathologic review according to the WHO classification. *Int J Radiat Oncol Biol Phys* 57:172, 2003

Hoang-Xuan T, Bodaghi B, Toublanc M *et al.*: Scleritis and mucosal-associated lymphoid tissue lymphoma: A new masquerade syndrome. *Ophthalmology* 103:631, 1996

Hsu MW, Chung CH, Chang CH *et al.*: Ptosis as an initial manifestation of orbital lymphoma: a case report. *Kaohsiung J Med Sci* 22:194, 2006

Hudock J, Chatten J, Miettinen M: Immunohistochemical evaluation of myeloid leukemia infiltrates (granulocytic sarcomas) in formaldehyde-fixed tissue. *Am J Clin Pathol* 105:55, 1994

Inghirami G, Frizzera G: Role of the bcl-2 oncogene in Hodgkin's disease. *Am J Clin Pathol* 101:681, 1994

Jaffe ES, Harris NL, Diebold J *et al.*: World Health Organization classification of neoplastic diseases of the hematopoietic and lymphoid tissues. *Am J Clin Pathol* 111(Suppl. 1):S8, 1999

Jaffe ES, Krenacs L, Kumar S *et al.*: Extranodal peripheral T-cell and NK-cell neoplasms. *Am J Clin Pathol* 111(Suppl. 1):S46, 1999

Jamal S, Picker LJ, Aquino DB *et al.*: Immunophenotypic analysis of peripheral T-cell neoplasms: A multiparameter flow cytometric approach. *Am J Clin Pathol* 116:512, 2001

Kadin ME: Primary Ki-1-positive anaplastic large cell lymphoma: A distinct clinicopathologic entity. *Ann Oncol* 5(Suppl. 1):S25, 1994

Kahwash SB, Qualman SJ. Cutaneous lymphoblastic lymphoma in children: report of six cases with precursor B-cell lineage. *Pediatr Dev Pathol* 5:45, 2002

Kim H: Composite lymphomas and related disorders. *Am J Clin Pathol* 99:445, 1993

Kinney MC: The role of morphologic features, phenotype, genotype, and anatomic site in defining extranodal T-cell or NK-cell neoplasms. *Am J Clin Pathol* 111(Suppl. 1):S104, 1999

Kinney MC, Kadin ME: The pathologic and clinical spectrum of anaplastic large cell lymphoma and correlation with ALK gene regulation. *Am J Clin Pathol* 111(Suppl. 1):S56, 1999

Kirsch LS, Brownstein S, Codere F: Immunoblastic T-cell lymphoma presenting as an eyelid tumor. *Ophthalmology* 97:1352, 1990

Kohno T, Uchida H, Inomata H *et al.*: Ocular manifestations of adult T-cell leukemia/lymphoma. *Ophthalmology* 100:1794, 1993

Kornstein MJ, Bonner H, Gee B *et al.*: Leu M1 and S100 in Hodgkin's disease and non-Hodgkin's lymphomas. *Am J Clin Pathol* 85:433, 1986

Kumar SR, Gill PS, Wagner DG *et al.*: Human T-cell lymphotropic virus type I-associated retinal lymphoma: A clinicopathologic report. *Arch Ophthalmol* 112:954, 1994

Kurtin PL: How do you distinguish benign from malignant extranodal small B-cell proliferations? *Am J Clin Pathol* 111(Suppl. 1):S119, 1999

Lai R, Weiss LM, Chang KL *et al.*: Frequency of CD43 expression in non-Hodgkin lymphomas: A survey of 742 cases and further characterization of rare CD43+ follicular lymphoma. *Am J Clin Pathol* 111:488, 1999

Lee JL, Kim MK, Lee KH *et al.*: Extranodal marginal zone B-cell lymphomas of mucosa-associated lymphoid tissue-type of the orbit and ocular adnexa. *Ann Hematol* 84:13, 2005

Leidenix MJ, Mamalis N, Olson RJ *et al.*: Primary T-cell immunoblastic lymphoma of the orbit in a pediatric patient. *Ophthalmology* 100:998, 1993

Liang R. Diagnosis and management of primary nasal lymphoma of T-cell or NK-cell origin. *Clin Lymphoma* 1:33, 2000

Looi A, Gascoyne RD, Chhanabhai M *et al.*: Mantle cell lymphoma in the ocular adnexal region. *Ophthalmology* 112:114, 2005

Lowen MS, Saraiva VS, Martins MC *et al.*: Immunohistochemical profile of lymphoid lesions of the orbit. *Can J Ophthalmol* 40:634, 2005

Macgrognan G, Vergier B, Dubois P: CD30-positivite cutaneous large-cell lymphomas: A comparative study of clinicopathologic and molecular features of 16 cases. *Am J Clin Pathol* 105:440, 1996

Mann RB: Are there site-specific differences among extranodal aggressive B-cell neoplasms? *Am J Clin Pathol* 111(Suppl. 1):S144, 1999

Matteucci C, Galieni P, Leoncini L *et al.*: Typical genomic imbalances in primary MALT lymphoma of the orbit. *J Pathol* 200:656, 2003

Matzkin DC, Slamovits TL, Rosenbaum PS: Simultaneous intraocular and orbital non-Hodgkin's lymphoma in the acquired immune deficiency syndrome. *Ophthalmology* 101:850, 1994

Meunier J, Lumbroso-Le RL, Vincent-Salomon A *et al.*: Ophthalmologic and intraocular non-Hodgkin's lymphoma: a large single centre study of initial characteristics, natural history, and prognostic factors. *Hematol Oncol* 22:143, 2004

Meyer D, Yanoff M, Hanno H: Differential diagnosis in Mikulicz's syndrome, Mikulicz's disease and similar disease entities. *Am J Ophthalmol* 71:516, 1971

Nowell PC, Croce CM: Chromosome translocations and oncogenes in human lymphoid tumors. *Am J Clin Pathol* 94:229, 1990

Ohtsuka K, Hashimoto M, Suzuki Y. High incidence of orbital malignant lymphoma in Japanese patients. *Am J Ophthalmol* 138:881, 2004

Ohtsuka K, Hashimoto M, Suzuki Y: A review of 244 orbital tumors in Japanese patients during a 21-year period: origins and locations. *Jpn J Ophthalmol* 49:49, 2005

O'Keefe JS, Sippy BD, Martin DF et al.: Anterior chamber infiltrates associated with systemic lymphoma. Report of two cases and review of the literature. *Ophthalmology* 109:253, 2002

Pangalis GA, Boussiotis VA, Kittas C: Malignant disorders of small lymphocytes. *Am J Clin Pathol* 99:402, 1993

Perkins SL: Immunophenotypic analysis of CD5 positivity in paraffin-embedded tissues: Still waiting for an effective diagnostic antibody. *Am J Clin Pathol* 106:273, 1996

Pileri S, Bocchia M, Baroni CD et al.: Anaplastic large cell lymphoma (CD30$^+$Ki-1$^+$) results of a prospective clinico-pathological study of 69 cases. *Br J Haematol* 86:513, 1994

Pinyol M, Campo E, Nadal A et al.: Detection of the bcl-1 rearrangement at the major translocation cluster in frozen and paraffin-embedded tissues of mantle cell lymphomas by polymerase chain reaction. *Am J Clin Pathol* 105:532, 1996

Quintanilla-Martínez L, Zukerberg LR, Ferry JA et al.: Extramedullary tumors of lymphoid or myeloid blasts: The role of immunohistology in classification. *Am J Clin Pathol* 104:431, 1995

Raderer M, Traub T, Formanek M et al.: Somatostatin-receptor scintigraphy for staging and follow-up of patients with extraintestinal marginal zone B-cell lymphoma of the mucosa associated lymphoid tissue (MALT)-type. *Br J Cancer* 85:1462, 2001

Salhany KE, Pietra GC: Extranodal lymphoid disorders. *Am J Clin Pathol* 99:472, 1993

Segal ZI, Cohen I, Szvalb S et al.: Solitary extranodal anaplastic large cell lymphoma, Ki-1$^+$, of the eyelid. *Am J Ophthalmol* 124:105, 1997

Sigudardoottir M, Sigurdsson H, Björk Bakardottir R et al.: Lymphoid tumors of the ocular adnexa: a morphologic and genotypic study of 15 cases. *Acta Ophthalmol Scand* 81:299, 2003

Sharara N, Holden JT, Wojo TH et al.: Ocular adnexal lymphoid proliferations. Clinical, histologic, flow cytometric, and molecular analysis of forty-three cases. *Ophthalmology* 110:1245. 2003

Shields CL, Shields JA, Caravlho C et al.: Conjunctival lymphoid tumors: clinical analysis of 117 cases and relationship to systemic lymphoma. *Ophthalmology* 108:979, 2001

Shields JA, Stopyra GA, Marr BP et al.: Bilateral orbital myeloid sarcoma as initial sign of myeloid leukemia: case report and review of the literature. *Arch Ophthalmol* 121:33, 2003

Shin SS, Sheibani K: Monocytoid B-cell lymphoma. *Am J Clin Pathol* 99:421, 1993

Streeten BW: Burkitt's lymphoma of the conjunctiva. Presented at the meeting of the Verhoeff Society, 1990

Streubel B, Simonitsch-Klupp I, Mullauer L et al.: Variable frequencies of MALT lymphoma-associated genetic aberrations in MALT lymphomas of different sites. *Leukemia* 18:1722, 2004

Suh CO, Shim SJ, Lee SW et al.: Orbital marginal zone B-cell lymphoma of MALT: radiotherapy results and clinical behavior. *Int J Radiat Oncol Biol Phys* 65:228, 2006

Suzuki J, Ohguro H, Satoh M et al.: Clinicopathologic and immunogenetic analysis of mucosa-associated lymphoid tissue lymphomas arising in conjunctiva. *Jpn J Ophthalmol* 43:155, 1999

Swerdlow S: Extranodal hematopoietic/lymphoid disorders: Pathology patterns. *Am J Clin Pathol* 111(Suppl. 1):S1–S152, 1999

Variakojis D, Anastasi J: Unresolved issues concerning Hodgkin's disease and its relationship to non-Hodgkin's lymphoma. *Am J Clin Pathol* 99:436, 1993

Watkins LM, Remulla HD, Rubin PAD: Orbital granulocytic sarcoma in an elderly patient. *Am J Ophthalmol* 123:854, 1997

Weisenburger DD: Progress in the classification of non-Hodgkin's lymphoma. *Am J Clin Pathol* 99:367, 1993

Weisenburger DD, Chan WC: Lymphomas of follicles: Mantle cell and follicle center cell lymphomas. *Am J Clin Pathol* 99:409, 1993

Weisenthal RW, Streeten BW, Dubansky AS et al.: Burkitt lymphoma presenting as a conjunctival mass. *Ophthalmology* 102:129, 1995

Wender A, Adar A, Maor E et al.: Primary B-cell lymphoma of the eyes and brain in a 3-year-old boy. *Arch Ophthalmol* 112:450, 1994

White WL, Ferry AP, Harris NL et al.: Ocular adnexal lymphomas: A clinicopathologic study with identification of lymphomas of mucosa-associated lymphoid tissue type. *Ophthalmology* 102:1994, 1995

Williams GC, Holz E, Lee AG et al.: T-cell lymphoproliferative disorder of vitreous associated with mycosis fungoides. *Arch Ophthalmol* 118:278, 2000

Winberg CD: Peripheral T-cell lymphoma. *Am J Clin Pathol* 99:426, 1993

Yaghouti F, Nouri M, Mannor GE: Ocular adnexal granulocytic sarcoma as the first sign of acute myelogenous leukemia relapse. *Am J Ophthalmol* 127:361, 1999

Yanoff M, Scheie HG: Malignant lymphoma of the orbit: Difficulties in diagnosis. *Surv Ophthalmol* 12:133, 1967

Yoshikawa T, Ogata N, Takahashi K et al.: Bilateral orbital tumor as initial presenting sign in human T-cell leukemia virus-1 associated adult T-cell leukemia/lymphoma. *Am J Ophthalmol* 140:327, 2005

Zucker JL, Doyle MF: Mycosis fungoides metastatic to the orbit. *Arch Ophthalmol* 109:688, 1991

Zukerberg LR, Medeiros JL, Ferry JA et al.: Diffuse low-grade B-cell lymphomas. *Am J Clin Pathol* 100:373, 1993

Tumors: Leukemia

Arber DA, Lopategui JR, Brynes RK: Chronic lymphoproliferative disorders involving blood and bone marrow. *Am J Clin Pathol* 99:494, 1993

Bhattacharjee K, Bhattacharjee H, Das D et al.: Chloroma of the orbit in a non-leukemic adult: A case report. *Orbit* 22:293, 2003

Chen E, Morrison DG, Donahue SP: Acute myeloid leukemia presenting as bilsteral proptosis from diffuse extraocular muscle infiltration. *Am J Ophthalmol* 137:948, 2004

Cook BE, Bartley GB: Acute lymphoblastic leukemia manifesting in an adult as a conjunctival mass. *Am J Ophthalmol* 124:104, 1997

Dickstein JI, Vardiman JW: Issues in the pathology and diagnosis of the chronic myeloproliferative disorders and the myelodysplastic syndromes. *Am J Clin Pathol* 99:513, 1993

Frizzera G, Wu CD, Inghirami G: The usefulness of immunophenotypic and genotypic studies in the diagnosis and classification of hematopoietic and lymphoid neoplasms. *Am J Clin Pathol* 111(Suppl. 1): S13, 1999

Jordan DR, Noel LP, Carpenter BF: Chloroma. *Arch Ophthalmol* 109:734, 1991

Jaffe ES, Harris NL, Diebold J et al.: World Health Organization classification of neoplastic diseases of the hematopoietic and lymphoid tissues. *Am J Clin Pathol* 111(Suppl. 1):S8, 1999

Locurto M, D'Angelo P, Lumia F et al.: Leukemic ophthalmopathy: A report of 21 pediatric cases. *Med Pediatr Oncol* 23:8, 1994

Ohta K, Kondoh T, Yasuo K et al.: Primary granulocytic sarcoma in the sphenoidal bone and orbit. *Childs Nerv Syst* 19:674, 2003

Porto L, Kieslich M, Schwabe D et al.: Granulocytic sarcoma in children. *Neuroradiology* 46:374, 2004

Quintanilla-Martínez L, Zukerberg LR, Ferry JA *et al.*: Extramedullary tumors of lymphoid or myeloid blasts: The role of immunohistology in classification. *Am J Clin Pathol* 104:431, 1995

Shome DK, Gupta NK, Prajapati NC *et al.*: Orbital granulocytic sarcomas (myeloid sarcomas) in acute nonlymphocytic leukemia. *Cancer* 70:2298, 1992

Traweek ST: Immunophenotypic analysis of acute leukemia. *Am J Clin Pathol* 99:504, 1993

Tumuluri K, Woo T, Crowston J *et al.*: Bilateral leukemic orbital infiltration presenting as proptosis and narrow-angle glaucoma. *Ophthalm Plast Reconstr Surg* 20:248, 2004

van Veen S, Kluin PM, de Keizer RJW *et al.*: Granulocytic sarcoma (chloroma). *Am J Clin Pathol* 95:567, 1991

Tumors: Monoclonal and Polyclonal Gammopathies

Alexanian R, Jagannath S: Plasma cell dyscrasias. *JAMA* 268:2946, 1992

Barlogie B, Alexanian R, Jagannath S: Plasma cell dyscrasias. *JAMA* 268:2946, 1992

Bullock JD, Bartley RJ, Campbell RJ *et al.*: Necrobiotic xanthogranuloma with paraproteinemia: Case report and a pathogenetic theory. *Ophthalmology* 93:1233, 1986

Ezra E, Mannor G, Wright JE *et al.*: Inadequately radiated solitary extramedulllary plasmocytoma of the orbit requiring exenteration. *Am J Ophthalmol* 120:803, 1995

Keren DF, Morrison N, Gulbranson R: Evolution of a monoclonal gammopathy. *Lab Med* 5:313, 1994

Lam S, Tessler HH: Iris crystals and hypergammaglobulinemia. *Am J Ophthalmol* 110:440, 1990

Peterson LC, Bradley AB, Crosson JT *et al.*: Application of the immunoperoxidase technic to bone marrow trephine biopsies in the classification of patients with monoclonal gammopathies. *Am J Clin Pathol* 85:688, 1986

Sen HN, Chan C-C, Caruso RC *et al.*: Waldenström's macroglobulinemia-associated retinopathy. *Ophthalmology* 111:535, 2004

Shaen DF, Fardeau C, Roberge FG *et al.*: Rearrangement of immunoglobulin gene in metastatic Waldenström macroglobulinemia. *Am J Ophthalmol* 129:395, 2000

Ugurlu S, Bartley GB, Gibson LE: Necrobiotic xanthogranuloma: Long-term outcome of ocular and systemic involvement. *Am J Ophthalmol* 129:651, 2000

Yanoff M, Nix R, Arvan D: Bilateral lacrimal gland enlargement associated with a diffuse gamma globulin elevation: A case report. *Ophthalmol Res* 1:245, 1970

Tumors: Melanotic

See Chapter 17.

Secondary Orbital Tumors

Albert DM, Rubenstein RA, Scheie HG: Tumor metastasis to the eye. Incidence in 213 adult patients with generalized malignancy: II. Clinical study in infants and children. *Am J Ophthalmol* 63:723, 727, 1967

Callejo SA, Kronish JW, Decker SJ *et al.*: Malignant granular cell tumor metastatic to the orbit. *Ophthalmology* 107:550, 2000

Fan JT, Buettner H, Bartley GB *et al.*: Clinical features and treatment of seven patients with carcinoid tumor metastatic to the eye and orbit. *Am J Ophthalmol* 119:211, 1995

Font RL, Ferry AP: Carcinoma metastatic to the eye and orbit: III. A clinicopathologic study of 28 cases metastatic to the orbit. *Cancer* 38:1326, 1976

Johnson LN, Krohel GB, Yeon EB *et al.*: Sinus tumors invading the orbit. *Ophthalmology* 91:209, 1984

Ormerod LD, Weber AL, Rauch SD *et al.*: Ophthalmic manifestations of maxillary sinus mucoceles. *Ophthalmology* 94:1013, 1987

Riddle PJ, Font RL, Zimmerman LE: Carcinoid tumors of the eye and orbit: A clinicopathologic study of 15 cases, with histochemical and electron microscopic observations. *Hum Pathol* 13:459, 1982

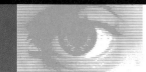
NATURAL HISTORY

I. Diabetes mellitus (DM) is a heterogeneous group of disorders characterized by elevated blood glucose and other metabolic abnormalities.

Elevated blood glucose levels cause an elevated retinal glucose level, resulting in a hypoxic-like redox imbalance that may contribute to the ischemia that precedes the development of diabetic retinopathy (DR).

A. The disorder may result from decreased circulating insulin or from ineffective insulin action in target cells.

Diabetes accompanied by renal disease (in the form of focal and segmental glomerulosclerosis) is found in adult individuals with mitochondrial tRNA (Leu) genetic mutation. In patients with the A3243G mutation, deafness is almost consistently found, and extrarenal manifestations also include neuromuscular, cardiac, and retinal disease. The latter is in the form of macular dystrophy. The extrarenal manifestations, including diabetes, tend to occur later in the course of the disease.

B. DM, which affects approximately 5% of the United States population and 29% of the population 65 years or older, is classified as either type 1 (previously called *insulin-dependent*) or type 2 (previously called *noninsulin-dependent*) DM.

Type 2 DM accounts for approximately 90% of diabetic patients. Target cell resistance occurs in both types, but is a central feature in type 2. Genetic defects in the cellular insulin receptor may account for the insulin resistance. In animal experiments, C-peptide, a cleavage product in the processing of proinsulin but retained in the secretory granule and cosecreted with insulin in response to glucose stimulation, seems to prevent the vascular and neural dysfunction in diabetic rats.

II. DR is a leading cause of blindness in the United States.
   A. Over three-fourths of the blind are women.
   B. There is a significantly higher prevalence of DR in individuals of black or latino descent compared to whites or Chinese.
   C. The most important factor in the occurrence of DR is how long the patient has been diabetic.
      1. Although approximately 60% of patients develop retinopathy after 15 years of diabetes, and almost 100% after 30 years, the risk of legal blindness in a given diabetic person is only 7% to 9% even after 20 to 30 years of DM.
         a. When the onset of type 1 DM is before 30 years of age and no DR is present at onset, approximately 59% of patients have developed DR 4 years later, and almost 100% 20 years later. In this group, the incidence of proliferative DR (PDR) stabilizes after 13 to 14 years of diabetes at between 14% and 17%.
         b. When the onset of type 1 DM is after 30 years of age and no DR is present at onset, approximately 47% of patients have developed DR 4 years later. Among patients older than 30 years of age who develop type 2 DM, 34% develop DR 4 years later. In this group of patients with type 1 DM, 7% who were free of PDR at onset of DM developed PDR 4 years later; 2% of the patients with type 2 DM developed PDR 4 years later.

2. Once blindness develops, the average life expectancy is less than 6 years.

3. Ocular symptoms occur in approximately 20% to 40% of diabetic patients at the clinical onset of the disease, but these symptoms are mainly caused by refractive changes, rather than by DR.

4. The low frequency of retinopathy in secondary diabetes (e.g., chronic pancreatitis, pancreatectomy, hemochromatosis, Cushing's syndrome, and acromegaly) may be due to the decreased survival among patients with secondary diabetes.

A positive correlation exists between the presence of DR and nephropathy (Kimmelstiel–Wilson disease).

---

5. It appears that the risk for developing DR in type 1 DM is reduced if glycemic control is achieved from the time of diagnosis; conversely, if DR is already present, early intensive insulin treatment can initially worsen the DR.

6. Among diabetic individuals, plasma lipid levels are associated with the presence of hard retinal exudates, and carotid artery intima–media wall thickness is associated with retinopathy; however, other manifestations of atherosclerosis and most of its risk factors are not associated with the severity of DR.

III. In juvenile DM, PDR is uncommon in patients younger than 20 years of age, and almost unheard of in patients younger than 16 years of age.

A. Background DR (BDR; especially microaneurysms), however, can be demonstrated on fluorescein angiography in juvenile diabetic patients as young as 3 years of age, and is present in most patients older than 10 years of age.

Evidence suggests that a virus, perhaps coxsackievirus B4, can cause some cases of juvenile-onset diabetes, probably by damaging the pancreatic cells. Autoimmune mechanisms may also play a role. Recently, DR has been found to have characteristics of chronic inflammatory disease and neurodegenerative disease. Elevated vitreous levels of interleukins-6 and 8 in PDR support immune or inflammatory mechanisms in the pathogenesis of PDR.

IV. Most diabetic patients never acquire PDR, and in those who do, it develops only after at least 15 years of DM.

Rarely, a patient presents with BDR, or even with PDR before any systemic evidence of DM (such as hyperglycemia) is discovered.

V. Other associations

A. Primary open- and closed-angle glaucoma occurs more often in diabetic patients than in nondiabetic individuals.

B. DR is approximately 6% more frequent in diabetic patients who have a diagonal earlobe crease than in those individuals who do not have a diagonal earlobe crease. A positive association exists between a diagonal earlobe crease and coronary artery disease in patients with diabetes.

C. A positive association also exists between DR and the presence of elevated blood pressure (especially increased diastolic blood pressure), glycosylated hemoglobin, and smoking.

Poor control in DM adversely impacts nerve fiber layer thickness as measured by the scanning laser polarimeter. This finding does not appear to be acute because it is not reversed by short-term blood glucose regulation.

D. Other risk factors for the development of DR include hypertension and abdominal obesity.

RETINAL VASCULATURE IN NORMAL SUBJECTS AND DIABETIC PATIENTS

Figure 15.1 shows examples of retinal vasculature in normal subjects and diabetic patients (see also section *Neurosensory Retina*, later in this chapter).

CONJUNCTIVA AND CORNEA

I. Conjunctival microaneurysms may be found in diabetic individuals, but they are of questionable diagnostic significance because they also occur in nondiabetic subjects.

II. Transmural lipid imbibition may occur in conjunctival capillaries in diabetic lipemia retinalis (Fig. 15.2). Histologically, lipid-laden cells, either endothelial cells or subintimal macrophages, are present projecting into and encroaching on conjunctival capillary lumens.

III. The conjunctiva may show decreased vascularity in the capillary bed, increased capillary resistance, and decreased area occupied by the microvessels.

Microvascular abnormalities have even been detected in the conjunctiva of pediatric diabetic patients. The severity of these findings correlates with hemoglobin A1c levels, but not with the duration of the disease. Such conjunctival microvascular changes correlate significantly with disease severity in type 2 diabetes, but not with disease duration since diagnosis.

IV. Corneal epithelium and its basement membrane may be abnormal, and epithelial erosions are common. Corneal sensation may be reduced, and the stroma may be thickened. Tear production is more frequently reduced in diabetic patients than in nondiabetics.

A. Diabetic ocular surface disease following cataract surgery is ameliorated with oral aldose reductase inhibitor treatment by improving ocular surface sensitivity.

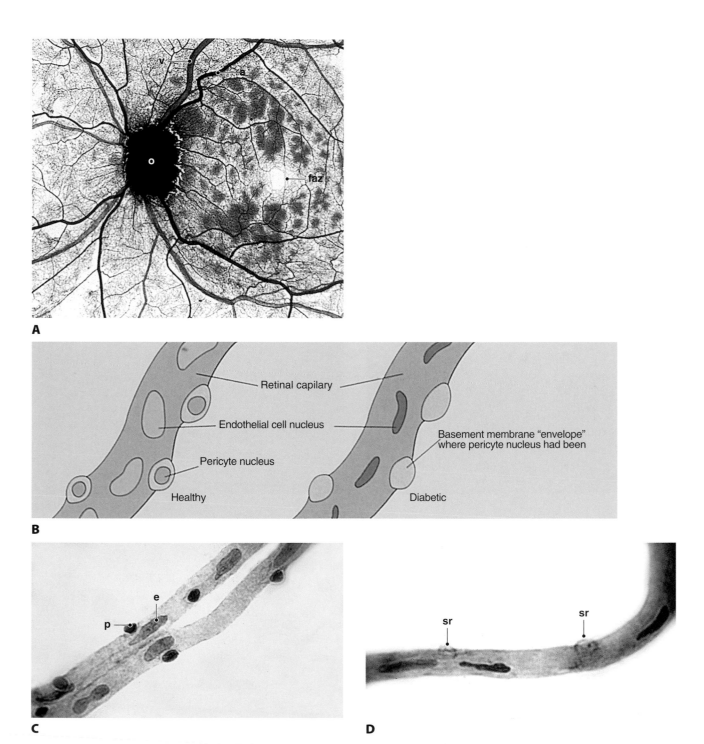

Fig. 15.1 Retinal vasculature (normal and diabetic). **A,** Periodic acid–Schiff- and hematoxylin-stained trypsin digest of normal neural retina shows the optic nerve (o) and major blood vessels. The arterioles (a), darker and slightly smaller than the venules (v) (ratio of vein to artery, 5:4), are surrounded by a narrow, characteristic, capillary-free zone. The foveal avascular zone (faz) is clearly seen. **B,** Diagram of healthy retinal capillary shows normal 1:1 ratio of pericyte to endothelial cell nuclei. The ratio is decreased in the diabetic patient because of a loss of pericyte nuclei, perhaps by apoptosis. **C,** Trypsin digest of normal neural retina shows retinal capillary with its normal 1:1 ratio of pericyte (p) to endothelial (e) cell nuclei. **D,** Trypsin digest of diabetic neural retina shows capillary with a decreased pericyte-to-endothelial cell nuclei ratio. Endothelial cell nuclei are present but appear pyknotic. Pericyte nuclei are absent from their basement membrane shells (sr).

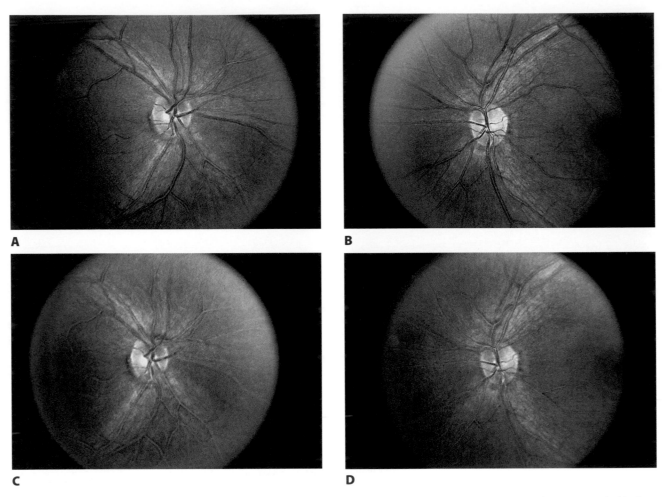

Fig. 15.2 Lipemia retinalis. Right eye (**A** and **C**) and left eye (**B** and **D**) of same patient taken 1 month apart. Lipemia retinalis is more marked in **C** and **D** than in **A** and **B**. Transmural lipid imbibition may also occur in conjunctival capillaries in diabetic lipemia retinalis.

Keratoepitheliopathy, conjunctival squamous metaplasia, and abnormal corneal sensitivity, tear break-up time, Schirmer test, and tear secretion level are all related to the status of metabolic control, diabetic neuropathy, and stage of DR. The prevalence of keratoepithelialiopathy is 22.8% in diabetic individuals, but 8.5% in nondiabetics, and is associated with tear film abnormalities, particularly nonuniformity of the tear lipid layer, in diabetic patients.

B. Decreased penetration of "anchoring" fibrils from the corneal epithelial basement membrane into the corneal stroma may be responsible for the loose adhesion between the corneal epithelium and the stroma.

The corneal epithelium in diabetic patients is much easier to wipe off, often in a single sheet (e.g., during vitrectomy procedures), than is the epithelium of nondiabetic patients. Approximately 50% of diabetic patients undergoing vitrectomy surgery have corneal complications following the procedure, with 44.6% having an epithelial disturbance, and 23.8% exhibiting corneal edema. These complications are significantly correlated with the degree of surgical invasion during the procedure.

Specular microscopic studies show corneal endothelial structural abnormalities reflected in an increased coefficient of variation of cell area, a decreased percentage of hexagonal cells, an increased corneal autofluorescence, and an increased intraocular pressure. The changes in corneal endothelium resemble those that occur with aging. In the Ocular Hypertension Treatment Trial* increased central corneal thickness was associated with younger age, female gender, and diabetes.

Decreased corneal endothelial cell density and increased coefficient of variability in cell size are noted in high-risk PDR patients undergoing cataract surgery by phacoemulsification, but not in normal individuals.

C. Contact lens studies in patients who have type 2 DM have demonstrated that the diabetic corneal endothelium shows significantly lower function than the nondia-

*Brandt JD, Beiser JA, Kass MA et al.: *Central corneal thickness in the Ocular Hypertension Treatment Study (OHTS)*. Ophthalmology *108*:1779, 2001.

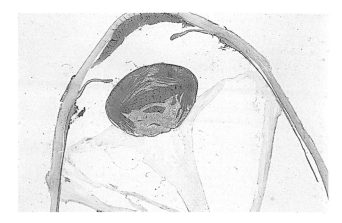

Fig. 15.3 Cataract. Histologic section shows marked cortical and nuclear cataractous changes in diabetic patient. The changes are nonspecific and, therefore, indistinguishable from those in nondiabetic patients.

betic corneal endothelium, even though the morphometry of corneal endothelial cells and central corneal thickness in diabetic patients who wear soft contact lenses are not appreciably different from the values found in contact lens-wearing control individuals.

 D. Corneal endothelial cells of diabetic individuals are more susceptible to damage during cataract surgery than nondiabetics, and exhibit a delay in recovering from postoperative corneal edema. Diabetes is also a significant risk factor for unsuccessful initial corneal transplant grafts because of endothelial failure.

 V. Corneal nerve tortuosity may relate to the severity of the neuropathy in diabetic patients.

Corneal confocal microscopy also demonstrates that corneal nerve fiber density and branch density are reduced in diabetic patients compared to control individuals, and these measures tend to be worse in individuals with more severe neuropathy.

LENS

 I. "Snowflake" cataract of juvenile diabetic patient
  A. The cataract consists of subcapsular opacities with vacuoles and chalky-white flake deposits.
  B. The whole lens may become a milky-white cataract (occasionally the process is reversible), and even may be bilateral.
  C. The histopathology has not been defined.
 II. Adult-onset diabetic cataract (Fig. 15.3)
  A. The cataract (cortical and nuclear) is indistinguishable clinically and histopathologically from the "usual" age-related cataracts. Diabetic patients, however, are at an increased risk for development of cataracts compared with nondiabetic subjects. Nevertheless, diabetes is not universally accepted as a risk factor for nuclear cataracts.

   1. Diabetes is a strong risk factor for the development of posterior subcapsular cataract.
   2. Apoptosis plays an important role in the development of cataracts in DR compared to senile cataract.
   3. Nuclear fiber compaction analysis demonstrates no difference in compaction between diabetic and nondiabetic cataracts, although diabetes does appear to accelerate the formation of cataracts that are similar to age-related nuclear cataracts.

Reversible lens opacities, even posterior subcapsular opacities, may be seen. Aldose reductase probably plays a key role in initiating the formation of lens opacities in diabetic patients, as it does in galactosemia. Calpains may be responsible for the unregulated proteolysis of lens crystallins, thereby contributing to diabetic cataract development.

 B. Patients with diabetes may have transient lens opacities and induced myopia during hyperglycemia.
 C. Cataract surgery and progression of DR
  1. The visual prognosis for patients who have pre-existing DR, both nonproliferative and proliferative, and who undergo cataract extraction and posterior-chamber lens implantation is less favorable than for patients who have no retinopathy.
  2. The poorer prognosis results from increased progression of DR, both background and proliferative, after cataract extraction.
  3. Posterior capsule opacification is greater in diabetic individuals following cataract surgery than in nondiabetic control patients; however, among diabetic individuals, neither the stage of DR nor the systemic status of the diabetes correlates with the degree of posterior capsule opacification.

IRIS

 I. Vacuolation of iris pigment epithelium (Fig. 15.4)
  A. Vacuolation of the iris pigment epithelium is present in 40% of enucleated diabetic eyes. The vacuoles contain glycogen.

Rupture of the vacuoles when the intraocular pressure is suddenly reduced, as in entering the anterior chamber during cataract surgery, results in release of pigment into the posterior chamber. The pigment is visible clinically as a cloud moving through the pupil into the anterior chamber. Lacy vacuolation and "damage" to the overlying dilator muscle may be the cause of delayed dilatation of the iris after instillation of mydriatics.

  B. Pinpoint "holes" may be seen clinically with the slit lamp when transpupillary retroillumination is used. The holes may be seen in at least 25% of known diabetic patients who have blue irises.

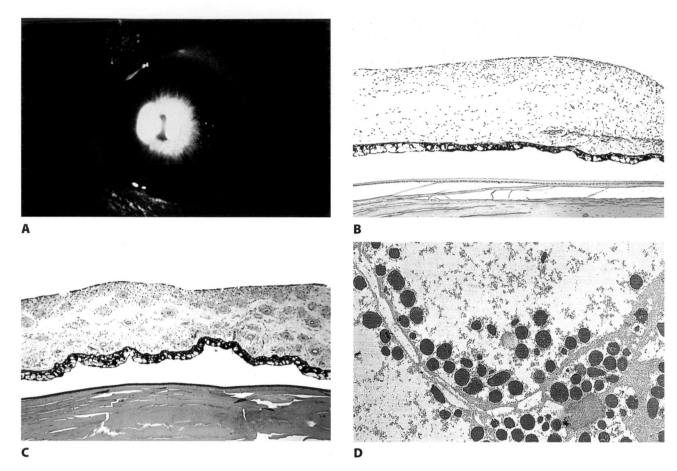

Fig. 15.4 Lacy vacuolation of iris pigment epithelium. **A,** Transpupillary retroillumination shows myriad pinholes of transillumination of the iris just to the right of pupil (light coming from left). Fine points of light tend to follow pattern of circumferential ridges of posterior pigment epithelial layer. Transmission caused by swelling of epithelial cells and displacement of pigment, not by loss of pigment from cells. **B,** Vacuolation involves both layers of iris pigment epithelium and ceases abruptly at the iris root. Vacuoles appear empty in sections stained with hematoxylin and eosin. **C,** Vacuoles stain positively with periodic acid–Schiff stain. Circumferential ridges (cut here meridionally) are greatly accentuated. **D,** Glycogen particles (very dark, tiny dots) present throughout pigment epithelial vacuoles, along with large melanin granules. Plasma membranes separate adjacent cells. (**A,** Modified from Fine BS *et al.: Am J Ophthalmol* 69:197. © Elsevier 1970. **B** and **C,** modified from Yanoff M *et al.: Am J Ophthalmol* 67:21, 1969. © Elsevier 1969.)

In autopsy eyes from diabetic patients, vacuolation of the iris pigment epithelium may be related to increased blood glucose levels before death. The vacuolation is also seen histologically in neonates and in patients who have systemic mucopolysaccharidoses (the vacuoles contain acid mucopolysaccharides), Menkes' syndrome, and multiple myeloma.

II. Neovascularization of iris (rubeosis iridis; Fig. 15.5; see also Figs 9.13 and 9.14)

    A. *Rubeosis iridis* is the clinical term for iris neovascularization.

        1. It is present in fewer than 5% of diabetic patients without PDR, but in approximately 50% of patients who have PDR.

        2. The new iris vessels arise from venules.

Neovascularization of the iris appears to be related to an angiogenic factor derived from hypoxic neural retina. The lens–zonular diaphragm and a vitreous antiangiogenic factor seem to decrease the anterior flow of the neural retinal angiogenic factor into the aqueous compartment; therefore, lensectomy and vitrectomy remove these barriers and facilitate the development of iris neovascularization in approximately 50% of cases. An alternative explanation for its development is a generalized hypoxic state of the anterior segment of the eye in diabetic patients.

    B. Neovascularization of the iris may arise from the anterior-chamber angle, the pupillary border, midway between, or all three.

Infrequently, the anterior iris stroma, between the pupil and the collarette, may show a very fine neovascularization that can remain stationary for years without the development of angle neovascularization.

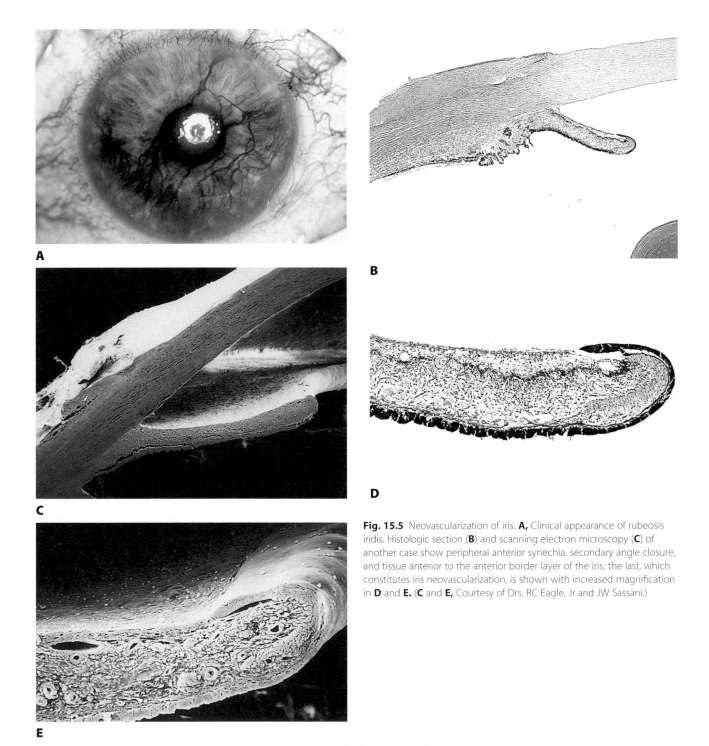

Fig. 15.5 Neovascularization of iris. **A,** Clinical appearance of rubeosis iridis. Histologic section (**B**) and scanning electron microscopy (**C**) of another case show peripheral anterior synechia, secondary angle closure, and tissue anterior to the anterior border layer of the iris; the last, which constitutes iris neovascularization, is shown with increased magnification in **D** and **E**. (**C** and **E,** Courtesy of Drs. RC Eagle, Jr and JW Sassani.)

C. Early, anterior chamber angle neovascularization causes a secondary open-angle glaucoma that progresses rapidly to a closed-angle glaucoma caused by peripheral anterior synechiae.

As the fibrovascular tissue on the anterior iris surface contracts, *ectropion uveae* may develop. The new blood vessels tend to bleed easily, hence the misused and poor term *hemorrhagic glaucoma*; *neovascular glaucoma* is the preferred term so as not to confuse the entity with glaucoma secondary to traumatic hemorrhage. Even without the development of iris neovascularization, an increased incidence of both primary open- and closed-angle glaucoma exists in diabetes.

CILIARY BODY AND CHOROID

I. Basement membrane of ciliary pigment epithelium (external basement membrane of ciliary epithelium; Fig. 15.6)

   A. The multilaminar basement membrane of the pigment epithelium is diffusely thickened in the region of the pars plicata.

   B. The diffuse thickening of the external basement membrane of ciliary pigment epithelium in diabetic patients is different from the "spotty" or "patchy" thickening that may be seen in nondiabetic subjects.

II. The multilaminar basement membrane of ciliary nonpigmented epithelium (internal basement membrane of ciliary epithelium) is not affected.

III. Fibrovascular core of ciliary processes (see Fig. 15.6)

   A. Fibrosis results in obliteration of capillaries in the "core" of the ciliary processes.

   B. The capillary basement membrane is often significantly thickened.

IV. Choriocapillaris, Bruch's membrane, and retinal pigment epithelium (Figs 15.7 and 15.8)

   A. Periodic acid-Schiff–positive material thickens and may partially obliterate the lumen of the choriocapillaris in the macula.

   B. The cuticular portion of Bruch's membrane (basement membrane of the retinal pigment epithelium; basal laminar-like deposits) may become thickened, and the lumen of the choriocapillaris narrowed by endothelial cell proliferation and basement membrane elaboration.

      The incidence of choriocapillaris degeneration is approximately fourfold greater in diabetic patients than in nondiabetic subjects.

   C. Drusen are common.

   D. Scanning electron microscopy of choroidal vascular casts shows increased tortuosity, dilatation and narrowing, hypercellularity, vascular loop, and microaneurysm formation, "dropout" of choriocapillaris, and formation of sinus-like structures between choroidal lobules.

V. Arteries and arterioles of choroid (see Figs 15.7 and 15.8)

    Arteriosclerosis occurs at a younger age in diabetic patients than in the general population.

    1. The incidence increases sharply beyond the 15th year of the disease.

    2. The change is reflected in atherosclerosis and arteriolosclerosis of the choroidal vessels.

NEUROSENSORY RETINA

I. The cause(s) of DR, Table 15.1 (see also discussion of PDR later in this section)

   A. Although DR is usually discussed relative to the characteristic and clinically apparent vascular changes, recent evidence suggests that DR involves alterations in all of the retinal cellular elements, including: vascular endothelial cells and pericytes, glial cells including macroglia (Müller cells and astrocytes) and microglia, and neurons, including photoreceptors, bipolar cells, amacrine cells, and ganglion cells (Table 15.2, p. 607). Each of these elements makes unique contributions to visual function, and participates in multiple homeostatic relationships to the other cellular elements.

   B. Damage to multiple retinal neuronal elements through apoptosis, and accompanying glial cell reactivity and microglial activation, suggests that DR might be classified as a neurodegenerative disorder, and not simply as a vasculopathy.

> Support for the concept of a neurodegenerative process in diabetes is found in the fact that neurovisual tests are abnormal in type 1 diabetic individuals prior to the onset of clinically apparent retinopathy. Viewed from this perspective, it is doubtful that the entity that we call "diabetic retinopathy" is the manifestation of a single pathophysiologic disturbance or of the malfunction of one cell type. Rather, as can be seen in Table 15.2, multiple pathophysiologic mechanisms come into play in DR, including structural alterations, cell death, inflammation, cellular proliferation, and atrophy. These apparent alterations must require the participation of numerous biologically active mediators. For example, in DR advanced glycation end products (AGEP) and/or lipoxidation end products form on the amino groups of proteins, lipids, and DNA, and may impact the retina by modifying the structure and function of proteins and/or cause intramolecular and intermolecular cross-link formation. AGEP not only alter structure and function of molecules, they also increase oxidative stress. AGEP with polyol pathway activation may mediate the direct impairment of retinal endothelial cell barrier function caused by high glucose levels.

   C. Apoptosis probably contributes to retinal ganglion cell death in DR and glial cells may modify the expression of such apoptosis.

   D. Given the multiple pathways contributing to the development of DR, gene therapy holds promise for modifying key contributing mechanisms.

II. The diagnosis of DR—the best way to diagnose DR is by means of a thorough fundus examination through a dilated pupil.

> Ancillary studies can be very helpful in demonstrating the scope of retinal involvement. For example, retinal thickness, as measured by the Retinal Thickness Analyzer, has been found to be abnormal diffusely in the retina and not just in the areas exhibiting clinically apparent retinopathy.

The vascular lesions in diabetes are not uniformly distributed across the retina. Microaneurysms, acellular capillaries, and pericyte ghosts are more numerous in the temporal retina than in the nasal retina; however, retinal capillary basement membrane thickness does not exhibit such regional variation.

III. Specific constellation of vascular findings—clinical BDR

   A. Loss of capillary pericytes (see Fig. 15.1)

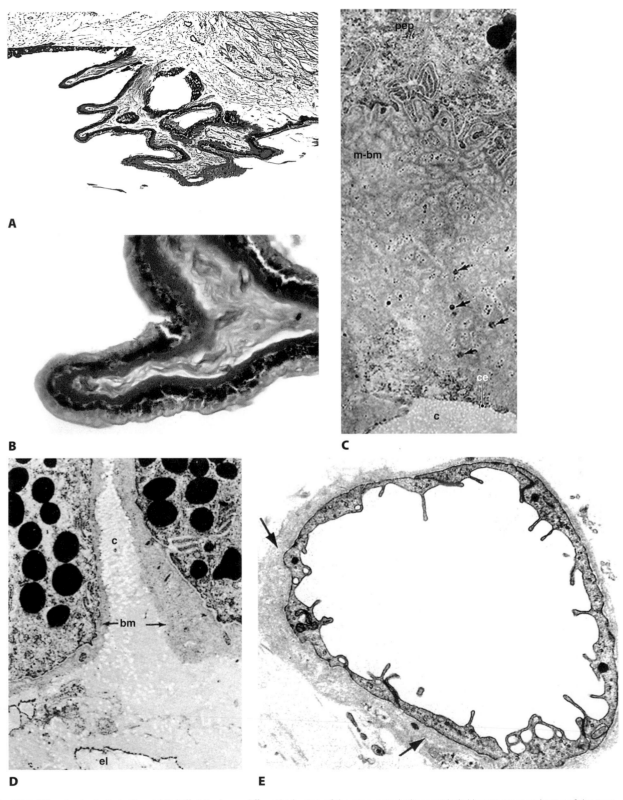

Fig. 15.6 Ciliary body. **A,** Periodic acid–Schiff stain shows diffuse thickening of the pigmented ciliary epithelial basement membrane of the pars plicata. **B,** Increased magnification shows the thickened basement membrane characteristic of diabetes. Note marked decrease in number of core capillaries. **C,** Multilaminar external basement membrane (m-bm) of ciliary epithelium in region of pars plicata thickened markedly. Distal edge demarcated by plane of attenuated nonpigmented uveal cells (ce). Numerous small granules (*arrows*), presumably calcific, present in distal parts of basement membrane (pep, bases of pigment epithelial cells; c, collagen). **D,** Normally thick homogeneous external basement membrane (bm) of ciliary epithelium in region of pars plana not altered; sample from same patient as in **C** (c, collagen; el, elastic lamina). **E,** Capillary in pars plicata shows diffuse and asymmetric homogeneous thickening of basement membrane (*arrows*).

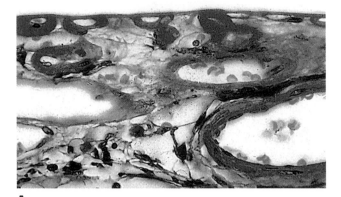

A

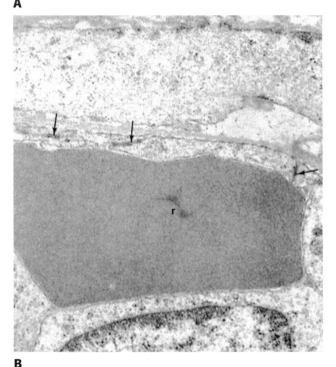

B

Fig. 15.7 Choroidopathy. **A,** Histologic section of the foveomacular region shows diffuse thickening of choroidal vessels, especially involving the choriocapillaris, which are partially occluded by periodic acid–Schiff-positive material. **B,** Electron micrograph shows choroidal arteriole apposed to characteristic basement membrane material of outer layer of Bruch's membrane. Note red blood cell (r) in small lumen of vessel. Endothelial cells swollen and junctional attachments (*arrows*) present. Smooth-muscle cells in arteriole wall also present.

Capillary pericytes probably contribute to the mechanical stability of the capillary wall.

---

1. In the normal retinal capillary, the pericyte-to-endothelial-cell ratio is 1:1.
2. In the diabetic retinal capillary, the pericyte-to-endothelial-cell ratio is less than 1:1 because of a selective loss of pericytes.

Pericytes have a contractile function, regulate microvascular retinal blood flow, are excitable cells, and react to several vasoactive substances (e.g., norepinephrine and histamine). Pericytes contain aldose reductase, and show the presence of the sorbitol pathway. They may influence the neural retinal microvasculature through their production and release of prostacyclin. The viability of cultured retinal capillary pericytes is decreased by high concentrations of glucose, probably by inhibiting phospholipase C activity of pericytes through a guanine nucleotide-dependent and pertussis toxin-insensitive regulatory pathway. Glycolytic metabolites activate three of the major biochemical pathways implicated in the pathogenesis of DR. These pathways are the hexosamine pathway, the advanced glycation end product formation pathway, and the diacylglycerol–protein kinase C pathway. Benfotiamine, a thiamine derivative, inhibits these three pathways simultaneously, and prevents DR in experimental animals.

3. Pericyte death is accompanied by morphologic nuclear changes and lack of inflammation characteristic of apoptosis (see p. 23 in Chapter 1).

Activation of nuclear factor-kappaB, induced by high glucose in diabetes, may regulate a proapoptotic program in retinal pericytes.

Evidence suggests that hyperglycemia followed abruptly by euglycemia triggers the process of apoptosis, resulting in retinal capillary pericyte death. This finding explains why DR sometimes develops, or accelerates rapidly, in patients who had been under poor or moderate control, and are placed rapidly on tight, excellent control.

B. Capillary microaneurysms (Figs 15.9 and 15.10)
1. Many more retinal capillary microaneurysms (RCMs) are detected microscopically and by fluorescein angiography than are seen clinically with the ophthalmoscope.

Optical coherence tomography (OCT) may provide a noninvasive tool for the detection of early diabetic retinal changes in patients lacking clinically apparent retinopathy. Mean macular thickness, as measured by OCT, correlates with visual acuity in DR. Retinal thickness is increased in diabetic individuals without clinically apparent retinopathy compared to nondiabetic control subjects. In individuals with type 2 diabetes and mild nonproliferative retinopathy, areas of increased retinal thickness are associated with retinal vascular leakage at those sites. Similarly, perimetry can provide more useful information than visual acuity testing relative to functional loss in diabetes.

---

2. An increase in the number of RCMs can be directly correlated with the loss of pericytes.
3. RCMs are formed in response to a hypoxic environment in which abortive attempts at neovascularization or regressed changes, or both, have been made in a previously proliferating vessel.

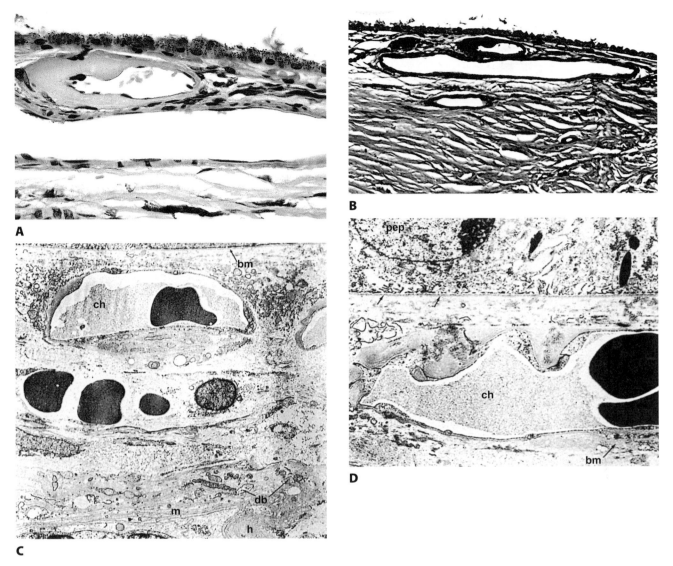

Fig. 15.8 Choroidopathy. **A,** Histologic section of foveal region shows choroidal artery partially occluded by eosinophilic material. Choriocapillaris occluded in this area. **B,** Periodic acid–Schiff (PAS) stain of same region shows PAS-positive material in walls of arterioles and choriocapillaris. **C,** Inner choroid, foveomacula. Segment of choriocapillaris (ch) is small. Thickening of the basement membrane is most apparent along the outer capillary wall. Masses of disordered banded (trilaminar) basement membrane form the intercapillary columns. Masses of multilaminar (m), homogeneous (h), and disordered banded (db) basement membrane lie along the inner wall of a deeper choroidal vessel. A moderately thickened basement membrane (*arrows*) lies along the vessel outer wall (bm, normally thin basement membrane of pigment epithelium). **D,** Region of choriocapillaris (ch), foveomacula. Thin basement membrane (*arrows*) of pigment epithelium (pep) is unaltered. Focal hyperproduction of choriocapillaris homogeneous basement membrane has occurred along the inner capillary wall ("drusen" of choriocapillaris). Segments of ordered banded basement membrane are present in the choriocapillaris drusen. Adjacent, to the left, are myriad fragments of disordered banded (trilaminar) basement membrane. The outer capillary basement membrane (bm) is also focally thickened. (**A** and **B,** Modified from Yanoff M: *Am J Ophthalmol* 67:21. © Elsevier 1969.)

a. RCMs, which are randomly distributed across the arteriolar and venular sides of the capillary network, start as thin outpouchings (saccular) from the wall of a capillary.

b. The retinal capillary endothelial cells proliferate and lay down increased amounts of basement membrane (Fig. 15.11).

c. Ultimately, all of the endothelial cells may disappear; ghost retinal capillaries result.

d. The lumen of the RCM may remain patent or may become occluded by the accumulated basement membrane material.

C. Thickening of retinal capillary basement membrane (see Figs 15.1, 15.10, and 15.11)

TABLE 15.1 Proposed Pathogenic Mechanisms for Diabetic Retinopathy

Proposed Mechanism	Putative Mode of Action	Proposed Therapy
Aldose reductase	Increases production of sorbitol (sugar alcohol produced by reduction of glucose) and may cause osmotic or other cellular damage	Aldose reductase inhibitors (clinical trials in retinopathy and neuropathy thus far have been unsuccessful)
Inflammation	Increases adherence of leukocytes to capillary endothelium, which may decrease flow and increase hypoxia; may also increase breakdown of blood–retinal barrier and enhance macular edema	Aspirin (ineffective in the Early Treatment Diabetic Retinopathy Sudy, but did not increase vitreous hemorrhage; therefore not contraindicated in patients with diabetes who require it for other reasons); corticosteroids (intravitreal injection or slow-release implants for macular edema now being tested)
Protein kinase C	Protein kinase C upregulates VEGF and is also active in "downstream" actions of VEGF following binding of the cytokine to its cellular receptor. Protein kinase C activity increased by diacylglycerol, which is accelerated by hyperglycemia	Clinical trials of a protein kinase Cβ isoform inhibitor in retinopathy have thus far been unsuccessful
Reactive oxygen species	Oxidative damage to enzymes and to other key cellular components	Antioxidants (limited evaluation in clinical trials)
Nonenzymatic glycation of proteins; advanced glycation end producs	Inactivation of critical enzymes; alteration of key structural proteins	Aminoguanidine (clinical trial for nephropathy halted by sponsor)
Inducible form of nitric oxide synthase	Enhances free-radical production; may upregulate VEGF	Aminoguanidine
Altered expression of critical gene or genes	May be caused by hyperglycemia in several poorly understood ways. May cause long-lived alteration of one or more critical cellular pathways	None at present
Apoptotic death of retinal capillary pericytes, endothelial cells	Reduces blood flow to retina, which reduces function and increases hypoxia	None at present
VEGF	Increased by retinal hypoxia and possibly other mechanisms; induces breakdown of blood–retinal barrier, leading to macular edema; induces proliferation of retinal capillary cells and neovascularization	Reduction of VEGF by extensive (panretinal) laser photocoagulation; several experimental medical therapies being tested
PEDF	Protein normally released in retina inhibits neovascularization; reduction in diabetes may eliminate this infection	PEDF gene in nonreplicating adenovirus introduced into eye to induce PEDF formation in retina (phase I clinical trial ongoing)
Growth hormone and IGF-1	Permissive role allows pathologic actions of VEGF; reduction in growth hormone or IGF-1 prevents neovascularization	Hypophysectormy (now abandoned); pegvisomant (growth hormone receptor blocker); (brief clinical trial failed); octreotide (somatostatin analogue, clinical trial now in progress)

For all the proposed mechanisms, hyperglycemia accelerates the progression to diabetic retinopathy.
VEGF, vascular endothelial growth factor; PEDF, pigment epithelium-derived factor; IGF-1, IGF, insulin-like growth factor-1. Modified from : Frank RN. Diabetic retinopathy. N Engl J Med 2004;350:48–58.

D. Arteriolovenular connections ("shunts": actually, collaterals; Fig. 15.12)
1. Arteriolovenular connections (collaterals) are secondary phenomena (i.e., secondary to the surrounding environmental hypoxic stimulus).
2. The arteriolovenular connections have a decreased rate of blood flow, unlike true shunts.
E. Other findings
1. Often, an irregular, large foveal avascular zone is present (its irregularity and greater size with BDR are even more pronounced with PDR).

TABLE 15.2 Diabetic Alterations in Retinal Cellular Elements

Cell Type	Changes
Vascular	Altered tight junctions Endothelial cell and pericyte death
Glial	Altered contacts with vessels Release inflammatory mediators Impaired glutamate metabolism
Microglial	Increased numbers Release inflammatory mediators
Neuronal	Death of ganglion cells, inner nuclear layer Axonal atrophy

Modified from Gardner TW et al. Diabetic retinopathy: More than meets the eye. Surv Ophthalmol 47 (Suppl 2):S253, © Elsevier, 2002.

2. Diabetic patients show an abnormal macular capillary blood flow velocity, and decreased entoptically perceived leukocytes, over age-matched nondiabetic subjects. Conversely, choroidal blood flow is significantly decreased in the foveal region, particularly in diabetic macular edema (DME).
   a. Pulsatile ocular blood flow is unaffected in early DR, increases significantly in eyes with moderate to severe nonproliferative DR, and decreases following laser treatment of PDR.
3. Partitions of the larger retinal venules by a double layer of endothelial cells anchored to a thin basement membrane are associated with the formation of venous loops and reduplications that are caused by gradual venous occlusion.

IV. Exudative retinopathy
   A. "Hard" or "waxy" exudates (Fig. 15.13; see also Figs 15.9 and 15.12)
      1. Hard or waxy discrete exudates are collections of serum and glial–neuronal breakdown products located predominantly in the outer plexiform (Henle) layer.

> One of the earliest changes in the neural retina in diabetic patients, often before BDR is evident clinically, is a breakdown of the blood–neural retinal barrier in the retinal capillaries. Fluorescein angiography and vitreous fluorophotometry can show "leakage" of fluorescein from retinal capillaries in diabetic patients who do not show signs of DR when examined by conventional clinical methods. In patients who have BDR, elevated serum lipids are associated with an increased risk of retinal hard exudates.

   2. The discrete exudates are removed by macrophages in 4 to 6 months; it may take a year or more if the exudates are confluent.
   3. When they are distributed around the fovea, hard exudates may form a macular "star."

> Although macular edema is common in diabetic patients, macular star formation is uncommon, unlike in grades III and IV hypertensive retinopathy, where a macular star is quite common.

B. Macular edema
   1. *Clinically significant macular edema* (CSME) is the greatest single cause of vision impairment in diabetic patients.
      a. The overall incidence of CSME is approximately 3% to 8% in the diabetic population after 4 years' follow-up from the baseline examination.
      b. The greater incidence is associated with younger age or more severe DR at the baseline examination, increased levels of glycosylated hemoglobin, increased duration of the diabetes, and an absence of posterior vitreous detachment.
      c. Systemic factors that can contribute to CSME in diabetes include poor metabolic control of the diabetes, elevated blood pressure, intravascular fluid overload, anemia, and hyperlipidemia. Fluid overload is relative, and may reflect decreased serum oncotic pressure, such as from decreased serum albumin.
   2. Morphologic evidence suggests that macular edema may be caused by functional damage to the retinal vascular endothelium (e.g., hypertrophy or liquefaction necrosis of endothelial cells of the retinal capillaries or venules; see Fig. 15.11); pericyte degeneration probably also plays a role.
      a. Fluid leaks out of the retinal vessels, enters Müller cells, and causes intracellular swelling.
      b. Mild to moderate amounts of intracellular fluid collections in Müller cells may result in macular edema (Fig. 15.14), a reversible process.
      c. Excessive swelling (ballooning) and rupture or death of Müller cells produces pockets of fluid and cell debris (i.e., cystoid macular edema), a process that may be irreversible.
      d. Adjacent neurons undergo similar changes secondarily.
      e. Intravitreal steroid injections hold promise for the treatment of CSME. The success of this therapy supports the possibility that inflammatory mechanisms may play a significant contributory role in the development of CSME. Nevertheless, other mechanisms are probably also pathogenic in CSME because vitrectomy with internal limiting membrane peeling can be an effective treatment.
   1. Support for hypoxia as a causative or contributing factor in the pathogenesis of CSME is found in the fact that supplemental inspired oxygen can improve DME.
   2. The presence of a cilioretinal artery may worsen DME.
C. Microcystoid degeneration of the neural retinal macula (see Fig. 15.14)

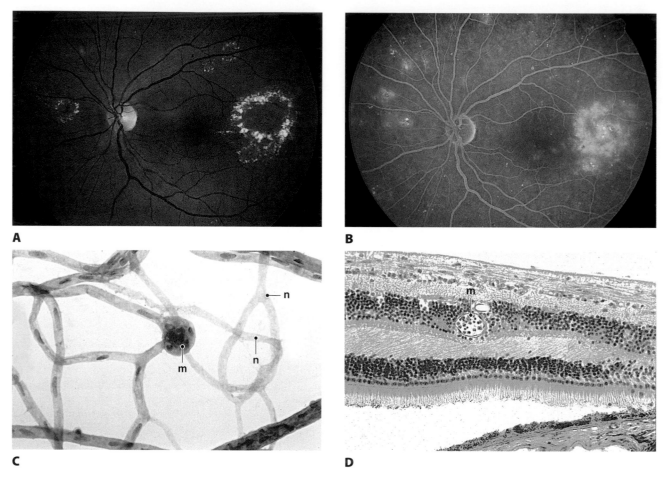

Fig. 15.9 Background diabetic retinopathy. **A,** Background diabetic retinopathy consists of retinal capillary microaneurysms (RCMs), hemorrhages, edema, and exudates (here in a circinate pattern). **B,** The RCMs are seen more easily with fluorescein. The areas of circinate retinopathy show leakage (see also Figs 15.12 and 15.13). **C,** Trypsin digest preparation shows that an RCM consists of a proliferation of endothelial cells (n, nonviable capillaries; m, microaneurysm). **D,** A histologic section shows a large blood-filled space lined by endothelium (m, microaneurysm). The caliber is approximately that of a venule. Venules, however, do not occur in this location (in the inner nuclear layer), but are mainly found in the nerve fiber layer. By a process of elimination, the "vessel" is therefore identified as a cross-section of an RCM. (**A** and **B,** Courtesy of Dr. GE Lang.)

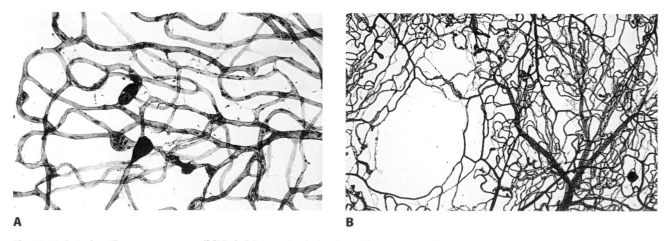

Fig. 15.10 Retinal capillary microaneurysm (RCM). **A,** RCMs randomly distributed between arterioles and venules. "Young" RCMs appear as saccular capillary outpouchings that contain a few proliferated endothelial cells. "Older" RCMs appear as larger sacs that contain numerous endothelial cells and increased periodic acid–Schiff (PAS) positivity (increased basement membrane deposition). "Oldest" RCMs appear as solid black balls with their lumina obliterated by PAS-positive material. **B,** Foveomacular area shows "broken" foveal capillary ring and scattered microaneurysms.

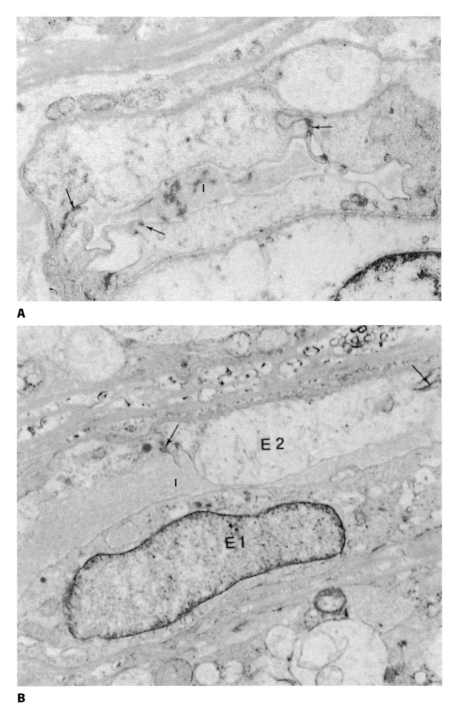

Fig. 15.11 Diabetic retinal vessels. **A,** Diabetic retinal capillary in nerve fiber layer of macula. Lumen (l) is exceedingly narrow and contains small amount of fibrinous, proteinaceous material. Endothelial cell junctional attachments (adherentes) present (*arrows*). Basement membrane of capillary wall is thickened. **B,** Small retinal vessel from foveomacular ganglion cell layer of diabetic patient. Lower endothelial cell (E1) hypertrophic, whereas upper endothelial cell (E2) necrotic (liquefaction). Vessel lumen (l) greatly narrowed. Adherentes of cell junctions present (*arrows*). Secondarily (age-related) vacuolated basement membrane of vessel wall probably normal thickness for age.

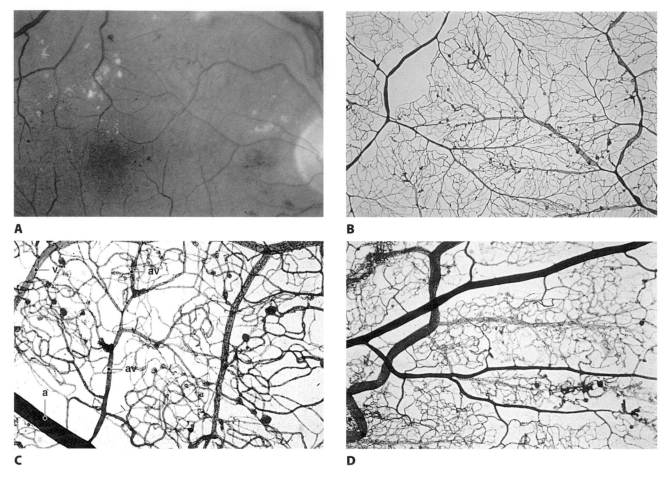

A

B

C

D

Fig. 15.12 Background and preproliferative diabetic retinopathy. **A,** Cotton-wool spot of recent onset is present just inferior to the superior arcade. Note also retinal "hard" exudates, capillary microaneurysms, and hemorrhages. **B,** Trypsin digest preparation shows sausage-shaped dilated venules. **C,** Arteriolovenular collateral vessel (av) is present (a, arteriole; v, venule). **D,** Intraretinal microvascular abnormalities are present in the form of dilated capillaries, capillary buds and loops, and areas of capillary closure.

1. Exudates or edema fluid, or both, may cause pressure atrophy of the neural retina or enlargement of the intercellular spaces, and result in microcystoid degeneration, especially in the macular area.
2. Microcystoid neural retinal degeneration may progress to macular retinoschisis (cyst), and even partial (inner layer of schisis) or complete macular hole formation.

D. "Soft" exudates or "cotton-wool" spots (see Figs 11.9, 11.11, 11.14, and 15.12)
   1. The cotton-wool spot observed clinically is a result of a microinfarct (coagulative necrosis) of the nerve fiber layer of the retina and is not a true exudate.
   2. They are present most commonly in the preproliferative or early part of the proliferative stage of DR, especially during a phase of rapid progression.
   3. Cotton-wool spots are formed at the edges of microinfarcts of the nerve fiber layer of the neural retina (see p. 404 in Chapter 11) and represent back-up of axoplasmic flow.
   4. Cytoid bodies are the characteristic histologic counterpart of the cotton-wool spot, and are caused by the swollen ends of ruptured axons in the nerve fiber layer in the infarcted area.
   5. Cotton-wool spots usually disappear from view in weeks to months.

V. Hemorrhagic retinopathy (Fig. 15.15). The clinical appearance of a retinal hemorrhage is determined by the microanatomy of the retinal layer in which the hemorrhage is located.
   A. Dot-and-blot hemorrhages
      1. Dot-and-blot hemorrhages are relatively small hemorrhages located in the inner nuclear layer that spread to the outer plexiform layer of the neural retina.
      2. In three-dimensional view, they appear serpiginous.
   B. Splinter (flame-shaped) hemorrhages are small hemorrhages located in the nerve fiber layer.
   C. Globular hemorrhages are caused by the spread of dot-and-blot hemorrhages in the middle neural retinal layers.
   D. Confluent hemorrhages are large and involve all of the neural retinal layers.
   E. Massive hemorrhages may break through the internal limiting membrane to extend beneath or into the

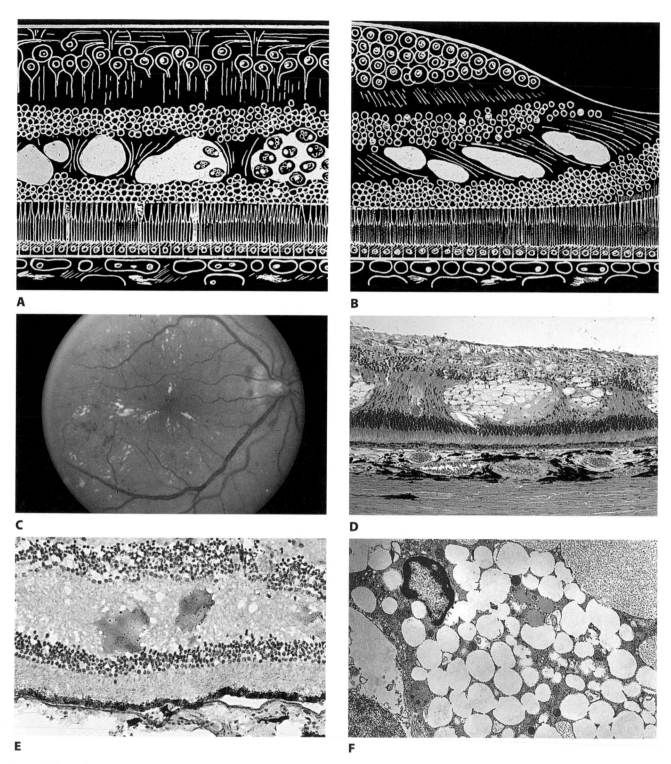

Fig. 15.13 Exudates. **A,** Diagram shows exudates predominantly in outer plexiform (Henle fiber) layer of macula. Exudates on right contain fat-filled (lipidic) histiocytes (gitter cells). **B,** Diagram shows exudates in outer plexiform layer (Henle fiber layer) of fovea. In foveal area, fibers run obliquely, resulting in clinically seen star figure. **C,** Fundus appearance of exudates, small hemorrhages, microaneurysms, and early neovascularization of temporal disc. Note star figure in fovea, an unusual finding in diabetic patients. **D,** Histologic section shows exudates present in outer plexiform layer. **E,** Oil red-O stain shows lipid-positivity of exudates. **F,** Electron microscopy shows exudates filled with foamy (lipidic) histiocytes. (**A** and **B,** Modified from drawings by Dr. RC Eagle, Jr.)

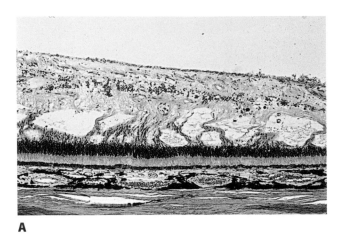

A

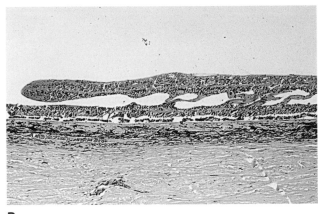

B

Fig. 15.14 Exudates. Microcystoid or macrocystoid (retinoschisis) macular degeneration may occur as a result of exudation. **A,** Small exudates can coalesce into larger ones. **B,** Eventually, coalescence of exudates can result in a macrocyst (macular retinoschisis), as occurred here. Note hole (smooth edge shows it is not an artifact) in inner wall of macrocyst.

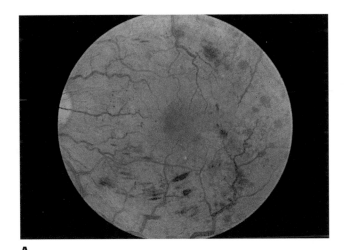

A

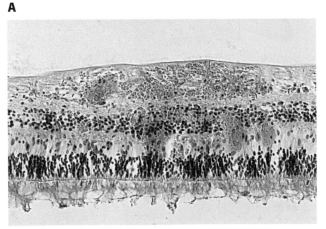

B

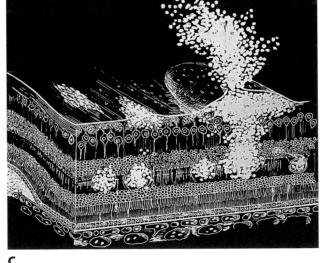

C

Fig. 15.15 Hemorrhagic retinopathy. **A,** Dot, blot, flame-shaped, and globular hemorrhages are present in the neural retina. **B,** Flame-shaped or splinter hemorrhages consist of small collections of blood in the nerve fiber layer. Dot-and-blot hemorrhages are caused by small hemorrhagic collections in the inner nuclear and outer plexiform layers. **C,** Diagram shows dot-and-blot and globular hemorrhages in middle layers, and splinter hemorrhage in nerve fiber layer of neural retina. Large hemorrhage under internal limiting membrane (submembranous intraneural retinal hemorrhage) has broken through neural retina into the vitreous compartment. (**C,** Modified from a drawing by Dr. RC Eagle Jr.)

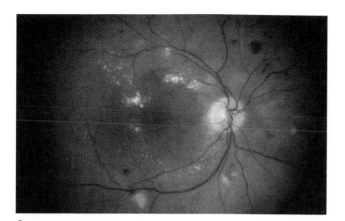

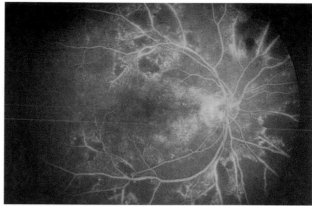

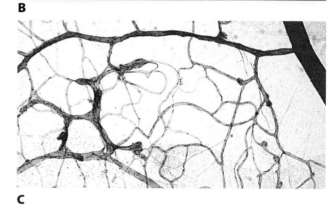

Fig. 15.16 Preproliferative retinopathy. Fundus (**A**) and fluorescein (**B**) appearance. Note numerous areas of nonperfusion. **C,** Trypsin digest of neural retina shows mainly nonviable capillaries. Some capillaries on left demonstrate endothelial cell proliferation and increased basement membrane deposition, representing intraretinal microvascular angiopathy. (**A** and **B,** Courtesy of Dr. GE Lang.)

vitreous body or, rarely, into the subneural retinal space.

F. Larger hemorrhages (i.e., globular and confluent) may herald the onset of the proliferative (malignant) phase of the disease.

VI. Preproliferative retinopathy (Fig. 15.16; see also 15.12) consists of:

A. Increased neural retinal hemorrhages

B. Cotton-wool spots

C. Venous dilatation

D. Venous beading

E. Intraretinal microangiopathy

VII. PDR ("malignant" stage; Figs 15.17 to 15.20)

A. Classically, PDR has been characterized as a vascular response to a hypoxic neural retinal environment. Recently, numerous factors have been cited as contributing to its pathobiology.

1. Some of these factors include hyperglycemia, retinal arteriolar and capillary closure; hemodynamic alterations in retrobulbar circulation and microcirculation; retinal capillary basement membrane alterations; immunogenic mechanisms related to insulin; pregnancy; absence of female hormones; altered plasma proteins that cause platelet and red cell aggregation; increased blood viscosity; altered ability of the blood to transport oxygen; virus induction of DM; and abnormal metabolic pathways in the retinal capillaries.

Development of anemia in a diabetic patient may cause background retinopathy to progress rapidly to PDR.

---

a. An adequate number of functioning photoreceptors appears to be required for the development of proliferative retinopathy because neonatal mice with hereditary retinal degeneration fail to develop reactive retinal neovascularization in a model of oxygen-induced proliferative retinopathy.

2. Table 15.3 (p. 617) lists some of the myriad vitreous and serum factors that are altered in PDR. They may be produced, in part, by retinal cellular elements, and in turn, probably help modify the behavior of these cellular retinal constituents.

3. Among the mediators acting during the development of PDR, vascular endothelial growth factor (VEGF) plays a key role.

VEGF is strongly expressed in the endothelial cells of the new blood vessels in fibrovascular membranes removed at vitrectomy for PDR. Conversely, pigment epithelium-derived factor (PEDF), which inhibits angiogenesis, is only weakly expressed in such membranes. VEGF levels are increased in the aqueous humor of diabetic patients, but PEDF levels are decreased in such individuals, particularly those with PDR. Moreover, lowered PEDF levels in aqueous

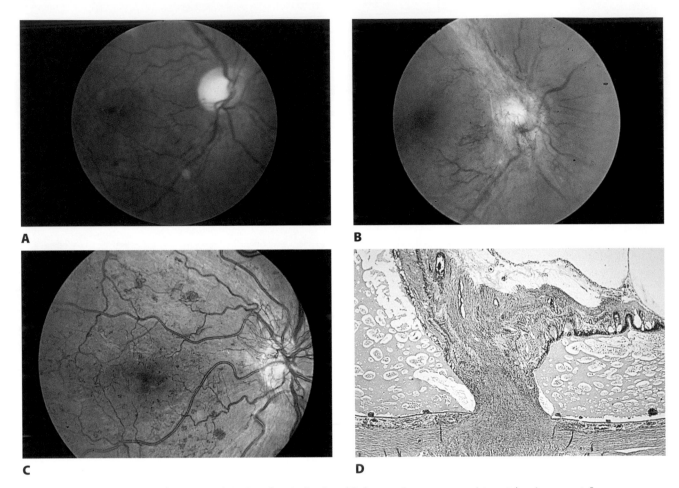

Fig. 15.17 Proliferative retinopathy. Neovascularization of optic disc. **A** and **B,** Same patient, same eye, pictures taken 1 year apart. Severe neovascularization of optic disc has developed. **C,** Moderate to severe neovascularization of optic disc. **D,** Histologic section of another case shows shrinkage and contracture of a preretinal fibroglial vascular membrane that had arisen from the optic disc and caused a total neural retinal detachment with fixed folds of the internal limiting membrane (see also Fig. 15.20D). Intraretinal cystic spaces are often present in long-standing detachments.

humor of diabetic patients strongly predicts those who will have progressive retinopathy. In a similar manner, levels of VEGF and endostatin, which is an inhibitor of angiogenesis, in aqueous humor and vitreous vary appropriately to reflect the severity of DR.

___

a. The VEGF family of growth factors utilizes several receptors that are selectively expressed in homeostasis and in disease. VEGF receptors (VEGFR)-2, -3, and -A may be particularly important in the development and progression of DR. Other contributing factors may be changes in the ratio of VEGF isoforms, and its interactions with various cellular regulators and factors.

b. Although the relationship between VEGF and PDR is well established, VEGF levels may also be elevated in other retinal disorders such as retinal detachment and proliferative vitreoretinopathy in nondiabetic patients.

4. Other factors that may contribute to the development of PDR that have been proposed, but still are speculative, include aldose reductase inhibition, nonenzymatic glycation (glycosylation) of proteins, dysproteinemia, basic or acidic fibroblastic growth factors, and the adhesion receptor integrin $\alpha_v\beta_3$. Erythropoietin levels are significantly elevated in the vitreous of patients with PDR. Multiple other stimulatory and inhibitory relationships with VEGF seem to be elucidated on an almost daily basis.

5. It is important that the constituents of PDR membranes be compared to those resulting from other forms of intraocular proliferation in order to determine the characteristics of PDR. For example, pro-

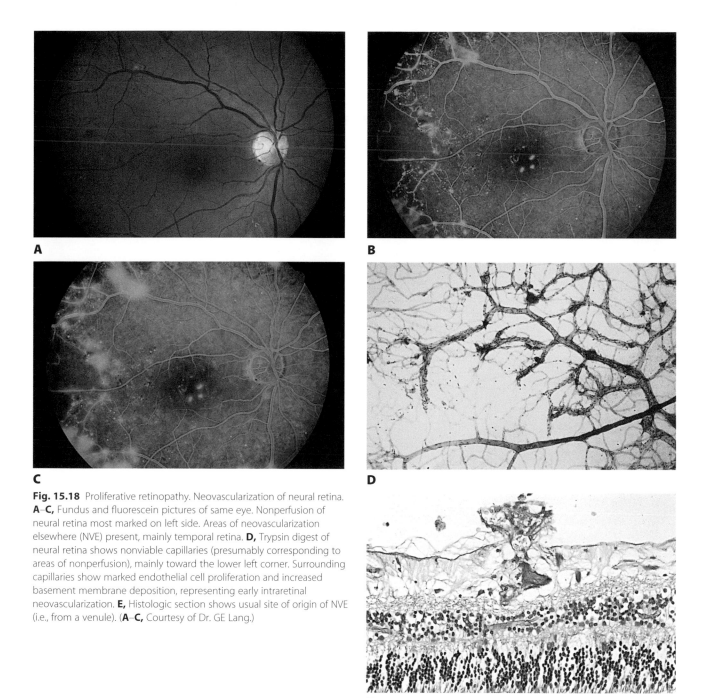

Fig. 15.18 Proliferative retinopathy. Neovascularization of neural retina. **A–C,** Fundus and fluorescein pictures of same eye. Nonperfusion of neural retina most marked on left side. Areas of neovascularization elsewhere (NVE) present, mainly temporal retina. **D,** Trypsin digest of neural retina shows nonviable capillaries (presumably corresponding to areas of nonperfusion), mainly toward the lower left corner. Surrounding capillaries show marked endothelial cell proliferation and increased basement membrane deposition, representing early intraretinal neovascularization. **E,** Histologic section shows usual site of origin of NVE (i.e., from a venule). (**A–C,** Courtesy of Dr. GE Lang.)

teolytic activation appears to be involved in extracellular matrix production in PDR and in nondiabetic membranes.

a. Neovascular membranes in retinopathy of prematurity are associated with the glucose transporter GLUT1, which is lacking in proliferative retinopathy.

6. Decreased serum insulin and high glucose levels have been postulated to contribute to decreased fibroblast growth factor-2 production in the RPE and increased glial cell activation in the diabetic retina.

7. PEDF may help protect against pericyte apoptosis. It is suppressed by angiotensin II, which may contribute to exacerbation of DR in hypertensive patients. Conversely, blockade of the renin–angiotensin system can confer retinal protection in experimental models of DR.

8. Elevated expression of matrix metalloproteinases in the diabetic retina may contribute to increased vascular permeability by a mechanism involving proteolytic degradation of the tight junction protein occludin and subsequent disruption of the tight junction complex.

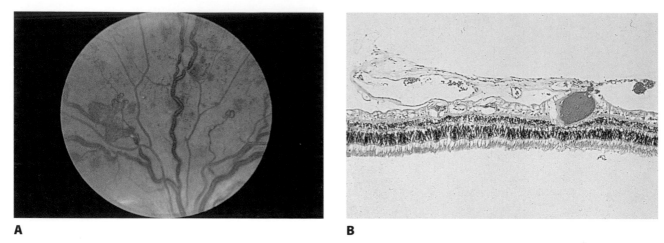

A   **B**

Fig. 15.19 Proliferative retinopathy. Neovascularization of neural retina. **A,** The superior venule is dilated and beaded. Neovascular tufts arise from the venules. **B,** A histologic section of another case shows new blood vessel arising from a retinal venule, perforating the internal limiting membrane, and spreading out on the internal surface of the retina between the internal limiting membrane and the vitreous body. In this location, the fragile new abnormal blood vessels may be subject to trauma (e.g., vitreous detachment), resulting in a subvitreal hemorrhage between the retinal internal limiting membrane and the posterior hyaloid of the separated vitreous body.

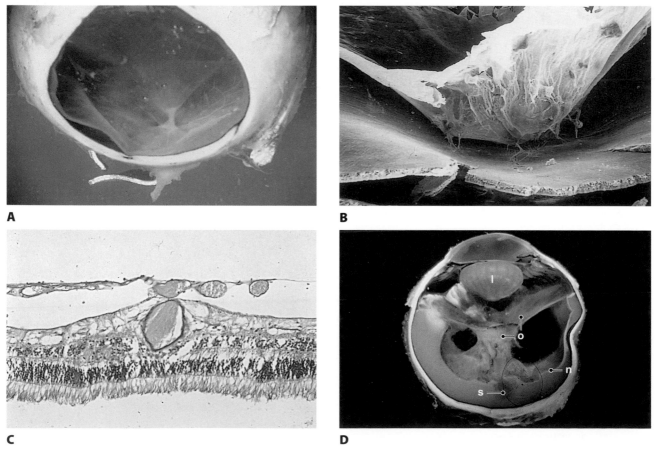

A   **B**

C   **D**

Fig. 15.20 Proliferative retinopathy. Neovascularization of optic disc and retina. **A,** Tuft of neovascularization arising from the optic nerve head is attached to the posterior surface of an otherwise detached vitreous body. **B,** Scanning electron micrograph shows blood vessels arising from the internal surface of the neural retina and attaching to the posterior surface of the partially detached vitreous. **C,** Periodic acid–Schiff-stained histologic section shows blood vessels originating from a retinal venule and attaching to the posterior surface of the vitreous. **D,** The gross specimen shows the end stage of diabetic retinopathy. Extensive neovascularization of the retina and the detached vitreous have resulted in a traction neural retinal detachment. The subneural retinal space is filled with a gelatinous material (l, lens; o, organized vitreous; n, neural retina; s, subneural retinal exudate). (**B,** Courtesy of Dr. RC Eagle, Jr.) The absence of similar material underlying a retinal detachment in any fixed specimen should raise the suspicion that the detachment is an artifact of sectioning and was not present *in vivo*.

TABLE 15.3 Vitreous and Serum Factors Altered in Human Proliferative Diabetic Retinopathy

Increased in vitreous and/or retina	**PROANGIOGENIC** Peptide growth factors: VEGF, HGF, FGF5, leptin, IGF1, IGF2, PDGFAB, SDF1, angiogenin Extracellular matrix adhesion molecules, ICAM1, oncofetal fibronectin Inflammatory cytokines: Il-6, IL-8, endothelin-1, TNF-α, TGF-β_1, AGEs Complement: complement C94) fragment Polyamines: spermine, spermidine Vasoactive peptides: endothelin-1, angiopoietin-2, angiotensin-2, adrenomedullin, ACE, nitrate Inflammatory cells: CD4 and CD8 (T lymphocytes), CD22 (B lymphocytes), macrophages, HLA-DR
Increased in vitreous and/or retina	**ANTIANGIOGENIC** Endostatin, angiostatin, PEDF, TGF-β_1 Undefined retinal function: α_1-antitrypsin, α_2-HS glycoprotein
Decreased in vitreous and/or retina	Angiopoietin-2, putrescine, kallistatin, chymase, TGF-β_2 activation, CD55, CD59
No change in vitreous and/or retina	ACE, C1q and C4
Increased in serum	NO, IL-2R, IL-8, TNF-α, VEGF, angiotensin-2, renin, endothelin
Decreased in serum	Soluble angiopoietin receptor Tie2, IL-1β, IL-6

(From: Gariano RF, Gardner TW. Retinal angiogenesis in development and disease. Nature 438:960, 2005.)
ACE, angiotensin-converting enzyme; AGE, advanced glycation end-products; FGF, fibroblast growth factor; HGF, hepatocyte growth factor (scatter factor); HLA, human leukocyte antigen; ICAM, intercellular adhesion molecule; IGF, insulin-like growth factor; IL, interleukin; NO, nitric oxide; PDGF, platelet-derived growth factor; PEDF, pigment epithelium-derived factor; SDF1, stromal-derived factor 1; sIL-2R, soluble interleukin-2 receptor; TGF-α_1, transforming growth factor α_1; TNF-β, tumor necrosis factor-β; VEGF, vascular endothelial growth factor.

9. The NH$_2$-terminal connective tissue growth factor fragment is increased in the vitreous in PDR and is found within myofibroblasts in active PDR membranes, suggesting a local paracrine mechanism for the induction of fibrosis and neovascularization.

10. Circulating systemic factors cannot be ignored. For example, growth hormone–sufficient diabetic patients have an increased prevalence of DR over growth hormone–deficient diabetic patients. Somatostatin analogs that block the local and systemic production of insulin-like growth factor and growth hormone may prevent DR progression to the proliferative stage.

a). Pregnant women are at particular risk for the development and progression of DR.

11. The new retinal vessels (neovascularization) in PDR tend to arise from retinal venules, usually at the edge of an area of capillary nonperfusion. Rarely, they may arise from retinal arterioles.

12. The new retinal vessels contain both endothelial cells and pericytes.

    a. Neovascular membranes that lie flat on the internal surface of the neural retina are called *epiretinal neovascular membranes.*

    b. Elevated neovascular membranes are called *preretinal neovascular membranes.*

B. The neovascularization, which is initially intraretinal, usually breaks through the internal limiting membrane, and lies between it and the vitreous. Endothelial cell-associated proteinases can locally disrupt basement membrane (internal limiting membrane) and facilitate angiogenesis.

Vitreous shrinkage (i.e., detachment) may tear the new vessels, leading to a hemorrhage. If a subvitreal hemorrhage results (the common type of diabetic "vitreous" hemorrhage between the posterior surface of the vitreous body and the internal limiting membrane of the neural retina), it clears rapidly in weeks to a few months. If a hemorrhage extending into the formed vitreous (vitreous framework) results, it may take from many months to years to clear. In such patients, vitrectomy may be indicated.

C. Pure neovascularization is eventually accompanied by a fibrous and glial (Müller cells and fibrous astrocytes) component; it is then called *retinitis proliferans.*

1. The membranes are composed of blood vessels, fibrous and glial matrix tissue, fibroblasts, glial cells, scattered B and T lymphocytes, and monocytes, along with immunoglobulin, complement deposits, and class II major histocompatibility complex antigens.

2. Shrinkage of the fibroglial component often leads to a neural retinal detachment, which is usually nonrhegmatogenous (i.e., without a neural retinal tear or hole).

3. Ultimately, the whole process of PDR tends to "burn out" and become quiescent.

D. Fewer than 40% of patients who have PDR, even if they are not blind, survive 10 years; fewer than 25% of diabetic blind patients survive 10 years.

E. Cataract surgery and progression of DR (see earlier in this chapter under section *Lens*)

VIII. Proposed international clinical DR (diabetic retinopathy) and DME (diabetic macular edema) severity scales*

A. DR severity scale

1. No apparent retinopathy (no abnormalities)

2. Mild nonproliferative DR (microaneurysms only)

Modified from Wilkinson CP, Ferris FL, Klein RE et al.: Proposed international clinical diabetic retinopathy and diabetic macular edema disease severity scales. Ophthalmology 110:1677, 2003.

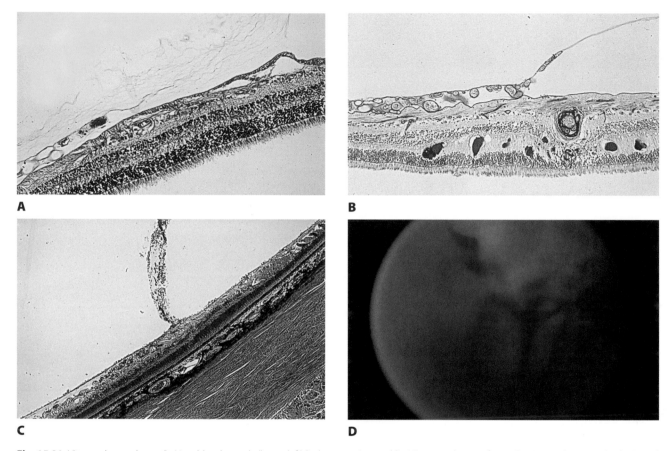

Fig. 15.21 Vitreous hemorrhage. **A,** New blood vessels (lower left) lie between internal limiting membrane of neural retina and vitreous body. Partial detachment of vitreous (upper right) has caused traction on neural retina. **B,** If no further detachment of the vitreous occurs, vessels may grow on to the posterior surface of the detached vitreous. **C,** With further vitreous detachment, the fragile new vessels can break, resulting in hemorrhage into the vitreous compartment (**D**).

3. Moderate nonproliferative DR (more than just microaneurysms but less than severe nonproliferative DR)
4. Severe nonproliferative DR (any of the following: greater than 20 intraretinal hemorrhages in each of four quadrants; definite venous beading in 2+ quadrants; prominent intraretinal microvascular abnormalities in 1+ quadrants)
5. PDR (neovascularization or vitreous/preretinal hemorrhage, or both)

B. DME severity scale
1. DME apparently absent
2. DME apparently present
   a. Mild DME (some retinal thickening or hard exudates in posterior pole but distant from center of macula)
   b. Moderate DME (retinal thickening or hard exudates approaching center of macula but not involving center)
   c. Severe DME (retinal thickening or hard exudates involving center of macula)

VITREOUS

I. Vitreous detachment (Fig. 15.21; see also Figs 12.8 and 12.9)

A. Vitreous detachment ("contracture") is more common in diabetic patients than in nondiabetic subjects and seems to occur at an earlier age.

B. The proliferating fibroglial vascular tissue from the optic nerve head or neural retina usually grows between the vitreous and the neural retina (i.e., along the inner surface of the internal limiting membrane of the neural retina), along the external surface of a detached vitreous, or into Cloquet's canal. The proliferating tissue does not grow directly into a formed vitreous. A preoptic disc canal-like structure, probably Cloquet's canal and the area of Martegiani, is associated with PDR.

In eyes with diffuse DME associated with vitreomacular traction and a thickened premacular cortical vitreous, ultrastructural examination demonstrates native vitreous collagen with single

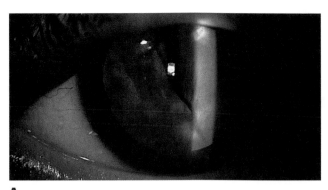

A

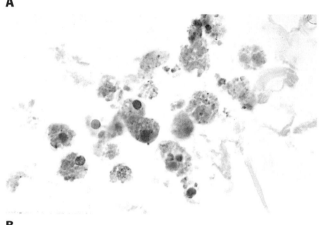

B

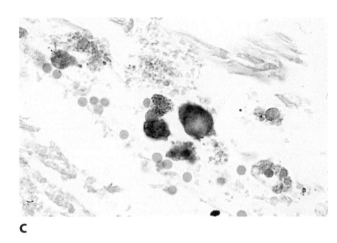

C

Fig. 15.22 Vitreous hemorrhage. **A,** Clinical appearance of vitreous hemorrhage. **B,** Hemosiderin-laden macrophages and red blood cells present in vitreous compartment. **C,** Macrophages stain positive for hemosiderin (blue) with iron stain, but red blood cells do not.

cells interspersed within the collagenous layer or a cellular monolayer. Eyes with tangential vitreomacular traction exhibit multilayered membranes on a layer of native vitreous collagen. The predominant cell types are fibroblasts and fibrous astrocytes, with some myofibroblasts and macrophages. Thus, the vitreomacular interface is characterized by a layer of native vitreous collagen and a varying cellular component in eyes with diffuse DME.

II. Hemorrhage into vitreous compartment (Fig. 15.22; see Fig. 15.21)
   A. A hemorrhage into the subvitreal space is more common than into the vitreous body.

> Vitreous hemorrhage does not seem to be related to activity. In fact, approximately 60% of vitreous hemorrhages follow sleep or resting. This fact may be related to an increased neural retinal blood flow that normally occurs in the dark (at night).

   B. Organization of the hemorrhage with fibroglial overgrowth may occur, usually along the external surface of the detached vitreous.
III. Asteroid hyalosis—some studies show a correlation between asteroid hyalosis and diabetes; others do not. If diabetes is correlated with asteroid hyalosis, it is probably a very weak correlation (see pp. 486–487 in Chapter 12).

OPTIC NERVE

I. Neovascularization (see Fig. 15.17)—the optic disc is a site of predilection for neovascularization, which often grows into Cloquet's canal.
II. Ischemic (nonarteritic) optic neuropathy
   A. Retrobulbar neuritis, papillitis, optic disc edema, and optic atrophy, all occurring infrequently, may be ischemic manifestations of diabetic microangiopathy in the optic nerve head when collateral circulation is inadequate.
   B. Transient bilateral optic disc edema and minimal impairment of function (diabetic papillopathy) may develop in patients with juvenile-onset diabetes.
      1. DR may be quite mild in those patients.
      2. The condition usually resolves without treatment.
      3. It should not be confused with neovascularization of the disc or central nervous system-induced papilledema.

4. It may also be found in older type II diabetics. DR and macular edema may be associated with it.

Diabetic papillopathy may rarely be associated with a rapidly progressive optic disc neovascularization. Transient optic disc edema secondary to vitreous traction in a quiescent eye with PDR may mimic diabetic papillopathy. The development of bilateral nonarteritic anterior ischemic optic neuropathy from diabetic papillopathy has been reported.

III. Central retinal vein occlusion (see pp. 406 and 407 in Chapter 11)
IV. Based on animal studies, diabetes is a risk factor for glaucomatous optic neuropathy. Diabetes is also among the risk factors for optic disc hemorrhages in glaucoma. Nerve fiber layer is decreased, particularly in the superior segment of the retina, in diabetic patients even before the development of clinical retinopathy. Nerve fiber layer thickness further decreases with the development of DR and with impairment of metabolic regulation. This finding may impact the evaluation of nerve fiber layer in glaucomatous diabetic patients.

BIBLIOGRAPHY

Natural History

Andresen AR, Christiansen JS, Jenson JK: Diagonal ear-lobe crease and diabetic retinal angiopathy (letter). *N Engl J Med* 294:1182, 1976

Canataroglu H, Varinli I, Ozcan AA et al.: Interleukin (IL)-6, interleukin (IL)-8 levels and cellular composition of the vitreous humor in proliferative diabetic retinopathy, proliferative vitreoretinopathy, and traumatic proliferative vitreoretinopathy. *Ocul Immunol Inflamm* 13:375, 2005

Chase HP, Garg SK, Jackson WE et al.: Blood pressure and retinopathy in type 1 diabetes. *Ophthalmology* 97:155, 1990

Davis MD, Hiller R, Magli YL et al.: Prognosis for life in patients with diabetes: relation to severity of retinopathy. *Trans Am Ophthalmol Soc* 77:144, 1979

Diabetes Control and Complications Trial Research Group: Early worsening of diabetic retinopathy in the Diabetes Control and Complications Trial. *Ophthalmology* 116:874, 1998

Dielemans I, deJong PTVM, Stolk R et al.: Primary open-angle glaucoma, intraocular pressure, and diabetes mellitus in the general population: The Rotterdam Study. *Ophthalmology* 103:1271, 1996

Goldstein DE, Blinder KJ, Ide CH et al.: Glycemic control and development of retinopathy in youth-onset insulin-dependent diabetes mellitus. *Ophthalmology* 100:1125, 1993

Guery B, Choukroun G, Noel LH et al.: The spectrum of systemic involvement in adults presenting with renal lesion and mitochondrial tRNA(Leu) gene mutation. *J Am Soc Nephrol* 14:2099, 2003

Ido Y, Vindigni A, Chang K et al.: Prevention of vascular and neural dysfunction in diabetic rats by C-peptide. *Science* 277:563, 1997

Klein R, Klein BEK, Moss SE et al.: The Wisconsin Epidemiologic Study of Diabetic Retinopathy: XIV. Ten-year incidence and progression of diabetic retinopathy. *Arch Ophthalmol* 112:1217, 1994

Klein R, Klein BEK, Moss SE et al.: The Wisconsin Epidemiologic Study of Diabetic Retinopathy: XV. The long-year incidence of macular edema. *Ophthalmology* 102:7, 1995

Klein R, Klein BEK, Moss SE et al.: The Wisconsin Epidemiologic Study of Diabetic Retinopathy: XVII. The 14-year incidence and progression of diabetic retinopathy and associated risk factors in type 1 diabetes. *Ophthalmology* 105:1801, 1998

Klein R, Meuer SM, Moss SE et al.: Retinal microaneurysm counts and progression of diabetic retinopathy. *Arch Ophthalmol* 113:1386, 1995

Klein R, Meuer SM, Moss SE et al.: Incidence of retinopathy and associated risk factors from time of diagnosis of insulin-dependent diabetes. *Arch Ophthalmol* 115:351, 1997

Klein R, Sharrett AR, Klein BE et al.: The association of atherosclerosis, vascular risk factors, and retinopathy in adults with diabetes: the atherosclerosis risk in communities study. *Ophthalmology* 109:1225, 2002

Leal EC, Santiago AR, Ambrosio AF: Old and new drug targets in diabetic retinopathy: from biochemical changes to inflammation and neurodegeneration. *Curr Drug Targets CNS Neurol Disord* 4:421, 2005

Lonneville YH, Ozdek SC, Onol M et al.: The effect of blood glucose regulation on retinal nerve fiber layer thickness in diabetic patients. *Ophthalmologica* 217:347, 2003

Marshall G, Garg SK, Jackson WE et al.: Factors influencing the onset and progression of diabetic retinopathy in subjects with insulin-dependent diabetes mellitus. *Ophthalmology* 100:1133, 1993

Miceli MV, Newsome DA: Cultured retinal pigment cells from donors with type I diabetes show an altered insulin response. *Invest Ophthalmol Vis Sci* 32:2847, 1991

Mitchell P, Smith W, Chey T et al.: Open-angle glaucoma and diabetes: The Blue Mountain Eye Study, Australia. *Ophthalmology* 104:712, 1997

Mohan R, Rajendran B, Mohan V et al.: Retinopathy in tropical pancreatic diabetes. *Arch Ophthalmol* 103:1487, 1985

Moss SE, Klein R, Klein BEK: Ten-year incidence of visual loss in a diabetic population. *Ophthalmology* 101:1061, 1994

Moss SE, Klein R, Meuer MB et al.: The association of iris color with eye disease in diabetes. *Ophthalmology* 94:1226, 1987

Sacks DA, McDonald JM: The pathogenesis of type II diabetes mellitus: A polygenic disease. *Am J Clin Pathol* 105:149, 1996

van de Enden M, Nyengaard JR, Ostrow E et al.: Elevated glucose levels increase retinal glycolysis and sorbitol pathway metabolism: Implications for diabetic retinopathy. *Invest Ophthalmol Vis Sci* 36:1675, 1995

Van Leiden HA, Dekker JM, Moll AC, et al: Risk factors for incident retinopathy in a diabetic and nondiabetic population. *Arch Ophthalmol* 121:245, 2003

Wong TY, Klein R, Islam FM et al.: Diabetic retinopathy in a multi-ethnic cohort in the United States. *Am J Ophthalmol* 141:446, 2006

Conjunctiva and Cornea

Arnarsson A, Jonasson F, Sasaki H et al.: Risk factors for nuclear lens opacification: the Reykjavik Eye Study. *Dev Ophthalmol* 35:12, 2002

Azar DT, Spurr-Michaud SJ, Tisdale AS et al.: Decreased penetration of anchoring fibrils into the diabetic stroma. *Arch Ophthalmol* 107:1520, 1989

Brandt JD, Beiser JA, Kass MA et al.: Central corneal thickness in the Ocular Hypertension Treatment Study (OHTS). *Ophthalmology* 108:1779, 2001

Cheung AT, Price AR, Duong PL et al.: Microvascular abnormalities in pediatric diabetic patients. *Microvasc Res* 63:252, 2002

Cheung AT, Ramanujam S, Greer DA *et al.*: Microvascular abnormalities in the bulbar conjunctiva of patients with type 2 diabetes mellitus. *Endocr Pract* 7:358, 2001

Fujishima H, Tsubota K: Improvement of corneal fluorescein staining in post cataract surgery of diabetic patients by an oral aldose reductase inhibitor, ONO-2235. *Br J Ophthalmol* 86:860, 2002

Hiraoka M, Amano S, Oshika T *et al.*: Factors contributing to corneal complications after vitrectomy in diabetic patients. *Jpn J Ophthalmol* 45:492, 2001

Inoue K, Kato S, Ohara C *et al.*: Ocular and systemic factors relevant to diabetic keratoepitheliopathy. *Cornea* 20:798, 2001

Jacques PF, Moeller SM, Hankinson SE *et al.*: Weight status, abdominal adiposity, diabetes, and early age-related lens opacities. *Am J Clin Nutr* 78:400, 2003

Kallinikos P, Berhanu M, O'Donnell C *et al.*: Corneal nerve tortuosity in diabetic patients with neuropathy. *Invest Ophthalmol Vis Sci* 45:418, 2004

Keoleian GM, Pach JM, Hodge DO *et al.*: Structural and functional studies of the corneal endothelium in diabetes mellitus. *Am J Ophthalmol* 113:64, 1992

Larson L-I, Bourne WM, Pach JM *et al.*: Structure and function of the corneal endothelium in diabetes mellitus type I and type II. *Arch Ophthalmol* 114:9, 1996

Lee JS, Lee JE, Choi HY *et al.*: Corneal endothelial cell change after phacoemulsification relative to the severity of diabetic retinopathy. *J Cataract Refract Surg* 31:742, 2005

Leske MC, Wu SY, Nemesure B *et al.*: Risk factors for incident nuclear opacities. *Ophthalmology* 109:1303, 2002

Malik RA, Kallinikos P, Abbott CA *et al.*: Corneal confocal microscopy: a non-invasive surrogate of nerve fibre damage and repair in diabetic patients. *Diabetologia* 46:683, 2003

Morikubo S, Takamura Y, Kubo E *et al.*: Corneal changes after small-incision cataract surgery in patients with diabetes mellitus. *Arch Ophthalmol* 122:966, 2004

Okamura N, Ito Y, Shibata MA *et al.*: Fas-mediated apoptosis in human lens epithelial cells of cataracts associated with diabetic retinopathy. *Med Electron Microsc* 35:234, 2002

Price MO, Thompson RW Jr, Price FW Jr: Risk factors for various causes of failure in initial corneal grafts. *Arch Ophthalmol* 121:1087, 2003

Sani JS, Mittal S: In vivo assessment of corneal endothelial function in diabetes mellitus. *Arch Ophthalmol* 114:649, 1996

Schultz RO, van Horn DL, Peters MA *et al.*: Diabetic keratopathy. *Trans Am Ophthalmol Soc* 74:180, 1981

Shetlar DJ, Bourne WM, Campbell RJ: Morphologic evaluation of Descemet's membrane and corneal endothelium in diabetes mellitus. *Ophthalmology* 96:247, 1989

Siribunkum J, Kosrirukvongs P, Singalavanija A: Corneal abnormalities in diabetes. *J Med Assoc Thai* 84:1075, 2001

Taylor HR, Kimsey RA: Corneal epithelial basement membrane changes in diabetes. *Invest Ophthalmol* 20:548, 1981

Yoon KC, Im SK, Seo MS: Changes of tear film and ocular surface in diabetes mellitus. *Korean J Ophthalmol* 18:168, 2004

Lens

Barber AJ: A new view of diabetic retinopathy: a neurodegenerative disease of the eye. *Prog Neuropsychopharmacol Biol Psychiatry* 27:283, 2003

Biswas S, Harris F, Singh J *et al.*: Role of calpains in diabetes mellitus-induced cataractogenesis: a mini review. *Mol Cell Biochem* 261:151, 2004

Chung SS, Chung SK: Genetic analysis of aldose reductase in diabetic complications. *Curr Med Chem* 10:1375, 2003

Cunliffe IA, Flanagan DW, George NDL *et al.*: Extracapsular cataract surgery with lens implantation in diabetics with and without proliferative retinopathy. *Br J Ophthalmol* 75:9, 1991

Datiles MB, Kador PF: Type I diabetic cataract. *Arch Ophthalmol* 117:284, 1999

Freel CD, al-Ghoul KJ, Kuszak JR *et al.*: Analysis of nuclear fiber cell compaction in transparent and cataractous diabetic human lenses by scanning electron microscopy. *BMC Ophthalmol* 3:1, 2003

Gardner TW, Antonetti DA, Barber AJ *et al.*: Diabetic retinopathy: more than meets the eye. *Surv Ophthalmol* 47 (Suppl. 2):S253, 2002

Hayashi K, Hayashi H, Nakao F *et al.*: Posterior capsule opacification after cataract surgery in patients with diabetes mellitus. *Am J Ophthalmol* 134:10, 2002

Jaffe GJ, Burton TC, Kuhn E *et al.*: Progression of nonproliferative diabetic retinopathy and visual outcome after extracapsular cataract extraction and intraocular lens implantation. *Am J Ophthalmol* 114:448, 1992

Klein BEK, Klein R, Moss SE: Prevalence of cataracts in a population-based study of persons with diabetes mellitus. *Ophthalmology* 92:1191, 1985

Lopes de Faria JM, Katsumi O, Cagliero E *et al.*: Neurovisual abnormalities preceding the retinopathy in patients with long-term type 1 diabetes mellitus. *Graefes Arch Clin Exp Ophthalmol* 239:643, 2001

Lorenzi M, Gerhardinger C: Early cellular and molecular changes induced by diabetes in the retina. *Diabetologia* 44:791, 2001

Pollack A, Dotan S, Oliver M: Course of diabetic retinopathy following cataract surgery. *Br J Ophthalmol* 75:2, 1991

Santiago AP, Rosenbaum AL, Masket S: Insulin-dependent diabetes mellitus appearing as bilateral mature diabetic cataracts in a child. *Arch Ophthalmol* 115:422, 1997

Schatz H, Atienza D, McDonald HR *et al.*: Severe diabetic retinopathy after cataract surgery. *Am J Ophthalmol* 117:314, 1994

Smith R: Diabetic retinopathy and cataract surgery. *Br J Ophthalmol* 75:1, 1991

Yanoff M: Ocular pathology of diabetes mellitus. *Am J Ophthalmol* 67:21, 1969

Iris

Aiello LM, Wand M, Liang G: Neovascular glaucoma and vitreous hemorrhage following cataract surgery in patients with diabetes mellitus. *Ophthalmology* 90:814, 1983

Fine BS, Berkow JW, Helfgott JA: Diabetic lacy vacuolation of iris pigment epithelium. *Am J Ophthalmol* 69:197, 1970

Smith ME, Glickman P: Diabetic vacuolation of the iris pigment epithelium. *Am J Ophthalmol* 79:875, 1975

Yanoff M: Ocular pathology of diabetes mellitus. *Am J Ophthalmol* 67:21, 1969

Yanoff M, Fine BS, Berkow JW: Diabetic lacy vacuolation of iris pigment epithelium. *Am J Ophthalmol* 69:201, 1970

Ciliary Body and Choroid

Cao J, McCeod DS, Merges CA *et al.*: Choriocapillaris degeneration and related pathologic changes in human diabetic eyes. *Arch Ophthalmol* 116:589, 1998

Fryczkowski AW, Sato SE, Hodes BL: Changes in the diabetic choroidal vasculature: Scanning electron microscopy findings. *Ann Ophthalmol* 20:299, 1988

Hidayat AA, Fine BS: Diabetic choroidopathy: Light and electron microscopic observations of seven cases. *Ophthalmology* 92:512, 1985

Rothova A, Meenken C, Michels RPJ *et al.*: Uveitis and diabetes mellitus. *Am J Ophthalmol* 106:17, 1988

Yanoff M: Ocular pathology of diabetes mellitus. *Am J Ophthalmol* 67:21, 1969

Retina

Adamis AP, Miller JW, Bernal M-T *et al.*: Increased vascular endothelial growth factor levels in the vitreous of eyes with proliferative diabetic retinopathy. *Am J Ophthalmol* 118:445, 1994

Aguilar E, Friedlander MF, Gariano RF *et al.*: Endothelial proliferation in diabetic retinal aneurysms. *Arch Ophthalmol* 121:740, 2003

Aiello LP, Northrup JM, Keyt BA *et al.*: Hypoxic regulation of vascular endothelial growth factor in retinal cells. *Arch Ophthalmol* 113:1538, 1995

Alzaid AA, Dinneen SF, Melton LJ III *et al.*: The role of growth hormone in the development of diabetic retinopathy. *Diabetes Care* 17:531, 1994

Ambati J, Chalam KV, Chawla DK *et al.*: Elevated γ-aminobutyric acid, glutamate, and vascular endothelial growth factor levels in the vitreous of patients with proliferative diabetic retinopathy. *Arch Ophthalmol* 115:1161, 1997

Ashton N: Vascular basement membrane changes in diabetic retinopathy. *Br J Ophthalmol* 58:344, 1974

Ballantyne AJ, Lowenstein A: Diseases of the retina: I. The pathology of diabetic retinopathy. *Trans Ophthalmol Soc UK* 63:95, 1943

Baudouin C, Gordon WC, Fredj-Reygrobellet D *et al.*: Class II antigen expression in diabetic preretinal membranes. *Am J Ophthalmol* 109:70, 1990

Bek T: A clinicopathological study of venous loops and reduplications in diabetic retinopathy. *Acta Ophthalmol Scand* 80:69, 2002

Bengtsson B, Heijl A, Agardh E: Visual fields correlate better than visual acuity to severity of diabetic retinopathy. *Diabetologia* 48:2494, 2005

Bloodworth JMB Jr: Diabetic microangiopathy. *Diabetes* 12:99, 1963

Boehm BO, Lang G, Feldmann B *et al.*: Proliferative diabetic retinopathy is associated with a low level of the natural ocular anti-angiogenic agent pigment epithelium-derived factor (PEDF) in aqueous humor. a pilot study. *Horm Metab Res* 35:382, 2003

Boehm BO, Lang G, Volpert O *et al.*: Low content of the natural ocular anti-angiogenic agent pigment epithelium-derived factor (PEDF) in aqueous humor predicts progression of diabetic retinopathy. *Diabetologia* 46:394, 2003

Bronson SK, Reiter CE, Gardner TW: An eye on insulin. *J Clin Invest* 111:1817, 2003

Brooks PC, Clark RAF, Cheresh DA: Requirement of vascular integrin for angiogenesis. *Science* 264:569, 1994

bu-El-Asrar AM, Dralands L, Missotten L *et al.*: Expression of apoptosis markers in the retinas of human subjects with diabetes. *Invest Ophthalmol Vis Sci* 45:2760, 2004

Chen YJ, Kuo HK, Huang HW: Retinal outcomes in proliferative diabetic retinopathy presenting during and after pregnancy. *Chang Gung Med J* 27:678, 2004

Chew EY, Klein ML, Ferris FL *et al.*: Association of elevated serum lipid levels with retinal hard exudate in diabetic retinopathy: Early Treatment Diabetic Retinopathy Study (ETDRS) report 22. *Arch Ophthalmol* 114:1079, 1996

Clermont AC, Aiello LP, Mori F *et al.*: Vascular endothelial growth factor and severity of nonproliferative diabetic retinopathy mediate retinal hemodynamics in vivo: A potential role for vascular endothelial growth factor in the progression of nonproliferative diabetic retinopathy. *Am J Ophthalmol* 124:433, 1997

Cogan DG, Toussaint D, Kuwabara T: Retinal vascular patterns: IV. Diabetic retinopathy. *Arch Ophthalmol* 66:366, 1961

Cussick M, Chew EY, Chan C-C *et al.*: Histopathology and regression of retinal hard exudates in diabetic retinopathy after reduction of elevated serum lipid levels. *Ophthalmology* 110:2126, 2003

Daria B, Maiello M, Lorenzi M: Increased incidence of micro thrombosis in retinal capillaries of diabetic individuals. *Diabetes* 50:1432, 2002

Diabetes Control and Complications Trial Research Group: Early worsening of diabetic retinopathy in the diabetes control and complications trial. *Ophthalmology* 116:874, 1998

Economopoulou M, Bdeir K, Cines DB *et al.*: Inhibition of pathologic retinal neovascularization by alpha-defensins. *Blood* 106:3831, 2005

Frank RN: On the pathogenesis of diabetic retinopathy: A 1990 update. *Ophthalmology* 98:586, 1991

Frank RN: Diabetic retinopathy. *N Engl J Med* 350:48, 2004

Fritsche P, van der HR, Suttorp-Schulten MS *et al.*: Retinal thickness analysis (RTA): an objective method to assess and quantify the retinal thickness in healthy controls and in diabetics without diabetic retinopathy. *Retina* 22:768, 2002

Funatsu H, Yamashita H, Noma H *et al.*: Stimulation and inhibition of angiogenesis in diabetic retinopathy. *Jpn J Ophthalmol* 45:577, 2001

Gargiulo P, Giusti C, Pietrobono D *et al.*: Diabetes mellitus and retinopathy. *Dig Liver Dis* 36(Suppl. 1):S101, 2004

Gariano RF, Gardner TW: Retinal angiogenesis in development and disease. *Nature* 438:960, 2005

Giebel SJ, Menicucci G, McGuire PG *et al.*: Matrix metalloproteinases in early diabetic retinopathy and their role in alteration of the blood–retinal barrier. *Lab Invest* 85:597, 2005

Goebel W, Kretzchmar-Gross T: Retinal thickness in diabetic retinopathy: a study using optical coherence tomography (OCT). *Retina* 22:759, 2002

Güven D, O*P4zdemir H, Hasanreisoglu B: Hemodynamic alterations in diabetic retinopathy. *Ophthalmology* 103:1245, 1996

Hammes HP, Du X, Edelstein D *et al.*: Benfotiamine blocks three major pathways of hyperglycemic damage and prevents experimental diabetic retinopathy. *Nat Med* 9:294, 2003

Hanneken A, de Juan E Jr, Lutty GA *et al.*: Altered distribution of basic fibroblast growth factor in diabetic retinopathy. *Arch Ophthalmol* 109:1005, 1991

Helbig H, Kornacker S, Berweck S *et al.*: Membrane potentials in retinal capillary pericytes: Excitability and effect of vasoactive substances. *Invest Ophthalmol Vis Sci* 33:2105, 1992

Hellstedt T, Immonen I: Disappearance and formation rates of microaneurysms in early diabetic retinopathy. *Br J Ophthalmol* 80:135, 1996

Hersh PS, Green WR, Thomas JV: Tractional venous loops in diabetic retinopathy. *Am J Ophthalmol* 92:661, 1981

Hinton DR, Spee C, He S *et al.*: Accumulation of NH2-terminal fragment of connective tissue growth factor in the vitreous of patients with proliferative diabetic retinopathy. *Diabetes Care* 27:758, 2004

Hussain A, Hussain N, Nutheti R: Comparison of mean macular thickness using optical coherence tomography and visual acuity in diabetic retinopathy. *Clin Exp Ophthalmol* 33:240, 2005

Ioachim E, Stefaniotou M, Gorezis S *et al.*: Immunohistochemical study of extracellular matrix components in epiretinal membranes of vitreoproliferative retinopathy and proliferative diabetic retinopathy. *Eur J Ophthalmol* 15:384, 2005

Kador PF, Akagi Y, Takahashi Y *et al.*: Prevention of retinal vessel changes associated with diabetic retinopathy in galactose-fed dogs by aldose reductase inhibitors. *Arch Ophthalmol* 108:1301, 1990

Karacorlu M, Ozdemir H, Karacorlu S *et al.*: Intravitreal triamcinolone as a primary therapy in diabetic macular oedema. *Eye* 19:382, 2005

Klein R, Klein BEK, Moss SE *et al.*: Retinal vascular abnormalities in persons with type 1 diabetes: The Wisconsin Epidemiologic Study of diabetic retinopathy: XVIII. *Ophthalmology* 110:2118, 2003

Klein R, Meuer SM, Moss SE *et al.*: The relationship of retinal micro-aneurysm counts to the 4-year progression of diabetic retinopathy. *Arch Ophthalmol* 107:1780, 1989

Klein R, Meuer SM, Moss SE *et al.*: Retinal microaneurysm counts and progression of diabetic retinopathy. *Arch Ophthalmol* 113:1386, 1995

Klein R, Moss SE, Klein BEK *et al.*: The Wisconsin Epidemiologic Study of Diabetic Retinopathy: XI. The incidence of macular edema. *Ophthalmology* 96:1501, 1989

Knudsen LL, Lervang HH: Can a cilio-retinal artery influence diabetic maculopathy? *Br J Ophthalmol* 86:1252, 2002

Kuhn F, Kiss G, Mester V *et al.*: Vitrectomy with internal limiting membrane removal for clinically significant macular oedema. *Graefes Arch Clin Exp Ophthalmol* 242:402, 2004

Lahdenranta J, Pasqualini R, Schlingemann RO *et al.*: An anti-angiogenic state in mice and humans with retinal photoreceptor cell degeneration. *Proc Natl Acad Sci U S A* 98:10368, 2001

Layton CJ, Becker S, Osborne NN: The effect of insulin and glucose levels on retinal glial cell activation and pigment epithelium-derived fibroblast growth factor-2. *Mol Vis* 12:43, 2006

Lee VS, Kingsley RM, Lee ET *et al.*: The diagnosis of diabetic retinopathy. *Ophthalmology* 100:1504, 1993

Leto G, Pricci F, Amadio L *et al.*: Increased retinal endothelial cell monolayer permeability induced by the diabetic milieu: role of advanced non-enzymatic glycation and polyol pathway activation. *Diabetes Metab Res Rev* 17:448, 2001

Li W, Liu X, Yanoff M *et al.*: Cultured retinal capillary pericytes die by apoptosis after an abrupt fluctuation from high to low glucose levels: A comparative study with retinal capillary endothelial cells. *Diabetologia* 39:537, 1996

Li W, Tao L, Yanoff M: Agonist-induced phosphatidylinositide breakdown and mitogenesis in retinal capillary pericytes. *Ophthalmic Res* 26:36, 1994

Li W, Tao L, Zhan Y *et al.*: Inhibitory effect of glucose on activation of phospholipase C by guanine nucleotide in retinal capillary pericytes. *Exp Eye Res* (*in press*)

Lindahl P, Johansson BR, Levéen P *et al.*: Pericyte loss and microaneurysm formation in PDGF-B-deficient mice. *Science* 277:242, 1997

Ljubimov AV, Caballero S, Aoki A *et al.*: Involvement of protein kinase CK2 in angiogenesis and retinal neovascularization. *Invest Ophthalm Vis Sci* 45:4583, 2004

Lobo CL, Bernardes RC, de A Jr *et al.*: One-year follow-up of blood–retinal barrier and retinal thickness alterations in patients with type 2 diabetes mellitus and mild nonproliferative retinopathy. *Arch Ophthalmol* 119:1469, 2001

Lyons TJ, Jenkins AJ, Zhen D *et al.*: Diabetic retinopathy and serum lipoprotein subclasses in the DCCT/EDIC cohort. *Invest Ophthalmol Vis Sci* 45:910, 2004

Mansour AM, Schachat A, Bodiford G *et al.*: Foveal avascular zone in diabetes mellitus. *Retina* 13:125, 1993

Massin P, Audren F, Haouchine B *et al.*: Intravitreal triamcinolone acetonide for diabetic diffuse macular edema: preliminary results of a prospective controlled trial. *Ophthalmology* 111:218, 2004

Matsuoka M, Ogata N, Minamino K *et al.*: Expression of pigment epithelium-derived factor and vascular endothelial growth factor in fibrovascular membranes from patients with proliferative diabetic retinopathy. *Jpn J Ophthalmol* 50:116, 2006

McFarland TJ, Zhang Y, Appukuttan B *et al.*: Gene therapy for proliferative ocular diseases. *Expert Opin Biol Ther* 4:1053, 2004

Nagaoka T, Kitaya N, Sugawara R *et al.*: Alteration of choroidal circulation in the foveal region in patients with type 2 diabetes. *Br J Ophthalmol* 88:1060, 2004

Nguyen QD, Shah SM, Van AE *et al.*: Supplemental oxygen improves diabetic macular edema: a pilot study. *Invest Ophthalmol Vis Sci* 45:617, 2004

Nicoletti VG, Nicoletti R, Ferrara N *et al.*: Diabetic patients and retinal proliferation: an evaluation of the role of vascular endothelial growth factor (VEGF). *Exp Clin Endocrinol Diabetes* 111:209, 2003

Nishiwaki H, Shahidi M, Vitale S *et al.*: Relation between retinal thickening and clinically visible fundus pathologies in mild nonproliferative diabetic retinopathy. *Ophthalmic Surg Lasers* 33:127, 2002

Noma H, Funatsu H, Yamashita H *et al.*: Regulation of angiogenesis in diabetic retinopathy: possible balance between vascular endothelial growth factor and endostatin. *Arch Ophthalmol* 120:1075, 2002

North PE, Anthony DC, Young TL *et al.*: Retinal neovascular markers in retinopathy of prematurity: aetiological implications. *Br J Ophthalmol* 87:275, 2003

Perrin RM, Konopatskaya O, Qiu Y *et al.*: Diabetic retinopathy is associated with a switch in splicing from anti- to pro-angiogenic isoforms of vascular endothelial growth factor. *Diabetologia* 48:2422, 2005

Poulaki V, Joussen AM, Mitsiades N *et al.*: Insulin-like growth factor-I plays a pathogenetic role in diabetic retinopathy. *Am J Pathol* 165:457, 2004

Romeo G, Liu WH, Asnaghi V *et al.*: Activation of nuclear factor-kappaB induced by diabetes and high glucose regulates a proapoptotic program in retinal pericytes. *Diabetes* 51:2241, 2002

Roy S, Cagliero E, Lorenzi M: Fibronectin overexpression in retinal microvessels of patients with diabetes. *Invest Ophthalmol Vis Sci* 37:258, 1996

Savage HI, Hendrix JW, Peterson DC *et al.*: Differences in pulsatile ocular blood flow among three classifications of diabetic retinopathy. *Invest Ophthalmol Vis Sci* 45:4504, 2004

Schneeberger SA, Hjelmeland LM, Tucker RP *et al.*: Vascular endothelial growth factor and fibroblastic growth factor 5 are colonized in vascular and avascular epiretinal membranes. *Am J Ophthalmol* 124:433, 1997

Schröder S, Palinski W, Schmid-Schönbein GW: Activated monocytes and granulocytes, capillary nonperfusion, and neovascularization in diabetic retinopathy. *Am J Pathol* 139:81, 1991

Sennlaub F, Valamanesh F, Vazquez-Tello A *et al.*: Cyclooxygenase-2 in human and experimental ischemic proliferative retinopathy. *Circulation* 108:198, 2003

Sinclair SH: Macular retinal capillary hemodynamics in diabetic patients. *Ophthalmology* 98:1580, 1991

Siren V, Immonen I: uPA, tPA and PAI-1 mRNA expression in periretinal membranes. *Curr Eye Res* 27:261, 2003

Sonkin PL, Sinclair SH, Hatchell DL: The effect of pentoxifylline on retinal capillary blood flow velocity and whole blood velocity. *Am J Ophthalmol* 115:775, 1993

Stitt AW, Frizzell N, Thorpe SR: Advanced glycation and advanced lipoxidation: possible role in initiation and progression of diabetic retinopathy. *Curr Pharm Des* 10:3349, 2004

Sugimoto M, Sasoh M, Ido M *et al.*: Detection of early diabetic change with optical coherence tomography in type 2 diabetes mellitus patients without retinopathy. *Ophthalmologica* 219:379, 2005

Tang J, Mohr S, Du YD *et al.*: Non-uniform distribution of lesions and biochemical abnormalities within the retina of diabetic humans. *Curr Eye Res* 27:7, 2003

Vinores SA, Gadegbeku C, Compochiaro PA *et al.*: Immuno histochemic localization of blood–retinal barrier breakdown in human diabetes. *Am J Pathol* 134:231, 1989

Vitale S, Maguire MG, Murphy RP *et al.*: Clinically significant macular edema in type I diabetes. *Ophthalmology* 102:1170, 1995

Vlassara H, Palace MR: Diabetes and advanced glycation endproducts. *J Intern Med* 251:87, 2002

Watanabe D, Suzuma K, Matsui S *et al.*: Erythropoietin as a retinal angiogenic factor in proliferative diabetic retinopathy. *N Engl J Med* 353:782, 2005

Wilkinson CP, Ferris FL, Klein RE *et al.*: Proposed international clinical diabetic retinopathy and diabetic macular edema disease severity scales. *Ophthalmology* 110:1677, 2003

Wilkinson-Berka JL: Angiotensin and diabetic retinopathy. *Int J Biochem Cell Biol* 38:752, 2006

Witmer AN, Blaauwgeers HG, Weich HA *et al.*: Altered expression patterns of VEGF receptors in human diabetic retina and in experimental VEGF-induced retinopathy in monkey. *Invest Ophthalmol Vis Sci* 43:849, 2002

Yamagishi S, Matsui T, Nakamura K *et al.*: Pigment epithelium-derived factor is a pericyte mitogen secreted by microvascular endothelial cells: possible participation of angiotensin II-elicited PEDF downregulation in diabetic retinopathy. *Int J Tissue React* 27:197, 2005

Yanoff M: Diabetic retinopathy. *N Engl J Med* 274:1344, 1966

Yanoff M: Ocular pathology of diabetes mellitus. *Am J Ophthalmol* 67:21, 1969

Yanoff M: Histopathogenesis of diabetic retinopathy. *Acta Diabetol Lat* 9:527, 1972

Vitreous

Anderson B Jr: Activity and diabetic vitreous hemorrhages. *Ophthalmology* 87:173, 1980

Bergren RL, Brown GC, Duker JS: Prevalence and association of asteroid hyalosis with systemic disease. *Am J Ophthalmol* 111:289, 1991

Feke GT, Zuckerman R, Green GJ *et al.*: Response of human retinal blood flow to light and dark. *Invest Ophthalmol Vis Sci* 24:136, 1983

Foos RY, Kreiger AE, Forsythe AB *et al.*: Posterior vitreous detachment in diabetic subjects. *Ophthalmology* 87:122, 1980

Foos RY, Kreiger AE, Nofsinger K: Pathologic study following vitrectomy for proliferative diabetic retinopathy. *Retina* 5:101, 1985

Gandorfer A, Rohleder M, Grosselfinger S *et al.*: Epiretinal pathology of diffuse diabetic macular edema associated with vitreomacular traction. *Am J Ophthalmol* 139:638, 2005

Jerdan JA, Michels RG, Glaser BM: Diabetic preretinal membranes: An immunohistochemical study. *Arch Ophthalmol* 104:286, 1986

Luxenberg M, Sime D: Relationship of asteroid hyalosis to diabetes mellitus and plasma lipid levels. *Am J Ophthalmol* 67:406, 1969

Nasrallah FP, Jalkh AE, Van Coppenolle F *et al.*: The role of the vitreous in diabetic macular edema. *Ophthalmology* 95:1335, 1988

Roy MS, Podgor MJ, Bungay P *et al.*: Posterior vitreous fluorophotometry in diabetic patients with minimal or no retinopathy. *Retina* 7:170, 1987

Yamakiri K, Yamashita T, Miyazaki M *et al.*: Fibrous proliferation of the pre-papillary canal in proliferative diabetic retinopathy: Cloquet's canal as a scaffold for proliferative diabetic retinopathy. *Graefes Arch Clin Exp Ophthalmol* 243:204, 2005

Yanoff M: Ocular pathology of diabetes mellitus. *Am J Ophthalmol* 67:21, 1969

Optic Nerve

Appen RE, Chandra SR, Klein R *et al.*: Diabetic papillopathy. *Am J Ophthalmol* 90:203, 1980

Barr CC, Glaser JS, Blankenship G: Acute disc swelling in juvenile diabetes: Clinical profile and natural history of 12 cases. *Arch Ophthalmol* 98:2185, 1980

Bayraktar Z, Alacali N, Bayraktar S: Diabetic papillopathy in type II diabetic patients. *Retina* 22:752, 2002

Ho AC, Maguire AM, Fisher YL *et al.*: Rapidly progressive optic disc neovascularization after diabetic papillopathy. *Am J Ophthalmol* 120:673, 1995

Lopes de Faria JM, Russ H, Costa VP: Retinal nerve fibre layer loss in patients with type 1 diabetes mellitus without retinopathy. *Br J Ophthalmol* 86:725, 2002

Nakamura M, Kanamori A, Negi A: Diabetes mellitus as a risk factor for glaucomatous optic neuropathy. *Ophthalmologica* 219:1, 2005

Ozdek S, Lonneville YH, Onol M *et al.*: Assessment of nerve fiber layer in diabetic patients with scanning laser polarimetry. *Eye* 16:761, 2002

Pavan PR, Aiello LM, Wafai Z *et al.*: Optic disc edema in juvenile-onset diabetes. *Arch Ophthalmol* 98:2193, 1980

Regillo CD, Brown GC, Savino PJ *et al.*: Diabetic papillopathy: Patient characteristics and fundus findings. *Arch Ophthalmol* 113:889, 1995

Saito Y, Ueki N, Hamanaka N *et al.*: Transient optic disc edema by vitreous traction in a quiescent eye with proliferative diabetic retinopathy mimicking diabetic papillopathy. *Retina* 25:83, 2005

Sato T, Fujikado T, Hosohata J *et al.*: Development of bilateral, nonarteritic anterior ischemic optic neuropathy in an eye with diabetic papillopathy. *Jpn J Ophthalmol* 48:158, 2004

Soares AS, Artes PH, Andreou P *et al.*: Factors associated with optic disc hemorrhages in glaucoma. *Ophthalmology* 111:1653, 2004

Yassur Y, Pickle LW, Fine SL *et al.*: Optic disc neovascularisation in diabetic retinopathy: II. Natural history and results of photocoagulation treatment. *Br J Ophthalmol* 64:77, 1980

16

Glaucoma

NORMAL ANATOMY (Figs 16.1–16.3)

I. The outermost or corneoscleral layer of the eye can be separated into corneal and scleral portions by two circumferential grooves, a shallow outer one, the *outer scleral sulcus*, and a deeper inner one, the *inner scleral sulcus*.

A. The posterior boundary of the inner scleral sulcus is a ridge, mainly composed of circumferentially oriented bundles of collagen fibrils, the *scleral roll* or *Schwalbe's posterior-border ring*.

B. After continuing a short distance posteriorly, the ridge or roll tapers and finally blends with the more predominant, obliquely arranged collagenous lamellae of the sclera.

C. Deep within this inner sulcus and applied closely to the collagenous tissue of the corneosclera lies the large vessel called the *canal of Schlemm*.

1. This circumferentially arranged branching vessel is formed by a continuous layer of nonfenestrated endothelial cells with a rather patchy or diffuse basement membrane.

2. The structure of the canal of Schlemm closely resembles the structure of a lymphatic.

3. It is called an *aqueous vessel* because *in vivo* it contains aqueous fluid alone.

4. The outer wall of the canal also rests on a basement membrane that is separated from the dense collagenous lamellae of cornea and sclera by a few loose cells.

5. The inner wall rests on a thinner or patchy basement membrane that is associated with a zone of delicate connective tissue, the juxtacanalicular connective tissue.

a. The *juxtacanalicular connective tissue* is a special zone of the corneoscleral trabecular meshwork and consists of cells surrounded by a variety of fibrous and mucinous extracellular materials. The juxtacanalicular connective tissue is irregular in thickness from front to back in any single meridional section; it is more delicate in the younger eye and more prominent in the adult eye.

b. Examination of trabeculectomy specimens containing the external portion of the trabecular meshwork reveals severely decreased cellularity in glaucoma.

6. Pores are present in the wall of Schlemm's canal. Their role, if any, in regulating aqueous outflow has not been established.

7. It is probable that a history of previous glaucoma filtration surgery and long-term high intraocular pressure (IOP) are associated with shortening of Schlemm's canal.

8. Ultrastructural analysis of ocular basement membrane components fails to demonstrate significant differences between the characteristics of these structures in normal and glaucomatous eyes.

D. Large endothelium-lined channels (collector channels) connect the canal of Schlemm either anteriorly or, more commonly, posterior to the *intrascleral venous plexus* that drains both the canal of Schlemm and the longitudinal ciliary muscle.

If the collector channels reach the surface of the sclera unconnected, they can be observed in vivo as the clear aqueous veins (Ascher).

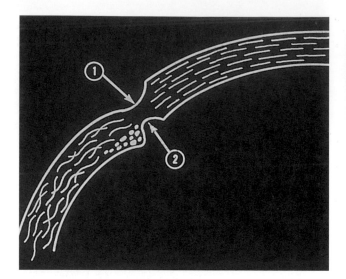

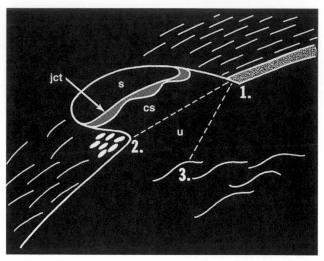

Fig. 16.1 Normal adult angle. Schematic representation of meridional section of corneoscleral coat. Circumferential shallow outer sulcus (1) and deeper, inner sulcus (2) are present in region of union of sclera with cornea. Posterior boundary of inner sulcus is thickened by scleral roll (posterior border ring of Schwalbe).

Fig. 16.2 Normal adult angle. The trabecular meshwork is a loose collagenous meshwork that fills the inner scleral sulcus and extends as an open fan to the root of the iris. The meshwork may be separated into two parts by an imaginary line extending from the end of Descemet's membrane (1) to the scleral roll (2). The meshwork lying external to the line and extending from cornea to sclera is known as the *corneoscleral* (cs) *meshwork*. The meshwork lying internal to the line and in continuity with the uveal tract posteriorly (3) is known as the *uveal* (u) *meshwork*. A third part, which rests on the inner wall of the canal of Schlemm (s), is a thin or patchy basement membrane associated with a zone of delicate connective tissue called the *juxtacanalicular connective tissue* (jct).

II. The trabecular meshwork

A. In meridional sections of a young eye, a loose collagenous meshwork can be seen filling the inner scleral sulcus and extending as an open fan to the root of the iris. The "handle" of this fan is located just anterior to the end of Descemet's membrane—Schwalbe's anterior-border ring—where a few layers of meshwork enter into and blend with the deep peripheral corneal stroma.

B. The meshwork may be easily and usefully separated into two parts by an imaginary line extending from the scleral roll to the end of Descemet's membrane (see Fig. 16.2).

    1. The meshwork lying external to the line and extending from cornea to sclera is known as the *corneoscleral meshwork*.

    2. The meshwork lying internal to the line and in continuity with the uveal tract posteriorly is known as the *uveal meshwork*.

C. A single trabecula of uveal meshwork consists of a collagenous core surrounded by a single layer of polarized cells ("endothelium"—in reality a mesothelium).

    1. A basement membrane separates the polarized endothelial cells from the underlying collagenous core and, not infrequently, patches of this basement membrane present a periodic structure (banded basement membrane) measuring 100 nm (1000 → A).

D. Lying within the tightly packed collagenous cores of the trabeculae are many aggregates of filamentous and homogenous elastic tissue whose density increases with age.

    1. The aggregates also take the stains for elastic tissue.

    2. As in other connective tissues, additional ground substance materials are probably present, but their identification and quantitation remain obscure.

E. The endothelial cells covering the connective tissue core have apical surfaces, line intertrabecular spaces, and therefore are bathed by aqueous.

F. The trabeculae of the meshwork are roughly arranged into circumferential sheets lying superimposed one on the other.

They can be fairly easily separated from one another mechanically, especially in the uveal meshwork. The spaces between adjacent sheets are called *intertrabecular spaces*. Large oval apertures traverse each trabecular sheet and may be called *transtrabecular spaces*. The transtrabecular apertures are not superimposed, and decrease in size in the direction of the corneoscleral meshwork. The corneoscleral sheets differ only slightly from the uveal in having somewhat flatter trabeculae as observed in cross-section and in lacking the staining characteristics for elastic fibers. The transtrabecular apertures here are more circular and smaller than those of the uveal meshwork. All intertrabecular and transtrabecular spaces thus may be considered extensions of the anterior chamber.

G. Spaces between individual sheets are well seen in proper meridional section, and here are termed the *intertrabecular spaces*.

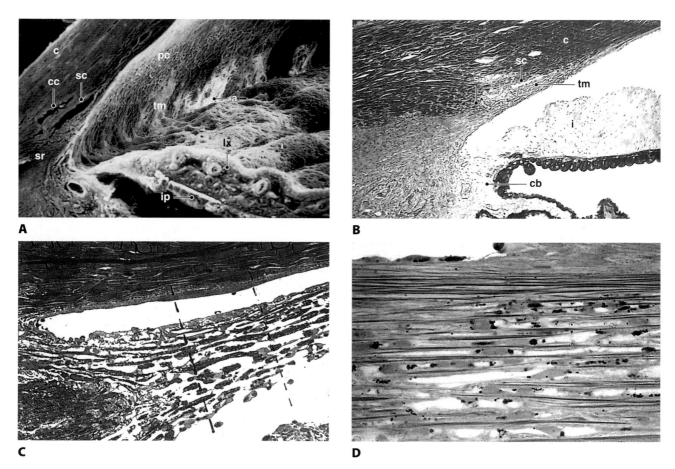

Fig. 16.3 Normal adult angle. **A,** Scanning electron microscopy shows the main aqueous drainage area [i.e., the angle (a) of the anterior chamber]. Aqueous drains through the trabecular meshwork (tm) into Schlemm's canal (sc), the collector channels (cc), and the aqueous veins, as well as into the uveal tract and out through the anterior ciliary and vortex veins. Some aqueous also drains into the iris and out through the iris vessels (c, cornea; pc, posterior surface of cornea; sr, scleral roll/spur; i, iris; ix, iris in cross-section; ip, iris pigment epithelium). **B,** In an adult, the scleral roll becomes thickened by compacting of the uveal meshwork to form the scleral spur (s), a bipartite structure. Between the scleral portion and the cornea lies the corneoscleral trabecular meshwork (tm). Just posterior lies the uveal trabecular meshwork and, just anterior, adjacent to Schlemm's canal (sc), lies the juxtacanalicular connective tissue (see Fig. 16.11A) (c, cornea; i, iris; cb, ciliary body). **C,** We usually view the transtrabecular and intertrabecular trabecular meshwork spaces meridionally. A section perpendicular to this plane, through the dotted lines, results in an anterior–posterior (coronal or frontal) view of the trabecular meshwork intertrabecular drainage spaces or canals, as seen in **D** (see Fig. 16.9A and C). (**A,** Courtesy of Dr. RC Eagle, Jr.)

In the uveal meshwork, the intertrabecular spaces pass the scleral roll to continue with the tissue spaces lying between the smooth-muscle cells of the ciliary muscles—especially those of the meridional (longitudinal) ciliary muscle. If serially sectioned in a frontal or coronal plane, the spaces can be seen as large-apertured, relatively straight, short tubes. Such a grouping of tubes with apertured walls might be termed a system of compound aqueous tubes. In the corneoscleral meshwork, which blends posteriorly with the region of the scleral roll, the intertrabecular spaces (tubes) abut the canalicular extensions of the canal of Schlemm. Such extensions are frequent in this region.

H. The blind inpouchings of the canal of Schlemm (canals of Sondermann), here termed *canaliculi*, are endothelium-lined, and do not appear to be in continuity with the intertrabecular spaces. Their function, presumably, is to drain off aqueous passing laterally along the corneoscleral trabecular meshwork (i.e., along the intertrabecular spaces).

I. The presence of adenylate cyclase subtypes II and IV in the human aqueous outflow pathway suggests that cholinergics may exert an effect on outflow facility, mediated by cyclic adenosine monophosphate (cAMP), that is independent of muscle contraction.

III. The roles of various genes in the development of the forms of glaucoma are beginning to be elucidated. Specific genes that may play such a role are *Bmp4*, *Cyp1b1*, *Foxc1*, *Foxc2*, *Pitx2*, *Lmx1b*, and *Tyr*. Similarly, specific gene products, such as growth factors, may be implicated in the development of glaucoma.

INTRODUCTION

Six genetic loci have been recognized to date (GLC1A–GLC1F) as contributing to glaucoma. A glaucoma-causing gene has been identified at two of these loci—GLC1A and GLC1E, and sequence variations in the optineurin (*OPTN*) gene on GLC1E have been found to be associated with the development of normal-tension glaucoma in at least nine separate families.

The E50K mutation in the optineurin gene is associated with increased severity of normal-tension glaucoma. There may be racial differences in glaucoma-associated optineurin genotypes.

In families with the GLC1A Gln368STOP mutation, age-related penetrance for ocular hypertension or primary open-angle glaucoma (POAG) was 72% at age 40 years, and 82% at age 65 years. In general, individuals with the mutation have an earlier age at onset, higher peak IOP, and are more likely to have undergone filtration surgery than nonmutation glaucoma patients.

I. Glaucoma is characterized by an IOP sufficient to produce ocular tissue damage, either transient or permanent.
   A. Glaucoma is a "family" of diseases having in common a type of optic atrophy called *optic nerve head cupping* or *excavation*.
      1. Various systemic abnormalities have been associated with glaucoma, including elevation of the 20S proteasome alpha-subunit of leukocytes.
      2. The appearance of the optic disc is an important diagnostic finding in glaucoma. The ratio of the optic cup : disc is moderately heritable.

A more appropriate name may be *glaucomatous optic neuropathy* because the primary defect, especially in chronic open-angle glaucoma, appears to be within the optic nerve head. High IOP (>25 mmHg), or the presence of glaucoma, is a marker for decreased life expectancy.

   B. Although most individuals associate glaucoma with an elevated IOP, the pressure may, in fact, be within the statistically "normal" range and still cause ocular tissue damage in *normal-tension* (improperly called *low-tension*) *glaucoma*.
      1. IOP is a risk factor for glaucoma, and the higher the pressure, the greater the probability of the development of the disorder.
         a. The accurate measurement of IOP is vital to the proper diagnosis and treatment of glaucoma.
         b. Central corneal thickness (CCT) impacts the validity of IOP measurements, particularly in the diagnosis of ocular hypertension. Thicker corneas, comprised of normal corneal tissue, produce an artificially high IOP measurement compared to manometrically measured "true" IOP. Conversely, corneas that are thinner than normal produce an inappropriately low pressure measurement. The impact of CCT on IOP measurement varies with the type of tonometer employed for the measurement. Refractive surgery can alter the validity of tonometry through several mechanisms, including change in corneal thickness and creating a fluid interface between the flap and the residual stroma. Corneal thickness also probably correlates with

glaucoma progression and visual field loss, although this relationship has been questioned.

Decreased CCT is present in normal-tension glaucoma and thinner than in POAG. Similarly, CCT is thinner in patients with vascular risk factors for glaucoma. Patients with congenital aniridia have CCT that is significantly thicker than normal. This abnormality is not secondary to corneal edema resulting from endothelial dysfunction.

         c. CCT is increased in children with ocular hypertension.
         d. There is considerable racial variation in CCT.
         e. Osteogenesis imperfecta may be associated with an abnormally thin CCT.
         f. Alterations in corneal thickness related to forkhead gene dosage can result in errors in IOP measurement. Increased CCT is associated with segmental gene duplication.
         g. In the past, individuals having thinner than normal corneas that have led to spuriously low IOP measurements have probably been included in the population said to have normal-pressure glaucoma. Conversely, some individuals with thicker than normal corneas that produced artificially elevated IOP measurements, but who had true IOP within the normal range, were probably included in the population classified as ocular hypertensives (see below).

Glaucoma, therefore, is not an IOP reading, it is a syndrome. In fact, the cause of the glaucoma may be due to factors (mostly poorly understood) other than IOP (i.e., IOP is simply one risk factor).

---

      2. Normal-tension glaucoma probably accounts for approximately one-third of all cases of POAG.

Disc hemorrhage is a significantly negative prognostic factor in normal-tension glaucoma.

---

      3. *OPA1* on chromosome 3 is the gene responsible for dominant optic atrophy. It encodes for a mitochondrial metabolic protein. Some cases of normal-tension glaucoma are associated with polymorphisms of the *OPA1* gene. This association raises the possibility that normal-tension glaucoma may result from mitochondrial dysfunction.
      4. Over 6% of patients with normal-tension glaucoma may have relevant intracranial compressive lesions. Such lesions are usually lacking in POAG.
      5. Predictive factors for progression of normal-tension glaucoma differ from those of POAG, possibly suggesting different pathobiologic mechanisms for these disorders.
      6. Plasma levels of the 20S proteasome alpha-subunit are significantly increased in glaucoma patients

compared to control patients, and is even more elevated in normal-tension glaucoma patients.

Papillorenal syndrome is associated with optic disc and visual field anomalies that may lead to an erroneous diagnosis of normal-tension glaucoma.

II. Glaucoma suspect
A. Increased IOP without detectable ocular tissue damage or visual functional impairment is called ocular hypertension. An individual who has some features of glaucoma, but in whom a definitive diagnosis has not yet been confirmed, is termed a *glaucoma suspect*.
B. Ocular hypertension may be tolerated by the person or, eventually, may lead to ocular tissue damage and hence to glaucoma.

The prevalence of glaucoma suspect is approximately 8%. The incidence of glaucoma among glaucoma suspects is approximately 1% per year.

III. Glaucoma is the leading cause of blindness among the 500 000 legally blind people in the United States—approximately 14% (1 in 7) of blind people.

The second leading cause of blindness is retinal disease (exclusive of diabetic retinopathy), mainly age-related macular degeneration, followed by cataract. Optic nerve disease is fourth; diabetic retinopathy, fifth; uveitis, sixth; and corneal and scleral disease, seventh. Leading causes of new cases of blindness, in order of importance, are macular degeneration, glaucoma, diabetic retinopathy, and cataract.

A. Glaucoma of all types affects approximately 0.5% to 1% of the general population, 2% of people age 35 years or older, and 3% of people age 65 years or older.
B. POAG accounts for approximately two-thirds of all glaucoma seen in white patients.
1. The prevalence of POAG in white patients ranges from approximately 0.9% in people 40 to 49 years of age to approximately 2.2% in those 80 years of age or older.
2. The prevalence of POAG in black patients ranges from approximately 1.2% in people 40 to 49 years of age to approximately 11.3% in those 80 years of age old or older.
3. The prevalence of POAG and ocular hypertension in adult Latinos ≥40 years is about 4.7% and 3.6%, respectively.
IV. Primary closed-angle glaucoma, which has a prevalence of less than 0.5%, is much less common in black patients than in white patients. A high percentage of black patients who develop angle closure, however, have chronic closed-angle glaucoma instead of the acute type.

The prevalence of primary closed-angle glaucoma is highest amongst Inuits (approximately 2% to 3%), followed by Asians (approximately 1%).

V. There is considerable racial variation in the incidence and prevalence of the various forms of glaucoma.

NORMAL OUTFLOW

Hypersecretion

I. Hypersecretion glaucoma is rare and has no antecedent cause.
II. Outflow facility is normal. The elevated IOP is presumed to be caused by an increased production of aqueous humor.
III. The glaucoma mainly affects middle-aged women, especially when they have neurogenic systemic hypertension.
IV. Histologically, the angle of the anterior chamber shows no abnormalities.

IMPAIRED OUTFLOW

Congenital Glaucoma

I. General information
A. The rate of congenital glaucoma is from 1:5000 to 1:10 000 live births.
B. It is usually inherited as an autosomal-recessive trait, but can have an infectious cause (e.g., rubella).
C. Approximately 60% to 70% of affected children are boys.
D. The disease is bilateral in 64% to 88% of cases.
E. Age of onset
1. Present at birth: 40%
2. Between birth and 6 months: 34%
3. Between 6 months and 1 year: 12%
4. Between 1 year and 6 years: 11%
5. Over 6 years: 2%
6. No information: 1%

Primary juvenile glaucoma can be arbitrarily defined as an autosomal-dominant syndrome, not associated with any other ocular or systemic abnormalities, and occurring between the ages of 3 and 20 years. One gene responsible for this condition, called the *GLC1A* gene, has been localized to the 1q21–q31 region of chromosome 1. The same mutation has been found in 2.9% of patients with open-angle glaucoma (see below).

II. Pathogenesis (many theories)
A. Barkan's membrane (mesodermal surface membrane or imperforate innermost uveal sheet) mechanically prevents the aqueous from leaving the anterior chamber (histologic proof for this theory is scarce).
B. Congenital absence of Schlemm's canal
1. Congenital absence of Schlemm's canal is very rare, if it exists at all.

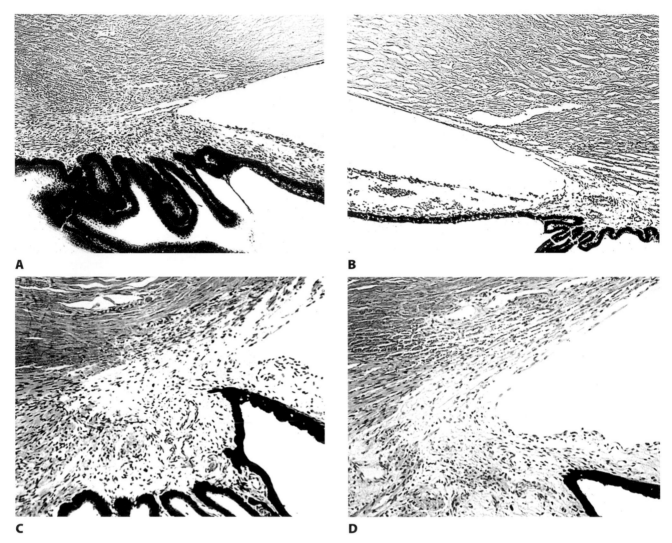

A

B

C

D

Fig. 16.4 Congenital glaucoma. **A** and **B** from premature infants (**A,** 700 g—died shortly after birth; **B,** 1050 g—lived 1 day); neither had clinical or histologic evidence of glaucoma. Note each has anterior "insertion" of iris root, anteriorly displaced ciliary processes, continuity of ciliary meridional muscles with uveal trabecular meshwork, and mesenchymal tissue in anterior-chamber angle. **C,** Eye obtained from 2-year-old child at time of accidental drowning but sectioned *tangentially*. Bilateral congenital glaucoma well documented; goniotomy and goniopuncture had been performed in another area of eye; pressure well controlled after surgery. Note similarity to nonglaucomatous premature eyes shown in **A** and **B.** **D,** However, when eye shown in **C** is sectioned properly (*meridionally*), the angle appears completely normal compared with other 2-year-olds.

2. Most often, the canal is compressed or collapsed as a secondary change resulting from chronically elevated IOP. The canal, therefore, may be difficult to find histologically.

C. An "embryonic" anterior-chamber angle that results from faulty cleavage of tissue during embryonic development of the eye prevents the aqueous from leaving the anterior chamber.

1. Histologically, the angle shows an anterior "insertion" of the iris root, anteriorly displaced ciliary processes, insertion of the ciliary meridional muscles into the trabecular meshwork instead of into (or over) the scleral roll, and mesenchymal tissue in the anterior-chamber angle (Fig. 16.4).

2. Many nonglaucomatous infant eyes show a similar anterior-chamber angle structure.

3. To interpret angle histology accurately, it is necessary to study truly meridional sections through the anterior-chamber angle.

a. Tangential sectioning makes interpretation difficult (see Fig. 16.4C and D).

b. Unfortunately, in the usual serial sectioning of a whole eye, because of the continuously curved surface, only a few sections from the center of the embedded tissue are truly meridional.

D. The true cause or causes of congenital glaucoma probably remain unknown.

The site or sites of impaired outflow may vary from eye to eye. The major obstruction may lie near the entrance to the meshwork, in the meshwork, near the efferent vessels of the drainage angle, or any combination thereof. Congenital glaucoma, therefore, will most probably be shown to have a number of causes. For example, a case of congenital glaucoma associated with the chromosomal defect of deletion of the short arm of the 10th chromosome (10ᵖ⁻) showed aberrant trabecular pillars* extending from the iris root toward Schwalbe's line. Also, as mentioned earlier, a form of autosomal-dominant juvenile glaucoma has been mapped to the long arm of chromosome 1 (1q21–q31).

III. Associated diseases and conditions
  A. Iris anomalies (see pp. 334–338 in Chapter 9)
    1. Hypoplasia of the iris ("aniridia") and iris coloboma may be associated with congenital glaucoma.
       a. The PAX6 point mutation defect (1630A > T) has been associated with some cases of aniridia.
       b. Aniridia may be found in *Brachmann–de Lange syndrome*, which may also include conjunctivitis, blepharitis, microcornea, and corectopia.
  B. Axenfeld's anomaly and Rieger's syndrome (see pp. 263 in Chapter 8)
  C. Peters' anomaly (see p. 260 in Chapter 8, and p. 45 in Chapter 2)
    1. Peters' anomaly and primary congenital glaucoma may share a common molecular pathophysiology. Both of these disorders can be associated with mutation in the cytochrome P4501B1 (*CYP1B1*) gene.
  D. Phakomatoses
    1. Sturge–Weber syndrome (see pp. 30–31 in Chapter 2)
       a. *Phakomatosis pigmentovascularis (PPV) types II A and B* are associated with melanosis bulbi and glaucoma. Ectodermal and mesodermal migration disorders have been postulated to be involved in the pathogenesis of this disorder. PPV II B is also associated with iris mamillations, Sturge–Weber syndrome, hemifacial, and hemicorporal, or limb hypertrophy without venous insufficiency.
    2. Neurofibromatosis (see pp. 31–34 in Chapter 2)
  E. Lowe's syndrome (see p. 367 in Chapter 10)
  F. Pierre Robin syndrome
    1. Pierre Robin syndrome consists of hypoplasia of the mandible, glossoptosis, cleft palate, and ocular anomalies.
    2. Ocular anomalies include glaucoma, high myopia, cataract, neural retinal detachment, and microphthalmos.
  G. Rubella (see pp. 43–44 in Chapter 2)
  H. Marfan's syndrome (see pp. 385–387 in Chapter 10)

  I. Homocystinuria (see p. 385 in Chapter 10)
  J. Microcornea (see p. 257 in Chapter 8)
  K. Spherophakia (see p. 387 in Chapter 10)
  L. Chromosomal abnormalities (e.g., trisomy 13; see pp. 38–39 in Chapter 2)
  M. Persistent hyperplastic primary vitreous (see p. 747 in Chapter 18)
  N. Retinopathy of prematurity (see p. 748 in Chapter 18)
  O. Retinoblastoma (see p. 733 in Chapter 18)
  P. Juvenile xanthogranuloma (see p. 343 in Chapter 9)
IV. Secondary histologic ocular effects in young eyes (<10 years of age)
  Q. Hennekam syndrome, which includes lymphedema, lymphangiectasis, and developmental delay.
       Other associated findings are dental anomalies, hearing loss, and renal anomalies.
  R. Nail–patella syndrome is characterized by dysplasia of the nails, patellar aplasia or hypoplasia, iliac horns, dysplasia of the elbows, and frequently glaucoma and progressive nephropathy.
       The underlying gene involved is *LMX1B*, which is a LIM-homeodomain transcription factor. The gene is located at 9q34.
  S. Congenital glaucoma can accompany Marshall–Smith syndrome, which is characterized by orofacial dysmorphism, failure to thrive, and accelerated osseous maturation.
  T. Subtelomeric deletion of chromosome 6p results in a syndrome characterized by ptosis, posterior embryotoxin, optic nerve abnormalities, mild glaucoma, Dandy–Walker malformation, hydrocephalus, atrial septal defect, patent ductus arteriosus, and mild mental retardation. This syndrome phenotypically overlaps Ritscher–Schinzel [or craniocerebellocardiac (3C) syndrome].
  U. A possible new autosomal-recessive syndrome phenotypically resembles Ivemark syndrome (hepatorenal–pancreatic syndrome) and is characterized by neonatal diabetes mellitus, congenital hypothyroidism, hepatic fibrosis, polycystic kidneys, and congenital glaucoma.
  V. Neurofibromatosis type 1 should be excluded in newborns with unilateral congenital glaucoma.
  W. Subepithelial amyloid deposits, in a recessive form of congenital hereditary endothelial dystrophy, can be associated with congenital glaucoma.
  X. Congenital glaucoma has occurred in a 28-year-old man with trisomy 7q34-qter and monosomy 15q26.3-qter caused by a paternal balanced chromosomal translocation t(7;15) (q34;q26.3). The patient had some features of the Silver–Russell syndrome, including short stature of prenatal onset, triangular face, clinodactyly of the fifth fingers, and body asymmetry. One copy of the insulin-like growth factor-1 receptor gene (IGF1R) at 15q25–q26 was deleted, which suggested a possible role for IGF1R in the Silver–Russell syndrome.
IV. Secondary histologic ocular effects in young eyes (<10 years of age)
  A. Buphthalmos ("large eye") is caused by an enlargement, stretching, and thinning of the coats of the eye,

---

Trabecular pillars are distinguished from iris processes by their collagenous core. Iris processes, which are extensions of the iris anterior-border layer, have no collagenous core.

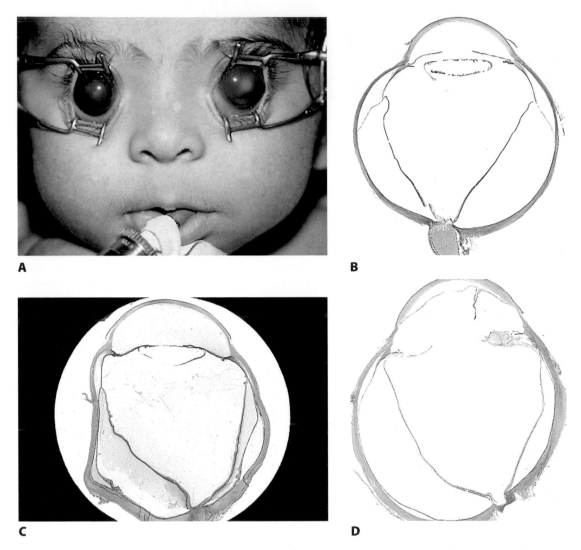

Fig. 16.5 Congenital glaucoma. **A,** Child with congenital glaucoma and enlarged eyes (buphthalmos) shows bilateral aniridia. The markedly enlarged corneas are caused by glaucoma. **B,** Histologic section shows that most of the enlargement of the globe in buphthalmos takes place in the anterior segment. Note stretching and thinning of cornea and sclera, especially in the limbal region (limbal ectasia). **C,** Anterior stretching and thinning of cornea, limbal region, and anterior sclera are quite marked. **D,** Deep glaucomatous optic nerve head excavation present in buphthalmic eye removed from a 7-year-old girl who had congenital glaucoma and multiple surgical procedures. Note that secondary anterior iris synchia has caused the ectatic limbus to be lined by iris (limbal staphyloma). (**A,** Courtesy of Dr. HG Scheie.)

especially marked in the anterior segment, resulting in a deep anterior chamber (Fig. 16.5).

Subluxated lenses may develop in these eyes.

B. Ruptures of Descemet's membrane (Haab's striae) may be found in the enlarged corneas (Fig. 16.6), are usually horizontal in the central cornea but concentric toward the limbus, mainly in the lower half, and are often associated with corneal edema.

Ruptures of Descemet's membrane secondary to birth trauma tend to be unilateral, most often in the left eye (most common fetal presentation is left occiput anterior), and usually run in a diagonal direction across the central cornea.

C. The limbal region becomes stretched and thin, with a resultant limbal ectasia (see Fig. 16.5).

When the limbal ectasia is lined by uvea (e.g., with peripheral anterior synechiae), it is called a *limbal staphyloma* (see Fig. 16.5). When it extends posteriorly to involve the sclera over the ciliary body, it is called an *intercalary staphyloma*.

D. Fibrosis of the iris root and trabecular meshwork is a late manifestation, as is disappearance of Schlemm's canal.

E. Continued high IOP may cause atrophy of the ciliary body, choroid, and retina, cupping of the optic disc (see Fig. 16.5), and atrophy of the optic nerve.

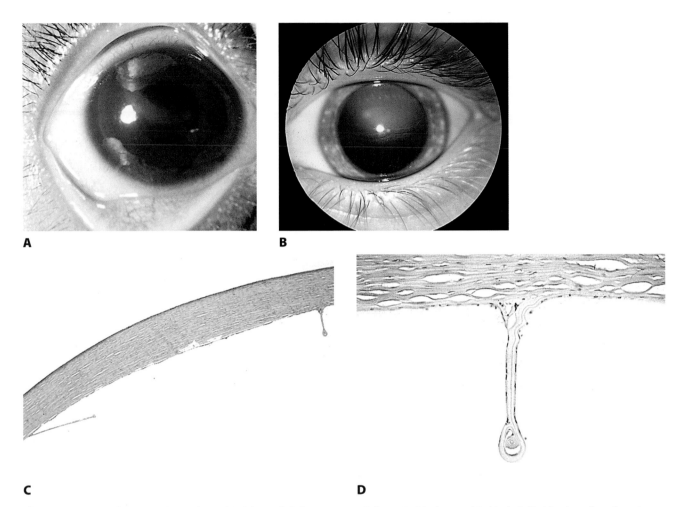

A   **B**

C   **D**

Fig. 16.6 Ruptures of Descemet's membrane (Haab's striae). **A,** Rupture extends from 10 o'clock toward 4 o'clock. **B,** Red fundus reflex of another case shows a horizontal Haab's stria. **C,** Histologic section shows two breaks in Descemet's membrane. The one on the right is shown with increased magnification in **D. D,** The ruptured end of Descemet's membrane has healed over. Scroll-like extension of Descemet's membrane, covered by endothelium, hangs into the anterior chamber. (**A,** Courtesy of Dr. HG Scheie; **B,** courtesy of Dr. DB Schaffer.)

Cupping of the optic nerve head secondary to glaucoma develops more rapidly in infant eyes than in adult eyes. Unlike in the adult eye, however, cupping in the infant eye is often reversible when the IOP normalizes. Restoration of a normal cup is most rare with glaucomatous cupping in adults.

Primary Glaucoma (Closed- and Open-Angle)

I. The classification of the various forms of glaucoma depends on the clinical examination of the anterior-chamber angle by gonioscopy. It is important that the clinician be able to correlate the clinical findings with their histologic counterparts.

II. Optical coherence tomography and ultrasound biomicroscopy can be utilized to evaluate the anatomic configuration of the anterior-chamber angle and adjacent structures for the classification of the pathophysiology of the glaucomas.

Primary open- and closed-angle glaucoma occur more often in diabetic patients than in nondiabetic subjects.

III. Closed-angle (narrow-angle; angle closure; acute congestive) glaucoma (Figs 16.7 and 16.8)

A. In anatomically predisposed eyes, primary closed-angle glaucoma develops.

1. The surface of the peripheral iris is close to the inner surface of the trabecular meshwork, causing a narrow or shallow anterior-chamber angle.

Plateau iris configuration is a much rarer cause of closed-angle glaucoma than is the typical narrow anterior-chamber angle configuration. In the former condition, closed-angle glaucoma occurs, but direct examination with a slit lamp shows a normal-depth central anterior chamber, and a flat iris plane except at the extreme periphery. A vertical section through the iris displays a "hockey-stick" configuration to the iris contour. Gonioscopic examination, during the acute glaucomatous

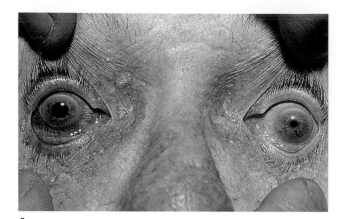

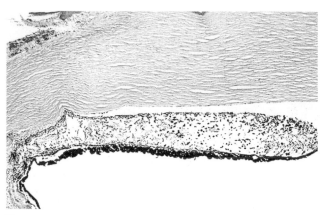

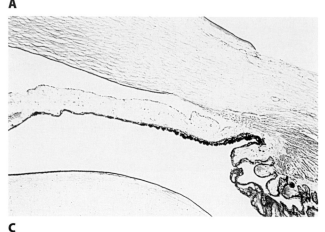

Fig. 16.7 Closed-angle glaucoma. **A,** Patient complained of pain, photophobia, and seeing halos around lights. Right eye shows a semidilated pupil and ciliary injection. **B,** Histologic section shows peripheral iris surface compressing trabecular meshwork. **C,** Histologic section of another case shows that eyes prone to acute attacks have a characteristic "crowded" anterior segment.

attack, shows a closed anterior-chamber angle. Rarely, multiple ciliary body cysts can cause a plateau iris configuration to the anterior-chamber angle.

2. Small, hypermetropic eyes are especially vulnerable to angle closure.

   A founder gene effect is probably related to two families of the Faroe Islands with hereditary high hyperopia, angle closure glaucoma, uveal effusion, cataract, esotropia, and amblyopia.

   Closed-angle glaucoma may be a prominent feature of the *oculodentodigital dysplasia* (ODDD) syndrome, associated with microcornea, and iris atrophy. It is a rare inherited disorder that impacts the development of the face, teeth, and limbs including narrow nose, hypoplastic alae nasi, anteverted nostrils, syndactyly, and hypoplasia and yellowing of the dental enamel. Other less common findings are intracranial calcification, and conductive deafness secondary to recurrent otitis media. This syndrome can be associated with a mutation (P59H) in the *GJ1A* gene. It can have an autosomal-recessive inheritance.

3. The lens is normal-sized or large.

   If the lens becomes large enough (e.g., a swollen, intumescent lens), it may push the iris diaphragm anteriorly so that an angle closure can result even though the anterior-chamber angle had been of normal or average depth.

4. Closed-angle glaucoma is usually a disorder affecting older individuals; however, it may be found even in individuals 40 years of age and younger. The most common causes (in decreasing order of frequency) in this age group are plateau iris syndrome, iridociliary cysts, retinopathy of prematurity, uveitis, isolated nanophthamlos, relative pupillary block, and Weil–Marchesani syndrome.

B. The trabecular meshwork is normal before an initial attack of acute primary closed-angle glaucoma. After repeated attacks (often at subclinical levels), the still-open anterior-chamber angle may become damaged (fibrotic) and, therefore, may simulate chronic simple (open-angle) glaucoma. Pigment accumulation within trabecular cells and loss of trabecular endothelial cells are also common findings following angle closure.

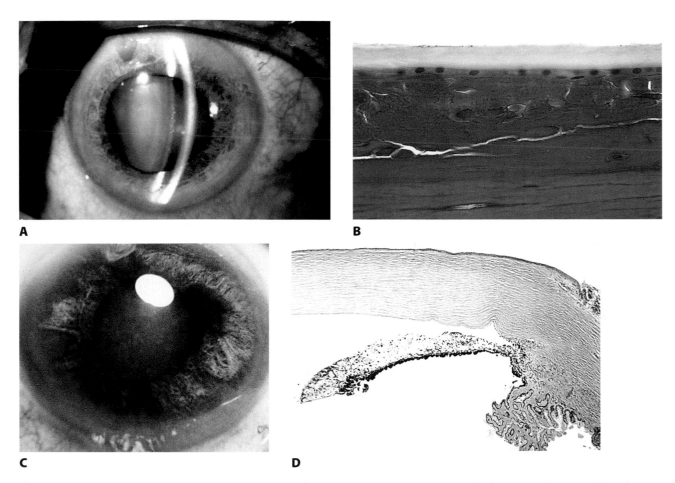

Fig. 16.8 Closed-angle glaucoma. **A,** After acute attack, glaukomflecken (i.e., tiny, white anterior subcapsular lens opacities) present. **B,** Histologic section shows that glaukomflecken are characterized by small areas of lens epithelial necrosis and tiny adjacent areas of subcapsular cortical degeneration. **C,** Another case demonstrates triad of irregular pupil, segmental iris atrophy (only brown iris from 5:30 to 9 o'clock relatively normal), and glaukomflecken. **D,** Histologic section of another case shows that loss of iris dilator muscle, absence of considerable amount of iris stroma in necrotic iris, and loss of pupillary iris pigment epithelium are responsible for clinically seen triad.

C. A sudden rise in IOP results from the peripheral iris being in apposition to the trabecular meshwork from the pupillary-block mechanisms except in the plateau iris syndrome, which in its pure form, does not involve pupillary block.

The association of typical acute closed-angle glaucoma with increasing age is due, in part, to progressive pupillary block from the increase in lens size as it adds layers of lens fibers over time.

Malignant glaucoma is a rare postoperative complication that follows ocular surgery to control glaucoma (or even after cataract surgery) in eyes that have shallow anterior chambers, often chronic angle closure, and usually peripheral anterior synechiae. Miotics tend to aggravate the condition and, rarely, may precipitate malignant glaucoma even without previous surgery. The condition results from misdirection of aqueous into the posterior segment of the globe, thereby shifting the iris lens diaphragm anteriorly and resulting in angle closure.

D. Histology
   1. Segmental iris atrophy
      a. Swelling of the iris root and occlusion of the greater arterial circle of the iris or its branches result in occlusion of the arterial supply to the iris stroma and subsequent necrosis.
      b. Segmental iris atrophy is usually seen in the upper half of the iris in a sector configuration.

Segmental iris atrophy following closed-angle glaucoma resembles that of herpes zoster iritis. Iris atrophy can also be seen in pseudoexfoliation syndrome and after trauma. The atrophy may be extreme, resulting in a through-and-through iris hole, thereby curing the acute attack of glaucoma.

      c. Histologically, there is marked atrophy of the iris stromal layer and, often, of iris pigment epithelium.

2. Irregular pupil results from necrosis of the dilator and sphincter muscles.

  b. Histologically, segments of the dilator muscle or its entire length are absent.

  c. The sphincter muscle shows varying degrees of atrophy.

3. Glaukomflecken (cataracta disseminata subcapsularis glaukomatosa; see Fig. 16.8)

  a. Glaukomflecken probably results from interference with the normal metabolism of the anterior lens cells owing to a stagnation of aqueous humor that contains toxic products of necrosis, or from foci of pressure necrosis (see p. 374 in Chapter 10).

  b. Anterior subcapsular, multiple, tiny gray-white lenticular opacities are seen.

  c. Histologically, small areas of epithelial cell necrosis together with tiny adjacent areas of subcapsular cortical degeneration are found.

4. Optic disc edema

  a. The nerve fibers in the optic nerve are more susceptible to an acute rise in IOP than are the retinal ganglion cells (RGC).

  b. Irreversible vision impairment after an acute attack is mainly caused by optic nerve damage.

Optic disc edema occurs early, probably from temporary obstruction of the venous return at the nerve head caused by the abrupt increase in IOP. If the associated corneal edema is cleared with glycerol during an acute attack, the optic disc edema can be seen ophthalmoscopically in many cases.

---

  c. Histology (see Fig. 13.7B)

5. Neovascularization of iris

  a. Neovascularization of iris (clinical rubeosis iridis) is usually secondary to a central retinal vein or artery thrombosis caused by elevated IOP during the acute attack.

  b. Histologically, fibrovascular tissue is found in the anterior-chamber angle and on the anterior surface of the iris.

Familial amyloidotic polyneuropathy type I (Met 30) has presented with neovascular glaucoma.

E. Failure to reverse the initial attack of angle closure can result in chronic angle closure glaucoma.

1. This entity can be confused clinically with chronic open-angle glaucoma unless careful gonioscopy is performed routinely on all suspected cases of glaucoma.

  a. Chronic angle-closure glaucoma is associated with the necessity of continued treatment and subsequent procedures even in the presence of a patent iridotomy.

2. Histology

  a. There is disorganization of the trabecular architecture, narrowing or loss of trabecular spaces, scarring of the trabecular beams, trabecular

endothelial cell loss, deposition of banded fibrillar material, and melanin pigment deposition.

IV. Chronic open-angle (chronic simple) glaucoma (POAG) (Figs 16.9 and 16.10)

A. The angle appears normal gonioscopically.

B. The site or sites of resistance to aqueous humor outflow lie within the structures of the drainage angle of the anterior chamber.

Widespread belief exists that the major site of obstruction lies near Schlemm's canal, but the belief has not been well supported by either experimental or histologic evidence.

C. The condition is most often bilateral.

1. Glaucoma may develop in one eye months to years before the fellow eye.

Patients who have POAG show a significantly higher prevalence of splinter hemorrhages on the optic nerve than do patients who do not have glaucoma. These splinter hemorrhages are associated with an increased incidence of field defects. Disc hemorrhages in glaucomatous or glaucoma suspect eyes are often associated with progressive changes of the optic nerves and of the visual fields.

---

2. One eye may be more severely affected than the other eye.

  a. Open-angle glaucoma with dilated episcleral vessels may be seen unilaterally in orbital and lid hemangioma (Sturge–Weber syndrome), or bilaterally in carotid cavernous fistula, familial cases, or idiopathic cases.

  b. Unilateral open-angle glaucoma may occur in association with lid thickening caused by neurofibromatosis.

D. Prevalence (see earlier, section *Introduction*)

E. Heredity and genetics

1. In most cases, the condition is probably inherited as an autosomal-recessive trait.

Probably at least six POAG genes are at fault. The POAG loci are named *GLC1*, and a letter is added to indicate each new locus (the first described is *GLC1A*). One, the juvenile-onset POAG *GLC1A* gene is on chromosome 1q21–31 [in the region of the trabecular meshwork protein gene (*TIGR*), also known as *myocilin*]. Glaucoma usually manifests in late childhood and early adulthood, and is moderately severe. The other five (at least) genes are related to adult-onset POAG and are milder than the juvenile form. These are *GLC1B* (2qcen–2q13, *GLC1C* (3q21–q24), *GLC1D* (8q23), *GLC1E* (10p), and *GLC1F* (7q35–q36).

---

2. Mutations in the myocilin/*TIGR* gene are present in 1% to 4% of POAG patients, but not in patients with pseudoexfoliation. Linkage analysis for maximum recorded IOP locates near marker D10S537 on 10q22 whereas maximum cup-to-disc ratio is near markers D1S197 to D1S220 on 1p32. Inclusion of the myocilin Q368X mutation as a covariate suggests an interaction between this mutation and the IOP and cup-to-disc ratio loci.

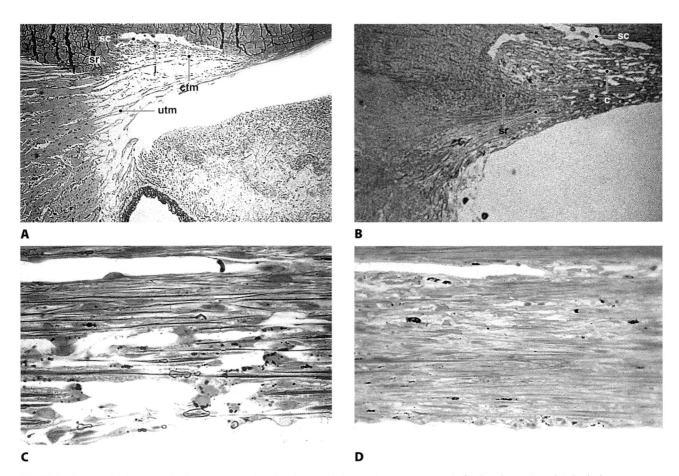

Fig. 16.9 Open-angle glaucoma. **A,** The normal anterior-chamber angle shows a loose arrangement of trabecular meshwork in both the corneoscleral and uveal components (ctm, corneoscleral trabecular meshwork; utm, uveal trabecular meshwork). The juxtacanalicular connective tissue (j) of the trabecular meshwork is adjacent to Schlemm's canal (sc) (sr, scleral roll). **B,** An eye removed from a patient who had chronic open-angle glaucoma shows the results of the aging process. The normally loose tissue in the uveal trabecular meshwork and angle recess has compacted (c, compressed trabecular meshwork), producing a prominent scleral roll/spur (sr) (sc, Schlemm's canal). **C,** A coronal section taken through normal trabecular meshwork shows that the loose beams of the meshwork form large tubes running in an anterior–posterior direction. **D,** Coronal sections through the trabecular meshwork in a patient who had chronic open-angle glaucoma show that the aging process has caused marked compaction of the trabecular meshwork beams, resulting in occlusion of most of the tubes. (**A,** Rhesus monkey; **A–D,** PD stain; case reported in Fine BS *et al.: Am J Ophthalmol* 91:88. © Elsevier 1981.)

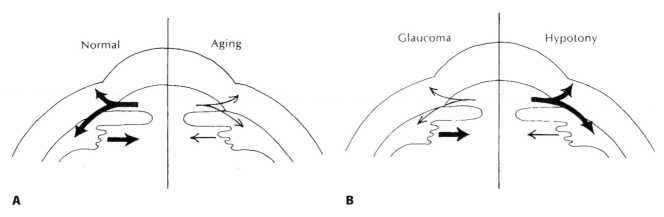

Fig. 16.10 A, Diagram shows theoretical situation of aqueous inflow and outflow in normal (*left*) and in aging (*right*) persons. **B,** If outflow facility decreases faster than does aqueous inflow, glaucoma results (*left*). Opposite situation results in hypotony (*right*).

The Thr377Met mutation in myocillin may represent a susceptibility allele for glaucoma. Other myocillin mutations, including Phe369Leu, Ile-360Asn, Ala363Thr, and Thr448Pro, have been associated with 2.9% of POAG in Japanese individuals. The nonsense mutation Gln368Stop is found in western populations but not in India or Japan. The Gln368STOP mutation is not associated with earlier onset or different clinical course of POAG or ocular hypertension than those disorders in individuals lacking the mutation.

   a. The GLC1A Thr377Met mutation in the myocilin gene has been associated with glaucoma that has a younger age of onset and higher peak IOP than in pedigrees with with the more common Gln368STOP mutation. Additionally, individuals with the Thr377Met mutation are more likely to undergo filtration surgery.

   b. In French patients, myocilin gene mutations other than Q368X are associated with a younger age at diagnosis than that of Q368X carriers or of patients with a normal MYOC. In Australia, a founder effect Q368STOP mutation in the myocilin gene has been detected in 15 families. The families, therefore, share a common ancestor who probably lived prior to the European settlement of Australia.

   c. The pathobiology of myocilin gene mutations is probably the result of gain of function rather than from haploinsufficiency.

   d. It is probable that accumulation of mutant myocilin in the rough endoplasmic reticulum in glaucoma stresses the endoplasmic reticulum and may produce cytotoxicity in the human trabecular meshwork cells. Most known myocilin mutations localize to the C-terminus, an olfactomedin-like domain. This material is probably not properly processed in the endoplasmic reticulum. Therefore the material accumulates into insoluble aggregates.

   e. In cultured trabecular cells, increased myocilin expression results in loss of actin stress fibers and focal adhesions. Cell adhesion to fibronectin and cell spreading are also compromised. The impact on cellular adhesion is similar to matricellular proteins. Increased sensitivity to apoptosis is also found in cells displaying enhanced myocilin expression.

     1). Frequently, a family history of POAG is reported.

     2). A high incidence of impaired facility of outflow is found in younger members of families with POAG.

A more appropriate name for POAG might be *glaucomatous optic neuropathy* because the primary defect is probably in the optic nerve.

F. Normal-tension (improperly called *low-tension*) glaucoma is a subdivision of POAG (see section *Introduction* in this chapter).

G. Histology and pathophysiology

   1. Optic nerve (see pp. 658–660 in this chapter)

   2. Little is known about the early histologic changes that take place in the region of the drainage angle because the number of human eyes that have well-characterized early open-angle glaucoma available for histologic examination is small (see Fig. 16.9).

   3. Very little meaningful information can be derived from long-standing, "end-stage" diseased eyes or from tiny biopsies taken during surgery for control of glaucoma.

Many reported histologic changes such as "sclerosis" of the trabecular meshwork, compression or absence of Schlemm's canal, or decrease in number of macrovacuoles in the endothelial lining of Schlemm's canal are probably end-stage changes, artifacts, or misinterpretations. Proteomic analysis of the trabecular meshwork in POAG demonstrates cochlin, which is a protein associated with the deafness disorder DFNA9 in patients with POAG but not in the normal trabecular meshwok. Deposits of cochlin and mucopolysaccharide are present in human trabecular meshwork around Schlemm's canal, similar to that observed in the cochlea in DFNA9 deafness. It is postulated that cochlin may disrupt trabecular meshwork architecture and render its components, like collagen, more susceptible to degradation and collapse. Thus, the cochlin would interact with the extracellular matrix (ECM), leading to a cascade of effects, resulting in decreased aqueous outflow.

---

   4. Aging changes in the drainage angle of the anterior chamber

     a. COAG is usually associated with a progressive decrease in the facility of outflow of aqueous humor from the anterior chamber.

     b. The resulting IOP becomes incompatible with the continued health of the tissues of the optic nerve head.

     c. Decreased facility of outflow results from an obstruction produced by excessive aging changes in the drainage angle.

     d. The degree of obstruction is a *quantitative* problem; two extremes of excessive obstruction are:

       1). Proliferation of the endothelium (and possibly of juxtacanalicular connective tissue cells) lining Schlemm's canal into its lumen for much of its circumference

       2). Compaction of the uveal meshwork against the scleral roll, producing a prominent scleral spur ("hyalinization" of adjacent ciliary muscle and atrophy of the iris root also occur)

     e. The two major aging changes—each may be seen in almost pure form, or may be combined.

       1). They may also be associated with proliferations of trabecular endothelial cells in the meshwork.

2). COAG depends on the amount of aqueous inflow and the degree of obstruction to outflow caused by the aging changes (see Fig. 16.10).

    f. Molecular analysis of human trabecular meshwork in glaucoma demonstrates oxidative DNA damage in glaucoma.

The aging changes listed here as occurring in the tissues of the drainage angle are mostly irreversible. Their obstructive nature may be circumvented for short or long periods with a variety of pharmacologic agents. Thus, whether glaucoma develops is a quantitative problem based on whether aging changes of decreased outflow exceed aging changes of decreased inflow.

---

5. Ischemia involving the aqueous outflow pathway has been postulated to contribute to the development of POAG.
6. Oculomedin is expressed in stretched trabecular cells in tissue culture. It is localized to the trabecular meshwork, Schlemm's canal endothelium, retinal photoreceptor cells, and corneal and conjunctival epithelium. Its gene is composed of two exons located within the intron of the *C1orf27* gene on chromosome 1q25, near and telomeric to myocilin.
7. Carbonic anhydrase (CA12) enzyme mRNA is increased in neural pigment epithelial cells in glaucoma patients, which may be a target for therapy in glaucoma.

Secondary Closed-Angle Glaucoma

Causes

I. Chronic primary angle-closure glaucoma
    A. Repeated attacks of primary closed-angle glaucoma may give rise either to peripheral anterior synechiae and secondary closed-angle glaucoma, or to trabecular damage and secondary COAG.

In black patients, the acute attacks may be subclinical while the closure of the angle progresses relentlessly.

    B. Histologically, peripheral anterior synechiae are seen, sometimes broad based.
II. Phacomorphic
    A. Swelling of the lens may cause peripheral anterior synechiae (through pupillary block and iris bombé).
    B. More frequently, a maturing cataractous lens swells rapidly and simulates primary closed-angle glaucoma.
III. Subluxated or anteriorly dislocated lens can cause a pupillary block that, if not relieved, leads to iris bombé, peripheral anterior synechiae, and secondary angle closure.

IV. Persistent flat chamber after surgical or nonsurgical trauma may lead to broad-based peripheral anterior synechiae, occasionally causing total anterior synechiae.
V. Iridocorneal endothelial (ICE) syndrome
    A. The ICE syndrome consists of a spectrum of changes that include the iris nevus (Cogan–Reese) syndrome, Chandler's syndrome, and essential iris atrophy.

Antibody titers to the Epstein–Barr virus are increased in patients who have the ICE syndrome; the significance of this increase remains to be clarified.

---

1. All three entities share a basic corneal endothelial defect and iris involvement.
    a. Specular microscopy shows abnormal cells, called *ICE cells*, that are larger and more pleomorphic than normal endothelial cells, and whose specular reflex shows light–dark reversal (i.e., the cell surface is dark instead of light, often with a central light spot, and the intercellular junctions are light instead of dark).

Electron microscopically, ICE cells show epithelial features (e.g., tonofilaments, desmosomes, multilayering, microvilli, and conspicuous "blebs").

---

    b. The abnormal endothelial cells may coexist with normal endothelial cells, a condition called *subtotal ICE*, when 25% to 75% of the total cells are ICE cells.

Immunohistochemical stains of the corneal endothelium are positive for AE1 and AE3 (epidermal keratins) and vimentin, which, along with electron microscopic observations, suggests an "epithelialization" of the endothelium, and may explain, at least in part, the aggressive proliferative nature of the corneal endothelium in the ICE syndrome.

---

    c. On specular microscopy, the clinically uninvolved contralateral eye often demonstrates subclinical corneal abnormalities such as a relatively low percentage of hexagonal cells and a relatively high coefficient of variation of cell area.
2. All ICE syndrome entities tend to be unilateral, occur in young women, and cause corneal edema when the IOP is only slightly elevated or even normal.
3. Glaucoma occurs in approximately 50% of cases.
4. Although in their pure forms the three entities are distinct clinicopathologic types, findings overlap so much in many cases that they are considered variants of the same process.
5. Each variant is described separately, but all are considered to belong to the ICE syndrome.

TABLE 16.1 Comparison of Posterior Polymorphous Dystrophy and Iridocorneal Endothelial Syndrome

	Posterior Polymorphous Dystrophy	Iridocorneal Endothelial Syndrome
CORNEA		
Edema	Common	Common
Endothelial surface	Vesicles, ridges, plaques, guttata	Fine guttatalike lesions common
IRIDOCORNEAL ADHESIONS	25%	100%
IRIS		
Stromal atrophy	Minimal or none	Marked (essential iris atrophy), moderate (iris nevus syndrome), or mild (Chandler's syndrome)
Ectropion uveae	Occasional	Occasional to common
GLAUCOMA	13%	~80%
HEREDITARY TRANSMISSION	Present (autosomal-dominant)	None
LATERALITY	Bilateral	Unilateral
SEX DISTRIBUTION	Equal	Women > men
ONSET OF SYMPTOMS	Any age, including congenital	Third and fourth decades
PROGRESSION	Corneal changes often progress to edema and degeneration; iridocorneal adhesions may progress very slowly	Fairly rapid formation of synechiae and severe glaucoma
HISTOPATHOLOGY		
Cornea	Thickened, multilayered Descemet's membrane; endothelial cells resemble epithelial cells (microvilli, desmosomes, cytoplasmic tonofilaments)	Thickened, multilayered Descemet's membrane; endothelial cells attenuated, reduced in number, and missing in areas
Chamber angle	Corneal endothelium and Descemet's membrane over trabecular meshwork and iris	Corneal endothelilum and Descemet's membrane over trabecular meshwork and iris

(Modified from Rodrigues MM et al.: Arch Ophthalmol 98:688, 1980. © American Medical Association. All rights reserved.)

Posterior polymorphous dystrophy (PPMD; see p. 307 in Chapter 8) shares some characteristics with the ICE syndrome (Table 16.1) such as endothelial degeneration, corneal edema, iridocorneal adhesions, endothelialization of the anterior-chamber angle, and glaucoma. Differences between the entities include the structure of the corneal endothelium (epithelial-like in PPMD), hereditary transmission (positive in PPMD), laterality (bilateral in PPMD), and progression (relatively stable in PPMD).

B. Iris nevus syndrome (Figs 16.11 and 16.12).
 1. The iris nevus syndrome mainly occurs in young women, and is characterized by several of the following signs: peripheral anterior synechiae, often associated with atrophic defects in adjacent iris stroma; matted appearance of iris stroma; a velvety, whorl-like iris surface; loss of iris crypts; fine iris nodules; pupillary eversion (ectropion uveae); heterochromia; secondary glaucoma; and corneal edema at only slightly elevated, or even normal, IOP.
 2. Histologically, the two main features are: (1) a diffuse or nodular, or both, nevus of the anterior surface of the iris; and (2) corneal endothelializa-tion of the anterior-chamber angle and anterior surface of the iris.

C. Chandler's syndrome (Fig. 16.13)
 1. The condition, probably the most common variant of the ICE syndrome, is unilateral and occurs mainly in young women.
 2. Endothelial dystrophy causes corneal edema to develop at a slightly elevated or normal IOP.

Patients with Chandler's syndrome tend to have worse corneal edema and less glaucoma than patients with the other two variants.

 3. Small peripheral anterior synechiae and mild pupillary distortion are found.
 4. Small areas of iris stromal thinning may be found, but through-and-through holes are rare.
 5. The glaucoma is usually mild.
 6. Histology
  a. The iris stroma is atrophic.
  b. In the areas of iris hole formation, the stroma and pigment epithelium are absent.

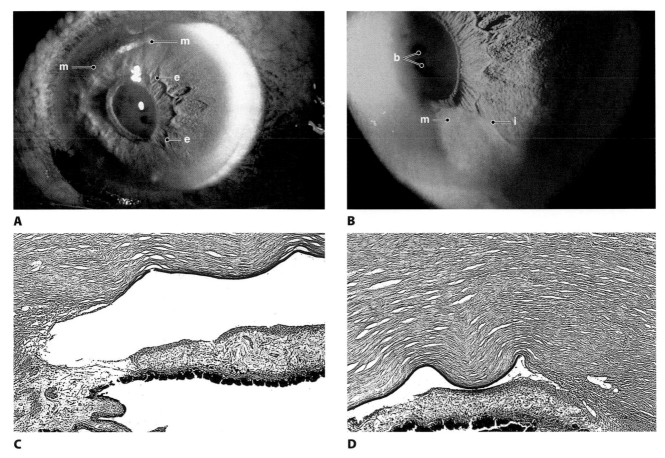

Fig. 16.11 Iridocorneal endothelial (ICE) syndrome (iris nevus syndrome variant). **A,** Patient had unilateral corneal edema and heterochromia iridum. Normal iris pattern on right side and effaced pattern on left caused by overgrowth of corneal endothelium Descemet's ("glass") membrane on left side (m, membrane over nasal iris; e, edge of membrane). **B,** Close-up view shows start of glass membrane inferiorly (b, corneal blebs; m, membrane; i, inferior temporal membrane edge). **C,** Periodic acid–Schiff (PAS)-stained histologic section of another eye shows a diffuse nevus on the anterior surface of the iris. Endothelium has partially grown over trabecular meshwork and laid down a new basement (Descemet's) membrane. **D,** Another PAS-stained section of the same case shows a diffuse iris nevus and a peripheral anterior synechia. Endothelium has migrated posteriorly over trabecular meshwork and has laid down new Descemet's membrane. (**C** and **D,** From Yanoff M: *Am J Ophthalmol* 70:898. © Elsevier 1970.)

c. Endothelialization of the anterior-chamber angle, often extending over the anterior surface of the iris, and formation of new Descemet's membrane are characteristic components.

> Iris nodules may appear late in the course of the disease. At first they appear small and yellow, but then increase in number and become dark brown.

D. Essential iris atrophy (Fig. 16.14)
  1. Essential iris atrophy is usually unilateral, is found most often in women, and is of unknown cause.
  2. The onset is usually in the third decade.
  3. Corneal edema often develops when IOP is slightly elevated or even normal.
     The corneal endothelium shows a fine, hammered-silver appearance, similar to cornea guttata but less coarse.
  4. The initial event is the formation of a peripheral anterior synechia distorting the pupil to that side.

a. The pupil becomes more distorted, sometimes with the development of an ectropion uveae.
b. Through-and-through holes develop in the iris, usually opposite to the distorted pupil.

> The holes seem to be caused by mechanical traction, related to sector corneal endothelial iris overgrowth.

  5. Peripheral anterior synechiae increase circumferentially, and an intractable glaucoma develops.
     Corneal endothelial overgrowth is a feature common to all three variants included in the ICE syndrome.
VI. Iridoschisis (Fig. 16.15)
  A. The condition starts mainly in the seventh decade of life and is usually bilateral; the sexes are equally affected.
  B. The pupil is not displaced and remains reactive.

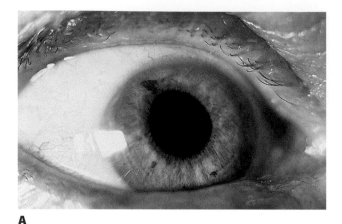

A

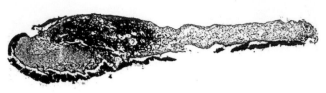

B

Fig. 16.12 Iridocorneal endothelial (ICE) syndrome (iris nevus syndrome variant). **A,** Small iris nevus at half past 10 o'clock in the right eye causes distortion of pupil, effacing of iris pattern around nevus, and ectropion uveae. A sector iridectomy was performed. **B,** Biopsy shows deep stromal pigmentation. Bleached sections demonstrated nevus cells. **C,** Another section of the same case shows a fragment of peripheral Descemet's membrane (on the right) adherent to the iris by means of a bridge. Endothelial cells have migrated and proliferated, cover both sides of the synechia, and have grown on to the anterior surface of the iris up to the pupil on the left, causing an ectropion uveae. Note normal stromal architecture and absence of inflammation or degeneration. (From Jakobiec FA *et al.*: *Am J Ophthalmol* 83:884. © Elsevier 1977.)

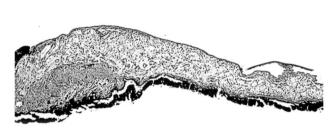

C

C. The anterior iris stromal layers separate widely from the deeper layers, resembling spaghetti.
  1. The lower half of the iris is most frequently involved.
  2. Initially, the loosened stromal fibers remain attached centrally and peripherally so that the delicate middle part of the fibers bows forward into the anterior chamber. Ultimately, the fibers break, and the free ends float in the aqueous.
D. Glaucoma develops in approximately 50% of affected eyes; it begins as peripheral anterior synechiae develop.
E. Cause
  1. Most cases seem to be a peculiar type of aging change.
  2. It may follow trauma.
  3. Rarely, it may occur with POAG.
VII. Anterior uveitis (see Figs 3.11 and 3.12)—Anterior uveitis from any cause [e.g., trauma, infection, "allergy," sympathetic uveitis (phacoanaphylactic endophthalmitis)] may result in posterior synechiae, iris bombé, and, finally, peripheral anterior synechiae.
VIII. Retinopathy of prematurity
A. The retrolental mass of neovascular tissue pushes the lens forward and causes "crowding" of the anterior-chamber angle.

B. Closed-angle glaucoma may result, sometimes years after the initial damage.
IX. Spherophakia (Weill–Marchesani syndrome; see p. 387 in Chapter 10)
X. Persistent hyperplastic primary vitreous (see p. 747 in Chapter 18)
A. Repeated hemorrhages result in organization and iridocorneal synechiae.
B. Less often, swelling of the lens or iris bombé can produce a closed angle.
XI. Epithelialization of anterior-chamber angle (see p. 119 in Chapter 5)
XII. Endothelialization of anterior-chamber angle (see Fig. 5.34).
A. Endothelialization of the anterior-chamber angle (or pseudoangle in the presence of peripheral anterior synechiae) is seen histologically in 20% of enucleated eyes.
B. Most of the eyes with endothelialization have peripheral anterior synechiae; a little less than half of the eyes are associated with neovascularization of iris.
C. Histologically, the endothelial cells possess junctional complexes, apical villi, prominent basement membranes, and myoblastic differentiation.
XIII. Neovascularization of anterior surface of the iris (clinically termed *rubeosis iridis*; see Figs 9.13, 9.14, and 15.5)

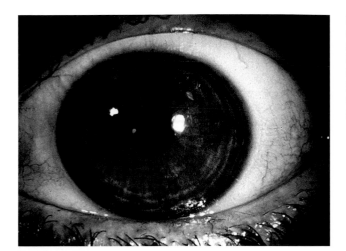

A

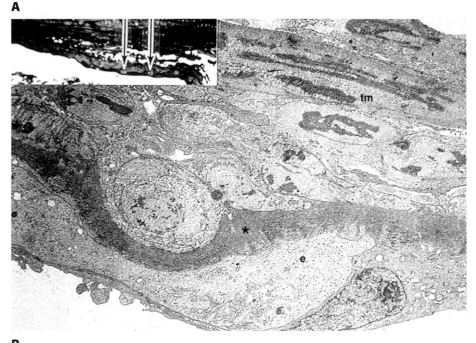

B

Fig. 16.13 Iridocorneal endothelial (ICE) syndrome (Chandler's syndrome variant). **A,** Left eye shows focal, peripheral, angle closure superonasally. **B,** Irregular layer of filamentous Descemet's membrane (*) between attenuated corneal endothelium (e) and trabecular meshwork (tm). **Inset,** thin (1.5 μm) section shows peripheral extension of Descemet's membrane (*arrows*) lining indentations of uveal meshwork. (From Rodrigues MM *et al.: Arch Ophthalmol* 96:643, 1978, with permission. © American Medical Association. All rights reserved.)

The many causes include diabetes mellitus, central retinal vein or artery occlusion, branch retinal artery occlusion, diffuse retinal vascular disease, carotid artery ischemia, retinoblastoma, malignant melanoma of uvea (Table 16.2), long-standing retinal detachment, any chronic retinal disease, penetrating or contusive ocular injuries, metastatic tumors to the retina and vitreous including cutaneous melanoma, and Fuchs' heterochromic iridocyclitis (see p. 65 in Chapter 3).

XIV. Cysts of iris and anterior ciliary body (see Figs 9.9 and 9.10)

    A. Multiple cysts of the iris and ciliary epithelium can cause both secondary acute and chronic closed-angle glaucoma.

        1. Congenital cysts of the iris are extremely rare but may cause secondary glaucoma when they enlarge, and can even be confused with iris melanoma.

    2. Primary angle closure glaucoma is uncommon in younger individuals, such as teenagers. Therefore, such individuals who present with angle closure should be evaluated to exclude secondary causes of angle closure such as ciliary body cysts.

The cysts may be idiopathic or may be associated with late syphilitic interstitial keratitis. Another cause of glaucoma in late syphilitic interstitial keratitis is secondary chronic angle closure due to peripheral anterior synechiae.

    B. Histologically, a proliferation of the posterior layer of the iris pigment epithelium or of the inner layer of ciliary epithelium lines the cyst (see pp. 339–341 in Chapter 9).

XV. Juvenile xanthogranuloma (see p. 343 in Chapter 9)

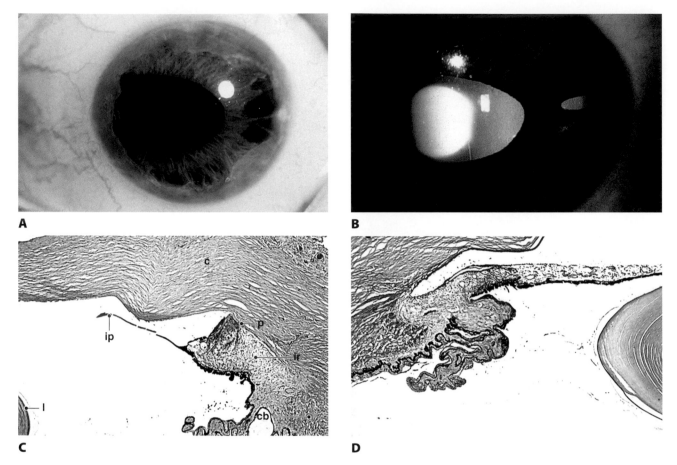

Fig. 16.14 Iridocorneal endothelial (ICE) syndrome (essential iris atrophy variant). **A,** Slit-lamp and (**B**) red-reflex views of the same eye show migration of the iris nasally toward the initial synechia and stretching of the iris temporally, causing holes clear through the iris. **C,** Histologic section of another eye with essential iris atrophy shows a peripheral anterior synechia (p), various degrees of degeneration and loss of the central iris stroma, and total loss of the central iris pigment epithelium (ip) (c, cornea; ir, iris root; cb, ciliary body; l, lens). **D,** In an area away from the peripheral anterior synechia, the anterior-chamber angle is open but the trabecular meshwork is covered by proliferated corneal endothelium and Descemet's membrane. (**A** and **B,** Courtesy of Dr. HG Scheie; **C** and **D,** reported in Scheie HG *et al.: Arch Ophthalmol* 94:1315, 1976. © American Medical Association. All rights reserved.)

XVI. Secondary to uveal malignant melanoma (Figs 16.16 to 16.18)
  A. Posterior synechiae and iris bombé (see Fig. 16.16)
    1. A large posterior malignant melanoma and a total neural retinal detachment may combine to displace the iris lens diaphragm anteriorly, resulting in posterior synechiae and iris bombé followed by secondary peripheral anterior synechiae.
    2. Similar changes may occur with a large posterior metastatic neoplasm.
  B. Neovascularization of iris (see Fig. 16.17)
    1. Neovascularization of the iris may occur with a large posterior choroidal malignant melanoma.
    2. The neovascularization causes peripheral anterior synechiae.
    3. Similar changes may occur with a large posterior metastatic neoplasm.
  C. Diffuse iris malignant melanoma (see Fig. 16.18)
    1. A diffuse iris malignant melanoma, or even a diffuse iris nevus, may induce peripheral anterior synechiae,

although diffuse melanomas do not usually present with such changes.
    2. The condition may simulate the ICE syndrome.

Rarely, an aggressive iris nevus can involve the angle, cause synechiae, and result in secondary angle closure glaucoma.

XVII. Immune recovery resulting from highly active antiretroviral therapy (HAART) has been associated with severe vitritis resulting in acute angle closure secondary to posterior synechias in a patient with inactive AIDS and inactive cytomegalovirus retinitis.
XVIII. Dense vitreous hemorrhage can result in angle closure, presumably from anterior displacement of the iris lens diaphragm.
XIX. Snake bite is an unusual cause of bilateral angle-closure glaucoma.

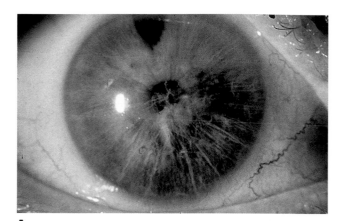

A

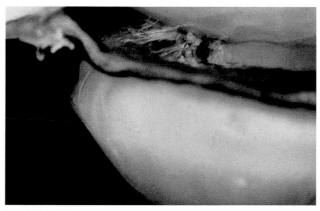

B

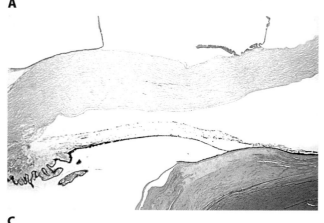

C

Fig. 16.15 Iridoschisis. **A,** The iris is in disarray, with long rolled strips from the 3 o'clock to the 6 o'clock position. **B,** The gross specimen from another eye shows separation and breakage of the collagenous columns of the iris stroma. **C,** Histologic section of the eye shown in **B** demonstrates epithelial blebs (bullous corneal edema) and separation of the iris stroma into elongated lamellae. (**A,** Courtesy of Prof. GOH Naumann.)

TABLE 16.2 Histopathologic Mechanisms Producing Secondary Glaucoma in Eyes Containing Uveal Malignant Melanomas

Mechanism	Underlying Cause
Peripheral anterior synechiae and angle closure	1. Posterior synechiae, iris bombé, and peripheral anterior synechiae 2. Iris neovascularization and peripheral anterior synechiae 3. Diffuse iris nevus or melanoma and peripheral anterior synechiae
Cellular obstruction of aqueous drainage area of an open angle	1. Seeding of neoplasm into anterior-chamber angle 2. Ring melanoma with invasion of anterior-chamber angle structures 3. Melanin phagocytosis by macrophages with obstruction of anterior-chamber angle (melanomalytic glaucoma)

(Modified from Yanoff M: Am J Ophthalmol 70:898. © Elsevier 1970.)

XX. Autosomal vitreoretinochoroidopathy can be associated with angle closure secondary to microcornea and shallow anterior chamber without microphthalmia.

Secondary Open-Angle Glaucoma

I. Secondary to cells or debris in angle
  A. Hyphema (see p. 135 in Chapter 5)
  B. Uveitis
    1. Cyclitis (or iridocyclitis) may lead to excessive cellular production that obstructs the open angle.

Anterior uveitis usually causes a decrease in aqueous inflow so that glaucoma rarely ensues. Glaucoma is also less likely if the cyclitis is segmental rather than circumferential. Glaucoma is most unlikely with a posterior cyclitis or pars planitis. Intractable glaucoma may complicate herpes simplex ocular infection even in the absence of obvious keratitis. Such infection can be confirmed by polymerase chain reaction analysis of aqueous humor.

---

    2. Glaucomatocyclitic crisis (*Posner–Schlossman syndrome*)
      a. The condition mainly occurs as a unilateral acute rise in IOP in people in their third through fifth decades; it may recur.

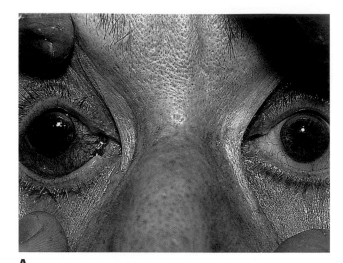

A

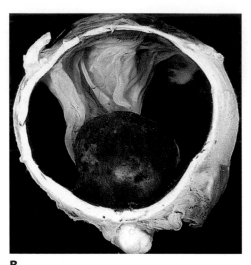

B

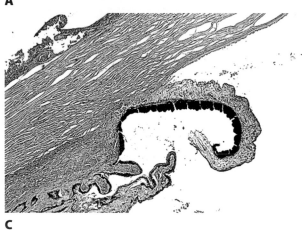

C

Fig. 16.16 Closed-angle glaucoma secondary to uveal melanoma. **A,** Patient presented with signs and symptoms of acute closed-angle glaucoma in right eye. Left eye had shallow anterior chamber and narrow angle. Ultrasonography showed solid tumor in choroid. **B,** Enucleated right eye shows large posterior melanoma and neural retinal detachment. **C,** Histologic section shows a closed angle secondary to iris bombé and secondary peripheral anterior synechia. Melanoma should be suspected in any glaucomatous eye that contains neural retinal detachment.

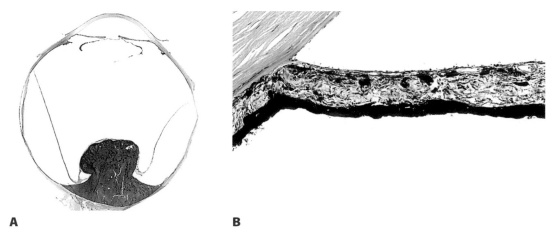

A   **B**

Fig. 16.17 Closed-angle glaucoma secondary to uveal melanoma. **A,** Histologic section shows large, mushroom-shaped melanoma and complete neural retinal detachment. **B,** Iris neovascularization and secondary peripheral anterior synechia have closed the angle. (From Yanoff M: *Am J Ophthalmol* 70:898. © Elsevier 1970.)

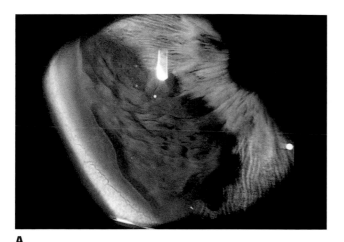

A

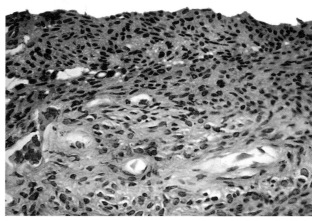

B

Fig. 16.18 Closed-angle glaucoma secondary to uveal melanoma. **A,** Diffuse iris malignant melanoma has involved the angle for 360°, resulting in secondary angle closure. Infiltration by melanoma also can produce a form of secondary open angle glaucoma (see Figs 16.23 and 16.24). **B,** Most iris melanomas show a rather bland cytology and can be considered as spindle nevi.

Although the cause is unknown, an abnormal instability of the ciliary vascular system may be related to the development of the acute glaucoma.

---

   b. Epithelial edema and one or more keratic precipitates (tiny and fine at first, but may become mutton-fat) are seen clinically.

Indirect evidence suggests that the herpes simplex virus may play a role in the origin of Posner–Schlossman syndrome.

---

   c. Little or no reaction occurs in the aqueous humor, and the angle usually appears normal.
   d. The disease is self-limited and subsides in 1 to 3 weeks.
   e. The histology is unknown.

Glaucomatocyclitic crisis appears to have a predilection for patients who have POAG or in whom it will develop.

---

  3. In oculodermal melanocytosis, in the involved eye, glaucoma may result from a low-grade chronic anterior uveitis of unknown cause.
C. Phacolytic glaucoma (see p. 384 in Chapter 10)
D. Nondenatured lens material-induced glaucoma usually follows a very recent traumatic rupture of the lens.
  1. If glaucoma develops after needling of a soft cataract, it occurs within the first week.
  2. After penetrating ocular injury
  3. The glaucoma is caused by occlusion of the open anterior-chamber angle by the swollen lens material, and is not related to phagocytic action.

The ruptured lens may not release its material, but may swell and result in pupillary block and a secondary acute or chronic closed-angle glaucoma.

E. Hemolytic (ghost-cell) glaucoma (Figs 16.19 and 16.20)
  1. Hemolytic (ghost cell) glaucoma presents as an acute open-angle glaucoma.
  2. The glaucoma results as a complication of long-standing vitreous or, rarely, anterior-chamber hemorrhage from any cause.

Glaucoma may be caused by macrophages and red blood cell (RBC) debris, especially hemoglobin aggregates, or by hemolyzed RBCs (ghost cells). Both RBC debris and ghost cells result from hemolysis; therefore, *hemolytic glaucoma* is a more accurate term than *ghost cell glaucoma*. Neither fresh RBCs nor ghost cells seem able to pass from the vitreous compartment through an intact anterior hyaloid face into the aqueous compartment; a rent or passageway is necessary.

---

  3. Histologically, the anterior-chamber angle is obstructed by debris, hemoglobin, ghost cells, and macrophages filled mainly with hemoglobin but also containing some hemosiderin.
F. Pigment dispersion syndrome (pigmentary "glaucoma"; Figs 16.21 and 16.22)
  1. The pigment dispersion syndrome is found most often in young, myopic, adult white men.
    a. Pigment dispersion may result from iris chafing secondary on foreign material such as an intraocular lens.

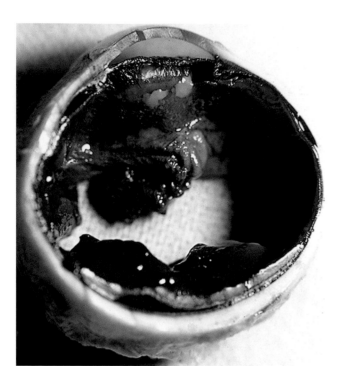

A

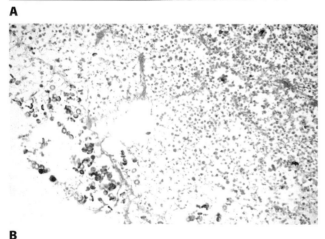

B

Fig. 16.19 Hemolytic (ghost-cell) glaucoma. **A,** Macroscopic appearance of fresh blood in subvitreal area (dark red) and old blood in vitreous (yellow-red). **B,** Histologic section shows intact erythrocytes (toward lower left). Hemolysis of the erythrocytes releases the hemoglobin particles and leaves empty shells ("ghost cells") behind.

The insertion of the iris into the ciliary body is more posterior in pigment dispersion syndrome than in control eyes. A low prevalence of pigment dispersion syndrome and pigmentary glaucoma occurs in blacks, Hispanics, and Asians. In black patients, pigmentary glaucoma tends to develop in an older age group (average, 73 years), mainly in hyperopes and women, shows no iris transillumination, and occurs in irises that have a relatively flat connection to the anterior face of the ciliary body.

2. Depigmentation of the iris epithelium, especially peripherally, results in circumferential foci of increased iris transillumination where the peripheral third of the iris meets the middle third.

The eye on the side of greatest increased iris transillumination may contain a larger pupil than the other eye (anisocoria). By slit-lamp biomicroscopy, a band of increased granular iris pigmentation can be seen overlying the ring of increased retroillumination (best seen in blue irises but also seen fairly easily in brown). The band is presumably caused by the many pigment-filled macrophages in this region of stroma. In predisposed eyes, because of a basic abnormality of the iris pigment epithelium, an important factor in the loss of posterior iris pigment may be the rubbing between anterior packets of zonules and peripheral iris.

3. Iridodonesis may be present.
4. Krukenberg's spindle consists of a vertical band of melanin pigment phagocytosed by the central and inferior corneal endothelium, most often bilateral.

Pigment may be released into the aqueous compartment after pupillary dilatation or after physical exercise. When a Krukenberg's spindle is present unilaterally, ocular trauma may be the cause.

5. The pigment is deposited on the iris surface, lens, zonules, and in the trabecular meshwork.

The disease seems to ameliorate with increasing age in some patients. In these patients, the corneal and trabecular meshwork pigmentation decreases. The picture resembles that of pseudoexfoliation of the lens. Rarely, the pigment dispersion syndrome can coexist with the pseudoexfoliation syndrome.

6. Incidence of neural retinal detachments is increased in patients who have pigment dispersion syndrome, and there is an increased incidence of retinal lattice degeneration.

Glaucoma seems to be present in approximately 10% of cases. Perhaps the relationship of the iris pigment epithelial defect to the glaucoma is a matter of two independent gene loci that are very close together on the same chromosome and tend to be inherited together, but not necessarily so. Furthermore, patients with pigment dispersion syndrome and glaucoma are the same age (approximately 49 years) as patients with the syndrome but without glaucoma. If glaucoma resulted from the dispersion of pigment, patients with glaucoma should have a higher average age than patients without glaucoma. The number of aqueous melanin granules (measured with the laser-flare cell meter) correlates with increased IOP.

7. Compared with normal eyes, pigment dispersion syndrome eyes have a larger iris, a mid peripheral posterior iris concavity that increases with accommodation, a more posterior iris insertion, increased

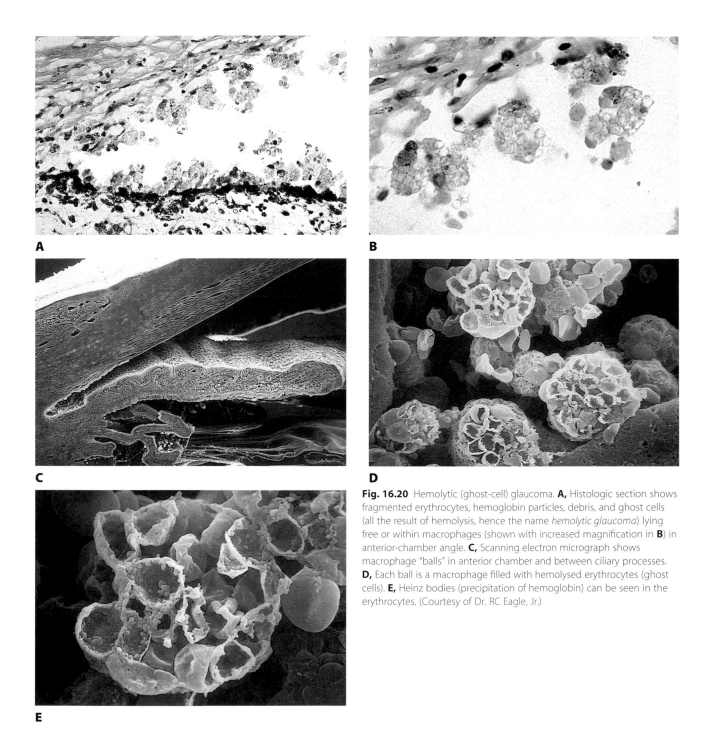

Fig. 16.20 Hemolytic (ghost-cell) glaucoma. **A,** Histologic section shows fragmented erythrocytes, hemoglobin particles, debris, and ghost cells (all the result of hemolysis, hence the name *hemolytic glaucoma*) lying free or within macrophages (shown with increased magnification in **B**) in anterior-chamber angle. **C,** Scanning electron micrograph shows macrophage "balls" in anterior chamber and between ciliary processes. **D,** Each ball is a macrophage filled with hemolysed erythrocytes (ghost cells). **E,** Heinz bodies (precipitation of hemoglobin) can be seen in the erythrocytes. (Courtesy of Dr. RC Eagle, Jr.)

iridolenticular contact that is reversed by inhibition of blinking, possibly an inherent weakness of iris pigment epithelium.

    a. The most likely cause of the aforementioned constellation of findings is a gene affecting some aspect of the development of the middle third of the eye.

8. Histologically, the posterior layer of iris pigment epithelium, mainly at the junction of middle and peripheral thirds of the iris, atrophies in foci that correspond to the clinically observed peripheral foci of increased iris transillumination.

    a. The dilator muscle may be dysplastic, present in excessive amounts, atrophic, or absent.

    b. The adjacent iris stroma contains pigment-filled macrophages.

    c. Neuroepithelial melanin granules are widely distributed in the endothelium of both the posterior cornea (Krukenberg's spindle) and the trabecular meshwork.

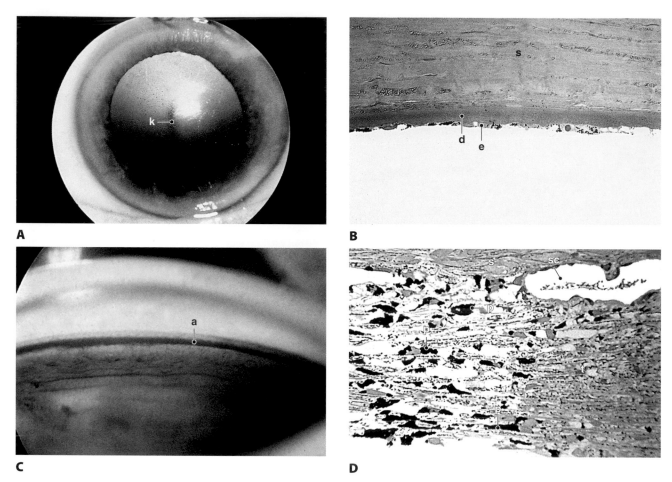

A **B**

C **D**

Fig. 16.21 Pigment dispersion syndrome. **A,** A Krukenberg's spindle (k) is seen as a vertical linear deposition of melanin pigment in the central inferior cornea. **B,** Granules of melanin pigment are present in corneal endothelial cells (s, stroma; d, Descemet's membrane; e, endothelium containing pigment). **C,** The anterior-chamber angle (a) is deeply pigmented. **D,** Melanin pigment (p) is present in the endothelial cells lining the beams of the trabecular meshwork (t) (s, stroma; sc, Schlemm's canal).

9. Mutations in the genes encoding for melanosomal proteins can cause pigmentary glaucoma and iris stromal atrophy in a DBA/2J mouse model. These findings suggest that pigment production and mutant melanosomal protein genes may contribute to human pigmentary glaucoma.
10. Familial occurrence of pigment dispersion syndrome has been reported.
11. The cause is uncertain, but the pigmentary changes may be coincidental to the glaucoma instead of its cause.

G. Pseudoexfoliation syndrome (see pp. 368–373 in Chapter 10)

H. Secondary to uveal malignant melanomas (Figs 16.23 to 16.25; see Table 16.2)
1. Seeded malignant melanoma cells (see Fig. 16.23) may block the anterior-chamber angle.

> Similar seeding can occur with metastatic neoplastic cells or juvenile xanthogranuloma cells. Rarely, an aggressive

nevus can infiltrate an open angle, resulting in secondary open-angle glaucoma.

2. A ring malignant melanoma (see Fig. 16.24) may directly invade the anterior-chamber angle structures and block the open angle. Therefore, glaucoma my be the presenting finding.

> A ring melanoma arises from the root of the iris and anterior ciliary body for 360° and should not be confused with a segmental iris or ciliary body melanoma that may seed the anterior-chamber angle for 360°.

3. Melanomalytic glaucoma (see Fig. 16.25)
   a. Necrosis (partial or complete) of a malignant melanoma (or a melanocytoma), usually of the ciliary body, causes the liberation of melanin pigment.

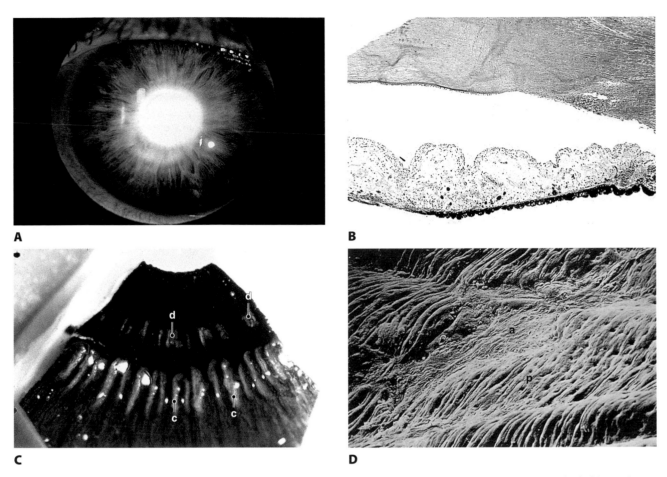

Fig. 16.22 Pigment dispersion syndrome. **A,** Extensive increased iris transillumination is present, predominantly in the middle third of the iris, best seen toward the left of the figure. **B,** The area of increased transillumination corresponds to the area of loss of pigment epithelium from the back of the iris. **C,** The gross specimen confirms this, as does **D,** a scanning electron microscopic view of the posterior surface of the iris (d, defects of pigment epithelium in iris; c, ciliary processes; a, area devoid of pigment epithelium; p, posterior surface of iris).

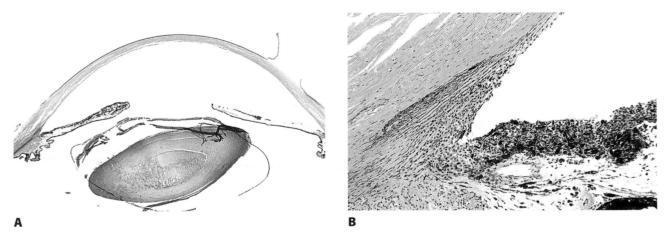

Fig. 16.23 Open-angle glaucoma secondary to uveal melanoma. **A,** Histologic section shows seeding of iris melanoma on to anterior surface of iris. **B,** Melanoma cells also cover angle recess and trabecular meshwork. (From Yanoff M: *Am J Ophthalmol* 70:898. © Elsevier 1970.)

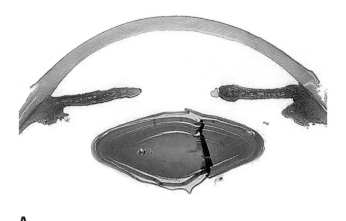

A

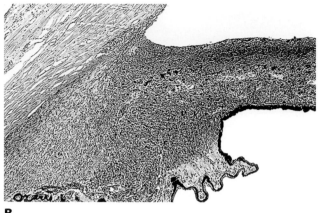

B

Fig. 16.24 Open-angle glaucoma secondary to uveal melanoma. **A,** Histologic section shows a ring melanoma involving the iris root and anterior ciliary body for 360° and invading the anterior-chamber angle structures. **B,** Increased magnification shows the melanoma cells invading the trabecular meshwork. (From Yanoff M: *Am J Ophthalmol* 70:898 © Elsevier 1970.)

A similar process, called *melanocytomalytic* glaucoma, has been reported with necrotic iris melanocytomas.

    b. The liberated melanin induces phagocytosis by macrophages.
    c. The melanin-laden macrophages then obstruct the open angle of the anterior chamber.
  4. Epithelialization or endothelialization of anterior-chamber angle (see pp. 119–120 in Chapter 5)
  5. Diffuse iris melanoma presents with glaucoma in 56% of cases, and 32% of cases have had laser or incisional glaucoma surgery at the time of presentation.
 II. Secondary to damaged outflow channels
  A. Old uveitis may result in "scarring" of the tissues in the drainage angle.
  B. Repeated attacks of acute closed-angle glaucoma may cause damage to the trabecular meshwork so that, even though the angle appears open, the facility of outflow is decreased.
  C. Repeated hyphema may damage the aqueous outflow tissue.
  D. In both siderosis and hemosiderosis bulbi, iron has a "toxic," sclerosing effect on tissues within the drainage angle.
  E. Trauma
    1. It may have a direct effect on the tissues of the drainage angle by inducing scarring (sclerosis) of the trabecular meshwork, or it may cause a postcontusion deformity of the anterior-chamber angle (see pp. 136–138 in Chapter 5).
    2. Iris melanocytes may proliferate over the trabecular meshwork and occlude an open anterior-chamber angle.
  F. Cornea guttata (see p. 305 in Chapter 8)
  G. In early iris neovascularization, before peripheral anterior synechiae form, an open anterior-chamber angle may be obstructed by an almost transparent, delicate fibrovascular membrane arising from vessels near the iris root or near the anterior face of the ciliary body.
 III. Secondary to corneoscleral and extraocular diseases such as interstitial keratitis, orbital venous thrombosis, cavernous sinus thrombosis, carotid–cavernous fistula, encircling band after retinal detachment surgery, retrobulbar mass, leukemia, and mediastinal syndromes

Carotid–cavernous fistula may also cause closed-angle glaucoma by a pupillary-block mechanism.

 IV. Unknown mechanisms (usually reversible)
  A. Corticosteroid-induced glaucoma (either oral or inhaled)
    1. Aqueous humor endothelin-1 concentration is increased in human and animal models of POAG. This increased concentration could result in increased release of nitric oxide, thereby resulting in increased contraction and decreased relaxation of the trabecular meshwork, and contribute to a decline in conventional aqueous outflow and the increased IOP seen in patients taking topical steroids.
    2. Glucocorticoids can induce myocilin production in human and monkey trabecular meshwork cells and tissues.
    3. Dexamethasone treatment does not enhance myocilin expression in corneal fibroblasts as it does in trabecular meshwork cells, and it is not associated with mitochondria in corneal fibroblasts. These differences may explain the differential impact of steroids on the trabecular meshwork compared to other ocular tissues, even though myocilin is expressed in those tissues.
  B. α-Chymotrypsin-induced glaucoma

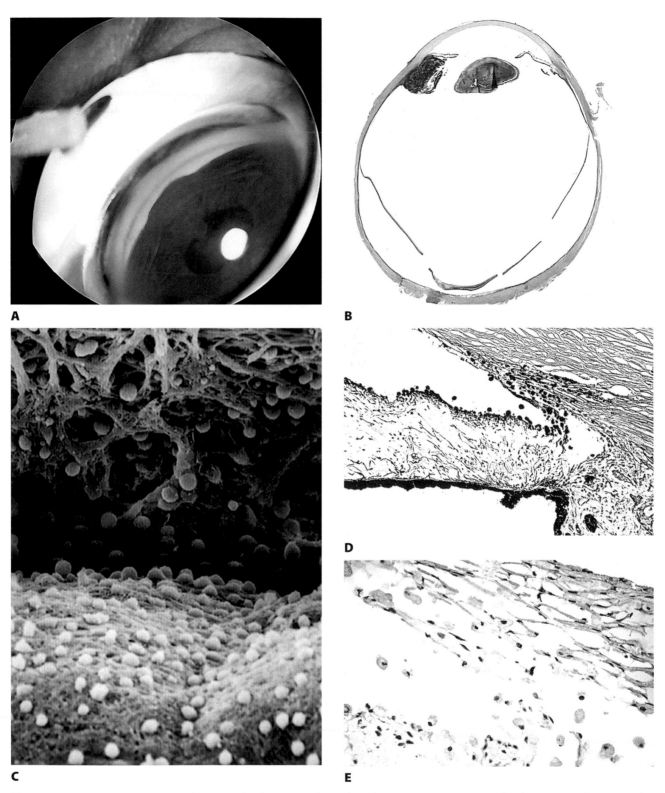

A

B

C

D

E

Fig. 16.25 Open-angle glaucoma secondary to uveal melanoma—melanomalytic glaucoma. **A,** Patient presented with symptoms of acute closed-angle glaucoma. By gonioscopy, angle wide open, except 8 to 9 o'clock, in area of tumor. Eye enucleated because intraocular pressure uncontrollable. **B,** Histologic section shows small, completely necrotic ciliary body melanoma. **C,** Scanning electron micrograph shows many round "balls" on trabecular meshwork (*top*), angle recess (middle dark groove), and anterior iris surface (*bottom*). **D,** Histologic section shows an open anterior-chamber angle heavily infiltrated by pigment-laden macrophages (balls seen in **C**). It is impossible to tell whether the large pigmented cells are melanoma cells or macrophages. **E,** Bleached section shows clearly that cells have macrophagic features (abundant cytoplasm and tiny, innocuous nuclei). (Modified with permission from Yanoff M, Scheie HG: *Arch Ophthalmol* 84:471, 1970. © American Medical Association. All rights reserved.)

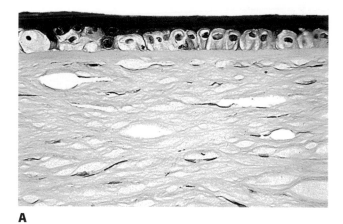

A

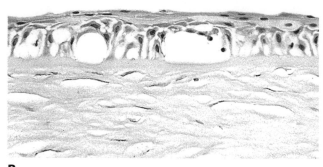

B

Fig. 16.26 *Corneal edema.* **A,** Fluid present in the basal layer of the corneal epithelium causes swelling of the cells. Clinically, this would appear as bedewing. **B,** The edema has spread both within and between the epithelial cells. **C,** Further collection of fluid has caused the entire epithelium to lift off from Bowman's membrane (b), forming a large bleb. The bleb may become ulcerated and even lead to corneal infection and perforation (see also Figs 16.27 and 16.28). (**A,** trichrome.)

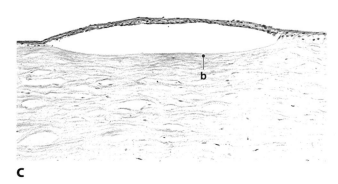

C

TISSUE CHANGES CAUSED BY ELEVATED INTRAOCULAR PRESSURE

Cornea (Figs 16.26 to 16.28; see also Fig. 8.50)

I. Edema of stroma and epithelium (see Fig. 16.26)
II. Epithelial bullae (bullous keratopathy; see Fig. 16.26)
III. Corneal ulcer
   A. The blebs of bullous keratopathy may rupture, causing the cornea to be susceptible to infection and corneal ulcer.
   B. The corneal ulcer can result in corneal perforation, and even in an expulsive hemorrhage (see Figs 10.5, 16.27, and 16.28).
   C. Corneal ulcer and associated sequelae are common findings in blind, painful, glaucomatous eyes that come to enucleation.
IV. Degenerative subepithelial pannus
   A. Histologically, the corneal edema is best seen in its earliest stage as a swelling and pallor of the basal layer of the epithelium.
   B. Increased edema causes the basal layer of cells to swell more (clinically observed as corneal bedewing), causing a form of microcystoid degeneration.
   C. The edema then spreads to overlying (anterior) epithelial cells.
   D. Further accentuation of the edema ruptures the cell membranes, and macrocysts result.
   E. At the same time, the epithelium is lifted off the underlying Bowman's membrane by collections of fluid.
      1. The overlying epithelium then appears irregular with areas of atrophy and hypertrophy.
      2. The basement membrane of the epithelium is usually irregular.
   F. With chronic edema, fibrous or fibrovascular tissue grows between epithelium and Bowman's membrane, and forms a pannus.
   G. Ultimately, the vascular component regresses completely, any inflammatory cells disappear, and a relatively acellular scar, a *degenerative pannus*, remains between epithelium and Bowman's membrane.
V. Atrophy of epithelium and endothelium
VI. Hypertrophy of corneal nerves
VII. Corneal vascularization (Fig. 16.29)

Anterior-chamber angle

I. "Scarring" (sclerosis) of the tissues of the drainage angle results from chronic glaucoma.

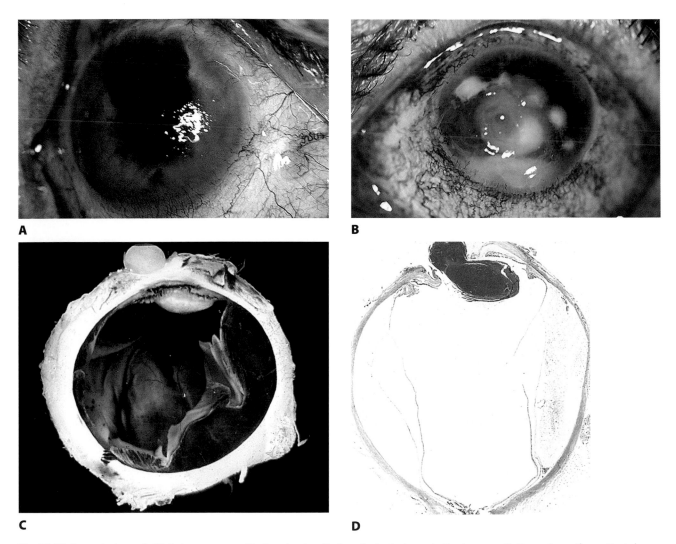

Fig. 16.27 Corneal edema. **A,** Clinical appearance of bullous keratopathy in patient who has aphakic glaucoma. **B,** Cornea in another patient shows that blebs have ruptured and have become infected. Note hypopyon. **C,** Gross specimen shows that infection of the ruptured corneal blebs has resulted in corneal perforation and lens prolapse. Sudden decrease in intraocular pressure after perforation has ruptured ciliary arteries and caused massive, expulsive choroidal hemorrhage. **D,** Histologic section shows lens prolapsed through the ulcerated and ruptured cornea; note elasticity of indented lens. A massive choroidal hemorrhage is seen. (**A** and **B,** Courtesy of Dr. HG Scheie.)

II. Proliferation of corneal endothelium over the anterior-chamber angle (e.g., in postcontusion deformity of the anterior-chamber angle) or over the pseudoangle formed by a peripheral anterior synechia is commonly seen in enucleated glaucomatous eyes.

Iris

I. Dispersion of pigment onto and from the iris

Melanin pigment liberated from pigment epithelium or uveal melanocytes does not usually exist "free" on surfaces but is present in cells (e.g., in macrophages in iris, or in endothelium on posterior cornea or trabecular meshwork).

II. Fibrosis of stroma

III. Atrophy or necrosis of stroma dilator muscle and pigment epithelium

IV. Ectropion uveae (usually secondary to neovascularization of iris*)

V. Iris hyperpigmentation is a side-effect of topical prostaglandin therapy for glaucoma. Histologic evaluation of involved irides demonstrates increased melanin production by melanocytes without melanocytic proliferation or atypia.

---

*Neovascularization of the iris is rare, if it occurs at all, in cases of primary open-angle glaucoma that have not had intraocular surgery or retinal vascular occlusion. It may occur in cases of primary closed-angle glaucoma, even without intraocular surgery, but with central retinal vein thrombosis.

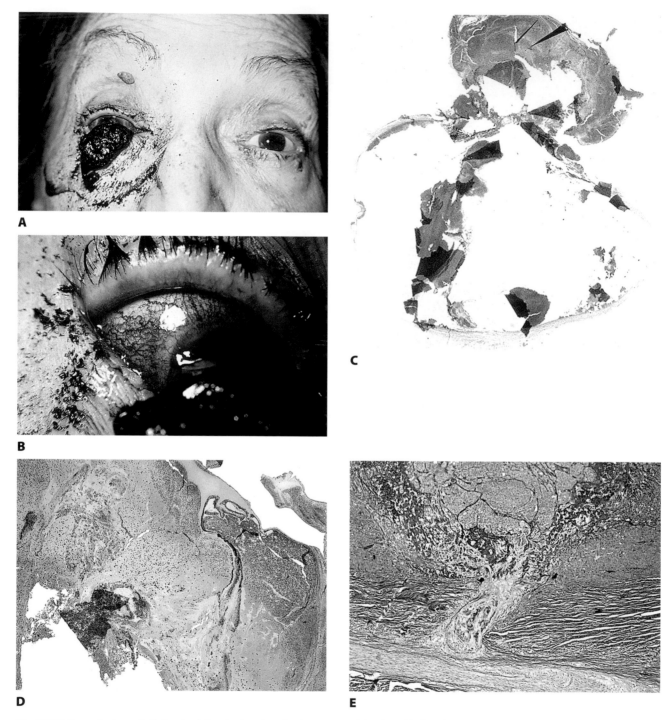

Fig. 16.28 Corneal edema. **A,** Patient had chronic closed-angle glaucoma, and developed bullous keratopathy and secondary infection. Infected cornea perforated, leading to massive expulsive hemorrhage. **B,** Hemorrhagic, mushroom-shaped mass comes through the ulcerated and perforated cornea, and protrudes between the lids. **C,** Enucleated eye is filled with blood that has ruptured through an extensive corneal perforation. **D,** Increased magnification shows retina in the hemorrhagic mass external to the eye. **E,** Elastic stain demonstrates that the posterior ciliary artery is seemingly torn as it enters the choroid from the suprachoroidal space. (From Winslow RL *et al.: Arch Ophthalmol* 92:33, 1974, with permission. © American Medical Association. All rights reserved.)

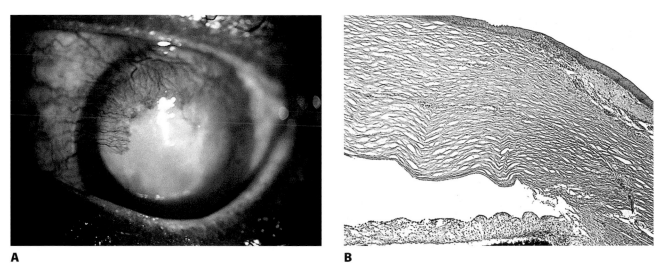

Fig. 16.29 Corneal vascularization. **A,** Marked corneal vascularization in eye that had glaucoma and infected bullous keratopathy. **B,** Histologic section shows a large blood vessel in the corneal mid-stroma.

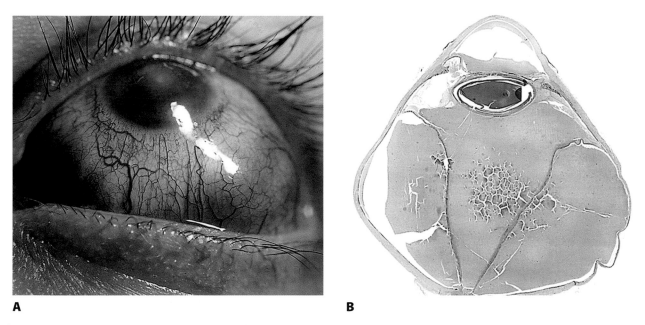

Fig. 16.30 Scleral staphyloma. **A,** Clinical appearance of equatorial staphyloma. **B,** Equatorial sclera is quite ectatic, especially on right side. Because ectatic sclera is lined by the underlying uvea (choroid), it is called a *scleral staphyloma*.

Ciliary Body

    I. Fibrosis and hyalinization of the core of fibrovascular tissue in the ciliary processes of the pars plicata

    II. Atrophy of pars plicata

Lens

Cataract, especially after glaucoma surgery or after an acute attack of glaucoma (e.g., glaukomflecken with acute closed-angle glaucoma)

Sclera

Ectasia (thinning) or, if lined by uvea, staphyloma (Fig. 16.30)

Neural Retina (Fig. 16.31)

    I. Degeneration of inner layers, predominantly nerve fiber and ganglion cell layer.

      A. Mechanisms that have been proposed for the apoptotic cell death of RGC in glaucoma include neurotrophic factor deprivation, glutamate excitotoxicity, ischemia, glial cell activation, and immune response.

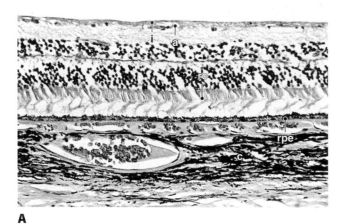
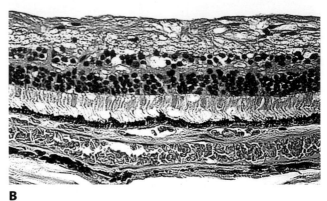

A **B**

Fig. 16.31 Retina. **A,** Histologic section of the nasal neural retina shows that only an occasional ganglion cell remains instead of the normally seen continuous single layer. The atrophic inner neural retinal layers are still identifiable, unlike the neural retina after central retinal artery occlusion, where the inner layers appear as a homogeneous scar (i, internal limiting membrane; a, atrophic nerve fiber and ganglion cell layers; rc, rods and cones; rpe, retinal pigment epithelium; c, choroid). **B,** Another case shows more marked glaucomatous atrophy of the inner layers (compare with the inner nuclear layer in **A**).

B. The presence of the proline form of *p53* codon 72 appears to be a significant risk factor for the development of POAG. The *p53* gene helps regulate apoptosis, which contributes to the pathobiology of glaucomatous optic neuropathy.

C. Blocking RGC apoptosis utilizing recombinant adeno-associated viral vector coding for human baculoviral IAP repeat-containing protein-4 (BIRC4), which is a potent caspase inhibitor, promotes optic nerve axon survival in a rat model for glaucoma.

II. Retinal ganglion cell loss (particularly affecting small ganglion cells and those directly adjacent to the optic nerve) may be present in glaucoma. The implications for these findings on the pathobiology of glaucoma are not known; however, these ganglion cells may influence blood flow regulation in the lamina cribrosa region of the optic nerve.

A link exists between apoptosis of RGC, matrix metalloproteinase (MMP-9), laminin degradation, and IOP. Abnormal ECM remodeling in the glaucomatous retina may relate to RGC death. Corpora amylacea in the RGC layer may decrease in number with advancing glaucoma. Autopsy eyes from one patient with normal-tension glaucoma showed immunoglobulins G and A deposition in the RGC, and inner and outer retinal layers, and apoptotic retinal cell death. The significance of these findings is not clear.

III. Photoreceptors are not lost in substantial numbers in POAG.

IV. There is gliosis, especially with secondary glaucoma.

V. Changes in macular thickness and volume correlate with the severity of glaucoma.

Optic Nerve

I. The normal optic nerve fiber count decreases with advancing age, with a mean annual loss of approximately 400 000 fibers; this process is accelerated by glaucoma.

II. Optic nerve atrophy results from a loss of the nerve fibers of the inner neural retina and optic nerve.

A. Whether the neural damage is caused by local or distant astrocytic damage or by vascular insufficiency is not known.

1. Astrocyte metabolism related to neurosteroids, MMP-9, myocilin/*TIGR* and other cellular products are altered in glaucoma or in cells cultured at elevated IOP.

B. Also unknown is the exact effect or role the blockage of axoplasmic transport (flow) has on the process.

C. Although optic nerve cupping and atrophy result from glaucoma, some cupping may not result from permanent axonal damage. For example, cupping may be reversible in congenital glaucoma following normalization of IOP, particularly in younger patients. Improved neural rim area can also be seen after IOP normalization, even in adults.

D. Polymorphisms in the *OPA1* gene may be associated with the optic neuropathy of normal-tension glaucoma. Nevertheless, phenotypic differences are not noted in normal-tension glaucoma patients with and without *OPA1* (IVS 8 +4 C/T; +32T/C) genotype. The *OPA1* locus is also associated with autosomal-dominant optic atrophy, which can be confused with normal-tension glaucoma.

E. Increased mRNA and protein levels for the iron-regulating proteins transferrin, ceruloplasmin, and fer-

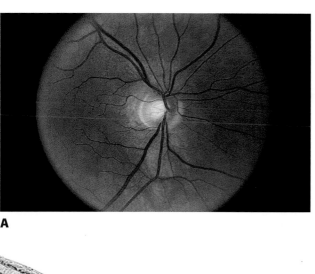

A

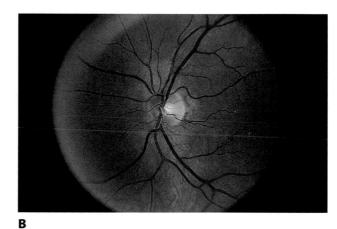

B

Fig. 16.32 Glaucoma cupping. Right (**A**) and left (**B**) eyes of the same patient. The right optic nerve is cupped, secondary to glaucoma. The left optic nerve is less involved (or "less cupped"). **C,** The optic nerve head is deeply cupped. Atrophy of the optic nerve is determined by comparing the diameter of the optic nerve at its internal surface and posteriorly, where it should double in size. Here it is the same size because of a loss of axons and myelin, which also causes an increase in size of the subarachnoid space and a proliferation of glial cells, resulting in an increased cellularity of the optic nerve.

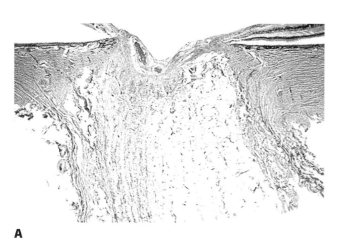

C

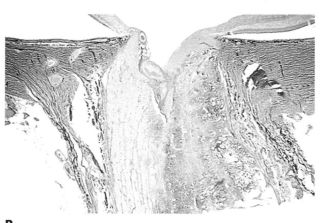

A

B

Fig. 16.33 Cavernous (Schnabel's) optic atrophy. **A,** The optic nerve head shows cupping of its surface and large cystic spaces in its parenchyma on right side. **B,** Special stain to test for the presence of acid mucopolysaccharides (AMP) shows that the cystic spaces are filled with a blue-staining material. Predigestion of the section with hyaluronidase produced empty spaces, demonstrating that they had contained hyaluronic acid. (**B,** AMP stain.)

ritin are present in glaucoma, suggesting a role for the involvement of iron, copper, and associated antioxidant systems in its pathogenesis.

III. Atrophy results in loss of substance from the optic nerve head, leading to cupping (Fig. 16.32) or, if the loss is extensive, to excavation of the optic nerve head. Cup enlargement, in turn, results in increased visibility of lamina cribrosa pores.

IV. Cavernous (Schnabel's) optic atrophy (Fig. 16.33) consists of cystoid spaces, usually posterior to scleral lamina cribrosa. The cystoid spaces are filled with hyaluronic acid (see p. 514 in Chapter 13).

Vitreous passes through the atrophic optic nerve head into the substance of the scleral portion of the optic nerve. Changes resembling Schnabel's optic atrophy have been seen in nonglaucomatous eyes that contain primary or metastatic melanomas.

V. Parapapillary chorioretinal atrophy is associated with glaucoma.
   A. Alpha parapapillary chorioretinal atrophy shows irregular hypopigmentation and hyperpigmentation.
   B. Beta parapapillary chorioretinal atrophy shows complete chorioretinal atrophy with visible large choroidal vessels and sclera.

BIBLIOGRAPHY

Normal Anatomy

Dietlein TS, Luke C, Jacobi PC *et al.*: Individual factors influencing trabecular morphology in glaucoma patients undergoing filtration surgery. *J Glaucoma* 11:197, 2002

Fine BS, Yanoff M: *Ocular Histology: A Text and Atlas*, 2nd edn. Hagerstown, PA, Harper & Row, 1979:251–269

Gould DB, Smith RS, John SW: Anterior segment development relevant to glaucoma. *Int J Dev Biol* 48:1015, 2004

Hamard P, Valtot F, Sourdille P *et al.*: Confocal microscopic examination of trabecular meshwork removed during ab externo trabeculectomy. *Br J Ophthalmol* 86:1046, 2002

Hann CR, Springett MJ, Wang X *et al.*: Ultrastructural localization of collagen IV, fibronectin, and laminin in the trabecular meshwork of normal and glaucomatous eyes. *Ophthalmic Res* 33:314, 2001

John SW, Anderson MG, Smith RS: Mouse genetics: a tool to help unlock the mechanisms of glaucoma. *J Glaucoma* 8:400, 1999

Johnson M, Chan D, Read AT *et al.*: The pore density in the inner wall endothelium of Schlemm's canal of glaucomatous eyes. *Invest Ophthalmol Vis Sci* 43:2950, 2002

Jonas JB, Budde WM, Panda-Jones S: Ophthalmoscopic evaluation of the optic nerve head. *Surv Ophthalmol* 43:293, 1999

Klenkler B, Sheardown H: Growth factors in the anterior segment: role in tissue maintenance, wound healing and ocular pathology. *Exp Eye Res* 79:677, 2004

Yanoff M, Fine BS: *Ocular Pathology: A Color Atlas*, 2nd edn. New York, Gower Medical Publishing, 1992:16.2, 16.5

Zhang X, Wang N, Schroeder A *et al.*: Expression of adenylate cyclase subtypes II and IV in the human outflow pathway. *Invest Ophthalmol Vis Sci* 41:998, 2000

Introduction

Aghaian E, Choe JE, Lin S *et al.*: Central corneal thickness of Caucasians, Chinese, Hispanics, Filipinos, African Americans, and Japanese in a glaucoma clinic. *Ophthalmology* 111:2211, 2004

Ahmed II, Feldman F, Kucharczyk W *et al.*: Neuroradiologic screening in normal-pressure glaucoma: study results and literature review. *J Glaucoma* 11:279, 2002

Aung T, Nolan WP, Machin D *et al.*: Anterior chamber depth and the risk of primary angle closure in 2 East Asian populations. *Arch Ophthalmol* 123:527, 2005

Aung T, Rezaie T, Okada K *et al.*: Clinical features and course of patients with glaucoma with the E50K mutation in the optineurin gene. *Invest Ophthalmol Vis Sci* 46:2816, 2005

Bashford KP, Shafranov G, Tauber S *et al.*: Considerations of glaucoma in patients undergoing corneal refractive surgery. *Surv Ophthalmol* 50:245, 2005

Bennett SR, Alward WLM, Folberg R: An autosomal dominant form of low-tension glaucoma. *Am J Ophthalmol* 108:238, 1989

Buono LM, Foroozan R, Sergott RC *et al.*: Is normal tension glaucoma actually an unrecognized hereditary optic neuropathy? New evidence from genetic analysis. *Curr Opin Ophthalmol* 13:362, 2002

Chang TC, Congdon NG, Wojciechowski R *et al.*: Determinants and heritability of intraocular pressure and cup-to-disc ratio in a defined older population. *Ophthalmology* 112:1186, 2005

Chauhan BC, Hutchison DM, Leblanc RP *et al.*: Central corneal thickness and progression of the visual field and optic disc in glaucoma. *Br J Ophthalmol* 89:1008, 2005

Collaborative Normal-Tension Glaucoma Study Group: Natural history of normal-tension glaucoma. *Ophthalmology* 108:247, 2001

Congdon N, Wang F, Tielsch JM: Issues in the epidemiology and population-based screening of primary angle-closure glaucoma. *Surv Ophthalmol* 36:411, 1992

Craig JE, Baird PN, Healey DL *et al.*: Evidence for genetic heterogeneity within eight glaucoma families, with the GLC1A Gln368STOP mutation being an important phenotypic modifier. *Ophthalmology* 108:1607, 2001

Dielemans I, Vingerling JR, Wolfs RCW *et al.*: The prevalence of primary open-angle glaucoma in a population-based study in the Netherlands: The Rotterdam Study. *Ophthalmology* 101:1851, 1994

Doyle A, Bensaid A, Lachkar Y: Central corneal thickness and vascular risk factors in normal tension glaucoma. *Acta Ophthalmol Scand* 83:191, 2005

Evereklioglu C, Madenci E, Bayazit YA *et al.*: Central corneal thickness is lower in osteogenesis imperfecta and negatively correlates with the presence of blue sclera. *Ophthalmic Physiol Opt* 22:511, 2002

Hewitt AW, Cooper RL: Relationship between corneal thickness and optic disc damage in glaucoma. *Clin Exp Ophthalmol* 33:158, 2005

Hiller R, Kahn HA: Blindness from glaucoma. *Am J Ophthalmol* 80:62, 1975

Hiller R, Pogdor MJ, Sperduto RD *et al.*: High intraocular pressure and survival: The Framingham Studies. *Am J Ophthalmol* 128:440, 1999

Ishida K, Yamamoto T, Sugiyama K *et al.*: Disc hemorrhage is a significantly negative prognostic factor in normal-tension glaucoma. *Am J Ophthalmol* 129:707, 2000

Jonas JB, Stroux A, Velten I *et al.*: Central corneal thickness correlated with glaucoma damage and rate of progression. *Invest Ophthalmol Vis Sci* 46:1269, 2005

Kim JW, Chen PP: Central corneal pachymetry and visual field progression in patients with open-angle glaucoma. *Ophthalmology* 111:2126, 2004

Klein BEK, Klein R, Sponsel WE *et al.*: Prevalence of glaucoma. *Ophthalmology* 99:1499, 1992

Lee GA, Khaw PT, Ficker LA *et al.*: The corneal thickness and intraocular pressure story: where are we now? *Clin Exp Ophthalmol* 30:334, 2002

Lehmann OJ, Tuft S, Brice G *et al.*: Novel anterior segment phenotypes resulting from forkhead gene alterations: evidence for cross-species conservation of function. *Invest Ophthalmol Vis Sci* 44:2627, 2003

Leske MC, Connell AMS, Wu S-Y *et al.*: Incidence of open-angle glaucoma: The Barbados Eye Studies. *Arch Ophthalmol* 119:89, 2001

Martus P, Stroux A, Budde WM *et al.*: Predictive factors for progressive optic nerve damage in various types of chronic open-angle glaucoma. *Am J Ophthalmol* 139:999, 2005

Muir KW, Jin J, Freedman SF: Central corneal thickness and its relationship to intraocular pressure in children. *Ophthalmology* 111:2220, 2004

Mukesh BN, McCarty CA, Rait JL *et al.*: Five-year incidence of open-angle glaucoma: the visual impairment project. *Ophthalmology* 109:1047, 2002

Parsa CF, Silva ED, Sundin OH *et al.*: Redefining papillorenal syndrome: an underdiagnosed cause of ocular and renal morbidity. *Ophthalmology* 108:738, 2001

Racette L, Wilson MR, Zangwill LM *et al.*: Primary open-angle glaucoma in blacks: a review. *Surv Ophthalmol* 48:295, 2003

Schumer RA, Podos SM: The nerve of glaucoma! *Arch Ophthalmol* 112:37, 1994

Shih CY, Graff Zivin JS, Trokel SL *et al.*: Clinical significance of central corneal thickness in the management of glaucoma. *Arch Ophthalmol* 122:1270, 2004

Sullivan-Mee M, Halverson KD, Saxon GB *et al.*: The relationship between central corneal thickness-adjusted intraocular pressure and glaucomatous visual-field loss. *Optometry* 76:228, 2005

Tielsch JM, Katz J, Quigley HA *et al.*: Diabetes, intraocular pressure, and primary open-angle glaucoma in the Baltimore Eye Study. *Ophthalmology* 102:48, 1995

Tielsch JM, Sommer A, Katz J *et al.*: Racial variations in the prevalence of primary open-angle glaucoma. *JAMA* 266:369, 1991

Toda Y, Tang S, Kashiwagi K *et al.*: Mutations in the optineurin gene in Japanese patients with primary open-angle glaucoma and normal tension glaucoma. *Am J Med Genet A* 125:1, 2004

Tonnu PA, Ho T, Newson T *et al.*: The influence of central corneal thickness and age on intraocular pressure measured by pneumotonometry, non-contact tonometry, the Tono-Pen XL, and Goldmann applanation tonometry. *Br J Ophthalmol* 89:851, 2005

Varma R, Ying-Lai M, Francis BA *et al.*: Prevalence of open-angle glaucoma and ocular hypertension in Latinos: the Los Angeles Latino Eye Study. Ophthalmology 111:1437, 2004

Walker JH, Buys Y, Trope G *et al.*: Association between corneal thickness, mean intraocular pressure, disease stability and severity, and cost of treatment in glaucoma: a Canadian analysis. *Curr Med Res Opin* 21:489, 2005

Whitson JT, Liang C, Godfrey DG *et al.*: Central corneal thickness in patients with congenital aniridia. *Eye Contact Lens* 31:221, 2005

Wilensky J: Racial influences in glaucoma. *Ann Ophthalmol* 9:1545, 1977

Wolfs RCW, Borger PH, Ramrattan RS *et al.*: Changing views on open-angle glaucoma: definitions and prevalences: The Rotterdam study. *Invest Ophthalmol Vis Sci* 41:3309, 2000

Wolfs RCW, Klaver CCW, Ramrattan RS *et al.*: Genetic risk of primary open-angle glaucoma: Population-based aggregation study. *Arch Ophthalmol* 116:1640, 1998

Wunderlich K, Golubnitschaja O, Pache M *et al.*: Increased plasma levels of 20S proteasome alpha-subunit in glaucoma patients: an observational pilot study. *Mol Vis* 8:431–5.:431, 2002

Yagci R, Eksioglu U, Midillioglu I *et al.*: Central corneal thickness in primary open angle glaucoma, pseudoexfoliative glaucoma, ocular hypertension, and normal population. *Eur J Ophthalmol* 15:324, 2005

Yamamoto T, Iwase A, Araie M *et al.*: The Tajimi Study report 2: prevalence of primary angle closure and secondary glaucoma in a Japanese population. *Ophthalmology* 112:1661, 2005

Zeppieri M, Brusini P, Miglior S: Corneal thickness and functional damage in patients with ocular hypertension. *Eur J Ophthalmol* 15:196, 2005

Normal Outflow: Hypersecretion

Becker B, Keaky GR, Christensen RE: Hypersecretion glaucoma. *Arch Ophthalmol* 56:180, 1956

Impaired Outflow: Congenital Glaucoma

Alward WLM, Kwon YH, Kawase K *et al.*: Evaluation of optineurin sequence variations in 1048 patients with open-angle glaucoma. *Am J Ophthalmol* 136:904, 2003

Angius A, De Giola E, Loi A *et al.*: A novel mutation in the GLCIA gene causes juvenile open-angle glaucoma in 4 families from the Italian region of Puglia. *Arch Ophthalmol* 116:793, 1998

Barkan O: Pathogenesis of congenital glaucoma: gonioscopic and anatomic observations of the anterior chamber in the normal eye and in congenital glaucoma. *Am J Ophthalmol* 40:1, 1955

Bongers EM, Gubler MC, Knoers NV: Nail–patella syndrome. Overview on clinical and molecular findings. *Pediatr Nephrol* 17:703, 2002

Broughton WL, Fine BS, Zimmerman LE: Congenital glaucoma associated with a chromosomal defect: A histologic study. *Arch Ophthalmol* 99:481, 1981

Broughton WL, Rosenbaum KN, Beauchamp GR: Congenital glaucoma and other abnormalities associated with pericentric inversion of chromosome 11. *Arch Ophthalmol* 101:594, 1983

Cibis GW, Tripathi RC: The differential diagnosis of Descemet's tears (Haab's striae) and posterior polymorphous dystrophy bands: A clinicopathologic study. *Ophthalmology* 89:614, 1982

De BI, Walter M, Noel LP: Phenotypic variations in patients with a 1630 A > T point mutation in the PAX6 gene. *Can J Ophthalmol* 39:272, 2004

Descipio C, Schneider L, Young TL *et al.*: Subtelomeric deletions of chromosome 6p: molecular and cytogenetic characterization of three new cases with phenotypic overlap with Ritscher–Schinzel (3C) syndrome. *Am J Med Genet A* 134:3, 2005

Edward D, Al RA, Lewis RA *et al.*: Molecular basis of Peters anomaly in Saudi Arabia. *Ophthalmic Genet* 25:257, 2004

Fine BS, Yanoff M: *Ocular Histology: A Text and Atlas*, 2nd edn. Hagerstown, PA, Harper & Row, 1979:251

Hoskins HD, Shaffer RN, Hetherington J: Anatomical classification of the developmental glaucomas. *Arch Ophthalmol* 102:1331, 1984

Hou JW: Long-term follow-up of Marshall–Smith syndrome: report of one case. *Acta Paediatr Taiwan* 45:232, 2004

Johnson AT, Richards JE, Boehnke M *et al.*: Clinical phenotype of juvenile-onset primary open-angle glaucoma linked to chromosome 1q. *Ophthalmology* 103:808, 1996

Kakiuchi T, Isashiki Y, Nakao K *et al.*: A novel truncating mutation of cytochrome P4501B1 (CYP1B1) gene in primary infantile glaucoma. *Am J Ophthalmol* 128:370, 1999

Kato R, Kishibayashi J, Shimokawa O *et al.*: Congenital glaucoma and Silver–Russell phenotype associated with partial trisomy 7q and monosomy 15q. *Am J Med Genet* 104:319, 2001

Lee WB, Brandt JD, Mannis MJ *et al.*: Aniridia and Brachmann–de Lange syndrome: a review of ocular surface and anterior segment findings. *Cornea* 22:178, 2003

Lichter PR, Richards JE, Boehnke M *et al.*: Juvenile glaucoma linked to the GLCIA gene on chromosome 1q in a Panamanian family. *Am J Ophthalmol* 123:413, 1997

Mullaney PB, Risco JM, Teichmann K *et al.*: Congenital hereditary endothelial dystrophy associated with glaucoma. *Ophthalmology* 102:186, 1995

Payne MS, Nadell JM, Lacassie Y *et al.*: Congenital glaucoma and neurofibromatosis in a monozygotic twin: case report and review of the literature. *J Child Neurol* 18:504, 2003

Rezaie T, Child A, Hitchings R *et al.*: Adult-onset primary open-agnle glaucoma caused by mutations in optineurin. *Science* 295:1077, 2002

Richards JE, Lichter PR, Boehnke M *et al.*: Mapping of a gene for autosomal dominant juvenile-onset open-angle glaucoma to chromosome 1q. *Am J Hum Genet* 54:62, 1994

Smith JL, Stowe FR: The Pierre Robin syndrome (glossoptosis, micrognathia, cleft palate): A review of 39 cases with emphasis on associated ocular lesions. *Pediatrics* 27:128, 1961

Stambolian D, Quinn G, Emanuel BS *et al.*: Congenital glaucoma associated with a chromosomal abnormality. *Am J Ophthalmol* 106:625, 1988

Sweeney E, Fryer A, Mountford R *et al.*: Nail patella syndrome: a review of the phenotype aided by developmental biology. *J Med Genet* 40:153, 2003

Taha D, Barbar M, Kanaan H *et al.*: Neonatal diabetes mellitus, congenital hypothyroidism, hepatic fibrosis, polycystic kidneys, and congenital glaucoma: a new autosomal recessive syndrome? *Am J Med Genet A* 122:269, 2003

Toulement PJ, Urvoy M, Coscas G *et al.*: Association of congenital microcoria with myopia and glaucoma: A study of 23 patients with congenital microcoria. *Ophthalmology* 102:186, 1995

Van BI, Alders M, Allanson J *et al.*: Lymphedema-lymphangiectasia-mental retardation (Hennekam) syndrome: a review. *Am J Med Genet* 112:412, 2002

Vemuganti GK, Sridhar MS, Edward DP *et al.*: Subepithelial amyloid deposits in congenital hereditary endothelial dystrophy: a histopathologic study of five cases. *Cornea* 21:524, 2002

Vidaurri-de la CH, Tamayo-Sanchez L, Duran-McKinster C *et al.*: Phakomatosis pigmentovascularis II A and II B: clinical findings in 24 patients. *J Dermatol* 30:381, 2003

Wiggs J, Auguste J, Allingham RR *et al.*: Lack of association of mutations in optineurin with disease in patients with adult-onset primary open-angle glaucoma. *Arch Ophthalmol* 121:1181, 2003

Wiggs JL, Del Bono EA, Schuman JS *et al.*: Clinical features of five pedigrees genetically linked to the juvenile glaucoma locus on chromosome 1q21-q31. *Ophthalmology* 102:1782, 1995

Impaired Outflow: Primary Closed-Angle

Azuara-Blanco A, Spaeth GL, Araujo SV *et al.*: Plateau iris syndrome associated with multiple ciliary body cysts. *Arch Ophthalmol* 114:666, 1996

Bruno CA, Alward WL: Gonioscopy in primary angle closure glaucoma. *Semin Ophthalmol* 17:59, 2002

Chandler PA: Narrow-angle glaucoma. *Arch Ophthalmol* 47:695, 1952

Chang BM, Liebmann JM, Ritch R: Angle closure in younger patients. *Trans Am Ophthalmol Soc* 100:201, 212, 2002

Dielemans I, deJong PTVM, Stolk R *et al.*: Primary open-angle glaucoma, intraocular pressure, and diabetes mellitus in the general population: The Rotterdam study. *Ophthalmology* 103:1271, 1996

Fine BS, Yanoff M: *Ocular Histology: A Text and Atlas*, 2nd edn. Hagerstown, PA, Harper & Row, 1979:251

Frasson M, Calixto N, Cronemberger S *et al.*: Oculodentodigital dysplasia: study of ophthalmological and clinical manifestations in three boys with probably autosomal recessive inheritance. *Ophthalmic Genet* 25:227, 2004

Fuchs J, Holm K, Vilhelmsen K *et al.*: Hereditary high hypermetropia in the Faroe Islands. *Ophthalmic Genet* 26:9, 2005

Kerman BM, Christensen RE, Foos RY: Angle-closure glaucoma: A clinicopathologic correlation. *Am J Ophthalmol* 76:887, 1973

Leung CK, Chan WM, Ko CY *et al.*: Visualization of anterior-chamber angle dynamics using optical coherence tomography. *Ophthalmology* 112:980, 2005

Shaffer RN, Hoskins HD Jr: Ciliary block (malignant) glaucoma. *Trans Am Acad Ophthalmol Otolaryngol* 85:215, 1978

Sihota R, Lakshmaiah NC, Walia KB *et al.*: The trabecular meshwork in acute and chronic angle closure glaucoma. *Indian J Ophthalmol* 49:255, 2001

Vasconcellos JP, Melo MB, Schimiti RB *et al.*: A novel mutation in the GJA1 gene in a family with oculodentodigital dysplasia. *Arch Ophthalmol* 123:1422, 2005

Wand M, Grant WM, Simmons RJ *et al.*: Plateau iris syndrome. *Trans Am Acad Ophthalmol Otolaryngol* 83:122, 1977

Impaired Outflow: Primary Open-Angle

Alvarado JA, Murphy CG: Outflow obstruction in pigmentary and primary open angle glaucoma. *Arch Ophthalmol* 110:1769, 1992

Alvarado JA, Yun AJ, Murphy CG: Juxtacanalicular tissue in primary open angle glaucoma and in nonglaucomatous normals. *Arch Ophthalmol* 104:1517, 1986

Alward WLM, Fingert JH, Coote MA *et al.*: Clinical features associated with mutations in the chromosome 1 open-angle glaucoma gene (GLC1A). *N Engl J Med* 338:1022, 1998

Anderson DR: Glaucoma: The damage caused by pressure. XLVI Edward Jackson Memorial Lecture. *Am J Ophthalmol* 108:485, 1989

Baird PN, Craig JE, Richardson AJ *et al.*: Analysis of 15 primary open-angle glaucoma families from Australia identifies a founder effect for the Q368STOP mutation of myocilin. *Hum Genet* 112:110, 2003

Bhattacharya SK, Rockwood EJ, Smith SD *et al.*: Proteomics reveal Cochlin deposits associated with glaucomatous trabecular meshwork. *J Biol Chem* 280:6080, 2005

Brubaker RF: Flow of aqueous humor in humans. *Invest Ophthalmol Vis Sci* 32:3145, 1991

Caballero M, Borras T: Inefficient processing of an olfactomedin-deficient myocilin mutant: potential physiological relevance to glaucoma. *Biochem Biophys Res Commun* 282:662, 2001

Charlesworth JC, Dyer TD, Stankovich JM *et al.*: Linkage to 10q22 for maximum intraocular pressure and 1p32 for maximum cup-to-disc ratio in an extended primary open-angle glaucoma pedigree. *Invest Ophthalmol Vis Sci* 46:3723, 2005

Dielemans I, deJong PTVM, Stolk R *et al.*: Primary open-angle glaucoma, intraocular pressure, and diabetes mellitus in the general population: The Rotterdam study. *Ophthalmology* 103:1271, 1996

Drance SM: Low-pressure glaucoma: Enigma and opportunity. *Arch Ophthalmol* 103:1131, 1985

Dunlop AA, Graham SL: Familial amyloidotic polyneuropathy presenting with rubeotic glaucoma. *Clin Exp Ophthalmol* 30:300, 2002

Fine BS: Observations on the drainage angle in man and rhesus monkey: A concept of the pathogenesis of chronic simple glaucoma. A light and electron microscopic study. *Invest Ophthalmol* 3:609, 1964

Fine BS, Yanoff M: *Ocular Histology: A Text and Atlas*, 2nd edn. Hagerstown, PA, Harper & Row, 1979:251

Fine BS, Yanoff M, Stone RA: A clinicopathologic study of four cases of primary open-angle glaucoma compared to normal eyes. *Am J Ophthalmol* 91:88, 1981

Fournier AV, Damjl KJ, Epstein DL *et al.*: Disc elevation in dominant optic atrophy: Differentiation from normal tension glaucoma. *Ophthalmology* 108:1595, 2002

Fujiwara N, Matsuo T, Ohtsuki H: Protein expression, genomic structure, and polymorphisms of oculomedin. *Ophthalmic Genet* 24:141, 2003

Graul TA, Kwon YH, Zimmerman MB *et al.*: A case-control comparison of the clinical characteristics of glaucoma and ocular hypertensive patients with and without the myocilin Gln368Stop mutation. *Am J Ophthalmol* 134:884, 2002

Huang EC, Barocas VH: Active iris mechanics and pupillary block: steady-state analysis and comparison with anatomical risk factors. *Ann Biomed Eng* 32:1276, 2004

Ishida K, Yamamoto T, Sugiyama K et al.: Disc hemorrhage is a significantly negative prognostic factor in normal-tension glaucoma. *Am J Ophthalmol* 129:707, 2000

Ishikawa K, Funayama T, Ohtake Y et al.: Novel MYOC gene mutation, Phe369Leu, in Japanese patients with primary open-angle glaucoma detected by denaturing high-performance liquid chromatography. *J Glaucoma* 13:466, 2004

Izzotti A: DNA damage and alterations of gene expression in chronic-degenerative diseases. *Acta Biochim Pol* 50:145, 2003

Izzotti A, Sacca SC, Cartiglia C et al.: Oxidative deoxyribonucleic acid damage in the eyes of glaucoma patients. *Am J Med* 114:638, 2003

Jansson M, Marknell T, Tomic L et al.: Allelic variants in the MYOC/TIGR gene in patients with primary open-angle, exfoliative glaucoma and unaffected controls. *Ophthalmic Genet* 24:103, 2003

Joe MK, Sohn S, Hur W et al.: Accumulation of mutant myocilins in ER leads to ER stress and potential cytotoxicity in human trabecular meshwork cells. *Biochem Biophys Res Commun* 19:592, 2003

Jonas JB, Naumann GOH: Parapapillary retinal vessel diameter in normal and glaucoma eyes: 11. Correlations. *Invest Ophthalmol Vis Sci* 30:1604, 1989

Jonas JB, Xu L: Optic disk hemorrhages in glaucoma. *Am J Ophthalmol* 118:1, 1994

Jonas JB, Budde WM, Panda-Jones S: Ophthalmoscopic evaluation of the optic nerve head. *Surv Ophthalmol* 43:293, 1999

Jonas JB, Nguyen XN, Naumann GOH: Parapapillary retinal vessel diameter in normal and glaucoma eyes: 1. Morphometric data. *Invest Ophthalmol Vis Sci* 30:1599, 1989

Kanagavalli J, Krishnadas SR, Pandaranayaka E et al.: Evaluation and understanding of myocilin mutations in Indian primary open angle glaucoma patients. *Mol Vis* 9:606, 2003

Kim BS, Savinova OV, Reedy MV et al.: Targeted disruption of the myocilin gene (Myoc) suggests that human glaucoma-causing mutations are gain of function. *Mol Cell Biol* 21:7707, 2001

Liao SY, Ivanov S, Ivanova A et al.: Expression of cell surface transmembrane carbonic anhydrase genes CA9 and CA12 in the human eye: overexpression of CA12 (CAXII) in glaucoma. *J Med Genet* 40:257, 2003

Mackey DA, Healey DL, Fingert JH et al.: Glaucoma phenotype in pedigrees with the myocilin Thr377Met mutation. *Arch Ophthalmol* 121:1172, 2003

Melki R, Belmouden A, Brezin A et al.: Myocilin analysis by DHPLC in French POAG patients: increased prevalence of Q368X mutation. *Hum Mutat* 22:179, 2003

Mitchell P, Cumming RG, Mackey DA: Inhaled corticosteroids, family history, and risk of glaucoma. *Ophthalmology* 106:2301, 1999

Mitchell P, Smith W, Chey T et al.: Open-angle glaucoma and diabetes: The Blue Mountain Eye Study, Australia. *Ophthalmology* 104:712, 1997

Murphy CG, Johnson M, Alvarado JA: Juxtacanalicular tissue in pigmentary and primary open angle glaucoma. *Arch Ophthalmol* 110:1779, 1992

Nakabayashi M: Review of the ischemia hypothesis for ocular hypertension other than congenital glaucoma and closed-angle glaucoma. *Ophthalmologica* 218:344, 2004

Puska P, Lemmela S, Kristo P et al.: Penetrance and phenotype of the Thr377Met Myocilin mutation in a large Finnish family with juvenile- and adult-onset primary open-angle glaucoma. *Ophthalmic Genet* 26:17, 2005

Rosman M, Aung T, Ang LP et al.: Chronic angle-closure with glaucomatous damage: long-term clinical course in a North American population and comparison with an Asian population. *Ophthalmology* 109:2227, 2002

Schulzer M, Drance SM, Carter CJ et al.: Biostatistical evidence for two distinct chronic open angle glaucoma populations. *Br J Ophthalmol* 74:196, 1990

Stone EM, Fingert JH, Alward WLM et al.: Identification of a gene that causes primary open angle glaucoma. *Science* 275:668, 1997

Trifan OC, Traboulsi EI, Stoilova D et al.: A third locus (GLC1D) for adult-onset primary open-angle glaucoma maps to the 8q23 region. *Am J Ophthalmol* 126:17, 1998

Trobe GE, Pavlin CJ, Baumal CR et al.: Malignant glaucoma: Clinical and ultrasound biomicroscopic features. *Ophthalmology* 101:1030, 1994

Wentz-Hunter K, Shen X, Okazaki K et al.: Overexpression of myocilin in cultured human trabecular meshwork cells. *Exp Cell Res* 297:39, 2004

Wirtz MK, Samples JR, Rust K et al.: GLC1F, a new primary open-angle glaucoma locus, maps to 7q35-q36. *Arch Ophthalmol* 117:237, 1999

Impaired Outflow: Secondary Closed-Angle

Agrawal S, Agrawal J, Agrawal TP: Iridoschisis associated with lens subluxation. *J Cataract Refract Surg* 27:2044, 2001

Alvarado JA, Murphy CG, Maglio M et al.: Pathogenesis of Chandler's syndrome, essential iris atrophy and the Cogan–Reese syndrome: I. Alterations of the corneal endothelium. *Invest Ophthalmol Vis Sci* 27:853, 1986

Alvarado JA, Murphy CG, Juster RP et al.: Pathogenesis of Chandler's syndrome, essential iris atrophy and the Cogan–Reese syndrome: II. Estimated age at disease onset. *Invest Ophthalmol Vis Sci* 27:873, 1986

Arthur SN, Mason J, Roberts B et al.: Secondary acute angle-closure glaucoma associated with vitreous hemorrhage after ruptured retinal arterial macroaneurysm. *Am J Ophthalmol* 138:682, 2004

Azuara-Blanco A, Wilson RP, Eagle RC Jr et al.: Pseudocapsulorrhexis in a patient with iridocorneal endothelial syndrome. *Arch Ophthalmol* 117:397, 1999

Badlani VK, Quinones R, Wilensky JT et al.: Angle-closure glaucoma in teenagers. *J Glaucoma* 12:198, 2003

Chandler PA: Atrophy of the stroma of the iris: endothelial dystrophy, corneal edema and glaucoma. *Am J Ophthalmol* 41:607, 1956

Colosi NJ, Yanoff M: Reactive corneal endothelialization. *Am J Ophthalmol* 83:219, 1977

Demirci H, Shields CL, Shields JA et al.: Diffuse iris melanoma: a report of 25 cases. *Ophthalmology* 109:1553, 2002

Doe EA, Budnez DL, Gedde SJ et al.: Long-term surgical outcome of patients with glaucoma secondary to the iridocorneal endothelial syndrome. *Ophthalmology* 108:1789, 2001

Drysler RM: Central retinal vein occlusion and chronic simple glaucoma. *Arch Ophthalmol* 73:659, 1965

Eagle RC Jr, Shields JA: Iridocorneal endothelial syndrome with contralateral guttate endothelial dystrophy: A light and electron microscopic study. *Ophthalmology* 94:862, 1987

Eagle RC Jr, Font RL, Yanoff M et al.: Proliferative endotheliopathy with iris abnormalities: The iridocorneal endothelial syndrome. *Arch Ophthalmol* 97:2104, 1979

Escalona-Benz E, Benz MS, Briggs JW et al.: Uveal melanoma presenting as acute glaucoma: report of two cases. *Am J Ophthalmol* 136:756, 2003

Gogos K, Tyradellis C, Spaulding AG et al.: Iris cyst simulating melanoma. *J AAPOS* 8:502, 2004

Goldberg DE, Freeman WR: Uveitic angle closure glaucoma in a patient with inactive cytomegalovirus retinitis and immune recovery uveitis. *Ophthalmic Surg Lasers* 33:421, 2002

Hirst LW, Bancroft J, Tamauchi K *et al.*: Immunohistochemical pathology of the corneal endothelium in iridocorneal syndrome. *Invest Ophthalmol Vis Sci* 36:820, 1995

Howell DN, Dammas T, Burchette JL Jr *et al.*: Endothelial metaplasia in the iridocorneal endothelial syndrome. *Invest Ophthalmol Vis Sci* 38:1896, 1997

Jakobiec FA, Yanoff M, Mottow L *et al.*: Solitary iris nevus with peripheral anterior synechias and iris endothelialization: A variant of the iris nevus syndrome. *Am J Ophthalmol* 83:884, 1977

Khawly JA, Shields MB: Metastatic carcinoma manifesting as angle-closure glaucoma. *Am J Ophthalmol* 118:1161, 1994

Lafaut BA, Loeys B, Leroy BP *et al.*: Clinical and electrophysiological findings in autosomal dominant vitreoretinochoroidopathy: report of a new pedigree. *Graefes Arch Clin Exp Ophthalmol* 239:575, 2001

Laganowski HC, Muir MGK, Hitchings RA: Glaucoma and the iridocorneal endothelial syndrome. *Arch Ophthalmol* 110:346, 1992

Levy SG, Kirkness CM, Fickler L *et al.*: On the pathology of the iridocorneal-endothelial syndrome: The ultrastructural appearances of "subtotal-ICE." *Eye* 9:318, 1995

Levy SG, McCartney ACE, Baghai MH *et al.*: Pathology of the iridocorneal syndrome: The ICE-cell. *Invest Ophthalmol Vis Sci* 36:2592, 1995

Lichter PR, Shaffer RN: Interstitial keratitis and glaucoma. *Am J Ophthalmol* 68:241, 1969

Lucas-Glass TC, Baratz KH, Nelson LR *et al.*: The contralateral corneal endothelium in the iridocorneal endothelial syndrome. *Arch Ophthalmol* 115:40, 1997

Makley TA, Kapetansky FM: Iris nevus syndrome. *Ann Ophthalmol* 20:311, 1988

Naumann GOH: Yanoff-Syndrom. In Naumann GOH, ed: *Pathologie des Auges.* Berlin, Springer, 1997:628

Rodrigues MM, Spaeth GL, Krachmer JH *et al.*: Iridoschisis associated with glaucoma and bullous keratopathy. *Am J Ophthalmol* 95:73, 1983

Rodrigues MM, Stulting RD, Waring GO III: Clinical, electron microscopic, and immunohistochemical study of the corneal endothelium and Descemet's membrane in the iridocorneal endothelial syndrome. *Am J Ophthalmol* 101:16, 1986

Scheie HG, Yanoff M: Iris nevus (Cogan–Reese) syndrome: A cause of unilateral glaucoma. *Arch Ophthalmol* 93:963, 1975

Scheie HG, Yanoff M, Kellogg WT: Essential iris atrophy: report of a case. *Arch Ophthalmol* 94:1315, 1976

Srinivasan R, Kaliaperumal S, Dutta TK: Bilateral angle closure glaucoma following snake bite. *J Assoc Physicians India* 53:46, 2005

Teekhasaenee C, Ritch R: Iridocorneal endothelial syndrome in Thai patients: Clinical variations. *Arch Ophthalmol* 118:187, 2000

Tester RA, Durcan FJ, Mamalis N *et al.*: Cogan–Reese syndrome: Progressive growth of endothelium over iris. *Arch Ophthalmol* 116:1126, 1998

Yanoff M: Glaucoma mechanisms in ocular malignant melanomas. *Am J Ophthalmol* 70:898, 1970

Yanoff M: Iridocorneal endothelial syndrome: Unification of a disease spectrum (editorial). *Surv Ophthalmol* 24:1, 1979

Yanoff M, Scheie HG, Allman MI: Endothelialization of filtering bleb in iris–nevus syndrome. *Arch Ophthalmol* 94:1933, 1976

Zografos L, Mirimanoff RO, Angeletti CA *et al.*: Systemic melanoma metastatic to the retina and vitreous. *Ophthalmologica* 218:424, 2004

Impaired Outflow: Secondary Open-Angle

Alvarado JA, Murphy CG: Outflow obstruction in pigmentary and primary open angle glaucoma. *Arch Ophthalmol* 110:1769, 1992

Anderson MG, Smith RS, Hawes NL *et al.*: Mutations in genes encoding melanosomal proteins cause pigmentary glaucoma in DBA/2J mice. *Nat Genet* 30:81, 2002

Bovell AM, Damji KF, Dohadwala AA *et al.*: Familial occurrence of pigment dispersion syndrome. *Can J Ophthalmol* 36:11, 2001

Breingan PJ, Esaki K, Ishikawa H *et al.*: Iridolenticular contact decreases following laser iridotomy for pigment dispersion syndrome. *Arch Ophthalmol* 117:325, 1999

Cameron JD, Havener VR: Histologic confirmation of ghost cell glaucoma by routine light microscopy. *Am J Ophthalmol* 96:251, 1983

Carlson DW, Alward WLM, Folberg R: Aggressive nevus of the iris with secondary glaucoma in a child. *Am J Ophthalmol* 119:367, 1995

Clark AF, Steely HT, Dickerson JE Jr *et al.*: Glucocorticoid induction of the glaucoma gene MYOC in human and monkey trabecular meshwork cells and tissues. *Invest Ophthalmol Vis Sci* 42:1769, 2001

Demirci H, Shields CL, Shields JA *et al.*: Ring melanoma of the ciliary body: report on twenty-three patients. *Retina* 22:698, 2002

Farrar SM, Shields MB: Current concepts in pigmentary glaucoma. *Surv Ophthalmol* 37:233, 1993

Feibel RM, Perlmutter JC: Anisocoria in the pigmentary dispersion syndrome. *Am J Ophthalmol* 110:657, 1990

Fine BS, Yanoff M, Scheie HG: Pigmentary "glaucoma": A histologic study. *Trans Am Acad Ophthalmol Otolaryngol* 78:314, 1974

Fineman MS, Eagle RC Jr, Shields JA *et al.*: Melanocytomalytic glaucoma in eyes with necrotic iris melanocytoma. *Ophthalmology* 105:402, 1998

Foulks GN, Shields MB: Glaucoma in oculodermal melanocytosis. *Ann Ophthalmol* 9:1299, 1977

Greenstein VC, Seiple W, Liebmann J *et al.*: Retinal pigment epithelial dysfunction in patients with pigment dispersion syndrome. *Arch Ophthalmol* 119:1291, 2001

Harris GJ, Rice PR: Angle closure in carotid-cavernous fistula. *Ophthalmology* 86:1521, 1979

Kozart DM, Yanoff M: Intraocular pressure status in 100 consecutive patients with exfoliation syndrome. *Ophthalmology* 89:214, 1982

Lichter PR, Shaffer RN: Interstitial keratitis and glaucoma. *Am J Ophthalmol* 68:241, 1969

Mardein CY, Küchle M, Nguyen NX *et al.*: Quantification of aqueous melanin granules, intraocular pressure and glaucomatous damage in primary pigment dispersion syndrome. *Ophthalmology* 107:435, 2000

McMenamin PG, Lee WR: Ultrastructural pathology of melanomalytic glaucoma. *Br J Ophthalmol* 70:895, 1986

Micheli T, Cheung LM, Sharma S *et al.*: Acute haptic-induced pigmentary glaucoma with an AcrySof intraocular lens. *J Cataract Refract Surg* 28:1869, 2002

Murphy CG, Johnson M, Alvarado JA: Juxtacanalicular tissue in pigmentary and primary open angle glaucoma. *Arch Ophthalmol* 110:1779, 1992

Pavlin CJ, Harasiewicz K, Foster FS: Posterior iris bowing in pigmentary dispersion syndrome caused by accommodation. *Am J Ophthalmol* 118:114, 1994

Phelps CD, Watzke RC: Hemolytic glaucoma. *Am J Ophthalmol* 80:690, 1975

Potash SD, Tello C, Liebmann J *et al.*: Ultrasound biomicroscopy in pigment dispersion syndrome. *Ophthalmology* 101:332, 1994

Raitta C, Vannas A: Glaucomatocyclitic crisis. *Arch Ophthalmol* 95:608, 1977

Rich R, Mudumbai R, Liebman JM: Combined exfoliation and pigment dispersion: Paradigm of an overlap syndrome. *Ophthalmology* 107:1004, 2000

Richards JE, Lichter PR, Herman S *et al.*: Probable exclusion of GLC1A as a candidate glaucoma gene in a family with middle-age-onset open-angle glaucoma. *Ophthalmology* 103:1035, 1996

Ritch R: A unification hypothesis of pigment dispersion syndrome. *Trans Am Ophthalmol Soc* 94:405, 1996

Ritch R, Steinberger D, Liebmann JM: Prevalence of pigment dispersion syndrome in a population undergoing glaucoma screening. *Am J Ophthalmol* 115:707, 1993

Santos C: Herpes simplex uveitis. *Bol Asoc Med P R* 96:71, 2004

Scheie HG, Cameron JD: Pigment dispersion syndrome: A clinical study. *Br J Ophthalmol* 65:264, 1981

Semple HC, Ball SF: Pigmentary glaucoma in the black population. *Am J Ophthalmol* 109:518, 1990

Siegner SW, Netland PA: Optic disc hemorrhages and progression of glaucoma. *Ophthalmology* 103:1014, 1996

Sokol J, Stegman Z, Liebmann JM et al.: Location of the iris insertion in pigment dispersion syndrome. *Ophthalmology* 103:289, 1996

Teichmann KD, Karcioglu ZA: Melanocytoma of the iris with rapidly developing secondary glaucoma. *Surv Ophthalmol* 40:136, 1995

Wentz-Hunter K, Shen X, Yue BY: Distribution of myocilin, a glaucoma gene product, in human corneal fibroblasts. *Mol Vis* 9:308–14:308, 2003

Yamamoto S, Pavan-Langston D, Yamamoto R et al.: Possible role of herpes simplex virus in the origin of Posner–Schlossman syndrome. *Am J Ophthalmol* 119:796, 1995

Yanoff M: Glaucoma mechanisms in ocular malignant melanomas. *Am J Ophthalmol* 70:898, 1970

Yanoff M: In discussion of Ritch R: A unification hypothesis of pigment dispersion syndrome. *Trans Am Ophthalmol Soc* 94:405, 1996

Yanoff M, Scheie HG: Cytology of human lens aspirate and its relationship to phacolytic glaucoma and phacoanaphylactic endophthalmitis. *Arch Ophthalmol* 80:166, 1968

Yanoff M, Scheie HG: Melanomalytic glaucoma: Report of patient. *Arch Ophthalmol* 84:471, 1970

Tissue Changes Caused by Elevated Intraocular Pressure

Agapova OA, Ricard CS, Salvador-Silva M et al.: Expression of matrix metalloproteinases and tissue inhibitors of metalloproteinases in human optic nerve head astrocytes. *Glia* 33:205, 2001

Agapova OA, Yang P, Wang WH et al.: Altered expression of 3 alpha-hydroxysteroid dehydrogenases in human glaucomatous optic nerve head astrocytes. *Neurobiol Dis* 14:63, 2003

Albert DM, Gangnon RE, Zimbric ML et al.: A study of iridectomy histopathologic features of latanoprost- and non-latanoprost-treated patients. *Arch Ophthalmol* 122:1680, 2004

Aung T, Okada K, Poinoosawmy D et al.: The phenotype of normal tension glaucoma patients with and without OPA1 polymorphisms. *Br J Ophthalmol* 87:149, 2003

Beck RW, Messner DK, Musch DC et al.: Is there a racial difference in physiologic cup size? *Ophthalmology* 92:873, 1985

Brownstein S, Font RL, Zimmerman LE et al.: Nonglaucomatous cavernous degeneration of the optic nerve: Report of two cases. *Arch Ophthalmol* 98:354, 1980

Caprioli J, Ortiz-Colberg R, Miller JM et al.: Measurements of peripapillary nerve fiber layer contour in glaucoma. *Am J Ophthalmol* 108:404, 1989

Carelli V, Ross-Cisneros FN, Sadun AA: Mitochondrial dysfunction as a cause of optic neuropathies. *Prog Retin Eye Res* 23:53, 2004

Colosi NJ, Yanoff M: Reactive corneal endothelialization. *Am J Ophthalmol* 83:219, 1977

Farkas RH, Chowers I, Hackam AS et al.: Increased expression of iron-regulating genes in monkey and human glaucoma. *Invest Ophthalmol Vis Sci* 45:1410, 2004

Giovannini A, Amato G, Mariotti C: The macular thickness and volume in glaucoma: an analysis in normal and glaucomatous eyes using OCT. *Acta Ophthalmol Scand Suppl* 236:34, 2002

Guo L, Moss SE, Alexander RA et al.: Retinal ganglion cell apoptosis in glaucoma is related to intraocular pressure and IOP-induced effects on extracellular matrix. *Invest Ophthalmol Vis Sci* 46:175, 2005

Healey PR, Mitchell P: Visibility of lamina cribrosa pores and open-angle glaucoma. *Am J Ophthalmol* 138:871, 2004

Hernandez MR, Agapova OA, Yang P et al.: Differential gene expression in astrocytes from human normal and glaucomatous optic nerve head analyzed by cDNA microarray. *Glia* 38:45, 2002

Hernandez MR, Andrzejewska WM, Neufeld AH: Changes in the extracellular matrix of the human optic nerve head in primary open-angle glaucoma. *Am J Ophthalmol* 109:180, 1990

Jonas JB, Fernàndez MC, Naumann GOH: Glaucomatous parapapillary atrophy. *Arch Ophthalmol* 110:214, 1992

Jonas JB, Naumann GOH: Parapapillary chorioretinal atrophy in normal and glaucoma eyes. *Invest Ophthalmol Vis Sci* 30:919, 1989

Jonas JB, Fernàndez MC, Naumann GOH: Parapapillary atrophy and retinal vessel diameter in nonglaucomatous optic nerve damage. *Invest Ophthalmol Vis Sci* 32:2942, 1991

Jonas JB, Nguyen NX, Gusek GC et al.: Parapapillary chorioretinal atrophy in normal and glaucoma eyes. *Invest Ophthalmol Vis Sci* 30:908, 1989

Jonas JB, Nguyen NX, Naumann GOH: The retinal nerve fiber layer in normal eyes. *Ophthalmology* 96:627, 1989

Jonas JB, Schmidt AM, Müller-Bergh JA et al.: Human optic nerve fiber count and optic disc size. *Invest Ophthalmol Vis Sci* 33:2012, 1992

Kendell KR, Quigley HA, Kerrigan LA et al.: Primary open-angle glaucoma is not associated with photoreceptor loss. *Invest Ophthalmol Vis Sci* 36:200, 1995

Kubota T, Naumann GOH: Reduction in number of corpora amylacea with advancing histological changes of glaucoma. *Graefes Arch Clin Exp Ophthalmol* 231:249, 1993

Kubota T, Holbach LM, Naumann GOH: Corpora amylacea in glaucomatous and non-glaucomatous optic nerve and retina. *Graefes Arch Clin Exp Ophthalmol* 231:7, 1993

Kuehn MH, Fingert JH, Kwon YH: Retinal ganglion cell death in glaucoma: mechanisms and neuroprotective strategies. *Ophthalmol Clin North Am* 18:383, 2005

Lin HJ, Chen WC, Tsai FJ et al.: Distributions of p53 codon 72 polymorphism in primary open angle glaucoma. *Br J Ophthalmol* 86:767, 2002

Ljubimov AV, Burgeson RE, Butkowski RJ et al.: Extracellular matrix alterations in human corneas with bullous keratopathy. *Invest Ophthalmol Vis Sci* 37:997, 1996

May CA, Lutjen-Drecoll E: Choroidal ganglion cell changes in human glaucomatous eyes. *J Glaucoma* 13:389, 2004

McKinnon SJ, Lehman DM, Tahzib NG et al.: Baculoviral IAP repeat-containing-4 protects optic nerve axons in a rat glaucoma model. *Mol Ther* 5:780, 2002

Miller KM, Quigley HA: The clinical appearance of the lamina cribrosa as a function of the extent of glaucomatous optic nerve damage. *Ophthalmology* 95:135, 1988

Radius RL: Anatomy of the optic nerve head and glaucomatous optic neuropathy. *Surv Ophthalmol* 32:35, 1987

Ricard CS, Agapova OA, Salvador-Silva M et al.: Expression of myocilin/TIGR in normal and glaucomatous primate optic nerves. *Exp Eye Res* 73:433, 2001

Schnabel J: Die Entwicklungsgeschichte der glaukomatosen Exkavation. *Z Augenheilkd* 14:1, 1905

Shin DH, Bielik M, Hong YJ et al.: Reversal of glaucomatous optic disc cupping in adult patients. *Arch Ophthalmol* 107:1599, 1989

Tan JC, Hitchings RA: Reversal of disc cupping after intraocular pressure reduction in topographic image series. *J Glaucoma* 13:351, 2004

Votruba M, Thiselton D, Bhattacharya SS: Optic disc morphology of patients with OPA1 autosomal dominant optic atrophy. *Br J Ophthalmol* 87:48, 2003

Wax MB, Tezel G: Neurobiology of glaucomatous optic neuropathy: diverse cellular events in neurodegeneration and neuroprotection. *Mol Neurobiol* 26:45, 2002

Wax MB, Tezel G, Edward PD: Clinical and ocular histopathologic findings in a patient with normal-pressure glaucoma. *Arch Ophthalmol* 116:993, 1998

Wu SC, Huang SC, Kuo CL *et al.*: Reversal of optic disc cupping after trabeculotomy in primary congenital glaucoma. *Can J Ophthalmol* 37:337, 2002

Yang P, Agapova O, Parker A *et al.*: DNA microarray analysis of gene expression in human optic nerve head astrocytes in response to hydrostatic pressure. *Physiol Genomics* 17:157, 2004

17

Ocular Melanocytic Tumors

NORMAL ANATOMY

Ocular Melanocytes

I. Conjunctival and uveal melanocytes (Fig. 17.1; see also Fig. 17.29D, top) are derived from the neural crest; pigment epithelial cells (PE) are derived from neuroepithelium or the layers of the optic cup.

II. Dermal and conjunctival melanocytes are solitary dendritic cells.

III. Uveal melanocytes are also solitary and dendritic, and their cytoplasm contains fine, dustlike, ovoid melanin granules of a size bordering on the limits of resolution of the light microscope.

> Cultured human melanocytes from different-colored eyes can produce melanin in vivo. The color of the iris is determined by the density of melanocytes in the most anterior portion of the iris.

IV. Pigment epithelium is neither solitary nor dendritic, but is epithelial, and exists as a sheet of cuboidal cells containing large, easily visualized pigment granules.

> The cytoplasm of PE cells contains two basic types of pigment granules: melanin granules, which are either ovoid or spherical, and lipofuscin granules, which are usually somewhat spherical.

V. Dermal, conjunctival, and uveal melanocytes tend to vary in size, number, and melanin content among the races.

VI. Normal PE tends to vary little, if at all, among the races, and always appears heavily pigmented.

VII. Dermal, conjunctival, and uveal melanocytes almost never undergo reactive (nonneoplastic) proliferation under normal circumstances. Neoplastic proliferation, however, does occur.

VIII. The PE readily undergoes reactive proliferation, but rarely becomes neoplastic.

IX. Dysplastic nevus syndrome is associated with an increased prevalence of conjunctival nevi, iris nevi, iris freckles, and choroidal nevi. It has been postulated that such individuals may have overstimulation of the melanocytic system not only in the skin, but also in ocular tissues, possibly increasing the risk for melanocytic malignancies.

MELANOTIC TUMORS OF EYELIDS

Ephelis (Freckle)

I. An ephelis (freckle) is a brown, circumscribed macule normally only found on areas of skin exposed to sunlight.

II. The color is due to increased pigmentation in the basal cell layer of the epidermis. The pigment (melanin) is derived from hyperactive melanocytes that "secrete" their pigment into epidermal basal cells.

III. The melanocytes are *fewer* in number, but larger and more functionally active than those in adjacent, surrounding, paler epidermis.

Lentigo

I. Lentigo

A. Lentigo is similar clinically to an ephelis but is somewhat larger.

B. In addition to hyperpigmentation of the basal cell layer of epithelium, *increased* numbers of melanocytes are

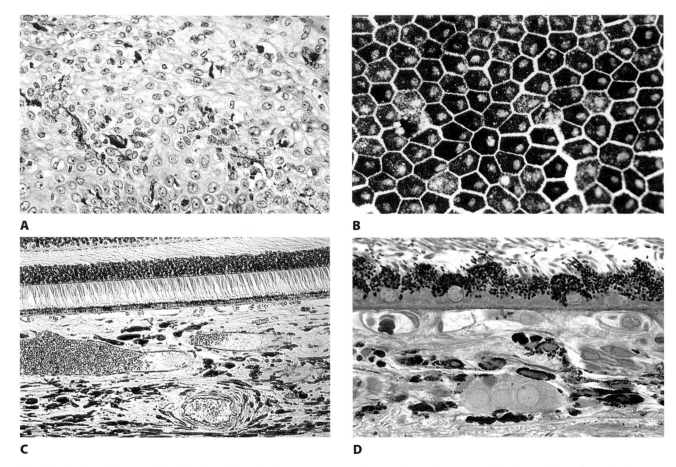

Fig. 17.1 Ocular melanocytes. Normally, the epidermal melanocytes appear in hematoxylin and eosin-stained sections as clear cells wedged between basal epithelial cells. Melanin is transferred by the dendritic processes of the melanocytes to the basal keratocytes, where it is stored and later degraded. **A,** In this tangential section of "reactive" epidermis, the usually clear melanocytes contain pigment around their nuclei and in their dendritic processes, making them easily visible (see Fig. 1.26C). **B,** A flat preparation of retinal pigment epithelium (RPE) of owl monkey shows the epithelial sheet configuration. RPE cells have a basement membrane (inner or cuticular portion of Bruch's membrane) and are attached to one another near their apexes by terminal bars that contain "tight junctions." **C,** Cross-section of the retina and choroid compares the epithelial nature of RPE with the nonepithelial individual and solitary choroidal melanocytes. The RPE cells have larger pigment granules than the choroidal melanocytes (see Fig. 9.2C). **D,** Thin section shows RPE pigment granules are considerably larger than those in choroidal melanocytes. Large nonpigmented cells in choroid (center toward bottom) are probably ganglion cells.

present. It may also be found on nonexposed skin in older people.

C. Multiple lentigines syndrome

1. Multiple lentigines syndrome also goes by the acronym LEOPARD (lentigines, multiple; electro-cardiographic conduction defects; ocular hyper-telorism; pulmonary stenosis; abnormal genitalia; retardation of growth; and deafness, sen-sorineural).

2. In addition to ocular hypertelorism (occurring in 40% of patients), other ocular findings include ptosis; microcornea; cortical punctate lenticular opacities and anterior subcapsular and zonular cata-racts; patches of myelinated nerve fibers; flat pig-mented spots of the iris; and glaucoma.

Multiple lentigines also occur in *Carney's syndrome* (complex; see p. 244 in Chapter 7). Carney's syndrome has

an autosomal-dominant inheritance pattern and consists of bilateral, primary, pigmented, nodular adrenocortical hyperplasia; multiple lentigines, especially of the head and neck, and blue nevi; cutaneous myxomata; large cell, calcifying Sertoli's cell tumor of testes; cardiac myxoma; myxoid fibroadenomas of breast; pituitary tumors (which may lead to Cushing's syndrome); and melanotic schwannomas.

D. Lentigo maligna (melanotic freckle of Hutchinson; cir-cumscribed precancerous melanosis of Dubreuilh; Fig. 17.2)

1. Lentigo maligna occurs as an acquired pigmented lesion, mostly in adults older than 50 years of age.

2. It appears as a brown or black flat lesion, usually on the face, sometimes with involvement of the eyelids and conjunctiva (see subsection *Primary Acquired Melanosis* in section *Melanotic Tumors of Conjunc-*

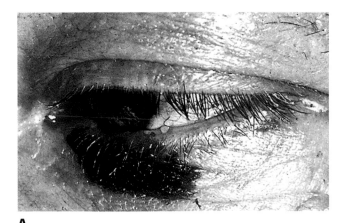

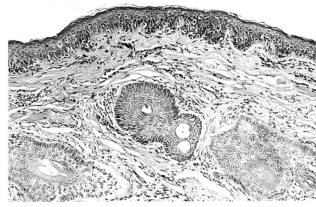

A

B

Fig. 17.2 Lentigo maligna (Hutchinson's freckle). **A,** Clinical appearance of acquired pigmented lesion of the left lower lid. **B,** Histologic section shows nevus cells in the junctional location, indistinguishable from a junctional nevus. (Case presented by Dr. VB Bernardino, Jr to the meeting of the Eastern Ophthalmic Pathology Society, 1975.)

tiva, later), enlarging slowly in an irregular manner.

3. Approximately one-third of all lentigo maligna eventuates in malignant melanoma, noted clinically by a thickening or infiltration that elevates into a papule or nodule.

Lentigo maligna melanoma is the most common type of melanoma of the eyelid.

---

4. Histologically, lentigo maligna is indistinguishable from a junctional nevus. An underlying, chronic, nongranulomatous inflammatory infiltrate is common.

Nevus*

I. General information
  A. A nevus is a congenital, hamartomatous tumor, a flat or elevated, usually well-circumscribed lesion.
    1. It may be pigmented early in life, or not until puberty or even early adulthood.
    2. The nevus is composed of nevus cells that are atypical but benign-appearing dermal melanocytes.

Congenital melanocytic nevus has occurred in association with ankyloblepharon. This lesion may be explained by a failure of eyelid separation, which should occur near the 20th week of gestation..

  B. Five types:
    1. Junctional
    2. Intradermal

A nevus is any congenital lesion composed of one of several types of cells found in the skin. A melanocytic nevus is composed of atypical but benign-appearing melanocytes (nevus cells). In this chapter (and elsewhere in the book), the term nevus always refers to the melanocytic nevus.

3. Compound (Fig. 17.3)
4. Blue (Fig. 17.5)
5. Congenital oculodermal melanocytosis (nevus of Ota) (Fig. 17.6)
  C. The familial atypical mole and melanoma (FAM-M) syndrome (*dysplastic nevus syndrome*; B-K mole syndrome)
    1. The FAM-M syndrome consists of multiple, large, typical and atypical cutaneous nevi of the upper part of the trunk, buttocks, and extremities.
    2. The nevi appear at an early age (usually during adolescence) and increase in number throughout life.
    3. Familial cases are inherited in an autosomal-dominant pattern; sporadic cases also occur.
    4. Patients who have the syndrome definitely carry an increased risk for development of cutaneous melanomas; melanomas develop in them at an earlier age than in the general population.

Unlike cutaneous melanomas, ocular (conjunctival and uveal) melanocytic lesions rarely occur, and may be no more common in patients with FAM-M syndrome than in the general population.

II. Junctional nevus
  A. A junctional nevus is flat, well circumscribed, and a uniform brown color.
  B. The nevus cells are located at the "junction" of the epidermis and dermis (Fig. 17.3C).
  C. The nevus has a low malignant potential.
III. Intradermal nevus (common mole; Fig. 17.4)
  A. Intradermal nevus is usually elevated, frequently is papillomatous, and is the most common type of nevus.
  B. It has a brown to black color when pigmented; often, however, it is almost flesh-colored.
  C. The nevus cells are entirely in the dermis.
    1. The nuclei of the nevus cells tend to become "mature" (i.e., smaller, thinner or spindle-shaped,

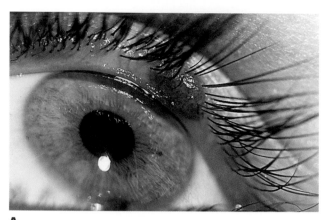

A

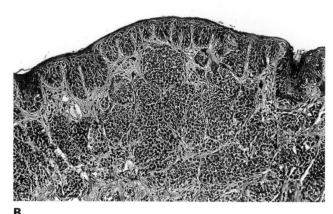

B

Fig. 17.3 Compound nevus. **A,** Moderately pigmented nevus at lid margin. **B,** Histologic section shows nevus cells at junction of epidermis and dermis as well as in dermis. **C,** Increased magnification demonstrates nevus cells in junctional and dermal locations.

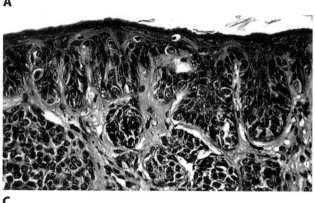

C

and darker) as they go deeper into the dermis. This orderly progression in structural change from superficial to deep layers is termed the *normal polarity* of the nevus.

2. No inflammatory cells are present unless the nevus is inflamed secondarily.

D. The nevus may be seen with proliferated Schwann elements (i.e., a neural nevus).

E. An unusual intradermal (or subepithelial) nevus is the peripunctal melanocytic nevus.

1. These involve the lower punctum, are dome-shaped and benign, and circumferentially surround the punctum, creating swollen punctal lips that result in a slitlike punctal orifice

2. The nevus cells are subepithelial and also infiltrate the orbicularis muscle fibers.

F. Intradermal nevus probably has no malignant potential.

IV. Compound nevus (see Fig. 17.3)

A. It combines junctional and dermal components, and is usually brown.

B. The dermal component shows a normal polarity (see Fig. 17.4C; i.e., cells closest to the epidermis are larger, plumper, rounder, and paler than the deeper cells).

C. The spindle cell nevus (juvenile "melanoma," Spitz nevus) is a special form of compound nevus that occurs predominantly in children, often as a solitary lesion on the face.

1. Histologically, it superficially resembles a malignant melanoma, but biologically it is benign.

2. It may contain spindle cells, "epithelioid" cells, and single-nucleus and multinucleated giant cells that contain abundant basophilic cytoplasm.

D. The compound nevus has a low malignant potential. The malignant melanoma arises from the junctional component.

V. Blue nevus

A. The blue nevus is usually flat and is almost always pigmented from birth; it appears blue to slate-gray.

Congenital pigmented (melanocytic) nevi are arbitrarily divided into small (<3 to 4 cm), large (up to 10 cm), and giant (>10 cm). The large and giant melanocytic nevi have an approximately 8.5% chance of undergoing malignant transformation during the first 15 years of life. Most primary orbital melanomas occur in white patients and are associated with blue nevi.

B. Nevus cells are present deep in the dermis in interlacing fasciculi.

1. The cells are located deeper than junctional, dermal, or compound nevus cells.

2. The nevus cells are more spindle-shaped, more elongated, and contain larger branching processes than other types of nevus cells. They more closely resemble uveal nevus cells than do other skin nevus cells.

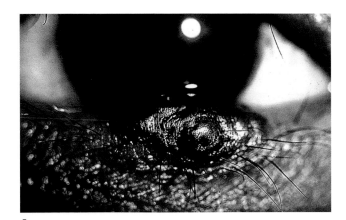

A

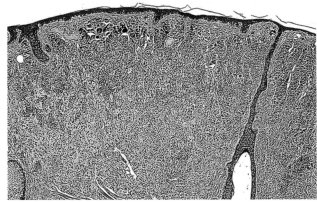

B

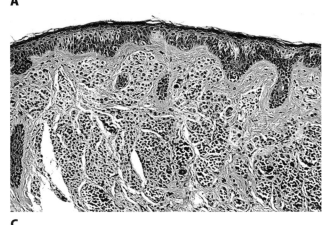

C

Fig. 17.4 Intradermal nevus. **A,** Large, deeply pigmented nevus at lid margin. **B,** Nests of nevus cells fill the dermis except for a narrow area just under the epithelium; shown with increased magnification in **C. C,** The nuclei of the nevus cells become smaller, thinner or spindle-shaped, and darker as they go deeper into the dermis (i.e., they show normal polarity).

3. It may be very cellular [i.e., a cellular blue nevus (Fig. 17.5), which has a low malignant potential].

C. Unless the nevus is the large or giant congenital cellular type, it has no malignant potential.

VI. Congenital oculodermal melanocytosis (nevus of Ota; Fig. 17.6; see also Fig. 17.36D)

A. The condition can be considered a type of blue nevus of the skin around the orbit (in the distribution of the ophthalmic, maxillary, and occasionally mandibular branches of the trigeminal nerve), associated with an ipsilateral blue nevus of the conjunctiva and a diffuse nevus of the uvea (i.e., ipsilateral congenital ocular melanocytosis).

1. Skin pigmentation is usually prominent, but may be quite subtle.

> Approximately 60% of patients have the complete syndrome of skin, conjunctival, and uveal involvement (congenital *oculodermal* melanocytosis); approximately 34% have only skin involvement (congenital *dermal* melanocytosis); and approximately 6% have only conjunctival and uveal involvement (congenital *ocular* melanocytosis).

2. It is quite common in black and Asian patients, but unusual in white patients.

3. Rarely, congenital oculodermal melanocytosis is bilateral.

4. Associated findings in the involved eye include glaucoma (which is common and may develop at any age), uveitis, and cataract.

> When congenital oculodermal melanocytosis and nevus flammeus (phakomatosis pigmentovascularis) occur together, especially when each extensively involves the globe, a strong predisposition exists for the development of congenital glaucoma.

B. The diffuse uveal involvement causes heterochromia iridum (i.e., the involved eye is darker than the uninvolved iris).

Heterochromia iridum (see Table 17.2, p. 694) is a difference in pigmentation between the two irises, as contrasted to *heterochromia iridis*, which is an alteration within a single iris (e.g., occasionally, ipsilateral segmental heterochromia is caused by segmental ocular involvement; the alteration of pigmentation in the single iris is properly called *heterochromia iridis*).

C. Congenital dermal melanocytosis may occur alone or concurrently with orbital melanocytosis, in which case it is called *congenital dermal orbital melanocytosis*. It may also occur concurrently with ocular melanocytosis, in which case it is called *congenital oculodermal melanocytosis* (nevus of Ota).

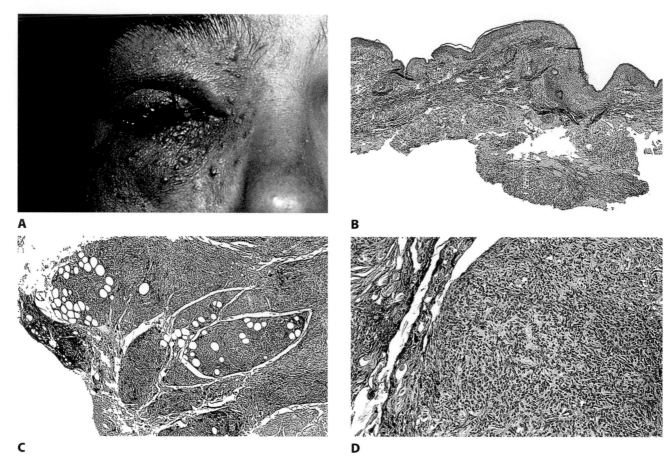

Fig. 17.5 Cellular blue nevus. **A,** Nevus involves lids, conjunctiva, and orbit. **B,** Histopathologic section of partially removed tumor shows nonpigmented and pigmented nevus cells in the deepest dermis. **C,** Another area shows nonpigmented and pigmented nevus cells involving orbital fat. **D,** Increased magnification of another region shows nonpigmented and pigmented dendritic nevus cells that contain abundant cytoplasm and small spindle nuclei. (Case presented by Dr. WC Frayer to the meeting of the Eastern Ophthalmic Pathology Society, 1975.)

D. Congenital ocular melanocytosis (see earlier)

E. Congenital oculodermal melanocytosis is potentially malignant only when it occurs in white patients.

Malignant melanomas have been reported in the skin, conjunctiva, uvea (most common), orbit (rarely), and even in the meninges.

> The lifetime prevalence of uveal melanomas in white patients who have congenital oculodermal melanocytosis has been estimated to be 1 in 400.

Malignant Melanoma

I. General information (Figs 17.7 and 17.8)

A. From the 1960s to the 1980s, the incidence of cutaneous malignant melanoma rose 3.5-fold in men and 4.6-fold in women.

> In the United States between 1973 and 1994, an increase in melanoma incidence and mortality rates of approximately 121% and 39%, respectively, occurred.

1. The rising incidence is probably attributable to increased voluntary exposure to sun and the depletion of the ozone layer.

2. An emerging epidemic of melanoma appears to be on the horizon.

B. Melanoma involves the lower lid two-thirds more often than the upper lid.

C. Associated histologic findings include solar elastosis, nevus, and basal cell carcinoma.

> Rarely, a primary choroidal melanoma can occur in a patient who has had a previous cutaneous melanoma.

D. Cuticular melanomas show a nonrandom alteration of chromosome 6.

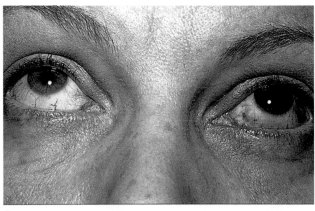

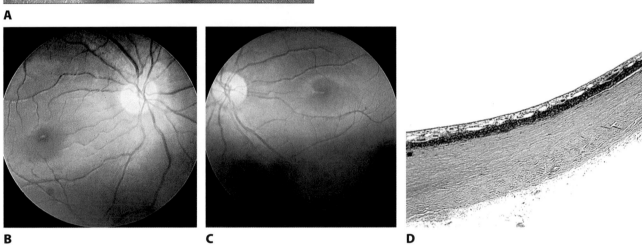

Fig. 17.6 Congenital oculodermal melanocytosis (nevus of Ota). **A,** Heterochromia iridum present; left iris darker than right. Slate-gray pigmentation of sclera is seen inferiorly in the left eye. Note hyperpigmentation of skin around left eye. Another patient who had congenital oculodermal melanocytosis in the left eye shows a normal-colored right (**B**) but a much darker left (**C**) fundus. **D,** Diffuse, maximally pigmented nevus cells fill the choroid, which is characteristic of the uveal lesion in congenital ocular melanocytosis.

II. Malignant melanoma may arise from a pre-existing junctional, compound, or, rarely, large or giant congenital melanocytic nevus, or it may arise de novo.

III. Skin melanomas are *not* classified according to cell type, as are uveal melanomas*

    A. Lentigo maligna melanoma

        1. The melanoma develops in a preinvasive lesion called *lentigo maligna* (see p. 668 in this chapter), also called *melanotic freckle of Hutchinson* or *circumscribed precancerous melanosis of Dubreuilh.*

        2. After a radial growth phase (intraepidermal spread), vertical growth phase (dermal invasion) may occur, elevating the lesion.

    B. Superficial spreading malignant melanoma

        1. Superficial spreading malignant melanoma has a prolonged radial growth phase before the vertical growth phase.

        2. Clinically, the lesion appears as a nodule or plaque with variable pigmentation and has a "surround component" caused by the intradermal spread.

    C. Nodular malignant melanoma

        1. This type has only a vertical growth phase, involves the dermis early, and has the worst prognosis.

        2. Clinically, the lesion appears as a nodule or plaque without a surround component because no radial growth phase occurs.

    D. *Acrolentiginous melanoma* occurs on the palms, soles, and terminal phalanges.

    E. The melanocytic neuroectodermal tumor (retinal anlage tumor, retinal choristoma) of infancy mainly involves the maxilla, but has been reported in many other locations.

    F. Mucous membrane malignant melanoma (see discussion of conjunctival melanoma, p. 682 in this chapter).

        Rarely, a primary lid melanoma can occur in conjunction with an ipsilateral primary conjunctival melanoma.

    G. Miscellaneous—malignant melanoma that arises in a large or giant congenital melanocytic nevus, in the central nervous system, and in the viscera

On the basis of gross appearance and biologic behavior, melanomas may be divided clinically into lentigo maligna melanoma, superficial spreading melanoma, and nodular melanoma.

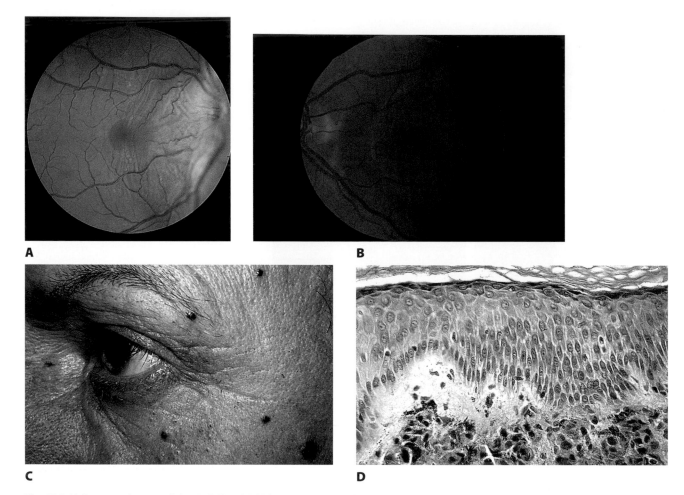

Fig. 17.7 Malignant melanoma of skin. **A** (OD) and **B** (OS), Patient presented with bilateral pigmented choroidal tumors. **C,** Same patient shows multiple pigmented skin tumors. **D,** Biopsy of skin tumor shows melanoma cells in dermis, sparing the junctional and epithelial locations, characteristic of metastatic melanoma—see Fig. 17.8. (Case referred by Drs. RC Lanciano, Jr and S Bresalier.)

IV. Histology
   A. Normal polarity is lost (i.e., the deep cells are indistinguishable from superficial cells).
   B. The overlying epithelium is invaded.

If only epithelial invasion is seen, it is called a *superficial spreading* or *incipient melanoma*. Pigmentation may or may not be present. If present, it may vary in different parts of the tumor. If pigmentation is not present, the tumor is called an *amelanotic melanoma*.

   Invasion of the underlying dermis occurs concurrently with (nodular malignant melanoma) or after (superficial spreading malignant melanoma) epithelial invasion.
   C. The cells of the neoplasm are atypical.
      1. The nuclear-to-cytoplasmic ratio is increased, and large abnormal cells may be seen.
      2. Mitotic figures may be present, but frequently are absent.

   D. Often, an underlying inflammatory infiltrate of round cells, predominantly lymphocytes, is present.
   E. Usually, a combination of the aforementioned criteria rather than any single criterion leads to the diagnosis of malignancy.

Immunohistochemical staining for versican, a major proteoglycan expressed by cutaneous malignant melanomas (CMM), may be helpful in differentiating benign melanocytic nevi (BMN), dysplastic nevi (DN), and CMM. Versican is generally negative in BMN, positive (ranging from weakly to intensively positive) in DN, and intensively positive in CMM. S-100 and NKI/C3 are helpful immunohistologic stains for determining the extent of melanocytic lesions in the conjunctiva. HMB45 immunoreactivity may be helpful in distinguishing benign from malignant melanocytic lesions, particularly those related to primary acquired melanosis (PAM).

   F. Radial growth
      1. Small clusters and single atypical melanocytes grow throughout the epidermis (pagetoid growth),

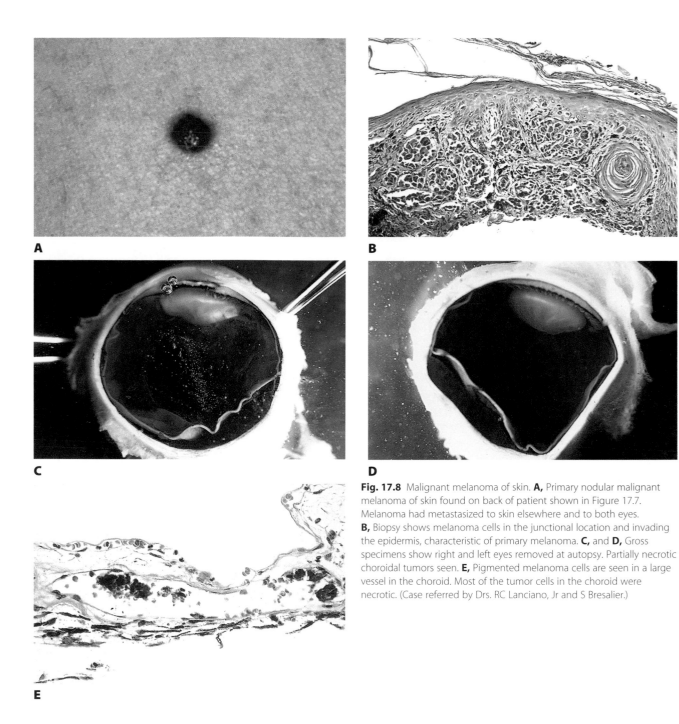

Fig. 17.8 Malignant melanoma of skin. **A,** Primary nodular malignant melanoma of skin found on back of patient shown in Figure 17.7. Melanoma had metastasized to skin elsewhere and to both eyes. **B,** Biopsy shows melanoma cells in the junctional location and invading the epidermis, characteristic of primary melanoma. **C,** and **D,** Gross specimens show right and left eyes removed at autopsy. Partially necrotic choroidal tumors seen. **E,** Pigmented melanoma cells are seen in a large vessel in the choroid. Most of the tumor cells in the choroid were necrotic. (Case referred by Drs. RC Lanciano, Jr and S Bresalier.)

or at the dermoepidermal junction (lentiginous growth), and may invade the dermis in a platelike fashion.

   2. Corium tumor cells tend to be small and of uniform size, similar to tumor cells in the epidermis or dermoepidermal junction.

  G. Vertical growth

   1. Vertical differs from radial growth mainly in cytoarchitectural heterogenicity (i.e., at least some of the tumor cells in the dermis have a different

appearance than those in the epidermis or at the dermoepidermal junction).

   2. Mitotic figures are usually present in the dermal component.

   3. Melanomas greater than 1.5 mm in depth carry a distinctly worse survival rate.

  V. Prognosis

  A. In general, involvement of the lid margin and conjunctiva is associated with a poorer survival rate than localization to the lid skin alone.

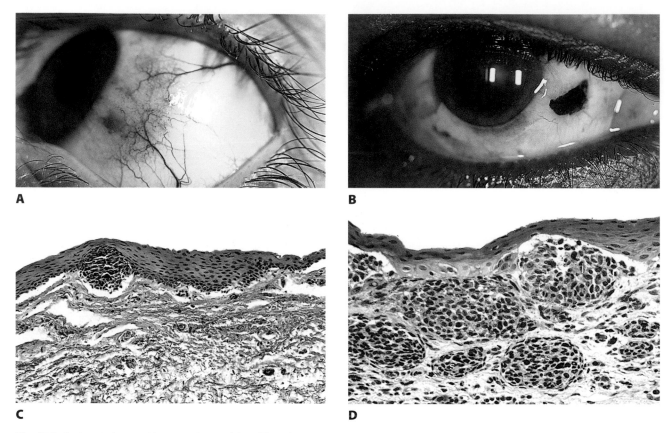

Fig. 17.9 Conjunctival nevus. Almost amelanotic (**A**) and heavily pigmented (**B**) nevi present in conjunctiva near limbus in two different patients. **C,** A junctional nevus is composed of nests of nevus cells at the junction of conjunctival epithelium and subepithelial tissue. **D,** A compound nevus contains nevus cells both at the junction of conjunctival epithelium and in subepithelial tissue (j, junctional nests of nevus cells; s, subepithelial nests of nevus cells). As in the skin, the nevus cells become smaller and darker the deeper they are in the substantia propria, representing the normal polarity of the nevus.

B. Superficial, spreading malignant melanoma has a 75% survival rate.

C. Deep malignant melanoma has a 10% to 39% survival rate (variability in survival rates is due to location of tumor and different authors' statistics).

D. The level of expression of at least three integrin subunits has been found to be correlated with melanoma progression.

> Breslow thickness is an important prognostic indicator for eyelid skin melanomas.

MELANOTIC TUMORS OF CONJUNCTIVA

Ephelis (Freckle)

I. An ephelis (freckle) is a brown, patchy, flat lesion with irregular borders.

   A. It most often involves the bulbar conjunctiva near the limbus, but it may involve the bulbar or palpebral conjunctiva.

B. The pigmented conjunctiva is movable over the sclera.

C. The lesion is present at birth.

II. Freckles are common in dark races.

III. The histology consists of increased pigmentation in the basal cell layer of the conjunctival epithelium; the number of melanocytes is normal or decreased.

> Histologically, the freckle and lentigo are similar, if not identical, to benign acquired melanosis that has no junctional activity.

Lentigo

I. A lentigo is somewhat larger than an ephelis.

II. Histologically, pigmentation of the basal cells of the conjunctival epithelium is increased and melanocytes are increased in number.

Nevus

I. General information (Figs 17.9 to 17.11)

   A. A nevus is a hamartomatous, congenital, flat or elevated, well-circumscribed lesion that may not become pigmented until puberty or early adulthood.

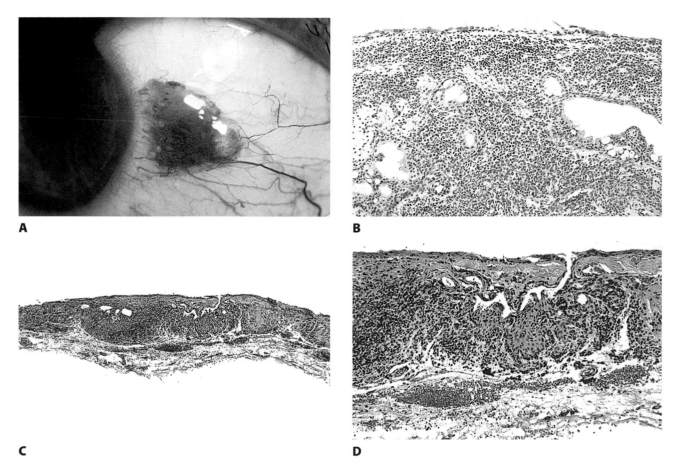

Fig. 17.10 Cystic nevus of conjunctiva. **A,** A variably pigmented nevus contains small and large cysts. **B,** A cystic nevus is composed of hamartomatous, epithelial, cystic structures admixed with nevus cells in the subepithelial tissue. Nevus cells are also present in the junctional position (compound nevus). Note collection of balloon cells in nevus. **C,** Histologic section of another compound cystic nevus shows one of the cysts opening to the surface; shown with increased magnification in **D.**

1. Conjunctival nevi are usually noted during the first two decades of life.
2. They are almost entirely restricted to the epibulbar surface, the plica, the caruncle (see Fig. 17.11), and the lid margin. The lesion is most commonly found at the nasal or temporal limbus.
3. Nevi are rarely located in the palpebral conjunctiva (1%), fornix (1%) , or cornea (<1%).
4. Over time, a change in color may be seen in 13% of lesions, and the size may change in 8%.

B. Nevi are primarily composed of nevus cells, but may also have epithelial elements (see later discussion of compound nevus).

C. A nevus is the most common conjunctival tumor and consists of five "classic" types:
1. Junctional
2. Subepithelial (analogous to intradermal nevus of skin)
3. Compound
4. Blue
5. Congenital melanocytosis

   a. Congenital ocular melanocytosis (melanosis oculi)
   b. Congenital oculodermal melanocytosis (nevus of Ota)
6. Unusual types of conjunctival nevi

II. Junctional nevus (Table 17.1; see Fig. 17.9C)
A. Similar in appearance to junctional nevus of the skin.
B. Nevus moves with conjunctiva over sclera.

> A junctional nevus (composed of nevocellular cells), not uncommonly, may be associated with a blue nevus (composed of blue nevus cells); the two together are called a *combined nevus* of the conjunctiva.

C. Histologically, nevus cells appear more "worrisome" than those of skin junctional nevi.
1. Cells tend to be larger and may reach the external surface of the epidermis.
2. The nevus cells are not necessarily limited to the junctional area of the epithelium and subepithelium, but may be found within the epithelial layers, simulating invasion.

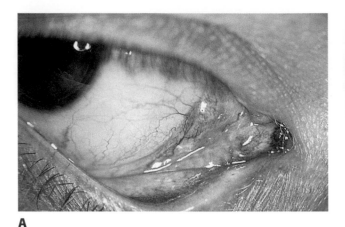

A

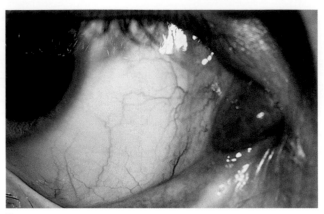

B

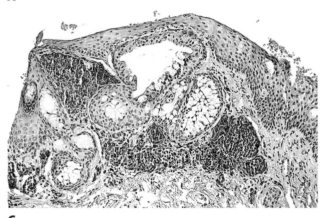

C

Fig. 17.11 Nevus of caruncle. Clinical appearance in two patients of a small (**A**) and a large (**B**) nevus of the caruncle. **C,** Histologic section of caruncular nevus shown in **A** demonstrates pigmented and nonpigmented nests of nevus cells mainly in the subepithelial area, but also in scattered junctional areas (i.e., compound nevus).

TABLE 17.1 Conjunctival Nevus, Congenital Ocular Melanocytosis, and Primary Acquired Melanosis Compared

	Conjunctival Nevus (Junctional, Subepithelial, and Compound)	**Congenital Ocular Melanocytosis (Melanosis Oculi)**	**Primary Acquired Melanosis (Precancerous and Cancerous Melanosis)**
Onset	Congenital (may not pigment until young adult)	Congenital	Middle age
Structure	Discrete	Diffuse	Diffuse
Color	Brown	Blue or slate-gray	Brown
Cysts	May be present (~50% of time)	None	None
Pigmentation	Variable pigmentation	Always pigmented	Always pigmented
With conjunctival movement	Lesion moves	Lesion does not move	Lesion moves
Growth	Stationary	Stationary	Tends to change
Uvea	Not involved	Heterochromia iridum	Not involved
Skin	Not involved	May be involved (nevus of Ota)	Not involved
Malignant potential	Conjunctival melanoma	Skin or uvea (rarely conjunctival melanoma)	Conjunctival melanoma only

3. Histologically, the junctional nevus, when maximally pigmented, is identical in appearance to benign acquired melanosis with junctional activity.

D. Malignant potential is low.

III. Subepithelial nevus (see Table 17.1)

A. Similar to intradermal nevus of the skin; appears flesh-colored to brown depending on the degree of pigmentation.

B. Nevus moves with conjunctiva over sclera.

C. It is not nearly as common as a junctional or compound nevus.

D. Histologically, the cells show normal polarity (i.e., smaller, darker, more spindle-shaped cells present in the deeper layers).

E. It probably has no malignant potential.

IV. Compound nevus (see Table 17.1 and Figs 17.9D and 17.10)

A. Quite similar to compound nevus of the skin; appears brown when pigmented.

B. Nevus moves with conjunctiva over sclera.

C. Histologically, the subepithelial component shows a normal polarity (i.e., cells found closest to the epithelium are plumper, larger, rounder, and paler).

D. The subepithelial hamartomatous component, in addition to containing nevus cells, frequently contains epithelial embryonic rests, which may develop into epithelial cysts (i.e., a cystic nevus; see Fig. 17.10).

1. The epithelial component is present in approximately 50% of conjunctival nevi.

2. Balloon cells, probably representing lipidized melanocytes, are often seen admixed with nevus cells and the epithelial component.

E. Spindle-cell nevus (Spitz nevus; juvenile melanoma)

1. This special form of compound nevus occurs predominantly in children.

2. Histologically, it is similar to "juvenile melanoma" of the skin.

F. Malignant potential is extremely low.

V. Blue nevus

A. Quite similar to blue nevus of the skin; appears diffuse, blue to slate-gray, and is pigmented from birth.

B. It does not move with the conjunctiva over the sclera.

A junctional nevus (composed of nevocellular cells) not uncommonly may be associated with a blue nevus (composed of blue nevus cells); the two together are called a *combined nevus* of the conjunctiva.

C. Histologically, nevus cells, mainly deeply pigmented, are seen deep in the subepithelial tissue in interlacing fasciculi.

1. The cells are deeper than the junctional, subepithelial, or compound nevus cells, and are more spindle-shaped and elongated, and contain larger branching processes than other types of nevus cells.

2. When very cellular, the nevus is called a *cellular blue nevus*.

a. It appears as a localized blue nodule.

b. It rarely becomes malignant.

D. A blue nevus may be difficult to differentiate from other lesions that cause episcleral pigmentation.

E. Only the cellular type is potentially malignant.

VI. Congenital melanocytosis (see Table 17.1)

A. Congenital ocular melanocytosis (melanosis oculi; see Fig. 17.6)

1. Probably it is best considered as a diffuse blue nevus of the conjunctiva.

It may occur as a cellular blue nevus.

---

2. The condition is usually unilateral and is mainly present in dark races (blacks and Asians).

3. The lesion is blue or slate-gray from birth, and does not move with the conjunctiva.

4. It is associated with an ipsilateral diffuse uveal nevus that causes heterochromia, which at times is subtle, especially in brown-eyed people.

Waardenburg's syndrome consists of heterochromia iridum or iridis (unilateral or bilateral; segmental or diffuse) usually with a similar (congenital hypopigmentation) involvement of the remainder of the uvea; lateral displacement of medial canthi, combined with dystopia of the lacrimal puncta and blepharophimosis; prominent, broad root of the nose; growing together of the eyebrows with hypertrichosis of the medial portions; white forelock, a form of partial albinism (early graying of the hair begins soon after puberty); defective pigmentation in any part of the body; and congenital deafness. The involved eye is the lighter eye. The defect resides on chromosome 2q32.

---

5. The ocular involvement may be segmental (i.e., limited to a quadrant).

When segmental, the diffuse uveal nevus usually involves the iris, ciliary body, and choroid in the same quadrant (more or less).

---

6. The condition is potentially malignant when it occurs in white patients; a uveal malignant melanoma results.

Rarely, the conjunctiva or orbit may be the primary site of malignancy.

B. Congenital oculodermal melanocytosis (nevus of Ota; see p. 671 in this chapter).

VII. Unusual types of conjunctival nevi

A. Recurrent nevus—recurrence of an incompletely excised nevus

B. Inflamed nevus—pseudoenlargement of a conjunctival nevus, secondary to inflammation, usually seen between the ages of 15 and 25 years

C. Dysplastic nevus (see p. 669 in this chapter)

D. Spindle-cell nevus (Spitz nevus; juvenile melanoma; see above in this chapter)

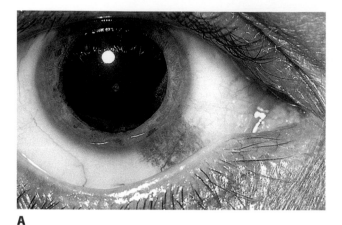

A

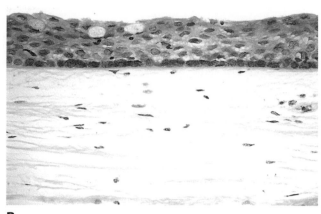

B

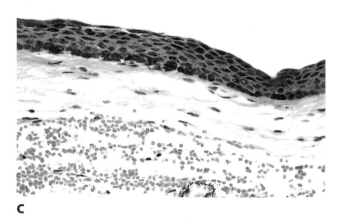

C

Fig. 17.12 Benign acquired melanosis. **A,** Clinical appearance of flat pigmented lesion of conjunctiva that developed in adulthood. The pigmentation also involved the cornea. **B,** Excisional biopsy shows stage IA (i.e., hyperpigmentation of basal layer of conjunctival epithelium). In other cases, pigmentation may extend into all layers of the epithelium, as shown in **C.**

E. Balloon cell nevus—probably represents lipidized melanocytes

F. Epithelioid cell nevus—composed entirely of epithelioid melanocytes

Primary Acquired Melanosis

I. PAM (Figs 17.12 and 17.13; see also Table 17.1)

A. Clinical characteristics

1. The melanosis consists of a unilateral, diffuse, brown pigmentation that moves with the conjunctiva over the sclera (analogous to lentigo maligna of the skin).

> Rarely, PAM may be amelanotic in both its benign and its malignant forms.

2. The condition has a variable and protracted course.

a. Rarely, it may remain stationary or even recede. It tends to remain benign, but slowly enlarges over the years.

b. Approximately 17% become malignant, usually 5 to 10 years after onset.

3. The age of onset is approximately 40 to 50 years of age.

4. Rarely, PAM may be associated with malignant melanomas of the nasal cavity and paranasal sinuses.

B. Classification of unilateral PAM*

1. Stage I: Benign acquired melanosis (precancerous melanosis)

a. Stage IA shows minimal melanocytic hyperplasia.

1). Hyperpigmentation of the epithelium may be the only finding (see Fig. 17.12).

2). Some increase in the number of enlarged melanocytes or a few scattered clusters of nevus cells along the basal layer may be seen.

b. Stage IB shows atypical melanocytic hyperplasia.

1). Stage IB1 shows mild to moderately severe atypical melanocytic hyperplasia (see Fig. 17.13C).

a). The lesions show enlarged melanocytes with enlarged nuclei, palisading of

Zimmerman LE: Criteria for management of melanosis: In correspondence. Arch Ophthalmol 76:307, 1966 (modified in Spencer WH, Zimmerman LE: Conjunctiva. In Ophthalmic Pathology, vol 1. An Atlas and Textbook. Philadelphia, WB Saunders, 1985:201).

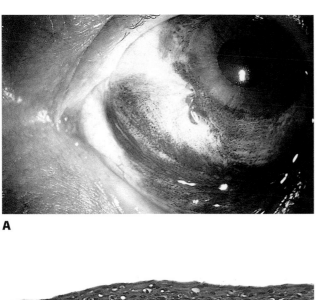

A

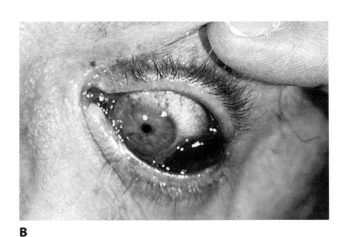

B

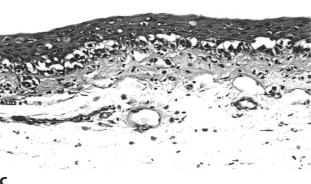

C

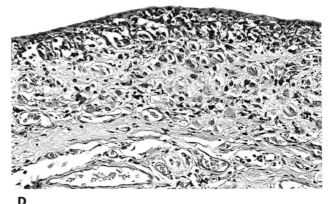

D

Fig. 17.13 Malignant acquired melanosis. **A,** Patient developed unilateral flat pigmentation of the conjunctiva and peripheral cornea as an adult. Completely flat pigmentation is rarely malignant. **B,** Another patient had adult-onset conjunctival pigmentation. A mass developed and excisional biopsy was performed. **C,** Biopsy of this area shows stage IB1 with moderately severe atypical melanocytic hyperplasia, appearing identical to a congenital conjunctival junctional nevus. **D,** Another area shows stage IIA with superficially invasive melanoma, almost complete replacement of the epithelium by atypical nevus cells, and invasion of the substantia propria by neoplastic cells. **E,** Still another area shows stage IIB (i.e., significantly invasive melanoma analogous to nodular melanoma of skin).

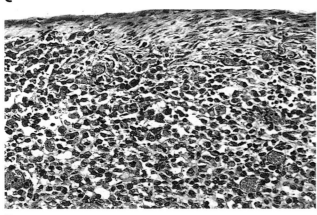

E

enlarged melanocytes along the basal layer, pagetoid "invasion" of the melanocytes into the conjunctival epithelium, and prominent nesting of melanocytes at various levels of the epithelium.

b). Histologically, it appears identical to a congenital, conjunctival, junctional nevus.

A clinical history of the age of onset is needed to differentiate between the two. Benign

acquired melanosis is a clinicopathologic diagnosis, not just a pathologic diagnosis.

2). Stage IB2 shows severe atypical melanocytic hyperplasia ("in situ" malignant melanoma).
   a). The lesions show mitotic activity and other cytologic features of malignancy, but no invasion of the substantia propria.
   b). Engorged vessels and inflammatory cells in the substantia propria are more apt to be present in IB2 than IB1.

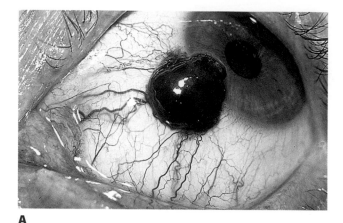

A

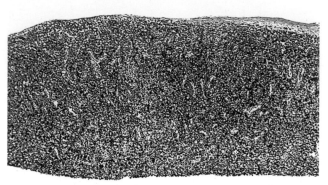

B

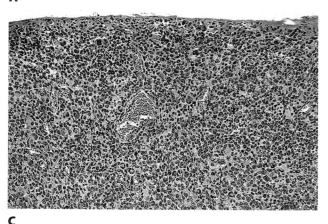

C

Fig. 17.14 Malignant melanoma. **A,** A pigmented conjunctival lesion near the limbus, present since childhood, had undergone recent rapid growth. **B,** A histological section of an incomplete excisional biopsy shows a heavily pigmented tumor. **C,** A bleached section shows a loss of normal polarity (i.e., the cells deep in the lesion are of the same size as those nearer the surface instead of being smaller). Usually, conjunctival melanomas not thicker than 1.5 mm have an excellent prognosis, whereas those thicker than 1.5 mm have a grave prognosis.

2. Stage II: Malignant acquired melanosis
   a. Stage IIA shows superficially invasive melanoma (tumor thickness <1.5 mm; see Fig. 17.13D).
      1). Minimal invasion of the substantia propria by neoplastic melanocytes is demonstrable somewhere in the lesion.
      2). The condition in stages IA, IB, and IIA is analogous to superficial spreading (radial growth phase) or incipient melanoma of skin.
   b. Stage IIB shows significantly invasive melanoma (tumor thickness >1.5 mm; see Fig. 17.13E). The condition in stage IIB is analogous to nodular melanoma of skin (vertical growth phase).

3. Prognosis
   a. The probability for development of a stage IA lesion into a malignant melanoma is quite low.
   b. The probability for development of a stage IB lesion into an invasive malignant melanoma is approximately 20% if individual atypical melanocytes are confined to the epithelial basal layer, and approximately 90% when they are arranged in nests or invade the epithelium in a pagetoid fashion.
   c. A thickness of the malignant melanoma of less than 1.5 mm (stage IIA) separates the mostly

nonlethal tumors (<1.5 mm) from the very lethal tumors (>1.5 mm—stage IIB).

II. Causes of secondary acquired melanosis*
   A. Radiation
   B. Metabolic disorders
      1. Addison's disease
      2. Pregnancy
   C. Chemical toxicity
      1. Arsenic
      2. Thorazine
   D. Chronic conjunctival disorders
      1. Trachoma
      2. Vernal conjunctivitis
      3. Keratomalacia
      4. Xeroderma pigmentosum
      5. Acanthosis nigricans

Malignant Melanoma

I. Primary (Fig. 17.14; see also Fig. 17.13)
   A. The incidence of primary conjunctival malignant melanoma is less than 5 cases per million in the United States. The 10-year mortality is about 10%.

*Modified from Henkind P, Friedman AH: External ocular pigmentation. Int Ophthalmol Clin 11:87, 1971.

About 1 in 20 primary conjunctival melanomas involve only the cornea ("corneally displaced conjunctival melanoma"), and have a favorable prognosis.

B. In 35% to 40% of cases, primary conjunctival malignant melanomas arise from junctional (rare) or compound nevi; in 25% to 30% of cases, they come from PAM; and in 25% to 30% of cases, they arise de novo or indeterminately.

A subset of conjunctival proliferations exists that cannot be classified as benign or malignant on purely cytologic criteria; these tumors should be called *intermediate melanocytic proliferation of the conjunctiva.*

C. Primary conjunctival malignant melanomas that arise from junctional or compound nevi are probably analogous to the cutaneous superficial spreading malignant melanoma.
D. Primary conjunctival malignant melanomas that arise de novo or indeterminately are probably analogous to the cutaneous nodular malignant melanoma.
E. It is rare for a melanoma to arise from congenital ocular melanocytosis.
F. Melanomas are rare in black people.
G. Histology (for histology of PAM, see pp. 680–681 in this chapter)
  1. Remnants of a conjunctival nevus may be found in or contiguous to the melanoma.
  2. Normal polarity is lost (i.e., deep cells are indistinguishable from superficial cells).
  3. The overlying epithelium is invaded.

Pigmentation may or may not be present. If present, it may vary in different parts of the tumor. If pigmentation is not present, the tumor is called an *amelanotic melanoma.*

  a. Invasion of the underlying subepithelial tissue occurs concurrently with epithelial invasion.
  4. The cells of the neoplasm are atypical.
    a. The nuclear-to-cytoplasmic ratio is increased, and large, abnormal cells may be seen.
    b. Mitotic figures may be present, but are frequently absent.
    c. The cells express S-100, tyrosinase, melan-A, HMB-45 and HMB-50 combination, and microphthalmia transcription factor at high levels. Pigment epithelium-derived growth factor can also be a a useful diagnostic marker for melanocytic tumors, especially malignant melanomas.
  5. Often, an underlying inflammatory infiltrate of round cells, predominantly lymphocytes, is present.
  6. Silver staining of the nuclear organizer regions is helpful in determining malignancy of pigmented conjunctival lesions.

  7. Usually, a combination of the aforementioned criteria rather than any single criterion leads to the diagnosis of malignancy.

Conjunctival melanomas and skin melanomas are not classified according to cell type, as are uveal melanomas. Probably, most, if not all, of the "primary malignant melanomas of the cornea" arise in the limbal conjunctiva primarily and invade the cornea secondarily. Most conjunctival melanomas are most closely analogous to superficial spreading melanomas of skin. It is not necessary, therefore, to use the classification for skin melanomas for the conjunctiva.

II. Secondary—these tumors may arise from intraocular melanomas or may be metastatic.

Rarely, a primary conjunctival malignant melanoma may extend through the anterior scleral canals to invade the eye. Differentiating between a uveal melanoma extending outward into the conjunctiva and a conjunctival melanoma invading inward to the uvea may be difficult.

III. Prognosis
A. Conjunctival melanoma arising from a junctional or compound nevus has a mortality rate of approximately 20%.
B. If it arises from PAM, the mortality rate is approximately 40%.
C. If it arises de novo or its origin is indeterminate, the mortality rate is approximately 40%.
D. An accurate parameter for predicting prognosis is tumor thickness at the time of extirpation.
  1. In general, if the thickness is no greater than 1.5 mm, the prognosis for life is excellent.
  2. If the tumor thickness is greater than 1.5 mm, however, the prognosis for life is extremely grave.

Sometimes, however, even flat conjunctival melanomas may be lethal.

  3. Prognosis also depends on "unfavorable" locations [i.e., the palpebral conjunctiva, fornices, plica, caruncle, and lid margins (2.2 times higher mortality rate than bulbar conjunctiva)].

In one series of 85 patients with conjunctival melanoma, 10-year survival rate based on tumor-related death was 77.7%. Higher local relapse rate was associated with unfavorable location (palpebral conjunctiva, fornix, caruncle, corneal stroma, and eyelid). Death from metastatic melanoma was associated with patient age greater than 55 years, higher tumor, node, metastasis (TNM) category, and unfavorable tumor location.

E. Patients who die of metastatic disease have significantly higher counts of cells positive for proliferating cell nuclear antigen than patients who survive a minimum of 5 years.

F. Adjunctive therapy for conjunctival melanoma, such as irradiation, cryotherapy, or local chemotherapy, has been suggested as a possible means to minimize local tumor recurrence.

Lesions That May Simulate Primary Conjunctival Nevus or Malignant Melanoma

I. See earlier discussion of secondary acquired melanosis in this chapter.
II. See preceding discussion of secondary malignant melanoma of conjunctiva in this chapter.
III. Nevus of sclera—blue nevus, cellular blue nevus, and melanocytoma can occur in the sclera.
IV. Pseudopigmentation
    A. Blue sclera (see p. 314 in Chapter 8)
    B. Ectatic sclera lined by choroid (i.e., staphyloma) may simulate a conjunctival melanoma.
    C. Scleromalacia perforans (see p. 317 in Chapter 8)
V. Endogenous pigmentations
    A. Blood, especially its oxidation product (i.e., hemosiderin), may simulate a conjunctival melanoma.
    B. Bile
        1. In acute icterus, bilirubin is deposited predominantly in the conjunctiva, not in the sclera.
        2. With chronic, long-standing icterus, the bilirubin, although mainly in the conjunctiva, is also deposited in the sclera.
VI. Metabolic disorders
    A. Ochronosis (alkaptonuria; see p. 314 in Chapter 8)
    B. Gaucher's disease shows conjunctival changes consisting of pigmented, triangular, brown pingueculae that contain Gaucher's cells. They appear in the second decade of life.
VII. Exogenous pigmentations
    A. Epinephrine plaques (see p. 235 in Chapter 7)
    B. Argyrosis (see Fig. 7.10)

Ocular argyrosis may occur secondary to the chronic self-application of eyelash tint. Silver deposition from this mechanism may be relatively extensive and involve the lid margin, caruncle, and conjunctiva as well as the eyelid.

    C. Mascara
    D. Industrial hazards
        1. Quinones
        2. Aniline dyes
    E. Iron
    F. Foreign bodies
VIII. Pigment spots of the sclera (Fig. 17.15)
    A. Pigment spots of the sclera are most commonly found with darkly pigmented irises.
    B. They consist of episcleral collections of uveal melanocytes 3 to 4 mm from the limbus and are always associated with a perforating anterior ciliary vessel, an intrascleral nerve loop of Axenfeld, or both.
    C. They decrease in frequency from superior to inferior to temporal to nasal quadrants.

D. The conjunctiva is freely movable over the pigment spot.
E. The associated intrascleral nerve loop remains painful to touch even after local instillation of a topical anesthetic.
F. Pigment spots of the sclera may be confused with conjunctival nevi, melanomas, and foreign bodies (see Fig. 17.15).

MELANOTIC TUMORS OF PIGMENT EPITHELIUM OF IRIS, CILIARY BODY, AND RETINA

The ultrasound biomicroscope (UBM) and similar devices are particularly useful in the evaluation of anteriorly located melanotic uveal and pigment epithelial tumors. UBM can be helpful in therapeutic planning and follow-up following treatment for such tumors.

Reactive Tumors

I. Congenital (see Fig. 9.10)
    A. Solid and cystic proliferation of the iris PE, especially the PE near the iris root, is a frequent congenital anomaly.

Although congenital, the anomaly may not be noted clinically until adult life. Most primary cysts of the iris PE have a benign clinical course that rarely necessitates treatment.

---

        1. The PE may break off and float freely in the anterior chamber, or lodge in the anterior-chamber angle, where it may be pigmented or clear and transparent.

Indications for surgical removal of such cysts include rapid enlargement or significant reduction in endothelial cell count. Visual symptoms from primary pupillary epithelial cysts have also necessitated cyst removal. Cysts in that location usually have an autosomal-dominant inheritance pattern, with occasional lack of penetrance.

---

        2. It may simulate a malignant melanoma of the anterior ciliary body. Conversely, cavitary melanoma simulating a cyst is an uncommon presentation for ciliary body melanoma.
        3. It may result from intrauterine inflammation, trauma, or unknown causes.
        4. Iris pigment epithelial cysts must be considered in the differential diagnosis of angle closure glaucoma in teenagers.
        5. Histologically, the PE proliferates in cords, tubes, or cystic structures.B. Congenital simple hamartoma of the RPE is usually a black, full-thickness mass, often adjacent to the fovea. Vision is usually well preserved.

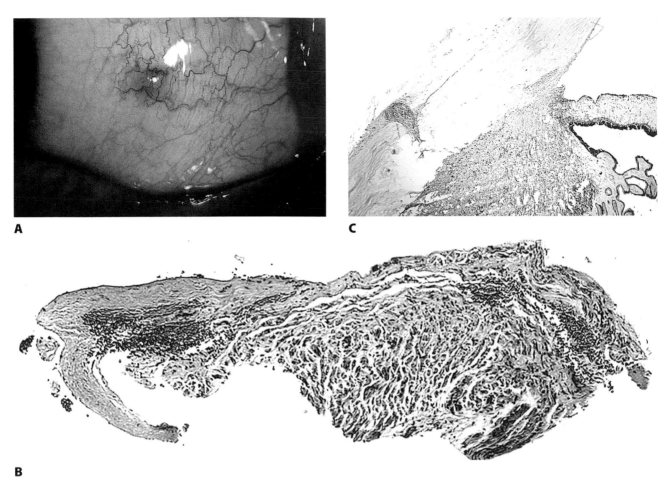

A

C

B

Fig. 17.15 Scleral pigment spot. **A,** Clinical appearance of pigment spot misdiagnosed as a foreign body in a 5-year-old boy. **B,** Biopsy shows ciliary nerve that contains scattered pigment. The nerve was an intrascleral nerve loop (of Axenfeld). **C,** The anterior scleral canal may also act as a conduit for a ciliary body melanoma to reach the epibulbar surface and simulate a conjunctival lesion. (**A** and **B,** Adapted from Crandall AS *et al.: Arch Ophthalmol* 95:497, 1977. © American Medical Association. All rights reserved.)

C. Combined hamartoma (idiopathic reactive hyperplasia) of the retina and retinal PE (Fig. 17.16)
1. The lesion is mainly juxtapapillary but may be located peripherally.

> The differential diagnosis includes cavernous hemangioma, capillary hemangioma (von Hippel's disease), astrocytic hamartoma (tuberous sclerosis), melanocytoma, malignant melanoma, choroidal osteoma, and retinoblastoma.

2. It is mostly seen in young men between the ages of 20 and 45 years (range, 12 to 63 years).

> It is not known whether these lesions are congenital or reactive, but they are most probably congenital.

3. Clinically, the lesion usually appears as a solitary grayish mass with variable pigmentation and vascularity.

a. Retinal contracture and subsequent impairment of vision (if the macula is involved) may occur.
b. Rarely, growth is documented.
c. Atypical findings include subneural retinal hemorrhage, fluid accumulation and neovascularization; intraneural retinal cystic spaces; arterioarterial anastomoses; vitreous hemorrhage; and inner-layer neural retinal holes in acquired retinoschisis.
d. Combined hamartoma may also be associated with retinal capillary nonperfusion and preretinal neovascularization presumably indicating associated retinal ischemia.
e. An association may exist between neurofibromatosis type-1 and combined hamartoma of the retina and retinal pigment epithelium (RPE). Combined hamartoma of the retina and RPE has been associated with juvenile nasopharyngeal angiofibroma, and has been reported involving the optic disc associated with choroidal neovascularization.

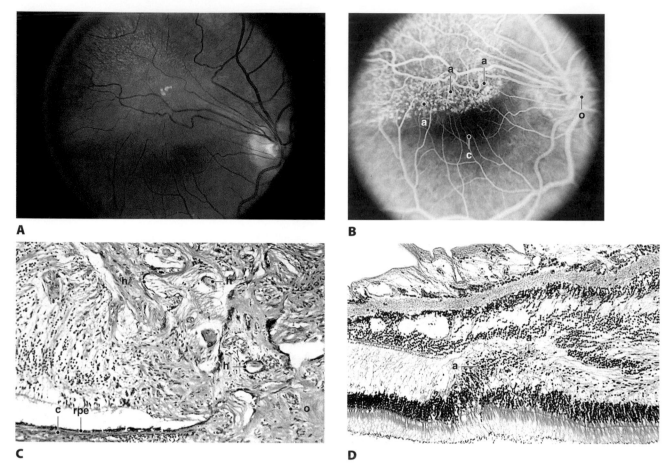

Fig. 17.16 Combined hamartoma of neural retina and retinal pigment epithelium (RPE). **A,** A 23-year-old nurse had esotropia of the right eye since childhood. Examination shows a thickened retina superior to the fovea. A few specks of what appears to be calcium are present in the lesion. **B,** Fluorescein angiography shows a highly vascularized lesion that contains abnormal blood vessels (a) (c, central fovea; o, optic nerve). **C,** A histologic section of another case shows that the RPE has proliferated into the retina in the juxtapapillary area. Both proliferating pigmented cells and abnormal retinal blood vessels are seen (h, RPE hamartoma; o, optic nerve; c, choroid). **D,** In another area, an abnormal, dysplastic, extension of the outer nuclear layer reaches into the outer plexiform layer, along with abnormally located small blood vessels (a, abnormal distribution of nuclei and blood vessels). (**C** and **D,** Courtesy of Dr. E Howes, reported by Vogel MH *et al.: Doc Ophthalmol* 26:461, 1969. Reproduced with kind permission of Springer Science and Business Media.)

Combined hamartoma of the retina and RPE may be indistinguishable from congenital RPE malformation or congenital simple hamartoma of the RPE. Congenital RPE malformation consists of RPE hypertrophy (not hyperplasia, as in the hamartoma) and abnormalities of the retina such as thickening, vascular tortuosity, and retinal capillary abnormalities. Congenital simple hamartoma of the RPE (also called RPE hamartoma, congenital or primary RPE hyperplasia, and congenital RPE adenoma) appears in the macula as a darkly pigmented, nodular mass involving full-thickness retina and containing sharp margins. Rarely, congenital simple RPE hamartoma may occur in the central fovea, and result in poor vision. Optical coherence tomography can be helpful in the evaluation of such lesions.

4. Histologically, combined hamartoma of the retina and RPE consists of an intraneural retinal proliferation of RPE associated with abnormal (hamar-tomatous) retinal blood vessels, and areas of dysplastic retina.

A 10-year-old girl with branchio-oculofacial (BOF) syndrome has been reported with an iris pigment epithelial cyst of the right eye, and a combined hamartoma of the retina and RPE. BOF syndrome is characterized by mild to severe craniofacial, auricular, oral, and ocular anomalies. The case reported also displayed lacrimal sac fistulas, and orbital dermoid cyst.

D. Medulloepithelioma (diktyoma)
   1. Medulloepithelioma is a unilateral, solitary ocular tumor.
      a. It arises from the ciliary epithelium as a well-circumscribed mass, or it may infiltrate the area around the lens.

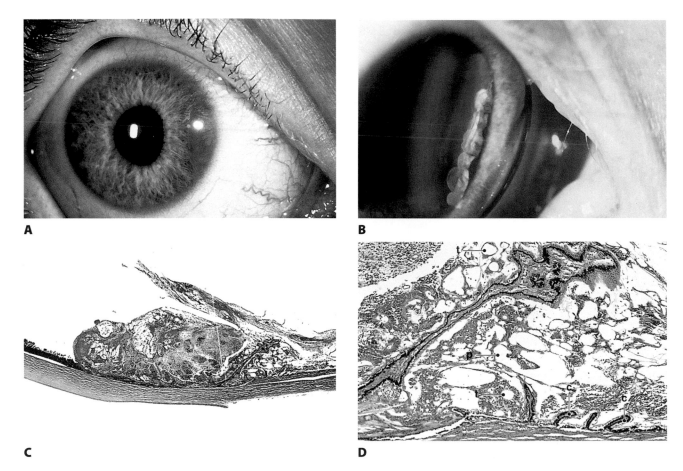

Fig. 17.17 Benign medulloepithelioma. **A,** The tumor seen in the anterior-chamber angle nasally had originated in the ciliary body, best seen in **B** (shown after pupillary dilatation). **C,** A histologic section of another case shows structures that resemble primitive medullary epithelium, ciliary epithelium, and retina. The tumor arises from nonpigmented ciliary epithelium. **D,** Increased magnification shows the cell tubules. Structures analogous to external limiting membrane of the retina appear on one surface of the tubules (in some areas forming lumina), whereas the less well-defined opposite surface is in contact with a primitive vitreous (p, primitive vitreous; c, ciliary process; t, tubules of cells containing lumina). (**A** and **B,** Courtesy of Dr. JA Shields; **C** and **D,** Courtesy of Dr. JS McGavic.)

Rarely, the tumor can arise from the iris or optic nerve in the region of the optic disc.

  b. Usually it presents during the first decade with a peculiar pupillary reflex, a characteristic lens notch and lens subluxation, and a tendency to cause a neoplastic cyclitic membrane and a secondary neovascular glaucoma.

Even more rarely, medulloepithelioma may present as a pigmented ciliary body tumor, instead of the usual fleshy pink appearance.

  c. The tumor grows slowly and is only locally aggressive.

Echographic findings of a highly reflective, irregularly structured tumor with associated cystic changes involving the ciliary body region may help establish the diagnosis of medulloepithelioma.

  d. Glaucoma may be the presenting sign.

2. Medulloepithelioma (*nonteratoid medulloepithelioma*) may be benign (Fig. 17.17) or malignant.

3. Heteroplastic elements may be present, in which case the tumor is termed a *teratoid medulloepithelioma*, benign or malignant (Fig. 17.18).

4. Histologically, nonteratoid medulloepithelioma consists of poorly differentiated neuroectodermal tissue that in some areas resembles embryonic retina.

  a. The cells are frequently arranged in a double layer, and the innermost layer secretes hyaluronic acid ("vitreous").

When heteroplastic elements are present [e.g., cartilage is present in 20% of cases; the tumor may also contain rhabdomyoblasts (see Fig. 17.18B and C), which are large globular cells that resemble ganglion cells], it is called a *teratoid medulloepithelioma*.

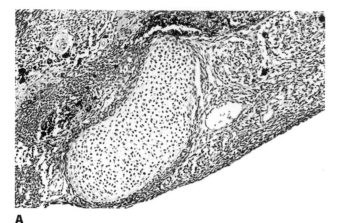

A

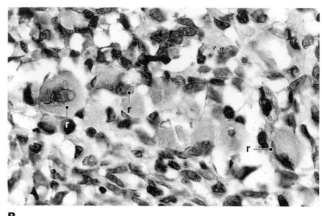

B

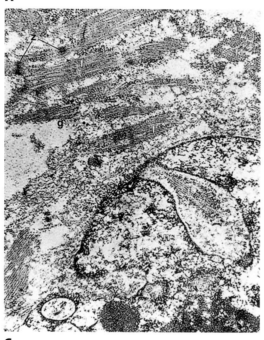

C

Fig. 17.18 Malignant teratoid medulloepithelioma. **A,** A heteroplastic element, namely, a large nodule of cartilage, is present in the tumor. Many atypical cells that simulate retinoblastoma surround the cartilage. **B,** In another area, rhabdomyoblasts (r) are present. **C,** Electron microscopy shows that rhabdomyoblast contains numerous bundles of thick and thin cytoplasmic filaments in longitudinal and cross-section. Note Z bands and numerous glycogen particles. Nucleus (right corner) shows infolding (f, filaments in longitudinal section; f1, filaments in cross-section; g, glycogen particles; n, nucleus). (**A** and **B,** Case presented by Dr. BW Streeten at the meeting of the Eastern Ophthalmic Pathology Society, 1973, and reported by Carrillo R, Streeten BW: *Arch Ophthalmol* 97:695, 1979. © American Medical Association. All rights reserved. **C,** from Zimmerman LE *et al.*: *Cancer* 30:817, 1979. © American Cancer Society. Modified by permission of Wiley-Liss, Inc., a subsidiary of John Wiley & Sons, Inc.)

b. The neuroepithelial cells are positive for neuron-specific enolase, vimentin, and often S-100 protein.

c. The neuroblastic cells are usually positive for neuron-specific enolase and synaptophysin.

Nonteratoid and teratoid medulloepithelioma, unlike retinoblastoma, appears to be a truly multipotential tumor.

---

d. Malignant nonteratoid tumors contain tightly packed neuroblastic cells that sometimes show marked mitotic activity and resemble retinoblastoma cells.

e. Malignant teratoid tumors often have sarcomatous changes in one or more of the heteroplastic

elements (e.g., rhabdomyosarcoma or chondrosarcoma).

Rarely, a congenital malignant teratoid tumor can involve both the eye and the orbit.

II. Drusen (see p. 425 in Chapter 11)
III. Pseudoneoplastic proliferations
  A. Pupillary—after miotic therapy (phospholine iodide for childhood accommodative esotropia), the iris PE may enlarge or proliferate into the pupillary area.
  B. Intraneural retinal (usually from RPE)
    1. Intraneural retinal reactive RPE proliferations may occur in abiotrophic diseases, e.g., retinitis pigmentosa (see Fig. 11.36).

In retinitis pigmentosa, the pigmented cells surrounding the blood vessels ("bone–corpuscular" pigmentation) may be pigment-filled macrophages, Müller cells, or migrated RPE cells.

2. Pseudoneoplastic proliferations may also occur in metabolic disorders such as homocystinuria; after trauma; as a senile change, especially in the region of the macula; after ocular inflammation; or in long-standing diabetes.
3. Ringschwiele or demarcation line (see p. 469 in Chapter 11)
4. Focal hyperplasia of the RPE can produce tumors that invade and replace the overlying sensory retina.
5. Optical coherence tomography can be helpful in evaluating RPE changes secondary to choroidal metastasis of nonocular tumors and for their follow-up after treatment.

C. Intravitreal (usually from ciliary PE or RPE, but may be from iris PE)
  1. Intravitreal pseudoneoplastic proliferations of the PE are most common after trauma.
  2. They may follow purulent endophthalmitis or other ocular inflammations.
  3. Histologically, proliferated epithelium, pigmented and nonpigmented, extends out in cords and sheets, surrounded by abundant basement membrane material.

D. Pseudoepitheliomatous hyperplasia of the ciliary body epithelium
  1. May simulate a malignant melanoma

IV. Metaplastic
  A. Disciform degeneration of the macula (i.e., macular scarring in age-related macular degeneration) represents fibrous metaplasia of the RPE.
  B. Bone formation (osseous metaplasia; see Fig. 3.14)
    1. It is not certain if the PE undergoes osseous metaplasia or acts as an inducer for surrounding mesenchymal tissue to undergo osseous metaplasia.
    2. Intraocular osseous metaplasia is not preceded by cartilage formation.
    3. It is common after trauma, long-standing uveitis, and endophthalmitis.

V. Atrophic changes other than as part of age-related macular degeneration.
  A. Green laser-induced retinopathy can result in a yellowish discoloration at the level of the RPE and RPE damage noted on histopathologic examination.
  B. Nummular changes at the level of the RPE may be found in bilateral diffuse uveal melanocytic proliferation (BDUMP) syndrome in which uveal melanocytic proliferation is usually the chief finding (see also below).

Nonreactive Tumors

I. Congenital
  A. Glioneuroma (Fig. 17.19)

1. Glioneuromas are rare, benign, choristomatous tumors.
2. Histologically, the tumor is composed only of brain tissue, containing neurons and glial cells and lacking the embryonic retina, ciliary epithelium, and primitive vitreous found in medulloepitheliomas.
  a. Immunohistochemistry shows positivity in the neuronal cells for neuron-specific enolase, synaptophysin, and neurofilaments; in the glial cells for vimentin, glial fibrillary acidic protein, and S-100 protein; and in the neuroepithelial cells for cytokeratins, vimentin, neuron-specific enolase, and S-100 protein (suggesting ciliary epithelial origin).

B. Grouped pigmentation (bear tracks; Fig. 17.20; see also p. 396 in Chapter 11)
C. RPE hypertrophy (melanotic RPE nevus; benign "melanoma" of the RPE of Reese and Jones; see Fig. 17.20)
  1. Congenital hypertrophy of the RPE (CHRPE) presents clinically as a round or oval, jet-black, flat (or slightly elevated) lesion usually surrounded by a halo (due to partial or complete RPE hypopigmentation).

The lesions may show enlargement over time, especially with lacunae formation and expansion.

  a. It may contain "punched-out," yellow, depigmented patches of irregular sizes and shapes, called *lacunae*.
  b. The depigmentation tends to enlarge or coalesce, or both, in approximately 80% of lesions and may lead to total depigmentation, leaving a recognizable, round or oval, well-circumscribed, orange hypopigmented or white (albinotic) amelanotic lesion.
  c. Often scotomata are found, corresponding to neural retinal photoreceptor degeneration overlying the lesion.

In some lesions, overlying retinal vascular changes can be demonstrated by fluorescein. The combination of CHRPE and abnormalities of the retina (such as a thickened retina, tortuosity of retinal vessels, and dilated abnormal capillaries) is called *congenital RPE malformation*.

  d. CHRPE can be divided into three forms: solid, grouped, and multiple; bilateral or multiple can be associated with *Gardner's syndrome*.
  2. It is a congenital lesion and has been found in a newborn.
  3. CHRPE may be associated with familial polyposis of the colon (Gardner's syndrome).
    a. Gardner's syndrome consists of familial adenomatous polyposis (FAP), which has an autosomal-dominant inheritance pattern, and

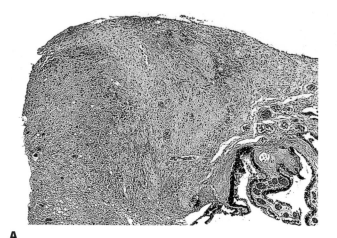

A

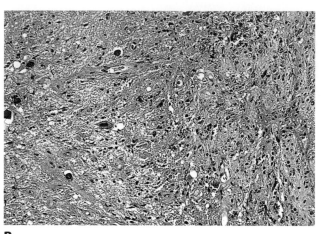

B

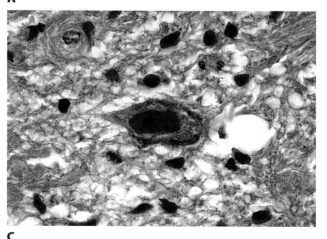

C

Fig. 17.19 Glioneuroma. **A,** Tumor in region of ciliary body, removed by iridocyclectomy, extends into iris root. **B,** Tumor shows tissue similar to brain tissue, containing ganglion cells; shown with increased magnification in **C.** (Case presented by Dr. DJ Addison at Meeting of the Association of Ophthalmic Alumni of the Armed Forces Institute of Pathology, Washington, DC, 1977.)

extracolonic manifestations, including hamartomas of the RPE, osteomas, epidermoid cysts, desmoid tumors, and infrequent malignant tumors of liver, thyroid, brain, and other organs.

b. In Slovakia, mutations within codons 1309 and 1060 were associated with a large number of colorectal polyps and CHRPE. Individuals with adenomatous polyposis and CHRPE, but lacking mutations in the adenomatous polyposis coli (APC) gene in patients in Hong Kong, suggest that these disorders can result from abnormalities not associated with APC coding region mutations.

A variant of this autosomal-dominant disorder is *Turcot's syndrome* (glioma–polyposis), which consists of FAP and neuroepithelial tumors of the central nervous system. Multiple regions of hamartomas of the RPE may be found on examination of the ocular fundi.

---

1). In patients with FAP, over 100 adenomatous colorectal polyps develop before early adulthood.

Without treatment, adenocarcinoma always develops.

---

2). Hamartomas of the RPE are divided into at least three types: a monolayer of hypertrophic RPE cells (CHRPE); a mound of pigmented cells interposed between Bruch's membrane and RPE basement membrane; and a small mound of hyperplastic RPE cells (nodular RPE hypertrophy).

b. Hamartomas of the RPE are most helpful in the diagnosis of Gardner's syndrome.
   1). Hamartomas of the RPE are detectable before the development of intestinal polyps.
   2). The presence of four or more hamartomas of the RPE is a highly specific phenotypic marker for Gardner's syndrome.

c. One or more genes on chromosome 5q21 are important for the development of colorectal cancers associated with FAP.

d. There is no association between CHRPE characteristics and specific FAP variants.

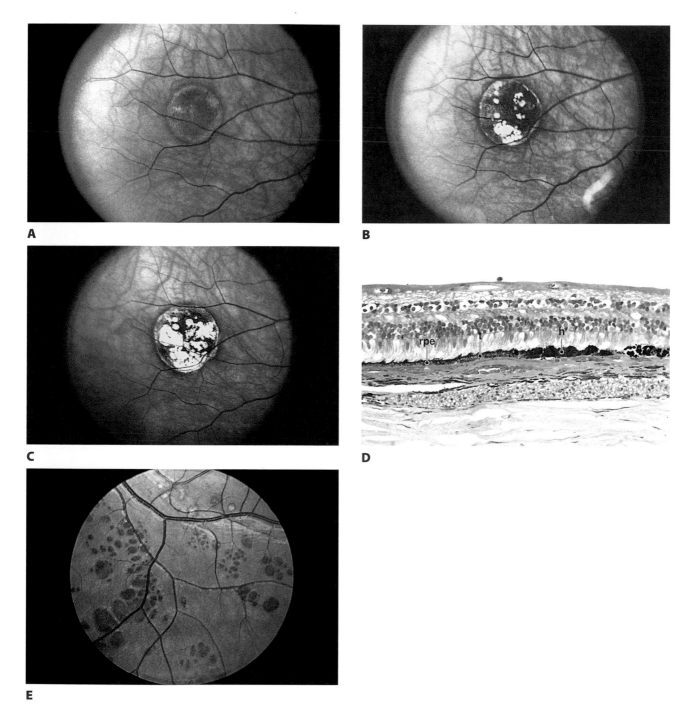

Fig. 17.20 Retinal pigment epithelium (RPE) hypertrophy. **A,** The characteristic jet-black lesion, surrounded by a halo, contains yellow patches of irregular size and shape. **B,** The same lesion, 6 years later, has increased in size and changed in appearance. **C,** After 12 years, most of the lesion is occupied by large yellow lacunae. **D,** A histologic section of another case shows a sudden transition (t) from normal RPE on the left to markedly enlarged cells (h, hypertrophied RPE). The enlarged cells contain enlarged pigment granules (macromelanosomes). Often, at the edge of such a lesion, the RPE cells are depigmented, giving rise to the halo seen clinically around the lesion. Congenital hypertrophy of the RPE may be found in familial adenomatous polyposis (Gardner's or Turcot's syndrome). **E,** Grouped pigmentation (bear tracks) usually affects a single sector-shaped retinal area whose apex points to the optic disc. The histology of grouped pigmentation is almost identical to that of congenital hypertrophy of the RPE and probably represents a clinical variant. (**D,** Presented by Dr. WR Lee at the meeting of the European Ophthalmic Pathology Society, 1982; **E,** courtesy of Dr. WE Benson.)

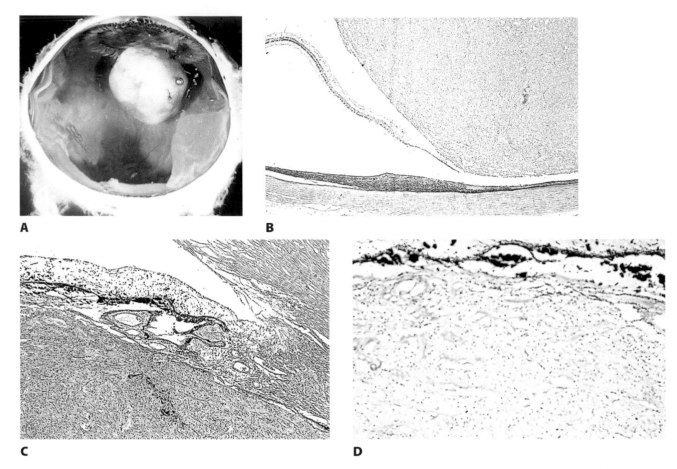

Fig. 17.21 Adenoma. **A,** Gross appearance of relatively amelanotic tumor (adenoma) of ciliary body. **B,** Histologic section shows two benign lesions: an adenoma of the ciliary epithelium and a choroidal nevus. **C,** The papillary adenoma of the ciliary epithelium is composed of chords of predominantly nonpigmented epithelial cells, along with occasional pigmented cells. **D,** Alcian blue stain demonstrates acid mucopolysaccharides in the tumor. The blue color disappeared when the sections were pretreated with hyaluronidase, signifying the presence of hyaluronic acid, which is secreted by the tumor.

4. Histologically, CHRPE consists of hypertrophy of RPE cells, and an increase in size (macromelanosomes) and number of their melanin granules.

Although RPE hypertrophy (increase in size of cells) is the predominant component, RPE hyperplasia (increase in number of cells) is also present in many lesions.

---

a. The surrounding halo is due to atrophy or loss of pigment from the adjacent RPE, or both.
b. Degeneration of the overlying neural retinal photoreceptor cells may be found.

The histology of CHRPE is almost identical to that of grouped pigmentation (bear tracks—see p. 396 in Chapter 11). Both can be considered variants of the same process. The former is a larger focal lesion, and the latter are smaller multifocal lesions.

---

5. Congenital hypertrophy of the RPE can give rise to adenocarcinoma.

Acquired Neoplasms

I. Fuchs' adenoma (proliferation rather than neoplasm; see Fig. 9.17)
II. Adenoma (epithelioma; Fig. 17.21)
  A. Adenomas may arise from the ciliary epithelium or RPE.
  B. Clinically, they tend to be darker and their margins more abruptly elevated than in ciliary body melanomas.

Adenoma of the ciliary body nonpigmented epithelium has been reported with concomitant neovascularization of the optic disc (NVD) and cystoid macular edema (CME). It was postulated that elevated vascular endothelial growth factors in intraocular fluids, which were determined in both aqueous and vitreous obtained at surgery, may have played a role the development of NVD and CME.

  C. Benign adenoma of the ciliary body pigment epithelium may exhibit progressive growth and undergo malignant change. These lesions may invade the anterior-chamber angle or cause pigment dispersion. Cataract, vitreous hemorrhage, and neovascular glaucoma have also been reported in association with these lesions.

D. Histologically, the epithelial cells appear polyhedral and have variable pigmentation.

1. They may show a tubular (papillary) pattern, a vacuolated (solid) pattern, or a mixture of both; the tumors may become cystic.

2. The heavily pigmented cells are frequently vacuolated.

The vacuoles contain a sialomucin that can be digested with neuraminidase (sialidase).

---

3. Nuclear atypia is common, but mitotic figures are rare.

4. Immunohistochemically, they show positivity for vimentin, S-100 protein, and low-molecular-weight cytokeratins. They are negative for vimentin.

5. In contrast to tumorlike hyperplastic lesions of the RPE, the RPE adenoma is sporadic melan-A-positive.

6. Histologically, adenoma may be difficult to differentiate from reactive proliferations of the PE.

   a. The cells of the adenoma are variably pigmented and are packed together tightly with little or no stroma, whereas the individual cells in pseudo-adenomatous hyperplasia tend to be separated by an amorphous basement membrane-like material, and show little atypia and no mitotic figures.

7. Transmission electron microscopy reveals tight junctions between cells.

III. Adenocarcinoma

A. Like adenomas, pleomorphic adenocarcinomas may have a vacuolated (solid) or tubular (papillary) pattern, or a mixture of both.

B. When the PE becomes malignant, it forms an incidentally pigmented adenocarcinoma, not a malignant melanoma.

Clinically, the tumors are locally invasive, but it is questionable whether they have the biologic ability to metastasize or even to undergo extrascleral extension.

C. Adenocarcinoma is a histologic diagnosis based on cellular atypia.

1. In addition to hyaluronic acid secretion, immunohistochemical staining shows strong positivity for vimentin, focal positivity for epithelial basement membrane antigen and S-100 protein, and weak positivity for neuron-specific enolase.

2. Adenocarcinoma of the nonpigmented ciliary epithelium has been reported to be immunohistochemically positive for AE1 and epithelial membrane antigen.

An imbalance of chromosome 6 has been found by comparative genomic hybridization in a patient with pleomorphic adenocarcinoma of the ciliary epithelium.

IV. Leiomyoepithelioma of iris PE

V. Melanotic neuroectodermal (retinal anlage) tumor of infancy

MELANOTIC TUMORS OF THE UVEA

Iris

I. Ephelis (freckle; Fig. 17.22)

A. A freckle shows increased pigmentation of anterior border layer melanocytes without increased number of melanocytes.

B. There is no discrete mass or nodule.

II. Nevus (see Fig. 17.22)

A. A nevus shows an increased number of atypical, benign-appearing melanocytes (i.e., nevus cells) with variable pigmentation.

B. A discrete mass or nodule is present, often on the iris anterior surface (i.e., within the anterior border layer of the iris).

C. An increased incidence of iris nevi occurs in people who have neurofibromatosis (see Fig. 2.4), but probably not in those who have ciliary body or choroidal malignant melanomas.

D. A diffuse (or rarely segmental) nevus of the iris (and the rest of the uvea) is present in congenital ocular or oculodermal melanocytosis.

Rarely, a diffuse nevus of the iris can cause glaucoma by direct involvement of the drainage area, or by synechiae and secondary closed-angle glaucoma.

E. An acquired, diffuse nevus of the iris may be associated with the iris nevus syndrome, part of the iridocorneal endothelial (ICE) syndrome (see p. 639 in Chapter 16).

Melanocytoma (magnocellular nevus; see p. 721 in this chapter) of the iris may occur. Necrosis of a melanocytoma may mislead the clinician to a diagnosis of malignant melanoma. Another unusual type of iris nevus is called the *benign epithelioid cell nevus*. A rare case of probable autosomal-dominant, "aggressive" iris nevus in childhood has been reported.

F. Malignant change is rare.

III. Heterochromia (Table 17.2)

IV. Malignant melanoma (Figs 17.23 and 17.24; see also Fig. 16.18)

A. Iris malignant melanomas have no sex predilection; the average age of involvement is 47 years.

B. They are the most common primary neoplasm of the iris and constitute approximately 5% to 8% of all uveal melanomas.

1. They usually arise from the anterior border layer tissue of the iris (as do iris nevi).

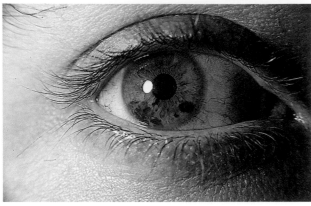

A

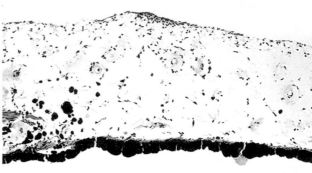

B

Fig. 17.22 Iris freckle and nevus. **A,** Clinical appearance of one iris nevus at 4 o'clock and numerous iris freckles. **B,** An iris freckle results from increased pigmentation of melanocytes of the anterior border layer without an increase of mass. **C,** An iris nevus is composed of nevus cells that result in increased mass—in this instance two nevi, one located near the pupillary border and the other slightly more peripheral.

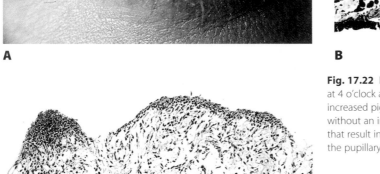

C

TABLE 17.2 Differential Diagnosis of Heterochromia

Involved Iris: Darker	Involved Iris: Lighter
1. Congenital ocular or oculodermal melanocytosis	1. Horner's syndrome (congenital or acquired)
2. Diffuse nevus of iris	2. Diffuse nevus (amelanotic nevus covering iris)
3. Diffuse melanoma of iris	3. Fuchs' heterochromic iridocyclitis
4. Siderosis of hemosiderosis bulbi	4. Chronic iritis (idiopathic or after trauma)
5. Paradoxical Fuchs' heterochromic iridocyclitis	5. Granulomatous iritis
6. Iridocorneal epithelial syndrome	6. Juvenile xanthogranuloma
	7. Metastatic carcinoma
	8. Waardenburg's syndrome

2. Most, if not all, iris malignant melanomas arise from pre-existing nevi of the iris.

3. The geographic sector distribution of iris malignant melanoma is, in descending frequency, pupillary zone, entire sector, pupillary and midzone, midzone, periphery, periphery and midzone.

4. The geographic quadrant distribution of iris malignant melanomas is, in descending frequency inferior, temporal, nasal, superior.

C. Clinically, an iris melanoma may present as a discrete mass, a diffuse mass, heterochromia (see Table 17.2), glaucoma, chronic uveitis, or spontaneous hyphema. The glaucoma is caused by direct invasion of the aqueous drainage area, synechiae and secondary angle closure glaucoma, or induction of neovascularization or melanomalytic glaucoma.

Diffuse iris melanomas most often present with unilateral glaucoma and heterochromia. Metastasis occurs in about 13% of cases.

D. The tumors may be deeply pigmented, partially pigmented, or nonpigmented, and frequently show increased vascularity and distortion of the pupil toward the iris quadrant of involvement.

E. Most iris malignant melanomas are composed of spindle cells and, therefore, are relatively benign.

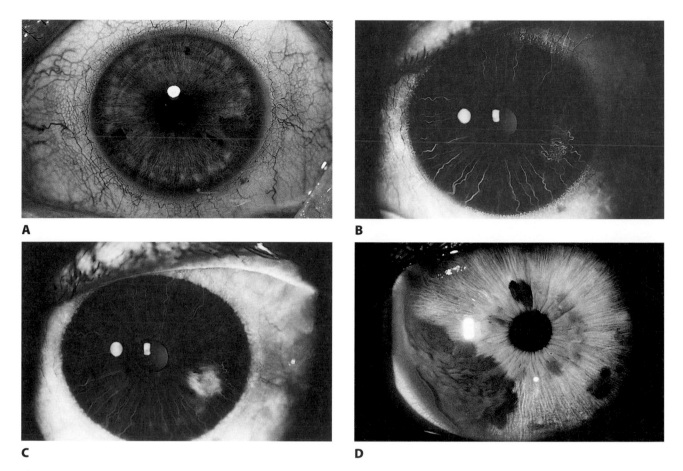

Fig. 17.23 Iris melanoma. **A–C,** Clinical (**A**) and fluorescein (**B** and **C**) appearance of probable iris melanoma. **D,** Another patient shows a definite iris "melanoma." Because of the smooth, wavy appearance to the surface, this type of tumor has been called a *tapioca melanoma.*

A spindle-A cell iris melanoma has no capacity to metastasize and can be considered a spindle cell nevus.

---

1. Only those tumors that have spindle-B or epithelioid cells, or involve the iris root or angle, have the ability to metastasize, and then they do so less than 10% of the time.

   Because most iris "melanomas" are spindle-cell nevi, the Callender classification is best applied to ciliary body and choroidal melanomas.

   ---

2. The mortality rate is 4% to 5%.

   On re-examination, 70% to 80% of previously diagnosed iris melanomas proved to be iris spindle-cell nevi, not melanomas.

F. Differential diagnosis
   1. Anterior staphyloma
   2. Exudative mass in anterior chamber
      a. Pigmented macrophages
      b. Phacoanaphylactic endophthalmitis
      c. Juvenile xanthogranuloma

3. Ocular penetration with uveal prolapse
4. "Postoperative confusion"
   a. Posterior- or anterior-chamber epithelial cyst

   Anterior-chamber cysts may also occur spontaneously without surgery. The postoperative and the spontaneous cysts have been confused with iris malignant melanomas.

   ---

   b. Iridencleisis (unplanned)
5. Miscellaneous
   a. Nodular iris thickening and scarring
   b. Foreign body in iris
   c. Ectropion uveae
   d. Segmental congenital ocular melanocytosis
   e. Intrairis hemorrhage
   f. Other iris tumors [e.g., nevus, ICE syndrome, leiomyoma, metastatic tumors (Fig. 17.25), rhabdomyosarcoma (Fig. 17.26), and ciliary body malignant melanoma]

1. Angioleiomyoma
   a. Tumor is composed of spindle cells with abundant cytoplasm

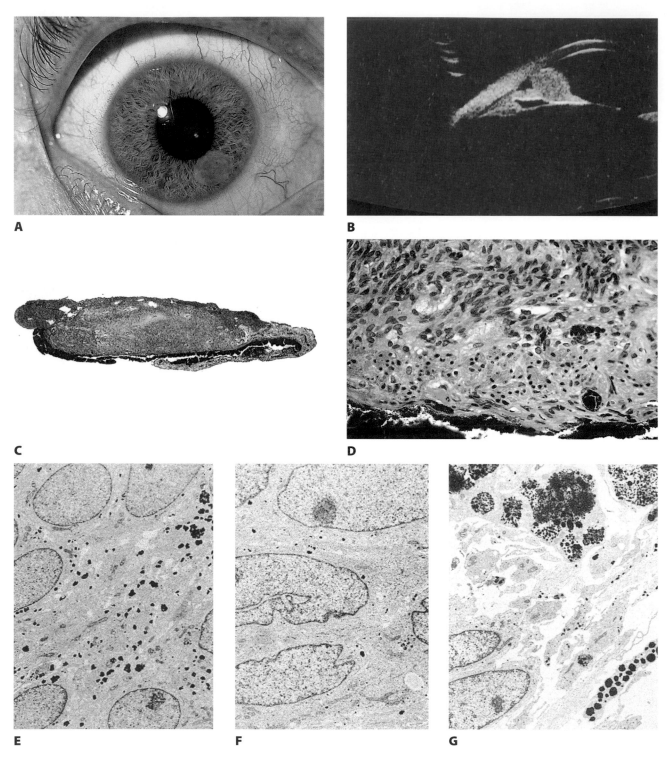

Fig. 17.24 Iris melanoma. **A,** Clinical appearance of iris tumor. **B,** Ultrasound biomicroscope appearance of iris malignant melanoma. (Courtesy of Drs. Carol and Jerry Shields). **C,** Histologic section shows tumor infiltrating the full thickness of the pupillary iris (on left). Note peripheral iris on right (and curled under the iris pigment epithelium) is free of tumor. **D,** Increased magnification shows spindle-cell nature of tumor (most of lower field is sphincter muscle). Although diagnosed as spindle-A melanoma in the past, it would now be diagnosed as spindle-cell nevus. **E** and **F,** Another case shows mostly spindled cells. Note in **F,** deep nuclear invagination in cell near center that accounts for "line of chromatin" in spindle-A melanoma cells (see Figs 17.37 and 17.38). **G,** Macrophages (above) contain pigment-filled phagosomes of melanin in varied sizes. Note normal iris melanocytes below and to the right. Two spindled tumor cells present on left.

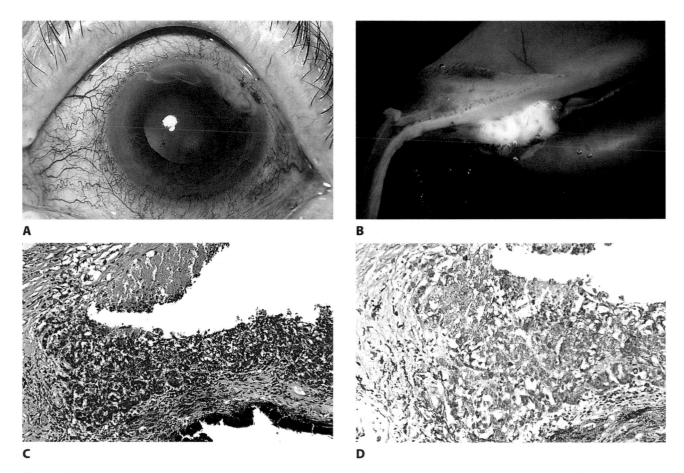

Fig. 17.25 Metastatic iris tumor. **A,** Clinical appearance of amelanotic metastatic tumor. A superior peripheral iris tumor, especially when amelanotic, should be thought of as metastatic until proven otherwise. **B,** Gross specimen shows appearance of tumor involving peripheral iris and anterior ciliary body. **C,** Histologic section shows carcinoma cells on surface of iris and infiltrating iris stroma and drainage angle. **D,** Many of the cells demonstrate periodic acid–Schiff-positivity.

b. Contains many blood vessels
c. Immunohistochemical stains positive for smooth-muscle actin, and desmin, and negative for S-100 and HMB-45.
d. Granulomatous inflammation with Busacca and Koeppe nodules
e. Iris varix

Ciliary Body and Choroid

I. Nevus (Figs 17.27 to 17.29; see also Fig. 17.21B)
  A. Incidence

1. Nevi of the ciliary body and choroid are found in at least 30% of people.

> At least one discrete, focal, pigmented nevus, 0.5 disc diameter (DD) or greater, is present in one eye in 30% of patients. Approximately 3% to 4% of patients have one or more nevi in both eyes, and 7% of patients have multiple nevi in the same eye. Approximately 55% of patients with choroidal nevi have iris freckles or nevi in the same eye, but only 20% of patients without choroidal nevi have iris freckles or nevi.

2. The nevi have no sex predilection.

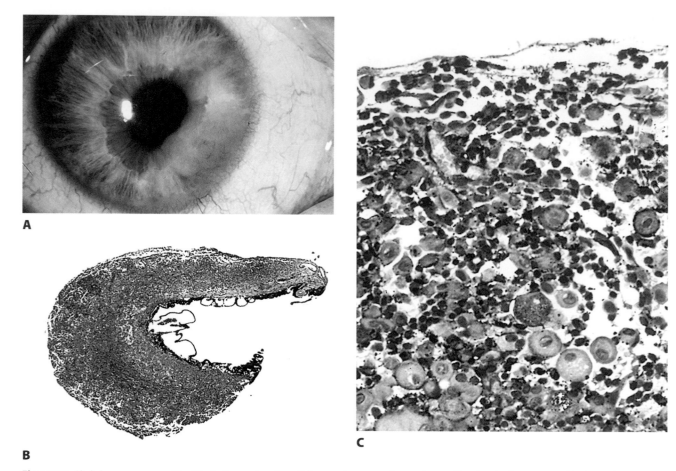

Fig. 17.26 Rhabdomyosarcoma of the iris. **A,** An amelanotic, mildly vascular tumor distorts the pupillary border from 3 to 6 o'clock. En bloc excision of tumor performed. **B,** Periodic acid–Schiff (PAS)-stained histologic section shows a cellular tumor replacing iris stroma. **C,** Large rhabdomyoblasts contain PAS-positive intracytoplasmic material. (Case courtesy of Prof. GOH Naumann and reported by Naumann GOH *et al.*: *Am J Ophthalmol* 74:110. © Elsevier 1972.)

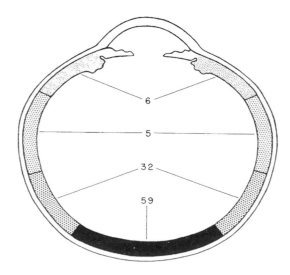

Fig. 17.27 Choroidal nevus. Distribution of 102 nevi in choroid and ciliary body. (From Naumann G *et al.*: *Arch Ophthalmol* 76:784, 1966. © American Medical Association. All rights reserved.)

3. The incidence in children is extremely low.

> The low incidence in children may be caused by delayed pigmentation of pre-existing nevi.

The incidence then increases progressively during the second, third, and fourth decades and levels off at approximately 35%.

B. Location (see Fig. 17.27)
1. The overwhelming majority (91%) occur in the posterior half of the eye; most (59%) occur in the posterior third.
2. An almost equal incidence occurs in the anterior third of the choroid and the ciliary body.

C. Size and shape (see Fig. 17.28)
1. Nevi range in diameter from 0.5 to 11.0 mm (i.e., 0.33 to 7 DD). Over 95% are 3 mm (2 DD) or less.
2. The lesions usually occupy the entire thickness of the choroid except for the choriocapillaris.
3. Typically, nevi are flat, discoid lesions, but 67% exceed the thickness of the adjacent choroid.

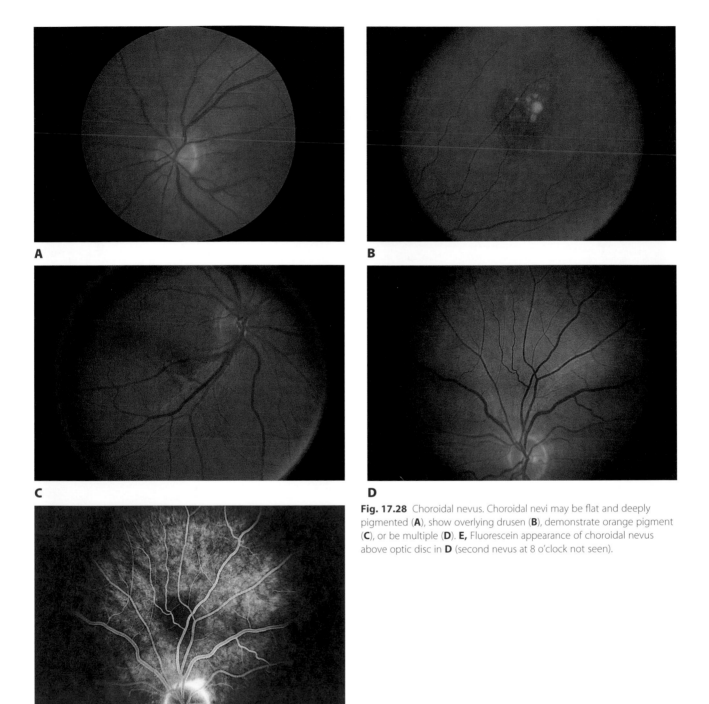

Fig. 17.28 Choroidal nevus. Choroidal nevi may be flat and deeply pigmented (**A**), show overlying drusen (**B**), demonstrate orange pigment (**C**), or be multiple (**D**). **E,** Fluorescein appearance of choroidal nevus above optic disc in **D** (second nevus at 8 o'clock not seen).

4. Nevi tend to be relatively avascular.

The relative avascularity helps to explain their fluorescein fundus picture, which is one of decreased fluorescence. An amelanotic nevus may be inadvertently detected when a fluorescein angiogram is being examined and shows a region of persistent choroidal hypofluorescence without the presence of a corresponding pigmented fundus. Melanomas, on the other hand, are highly vascular with abnormal vessels that readily leak fluorescein. Rarely, however, nevi leak fluorescein and melanomas do not.

D. Cytology and pigmentation (Figs 17.30 and 17.31; see also Figs 17.28 and 17.29)

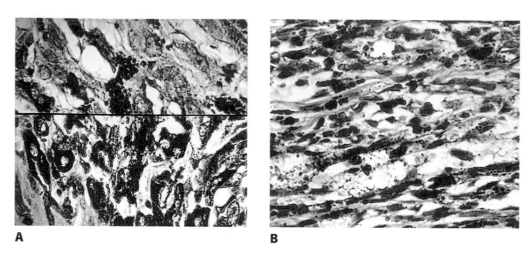

A **B**

Fig. 17.29 Cell types in nevus. **A,** Histologic section shows (*top*) plump polyhedral and plump fusiform nevus cells with rather small, uniform nuclei, and (*bottom*) plump fusiform and dendritic nevus cells. **B,** Section shows mainly balloon cells with, in the lower right corner, slender spindled nevus cells. (Modified from Naumann G *et al.: Arch Ophthalmol* 76:784, 1966. © American Medical Association. All rights reserved.)

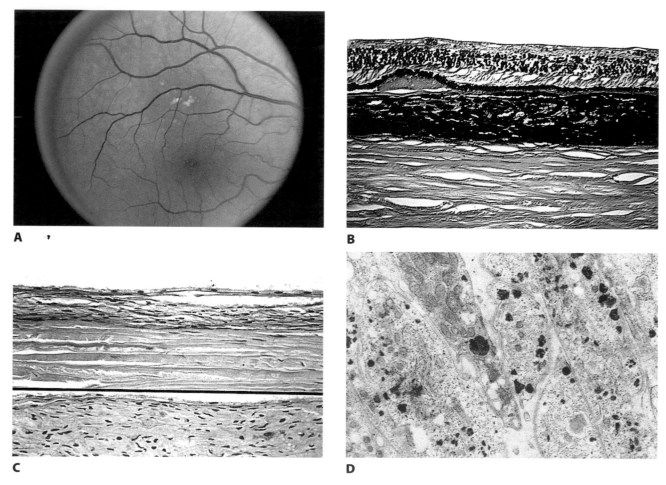

A **B**

C **D**

Fig. 17.30 Choroidal nevus. **A,** Clinical appearance of choroidal nevus with overlying drusen. **B,** Histologic section of another case shows a druse overlying a heavily pigmented choroidal nevus composed almost completely of plump polyhedral nevus cells. **C,** Top shows a bleached section of normal choroid. Note normal spindle nuclei of choroidal melanocytes. Bottom shows a bleached section of a choroidal nevus. Although the cells are larger than normal melanocytes, the nuclei are quite similar, hence nevus cells are benign-appearing, atypical melanocytes. **D,** Electron microscopy of a choroidal nevus shows tightly packed plump dendritic cells, which contain moderate pigmentation. (**B** and **C,** Modified from Naumann G *et al.: Arch Ophthalmol* 76:784, 1966. © American Medical Tussociation. All rights reserved.)

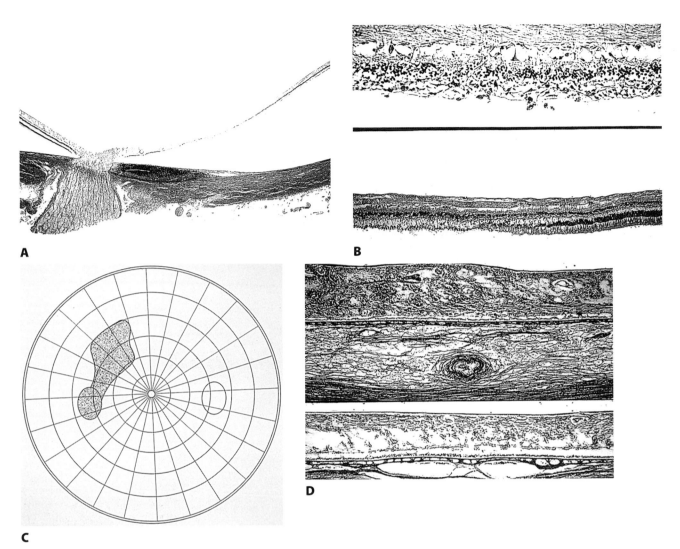

Fig. 17.31 Effects of choroidal nevus on overlying retina. **A,** Juxtapapillary nevus with marked degeneration of overlying retina. **B,** Bottom demonstrates transitional area between normal neural retina (right side) and degenerated retina (left side). Top shows degenerated neural retina at increased magnification. **C,** Neural retinal changes caused patient to have absolute scotoma, rare with nevus. **D,** Wilder elastic stain shows effects of nevus on choriocapillaris; bottom: choriocapillaris shows large lumina in normal choroid; top: choroidal nevi has markedly narrowed the lumina. (**A–C,** Modified from Naumann G *et al.: Am J Ophthalmol* 62:914. © Elsevier 1966. **D,** modified from Naumann G *et al: Arch Ophthalmol* 76:784, 1966. © American Medical Association. All rights reserved.)

1. In general, nevus cells are plumper than normal melanocytes of the choroid and ciliary body (i.e., they are atypical benign-appearing melanocytes).
2. The four types of uveal nevus cells are (see Fig. 17.29):
   a. Plump, polyhedral (see also Fig. 17.51C)
      1). This is the most common type and the "typical" nevus contains a majority of these cells.
      2). The cell is maximally pigmented.
      3). A nevus made up exclusively of this cell is called a *melanocytoma* (*magnocellular nevus*).
   b. Slender, spindled
      1). This is the second most common cell type.
      2). It contains little or no pigment.

Often, slender, spindled nevus cells may be seen mixed with the plump cells, or separate from them in a location next to the sclera.

   c. Plump, fusiform, and dendritic—these are less pigmented than plump, polyhedral nevus cells, but more pigmented than slender, spindled nevus cells.
   d. Balloon cells
      1). Balloon cells are large cells with abundant, foamy cytoplasm.
      2). Similar cells may be found in cutaneous and conjunctival nevi.

3. Congenital ocular or oculodermal melanocytosis is a diffuse nevus of the uvea composed primarily of plump, polyhedral nevus cells.

   Rarely, the melanocytosis may have a segmental distribution (see p. 671 in this chapter).

E. Microcirculation—the only vascular pattern present in nevi is that of normal vessels.

Vascular patterns seen in melanomas (see Figs 17.42 and 17.43), that is, zones of avascularity (silent pattern), straight pattern, parallel pattern with cross-linking, arcs (fragments of curved vessels or incompletely closed loops), loops (island of tumor surrounded by a large, closed vascular loop), and networks (back-to-back adjacent loops), are not present in nevi.

F. Effects of nevus on neighboring tissues
   1. Nevi frequently narrow the overlying choriocapillaris, and, rarely, may completely obliterate it (see Fig. 17.31).

      Slight degeneration, proliferation, or reactive deposition by RPE may occur. Frequently (approximately 40%), they induce overlying drusen formation (see Fig. 17.30).
   2. They may cause overlying outer neural retinal changes that are usually minimal.

      Rarely, they cause definite disturbances of rod and cone, or outer nuclear layer (see Fig. 17.31).
   3. Central serous choroidopathy (retinopathy) and subretinal neovascularization may rarely occur.

G. Uveal nevi are probably the precursor of most uveal melanomas (see later)

H. Uveal nevi are increased in eyes that contain uveal melanomas.

II. Bilateral diffuse melanocytic proliferations (BDUMP)
   A. BDUMP is associated with systemic malignant neoplasms, mainly poorly differentiated ovarian or uterine carcinomas in women, and lung carcinomas in men.
   B. Severe visual loss may occur, sometimes antedating the development of the uveal tumors.
   C. The signs of BDUMP are:
      1. Multiple, round or oval, subtle red patches at the level of the RPE, mainly in women, with a mean age of 63 years.
      2. A striking fluorescein angiography pattern of multifocal areas of early hyperfluorescence corresponding to the red patches
      3. Development of multiple, slightly elevated uveal melanotic tumors, plus diffuse thickening of the uvea
      4. Exudative neural retinal detachment
      5. Rapid progression of cataracts

III. Mesectodermal leiomyoma (see p. 350 in Chapter 9)

IV. Malignant melanoma
   A. General information
      1. The median age is 60.4 years (it is rare in children, but may even be congenital).
      2. There is a slight preponderance of melanomas in men.

3. White patients have intraocular melanomas more frequently than black patients in a ratio of 15:1.
   a. In addition, patients of Japanese, Chinese, Hispanic, and Native American origin have a lower incidence of choroidal melanoma than do white patients.
   b. A case of a choroidal melanoma has been reported in an African-American albino.
4. Bilaterality or multifocal origin is extremely rare.
5. Uveal melanomas are slightly more prevalent in individuals with blue or gray irises than in those with brown irises.
   a. Increased choroidal pigmentation secondary to increased density of pigmented choroidal melanocytes may be a risk factor for the development of posterior uveal melanoma. Similarly, melanoma patients with light iris color are more likely to have darker choroidal pigmentation than control patients.

In an Australian population, nonbrown eye color has been associated with increased risk of iris melanoma. Eye color is also the strongest constitutional predictor of choroidal and ciliary body melanoma in that population.

---

6. An increased risk factor for uveal melanoma is an occupation that involves intense exposure to ultraviolet light. Sun exposure has been associated with increased risk of choroidal and ciliary body melanoma in Auatralia.
7. The overall incidence of uveal melanomas in a white population is approximately 5 to 7 per million per year. For the age group beyond 20 years, an annual incidence rate of approximately 7.5 per million per year, and beyond 50 years an annual incidence rate of approximately 21 per million per year is expected. Therefore, approximately 1 of 2500 white patients will have a uveal melanoma during his or her lifetime.

The overall mean age-adjusted incidence of uveal melanomas in the United States is 4.3 per million with a greater rate in men and a preponderance in the white population (97.8%).

---

8. Heredity and bilaterality are not important factors.
9. Bilateral primary melanoma may occur in approximately 1.8% of all patients who have primary uveal melanoma. Extremely rarely, more than one primary uveal melanoma can occur in one eye.
10. Familial cases have also been reported.
11. Primary choroidal melanoma can occur in a patient who has had a previous cutaneous melanoma.
12. For sites of malignant melanoma within the eye, see Table 17.3.
13. Classification of tumors as to size is shown in Table 17.4.
14. The finding of activation of extracellular-regulated kinase in uveal melanoma suggests a causative role

TABLE 17.3 Site of Malignant Melanomas in the Eye

Location	Anterior*	Equatorial	Posterior	Anterior–Posterior†	Total
Superior	3		3	2	8
Inferior	2		2	1	5
Temporal	2	1	9	5	17
Inferotemporal	5	3	2		10
					51
Superotemporal	2		12	1	15
Macula			9		9
Nasal	3	2	7	3	15
Inferonasal	1		3	1	5
					31
Superonasal	5		4	2	11
Peripapillary			2		2
Whole eye				3	3
Total	23	6	53	18	100

*Includes ciliary body and choroid anterior to equator; does not include iris.
†Diffuse or large neoplasms extending from ciliary body or ora serrata to posterior choroid.
(From Yanoff M, Zimmerman LE: Cancer 20:493, 1967. © American Cancer Society. Adapted by permission of Wiley-Liss, Inc, a subsidary of John Wiley & Sons. Inc.)

TABLE 17.4 Classification of Tumor as to Size*

	Largest Diameter (mm)	Largest Elevation (mm)
Very small	≤7.0	≤2.0
Small	7.7–10.0	2.1–3.0
Medium	10.1–15.0	3.1–5.0
Large	>15.0	>5.0

*The largest dimension of a tumor is the most important measurement (i.e., a tumor 15.5 × 14.0 × 4.0 mm would be classified as "large").

for mitogen-activated protein kinase (MAPK) activation in uveal melanoma independent of activating v-raf murine sarcoma viral homolog or RAS mutations.

B. Clinical presentation

1. A mass found on routine examination or after a complaint of blurred vision is the most frequent presentation (Fig. 17.32).

Fluorescein angiography, ultrasonography, computed tomography, and magnetic resonance imaging, and, less often, ^{32}P tests may help to identify and clarify intraocular masses.

---

2. Episcleral vascular injection may occur overlying a ciliary body melanoma (Fig. 17.33A and B).

Some patients with the condition have been treated for chronic conjunctivitis until the melanoma was discovered by adequate ophthalmoscopy.

---

3. A ciliary body melanoma may cause decreased intraocular pressure. Conversely, tumors that infiltrate the anterior-chamber angle or tumors undergoing necrosis resulting in liberation of pigment (melanomalytic glaucoma) may present with elevated intraocular pressure.

a. Ring melanoma
1). This condition has a poor prognosis.
2). The mean is 8 clock-hours of ciliary body involvement at presentation, with 30% having 360° of involvement.
3). Mean tumor thickness: 8 mm.
4). Shallow anterior chamber present in 48%, anterior-chamber inflammation in 22%, cataract in 39%, lens indentation in 35%, and lens subluxation in 13%. A "sentinel" episcleral blood vessel is found in 74%.
5). Multilobulation present in 83%.

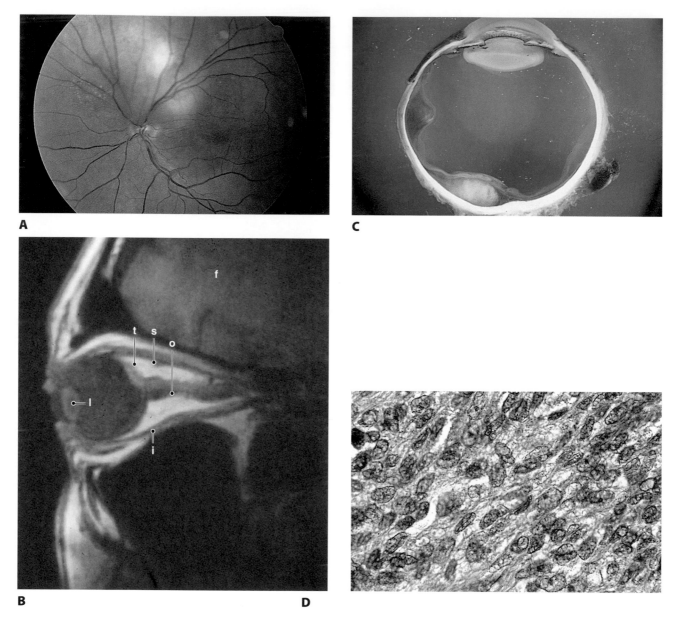

Fig. 17.32 Choroidal malignant melanoma. **A,** The patient had a slowly enlarging choroidal tumor, followed over a 9-year period. Tumor initially found on routine examination. **B,** Magnetic resonance imaging (T_1-weighted) shows the choroidal tumor just above the optic nerve. T_2-weighted imaging showed that the tumor became less white, characteristic of a malignant melanoma (hemangioma of the choroid, for example, becomes whiter with T_2 imaging) (f, frontal lobe; t, thickened choroid; s, superior rectus muscles; o, optic nerve; i, inferior rectus muscles; l, lens). **C,** The enucleated eye shows the gross appearance of the tumor. **D,** A histologic section demonstrates a malignant melanoma of the spindle-B type.

6). There is ultrasonic hollowness with intrinsic pulsations in 100% of cases.

7). The most common histopathologic type is mixed (74%), and metastasis develop in 52% of all patients after a mean follow-up of 55 months.

8). Regional lymph node metastasis may occur following filtration surgery for glaucoma associated with ring melanoma. Therefore, such tumors should be excluded before filtra-

tion surgery is performed for unilateral "pigmentary glaucoma."

b). Subconjunctival spread of ciliary body melanoma has been found after glaucoma filtration surgery in a patient with an underlying ciliary body melanoma.

4. The patient may present with an episcleral extension of a uveal malignant melanoma that may simulate a conjunctival lesion (see Fig. 17.33C, D, and E).

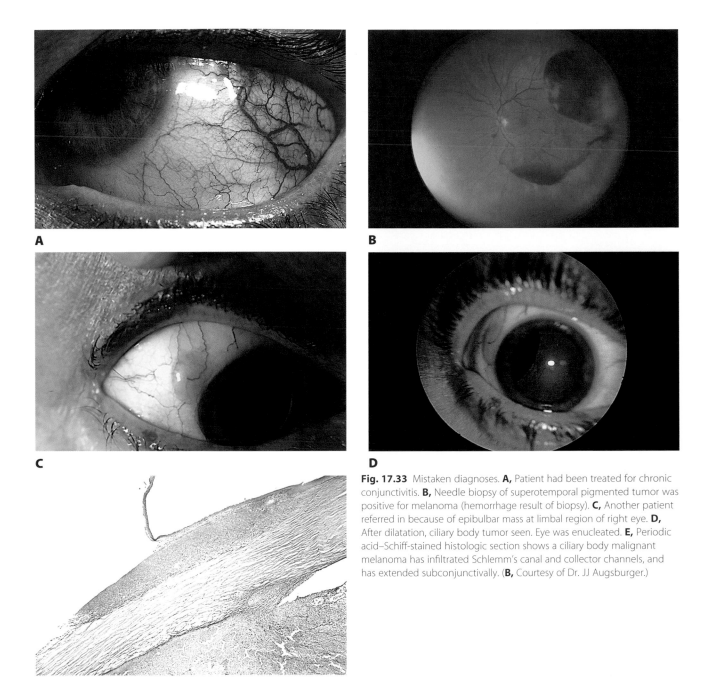

Fig. 17.33 Mistaken diagnoses. **A,** Patient had been treated for chronic conjunctivitis. **B,** Needle biopsy of superotemporal pigmented tumor was positive for melanoma (hemorrhage result of biopsy). **C,** Another patient referred in because of epibulbar mass at limbal region of right eye. **D,** After dilatation, ciliary body tumor seen. Eye was enucleated. **E,** Periodic acid–Schiff-stained histologic section shows a ciliary body malignant melanoma has infiltrated Schlemm's canal and collector channels, and has extended subconjunctivally. (**B,** Courtesy of Dr. JJ Augsburger.)

5. Vitreous hemorrhage (see p. 716 in this chapter)

The *Knapp–Ronne* type of malignant melanoma of the choroid is characterized by a location near the optic disc, early growth through the neural retina, and a structure showing both bloodless and blood-filled cavernous spaces. It presents with a massive hemorrhage into the vitreous that may result in hemosiderosis bulbi and heterochromia iridum.

---

6. An RPE detachment or central serous choroidopathy (retinopathy; Fig. 17.34) may accompany a peripheral uveal malignant melanoma.
7. CME (see Fig. 17.34; almost identical to that seen in Irvine–Gass syndrome, diabetic retinopathy, hypotony, and uveitis) may be found.
8. Neural retinal detachment, present in approximately 75% of cases (see p. 716 in this chapter), and occasionally, may mask the underlying melanoma.

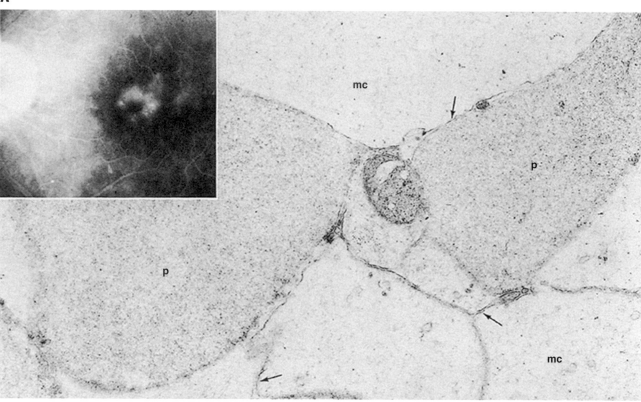

A

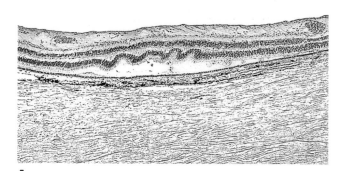

B

Fig. 17.34 Mistaken diagnoses. **A,** Patient presented with blurred vision caused by central serouslike choroidopathy. The eye was enucleated because of a peripheral choroidal melanoma. Histologic section shows serous fluid under the macular retina. **B,** Another patient had a peripheral choroidal melanoma and clinical and fluorescein appearance characteristic of cystoid macular edema (*inset*). Electron micrograph from Henle fiber layer of same eye shows swollen Müller cells (mc). Intercellular spaces (*arrows*) are normal. Adjacent photoreceptor (p) axons (Henle fibers) appear relatively normal. (Modified from Fine BS, Brucker AJ Jr: *Am J Ophthalmol* 92:466. © Elsevier 1981.)

Extremely rarely, a horseshoe retinal tear may accompany the retinal detachment.

---

   9. An unusual presentation is with a choroidal detachment.
10. Ocular inflammation may occur (Fig. 17.35), but is much less common than with retinoblastoma.
11. Glaucoma (see pp. 644 and 650 in Chapter 16).

    a. Acute angle closure glaucoma may result from choroidal melanoma.
12. Opaque media (see p. 720 in this chapter)
13. A uveal melanoma may originate in or invade the iris and produce heterochromia iridum.

Heterochromia iridum may also result from hemosiderosis bulbi after a vitreous hemorrhage associated with a uveal melanoma.

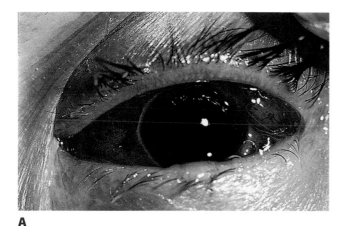

A

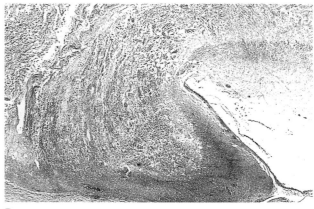

B

Fig. 17.35 Necrotic uveal melanoma. **A,** The patient presented with recent onset of blindness, pain, redness, and chemosis. Examination by ultrasonography showed a solid tumor. The eye was enucleated. **B,** A histologic section shows that the typical "mushroom" tumor had undergone spontaneous and complete necrosis, making identification of the melanoma cell type almost impossible. This type, therefore, is called the *necrotic cell melanoma*. Completely necrotic melanomas often present clinically, as this patient's did, with the appearance of inflammation.

14. A malignant melanoma may simulate a postoperative choroidal detachment.

15. Metastases are usually a late manifestation of uveal melanomas, whereas frequently, they are an early manifestation of skin melanomas (see Fig. 17.7).

16. Factors associated with a worse prognosis for survival following enucleation for choroidal and ciliary body melanomas are largest basal diameter (LBD), nonspindle cell type, and anterior location.

17. During the period 1955 to 2000 there was no apparent change in the clinical and histopathological presentation of choroidal or ciliary body melanomas.

18. The manner in which suspected melanomas of the choroid and ciliary body are managed has changed significantly over the past 30 years. During this period, an increased emphasis has been placed on the importance of tumor growth as an indication of a possible aggressive character for the lesion. Conversely, such lesions are not viewed as "ocular emergencies," thereby providing time for sober clinical deliberation and thorough evaluation before a course of therapy is chosen.

For example, in one study by Gass,* 116 suspected choroidal or ciliary body melanomas were observed for evidence of tumor growth. During a minimum observation period of 5 years, no tumor growth was observed in 69 patients, and none displayed evidence of metastatic disease. The tumor grew in 47 patients, resulting in enucleation in 35 individuals. In general, death from metastasis was associated with tumors that were observed to grow, particularly those having epithelioid cells. The period of observation was not judged to contribute to increased tumor mortality.

*Gass JD: Observation of suspected choroidal and ciliary body melanomas for evidence of growth prior to enucleation. Retina 23:523, 2003.

C. Histogenesis (theories)
1. Mesodermal: the tumor arises from mesodermal elements in the uvea, hence the old name *melanosarcoma*.
2. RPE: the melanoma arises from the RPE.
3. Neural: the melanoma arises from Schwann's cells associated with the ciliary nerves.
4. Nevoid: the melanoma arises from a pre-existing nevus. Most evidence points to this theory (i.e., the vast majority of uveal malignant melanomas arise from pre-existing nevi; Fig. 17.36).

   Five risk factors for growth of small (≤3 mm in thickness) melanocytic choroidal tumors are:

   1). Tumor thickness greater than 2 mm
   2). Posterior tumor margin touching disc
   3). Visual symptoms
   4). Orange pigment

   a. An apparently stable and nonmalignant choroidal nevus can produce overlying orange pigment that can even result in massive pigment accumulation, which can form a pseudohypopyon.
   5). Subretinal fluid
   b. Optical coherence tomography can be helpful in assessing for subretinal fluid in ocular melanocytic tumors, and in distinguishing from chronic retinal changes that may overly such lesions.
5. De novo (i.e., the melanoma arises in the uvea without any obvious antecedent cause)

D. Callender classification and prognosis (Figs 17.37 to 17.40)

The classification is used specifically for ciliary body and choroidal malignant melanomas; it may be applied to iris but not to conjunctival or skin malignant melanomas. Japanese patients have a worse prognosis than that reported in the

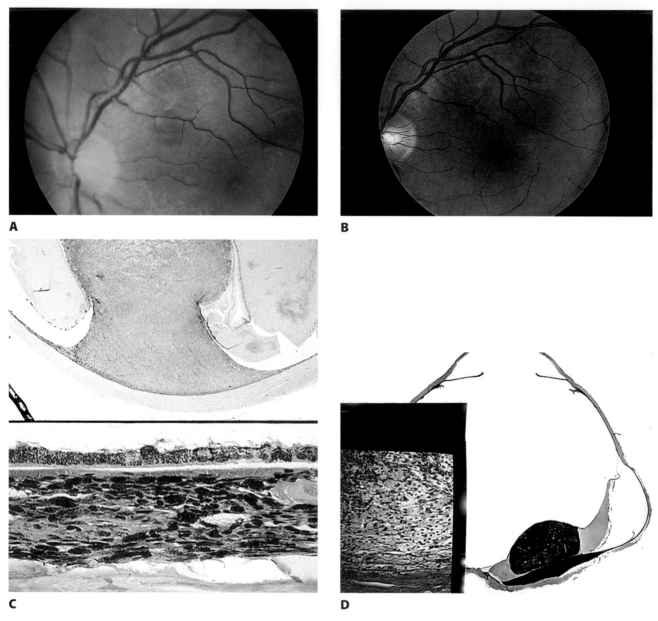

A

B

C

D

Fig. 17.36 Histogenesis. **A,** Choroidal nevus just above the central fovea of the left eye was noted in 1969. **B,** Rapid growth occurred almost 4 years later. Eye enucleated. Histology showed a heavily pigmented choroidal melanoma. **C,** Histologic section of another eye (*top*) shows a mushroom-shaped choroidal melanoma with a long "tail" extending to the right. Increased magnification of the tail (*bottom*) demonstrates cytology indistinguishable from a choroidal nevus. **D,** A mushroom-shaped choroidal melanoma is present in an eye with congenital ocular melanocytosis (i.e., a maximally pigmented, diffuse nevus of the uvea). The *inset* (bleached section) shows the innocuous nevus cells at the base of the melanoma. (**C,** Reproduced from Yanoff M, Zimmerman LE: *Cancer* 20:493, 1967. © American Cancer Society. Adapted by permission of Wiley-Liss, Inc, a subsidiary of John Wiley & Sons, Inc; **D,** Adapted from Yanoff M, Zimmerman LE: *Arch Ophthalmol* 77:331, 1967. © American Medical Association. All rights reserved.)

white population. Melanomas may have a poor prognosis because the melanoma cells seem capable of killing the body's immune cells (activated T lymphocytes) that attack them. The melanoma cells bear on their surface Fas (also called Apo-1), which can initiate cells to commit suicide by a process called apoptosis. When Fas binds to another molecule called Fas ligand (FasL), which occurs mainly on activated T lymphocytes, Fas triggers a series of events inside the immune cell that leads to its suicide (i.e., apoptosis).

Decreased expression of human leukocyte antigen (HLA) class I antigen is usually associated with nonuveal melanoma tumor progression. Paradoxically, loss of HLA I antigen in uveal melanoma is not associated with tumor cell escape and a worse survival.

1. Spindle-A (see Figs 17.37A, 17.38A, and 17.39B)
   a. Spindle-A is the second rarest type of melanoma (5%), and is made up of cohesive cells that

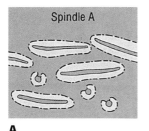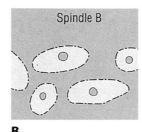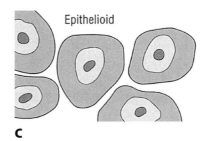

Fig. 17.37 Callender classification. **A,** Spindle-A cells are shown in longitudinal and transverse cross-sections. The cells are cohesive and have poorly defined cell borders. The nuclei contain nuclear folds that appear as dark stripes parallel to the long axis of the nuclei. The stripe is caused by infolding of the nucleus, as noted in the cross-section. **B,** Spindle-B nuclei are larger and plumper than spindle-A nuclei and contain prominent nucleoli rather than nuclear folds. The cells, similar to spindle-A, are cohesive and have poorly defined cell borders. **C,** Epithelioid cells are not cohesive, have distinct cell borders, and show large oval nuclei that contain prominent nucleoli. The cells are larger than spindle-A and spindle-B cells.

contain small, spindled nuclei having a central dark stripe (caused by a nuclear fold) but no distinct nucleoli; the cytoplasm is indistinct and has no easily identifiable cell borders.

The dark stripe does not always occur, but when it does, it is quite helpful in classification. A tumor is classified as spindle-A when it is estimated to contain no more than 5% spindle-B cells and no epithelioid cells. Some, if not all, of the tumors previously classified as spindle-A are benign, and really should be called *spindle cell nevi*.

---

b. Mitotic figures are extremely rare.
c. The survival rate is approximately 92%.
2. Spindle-B and fascicular (see Figs 17.37B, 17.38B and D, 17.39C, and 17.40A and B)
   a. Spindle-B is common (39%), and is made up of cohesive cells that contain prominent spindled nuclei with distinct nucleoli; the cytoplasm is indistinct and has no easily identifiable cell borders.
   b. Spindle-B cells have decreased pleomorphism, and nuclear area compared with epithelioid cells.

A tumor is classified as spindle-B when it contains more than 5% spindle-B cells, but no epithelioid cells. Because if enough sections are studied, most tumors composed of spindle cells contain both A and B cells, the tumors should probably simply be called *spindle cell type*.

---

c. In approximately 6% of spindle-B cell malignant melanomas, the spindled cells form a palisaded arrangement called a *fascicular* pattern.

The cell type of the fascicular pattern, however, remains spindle-B. Rarely, epithelioid cells are admixed within the fascicular pattern; the tumor should then be diagnosed as a mixed-cell type.

---

d. Mitotic figures are rare.
e. The survival rate is approximately 75%.
3. Epithelioid (see Figs 17.37C, 17.38C, 17.39D, and 17.40C and D)
   a. Epithelioid is the rarest type (3%), and is made up of noncohesive cells that contain large, round nuclei with prominent nucleoli (frequently pink) and abundant eosinophilic cytoplasm with distinct cell borders.
   b. Epithelioid cells have increased pleomorphism and nuclear area compared with spindle-B cells.

A small type of epithelioid cell that contains less cytoplasm, a smaller nucleus, and less distinct cell borders than the classic epithelioid cell is now recognized. This small *intermediate epithelioid* cell should not be confused with a "plump" spindle-B melanoma cell.

---

c. Mitotic figures are common.
d. The survival rate is approximately 28%.
4. Mixed (see Fig. 17.38D)
   a. Mixed cell, the most common type (45%), contains both a significant spindle-cell component (usually spindle-cell B), and an epithelioid cell component.

Mixed cell is not a mixture of spindle-A and spindle-B cells, but of spindle cells and epithelioid cells. A tumor is classified as mixed if only one large, unequivocal epithelioid cell is seen in approximately five fields at a magnification of 400.

---

b. The survival rate is approximately 41%.
5. Necrotic (Fig. 17.41; see also Fig. 17.35)
   a. Necrotic is an uncommon type (7%); the tumor is so necrotic that the cell type is not identifiable.

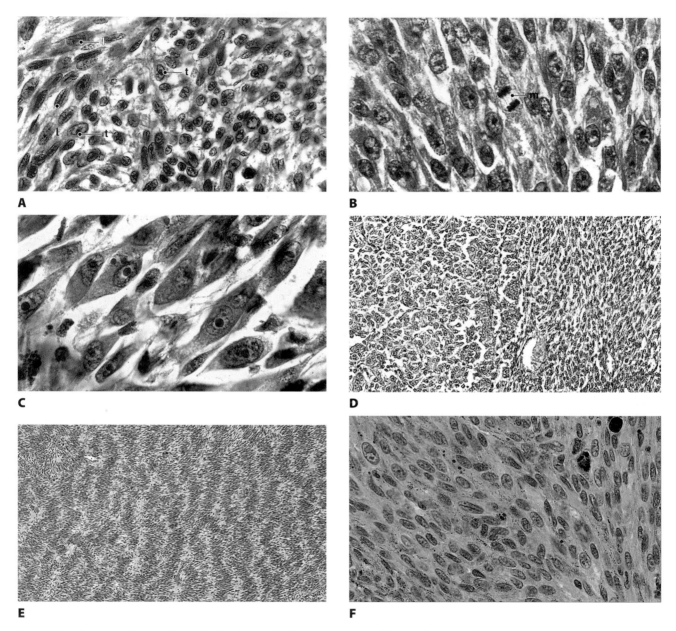

Fig. 17.38 Callender classification. **A,** Spindle-A cells, identified by a dark stripe parallel to the long axis of the nucleus, are seen in longitudinal section (l). They are identified in transverse cross-section (t) by the infolding of the nuclear membrane that causes the dark stripe. **B,** Spindle-B cells are identified by their prominent nucleoli. Note the mitotic figure (m). Both spindle-A and spindle-B cells tend to be quite cohesive and have poorly defined cell borders. **C,** Epithelioid cells are the largest of the melanoma cells, tend not to be cohesive, and have irregular shapes and sizes as well as very prominent nucleoli in the large nuclei. **D,** Some melanomas contain a mixture of spindle cells and epithelioid cells. The left half of this figure is occupied by epithelioid cells and the right half by spindle cells (this is called a mixed-cell melanoma). **E,** Fascicular pattern always consists of spindle-B cells. **F,** Higher magnification of another case shows spindle-A and B, and epithelioid cells. Note characteristic nuclear infolding of spindle-A cell. (Courtesy of Dr. Morton Smith.)

Necrosis may lead to large cystic spaces in the tumor or to a large accumulation of eosinophilic debris, sometimes containing cholesterol clefts. Clear cells may occur in necrotic melanomas. Clear cells may also be a predominant component of the melanoma, called a *clear-cell variant*, and should not be confused with other clear-cell neoplasms metastatic to the uvea (e.g., hypernephroma).

b. Tumor necrosis may be caused by an autoimmune mechanism (a large population of plasma cells in the tumor supports this hypothesis).

c. The survival rate is approximately 41%.

d. Scleritis and episcleritis are statistically associated with total tumor necrosis of choroidal and ciliary body melanomas.

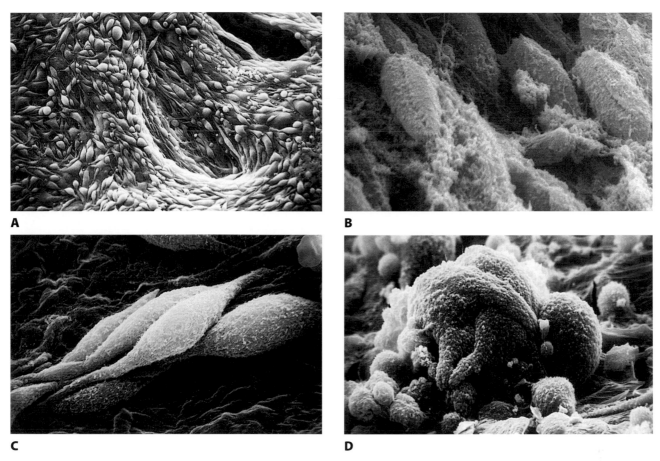

Fig. 17.39 Callender classification—scanning electron microscopy (SEM). **A,** Low-magnification SEM shows mostly spindle-B cells with a few epithelioid cells. **B,** SEM of spindle-A cells. Note nuclear infoldings. **C,** SEM of spindle-B cells. Note the single process coming out of each end of the spindle cell. **D,** SEM of epithelioid cells. Note larger round cell containing multiple processes. (Courtesy of Dr. RC Eagle, Jr.)

6. Classification and prognosis summary
    a. A little less than 50% of ciliary body and choroidal malignant melanomas are of the spindle-cell variety with an excellent prognosis (i.e., approximately 73% survival).
    b. A little more than 50% are of the nonspindle-cell variety (epithelioid, mixed, or necrotic) and have a poor prognosis (i.e., approximately 35% survive).
E. Other classifications and prognosis
    1. Wilder's stain for reticulum: in general, heavily fibered malignant melanomas have a better prognosis than lightly fibered ones, but this is not a very reliable criterion.
    2. Degree of pigmentation
        a. In general, lightly pigmented tumors have a better prognosis than heavily pigmented ones, but this is not a very reliable criterion.
        b. The pigmentation may vary greatly from cell to cell, region to region, and tumor to tumor.
            1). Unless serial sections are made, one may see only the pigmented part of the tumor or the nonpigmented (amelanotic) part.

            2). Some tumors are completely amelanotic,* others are maximally pigmented, and others show variable pigmentation.
3. Size of tumor
    a. Size seems to be the most reliable prognostic sign, even more reliable than cell type.

    Posterior choroidal melanomas with ciliary body involvement have a greater mortality than "pure" choroidal melanomas, most likely because of their greater size.

    b. The four factors for predicting prognosis best appear to be size (dimension), cell type, scleral extension, and mitotic activity.

    Size of tumors based on echographic tumor elevation differs from that based on measurements from histologic slides because of variable shrinkage in the latter.

Even in tumor cells considered completely amelanotic by light microscopy, some poorly formed, immature melanosomes are frequently found by electron microscopy.

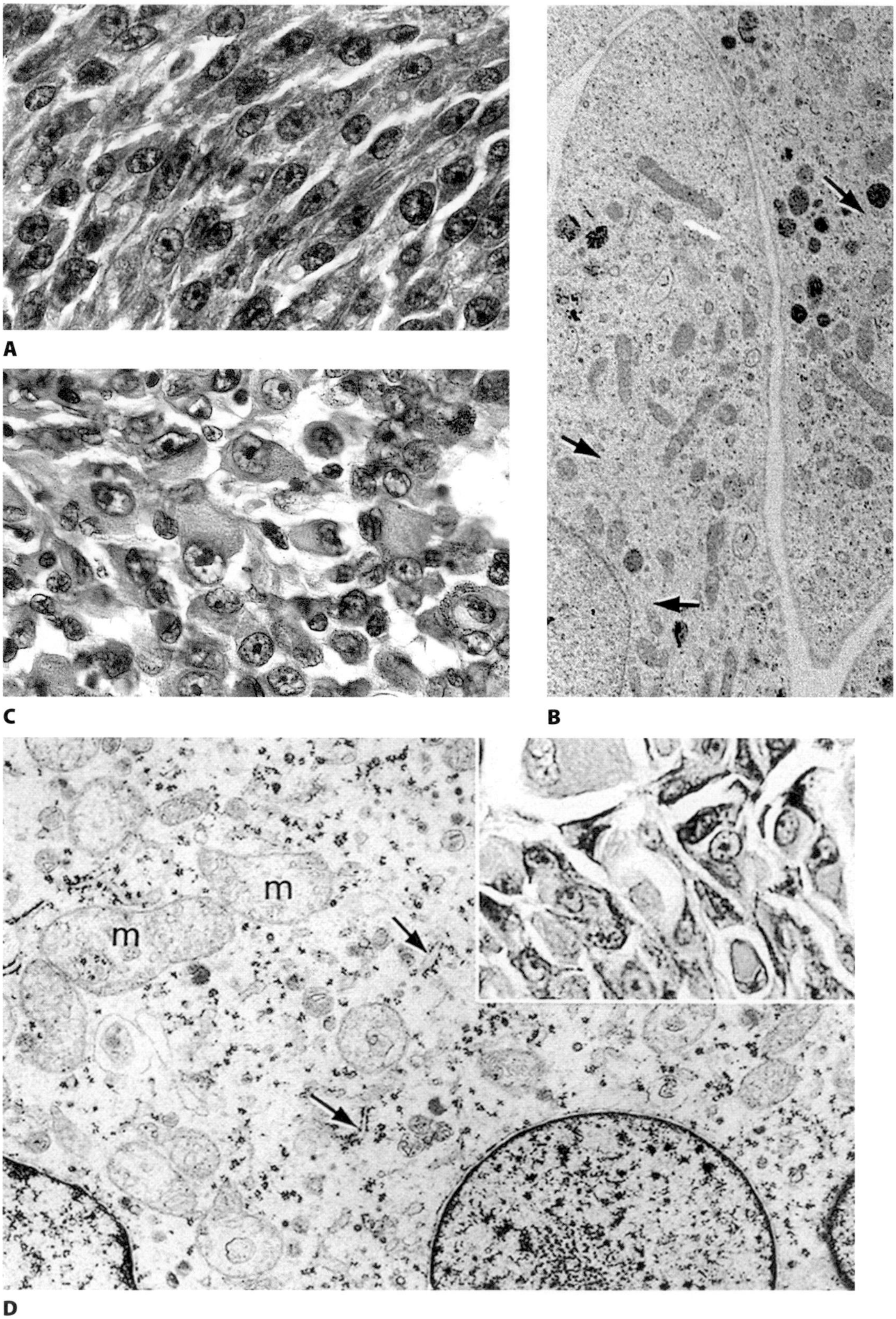

Fig. 17.40 Callender classification—light and transmission electron microscopy (EM). **A,** Histologic section of spindle-B cells. **B,** EM shows relatively amelanotic spindle-B melanoma cells with few intracytoplasmic filaments (*arrows*); mitochondria elongated and partially oriented along long axis of cell. Melanosomes all immature. **C,** Histologic section of epithelioid cells. **D,** EM of epithelioid cells shows large, watery cytoplasm, lack of cytoplasmic filaments, and loose (nonaligned) arrangement of cell organelles (e.g., m, mitochondria). Note widespread dispersion of ribosomal clusters (polysomes); some, however, remain attached to fragments of endoplasmic reticulum (*arrows*). *Inset* shows loss of cohesiveness of epithelioid cells.

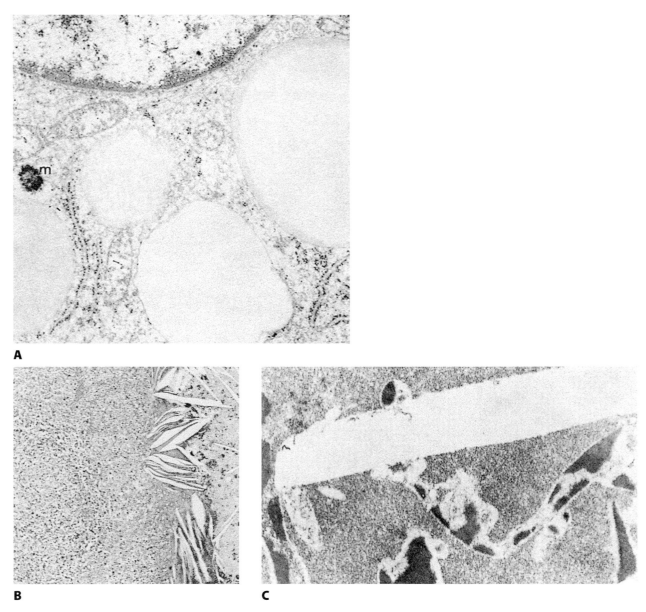

Fig. 17.41 Necrotic and degenerative changes in melanoma. **A,** Electron micrograph shows lipidic content of vacuoles still intact in vesicles on left (m, near-mature melanosome). **B,** Necrotic material on right filled with cell debris, pigment-filled macrophages (both melanin and hemosiderin), and cholesterol clefts. Some calcium present in necrotic region. **C,** Electron micrograph shows cholesterol clefts in mass of necrotic cellular debris.

   c. Malignant melanomas under 1 cm³ (approximately 6 × 6 × 6 DD or smaller clinically) have a very favorable prognosis.

     Of this group of small tumors, 69% are of the spindle-cell types.

   d. Malignant melanomas over 1 cm³ (10 × 10 × 10 mm) have a poor prognosis.

     Of this group of large tumors, 57% are of the nonspindle-cell types. The poor prognosis in the large tumor group reflects the preponderance of epithelioid cell-containing melanomas.

   e. For practical clinical purposes, a solid uveal tumor *under 6 DD in greatest diameter* and less than 3 mm in height has a favorable prognosis, with a survival rate of approximately 73%.

   f. Clinical features that may help predict metastases in small choroidal melanocytic tumors include posterior tumor location touching the optic nerve, increased tumor thickness, symp-

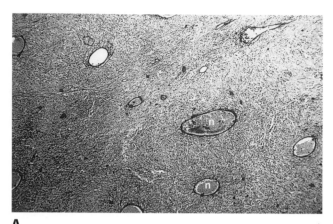

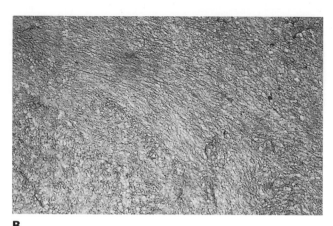

A

B

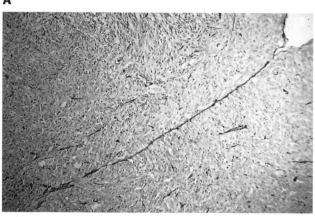

C

Fig. 17.42 Seven morphologic vascular patterns in uveal melanoma (see Fig. 17.43). **A,** Normal: tumor cells grow around normal choroidal vessels that are either filled with blood (n) or vacant (N). **B,** Silent (zones of avascularity): no normal vessels or new vessels are identified. **C,** Straight pattern: a straight vessel connects with a normal vessel (n). Straight vessels can also run in a parallel array. (From Folberg R *et al: Ophthalmology* 100:1389. © Elsevier 1993.)

toms of blurred vision, and documented tumor enlargement.

4. Nucleolar area
   a. Different techniques can measure the nucleolar area of melanoma cells directly from paraffin-embedded microsections.
   b. The standard deviation of nucleolar area is an extremely accurate predictor of death from tumor.

Automated image analysis may be more sensitive than flow cytometry in detecting euploidy in determining DNA quantification. Also, cytomorphometric analysis of nuclear characteristics may be easier than determining nucleolar characteristics, and equally accurate.

---

5. Vascular patterns in melanoma (Figs 17.42 and 17.43)

Different vascular patterns can be seen in melanomas, including zones of avascularity (silent pattern), straight pattern, parallel pattern with cross-linking, arcs (fragments of curved vessels or incompletely closed loops), loops (island of tumor surrounded by a large, closed vascular loop), and networks (back-to-back adjacent loops). The presence of vascular arcs with or without branching on

---

histopathologic examination implies that loops or networks will be detected in the same section plane, reflecting the architectural potential in aggressive tumors.

---

a. A closed vascular loop is a large vascular space occluded (closed) by melanoma cells.
b. A network is composed of at least three back-to-back closed vascular loops.
c. The presence of vascular networks provides a most significant association with death from metastatic melanoma.
d. It is important to distinguish vasculogenic mimicry patterns from fibrovascular septa when examining tumors for vascular patterns.
e. Alterations in p53 expression in uveal melanoma are associated with the expression of the cellular proliferation marker, Ki-67, but not with the presence of microvascular patterns.

Ezrin, radixin, and moesin form the ERN protein family, which mediates interaction between actin filaments and cell membranes. Ezrin immunoreactivity in uveal melanomas is associated with higher mortality and two independent high-risk characteristics: microvascular density and number of infiltrating macrophages.

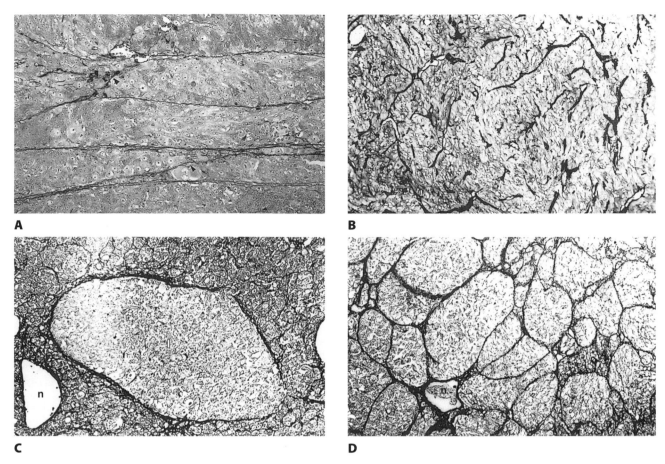

Fig. 17.43 Seven morphologic vascular patterns (see Fig. 17.42). **A,** Parallel with cross-linking: the cross-links are identified by arrowheads. **B,** Arcs: arcs are fragments of curved vessels or incompletely closed loops. Here, arcs with branching: dichotomous branching form fragments of incompletely closed loops. **C,** Loops: an island of tumor is surrounded by a large, closed vascular loop (l) which is to the right of a vacant, normal vessel (n). **D,** Networks: back-to-back adjacent loops. Notice the relationship of the network to a normal vessel (n). (From Folberg R *et al.:* *Ophthalmology* 100:1389. © Elsevier 1993.)

6. Nucleolar organizer region
   a. Nucleolar organizer regions are outpouchings of nucleolar DNA that direct ribosomal RNA transcription.
   b. Silver staining of nucleolar organizer regions can be helpful in differentiating benign from malignant pigmented uveal tumors.
7. Iris color

Patients who have blue or gray irises appear to be at increased risk of metastatic death from choroidal melanomas, independent of other risk factors.

---

8. Diffuse melanomas carry a metastatic potential of 24% at 5 years.
   a. Iris pigment and texture changes secondary to topically applied prostaglandin analogues may simulate a diffuse iris melanoma.
9. Epidermal growth factor receptor (EGFR)
   a. EGFR is a transmembrane glycoprotein that is correlated with the development of metastases in various human malignancies.
   b. Expression of EGFR is significantly correlated with death caused by metastases (strong preference for liver metastases) from primary uveal melanoma.
10. Tumors, Nodes Metastases (TNM) classification
    a. The TNM classification takes into consideration standardized definitions of different-size melanomas (small, medium, and large) based on LBD, height, and extraocular extension.
    b. The TNM is still a work in progress.
F. Prognosis without enucleation
   1. Because the natural history of uveal melanomas is not known, the prognosis is speculative when based on data after therapy.
   2. The mortality rate before enucleation, as extrapolated from incomplete data, seems to be 1% per year.

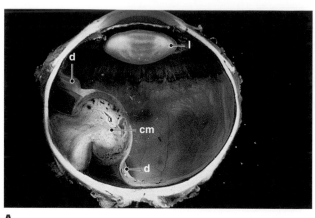

A

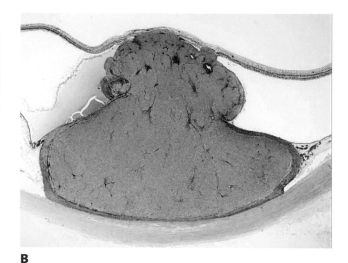

B

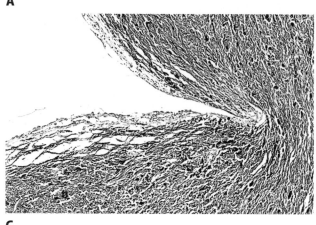

C

Fig. 17.44 Uveal "mushroom" melanoma. **A,** The melanoma has ruptured through Bruch's membrane, causing a mushroom configuration. The elastic Bruch's membrane remains around the base of the mushroom, acting as a tourniquet. Arteriolar blood gains access to the head of the mushroom, but venous blood has difficulty leaving, giving rise to dilated and engorged blood vessels in the head of the mushroom, as shown here (l, lens; d, detached retina; cm, choroidal melanoma). **B,** A histologic section shows the ruptured ends of Bruch's membrane (seen with increased magnification in **C**) and the dilated engorged blood vessels in the head of the tumor (r, ruptured end of Bruch's membrane; b, base of tumor). (**A,** Courtesy of Dr. RC Eagle, Jr.; **B,** Courtesy of Dr. Morton Smith)

3. The mortality rate after enucleation reaches a peak of approximately 8% during the second year after enucleation.

Based on the preceding statistical analysis, two-thirds of the fatalities could be attributed to tumor emboli being disseminated at the time of enucleation. Only a long-term follow-up study of untreated patients with uveal melanomas can clarify the situation.

G. Associated findings
1. Invasion of Bruch's membrane occurs in approximately 63% of tumors (Fig. 17.44).
   a. When Bruch's membrane is intact, the tumor usually has an oval shape.
   b. When Bruch's membrane is ruptured, the tumor assumes a mushroom shape.
   c. When the elastic Bruch's membrane is ruptured, it acts as a tourniquet around the base of the tumor so that:
      1). Arterial blood can easily be pumped into the mushroom head, but the venous return is obstructed, thereby leading to dilated, tortuous venous channels.
      2). The vascular abnormalities account for prolonged fluorescein staining, and the dilated,

thin veins may also lead to intravitreal hemorrhage (see p. 705 in this chapter).
2. Invasion of the scleral canals (Fig. 17.45A and B) occurs in approximately 32% of tumors and provides one route for tumor access to the orbit.
3. Invasion of scleral tissue occurs directly in approximately 15% of tumors.
4. Invasion of the optic nerve (see Fig. 17.45C and D) occurs in approximately 5% of tumors.

Peripapillary uveal melanomas tend to invade the optic nerve. Therefore, a long piece of optic nerve should be excised when an eye with such a tumor is enucleated.

---

5. Invasion of the vortex veins (Fig. 17.46) occurs in approximately 13% of tumors.
   a. Sampling of the vortex veins should be taken routinely for histology on all enucleated globes suspected of harboring an intraocular tumor.
   b. Vortex vein invasion carries an extremely unfavorable prognosis.
6. A neural retinal detachment (Fig. 17.47) is present in approximately 75% of cases, but in approximately 83% of those cases, the detachment is localized rather than total.

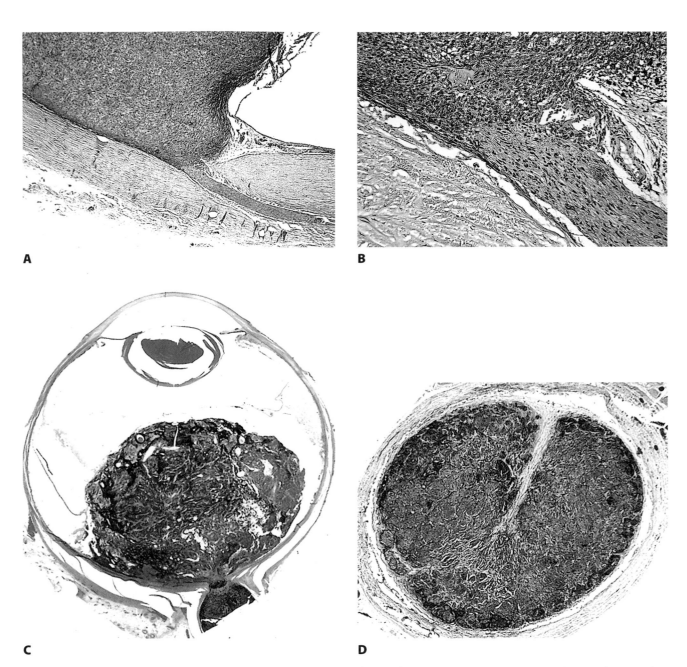

Fig. 17.45 Melanoma extension and invasion. **A,** Choroidal melanoma extends into scleral canal, surrounding ciliary nerve (shown with increased magnification in **B**). Cases like this have led, in the past, to the erroneous conclusion that melanomas arose from ciliary nerves. **C,** Choroidal melanoma has invaded and completely replaced this segment of optic nerve (shown in cross-section in **D**).

7. Extraocular extension (Fig. 17.48) occurs in approximately 13% of tumors.
   a. Following failed transpupillary thermotherapy, the melanoma may continue to grow along the paths of least resistance to extend laterally in the choroid or through scleral emissary canals, resulting in extrascleral extension, which may be difficult to detect by ultrasonography. Nevertheless, ultrasonography should be performed periodically to attempt to detect such extrascleral extension. Similarly, extrascleral extension of uveal melanoma may occur following failed proton beam therapy. Factors associated with local failure of proton beam radiotherapy for uveal melanoma include reduced safety margins, large ciliary body tumors, eyelids within the treatment field, inadequate positioning of tantalum clips, and male gender. Viable tumor cells may remain even in apparently nonrecurrent uveal melanoma treated with Ru-106 brachytherapy. A combination of plaque radiotherapy and transpupillary thermography has resulted in

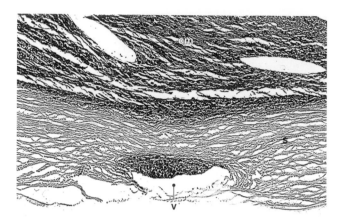

Fig. 17.46 Invasion of vortex vein. A large pigmented choroidal melanoma (cm) is present in the eye and is filling most of an intrascleral vortex vein (v). Obviously, vortex vein invasion, like extraocular extension into the orbit, carries a life-threatening prognosis (s, sclera).

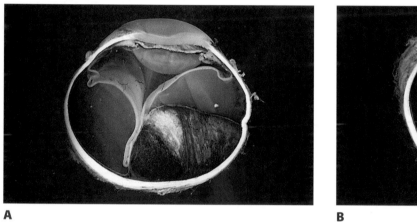

A   **B**

Fig. 17.47 Neural retinal detachment. **A** and **B,** Two different eyes with tumor and neural retinal detachment. Both proved to be choroidal melanomas by histopathologic examination. Note variation in pigmentation and shape of melanomas.

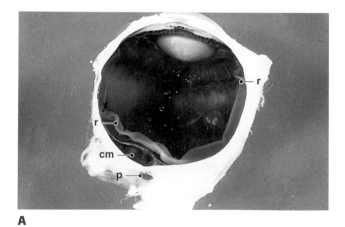
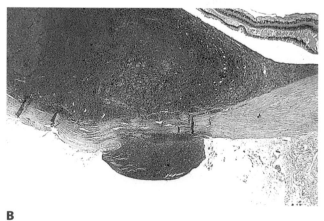

A   **B**

Fig. 17.48 Extraocular extension. **A,** Note the oval pigmented melanoma (cm, choroidal melanoma) of the choroid in the eye and the small pigmented lesion (p) on the surface of the sclera (r, retina). **B,** Histologic section shows the uveal melanoma in the eye and a nodule of extrascleral extension.

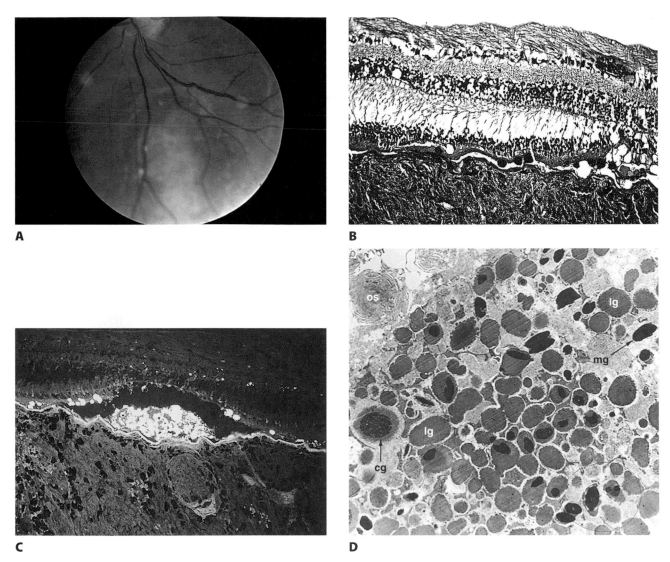

Fig. 17.49 Orange pigment. **A,** Fundus appearance of orange-colored material overlying melanoma. **B,** Periodic acid–Schiff-stained histologic section shows pigment-laden enlarged cells under the neural retina. **C,** Lipofuscin accumulated in pigment epithelium shows intense autofluorescence when examined by ultraviolet light. **D,** Electron micrograph shows myriad lipofuscin granules (lg) within pigment-laden macrophage (os, photoreceptor outer segments; mg, melanin granule; cg, compound granule). (Modified with permission from Font RL *et al.: Arch Ophthalmol* 91:359, 1974. © American Medical Association. All rights reserved.)

only a 3% local recurrence rate in choroidal melanoma at 5-year follow-up. Transpupillary thermotherapy is not the therapy of choice for diffuse choroidal melanoma. Subretinal pigment dispersion is an uncommon complication of the procedure.

b. After extraocular extension, the tumor orbital recurrence rate is 18%, compared with 0.7% in the absence of detectable extraocular extension.

c. If the extraocular portion of the tumor is incised or transected (rather than small or well encapsulated) at the time of enucleation, or if it is nonencapsulated, the tumor orbital recurrence rate is at least 50%.

d. Frequently, discovery of an orbital recurrence precedes the discovery of a metastatic lesion.

Because the orbital recurrence often precedes the metastasis, exenteration seems to be the treatment of choice when extraocular extension is significant, especially in cases that have nonencapsulated or surgically transected tumors. However, the efficacy of orbital exenteration for primary extraocular extension or for orbital recurrence of a uveal melanoma is still not known.

8. Reaction of overlying RPE
   a. Secondary drusen

b. Orange pigment overlying choroidal melanomas is seen clinically in approximately 47% of cases (Fig. 17.49).

Fluorescein angiography shows that the orange pigment is hypofluorescent. Orange pigment may also occur over a choroidal nevus. Histologically, the orange appearance results from aggregates of RPE cells and lipofuscin-containing macrophages overlying the melanoma.

---

c. Placoid or adenomatous proliferations are often accompanied by degenerative changes in the overlying retina.

H. Associated cytology

1. Cytogenetic studies show a consistent occurrence of monosomy 3 and trisomy 8q (i.e., the loss of gene sequences on chromosome 3 and the duplication of gene sequences on chromosome 8).
   a. Monosomy for chromosome 3, particularly as detected by fine-needle aspiration biopsy of uveal melanoma and analyzed by fluorescent in situ hybridization (FISH) analysis, may provide important information regarding prognosis for these tumors. Moreover, indicative chromosomal studies for monosomy of chromosome 3 can also be performed on glutaraldehyde or formalin-fixed, paraffin-embedded tissue using chromosome in situ hybridization (CISH). Loss of chromosome 3 may be associated with a reduction of 5-year survival from 95% to less than 50%.
   b. Several tumor suppressor loci on chromosome 3 are targets of specific deletions associated with uveal melanoma.
2. Uveal melanoma cells are positive for S-100 protein, HMB-45, and Ki-67.
3. Lymphocytes found in uveal melanomas (tumor-infiltrating lymphocytes) are predominantly T-suppressor/cytotoxic cells; B-cell lymphocytes are scarce.

I. Unsuspected malignant melanomas

1. Approximately 12% of ciliary body and choroid malignant melanomas proven histologically were unsuspected before surgery; most were in glaucoma eyes with opaque media.

Many of the eyes have a total neural retinal detachment. A patient who has a neural retinal detachment plus glaucoma, especially with no prior history of glaucoma and no glaucoma in the other eye, should be considered to have a uveal malignant melanoma until proven otherwise.

---

2. Approximately 4% of eyes that have opaque media and are enucleated from white patients (blind for at least 6 months) harbor a malignant melanoma.

This does not mean that 4% of enucleated blind eyes that have opaque media harbor a malignant melanoma, because the statistics are derived from a study done on enucleated eyes. The eyes were obviously enucleated for some reason. Therefore, if a blind eye that has opaque media becomes clinically symptomatic, a malignant melanoma should be considered. Ultrasonography is helpful in this situation.

J. Differential diagnosis of malignant melanomas of ciliary body and choroid

1. Hemorrhages: choroidal, sub-RPE, neural retinal or subneural retinal, and vitreous
2. Cysts: congenital, retinoschisis, solitary, and parasitic

Ciliary body melanomas can acquire an intralesional cavity (cavitary melanomas) and mimic a ciliary body cyst.

---

3. Serous detachment: neural retinal and choroidal
4. Subretinal neovascularization, especially with hemorrhage
5. Tumors: hemangioma, nevus, metastatic carcinoma (Fig. 17.50), lymphoma, and lesions of PE
   a. The typical "mushroom" or "collar button" configuration of an expanding choroidal melanoma has been simulated by metastatic adenocarcinoma to the choroid that ruptured through Bruch membrane.
6. Ultrasonography, fluorescein angiography, transillumination, and, to a much lesser extent, ^{32}P uptake are helpful methods of determining the correct diagnosis.

K. Primary, bilateral, diffuse, uveal, melanocytic lesions may occur along with another systemic primary tumor.

L. Melanoma-associated spongiform scleropathy

1. This condition is characterized by areas within the sclera where collagen bundles appear to have disintegrated into loose fibres
2. The extent of these scleral changes is proportional to the extent of direct contact between the tumor and sclera
3. It has been observed in 33% to 38.5% of cases examined, and is particularly common in eyes with tumor scleral extension (91.5%)
4. There is a significantly higher incidence in older patients
5. The incidence is reduced by pre-enucleation radiation
6. It is not correlated with tumor cell type
7. There are significantly lower levels of major amino acids of scleral collagen and total proteins in the involved areas, presumably indicating collagen degradation
8. Specific glycosaminoglycans (GAGs) and total GAGS are increased in these regions, resulting in localized water accumulation, which may further separate collagen bundles

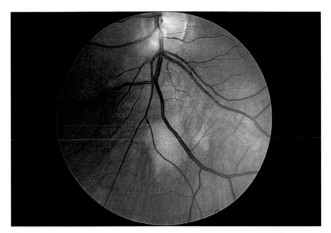

A

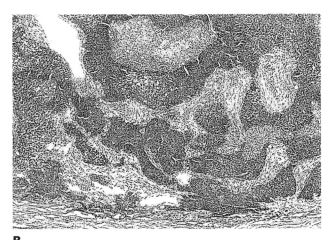

B

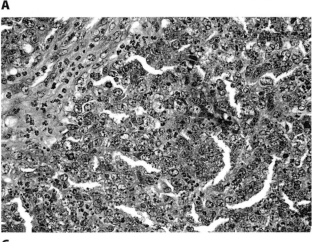

C

Fig. 17.50 Metastatic uveal tumors. **A,** Clinical appearance of metastatic carcinoma from breast. Usually, metastatic tumors are easily recognized clinically. **B,** Occasionally metastatic carcinoma is mistaken for melanoma, resulting in enucleation of the eye. The presence of significant stroma (pink areas between collections of tumor cells) is a tip-off that a tumor is metastatic. **C,** Increased magnification shows sheets of malignant epithelial cells.

9. The net result of the changes associated with melanoma-associated spongiform scleropathy may be to facilitate tumor extension

MELANOTIC TUMORS OF THE OPTIC DISC AND OPTIC NERVE

Melanocytoma (Magnocellular Nevus of the Nerve Head)

I. A melanocytoma (Fig. 17.51A) is a nevus composed entirely of maximally pigmented, plump, polyhedral nevus cells that contain giant melanosomes (macromelanosomes).

Rarely, melanocytomas may be associated with bone formation.

A. They may be found in any part of the uvea (Fig. 17.52; see also Fig. 17.51B and C) in addition to the optic disc, and even in the sclera.

B. Because a melanocytoma is a type of nevus, a more appropriate term for the tumor is *magnocellular* nevus.

C. When in the anterior uvea, a melanocytoma can present with glaucoma.

II. Usually, the tumor is located at the inferior temporal aspect of the optic disc in patients who have "dark" fundi.

A. The tumor usually fills less than half the optic disc, but rarely, it may fill the whole disc and may even "spill out" into the adjacent choroid and retina.

Rarely, a melanocytoma of the optic disc may cause a central retinal vascular obstruction. A bilateral case in a 10-month-old infant has been reported.

B. It may extend into the vitreous to an alarming degree, either directly or as a dispersion of pigment.

III. Whereas the ratio of white patients to black patients affected with uveal malignant melanoma is 15:1, the white-to-black ratio for melanocytoma of the optic disc is 0.1:1.

Even when a melanocytoma is present in white patients, it is usually seen in patients who have dark fundi. The melanocytoma

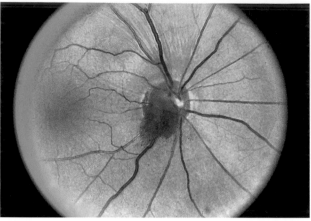

A

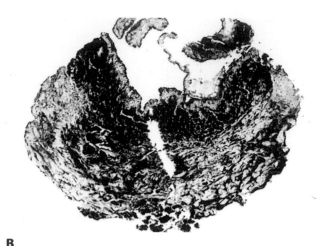

B

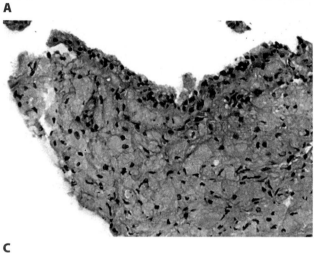

C

Fig. 17.51 Melanocytoma of optic disc. **A,** Characteristic black color and inferior temporal location of tumor in 37-year-old black woman. **B,** A histologic section of a ciliary body melanocytoma shows that the tumor is composed of maximally pigmented nevus cells. **C,** Bleached section demonstrates benign, plump, polyhedral nevus cells. A melanocytoma is simply a nevus that is entirely composed of maximally pigmented, plump, polyhedral nevus cells. (Modified with permission from Scheie HG, Yanoff M: *Arch Ophthalmol* 77:781, 1967. © American Medical Association. All rights reserved.)

frequently involves the adjacent neural retina for a short distance and clinically is seen to end in the neural retina with feathered edges.

IV. It is a benign lesion.
   A. In about 11% of cases it may enlarge.
   B. It probably has the same very low malignant potential of any nevus, and when it occurs in a white person, it has a higher potential for malignant change than in a black person.
   V. Melanocytoma may undergo necrosis resulting in such atypical features as opaque media, pain, and inflammation, thereby mimicking a necrotic malignant melanoma.

Malignant Melanoma

   I. Primary malignant melanomas of the optic disc are exceedingly rare.
   II. Most malignant melanomas thought to be primary in the nerve head are actually primary in the juxtapapillary choroid with secondary invasion of the optic disc.

III. Approximately 5% of choroidal malignant melanomas invade the optic disc and nerve (see Fig. 17.45C and D).

MELANOTIC TUMORS OF THE ORBIT

   I. Primary melanoma of the orbit is quite rare.

Most primary orbital melanomas occur in white patients and are associated with blue nevi.

   II. Malignant melanoma of the orbit may be associated with congenital oculodermal melanocytosis (the nevus of Ota) or with a primary melanoma of the lacrimal sac.

Primary melanoma of the orbit should be differentiated from *clear-cell sarcoma* (melanoma of soft parts), which produces melanin, is S-100-positive, and is probably a member of the family of malignant peripheral nerve cell tumors.

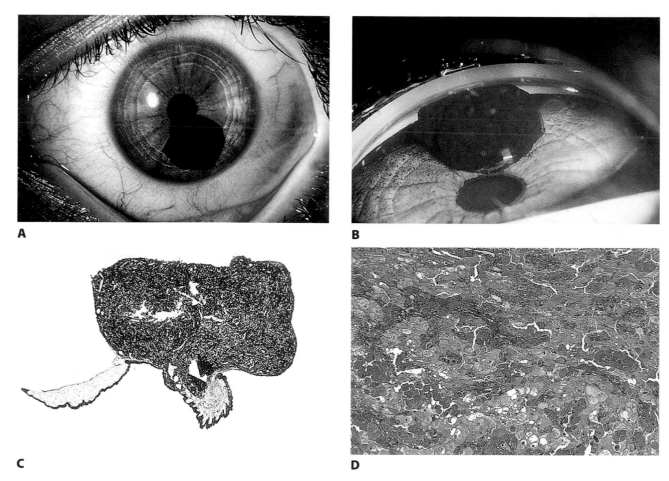

Fig. 17.52 Melanocytoma of iris and ciliary body. **A,** Black iris tumor in a 17-year-old patient (shown gonioscopically in **B**). **C,** Histologic section shows maximally pigmented tumor of iris root and ciliary body. **D,** Partially bleached section demonstrates large cells that contain bland nuclei. (Case presented by Prof. GOH Naumann at combined meeting of European Ophthalmic Pathology and Verhoeff Societies, 1996.)

BIBLIOGRAPHY

Normal Anatomy

Fine BS, Yanoff M: *Ocular Histology: A Text and Atlas*, 2nd edn. Hagerstown, PA, Harper & Row, 1979:61–70, 216–217

Fuchs U, Kivellä T, Tarkkanen A: Cytoskeleton in normal and reactive human retinal pigment epithelial cells. *Invest Ophthalmol Vis Sci* 32:3178, 1991

Hu D-N, McCormick SA, Orlow SJ *et al.:* Melanogenesis by human uveal melanocytes in vitro. *Invest Ophthalmol Vis Sci* 36:931, 1995

Imesch PD, Bindley CD, Khademian Z *et al.:* Melanocytes and iris color: Electron microscopic findings. *Arch Ophthalmol* 114:443, 1996

Panda-Jonas S, Jonas JB, Jakobczyk-Zmija M: Retinal pigment epithelial cell count, distribution, and correlations in normal human eyes. *Am J Ophthalmol* 121:181, 1996

Toth-Molnar E, Olah J, Dobozy A *et al.:* Ocular pigmented findings in patients with dysplastic naevus syndrome. *Melanoma Res* 14:43, 2004

Wilkerson CL, Syed NA, Fisher MR *et al.:* Melanocytes and iris color: Light microscopic findings. *Arch Ophthalmol* 114:437, 1996

Yanoff M, Fine BS: *Ocular Pathology: A Color Atlas*, 2nd edn. New York, Gower Medical Publishing, 1992:7.1–7.2

Melanotic Tumors of the Eyelids

Albert DM, Chang MA, Lamping K *et al.:* The dysplastic nevus syndrome: A pedigree with primary malignant melanomas of the choroid and skin. *Ophthalmology* 92:1728, 1985

Balmaceda CM, Fetell MR, Powers J *et al.:* Nevus of Ota and leptomeningeal melanocytic lesions. *Neurology* 43:381, 1993

Bowman CB, Guber D, Brown CH III *et al.:* Cutaneous malignant melanoma with diffuse intraocular metastases. *Arch Ophthalmol* 112:1213, 1994

Busam KJ: Lack of relevant information for tumor staging in pathology reports of primary cutaneous malignant melanoma. *Am J Clin Pathol* 115:743, 2001

Busam KJ, Antonescu CR, Marghoob AA *et al.:* Histologic classification of tumor-infiltrating lymphocytes in primary cutaneous malignant melanoma. A study of interobserver agreement. *Am J Clin Pathol* 115:856, 2001

Cole EL, Zakov ZN, Meisler DM *et al.:* Cutaneous malignant melanoma metastatic to the vitreous. *Arch Ophthalmol* 104:98, 1986

de German-Ribon RI, Singh AD, Arevalo JF *et al.:* Choroidal melanoma with oculodermal melanocytosis in Hispanic patients. *Am J Ophthalmol* 128:251, 1999

Duke-Elder S: Heterochromia. In *System of Ophthalmology*, vol. III, part 2. St. Louis, CV Mosby, 1964:813–818

Fine BS, Yanoff M: *Ocular Histology: A Text and Atlas*, 2nd edn. Hagerstown, PA, Harper & Row, 1979:61, 197, 198, 210

Giblin ME, Shields CL, Shields JA: Primary eyelid malignant melanoma associated with primary conjunctival malignant melanoma. *Aust N Z J Ophthalmol* 16:127, 1988

Glass AG, Hoover RN: The emerging epidemic of melanoma and squamous cell skin cancer. *JAMA* 262:2097, 1989

Goldberg M: Waardenburg's syndrome with fundus and other abnormalities. *Arch Ophthalmol* 76:797, 1966

Grossniklaus HE, McLean IW: Cutaneous melanoma of the eyelid. *Ophthalmology* 98:1867, 1991

Gündüz K, Shields JA, Shields CL et al.: Choroidal melanoma in a 14-year-old patient with ocular melanocytosis. *Arch Ophthalmol* 116:1112, 1998

Gündüz K, Shields JA, Shields CL et al.: Periorbital cellular blue nevus leading to orbitopalpebral and intracranial melanoma. *Ophthalmology* 105:2046, 1998

Hall IH, Miller DR, Rogers JD et al.: Update on the incidence and mortality from melanoma in the United States. *J Am Acad Dermatol* 40:35, 1999

Hiscott P, Seitz B, Naumann GOH: Epithelioid cell Spitz nevus of the eyelid. *Arch Ophthalmol* 126:735, 1998

Kincaid MC: Multiple lentigines syndrome. Presented at the meeting of the Verhoeff Society, 1993

Luxenberg MN: Periorbital giant congenital melanocytic nevus. *Arch Ophthalmol* 110:562, 1992

Margo CE, Habal MB: Large congenital melanocytic nevus: Light and electron microscopic findings. *Ophthalmology* 94:960, 1987

Martin-Reay DG, Shattuck MC, Guthrie FW: Psammomatous melanotic schwannoma: an additional component of Carney's complex. *Am J Clin Pathol* 95:484, 1991

McCarthy JM, Rootman J, Horsman D et al.: Conjunctival and uveal melanoma in the dysplastic nevus syndrome. *Surv Ophthalmol* 37:377, 1993

McDermott NC, Hayes DP, Al-Sader MH et al.: Identification of vertical growth phase in malignant melanoma: A study of interobserver agreement (editorial). *Am J Clin Pathol* 110:753, 1998

Paik JH, Lee MH, Lee MA: Periorbital congenital melanocytic nevus associated with ankyloblepharon. *Pediatr Dermatol* 18:31, 2001

Ruiz-Villaverde R, Blasco MJ, Buendia EA et al.: Bilateral Ota naevus. *J Eur Acad Dermatol Venereol* 17:437, 2003

Rumelt S, Pe'er J, Rubin PA: The clinicopathological spectrum of benign peripunctal tumours. *Graefes Arch Clin Exp Ophthalmol* 243:113, 2005

Scheie HG, Yanoff M, Sassani JW: Inverted follicular keratosis clinically mimicking malignant melanoma. *Ann Ophthalmol* 8:949, 1977

Scott KR, Jakobiec FA, Font RL: Peripunctal melanocytic nevi. *Ophthalmology* 96:994, 1989

Scull JJ, Alcocer CE, Deschênes J et al.: Primary choroidal melanoma in a patient with previous cutaneous melanoma. *Arch Ophthalmol* 115:796, 1997

Seregard S, af Trampe E, Mansson-Brahme E et al.: Prevalence of primary acquired melanosis and nevi of the conjunctiva and uvea in the dysplastic nevus syndrome: A case-control study. *Ophthalmology* 102:1524, 1995

Shah KD, Tabibzadeh SS, Gerber MA: Immunohistochemical distinction of Paget's disease from Bowen's disease and superficial spreading melanoma with the use of monoclonal cytokeratin antibodies. *Am J Clin Pathol* 88:689, 1987

Sharara NA, Alexander RA, Luthert PJ et al.: Differential immunoreactivity of melanocytic lesions of the conjunctiva. *Histopathology* 39:426, 2001

Shivers SC, Wang X, Li W et al.: Molecular staging of malignant melanomas correlation with clinical outcome. *JAMA* 280:1410, 1998

Singh AD, dePotter Pfilal BA et al.: Lifetime prevalence of uveal melanoma in white patients with oculo(dermal) melanocytosis. *Ophthalmology* 105:195, 1998

Tahery DP, Goldberg R, Moy RL: Malignant melanoma of the eyelid: A report of eight cases and a review of the literature. *J Am Acad Dermatol* 27:17, 1992

Taub M, Arumi-Uría M, Barranco C et al.: Expression of the proteoglycans versican and mel-CSPG in dysplastic nevi. *Am J Clin Pathol* 119:587, 2003

Teekhasaenee C, Ritch R: Glaucoma in phakomatosis pigmentovascularis. *Ophthalmology* 104:150, 1997

Teekhasaenee C, Ritch R, Rutnin U et al.: Glaucoma in oculodermal melanocytosis. *Ophthalmology* 97:562, 1990

Teekhasaenee C, Ritch R, Rutnin U et al.: Ocular findings in oculodermal melanocytosis. *Arch Ophthalmol* 108:1114, 1990

ten Berge P, Danen EHJ, van Muijen GNP et al.: Integrin expression in uveal melanoma differs from cutaneous melanoma. *Invest Ophthalmol Vis Sci* 34:3635, 1993

Trent JM, Stanbridge EJ, McBride HL et al.: Tumorigenicity in human melanoma cell lines controlled by introduction of human chromosome 6. *Science* 247:568, 1990

Vaziri M, Buffam FV, Martinka M et al.: Clinicopathologic features and behavior of cutaneous euelid melanomas. *Ophthalmology* 109:901, 2002

Vaziri M, Buffam FV, Martinka M et al.: Clinicopathologic features and behavior of cutaneous eyelid melanoma. *Ophthalmology* 109:901, 2002

Wick MR: Prognostic factors for cutaneous melanomas (editorial). *Am J Clin Pathol* 110:713, 1998

Melanotic Tumors of Conjunctiva

Baroody M, Holds JB, Kokoska MS et al.: Conjunctival melanoma metastasis diagnosed by sentinel lymph node biopsy. *Am J Ophthalmol* 137:1147, 2004

Bobic-Radovanovic A, Latkovic Z, Marinkovic J et al.: Predictors of survival in malignant melanoma of the conjunctiva: A clinico-pathologic and follow-up study. *Eur J Ophthalmol* 8:4, 1998

Buckman G, Jakobiec FA, Folberg R et al.: Melanocytic nevi of the palpebral conjunctiva. *Ophthalmology* 95:1053, 1988

Crandall AS, Yanoff M, Schaffer DB: Intrascleral nerve loop mistakenly identified as a foreign body. *Arch Ophthalmol* 95:497, 1977

Crawford JB, Howes EL, Char DH: Combined nevi of the conjunctiva. *Trans Am Ophthalmol Soc* 97:171, 1999

de Potter P, Shields CL, Shields JA et al.: Clinical predictive factors for development of recurrence and metastasis in conjunctival melanoma: A review of 68 cases. *Br J Ophthalmol* 77:624, 1993

Demirci H, McCormick SA, Finger PT: Topical mitomycin chemotherapy for conjunctival malignant melanoma and primary acquired melanosis with atypia: Clinical experience with histopathologic observations. *Arch Ophthalmol* 118:885, 2000

Demirci H, Shields CL, Shields JA et al.: Malignant melanoma arising from unusual conjunctival blue nevus. *Arch Ophthalmol* 118:1581, 2000

Esmaeli B, Reifler D, Prieto VG et al.: Conjunctival melanoma with a positive sentinel lymph node. *Arch Ophthalmol* 121:1779, 2003

Esmaeli B, Wang X, Youssef A et al.: Patterns of regional and distant metastasis in patients with conjunctival melanoma: Experience at a cancer center over four decades. *Ophthalmology* 108:2101, 2001

Folberg R, Jakobiec FA, Bernardino VB et al.: Benign conjunctival melanocytic lesions. *Ophthalmology* 96:436, 1989

Folberg R, McLean IW, Zimmerman LE: Conjunctival malignant melanoma. *Hum Pathol* 16:136, 1985

Folberg R, McLean IW, Zimmerman LE: Primary acquired melanosis of the conjunctiva. *Hum Pathol* 16:129, 1985

Folberg R, Yanoff M: Ocular melanotic tumors. In Tasman W, Jaeger EA, eds: *Duane's Foundations of Clinical Ophthalmology*, vol. 3, Chapter 20. Philadelphia, JB Lippincott, 1992:1–33

Gallardo MJ, Randleman JB, Price KM et al.: Ocular argyrosis after long-term self-application of eyelash tint. *Am J Ophthalmol* 141:198, 2006

Gilbert CM, El Baba F, Schachat AP et al.: Nonsimultaneous primary choroidal and cutaneous melanomas: Report of a case. *Ophthalmology* 94:1169, 1987

Glasgow BJ, McCall LC, Foos RY: HMB-45 antibody reactivity in pigmented lesions of the conjunctiva. *Am J Ophthalmol* 109:696, 1990

Gloor P, Alexandrkis G: Clinical characteristics of primary acquired melanosis. *Invest Ophthalmol Vis Sci* 36:1721, 1995

Grossniklaus HE, Margo CE, Solomon AR: Indeterminate melanocytic proliferations of the conjunctiva. *Trans Am Ophthalmol Soc* 97:157, 1999

Iwamoto T, Burrows RC, Grossniklaus HE et al.: Immunophenotype of conjunctival melanomas. Comparisons with uveal and cutaneous melanomas. *Arch Ophthalmol* 120:1625, 2002

Jakobiec FA, Folberg R, Iwamoto T: Clinicopathologic characteristics of premalignant and malignant melanocytic lesions of the conjunctiva. *Ophthalmology* 96:147, 1989

Jay V, Font RL: Conjunctival amelanotic malignant melanoma arising in primary acquired melanoma sine pigmento. *Ophthalmology* 105:191, 1998

Ko KW, Rabinowitz SM, Friedman AH et al.: Neurofibromatosis and neural crest neoplasms: Primary acquired melanosis and malignant melanoma of the conjunctiva. *Surv Ophthalmol* 33:373, 1989

Lieb WE, Shields JA, Shields CA et al.: Postsurgical hematic cyst simulating a conjunctival melanoma. *Retina* 10:63, 1990

McDonnell JM, Carpenter JD, Jacobs P et al.: Conjunctival melanocytic lesions in children. *Ophthalmology* 96:986, 1989

Morris DA, Jakobiec FA, Henkind P et al.: Recurrent conjunctival melanoma with neuroidal spindle cell features. *Ophthalmology* 94:56, 1987

Nawa Y, Hara Y, Saishin M et al.: Conjunctival melanoma associated with extensive congenital nevus and split nevus of eyelid. *Arch Ophthalmol* 117:269, 1999

Paridaens ADA, Minasian DC, McCartney ACE et al.: Prognostic factors in primary malignant melanoma of the conjunctiva: A clinicopathological study of 256 cases. *Br J Ophthalmol* 78:252, 1994

Puk DE, Ketcham JM, Probst LE et al.: Conjunctival malignant melanoma. *Arch Ophthalmol* 114:100, 1996

Saornil MA, Marcus DM, Doepner D et al.: Nucleolar organizer regions in determining malignancy of pigmented conjunctival lesions. *Am J Ophthalmol* 115:800, 1993

Seregard S: Cell proliferation as a prognostic indicator in conjunctival malignant melanoma. *Am J Ophthalmol* 116:93, 1993

Seregard S: Conjunctival melanoma. *Surv Ophthalmol* 42:321, 1998

Shields CL, Shields JA: Tumors of the conjunctiva and cornea. *Surv Ophthalmol* 49:1, 2004

Shields CL, Demirci H, Karatza E et al.: Clinical survey of 1643 melanocytic and nonmelanocytic conjunctival tumors. *Ophthalmology* 111:1747, 2004

Shields CL, Fasiudden A, Mashayekhi A et al.: Conjunctival nevi: clinical features and natural course in 410 consecutive patients. *Arch Ophthalmol* 122:167, 2004

Shields CL, Shields JA, Gündüz K et al.: Conjunctival melanoma: Risk factors for recurrence, exenteration, metastasis, and death in 150 consecutive patients. *Arch Ophthalmol* 118:1497, 2000

Shields JA, Shields CL, Eagle RC Jr et al.: Compound nevus of the cornea simulating a foreign body. *Am J Ophthalmol* 130:235, 2000

Singh AD, Campos OE, Rhatigan RM et al.: Conjunctival melanoma in the black population. *Surv Ophthalmol* 43:127, 1998

Tsuru M, Arima N, Toyozumi Y et al.: Pigment epithelium-derived factor as a new diagnostic marker for melanocytic tumors. *Kurume Med J* 52:81, 2005

Tuomaala S, Aine E, Saari M et al.: Corneally displaced malignant conjunctival melanomas. *Ophthalmology* 109:914, 2002

Wenkel H, Rummelt V, Naumann GOH: Malignant melanoma of the conjunctiva with intraocular extension. *Arch Ophthalmol* 118:557, 2000

Werschnik C, Lommatzsch PK: Long-term follow-up of patients with conjunctival melanoma. *Am J Clin Oncol* 25:248, 2002

Yanoff M: Pigment spots of the sclera. *Arch Ophthalmol* 81:151, 1969

Yanoff M, Scheie HG: Argyrosis of conjunctiva and lacrimal sac. *Arch Ophthalmol* 71:57, 1964

Yanoff M, Zimmerman LE: Histogenesis of malignant melanomas of the uvea: III. The relationship of congenital ocular melanocytosis and neurofibromatosis to uveal melanomas. *Arch Ophthalmol* 77:331, 1967

Zimmerman LE: Criteria for management of melanosis: in correspondence. *Arch Ophthalmol* 76:307, 1966

Melanotic Tumors of Pigment Epithelium of Iris, Ciliary Body, and Retina

Aiello LP, Traboulsi EI: Pigmented fundus lesions in a preterm infant with familial adenomatous polyposis. *Arch Ophthalmol* 111:302, 1993

Arevalo JF, Fernandez CF, Garcia RA: Optical coherence tomography characteristics of choroidal metastasis. *Ophthalmology* 112:1612, 2005

Badlani VK, Quinones R, Wilensky JT et al.: Angle-closure glaucoma in teenagers. *J Glaucoma* 12:198, 2003

Broughton WL, Zimmerman LE: A clinicopathologic study of 56 cases of intraocular medulloepitheliomas. *Am J Ophthalmol* 85:407, 1978

Capeans C, Pineiro A, Blanco MJ et al.: Ultrasound biomicroscopic findings in a cavitary melanocytoma of the ciliary body. *Can J Ophthalmol* 38:501, 2003

Carrillo R, Streeten BW: Malignant teratoid medulloepithelioma in an adult. *Arch Ophthalmol* 97:695, 1979

Chamot L, Zografos L, Klainguti G: Fundus changes associated with congenital hypertrophy of the retinal pigment epithelium. *Am J Ophthalmol* 115:154, 1993

Coden DJ, Hornblass A: Photoreceptor cell differentiation in intraocular medulloepithelioma: an immunohistopathologic study. *Arch Ophthalmol* 108:481, 1990

Coffey AJH, Brownstein S: The prevalence of macular drusen in post-mortem eyes. *Am J Ophthalmol* 102:164, 1986

Coleman DJ, Silverman RH, Chabi A et al.: High-resolution ultrasonic imaging of the posterior segment. *Ophthalmology* 111:1344, 2004

Conway RM, Chew T, Golchet P et al.: Ultrasound biomicroscopy: role in diagnosis and management in 130 consecutive patients evaluated for anterior segment tumours. *Br J Ophthalmol* 89:950, 2005

Cursiefen C, Schlötzer-Schrehardt U, Holbach LM et al.: Adenoma of the nonpigmented ciliary epithelium mimicking a malignant melanoma of the iris. *Arch Ophthalmol* 117:113, 1999

Demirci H, Shields CL, Shields JA: New ophthalmic manifestations of branchio-oculo-facial syndrome. *Am J Ophthalmol* 139:362, 2005

Diesenhouse MC, Palay DA, Newman NJ et al.: Acquired heterochromia with Horner syndrome in two adults. *Ophthalmology* 99:1815, 1992

Dinakaran S, Rundle PA, Parsons MA et al.: Adenoma of ciliary pigment epithelium: a case series. *Br J Ophthalmol* 87:504, 2003

Eagle RC: Iris pigmentation and pigmented lesions: an ultrastructural study. *Trans Am Ophthalmol Soc* 86:581, 1988

Edelstein C, Shields CL, Shields JA et al.: Presumed adenocarcinoma of the retinal pigment epithelium in a blind eye with a staphyloma. *Arch Ophthalmol* 116:525, 1998

Fan JT, Robertson DM, Campbell RJ: Clinicopathologic correlation of a case of adenocarcinoma of the retinal pigment epithelium. *Am J Ophthalmol* 119:243, 1995

Figus M, Ferretti C, Benelli U et al.: Free-floating cyst in the anterior chamber: ultrasound biomicroscopic reports. *Eur J Ophthalmol* 13:653, 2003

Fine BS: Free floating pigmented cyst in the anterior chamber: A clinicopathologic report. *Am J Ophthalmol* 67:493, 1969

Fine BS: Lipoidal degeneration of the retinal pigment epithelium. *Am J Ophthalmol* 91:469, 1981

Fine BS, Yanoff M: *Ocular Histology: A Text and Atlas*, 2nd edn. Hagerstown, PA, Harper & Row, 1979:214, 240

Fonesca RA, Dantes MA, Kaga T et al.: Combined hamartoma of the retina and retinal pigment epithelium associated with juvenile nasopharyngeal angeofibroma. *Am J Ophthalmol* 132:131, 2001

Fonseca RA, Dantas MA, Kaga T et al.: Combined hamartoma of the retina and retinal pigment epithelium associated with juvenile nasopharyngeal angiofibroma. *Am J Ophthalmol* 132:131, 2001

Font RL, Moura RA, Shetlar DJ et al.: Combined hamartoma of sensory retina and retinal pigment epithelium. *Retina* 9:302, 1989

Foster RE, Murray TG, Byrne SF et al.: Echographic features of medulloepithelioma. *Am J Ophthalmol* 130:364, 2000

Gass JDM: Focal congenital anomalies of the retinal pigment epithelium. *Eye* 3:1, 1989

Greenberg PB, Haik BG, Martin PC: A pigmented adenoma of the ciliary epithelium examined by magnetic resonance imaging. *Am J Ophthalmol* 120:679, 1995

Grossniklaus HE, Zimmerman LE, Kachmer ML: Pleomorphic adenocarcinoma of the ciliary body. *Ophthalmology* 97:763, 1990

Harbour JW, Augsburger JJ, Eagle RC Jr: Initial management and follow-up of melanocytic iris tumors. *Ophthalmology* 102:1987, 1995

Heegaard S, Larsen JN, Fledelius HC et al.: Neoplasia versus hyperplasia of the retinal pigment epithelium. A comparison of two cases. *Acta Ophthalmol Scand* 79:626, 2001

Helbig H, Niederberger H: Presumed combined hamartoma of the retina and retinal pigment epithelium with preretinal neovascularization. *Am J Ophthalmol* 136:1157, 2003

Holbach L, Völcker HE, Naumann GOH: Malignes teratoides Medulloepitheliom des Ziliarkörpers und saures Gliafaserprotein: Klinische, histochemische und immunhistochemische Befunde. *Klin Monatsbl Augenheilkd* 187:282, 1985

Hunt LM, Robertson MHE, Hugkulstone CE et al.: Congenital hypertrophy of the retinal pigment epithelium and mandibular osteomata as markers in familial colorectal cancer. *Br J Cancer* 70:173, 1994

Husain SE, Husain N, Boniuk M et al.: Malignant nonteratoid medulloepithelioma of the ciliary body in an adult. *Ophthalmology* 105:596, 1998

Inoue M, Noda K, Ishida S et al.: Successful treatment of subfoveal choroidal neovascularization associated with combined hamartoma of the retina and retinal pigment epithelium. *Am J Ophthalmol* 138:155, 2004

Johnson MW, Skuta GL, Kincaid MC et al.: Malignant melanoma of the iris in xeroderma pigmentosum. *Arch Ophthalmol* 107:402, 1989

Kasner L, Traboulsi EI, Delacruz Z et al.: A histopathologic study of the pigmented fundus lesions in familial adenomatous polyposis. *Retina* 12:35, 1992

Kawana K, Okamoto F, Nose H et al.: Ultrasound biomicroscopic findings of ciliary body malignant melanoma. *Jpn J Ophthalmol* 48:412, 2004

Kinzler KW, Nilbert MC, Su L et al.: Identification of FAP locus genes from chromosome 5q21. *Science* 253:661, 1991

Kivela T, Kauniskangas L, Miettinen P et al.: Glioneuroma associated with colobomatous dysplasia of the anterior uvea and retina. *Ophthalmology* 96:1799, 1989

Laver NM, Hidayat AA, Croxatto JO: Pleomorphic adenomas of the ciliary epithelium: Immunohistochemical and ultrastructural features of 12 cases. *Ophthalmology* 106:103, 1999

Lewis H, Straatsma BR, Foos RY: Chorioretinal juncture: Multiple extramacular drusen. *Ophthalmology* 93:1098, 1986

Li Z-Y, Tso MOM, Sugar J: Leiomyoepithelioma of iris pigment epithelium. *Arch Ophthalmol* 105:819, 1987

Lloyd WC, Eagle RC, Shields JA et al.: Congenital hypertrophy of the retinal pigment epithelium. *Ophthalmology* 97:1052, 1990

Lois N, Shields CL, Shields JA et al.: Primary cysts of the iris pigment epithelium. *Ophthalmology* 105:1879, 1998

Loose IA, Jampol LM, O'Grady R: Pigmented adenoma mimicking a juxtapapillary melanoma: A 20-year follow-up. *Arch Ophthalmol* 117:120, 1999

Lumbroso L, Desjardins L, Coue O et al.: Presumed bilateral medulloepithelioma. *Arch Ophthalmol* 119:449, 2001

Lyons LA, Lewis RA, Strong LC et al.: A genetic study of Gardner syndrome and congenital hypertrophy of the retinal pigment epithelium. *Am J Hum Genet* 42:290, 1988

Meyer CH, Rodrigues EB, Mennel S et al.: Grouped congenital hypertrophy of the retinal pigment epithelium follows developmental patterns of pigmentary mosaicism. *Ophthalmology* 112:841, 2005

Mohamed MD, Gupta M, Parsons A et al.: Ultrasound biomicroscopy in the management of melanocytoma of the ciliary body with extrascleral extension. *Br J Ophthalmol* 89:14, 2005

Munden PM, Sobol WM, Weingeist TA: Ocular findings in Turcot syndrome (glioma-polyposis). *Ophthalmology* 98:111, 1991

Nicolo M, Nicolo G, Zingirian M: Pleomorphic adenocarcinoma of the ciliary epithelium: a clinicopathological, immunohistochemical, ultrastructural, DNA-ploidy and comparative genomic hybridization analysis of an unusual case. *Eur J Ophthalmol* 12:319, 2002

Nishisho I, Nakamura Y, Miyoshi Y et al.: Mutations of chromosome 5q21 genes in FAP and colorectal cancer patients. *Science* 253:665, 1991

Nussbaum JJ, Pruett RC, Delori FC: Historic perspectives. Macular yellow pigment: The first 200 years. *Retina* 1:296, 1981

Ohguro H, Maruyama I, Nakazawa M: A case of pseudoadenomatous hyperplasia of ciliary body epithelium successfully treated by local resection. *Tohoku J Exp Med* 197:41, 2002

O'Keefe M, Fulcher T, Kelly P et al.: Medulloepithelioma of the optic nerve head. *Arch Ophthalmol* 115:1325, 1997

Olsen TW, Frayer WC, Myers FL et al.: Idiopathic reactive hyperplasia of the retinal pigment epithelium. *Arch Ophthalmol* 117:50, 1999

Pang CP, Fan DS, Keung JW et al.: Congenital hypertrophy of the retinal pigment epithelium and APC mutations in Chinese with familial adenomatous polyposis. *Ophthalmologica* 215:408, 2001

Robertson DM, McLaren JW, Salomao DR et al.: Retinopathy from a green laser pointer: a clinicopathologic study. *Arch Ophthalmol* 123:629, 2005

Roseman RL, Gass JD: Solitary hypopigmented nevus of the retinal pigment epithelium in the macula. *Arch Ophthalmol* 110:1358, 1992

Sallo FB, Hatvani I: Recurring transitory blindness caused by primary marginal pigment epithelial iris cysts. *Am J Ophthalmol* 133:407, 2002

Santos A, Morales L, Hernandez-Quintela E *et al.*: Congenital hypertrophy of the retinal pigment epithelium associated with familial adenomatous polyposis. *Retina* 14:6, 1994

Shields CL, Mashayekhi A, Ho T *et al.*: Solitary congenital hamartoma of the retinal pigment epithelium: clinical features and frequency of enlargement in 330 patients. *Ophthalmology* 110:1968, 2003

Shields CL, Shields JA, Marr BP *et al.*: Congenital simple hamartoma of the retinal pigment epithelium: a study of five cases. *Ophthalmology* 110:1005, 2003

Shields JA, Eagle RC Jr, Barr CC *et al.*: Adenocarcinoma of retinal pigment epithelium arising from a juxtapapillary histoplasmosis scar. *Arch Ophthalmol* 112:650, 1994

Shields JA, Eagle RC Jr, Shields CL *et al.*: Acquired neoplasms of the nonpigmented ciliary epithelium (adenoma and adenocarcinoma). *Ophthalmology* 103:2007, 1996

Shields JA, Eagle RC Jr, Shields CL *et al.*: Congenital neoplasms of the nonpigmented ciliary epithelium (medulloepithelioma). *Ophthalmology* 103:1998, 1996

Shields JA, Eagle RC Jr, Shields CL: Adenoma of nonpigmented ciliary epithelium with smooth muscle differentiation. *Arch Ophthalmol* 117:50, 1999

Shields JA, Eagle RC Jr, Shields CL *et al.*: Clinicopathologic reports, case reports, and small case series: progressive growth of benign adenoma of the pigment epithelium of the ciliary body. *Arch Ophthalmol* 119:1859, 2001

Shields JA, Eagle RC Jr, Shields CL *et al.*: Pigmented medulloepithelioma of the ciliary body. *Arch Ophthalmol* 120:207, 2002

Shields JA, Materin M, Shields CL: Adenoma of the retinal pigment epithelium simulating a juxtapapillary choroidal neovascular membrane. *Arch Ophthalmol* 119:289, 2001

Shields JA, Shields CL, Eagle RC Jr *et al.*: Adenocarcinoma arising from congenital hypertrophy of retinal pigment epithelium. *Arch Ophthalmol* 119:597, 2001

Shields JA, Shields CL, Gündüz K *et al.*: Adenoma of the ciliary body pigment epithelium: The 1998 Albert Ruedermann, Sr, Memorial Lecture, Part 1. *Arch Ophthalmol* 117:392, 1999

Shields JA, Shields CL, Gündüz K *et al.*: Neoplasms of the retinal pigment epithelium: The 1998 Albert Ruedermann, Sr, Memorial Lecture, Part 2. *Arch Ophthalmol* 117:392, 1999

Shields JA, Shields CL, Kiratli H *et al.*: Adenoma of the iris pigment epithelium: A report of 20 cases. The 1998 Pan-American lecture. *Arch Ophthalmol* 117:736, 1999

Shields JA, Shields CL, Singh AD: Acquired tumors arising from congenital hypertrophy of the retinal pigment epithelium. *Arch Ophthalmol* 118:637, 2000

Shields JA, Shields CL, Slakter J *et al.*: Locally invasive tumors arising from hyperplasia of the retinal pigment epithelium. *Retina* 21:487, 2001

Shukla D, Ambatkar S, Jethani J *et al.*: Optical coherence tomography in presumed congenital simple hamartoma of retinal pigment epithelium. *Am J Ophthalmol* 139:945, 2005

Simpson ER: Ciliary body melanoma: a special challenge. *Can J Ophthalmol* 39:365, 2004

Steinkuller PG, Font RL: Congenital malignant teratoid neoplasm of the eye and orbit: A case report and review of the literature. *Ophthalmology* 104:38, 1997

Suzuki J, Goto H, Usui M: Adenoma arising from nonpigmented ciliary epithelium concomitant with neovascularization of the optic disk and cystoid macular edema. *Am J Ophthalmol* 139:188, 2005

Terasaki H, Nagasaka T, Arai M *et al.*: Adenocarcinoma of the nonpigmented ciliary epithelium: report of two cases with immunohistochemical findings. *Graefes Arch Clin Exp Ophthalmol* 239:876, 2001

Theodossiadis PG, Panagiotidis DN, Baltatzis SG *et al.*: Combined hamartoma of the sensory retina and retinal pigment epithelium involving the optic disk associated with choroidal neovascularization. *Retina* 21:267, 2001

Torres VL, Allemann N, Erwenne CM: Ultrasound biomicroscopy features of iris and ciliary body melanomas before and after brachytherapy. *Ophthalmic Surg Lasers Imaging* 36:129, 2005

Tourino R, Conde-Freire R, Cabezas-Agricola JM *et al.*: Value of the congenital hypertrophy of the retinal pigment epithelium in the diagnosis of familial adenomatous polyposis. *Int Ophthalmol* 25:101, 2004

Traboulsi EI: Ocular manifestations of familial adenomatous polyposis (Gardner syndrome). *Ophthalmol Clin North Am* 18:163, 2005

Traboulsi EI, Maumenee IH, Krush AJ *et al.*: Congenital hypertrophy of the retinal pigment epithelium predicts colorectal polyposis in Gardner's syndrome. *Arch Ophthalmol* 108:525, 1990

Traboulsi EI, Murphy SF, de la Cruz, ZC *et al.*: A clinicopathologic study of the eyes in familial adenomatous polyposis with extracolonic manifestations (Gardner's syndrome). *Am J Ophthalmol* 110:550, 1990

Ulshafer RJ, Allen CB, Nicolaissen B Jr *et al.*: Scanning electron microscopy of human drusen. *Invest Ophthalmol Vis Sci* 28:683, 1987

Vianna RN, Pacheco DF, Vasconcelos MM *et al.*: Combined hamartoma of the retina and retinal pigment epithelium associated with neurofibromatosis type-1. *Int Ophthalmol* 24:63, 2001

Vogel MH, Zimmerman LE, Gass JDM: Proliferation of the juxtapapillary retinal pigment epithelium simulating malignant melanoma. *Doc Ophthalmol* 26:461, 1969

Wu S, Slakter JS, Shields JA *et al.*: Cancer-associated nummular loss of the pigment epithelium. *Am J Ophthalmol* 139:933, 2005

Yanoff M, Zimmerman LE: Pseudomelanoma of anterior chamber caused by implantation of iris pigment epithelium. *Arch Ophthalmol* 74:302, 1965

Zajac V, Kovac M, Kirchhoff T *et al.*: The most frequent APC mutations among Slovak familial adenomatous polyposis patients. Adenomatous polyposis coli. *Neoplasma* 49:356, 2002

Zhang J, Demirci H, Shields CL *et al.*: Cavitary melanoma of ciliary body simulating a cyst. *Arch Ophthalmol* 123:569, 2005

Zhang P, Feng G, Yue T *et al.*: Pathological, ultrastructural and immunohistochemical observations of adenoma of retinal pigment epithelium. *Yan Ke Xue Bao* 17:168, 2001

Zimmerman LE: Melanocytes, melanocytic nevi and melanocytomas. *Invest Ophthalmol* 4:11, 1965

Zimmerman LE: Verhoeff's "terato-neuroma": A critical reappraisal in light of new observations and current concepts of embryonic tumors. *Am J Ophthalmol* 72:1039, 1971

Melanotic Tumors of the Uvea: Iris

Bard LA: Heterogeneity in Waardenburg's syndrome: Report of a family with ocular albinism. *Arch Ophthalmol* 96:1193, 1978

Brown D, Boniuk M, Font RL: Diffuse malignant melanoma of iris with metastases. *Surv Ophthalmol* 34:357, 1990

Callanan DG, Lewis ML, Byrne SF *et al.*: Choroidal neovascularization associated with choroidal nevi. *Arch Ophthalmol* 111:789, 1993

Canning CR, Hungerford J: Familial uveal melanoma. *Br J Ophthalmol* 72:241, 1988

Capeáns C, Santos L, Sánchez-Salorio M *et al.*: Iris metastasis from endometrial carcinoma. *Am J Ophthalmol* 125:729, 1998

Carlson DW, Alward WLM, Folberg R: Aggressive nevus of the iris with secondary glaucoma in a child. *Am J Ophthalmol* 119:367, 1995

Char DH, Crawford JB: Iris melanomas: Diagnostic problems. *Ophthalmology* 103:251, 1996

Char DH, Crawford JB, Gonzales J *et al.*: Iris melanoma with increased intraocular pressure. *Arch Ophthalmol* 107:548, 1989

Chaudrey IM, Moster MR, Augsburger JJ: Iris ring melanoma masquerading as pigmentary glaucoma. *Arch Ophthalmol* 115:1480, 1997

Demirci H, Shields CL, Shields JA *et al.*: Diffuse iris melanoma: a report of 25 cases. *Ophthalmology* 109:1553, 2002

Duke-Elder S: Heterochromia. In *System of Ophthalmology*, vol. III, part 2. St. Louis, CV Mosby, 1964:813–818

Ferry AP: Lesions mistaken for malignant melanomas of the iris. *Arch Ophthalmol* 74:9, 1965

Fine BS, Yanoff M: *Ocular Histology: A Text and Atlas*, 2nd edn. Hagerstown, PA, Harper & Row, 1979:197

Greven CM, Stanton C, Yeatts RP *et al.*: Diffuse iris melanoma in a young patient. *Arch Ophthalmol* 115:682, 1997

Grossniklaus HE, Brown RH, Stulting RD *et al.*: Iris melanoma seeding through a trabeculectomy site. *Arch Ophthalmol* 108:1287, 1990

Harbour JW, Augsburger JJ, Eagle RC Jr: Initial management and follow-up of melanocytic iris tumors. *Ophthalmology* 102:1987, 1995

Honavar SG, Singh AD, Shields CL *et al.*: Iris melanoma in a patient with neurofibromatosis. *Surv Ophthalmol* 45:231, 2000

Jakobiec FA, Silbert G: Are most iris "melanomas" really nevi? A clinicopathologic study of 189 lesions. *Arch Ophthalmol* 99:2117, 1981

Jakobiec FA, Yanoff M, Mottow L *et al.*: Solitary iris nevus associated with peripheral anterior synechiae and iris endothelialization. *Am J Ophthalmol* 83:884, 1977

Katz NR, Finger PT, McCormick EA *et al.*: Ultrasound biomicroscopy in the management of malignant melanoma of the iris. *Arch Ophthalmol* 113:1462, 1995

Naumann GOH, Font RL, Zimmerman LE: Primary rhabdomyosarcoma of the iris. *Am J Ophthalmol* 74:110, 1972

Paridaens D, Lyons CJ, McCartney A *et al.*: Familial aggressive nevi of the iris in childhood. *Arch Ophthalmol* 109:1551, 1991

Rehany U, Rumeldt S: Iridocorneal melanoma associated with type 1 neurofibromatosis: A clinicopathologic study. *Ophthalmology* 106:614, 1999

Rootman J, Gallagher RP: Color as a risk factor in iris melanoma. *Am J Ophthalmol* 98:558, 1984

Scheie HG, Yanoff M: Iris nevus (Cogan–Reese) syndrome. *Arch Ophthalmol* 93:963, 1975

Shields CL, Eagle RC Jr, Shields JA *et al.*: Progressive growth of an iris melanocytoma in a child. *Am J Ophthalmol* 133:287, 2002

Shields CL, Shields JA, Materin M *et al.*: Iris melanoma: risk for metastasis in 169 consecutive patients. *Ophthalmology* 108:172, 2001

Shields JA, Shields CL, Mercado G *et al.*: Metastatic tumors to the iris in 40 patients. *Am J Ophthalmol* 119:422, 1995

Shields JA, Shields CL, Pulido J *et al.*: Iris varix simulating an iris melanoma. *Arch Ophthalmol* 118:707, 2000

Ticho BH, Rosner M, Mets MB *et al.*: Bilateral diffuse iris nodular nevi: Clinical and histopathologic characterization. *Arch Ophthalmol* 102:419, 1995

Yan J, Wu Z, Li Y *et al.*: Angioleiomyoma of the ciliary body: a case report. *Yan Ke Xue Bao* 20:19, 2004

Yanoff M, Zimmerman LE: Pseudomelanoma of anterior chamber caused by implantation of iris pigment epithelium. *Arch Ophthalmol* 74:302, 1965

Melanotic Tumors of the Uvea: Ciliary Body and Choroid

Aalto Y, Eriksson L, Seregard S *et al.*: Concomitant loss of chromosome 3 and whole arm losses and gains of chromosome 1, 6, or 8 in metastasizing primary uveal melanoma. *Invest Ophthalmol Vis Sci* 42:313, 2001

Albert DM: The ocular melanoma story: LII Edward Jackson Memorial Lecture: Part II. *Am J Ophthalmol* 123:729, 1997

Alyahya GA, Heegaard S, Prause JU: Characterization of melanoma associated spongiform scleropathy. *Acta Ophthalmol Scand* 80:322, 2002

Alyahya GA, Ribel-Madsen SM, Heegaard S *et al.*: Melanoma-associated spongiform scleropathy: biochemical changes and possible relation to tumour extension. *Acta Ophthalmol Scand* 81:625, 2003

Ardjomand N, Komericki P, Langmann G *et al.*: Lymph node metastases arising from uveal melanoma. *Wien Klin Wochenschr* 117:433, 2005

Augsburger JJ: Is observation really appropriate for small choroidal melanomas? *Trans Am Ophthalmol Soc* 91:147, 1993

Augsburger JJ, Schroeder RP, Territo C *et al.*: Clinical parameters predictive of enlargement of melanocytic choroidal lesions. *Br J Ophthalmol* 73:911, 1989

Bataille V, Pinney E, Hungerford JL *et al.*: Five cases of coexistent primary ocular and cutaneous melanoma. *Arch Dermatol* 129:198, 1993

Biswas J, D'Souza C, Shanmugam MP: Diffuse melanotic lesion of the iris as a presenting feature of ciliary body melanocytoma: Report of a case and review of the literature. *Surv Ophthalmol* 123:729, 1998

Blumenthal EZ, Pe'er J: Multifocal choroidal malignant melanoma: At least 3 melanomas in one eye. *Arch Ophthalmol* 117:255, 1999

Butler P, Char DH, Zarbin M *et al.*: Natural history of indeterminate pigmented choroidal tumors. *Ophthalmology* 101:710, 1994

Callender GR: Malignant melanotic tumors of the eye: A study of histologic types in 111 cases. *Trans Am Acad Ophthalmol Otolaryngol* 36:131, 1931

Chaudrey IM, Moster MR, Augsburger JJ: Iris ring melanoma masquerading as pigmentary glaucoma. *Arch Ophthalmol* 115:1480, 1997

Chowers I, Folberg R, Livni N *et al.*: p53 Immunoreactivity, Ki-67 expression, and microcirculation patterns in melanoma of the iris, ciliary body, and choroid. *Curr Eye Res* 24:105, 2002

Coleman K, Baak JPA, van Diest PJ *et al.*: DNA ploidy status in 84 ocular melanomas: A study of DNA quantitation in ocular melanomas by flow cytometry and automated and interactive static image analysis. *Hum Pathol* 26:99, 1995

Coleman K, Baak JPA, van Diest PJ *et al.*: Prognostic value of morphometric features and the Callender classification in uveal melanomas. *Ophthalmology* 103:1634, 1996

Collaborative Ocular Melanoma Study Group: Ten-year follow-up of fellow eyes of patients enrolled in Collaborative Ocular Melanoma Study Radomized Trials: COMS Repoirt No. 22. *Ophthalmology* 111:966, 2004

Connolly BP, Regillo CD, Eagle RC Jr *et al.*: The histopathologic effects of transpupillary thermotherapy in human eyes. *Ophthalmology* 110:415, 2003

Coupland SE, Sidiki S, Clark BJ *et al.*: Metastatic choroidal melanoma to the contralateral orbit 40 years after enucleation. *Arch Ophthalmol* 114:751, 1996

Cross NA, Ganesh A, Parpia M *et al.*: Multiple locations on chromosome 3 are the targets of specific deletions in uveal melanoma. *Eye* 20:476, 2006

Damato B: Treatment of primary intraocular melanoma. *Exp Rev Anticancer Ther* 6:493, 2006

de German-Ribon RI, Singh AD, Arevalo JF *et al.*: Choroidal melanoma with oculodermal melanocytosis in Hispanic patients. *Am J Ophthalmol* 128:251, 1999

Demirici H, Shields CS, Shields JA *et al.*: Ring melanoma of the anterior chamber angle: a report of fourteen cases. *Am J Ophthalmol* 132:336, 2001

Demirci H, Shields CL, Shields JA *et al.*: Ring melanoma of the ciliary body: report on twenty-three patients. *Retina* 22:698, 2002

Diener-West M, Hawkins BS, Markowitz JA et al.: A review of mortality from choroidal melanoma. *Arch Ophthalmol* 110:245, 1992

Dithmar S, Völcker HE, Grossniklaus HE: Multifocal intraocular malignant melanoma: Report of two cases and review of the literature. *Ophthalmology* 106:1345, 1999

Due EJ, Schachat AP, Albert DM et al.: Long-term survival in a patient with uveal melanoma and liver metastasis. *Arch Ophthalmol* 122:285, 2004

Duke-Elder S: Heterochromia. In *System of Ophthalmology*, vol. III, part 2. St. Louis, CV Mosby, 1964:813–818

Eagle RC Jr, Shields JA: Pseudoretinitis pigmentosa secondary to pre-retinal malignant melanoma cells. *Retina* 2:51, 1982

Egger E, Schalenbourg A, Zografos L et al.: Maximizing local tumor control and survival after proton beam radiotherapy of uveal melanoma. *Int J Radiat Oncol Biol Phys* 51:138, 2001

Ericsson C, Seregard S, Bartolazzi A et al.: Association of HLA class I and class II antigen expression and mortality in uveal melanoma. *Invest Ophthalmol Vis Sci* 42:2153, 2001

Espinoza G, Rosenblatt B, Harbour JW: Optical coherence tomography in the evaluation of retinal changes associated with suspicious choroidal melanocytic tumors. *Am J Ophthalmol* 137:90, 2004

Ferry AP: Lesions mistaken for malignant melanoma of posterior uvea. *Arch Ophthalmol* 72:463, 1964

Fine BS, Yanoff M: *Ocular Histology: A Text and Atlas*, 2nd edn. Hagerstown, PA, Harper & Row, 1979:215

Flocks M, Gerende JH, Zimmerman LE: The size and shape of malignant melanomas of the choroid and ciliary body in relation to prognosis and histologic characteristics. *Trans Am Acad Ophthalmol Otolaryngol* 59:740, 1955

Folberg R, Yanoff M: Ocular melanotic tumors. In Tasman W, Jaeger EA, eds: *Duane's Foundations of Clinical Ophthalmology*, vol. 3, Chapter 20. Philadelphia, JB Lippincott, 1992:1–33

Folberg R, Chen X, Boldt HC et al.: Microcirculation patterns other than loops and networks in choroidal and ciliary body melanomas. *Ophthalmology* 108:996, 2001

Folberg R, Pe'er J, Gruman LM et al.: The morphologic characteristics of tumor blood vessels as a marker of tumor progression in primary human uveal melanoma: A matched case-control study. *Hum Pathol* 23:1298, 1992

Folberg R, Rummelt V, Parys-Van Ginderdeuren R et al.: The prognostic value of tumor blood vessel morphology in primary uveal melanoma. *Ophthalmology* 100:1389, 1993

Font RL, Zimmerman LE, Armaly MF: The nature of the orange pigment over a choroidal melanoma: Histochemical and electron microscopic observations. *Arch Ophthalmol* 91:359, 1974

Gamel JW, McCurdy JB, McLean IW: A comparison of prognostic covariates for uveal melanoma. *Invest Ophthalmol Vis Sci* 33:1919, 1992

Gass JD: Observation of suspected choroidal and ciliary body melanomas for evidence of growth prior to enucleation. *Retina* 23:523, 2003

Gass JDM, Gieser RG, Wilkinson CP et al.: Bilateral diffuse uveal melanocytic proliferation in patients with occult carcinoma. *Arch Ophthalmol* 108:527, 1990

Gragoudas ES, Lane AM, Munzenrider J et al.: Long-term risk of local failure after proton therapy for choroidal/ciliary body melanoma. *Trans Am Ophthalmol Soc* 100:43, 2002

Grossniklaus HE, Albert DM, Green WR et al.: Clear cell differentiation in choroidal melanoma: COMS report no. 8. *Arch Ophthalmol* 115:894, 1997

Gündüz K, Shields JA, Shields CL et al.: Choroidal melanoma in a 14-year-old patient with ocular melanocytosis. *Arch Ophthalmol* 116:1112, 1998

Guyer DR, Mukai S, Egan KM et al.: Radiation maculopathy after proton beam irradiation for choroidal melanoma. *Ophthalmology* 99:1278, 1992

Hahne M, Rimoldi D, Schröter M et al.: Melanoma cell expression of Fas (Apo-1/CD95) ligand: Implications for tumor immune escape. *Science* 274:1363, 1996

Hammer ME, Margo CE: Unilateral multifocal melanoma with occult ring melanoma. *Arch Ophthalmol* 120:1090, 2002

Harbour JW, Brantley MA Jr, Hollingsworth H et al.: Association between choroidal pigmentation and posterior uveal melanoma in a white population. *Br J Ophthalmol* 88:39, 2004

Hiscott P, Campbell RJ, Robertson DM et al.: Intraocular melanocytoma in association with bone formation. *Arch Ophthalmol* 121:1791, 2003

Hoglund M, Gisselsson D, Hansen GB et al.: Dissecting karyotypic patterns in malignant melanomas: temporal clustering of losses and gains in melanoma karyotypic evolution. *Int J Cancer* 108:57, 2004

Holly EA, Aston DA, Ahn DK et al.: Intraocular melanoma linked to occupations and chemical exposure. *Epidemiology* 7:55, 1996

Honavar SG, Singh AD, Shields CL et al.: Iris melanoma in a patient with neurofibromatosis. *Surv Ophthalmol* 45:231, 2000

Horsman DE, White VA: Cytogenetic analysis of uveal melanoma: Consistent occurrence of monosomy 3 and trisomy 8q. *Cancer* 71:811, 1993

Hovland PG, Trempe C: Genomic investigations of posterior uveal melanoma. *Semin Ophthalmol* 20:231, 2005

Hurks HM, Metzelaar-Blok JAW, Barthen ER et al.: Expression of epidermal growth factor receptor: Risk factor in uveal melanoma. *Invest Ophthalmol Vis Sci* 41:2023, 2000

Isager P, Ehlers N, Overgaard J: Have choroidal and ciliary body melanomas changed during the period 1955–2000? *Acta Ophthalmol Scand* 82:509, 2004

Isager P, Ehlers N, Overgaard J: Prognostic factors for survival after enucleation for choroidal and ciliary body melanomas. *Acta Ophthalmol Scand* 82:517, 2004

Jager MJ, Hurks HM, Levitskaya J et al.: HLA expression in uveal melanoma: there is no rule without some exception. *Hum Immunol* 63:444, 2002

Jensen OA: Malignant melanomas of the human uvea: 25-year follow-up of cases in Denmark, 1943–1952. *Acta Ophthalmol* 60:161, 1982

Jürgens I, Roca G, Sedo S et al.: Presumed melanocytoma of the macula. *Arch Ophthalmol* 112:305, 1994

Kan-Mitchell J, Rao N, Albert DM et al.: S100 immunophenotypes of uveal melanomas. *Invest Ophthalmol Vis Sci* 31:1492, 1990

Karlsson M, Boeryd B, Carstensen J et al.: DNA ploidy and S-phase fraction as prognostic factors patients with ocular melanomas. *Br J Cancer* 71:177, 1995

Kath R, Hayungs J, Bornfeld N et al.: Prognosis and treatment of disseminated uveal melanoma. *Cancer* 72:2219, 1993

Kheterpal S, Shields JA, Shields CL et al.: Choroidal melanoma in an African-American albino. *Am J Ophthalmol* 122:901, 1996

Kilic E, Naus NC, van GW et al.: Concurrent loss of chromosome arm 1p and chromosome 3 predicts a decreased disease-free survival in uveal melanoma patients. *Invest Ophthalmol Vis Sci* 46:2253, 2005

Kilic E, van GW, Lodder E et al.: Clinical and cytogenetic analyses in uveal melanoma. *Invest Ophthalmol Vis Sci* 47:3703, 2006

Kiratli H, Bilgic S: Subretinal pigment dispersion following transpupillary thermotherapy for choroidal melanoma. *Acta Ophthalmol Scand* 80:401, 2002

Kujala E, Kivelä T: Tumor, node, metastasis classification of malignant ciliary body and choroidal melanoma. *Ophthalmology* 112:1135, 2005

LaRusso FL, Bomiuk M, Font RL: Melanocytoma (magnocellular nevus) of the ciliary body: Report of 10 cases and review of the literature. *Ophthalmology* 107:795, 2000

Leys AM, Dierick HG, Sciot RM: Early lesion of bilateral diffuse melanocytic proliferation. *Arch Ophthalmol* 109:1590, 1991

Lin AY, Maniotis AJ, Valyi-Nagy K et al.: Distinguishing fibrovascular septa from vasculogenic mimicry patterns. *Arch Pathol Lab Med* 129:884, 2005

Loeffler KU, Tecklenborg H: Melanocytoma-like growth of a juxtapapillary malignant melanoma. *Retina* 12:29, 1992

Lois N, Shields CL, Shields JA et al.: Trifocal uveal melanoma. *Am J Ophthalmol* 124:848, 1997

Lois N, Shields CL, Shields JA et al.: Cavitary melanoma of the ciliary body: A study of eight cases. *Ophthalmology* 105:1091, 1998

Magauran RG, Gray B, Small KW: Chromosome 9 abnormality in choroidal melanoma. *Am J Ophthalmol* 117:109, 1994

Mäkitie T, Summanen P, Tarkkanen A et al.: Tumor-infiltrating macrophages (CD68⁺ cells) and prognosis in malignant uveal melanoma. *Invest Ophthalmol Vis Sci* 42:1414, 2001

Mäkitte T, Carpén O, Vaheri A et al.: Ezrin as a prognostic indicator and its relationship to tumor characteristics in uveal malignant melanoma. *Invest Ophthalmol Vis Sci* 42:2442, 2001

Manschot WA, Lee WR, van Strik R: Uveal melanoma: Updated considerations on current management modalities. *Int Ophthalmol* 19:203, 1996

Marcus DM, Minkovitz JB, Wardwell SD et al.: The value of nucleolar organizer regions in uveal melanoma. *Am J Ophthalmol* 110:527, 1990

Margo CE, McLean IW: Malignant melanoma of the choroid and ciliary body in black patients. *Arch Ophthalmol* 102:77, 1984

Margo C, Pautler SE: Granulomatous uveitis after treatment of a choroidal melanoma with proton-beam irradiation. *Retina* 10:140, 1990

Margo CE, Pusateri TJ, Ulshafer RJ et al.: Lipid crystals in malignant melanoma of the choroid. *Retina* 10:68, 1990

McClean IW, Keefe KS, Burnier MN: Uveal melanoma: Comparison of the prognostic value of fibrovascular loops, mean of the ten largest nucleoli, cell type, and tumor size. *Ophthalmology* 104:777, 1997

McLean IW, Ainbinder DJ, Gamel JW et al.: Choroidal-ciliary body melanoma: A multivariate survival analysis of tumor location. *Ophthalmology* 102:1060, 1995

McLean IW, Foster WD, Zimmerman LE et al.: Inferred natural history of uveal melanoma. *Invest Ophthalmol* 19:760, 1980

McLean IW, Foster WD, Zimmerman LE: Uveal melanoma: location, size, cell type, and enucleation as risk factors in metastasis. *Hum Pathol* 13:123, 1982

McLean IW, Foster WD, Zimmerman LE et al.: Modifications of Callender's classification of uveal melanoma at the Armed Forces Institute of Pathology. *Am J Ophthalmol* 96:502, 1983

McNamara M, Felix C, Davison EV et al.: Assessment of chromosome 3 copy number in ocular melanoma using fluorescence in situ hybridization. *Cancer Genet Cytogenet* 98:4, 1997

Mehaffey MG, Folberg R, Meyer M et al.: Relative importance of quantifying area and vascular patterns in melanomas. *Am J Ophthalmol* 123:798, 1997

Mehaffey MG, Gardner LM, Folberg R: Distribution of prognostically important vascular patterns in ciliary body and choroidal melanomas. *Am J Ophthalmol* 126:373, 1998

Michael JC, de Venecia G: Retinal trypsin digest study of cystoid macular edema associated with choroidal melanoma. *Am J Ophthalmol* 119:152, 1995

Midena E, Bonaldi L, Parrozzani R et al.: In vivo detection of monosomy 3 in eyes with medium-sized uveal melanoma using transscleral fine needle aspiration biopsy. *Eur J Ophthalmol* 16:422, 2006

Mooy CM, de Jong PTVM: Prognostic parameters in uveal melanoma: A review. *Surv Ophthalmol* 41:215, 1996

Moshari A, Cheeseman EW, McLean IW: Totally necrotic choroidal and ciliary body melanomas: associations with prognosis, episcleritis, and scleritis. *Am J Ophthalmol* 131:232, 2001

Murthy R, Honavar SG, Naik M et al.: Clinicopathologic findings in choroidal melanomas after failed transpupillary thermotherapy. *Am J Ophthalmol* 137:594, 2004

Nakhleh RE, Wick MR, Rocamora A et al.: Morphologic diversity in malignant melanomas. *Am J Clin Pathol* 93:731, 1990

Nareyeck G, Zeschnigk M, Prescher G et al.: Establishment and characterization of two uveal melanoma cell lines derived from tumors with loss of one chromosome 3. *Exp Eye Res* 83:858, 2006

Naseripour M, Shields CL, Shields JA et al.: Pseudohypopyon of orange pigment overlying a stable choroidal nevus. *Am J Ophthalmol* 132:416, 2001

Naumann GOH, Hellner K, Naumann LR: Pigmented nevi of the choroid: Clinical study of secondary changes in the overlying tissues. *Trans Am Acad Ophthalmol Otolaryngol* 75:110, 1971

Naumann G, Yanoff M, Zimmerman LE: Histogenesis of malignant melanomas of the uvea: I. Histopathologic characteristics of nevi of the choroid and ciliary body. *Arch Ophthalmol* 76:784, 1966

Naumann G, Zimmerman LE, Yanoff M: Visual field defect associated with choroidal nevus. *Am J Ophthalmol* 62:914, 1966

Nitta T, Oksenberg JR, Rao NA et al.: Predominant expression of T cell receptor V7 in tumor-infiltrating lymphocytes of uveal melanoma. *Science* 249:672, 1990

Onken MD, Worley LA, Ehlers JP et al.: Gene expression profiling in uveal melanoma reveals two molecular classes and predicts metastatic death. *Cancer Res* 64:7205, 2004

Pach JM, Robertson DM, Taney BS et al.: Prognostic factors in choroidal and ciliary body melanomas with extrascleral extension. *Am J Ophthalmol* 101:325, 1986

Pasternak S, Erwenne CM, Nicolela MT: Subconjunctival spread of ciliary body melanoma after glaucoma filtering surgery: a clinicopathological case report. *Can J Ophthalmol* 40:69, 2005

Paul EV, Parnell BL, Fraker M: Prognosis of malignant melanomas of the choroid and ciliary body. *Int Ophthalmol Clin* 2:387, 1962

Pe'er J, Rummelt V, Mawn L et al.: Mean of the ten largest nucleoli, microcirculation architecture, and prognosis of ciliochoroidal melanomas. *Ophthalmology* 101:1227, 1994

Pe'er J, Stefani FH, Seregard S et al.: Cell proliferation activity in posterior uveal melanoma after Ru-106 brachytherapy: an EORTC ocular oncology group study. *Br J Ophthalmol* 85:1208, 2001

Pitts RE, Awan KJ, Yanoff M: Choroidal melanoma with massive retinal fibrosis and spontaneous regression of retinal detachment. *Surv Ophthalmol* 20:273, 1976

Pizzuto D, deLuise V, Zimmerman N: Choroidal malignant melanoma appearing as acute panophthalmitis. *Am J Ophthalmol* 101:249, 1986

Prescher G, Bornfeld N, Hirche H et al.: Prognostic implications of monosomy 3 in uveal melanoma. *Lancet* 347:1222, 1996

Read RW, Green RL, Rao NA: Metastatic adenocarcinoma with rupture through the Bruch membrane simulating a choroidal melanoma. *Am J Ophthalmol* 132:943, 2001

Robertson DM, Campbell RJ, Salomào DR: Mushroom-shaped melanocytoma mimicking malignant melanoma. *Arch Ophthalmol* 120:82, 2002

Rohrbach JM, Roggendorf W, Thanos S et al.: Simultaneous bilateral diffuse melanocytic uveal hyperplasia. *Am J Ophthalmol* 110:49, 1990

Rosenbaum PS, Boniuk M, Font RL: Diffuse uveal melanoma in a 5-year-old child. *Am J Ophthalmol* 106:601, 1988

Rummelt V, Folberg R, Rummelt C et al.: Microcirculation architecture of melanocytic nevi and malignant melanomas of the ciliary body and choroid. *Ophthalmology* 101:718, 1994

Rummelt V, Folberg R, Woolson RF *et al.*: Relation between the microcirculation architecture and the aggressive behavior of ciliary body melanomas. *Ophthalmology* 102:844, 1995

Rummelt V, Naumann GOH, Folberg R *et al.*: Surgical management of melanocytoma of the ciliary body with extrascleral extension. *Am J Ophthalmol* 117:169, 1994

Sakamota T, Sakamota M, Yoshikawa H *et al.*: Histologic findings and prognosis of uveal malignant melanoma in Japanese patients. *Am J Ophthalmol* 121:276, 1996

Sandinha MT, Farquharson MA, McKay IC *et al.*: Monosomy 3 predicts death but not time until death in choroidal melanoma. *Invest Ophthalmol Vis Sci* 46:3497, 2005

Sandinha MT, Farquharson MA, Roberts F: Identification of monosomy 3 in choroidal melanoma by chromosome in situ hybridisation. *Br J Ophthalmol* 88:1527, 2004

Sassani JW, Blankenship G: Disciform choroidal melanoma. *Retina* 14:177, 1994

Scheie HG, Yanoff M: Pseudomelanoma of ciliary body, report of a patient. *Arch Ophthalmol* 77:81, 1967

Schwartz GP, Schwartz LW: Acute angle closure glaucoma secondary to a choroidal melanoma. *CLAO J* 28:77, 2002

Scull JJ, Alcocer CE, Deschênes J *et al.*: Primary choroidal melanoma in a patient with previous cutaneous melanoma. *Arch Ophthalmol* 115:796, 1997

Seddon JM, Gragoudas ES, Glynn RJ *et al.*: Host factors, UV radiation, and risk of uveal melanoma. *Arch Ophthalmol* 108:1274, 1990

Seregard S, Daunius C, Kock E *et al.*: Two cases of primary bilateral malignant melanoma of the choroid. *Br J Ophthalmol* 72:244, 1988

Shields CL, Cater J, Shields JA *et al.*: Combination of clinical factors predictive of growth of small choroidal melanocytic lesions. *Arch Ophthalmol* 118:360, 2000

Shields CL, Cater J, Shields JA *et al.*: Combined plaque radiotherapy and transpupillary thermotherapy for choroidal melanoma: tumor control and treatment complications in 270 consecutive patients. *Arch Ophthalmol* 120:933, 2002

Shields CL, Shields JA, dePotter P *et al.*: Diffuse choroidal melanoma: Clinical features predictive of metastasis. *Arch Ophthalmol* 114:956, 1996

Shields CL, Shields JA, Eagle RC *et al.*: Uveal melanoma and pregnancy. *Ophthalmology* 98:1667, 1991

Shields CL, Shields JA, Kiratli H *et al.*: Risk factors for growth and metastasis of small choroidal melanocytic lesions. *Ophthalmology* 102:1351, 1995

Shields CL, Shields JA, Milite J *et al.*: Uveal melanoma in teenagers and children. *Ophthalmology* 98:1662, 1991

Shields CL, Shields JA, Perez N *et al.*: Primary transpupillary thermotherapy for small choroidal melanoma in 256 consecutive cases: outcomes and limitations. *Ophthalmology* 109:225, 2002

Shields CL, Shields JA, Shields MB *et al.*: Prevalence and mechanisms of secondary intraocular pressure elevation in eyes with intraocular tumors. *Ophthalmology* 94:839, 1987

Shields JA, McDonald PR, Leonard BC *et al.*: The diagnosis of uveal malignant melanomas in eyes with opaque media. *Am J Ophthalmol* 83:95, 1977

Shields JA, Shields CL, Eagle RC *et al.*: Malignant melanoma arising from a large uveal melanocytoma in a patient with oculodermal melanocytosis. *Arch Ophthalmol* 118:990, 2000

Singh AD, Eagle RC Jr, Shields CL *et al.*: Clinicopathologic reports, case reports, and small case series: enucleation following transpupillary thermotherapy of choroidal melanoma: clinicopathologic correlations. *Arch Ophthalmol* 121:397, 2003

Singh AD, Shields CL, dePotter P *et al.*: Familial uveal melanomas: Clinical observations on 56 patients. *Arch Ophthalmol* 114:392, 1996

Singh AD, Shields CL, Shields JA *et al.*: Bilateral primary uveal melanoma: Bad luck or bad genes? *Ophthalmology* 103:256, 1996

Singh AD, Shields CL, Shields JA *et al.*: Uveal melanoma in young patients. *Arch Ophthalmol* 118:918, 2000

Singh AD, Topham A: Incidence of uveal melanomas in the United States: 1973–1997. *Ophthalmology* 110:956, 2003

Singh AD, Topham A: Survival rates with uveal melanomas in the United States: 1973–1997. *Ophthalmology* 110:962, 2003

Sneed SR, Byrne SF, Mieler WF *et al.*: Choroidal detachment associated with malignant choroidal tumors. *Ophthalmology* 98:963, 1991

Steuhl KP, Rohrbach JM, Knorr M *et al.*: Significance, specificity, and ultrastructural localization of HMB-45 antigen in pigmented ocular tumors. *Ophthalmology* 100:208, 1993

Sumich P, Mitchell P, Wang JJ: Choroidal nevi in a white population: The Blue Mountain Eye Study. *Arch Ophthalmol* 116:645, 1998

Tabassian A, Zuravleff JJ: Necrotic choroidal melanoma with orbital inflammation. *Arch Ophthalmol* 113:1576, 1995

Teichmann KD, Karcioglu ZA: Melanocytoma of the iris with rapidly developing secondary glaucoma. *Surv Ophthalmol* 40:136, 1995

ten Berge PJM, Danen EHJ, van Muijen GNP *et al.*: Integrin expression in uveal melanoma differs from cutaneous melanoma. *Invest Ophthalmol Vis Sci* 34:3635, 1993

The Collaborative Ocular Melanoma Study Group: Accuracy of diagnosis of choroidal melanomas in the collaborative ocular melanoma study. *Arch Ophthalmol* 108:1268, 1990

The Collaborative Ocular Melanoma Study Group: The COMS randomixed trial of iodine 125 brachytherapy for choroidal melanoma, III: Initial mortality findings. COMS report no. 18. *Arch Ophthalmol* 118:969, 2001

Toivonen P, Mäkitie T, Kujala E *et al.*: Microcirculation and tumor-infiltrating macrophages in choroidal and ciliary body melanoma and corresponding metastases. *Invest Ophthalmol Vis Sci* 45:1, 2004

Tsai JC, Sivak-Callcott JA, Haik BG *et al.*: Latanoprost-induced iris heterochromia and open-angle glaucoma: a clinicopathologic report. *J Glaucoma* 10:411, 2001

Tschentscher F, Husing J, Holter T *et al.*: Tumor classification based on gene expression profiling shows that uveal melanomas with and without monosomy 3 represent two distinct entities. *Cancer Res* 63:2578, 2003

Tschentscher F, Prescher G, Zeschnigk M *et al.*: Identification of chromosomes 3, 6, and 8 aberrations in uveal melanoma by microsatellite analysis in comparison to comparative genomic hybridization. *Cancer Genet Cytogenet* 122:13, 2000

Vajdic CM, Kricker A, Giblin M *et al.*: Eye color and cutaneous nevi predict risk of ocular melanoma in Australia. *Int J Cancer* 92:906, 2001

Vajdic CM, Kricker A, Giblin M *et al.*: Sun exposure predicts risk of ocular melanoma in Australia. *Int J Cancer* 101:175, 2002

Warwar RE, Bullock JD, Shields JA *et al.*: Coexistence of 3 tumors of neural crest origin: Neurofibroma, meningioma, and uveal melanoma. *Arch Ophthalmol* 116:1241, 1978

Weber A, Hengge UR, Urbanik D *et al.*: Absence of mutations of the BRAF gene and constitutive activation of extracellular-regulated kinase in malignant melanomas of the uvea. *Lab Invest* 83:1771, 2003

Weiss E, Shah CP, Lajous M *et al.*: The association between host susceptibility factors and uveal melanomas. *Arch Ophthalmol* 124:54, 2006

Whelchel JC, Farah SE, McLean IW *et al.*: Immunohistochemistry of infiltrating lymphocytes in uveal malignant melanoma. *Invest Ophthalmol Vis Sci* 34:2603, 1993

White JS, Becker RL, McLean IW *et al.*: Molecular cytogenetic evaluation of 10 uveal melanoma cell lines. *Cancer Genet Cytogenet* 168:11, 2006

White VA, Chambers JD, Courtright PD *et al.*: Correlation of cytogenetic abnormalities with the outcome of patients with uveal melanoma. *Cancer* 83:354, 1998

White VA, McNeil BK, Horsman DE: Acquired homozygosity (isodisomy) of chromosome 3 in uveal melanoma. *Cancer Genet Cytogenet* 102:40, 1998

White VA, McNeil BK, Thiberville L *et al.*: Acquired homozygosity (isodisomy) of chromosome 3 during clonal evolution of a uveal melanoma: association with morphologic heterogeneity. *Genes Chromosomes Cancer* 15:138, 1996

Wilkes SR, Robertson DM, Kurland LT *et al.*: Incidence of uveal malignant melanoma in the resident population of Rochester and Olmsted County, Minnesota. *Am J Ophthalmol* 87:639, 1979

Yanoff M: Melanomas and the incidence of neoplastic disease (letter). *N Engl J Med* 273:284, 1965

Yanoff M: Glaucoma mechanisms in ocular malignant melanomas. *Am J Ophthalmol* 70:898, 1970

Yanoff M: In discussion of Kersten RC, Tse DT, Anderson RL *et al.*: The role of orbital exenteration in choroidal melanoma with extrascleral extension. *Ophthalmology* 92:442, 1985

Yanoff M, Scheie HG: Melanomalytic glaucoma: Report of patient. *Arch Ophthalmol* 84:471, 1970

Yanoff M, Zimmerman LE: Histogenesis of malignant melanomas of the uvea: II. Relationship of uveal nevi to malignant melanomas. *Cancer* 20:493, 1967

Yanoff M, Zimmerman LE: Histogenesis of malignant melanomas of uvea: III. The relationship of congenital ocular melanocytosis and neurofibromatosis to uveal melanomas. *Arch Ophthalmol* 77:331, 1967

Young TA, Rao NP, Glasgow BJ *et al.*: Fluorescent in situ hybridization for monosomy 3 via 30-gauge fine-needle aspiration biopsy of choroidal melanoma in vivo. *Ophthalmology* 114:142, 2007

Zaldivar RA, Aaberg TM, Sternberg P Jr *et al.*: Clinicopathologic findings in choroidal melanomas after failed transpupillary thermotherapy. *Am J Ophthalmol* 135:657, 2003

Zimmerman LE, McLean IW, Foster WD: Statistical analysis of follow-up data concerning uveal melanomas and the influence of enucleation. *Ophthalmology* 87:557, 1980

Melanotic Tumors of the Optic Disc and Optic Nerve

de Potter D, Shields CL, Eagle RC Jr *et al.*: Malignant melanoma of the optic nerve. *Arch Ophthalmol* 114:608, 1996

Demirci H, Shields CL, Shields JA: Bilateral optic disc melanocytoma in a 10-month-old infant. *Am J Ophthalmol* 136:190, 2003

García-Arumí J, Salvador F, Corcostegui B *et al.*: Neuroretinitis associated with a melanocytoma of the optic disk. *Retina* 14:173, 1994

Haas BD, Jakobiec FA, Iwamoto T *et al.*: Diffuse choroidal melanocytoma in a child: A lesion extending the spectrum of melanocytic hamartomas. *Ophthalmology* 93:1632, 1986

Hiscott P, Campbell RJ, Robertson DM *et al.*: Intraocular melanocytoma in association with bone formation. *Arch Ophthalmol* 121:1791, 2003

Kurli M, Finger PT, Manor T *et al.*: Finding malignant change in a necrotic choroidal melanocytoma: a clinical challenge. *Br J Ophthalmol* 89:921, 2005

LaRusso FL, Bomiuk M, Font RL: Melanocytoma (magnocellular nevus) of the ciliary body: Report of 10 cases and review of the literature. *Ophthalmology* 107:795, 2000

Lauritzen K, Augsburger JJ, Timmes J: Vitreous seeding associated with melanocytoma of the optic disc. *Retina* 10:60, 1990

Meyer D, Ge J, Blinder KI *et al.*: Malignant transformation of an optic disk melanocytoma. *Am J Ophthalmol* 127:710, 1999

Robertson DM, Campbell RJ, Salomào DR: Mushroom-shaped melanocytoma mimicking malignant melanoma. *Arch Ophthalmol* 120:82, 2002

Scheie HG, Yanoff M: Pseudomelanoma of ciliary body, report of a patient. *Arch Ophthalmol* 77:81, 1967

Shields CL, Eagle RC Jr, Shields JA *et al.*: Progressive growth of an iris melanocytoma in a child. *Am J Ophthalmol* 133:287, 2002

Shields JA, Demirci H, Mashayekhi A *et al.*: Melanocytoma of optic disc in 115 cases: The 2004 Samuel Johnson Memorial Lecture, Part 1. *Ophthalmology* 111:1739, 2004

Shields JA, Shields CL, Eagle RC *et al.*: Malignant melanoma associated with melanocytoma of the optic disc. *Ophthalmology* 97:225, 1990

Shields JA, Shields CL, Eagle RC *et al.*: Malignant melanoma arising from a large uveal melanocytoma in a patient with oculodermal melanocytosis. *Arch Ophthalmol* 118:990, 2000

Shields JA, Shields CL, Eagle RC *et al.*: Central retinal vascular obstruction secondary to melanocytoma of the optic disc. *Arch Ophthalmol* 119:12, 2001

Teichmann KD, Karcioglu ZA: Melanocytoma of the iris with rapidly developing secondary glaucoma. *Surv Ophthalmol* 40:136, 1995

Zimmerman LE: Melanocytes, melanocytic nevi and melanocytomas. *Invest Ophthalmol* 4:11, 1965

Zografos L, Othenin-Girard CB, Desjardin L *et al.*: Melanocytoma of the optic disk. *Am J Ophthalmol* 138:964, 2004

Melanotic Tumors of the Orbit

Delaney YM, Hague S, McDonald B: Aggressive primary orbital melanoma in a young white man with no predisposing ocular features. *Arch Ophthalmol* 122:118, 2004

Dutton JJ, Anderson RL, Schelper RL *et al.*: Orbital malignant melanoma and oculodermal melanocytosis: Report of two cases and review of the literature. *Ophthalmology* 91:497, 1984

Lloyd WC III, Leone CR Jr: Malignant melanoma of the lacrimal sac. *Arch Ophthalmol* 102:104, 1984

Mandeville JT, Grove AS JR, Dadras SS *et al.*: Primary orbital melanoma associated with an occult episcleral nevus. *Arch Ophthalmol* 122:287, 2004

Rice CD, Brown H: Primary orbital melanoma associated with orbital melanocytosis. *Arch Ophthalmol* 108:1130, 1990

Tellado M, Specht CS, McLean IW *et al.*: Primary orbital melanomas. *Ophthalmology* 103:929, 1996

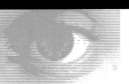

18

Retinoblastoma and Pseudoglioma

RETINOBLASTOMA

General Information

I. Retinoblastoma, along with leukemia and neuroblastoma, is one of the most common childhood malignancies and is the most common childhood intraocular neoplasm.

II. It is third to uveal malignant melanoma and metastatic carcinoma as the most common intraocular malignancy in humans of any age.

III. The incidence is approximately 1 in 18 000 live births in the United States, with a trend toward a higher prevalence than historically found (because of increased survival rate).

> The average annual incidence of retinoblastoma is 5.8 per million for children younger than 10 years and 10.9 per million for children younger than 5 years of age.

A. Reese–Ellsworth system relates clinical tumor characteristics to visual prognosis.

> Group I: very favorable for maintenance of sight

1. Solitary tumor, smaller than 4 disc diameters, at or behind the equator.
2. Multiple tumors, none larger than 4 disc diameters, all at or behind the equator.

> Group II: favorable for maintenance of sight

1. Solitary tumor, 4 to 10 disc diameters at or behind the equator.
2. Multiple tumors, 4 to 10 disc diameters behind the equator.

> Group III: possible for maintenance of sight

1. Any lesion anterior to the equator.
2. Solitary tumor, larger than 10 disc diameters behind the equator.

> Group IV: unfavorable for maintenance of sight

1. Multiple tumors, some larger than 10 disc diameters.
2. Any lesion extending anteriorly to the ora serrata.

> Group V: very unfavorable for maintenance of sight

1. Massive tumors involving more than one-half the retina.
2. Vitreous seeding.

B. Other classification systems predicting visual and ocular prognosis have been reported.

IV. No significant race or sex predilection exists.

V. Bilaterality occurs in 20% to 35% of all cases and is a useful marker for patients with hereditary retinoblastoma.

VI. The eye is a normal size at birth, but later may become phthisical or buphthalmic.

> A rare exception to the normal size at birth is a microphthalmic eye that contains both a retinoblastoma and persistent hyperplastic primary vitreous (PHPV). Microphthalmia, retinoblastoma, and 13q deletion syndrome can also occur and have been accompanied by colobomas.

VII. Age at initial diagnosis

A. Average age is 13 months, with 89% diagnosed before 3 years of age.

B. It is rare after 7 years of age, but has been reported in patients past 50 years of age.

Approximately 8.5% of patients are older than 5 years of age at the time of diagnosis. It is quite rare after the age of 20 years.

VIII. Children with retinoblastoma may have other congenital abnormalities such as the 13q deletion (deletion of chromosomal region 13q14) syndrome, 13qXp translocation, 21 trisomy, 47,XXX, 47,XXY, PHPV, the Pierre Robin syndrome, or hereditary congenital cataracts.

All children with 13q14 deletions should have an ophthalmologic examination to rule out retinoblastoma.

IX. Immune complexes may be present in the serum of patients with retinoblastoma. Populations of major histocompatibility complex (MHC)-II-positive cells are also found within the tumor, which may have significance for possible immunomodulation of these tumors.

Extraocular muscle biopsies obtained at enucleation for retinoblastoma in patients who had clinical signs of slight limitation of extraocular movements or strabismus exhibited muscle fibers with slight to severe atrophy and myopathic structures such as nemaline, filamentous and zebra bodies. Fiber necrosis and capillary abnormalities accompanied by inflammation were also noted. No direct tumor invasion was present. An extraocular paraneoplastic process related to the retinoblastoma was postulated as the cause of the findings. Also, DNA from oncogenic papilloma viruses 16 and 35 has been detected in 27.9% of 43 sporadic retinoblastoma specimens examined. Viral DNA was found in 63.3% of the more differentiated tumors.

X. Genetic cases have an increased prevalence of nonocular cancers, especially of the pineal gland (bilateral retinoblastoma plus pineal tumor comprise trilateral retinoblastoma), and sarcomas.

XI. Trilateral retinoblastoma
1. As noted above, the association of a midline intracranial neoplasm with bilateral retinoblastomas is known as *trilateral retinoblastoma* and is found in 4% to 8% of patients with hereditary retinoblastoma.
2. The intracranial neoplasm is most often an undifferentiated neuroblastic pineal tumor, or suprasellar or parasellar neuroblastoma.
   Pineal cysts are significantly more common in patients who have bilateral retinoblastoma than in those with unilateral tumor, thereby suggesting a benign variant of trilateral retinoblastoma, or possibly a hereditary influence.
3. Loss of the retinoblastoma "genes" is thought to confer an increased susceptibility to the development of an intracranial neoplasm.
   About 95% of patients who have trilateral retinoblastoma have a positive family history of retinoblastoma, bilateral retinoblastoma, or both.

XII. Retinoblastoma, which behaves as an autosomal-dominant trait with 90% penetrance, represents a prototype of a class of human cancers characterized by a loss of genetic

information at the constitutional or tumor level. Other cancers in this class include Wilms' tumor, neuroblastoma, small cell carcinoma of the lung, pulmonary carcinoid, breast and bladder cancer, osteosarcoma, and renal cell carcinoma.

Two leiomyosarcomas of the bladder at ages 17 and 39 years developed in a twin with bilateral retinoblastoma.

Heredity

I. "Two-hit" model
   Knudson's two-hit model states that retinoblastoma arises as a result of two mutational events (see discussion of chromosomal region 13q14, later).

Inactivation of both retinoblastoma 1 alleles may not be sufficient in itself to cause tumors in patients with hereditary retinoblastoma. On the other hand, some tumors that develop in patients with tuberous sclerosis complex or neurofibromatosis-1 may not require the "second hit". Retinoblastoma has developed in a boy diagnosed with macrocephaly–cutis marmorata telangiectatica congenita (M-CMTC). The child had macrosomy, body asymmetry, cutis marmorata, and tall stature. The diagnosis of M-CMTC was made even though macrocephaly was not noted. Retinoblastoma is usually said not to be associated with overgrowth syndromes; however, it has been suggested that M-CMTC may be a tumor-prone syndrome. Similarly, there is an increased incidence of multiple cutaneous malignant melanomas among individuals with retinoblastoma and dysplastic nevus syndrome, and among their family members. It has been recommended that survivors of inherited retinoblastoma and their families be screened for dysplastic nevus syndrome.

Speculation, with some preliminary evidence, suggests that inactivation of the chromosomal region 13q14 (the "retinoblastoma gene" that regulates normal development) by an oncogenic virus can produce the mutation.

1. If both mutations occur in the same somatic (postzygotic) cell, a single, unifocal, unilateral retinoblastoma results. Because the mutations occur in a somatic cell, the resultant condition is nonheritable.

The nonheritable form arises through two unrelated events occurring at homologous loci in a single neural retinal cell. Double such sporadic mutations are highly unlikely; hence, a unifocal, unilateral retinoblastoma results.

---

2. In the hereditary form, the first mutation occurs in a germinal (prezygotic) cell (which, therefore, would mean that the mutation would be present in all resulting somatic cells), and the second mutation occurs in a somatic (postzygotic) neural retinal cell, resulting in multiple neural retinal tumors (multifocal in one eye, bilateral, or both), as well as in

primary tumors elsewhere in the body (e.g., pineal tumors and sarcomas).

The heritable form arises through transmission of a mutant allele from a carrier parent or through a new mutation, which appears in the germline of the child, and is then carried in every cell. A second, somatic mutation occurs in the neural retina at a locus homologous to the mutant locus, triggering tumorigenesis (retinoblastoma) in different areas in the same eye as well as in the other eye (multifocal and bilateral).

---

    a. The probability that in the inherited form the tumor will develop in the patient (i.e., genotypically and phenotypically abnormal) is 90 in 100 (penetrance is estimated at 90%).

    b. Occasionally, a generation may be skipped, and the retinoblastoma may be transmitted to a genotypically abnormal but phenotypically normal family member.

II. The chromosomal region 13q14 (the retinoblastoma gene—*Rb* gene) regulates the development of normality (i.e., the region acts as an antioncogene).

Tumor suppressor genes, of which the *Rb* gene is one, are the "opposite numbers" of oncogenes, because their normal role is to inhibit cell growth; oncogenes, conversely, stimulate cell growth.

    A. If both chromosomal 13q14 regions are normal, no retinoblastoma will develop.

    B. If one of the two 13 chromosomes has a 13q14 deletion, duplication, or point mutation (a heterozygous condition), a retinoblastoma will still not result.

    C. If both 13 chromosomes have a 13q14 deletion, duplication, or point mutation (a homozygous condition), retinoblastoma results.

    D. Therefore, retinoblastoma is inherited as an autosomal-recessive trait at the cellular level; nevertheless, retinoblastoma behaves clinically as if it has an autosomal-dominant inheritance pattern with 90% penetrance.

    E. Gain of chromosome 1q31–1q32 is found in >50% of retinoblastoma, and also is common in other tumors. A determination of the minimal 1q region of gain reveals that 71% of retinoblastoma gained sequence-tagged sites (STS) at 1q32.1, which defines a 3.06 Mbp minimal region of gain between flanking markers and contained 14 genes. Of these genes, only *KIF14*, which is a putative chromokinesin, was overexpressed in various cancers.

    F. "Fragile-site" loci probably contribute synergistically to the development and progression of the cytogenetics of retinoblastoma malignancy.

    G. A facial phenotype for retinoblastoma patients having interstitial 13q14 deletions has been described in Japanese and then in Caucasian individuals, and includes cranial anomalies, frontal bossing, deeply grooved and long philtrum, depressed and broad nasal bridge, bulbous tip of the nose, thick lower lip, thin upper lip, broad cheeks, and large ears and lobules. Its recognition in newborns with no known family history of retinoblastoma may be helpful in making the diagnosis.

Retinoblastoma has recurred 12 years following multiple therapies for retinoblastoma in the second eye of a 25-year-old man with a g.153211T > A (p.Tyr606X) mutation in the retinoblastoma 1 gene whose fellow left eye was enucleated at age 2 years for two retinoblastomas. The patient was alive and without recurrence 11 years after the second eye was enucleated.

III. Hereditary cases (approximately 40% of cases)

    A. Approximately 10% of all retinoblastomas are inherited (familial). All are multifocal in one eye, bilateral, or both.

The clinical characteristics of patients who have retinoblastoma and a unilaterally affected parent are similar to those in all patients who have retinoblastoma and a positive family history.

    B. Another 30% are caused by a new germline mutation (see later discussion of sporadic cases). Although most of these mutations are multifocal in one eye, bilateral, or both, unilateral retinoblastoma, lack of family history, and older age do not exclude the possibility of a germline retinoblastoma 1 gene mutation.

    C. Retinoblastoma and hypochondroplasia have occurred as two clinically distinct heritable germline mutations arising de novo in a single individual.

IV. Sporadic cases

    A. Approximately 90% of all retinoblastomas develop by mutation (sporadic cases).

The mutation rate is approximately 2×10^{-5} (1 in 36 000 births), with, perhaps, a third representing a genetic mutation in a germinal cell capable of transmitting the retinoblastoma to offspring. The remaining two-thirds represent a somatic mutation incapable of transmitting the tumor.

    B. The retinoblastoma in sporadic somatic mutation cases is unifocal and unilateral (approximately 60% of the total cases); in the sporadic genetic mutation cases, it is usually multifocal in one eye, bilateral, or both (approximately 30% of the total cases).

The other 10% are the inherited familial cases.

V. Genetic counseling

    A. Healthy parents with one affected child run approximately a 6% risk of producing more affected children (the parent may be genotypically abnormal but phenotypically normal).

    B. If two or more siblings are affected, approximately a 50% risk exists that each additional child will be affected.

    C. A retinoblastoma survivor with the hereditary type has approximately a 50% chance of producing affected children.

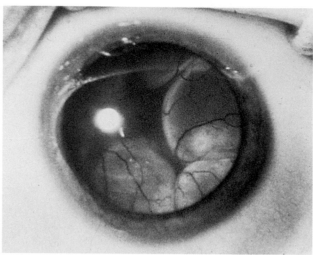

A

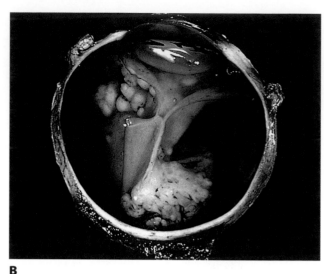

B

Fig. 18.1 Exophytic retinoblastoma. **A,** Clinical appearance of exophytic retinoblastoma, which grows predominantly toward the subneural retinal space, causing a neural retinal detachment that results in leukokoria. **B,** Gross specimen shows retinoblastoma growing into subneural retinal region, inducing a neural retinal detachment. Note multifocal growth of tumor. (**A,** Courtesy of Dr. HG Scheie; **B,** Armed Forces Institute of Pathology account no. 117729.)

Phetotypically normal children of an affected parent may be genetically abnormal.

D. A patient with sporadic disease has approximately a 12.5% chance of producing affected children.

E. Preimplantation genetic diagnosis has been helpful in genetic counseling in heritable retinoblastoma.

Clinical Features

I. Strabismus and leukokoria are the most common clinical manifestations of retinoblastoma in the typical tumor-prone age group

II. Early lesions may present with visual difficulties or strabismus. They may also be completely asymptomatic, as are small fundus lesions found on routine eye examination.

III. Moderate lesions may present as:
A. Leukokoria (i.e., "cat's-eye reflex"; Figs 18.1 and 18.2)

The term *leukokoria* is derived from the Greek *leukos*, meaning "white," and *kor*, meaning "pupil."

---

1. Computed tomography (CT) and magnetic resonance imaging (MRI):
   a. CT detects intraocular calcium with a high level of accuracy.
   b. MRI has superior contrast resolution to CT and, therefore, although not as specific as CT (MRI does not detect calcium), offers more information than CT on the different pathologic intraocular conditions that cause leukokoria.

MRI can also be helpful in tumor staging and detection of metastatic risk factors; however, detection of intraocular

---

tumor infiltration is difficult. Some MRI techniques may be particularly helpful in detecting optic nerve or scleral infiltration. Three-dimensional high-resolution MRI provides superior resolution for intraocular and orbital structures, and can be very useful in the evaluation of intraocular tumors and the nerve sheath complex. High-frequency ultrasound may be particularly helpful in evaluating anteriorly located tumors. Three-dimensional ultrasound may have some advantages for patient care, teaching, tumor volume analysis, and telemedicine. Rarely is fine-needle aspiration biopsy indicated to rule out retinoblastoma.

B. "Pseudoinflammation," i.e., simulating uveitis, endophthalmitis, or panophthalmitis with or without pseudohypopyon (Fig. 18.3)
   1. *Any childhood intraocular inflammation should be considered retinoblastoma until proven otherwise.*
   2. Orbital inflammation can occur even when the retinoblastoma is confined to the eye; signs of orbital cellulitis therefore do not necessarily mean orbital extension of the tumor.

C. Iris neovascularization (rubeosis iridis; Fig. 18.4A and B) with a hyphema, chronic secondary closed-angle glaucoma, or both
   1. Vascular endothelial growth factor, secreted by hypoxic retina, may play a role in the development of iris neovascularization. The glaucoma may lead to symptoms of photophobia and, if prolonged, buphthalmos may develop.
   2. Glaucoma and secondary hyphema may result from the iris neovascularization.
   3. Spontaneous hyphema in a child should always alert the physician to suspect retinoblastoma, juvenile xanthogranuloma, or nonaccidental trauma.

D. Phthisis bulbi

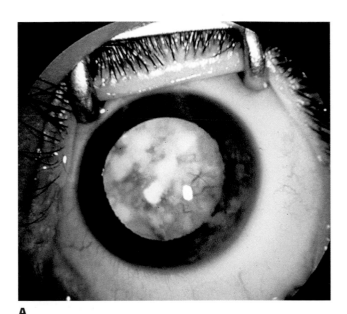 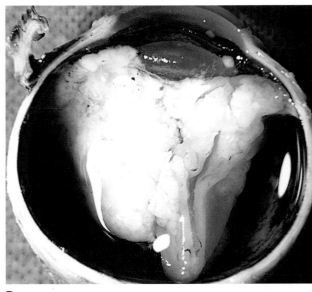

A **B**

Fig. 18.2 Endophytic retinoblastoma. **A,** Retinoblastoma grows mostly inward (endophytum). Note resemblance of tumor to brain tissue. **B,** Retinoblastoma grows inward from neural retina and fills vitreous compartment of eye. (**A,** Courtesy of Dr. HG Scheie.)

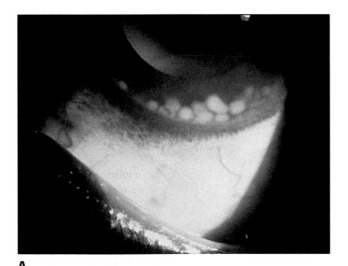 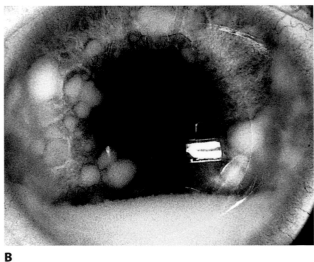

A **B**

Fig. 18.3 Spread of tumor. **A,** Retinoblastoma cells have formed balls of tumor in the anterior chamber inferiorly, simulating a hypopyon, thus "pseudohypopyon." **B,** In another case, clusters of retinoblastoma cells have spread from the neural retina into the anterior chamber and are present inferiorly as a pseudohypopyon and elsewhere float freely. (**A,** Courtesy of Dr. JA Shields; **B,** courtesy of Prof. GOH Naumann.)

IV. Advanced lesions may present with proptosis (see Fig. 18.4C and D), distant metastases, or both.

An advanced tumor at presentation in uncommon in the United States; however, it is a tragic fact of international ophthalmology that advanced tumors are relatively common at the time of diagnosis in many nonwestern countries. Proptosis is the most common presentation of retinoblastoma in eastern Nepal and is associated with orbital extension and tumor at the cut end of the optic nerve. In Ethiopia, retinoblastoma is the most common orbital tumor in children. Similarly, an Indian study reported a higher incidence of choroidal and optic nerve invasion in Asian Indian children than among children from the west. Whether this finding was secondary to delay in diagnosis or to ethnic differences in the tumor biology could not be determined. Advanced tumor at presentation and increased mortality appear to be common problems in countries such as Taiwan compared to western countries and to Japan, and in more rural areas of countries such as Mexico.

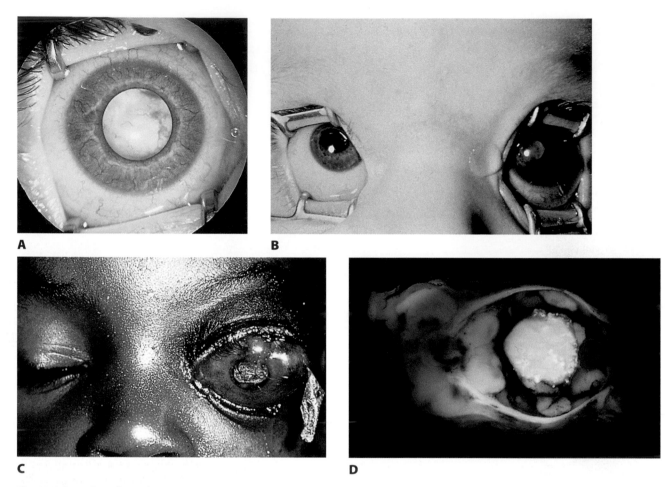

Fig. 18.4 Secondary effects of tumor. **A,** Iris neovascularization prominent in eye that shows leukokoria caused by retinoblastoma. **B,** Left eye in another case shows leukokoria caused by retinoblastoma. Eye buphthalmic because of secondary closed-angle glaucoma. **C,** Proptosis of left eye caused by posterior extraocular extension of retinoblastoma. **D,** Enucleated eye shows retinoblastoma in the eye with massive extension posteriorly behind the eye (to left). The cornea is to the right. (**A,** Courtesy of Dr. JA Shields; **B,** courtesy of Dr. HG Schele; **C,** courtesy of Dr. RE Shannon.)

Histology

I. Growth pattern
  A. Multifocal growth (i.e., spontaneous development from more than one region of the same neural retina; Fig. 18.5)
  B. Bilateral involvement is, itself, a reflection of multifocal neural retinal involvement.
  C. Exophytic retinoblastoma (see Fig. 18.1) grows predominantly toward the subneural retinal space and detaches the neural retina.
  D. Endophytic retinoblastoma (see Fig. 18.2) grows predominantly toward the vitreous. The neural retina is not detached.

Most retinoblastomas have both endophytic and exophytic components. Diffuse infiltrating retinoblastoma is a rare subtype of retinoblastoma, comprising approximately 1.5% of the total.

E. Rarely, retinal neovascularization may be found with retinoblastoma.

The histopathology of retinoblastoma can be helpful in suggesting in vitro drug resistance. Undifferentiated tumors are more sensitive to several cytostatic drugs. Calcification and apoptosis reflect an inverse relation to in vitro drug resistance to ifosfamide and vincristine. Extreme drug resistance to cytarabine has been observed.

II. The basic cell type is the radiosensitive undifferentiated retinoblastoma cell (Fig. 18.6).
  A. Retinoblastoma cells seem to be neuron-committed cells that arise from photoreceptor progenitor cells or from primitive stem cells that are capable of differentiation along both neuronal and glial cell lines. Mucin-like glycoprotein associated with photoreceptor cells is an immunohistochemical marker that is specific for retinal photoreceptor cells. Its use demonstrates photoreceptor differentiation even in apparently "undifferentiated" retinoblastomas.

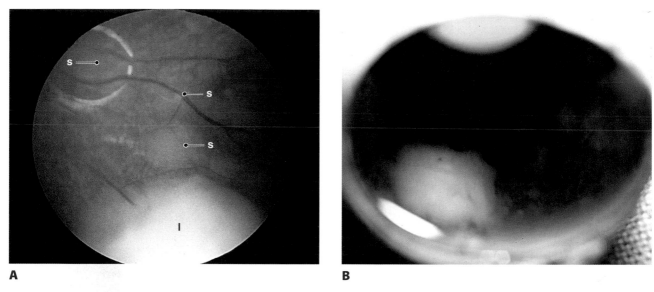

Fig. 18.5 Multifocal origin. **A,** Three small retinoblastoma (s) tumors and one large inferior tumor (l) are present in the same eye. **B,** Gross specimen of same eye after enucleation (see Fig. 18.9 for histology). (**A,** Courtesy of Dr. DB Schaffer.)

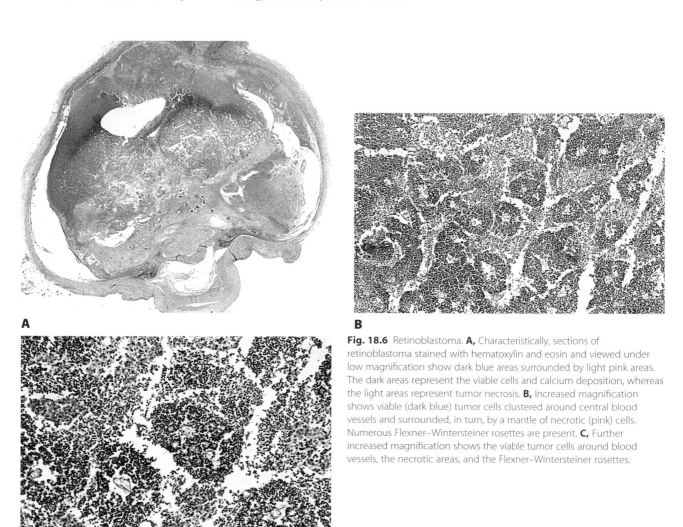

Fig. 18.6 Retinoblastoma. **A,** Characteristically, sections of retinoblastoma stained with hematoxylin and eosin and viewed under low magnification show dark blue areas surrounded by light pink areas. The dark areas represent the viable cells and calcium deposition, whereas the light areas represent tumor necrosis. **B,** Increased magnification shows viable (dark blue) tumor cells clustered around central blood vessels and surrounded, in turn, by a mantle of necrotic (pink) cells. Numerous Flexner–Wintersteiner rosettes are present. **C,** Further increased magnification shows the viable tumor cells around blood vessels, the necrotic areas, and the Flexner–Wintersteiner rosettes.

B. The cell of origin of retinoblastoma is not known with certainty. Evidence suggests that it may be the rod photoreceptor cell; however, polymerase chain reaction for interphotoreceptor retinoid-binding protein gene transcript is a useful method for detecting metastatic retinoblastoma cells, but rod beta-subunit of cyclic guanosine monophosphate (cGMP) was not found. Retinoblastomas can also express markers for other retinal nuclear cells, suggesting that the tumor may develop from visual stem cells that are progenitors of photoreceptor cells, intermediate neurons, and ganglion cells.

C. The primitive cells may be difficult to differentiate from other soft-tissue sarcomas. Immunohistochemistry, electron microscopy, and molecular assays for specific gene fusion may all be helpful in establishing the diagnosis.

D. The cells (bipolar-like) are positive for neuron-specific enolase, class III β-tubulin isotype (hβ4), microtubule-associated protein 2 (MAP2), and synaptophysin; they are negative for glial fibrillary acidic protein and S-100 protein.

 Neuron-specific enolase is present in the aqueous humor of patients who have intraocular retinoblastomas.

E. The product of the retinoblastoma susceptibility gene, $p110^{RB1}$, can be identified in paraffin-embedded tissues with commercially available techniques.

F. The Y79 retinoblastoma cell line, a prototype for retinoblastoma cells, shows decreased adhesion of the cells to extracellular matrix because of a deficit of integrin receptors; this may explain, in part, how the cells metastasize.

G. Apoptosis is more frequently found in tumors of young patients and to be distributed within rosettes.

III. Rosettes are of two types:
 A. Flexner–Wintersteiner rosettes (Figs 18.7 and 18.8; see also Fig. 18.6C) are the characteristic rosettes of retinoblastoma, but are not always present.
  1. In the rosettes, the cells line up around an apparently empty central lumen.
  2. Special stains show that the lumen contains a hyaluronidase-resistant acid mucopolysaccharide.
 B. Homer Wright rosettes (see Fig. 18.7) are found in medulloblastomas and neuroblastomas, and occasionally, in retinoblastomas.
  1. In 1910, John Homer Wright described the structure that bears his name in a series of cases of adrenal gland tumors that he called *neurocytoma* or *neuroblastoma*.
  2. In Homer Wright rosettes, the cells line up around an area containing cobweb-like material but no acid mucopolysaccharides.

IV. Pseudorosette—this very poor and confusing term is often used to refer to arrangements in the tumor that on cursory examination may resemble the aforementioned rosettes.
 The structures are formed by:
 A. Viable tumor cells that cluster around blood vessels

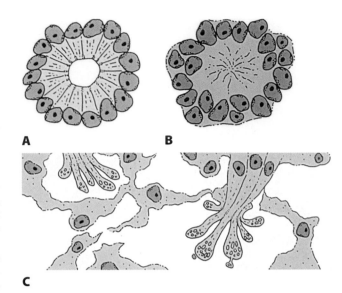

Fig. 18.7 Types of rosettes. **A,** A Flexner–Wintersteiner rosette consists of a central lumen lined by cuboidal tumor cells that contain nuclei positioned basally (away from the lumen). Delicate limiting membranes are seen at the apices of the cells that surround the lumen. **B,** Homer Wright rosettes are found more frequently in medulloblastomas and neuroblastomas than in retinoblastomas. In these rosettes, the cells line up around an acellular area that contains cobweb-like material. **C,** Fleurettes are flower-like groupings of tumor cells in the retinoblastoma. The cells of fleurettes show clear evidence of differentiation into photoreceptor elements.

 The cuff of retinoblastoma cells surrounding the blood vessels is rather uniform within the tumor, and from tumor to tumor, with a mean thickness of 98.7 μm.
 B. Small foci of necrotic cells between larger masses of viable tumor cells
 C. Incompletely formed Flexner–Wintersteiner or Homer Wright rosettes

V. Fleurettes and retinocytoma (Fig. 18.9; see also Figs 18.7 and 18.8)
 A. Fleurettes are flower-like groupings of tumor cells in the retinoblastoma that clearly show evidence of differentiation into photoreceptor elements.
 B. Fleurettes may be absent, may be present in small nodules, or rarely, may be present as the only cells in the tumor, so that the entire tumor has differentiated into photoreceptor-like elements.
  1. The fully differentiated retinoblastoma is called a *retinocytoma (retinoma)*.
  2. Retinocytomas have a uniformly bland cytology, photoreceptor differentiation, abundant fibrillar eosinophilic stroma, absence of mitotic activity, and occasional foci of calcification.
  3. Cells in the differentiated part of the tumor show immunoreactivity for retinal S antigen, S-100 protein, and glial fibrillary acidic protein.
  The histopathology and immunocytohistochemistry support the concept that retinocytomas arise de novo rather than from retinoblastomas that have undergone spontaneous regression.

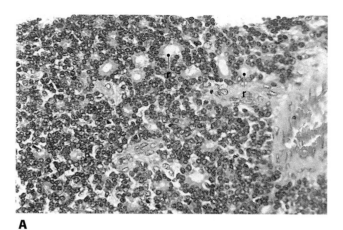
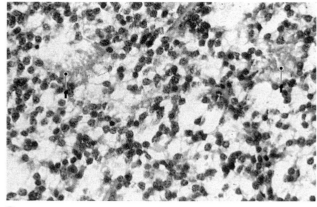

A

B

Fig. 18.8 Types of rosettes. **A,** Flexner–Wintersteiner rosettes (r) show clear lumina lined by a delicate limiting membrane and cuboidal retinoblastoma cells that contain basally located nuclei. **B,** In this histologic section of a retinoblastoma, almost all of the cells show photoreceptor differentiation, indicated by the pale eosinophilic cellular regions. The differentiated areas are forming fleurettes (f).

4. Multinucleated tumor cells may be found in retinocytomas.
5. Very rarely, a retinocytoma may undergo malignant transformation.

C. Those areas that show photoreceptor differentiation usually lack evidence of necrosis and show only occasional calcification.
   1. Retinocytoma is most likely to be found in the inherited form, the mutation presumably taking place in a relatively mature retinoblast.
   2. There may be an increased possibility of a second primary tumor following the development of retinoma.

D. Developing photoreceptors have apical adherens junctions, mitochondria-filled inner-segment regions, occasional fragments of membranous outer segments, and cilia that contain a 9 + 0 tubular arrangement.

VI. Other histologic features

A. Most tumors show significant areas of necrosis (Fig. 18.10; see also Fig. 18.6).
   1. Advanced necrotic retinoblastoma may present as orbital cellulitis.
   2. Total necrosis may lead to spontaneous and complete regression in a shrunken, scarred, calcific eye—a rare occurrence.
   3. After complete regression, the eye sometimes retains useful vision (Fig. 18.11).
   4. The necrosis of the retinoblastoma may be caused by tumor ischemia or host immunologic response to the tumor.
   5. Another group of "regressed" retinoblastomas, not found in scarred, calcified eyes, probably represents de novo origin of neural retinal lesions called *retinocytomas* (see earlier discussion of fleurettes and retinocytoma).

B. Calcification (see Fig. 18.10) is a frequent and important diagnostic feature. It is mainly present in areas of necrosis and may be detected clinically by CT.
   Calcification begins in nonviable cells or cells that are undergoing necrosis. The calcification is intracel-

lular and begins in the cytoplasm, probably in the mitochondria.

C. Basophilic areas around blood vessels (Fig. 18.12), and also lying freely within the tumor and on the lens capsule represent deposition of DNA liberated from necrotic retinoblastoma cells.

D. Approximately 1.5% of cases have a diffuse, infiltrating type of tumor but without a discrete neural retinal mass. It occurs in a slightly older age group than the usual type, tends not to be bilateral, and is frequently accompanied by a simulated hypopyon.

VII. Mode of extension

A. Local spread
   1. Anteriorly by seeding, into the vitreous and aqueous (see Figs 18.2B and 18.3)

Aqueous seeding may simulate a hypopyon. Deposits may appear on the iris and in the anterior-chamber angle, and may produce a secondary open-angle glaucoma. Aqueous lactate dehydrogenase (LDH) and neuron-specific enolase levels may be elevated in eyes containing retinoblastoma, especially if the tumor is in the anterior chamber. LDH may also be elevated in Coats' disease. It is not clear what the neuron-specific enolase level is in normal eyes in children or in eyes that have lesions simulating retinoblastoma (pseudogliomas).

---

   2. Posteriorly (see Fig. 18.4C and D) by direct extension into the subneural retinal space (Fig. 18.13)

After invasion into the choroid, the tumor may gain access to the systemic circulation. By spread into the optic nerve, the tumor may gain access to the subarachnoid space through passage alongside the central retinal vessels to their exit from the nerve into the subarachnoid space.

B. Extraocular extension
   1. Orbit (see Fig. 18.4C and D)
   2. Brain

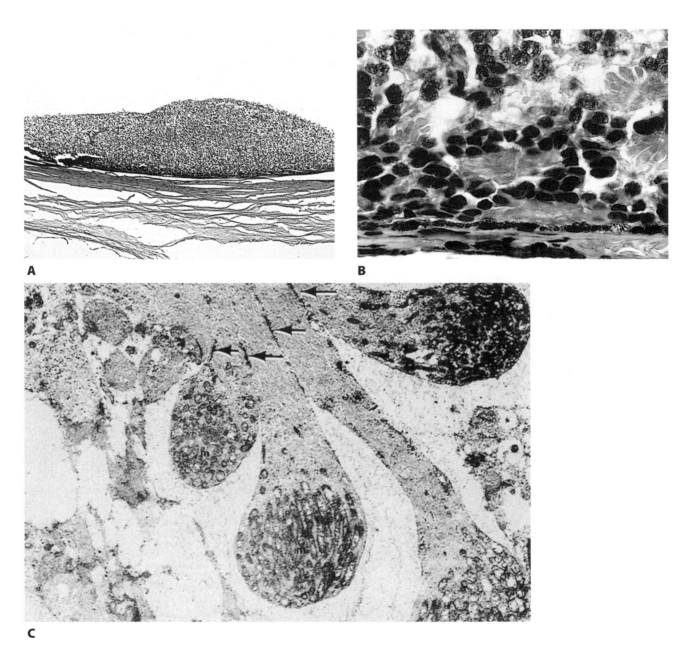

Fig. 18.9 Fleurettes. **A,** Retinoblastoma shows complete photoreceptor differentiation (see Fig. 18.5 for fundus and gross appearance). **B,** Note arrangement (fleurettes) of cells that have undergone photoreceptor differentiation. **C,** Photoreceptor inner segments resemble those of cone cells. They radiate from attachment girdle (zonulae adherentes) (*arrows*) of external limiting membrane, partly because intervening Müller cell processes are lacking (m, mitochondria). (**C,** Modified from Tso MOM *et al.: Am J Ophthalmol* 69:339, 350. © Elsevier 1970.)

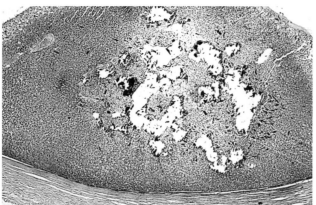

Fig. 18.10 Tumor necrosis. **A,** Retinoblastoma shows central area of necrosis and calcification. **B,** Electron microscopy of another case demonstrates transition between viable cell (above) and necrotic cell (below). Note nuclear chromatin clumping and focal densification of cytoplasmic component in necrotic cell. **C,** Radiograph of retinoblastoma-containing eye shows calcification. **D,** Early calcification in cytoplasm of necrotic retinoblastoma cell appears in mitochondria. Nucleus free of calcification. The arrows point to intact cell plasmalemma. Inset shows large foci of cytoplasmic calcification in another necrotic cell.

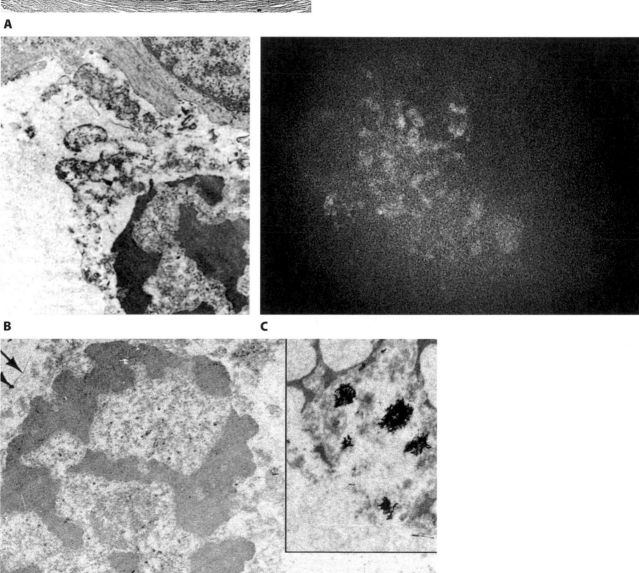

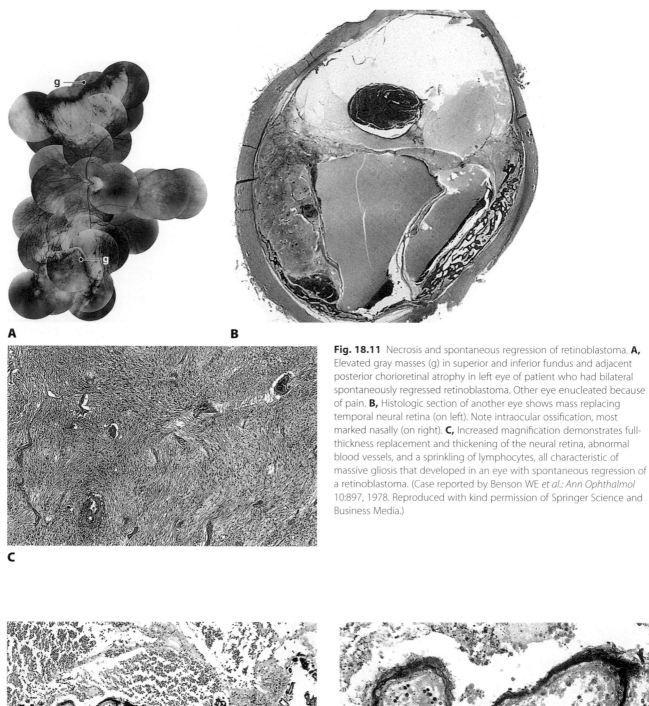

Fig. 18.11 Necrosis and spontaneous regression of retinoblastoma. **A,** Elevated gray masses (g) in superior and inferior fundus and adjacent posterior chorioretinal atrophy in left eye of patient who had bilateral spontaneously regressed retinoblastoma. Other eye enucleated because of pain. **B,** Histologic section of another eye shows mass replacing temporal neural retina (on left). Note intraocular ossification, most marked nasally (on right). **C,** Increased magnification demonstrates full-thickness replacement and thickening of the neural retina, abnormal blood vessels, and a sprinkling of lymphocytes, all characteristic of massive gliosis that developed in an eye with spontaneous regression of a retinoblastoma. (Case reported by Benson WE *et al.: Ann Ophthalmol* 10:897, 1978. Reproduced with kind permission of Springer Science and Business Media.)

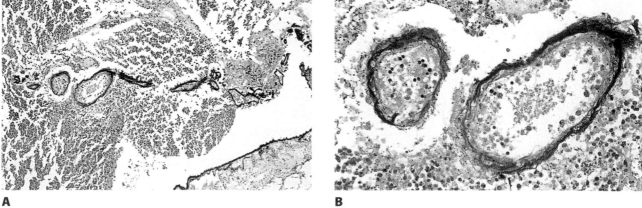

Fig. 18.12 Blood vessel basophilia. **A,** Basophilia present around retinal blood vessels probably represents DNA. Choroid in lower right corner. **B,** Increased magnification of basophilic blood vessel walls.

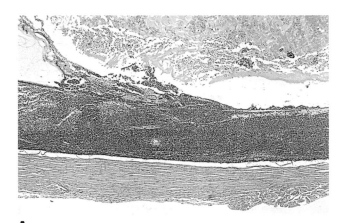

A

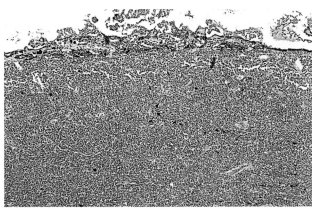

B

Fig. 18.13 Subneural retinal and choroidal invasion. **A,** Necrotic (pink) retinoblastoma present between neural retina (out of field above) and retinal pigment epithelium (RPE). Viable (blue) retinoblastoma fills the choroid. **B,** Increased magnification shows RPE changes over choroidal retinoblastoma.

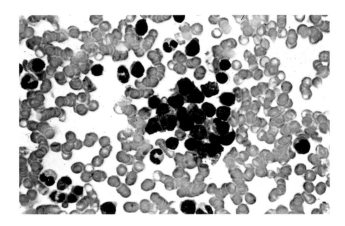

Fig. 18.14 Metastases. Retinoblastoma cells are present in bone marrow aspirate.

a. The most common site of metastasis is the central nervous system, and has an extremely poor prognosis, particularly if radiotherapy is not utilized in the treatment.

C. Metastases (Fig. 18.14; see section *Prognosis*, later)

Prognosis

I. Metastases—four factors appear to be independently associated with the development of metastases:

A. Invasion of the cut end of the optic nerve: 5-year metastatic risk, 67%

B. Invasion of the optic nerve (but not of the cut end): 5-year metastatic risk, 13%

C. Invasion of the choroid: 5-year metastatic risk, 8%
Choroidal invasion is a risk for metastases, especially if the invasion is associated with iris neovascularization, increased intraocular pressure, or optic nerve invasion.

D. Enucleation of the globe more than 120 days after initial diagnosis: 5-year metastatic risk, 4%.

The K-*ras* oncogene may undergo mutation in one-third of retinoblastomas, probably causing a selective growth advantage. The mutations seem to occur in, or cause, undifferentiated tumors. Mutations of the K-*ras* gene, therefore, may cause increased aggressiveness of retinoblastomas in which the mutations take place (i.e., increased malignancy).

II. Over the last two decades, the prognosis for life has improved considerably because of earlier diagnosis and improved methods of treatment. Nevertheless, a 2005 study of childhood cancer survival trends in Europe found no improvement for 5-year survival for retinoblastoma diagnosed under the age of 15 years during the period 1983 to 1994
Bilateral and unilateral cases have the same fatality rate.

III. Histologic correlation

A. Cellular differentiation

1. A patient whose tumor has abundant Flexner–Wintersteiner rosettes has approximately a sixfold better prognosis than one whose tumor has no rosettes.

2. A tumor that is completely differentiated (retinocytoma) is believed to augur a better prognosis than an undifferentiated retinoblastoma; the prognosis is even better than for a tumor with abundant Flexner–Wintersteiner rosettes but no differentiation (i.e., no fleurettes).

B. When choroidal invasion is slight (most cases with choroidal invasion), the mortality rate appears not to be affected; when the invasion is massive (Fig. 18.15), the mortality rate is approximately 60%.

C. Optic nerve involvement (see Fig. 18.15B)

1. When the optic nerve is not invaded, the mortality rate is approximately 8%.

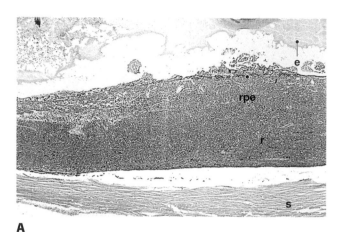
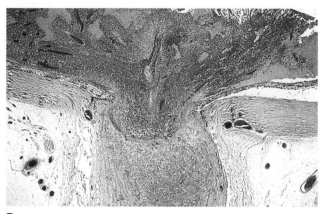

A

B

Fig. 18.15 Prognosis. **A,** The retinoblastoma has invaded through Bruch's membrane, massively replacing the choroid (r, choroid replaced by retinoblastoma cells; e, subneural retinal exudate containing necrotic retinoblastoma cells; rpe, retinal pigment epithelium; s, sclera). Patients who have massive invasion, as shown here, have a mortality rate of approximately 60%. **B,** The retinoblastoma has invaded the optic nerve up to the cut end. For those patients in whom the substance of the optic nerve has been invaded posterior to the lamina cribrosa, the mortality rate is approximately 42%. If retinoblastoma is present at the cut end of the optic nerve, the mortality rate increases to approximately 67%.

2. Grade I: when it is invaded up to, but not involving, the lamina cribrosa (superficial involvement of the optic nerve head only), the mortality rate is approximately 10%.
3. Grade II: when the invasion is up to and including the lamina cribrosa, the mortality rate is approximately 29%.
4. Grade III: when the invasion is beyond the lamina cribrosa, but not to the surgical margin, the mortality rate is approximately 42%.
5. Grade IV: when the invasion is to the line of transection or to the posterior point of exit of the central retinal vessels from the optic nerve, the mortality rate is approximately 67%.

D. The presence of iris neovascularization (rubeosis iridis) is a poor prognostic sign.

E. The clinical prognosis is determined by the location and size of the tumor.

F. Probably only retinoblastoma patients with the genetic (familial) tumor or sporadic tumors with germinal cell gene mutations have a definite predilection for the development of fatal second malignancies (with or without radiation therapy for the initial lesion) despite adequate control of their original eye tumor.
1. Patients who have bilateral retinoblastomas have a 26% chance of dying from a second primary neoplasm after 40 years; the risk is increased if the patient received radiation therapy for the initial lesion.
2. Osteosarcoma of the femur is the most common second malignancy; other tumors include fibrosarcoma, skin carcinoma, cutaneous melanoma, rhabdomyosarcoma, leukemia, Ewing's sarcoma, peripheral neuroepithelioma, benign and malignant neoplasms of brain and meninges, Langerhans' granulomatosis, and sinonasal carcinoma. Sebaceous carcinoma of the eyelid may occur in patients with hereditary retinoblastoma regardless of the primary treatment, especially within the field 5 to 15 years after radiotherapy.

> A primary osteosarcoma displaying a rosette-like appearance has developed 24 years after bilateral retinoblastoma at age 1 year. Also, orbital malignant fibrous histiocytoma has occurred 17 years following radiation therapy and systemic chemotherapy for retinoblastoma at age 5 months.

4. A pineal gland tumor plus bilateral retinoblastoma is called *trilateral retinoblastoma*.
   Pineal cyst may simulate pinealoblastoma in patients with retinoblastoma.
5. The second tumor is not necessarily related to prior radiation therapy of the primary retinoblastoma.
6. Cell proliferation may be more important than apoptosis and angiogenesis in determining tumor size. Higher apoptotic index (over 2.4%) appears to be related to decreased metastasis and lower proliferative index.

G. Angiogenesis is important in tumor survival. There is no difference in blood vessel density between unilateral and bilateral tumors; however, higher vessel density is associated with choroid and/or optic nerve invasion, and with metastasis at the time of presentation. The relative vascular area of a retinoblastoma may help to identify patients at higher risk for disease metastasis after enucleation.

PSEUDOGLIOMA

General Information

I. Terminology
A. The term *pseudoglioma*, introduced by Collins in 1892, designates a heterogeneous group of pathologic entities that may be confused with retinoblastomas.

TABLE 18.1 Classification of Conditions That Can Simulate Retinoblastoma

HEREDITARY CONDITIONS

Norrie's disease
Juvenile retinoschisis
Incontinentia pigmenti
Dominant exudative vitreoretinopathy

DEVELOPMENTAL ABNORMALITIES

Persistent hyperplastic primary vitreous
Congenital cataract
Coloboma
Retinal dysplasia
Congenital retinal fold
Myelinated nerve fibers
Morning-glory syndrome
Congenital corneal opacity
Congenital nonattachment of retina
Retinal heterotopic brain tissue

INFLAMMATORY DISORDERS

Ocular toxocariasis
Congenital toxoplasmosis
Congenital cytomegalovirus retinitis
Herpes simplex retinitis
Peripheral uveoretinitis
Metastatic endophthalmitis
Orbital cellulites

TUMORS

Retinal astrocytic hamartoma
Medulloepithelioma
Glioneuroma
Choroidal hemangioma
Retinal capillary hemangioma
Combined hamartoma
Leukemia

MISCELLANEOUS

Coats' disease
Retinopathy of prematurity
Rhegmatogenous retinal detachment
Vitreous hemorrhage
Perforating ocular injury

(Adapted from Shields JA et al.: Retina 11:232, 1991.)

    B. The term *pseudoretinoblastoma* is preferred, but has not gained wide acceptance.
  II. The clinical presentation of pseudoglioma is similar to retinoblastoma in that it may present with leukokoria (whitish pupil) or with a small endophytic or exophytic tumor.

Leukokoria (Table 18.1)

    I. Persistent hyperplastic primacy vitreous (PHPV) (Fig. 18.16)
      A. PHPV [also called persistent fetal vasculature (PFV)] is a congenital, unilateral condition recognizable at birth; rarely, it is bilateral.

        1. PHPV has been found in association with chromosome 6p25 terminal deletion resulting in karyotype 46,XX, del (6) (p25.1) and associated with Axenfeld–Rieger syndrome. It has occurred with neurofibromatosis-2, and with urogenital anomalies accompanying varicella syndrome. Focal dermal hypoplasia or Goltz syndrome, which has cutaneous, skeletal, dental, ocular, central nervous system, and soft-tissue defects, has been reported with sclerocornea in one eye and anterior PHPV in the fellow eye.

Bilateral PHPV has been reported in association with protein C deficiency, an autosomal-recessive disorder. Nonsyndromic, autosomal-recessive PHPV was studied in a six-generation consanguineous family and localized to chromosome 10q11–q21. It can also be an isolated finding.

---

        2. PHPV is the most common lesion simulating retinoblastoma.
      B. It is unrelated to prematurity.
      C. PHPV exists in a microphthalmic eye having a shallow anterior chamber. Long ciliary processes are frequently seen around the periphery of a small lens.

Buphthalmos may accompany PHPV if the eye becomes glaucomatous.

      D. Rarely, PHPV and retinoblastoma have been reported together in microphthalmic eyes.
      E. A lens capsule dehiscence is often present posteriorly. Rarely, the lens is cataractous.

Lenticular fibroxanthomatous nodule consisting of vascularized collections of foamy histiocytes, multinucleated cells, lens capsule, and lens epithelium that had undergone fibrous metaplasia has been found in one patient with PHPV and another with a history of trauma.

      F. The condition is the result of persistence of the embryonic primary vitreous and hyaloid vasculature system.
        Preretinal glial nodules may occur with PHPV. The preretinal nodules are thought to represent neuroectodermal proliferations.
      G. PHPV may cause angle closure glaucoma even in individuals 40 years of age or younger.
  II. Retinal dysplasia (see Fig. 2.9)
      A. Retinal dysplasia is congenital, usually bilateral, and recognizable at birth but is unrelated to prematurity.
      B. Bilateral retinal dysplasia is most often part of trisomy 13 (see p. 38 in Chapter 2). It may be unilateral and then is not associated with systemic anomalies and trisomy 13.
      C. Histologically, tubular and rosette-like structures form the dysplastic neural retina; four general types of rosettes are recognized.

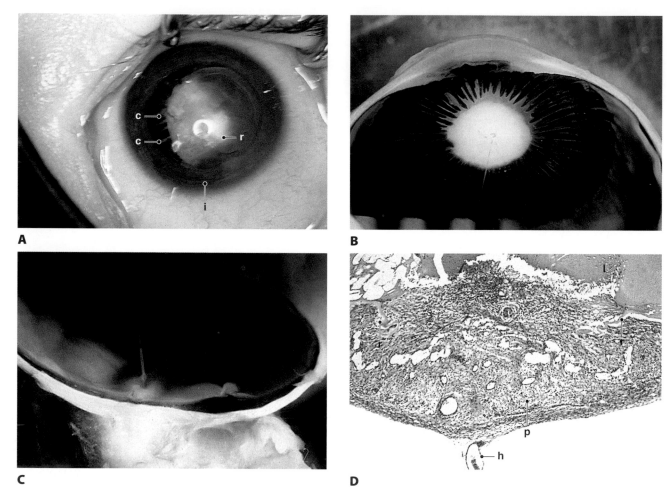

Fig. 18.16 Persistent hyperplastic primary vitreous. **A,** Clinically, the ciliary processes are characteristically drawn inward and a posterior lens opacity is noted (c, indrawn ciliary processes; r, retrolental mass; i, iris). **B** and **C,** Gross specimens of another case show a persistent hyaloid vessel and the ciliary processes stretched inward toward a posterior lens plaque (**B**); in **C** the hyaloid vessel extends to the optic nerve. **D,** A histologic section shows abundant mesenchymal fibrovascular tissue just behind and within the posterior lens (l). Note the ends of the ruptured lens capsule (r). A persistent hyaloid vessel (h) is also present (p, posterior plaque). (**B–D,** Courtesy of Dr. BW Streeten and reported in Caudill JW *et al.: Ophthalmology* 92:1153. © Elsevier 1985.)

1. Three-layer rosettes, that have the appearance of mature neural retina that has been thrown into folds secondarily
2. Two-layer rosettes, in which the innermost layer resembles a photoreceptor cell layer with an external limiting membrane and a relatively large lumen that often contains undifferentiated cells. Surrounding the rosette is a more peripheral layer of bipolar-like cells or poorly differentiated cells.
3. One-layer rosettes with a single layer of moderately well-differentiated neural cells, usually several cells in thickness, having an external limiting membrane-like structure and surrounding a lumen. In the lumen, larger undifferentiated cells are usually observed.
4. Primitive unilayer rosettes in which a single layer of undifferentiated neural retinal cells surrounds a lumen with a tangle of fibrils seen centrally.

III. Retinopathy of prematurity (ROP; retrolental fibroplasia; Figs 18.17 and 18.18): ROP is the fourth most common lesion simulating retinoblastoma.

Despite a decrease in mean gestational age and birth weight, a British survey found a reduced incidence of ROP from 1989 to 1998 and attributed the finding to improvements in ventilation techniques and overall care of the neonate, in particular, the use of steroids and surfactant.*

A. ROP is bilateral and not present at birth.

A number of cases of "congenital ROP" (e.g., in Potter's syndrome) have been reported. Although ROP is rare in children who have not had oxygen therapy or who were

*Rowlands E, Ionides AC, Chinn S et al. *Reduced incidence of retinopathy of prematurity.* Br J Ophthalmol *85:933, 2001.*

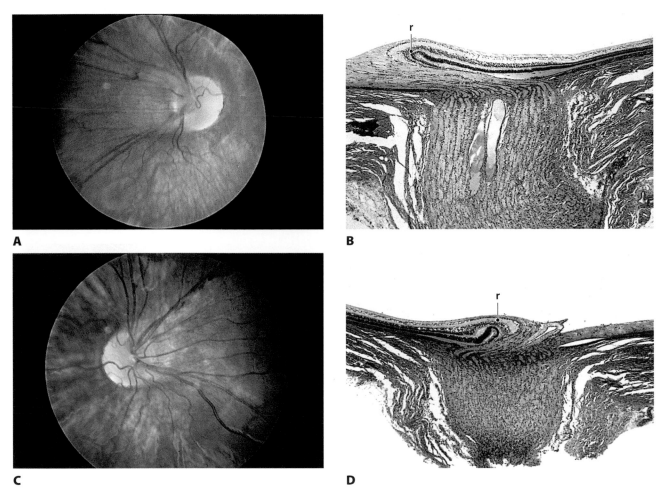

Fig. 18.17 Retinopathy of prematurity. **A,** The fundus picture shows the blood vessels in this right eye pulled temporally. **B,** A histologic section of another right eye shows the nasal retina (r, "pulled retina") displaced temporally over the optic nerve head. **C,** This is the clinical appearance of the left eye of the patient shown in **A. D,** A histologic section of another left eye (from the patient shown in **B**) demonstrates the temporal pulling of the nasal retina (r).

not premature, it does seem to occur. In some conditions, retinal neovascularization can simulate ROP. Missense mutations in the Norrie's disease gene may play a role in the development of severe ROP in premature infants.

B. It occurs in premature infants, most weighing less than 1.5 kg, who have a history of oxygen therapy.

    1. The degrees of early retinal vessel development and iris vessel dilatation are significant predictors of outcome from ROP.

> The retinal vessels must be immature to be affected by increased oxygen tension. If the infant is premature but the retinal vessels are mature, oxygen therapy will not cause ROP; conversely, if the infant is full-term but the retinal vessels are immature, oxygen therapy may cause ROP.

    2. ROP develops in approximately 66% of infants weighing less than 1251 g at birth, and in approximately 82% weighing less than 1000 g.

    3. An association exists between the incidence and severity of ROP, and the duration of exposure to arterial oxygen levels of 80 mmHg or higher, as measured transcutaneously.

    4. Hyperoxia causes neural retinal vascular closure, obliteration, and hypoxia, then induces neural retinal vasoproliferation; finally, after relief of hypoxia, normalization occurs.

    5. Based on data such as racial and sexual differences in the incidence of ROP, it has been suggested that genetic factors may predispose some individuals to develop ROP.

    6. In neonatal cats, the interaction of vascular endothelial growth factor and degenerating retinal astrocytes creates conditions for the growth of preretinal blood vessels.

C. The eyes are normal in size at birth but may become microphthalmic with development of shallow anterior chambers.

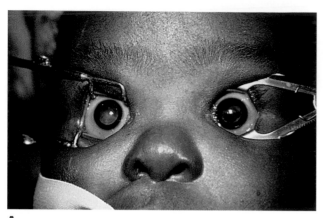

A

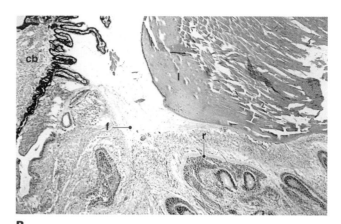

B

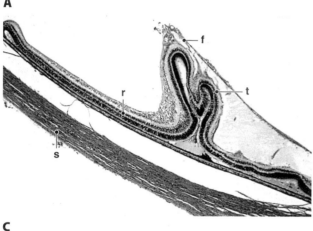

C

Fig. 18.18 Retinopathy of prematurity. **A,** A 6-month-old child shows bilateral leukokoria secondary to retinopathy of prematurity. **B,** A histologic section of another eye shows the detached neural retina (r) drawn by fibrovascular tissue (f) into a mass behind the lens (l) (hence the old term *retrolental fibroplasia*) (cb, ciliary body). **C,** Neovascularization of the neural retina has occurred anterior to the equator, forming fibrovascular bands (f) and causing a traction detachment (t) of the neural retina (r, retina; s, sclera).

D. Ciliary processes may be seen in the periphery of the retrolental mass.

E. The classification includes five stages (the process can arrest at any stage):

1. Stage 1: demarcation line
   a. The demarcation line separates the avascular neural retina anteriorly from the vascular neural retina posteriorly.
   b. The retinal vessels leading to the line have brush-like endings.
2. Stage 2: ridge
   a. Extraretinal neovascularization results from growth in width and height of the demarcation line.
   b. Small, isolated tufts of new vessels may be seen lying on the surface posterior to the ridge.
3. Stage 3: ridge with extraneural retinal fibrovascular proliferation
   a. Fibrovascular proliferation occurs posterior to the ridge.
   b. Mild, moderate, and severe grades exist.
4. Stage 4: partial neural retinal detachment
   a. Stage 4a: partial extrafoveal neural retinal detachment
   b. Stage 4b: partial neural retinal detachment involving fovea

   c. Progressive stage 4 retinopathy requiring surgical intervention is predicted by the absence of clear vitreous, ridge elevation of six or more clock-hours, and two or more quadrants of plus disease, but not by neovascularization.
5. Stage 5: total neural retinal detachment

> Subretinal organization in stage 5 retinopathy is most frequently identified as subretinal band formation, has been found in about 10% of stage 5 eyes, and is associated with incomplete retinal reattachment.

F. Plus disease is typified by increasing dilatation and tortuosity of the retinal vessels, iris engorgement, pupillary rigidity, and vitreous haze or hemorrhage, or both.

G. Regressed ROP is the common outcome of ROP.

H. A fulminant type of ROP may occur.

I. Histology
   1. Early, a sheet of spindle cells of mesenchymal origin—the precursors of the inner retinal endothelial cells—proliferate in the peripheral neural retina, associated with the development of retinal vessels.
   2. Behind the proliferating spindle cells are newly formed capillaries in an area of differentiating endothelium.

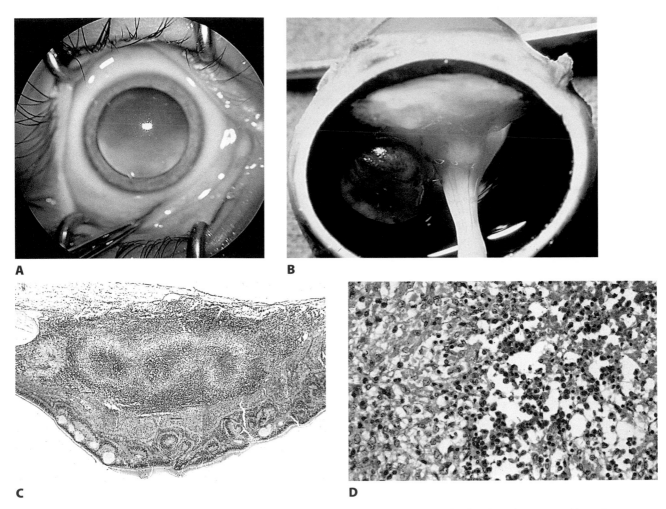

A   **B**

C   **D**

Fig. 18.19 Toxocariasis. **A,** This 8-year-old boy presented with leukokoria. The eye was white, and other than loss of vision, no additional symptoms were present. **B,** Another eye displaying leukokoria was enucleated to rule out retinoblastoma. A total neural retinal detachment and a peripheral neural retinal mass are seen. **C,** A histologic section shows the peripheral neural retinal mass that contains an eosinophilic abscess. **D,** Increased magnification shows a collection of eosinophils surrounded by a chronic granulomatous inflammatory reaction. Often, the worm itself is not found, but the eosinophils are evidence of its presence before dissolution. Granulomas (called Splendore–Hoeppli phenomona) may develop in the eyelid, the episclera, or the conjunctiva, and are caused by different agents, including toxocariasis.

Early in the acute phase, a demarcation line is seen clinically that separates the peripheral avascular neural retina from the vascular. Functioning arteriovenous collaterals occur in the region of the demarcation line. Microvascular abnormalities in the area include capillary tufts, collaterals, capillary-free zones, and neovascular membranes. Regression is evidenced by capillaries from the collaterals growing into the avascular neural retina. Cicatrization is characterized by both persistence of the vascular abnormalities of the proliferative phase and organization of the avascular neural retina into a contracting scar.

3. The young vessels break through the internal limiting membrane and grow into the subvitreal space.
4. A glial fibrocellular component develops; as it shrinks or contracts, a neural retinal detachment takes place.

The neural retinal detachment may be rhegmatogenous (usually with round or oval neural retinal breaks without opercula near the equator) or nonrhegmatogenous. Least common is an exudative type of neural retinal detachment that may occur secondary to peripheral vascular changes associated with ROP.

> Clinically important vitreous organization and vitreous hemorrhage are predictive for the development of retinal detachment.

5. The macula and posterior retinal vessels are displaced temporally.
6. The earliest neural retinal changes are seen in the periphery of the temporal neural retina.
7. Hemorrhagic areas may be seen.
8. Glaucoma, usually a chronic secondary closed-angle type, may occur in later years.

IV. *Toxocara* endophthalmitis (Fig. 18.19; see also p. 90 in Chapter 4): *Toxocara* endophthalmitis is the third most common lesion simulating retinoblastoma.

V. Coats' disease (Fig. 18.20)

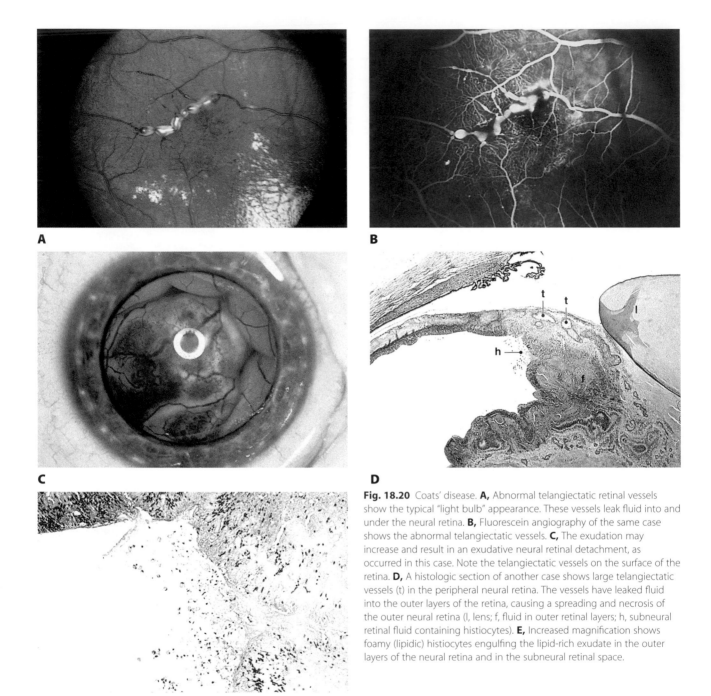

Fig. 18.20 Coats' disease. **A,** Abnormal telangiectatic retinal vessels show the typical "light bulb" appearance. These vessels leak fluid into and under the neural retina. **B,** Fluorescein angiography of the same case shows the abnormal telangiectatic vessels. **C,** The exudation may increase and result in an exudative neural retinal detachment, as occurred in this case. Note the telangiectatic vessels on the surface of the retina. **D,** A histologic section of another case shows large telangiectatic vessels (t) in the peripheral neural retina. The vessels have leaked fluid into the outer layers of the retina, causing a spreading and necrosis of the outer neural retina (l, lens; f, fluid in outer retinal layers; h, subneural retinal fluid containing histiocytes). **E,** Increased magnification shows foamy (lipidic) histiocytes engulfing the lipid-rich exudate in the outer layers of the neural retina and in the subneural retinal space.

A. Coats' disease is a unilateral (rarely bilateral) exudative neural retinal detachment that mainly affects boys between 18 months and 18 years of age, but with most cases occurring in an older age group than retinoblastoma.

In bilateral cases, long-term follow-up of the least affected eye is necessary so that late complications can be identified and treated adequately in order to prevent visual loss. Presentation in middle age can occur with typical Coats' disease findings, including unilateral disease, male preponderance, vascular tel-

angiectasis, lipid exudation, macular edema, and areas of capillary nonperfusion with adjacent filigree-like capillaries. In adult-onset disease; however, there tends to be a limited area of involvement, slower apparent progression of disease, and hemorrhage near larger vascular dilations compared to the childhood disease.

1. The clinical spectrum of Coats' disease may be classified as a subtype of idiopathic retinal telangiectasis with exudation.

a. Patients with typical and atypical Coats' disease are classified as severe, focal, juxtafoveal, or associated (with another disease) forms of idiopathic retinal telangiectasis with exudation.

b. Idiopathic retinal telangiectasis with exudation can be viewed as a spectrum of disease, synonymous with Coats' disease.

It has been postulated that the spectrum of disease severity seen in idiopathic retinal telangiectasis with exudation may be due to second somatic mutations in genes with an existing germline mutation (the two hit theory) and a mosaic phenotype.

Coats' plus encompasses a progressive familial syndrome of bilateral Coats' disease, characteristic cerebral calcification, leukoencephalopathy, slow pre- and postnatal linear growth, and defects of bone marrow and integument.

3. Coats' disease is the second most common lesion simulating retinoblastoma.

4. Clinically, Coats' disease may often be confused with retinoblastoma and presents as a pseudoglioma; rarely, retinoblastoma may simulate Coats' disease. Aqueous LDH may be elevated in both Coats' disease and retinoblastoma.

Bilateral cataract and Coats' disease have been reported in a child with Turner's syndrome and in a 3-month-old low-birth-weight infant.

B. *Leber's miliary aneurysms* (retinal telangiectasis) consists of fusiform and saccular dilatations (macroaneurysms) of venules and arterioles that surround a diffusely dilated capillary bed, and represents the earliest stage of Coats' disease.

1. The lesion tends to be unilateral in male patients and shows a propensity for a temporal (especially superior temporal) and parafoveal location, although any retinal quadrant can be affected.

2. The capillary bed shows coarse dilatation (telangiectasis), microaneurysms, and areas of nonperfusion. Arteriovenous communications may be seen.

3. The telangiectatic vessels leak fluid.

a. Leakage of fluid varies in amount from patient to patient, and even in the same patient at different times.

b. Coats' disease occurs when sufficient leakage of fluid results in subneural retinal exudation.

c. The affected globe tends to be significantly smaller than the uninvolved eye, unlike patients with retinoblastoma.

Acute open-angle glaucoma secondary to lipid crystals in the anterior chamber accompanying retinal detachment in Coats' disease may occur. Coats'-type retinal telangiectasis has accompanied Kabuki make-up syndrome or Niikawa–Kuroki syndrome. Coats' disease

---

may present as a prominent subfoveal nodule with peripheral retinal exudates in a 6-year-old boy.

C. Histologic characteristics are telangiectatic retinal vessels, an eosinophilic transudate (predominantly in a partially necrotic outer neural retinal layer), and a rich subneural retinal exudate containing foamy macrophages and evidence of cholesterol crystals.

Rarely, the cholesterol can be seen in the anterior chamber (cholesterolosis). Large, foamy cells in the neural retina and subneural retinal fluid probably arise from retinal pigment epithelial cells and macrophages. Rarely, intraocular bone formation in Coats' disease can cause confusion with retinoblastoma when calcium is seen by ultrasonography or CT.

D. Differential diagnosis

1. Idiopathic juxtafoveolar retinal telangiectasis (IJRT)

a. IJRT may be divided into four groups: (1) men with uniocular involvement, intraneural retinal lipid exudation, and telangiectasis largely confined to the temporal half of the juxtafoveolar area; (2) mostly men with symmetric areas of telangiectasis affecting the temporal half of the juxtafoveolar areas and minimal intraneural retinal exudation; (3) both sexes with symmetric involvement of all of the parafoveolar capillary bed and minimal exudation; and (4) telangiectasis with occlusive perifoveolar capillary changes and familial optic disc pallor.

b. The visual acuity prognosis in groups 1 to 3 is relatively good.

c. Ultrahigh-resolution optical coherence tomography (OCT) demonstrates: lack of correlation between retinal thickening on OCT and leakage on intravenous fluorescein angiography, loss and disruption of the photoreceptor layer, cyst-like structures in the foveola and within internal retinal layers such as the inner nuclear or ganglion cell layers, a unique internal limiting membrane draping across the foveola related to an underlying loss of tissue, intraretinal neovascularization near the fovea, and central intraretinal deposits and plaques.

d. Visual prognosis in IJRT depends upon type and clinical features; however, long-term prognosis for central vision is poor. Nevertheless, some therapies, such as combined treatment with photodynamic therapy and intravitreal triamcinolone, have resulted in regression of subfoveal neovascular membrane associated with IJRT.

2. A subgroup of familial retinal telangiectasis affects men and women, tends to be bilateral, and has a temporal parafoveal location.

3. Other forms of unilateral neural retinal telangiectasis may be associated with neural retinal angiomatosis, neural retinal capillary and cavernous

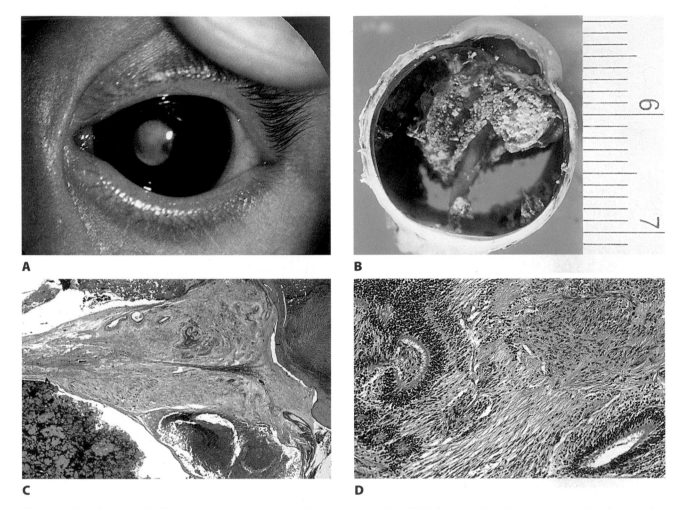

Fig. 18.21 Norrie's disease. **A,** Clinical appearance showing leukokoria in 5-month-old child. **B,** Gross specimen shows thickened, detached neural retina. **C,** Histologic section shows a detached gliotic neural retina with dysplastic areas. **D,** Areas of retinal dysplasia present. (Case presented by Dr. TP Dryja to the meeting of the Verhoeff Society, 1994.)

hemangioma, combined hamartoma of neural retina and retinal pigment epithelium, radiation retinopathy and branch retinal vein occlusion (both of which can produce an identical clinical appearance to Coats' disease), and retinal arterial macroaneurysm.

    4. Other forms of bilateral neural retinal telangiectasis may occur with ROP, retinitis pigmentosa, diabetic retinopathy, sickle-cell (SC) disease, sarcoidosis, hypogammaglobulinemia, muscular dystrophy, or Eales' disease.

VI. Norrie's disease (Fig. 18.21)

    A. It is a bilateral condition that starts in early childhood.

    B. Norrie's disease is transmitted in an X-linked recessive inheritance pattern.

        1. A putative gene for Norrie's disease has been isolated on chromosome Xp11.1.

Many disease-causing sequence variants have been identified; however a report of 14 French families with the disease has raised the question whether there has been misdiagnosis, phenocopies, or the existence of other X-linked or autosomal genes, the mutations of which would mimic the Norrie phenotype.

---

        a. Most mutations that cause Norrie's disease are deletions, frameshifts, or nonsense (premature stop) mutations, all null mutations producing no functional protein.

        b. The retinal dysplasia and gliosis found in Norrie's disease most probably result from the lack of a functional protein product.

    2. Sons of female carriers have a 50% risk for expressing the gene.

An extremely rare case of Norrie's disease has been reported in a girl who showed a mutation in the third exon (T776-A; Ile 123-Asn) identical to the mutation found in her two uncles, in whom Norrie's disease had been diagnosed.

---

    3. The prevalence of Norrie's disease is approximately 0.001%.

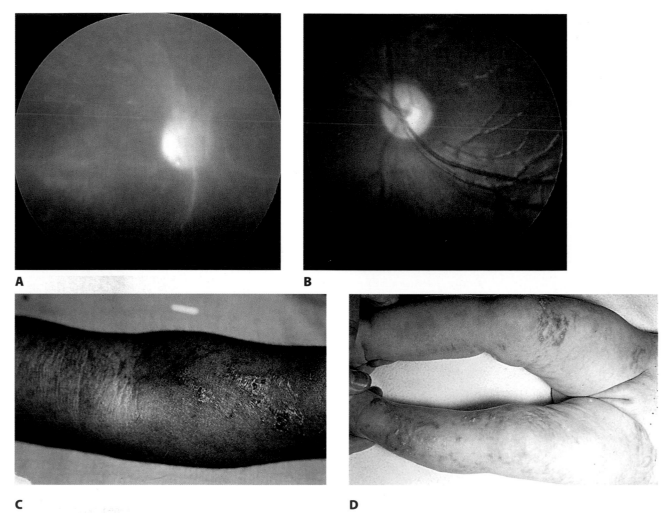

Fig. 18.22 Incontinentia pigmenti. **A** and **B,** Right and left fundi of patient who had incontinentia pigmenti. Fluorescein angiography showed stoppage of flow in both eyes just beyond four disc diameters from optic disc. Verrucous and nonelevated pigmented dermal lesions are present on the arms (**C**) and legs (**D**). The ocular histology is nonspecific.

C. It is characterized by deafness (approximately one-third of patients), mental retardation (approximately one-half to two-thirds of patients), cataract, and pseudoglioma.
   1. In infancy, a gray, vascularized mass is seen behind the lens in each eye.
   2. At approximately 1 year of age, corneal degeneration starts; cataracts follow by 2 years of age.
   3. In early childhood, the eyes, which were of normal size, start to shrink and become atrophic.
   4. The major pathologic event in the neural retina appears to occur before 25 weeks of gestation.
D. The histology is nonspecific, but hemorrhagic neural retinal detachment and neural retinal necrosis are common.

The cause may be neural retinal dysgenesis occurring early in the embryo (third to fourth gestational month) and involving the inner wall of the optic cup.

Norrin is the protein product of the Norrie disease gene. Norrin appears to play a crucial role in hyaloid vessel regression and in sprouting angiogenesis during retinal vasculature development, especially in the development of deep capillary networks. Ectopic norrin induces growth of ocular capillaries and restores normal angiogenesis in Norrie disease mutant mice. Norrin and Frizzled-4 (Fz4) function as a ligand-receptor pair and play a vital role in the vascular development of the eye and ear. Therefore, they may play an important role in the development of Norrie's disease.

VII. Incontinentia pigmenti (Bloch–Sulzberger syndrome; Fig. 18.22)
   A. Incontinentia pigmenti starts in infancy.
      It is a rare X chromosome-linked disorder, which is usually lethal in most male embryos so that the female-to-male ratio ranges from 20 to 37:1 (see later).
      a. The most frequent mutation, which accounts for >80% of new mutations, has been mapped

to Xq28 and is a deletion of part of the nuclear factor-kappaB essential modulator (NEMO) gene (NEMODelta4–10), although other mutations have been reported. Mutations of NEMO that do not abolish nuclear factor-kappaB activity permit male survival, causing an allelic variant of incontinentia pigmenti called hypohidrotic ectodermal dysplasia. A mutation in exon 7 of NEMO gene has been reported, which results in selection against the mutated X chromosome in this X-linked disease.

b. Molecular studies are required, in particular, of families with affected males lacking supernumerary X chromosomes to determine the exact mutation of the NEMO gene involved.

c. Incontinentia pigmenti associated with Klinefelter's syndrome (47,XXY), hypomorphic alleles, and somatic mosaicism are three mechanisms for survival of males carrying a NEMO mutation.

The identification of an incontinentia pigmenti patient with a 650-kb duplication at the X chromosome breakpoint in a patient with 46,X,t (X;8) (q28;q12) and non-syndromic mental retardation is further evidence for Xq28 being an unstable region of the human chromosome.

B. The dermal lesions can be divided into four stages:

1. An initial vesiculobullous stage of inflammatory papules, blisters, and pustules that are characterized histopathologically by acanthosis, keratocyte necrosis, epidermal spongiosis, and massive epidermal eosinophil infiltration.

The cause for the eosinophil accumulation has not yet been determined; however, it has been suggested that the release of cytokines during the initial inflammatory stage of incontinentia pigmenti induces epidermal expression of eotaxin, which may play a role in the epidermal accumulation of eosinophils. Late recurrence of the inflammatory first stage of incontinentia pigmenti may occur, suggesting that mutated cells can persist a long time in the epidermis. These recurrences may be triggered by infections.

---

2. A verrucous pigmented stage (noted at a few months of life and lasting several months)

Painful subungual tumors consistent with the late verrucous stage of incontinentia pigmenti have been reported, including involvement of more than one generation of the same family.

---

3. A pigmented nonelevated stage (noted at approximately 4 to 6 months of life)
4. An atrophic stage.

Whorled scarring alopecia corresponds to the lines of Blaschko, is permanent, and can be used as a marker for affected adult women who may no longer have other cutaneous manifestations.

C. Central nervous system involvement consists of calvarial deformities, microcephaly, convulsions, paresis, and mental retardation

D. Ocular findings are strabismus, nystagmus, vortex (whorl-like) keratitis, blue sclera, myopia, and pseudoglioma.
   1. Intraocular calcification and retinal detachment in this disorder have suggested the misdiagnosis of retinoblastoma; however, the presence of characteristic skin lesions can be helpful in making the correct diagnosis.

E. Dental abnormalities (e.g., delayed dentition and missing and peg-shaped teeth) are usually present. Permanent anterior teeth with a longer crown and a shorter root may be related to incontinentia pigmenti.

   Cardiovascular anomalies and cerebral infarction are also rare complications.

G. The inheritance pattern is X-linked dominant, but girls predominate.

Boys are hemizygous (i.e., they have only one of any of the genes found in the X chromosome). Thus, a mutant X chromosomal gene that codes for a structural protein (hence a dominant gene) would be the equivalent of a homozygous autosomal-dominant mutation that is usually lethal or sublethal for boys. It is thought that male fetuses with incontinentia pigmenti are aborted spontaneously, which is why the condition occurs almost exclusively in girls.

H. The histology is nonspecific.
   1. The RPE may show nodular proliferation and contain increased lipofuscin.
   2. Nonrhegmatogenous neural retinal detachment, foveal hypoplasia, intraocular hemorrhage, and neural retinal necrosis are common.

The neural retinal changes are similar to those seen in ROP and familial exudative retinopathy. Fluorescein studies of incontinentia pigmenti have shown changes consistent with an initial obliterative endarteritis starting peripherally and proceeding centrally. The arterioles ultimately become occluded. The differential diagnosis of incontinentia pigmenti includes conditions that cause peripheral neural retinal nonperfusion, preneural retinal neovascularization, infantile neural retinal detachment, and foveal hypoplasia.

VIII. Massive neural retinal fibrosis is caused by organization of a massive neural retinal hemorrhage in the newborn. Organization, fibrogliosis, and contracture may simulate growth of a retinoblastoma.

IX. Metastatic retinitis

X. Endogenous endophthalmitis
   A. Rarely, endogenous endophthalmitis presents clinically in such a fashion as to simulate retinoblastoma.

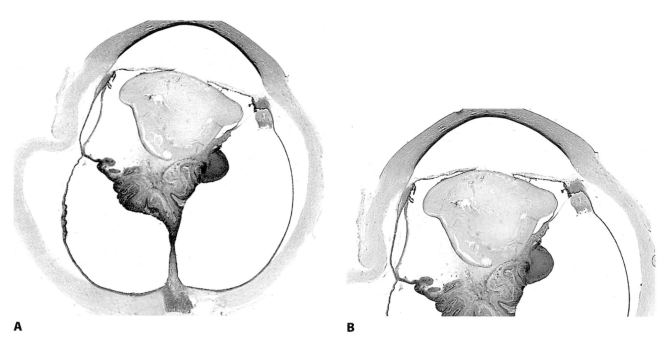

A   **B**

Fig. 18.23 Congenital nonattachment of neural retina. **A,** Periodic acid–Schiff-stained histologic section shows posterior lenticonus and congenital nonattachment of neural retina in infant eye enucleated because of suspected retinoblastoma (increased magnification in **B**).

B. The ocular findings are usually the primary findings and overshadow the systemic infection.

C. Causes include streptococcal, cytomegalovirus, *Candida*, and idiopathic endophthalmitis.

XI. Congenital nonattachment of neural retina (Fig. 18.23; see p. 398 in Chapter 11)

XII. Secondary neural retinal detachment

XIII. Juvenile retinoschisis (see Fig. 11.33)

XIV. Medulloepithelioma ("diktyoma"; see Figs 17.17 and 17.18)

XV. Melanogenic neuroectodermal tumor of the retina (primary malignant melanoma of the retina) may simulate retinoblastoma in infants.

XVI. Leukocoria may be caused by congenital cataract and be confused with a retinoblastoma.

XVII. Solitary, large retinal astrocytoma may mimic retinoblastoma both clinically and ultrasonographically without clinical findings of tuberous sclerosis or neurofibromatosis.

    A. Retinal astrocytomas may enlarge, and be accompanied by retinal detachment and vitreous seeding, which can lead to the erroneous diagnosis of retinoblastoma or melanoma.

    B. Further complicating the diagnostic picture, retinoblastoma and retinal astrocytoma have been reported to occur in the same eye.

XVIII. Intraocular heterotopic brain tissue can produce leukocoria.

XIX. *Osteoporosis–pseudoglioma syndrome* is characterized by severe juvenile-onset osteoporosis and congenital or early-onset blindness. It is a rare disorder that is autosomal recessive in inheritance. It can be accompanied by muscular hypotonia, ligament laxity, mild mental retardation, and seizures. The involved gene is the low-density lipoprotein receptor-related family member *LRP5* located on chromosome 11q11–12.

XX. Inflammatory pseudotumor in a 1-year-old girl has simulated retinoblastoma, resulting in enucleation.

Discrete Retinal or Chorioretinal Lesions

I. Small endophytic tumors

    A. Retinal hamartomas

        1. Tuberous sclerosis (see Chapter 2)

        2. Neurofibromatosis (see Chapter 2)

    B. Myelinated (medullated) nerve fibers (see Fig. 11.6)

    C. Coloboma of choroid (see pp. 338–339 in Chapter 9)

    D. Retinochoroiditis—when deposits of white exudates are present on the neural retina, retinochoroiditis is easily confused with retinoblastoma.

II. Small exophytic tumors

    A. Coats' disease may occur as a localized posterior lesion.

    B. Larval (*Toxocara canis*) granulomas may present in posterior locations.

    C. Choroiditis or acute exudative retinitis with subneural retinal exudate

    D. von Hippel–Lindau angiomatosis (see p. 29 in Chapter 2)

    E. Proliferative lesions of retinal pigment epithelium

BIBLIOGRAPHY

Retinoblastoma

General Information

Abramson DH, Frank CM: Second nonocular tumors in survivors of bilateral retinoblastoma: A possible age effect on radiation-related risk. *Ophthalmology* 105:573, 1998

Abramson DH, Melson M, Dunkel IJ *et al.*: Third (fourth and fifth) nonocular tumors in survivors of retinoblastoma. *Ophthalmology* 108:1868, 2001

Albert DM: Historic review of retinoblastoma. *Ophthalmology* 94:654, 1987

Bach LE, McCormick B, Abramson DH *et al.*: Trilateral retinoblastoma—incidence and outcome: A decade of experience. *Int J Radiat Oncol Biol Phys* 29:729, 1994

Beck PM, Balmer A, Maeder P *et al.*: Benign pineal cysts in children with bilateral retinoblastoma: a new variant of trilateral retinoblastoma? *Pediatr Blood Cancer* 46:755, 2006

Biswasm J, Manim B, Shanmugam MP *et al.*: Retinoblastoma in adults: Report of three cases and review of the literature. *Surv Ophthalmol* 44:409, 2000

Brinkert AW, Jager MJ, Otter WD *et al.*: Distribution of tumors in the retina in hereditary retinoblastoma patients. *Ophthalmic Genet* 19:63, 1998

Brucker B, Ernst L, Meadows A *et al.*: A second leiomyosarcoma in the urinary bladder of a child with a history of retinoblastoma 12 years following partial cystectomy. *Pediatr Blood Cancer* 46:811, 2006

Dunphy EB: The story of retinoblastoma. *Trans Am Acad Ophthalmol Otolaryngol* 68:249, 1964

Finol HJ, Marquez A, Navas E *et al.*: Extraocular muscle ultrastructural pathology in the paraneoplastic phenomenon associated with retinoblastoma. *J Exp Clin Cancer Res* 20:281, 2001

Harbour JW: Overview of RB gene mutations in patients with retinoblastoma: Implications for clinical genetic screening. *Ophthalmology* 105:1442, 1998

Irvine AR, Albert DM, Sang DN: Retinal neoplasia and dysplasia: II. Retinoblastoma occurring with persistence and hyperplasia of the primary vitreous. *Invest Ophthalmol Vis Sci* 16:403, 1977

Jain IS, Mohan K, Jain S: Retinoblastoma: Clinical and pathologic correlations. *J Ocul Ther Surg* 4:86, 1985

Jain IS, Mohan K, Jain S *et al.*: Retinoblastoma: Modes of presentation. *J Ocul Ther Surg* 4:83, 1985

Kivelä T, Tupperman K, Riikonen P *et al.*: Retinoblastoma associated with chromosome 13q14 deletion mosaicism. *Ophthalmology* 110:1983, 2003

Lueder GT, Judisch GF, Wen BC: Heritable retinoblastoma and pinealoma. *Arch Ophthalmol* 109:1707, 1991

Madigan MC, Penfold PL, King NJ *et al.*: Immunoglobulin superfamily expression in primary retinoblastoma and retinoblastoma cell lines. *Oncol Res* 13:103, 2002

Marcus DM, Brooks SE, Leff G *et al.*: Trilateral retinoblastoma: Insights into histogenesis and management. *Surv Ophthalmol* 43:59, 1998

Mietz H, Hutton WL, Font RL: Unilateral retinoblastoma in an adult: Report of a case and review of the literature. *Ophthalmology* 104:43, 1997

Mohney BG, Robertson DM, Schomberg PJ *et al.*: Second nonocular tumors in survivors of heritable retinoblastoma and prior radiation therapy. *Am J Ophthalmol* 126:269, 1998

Moll CL, Imhof SM, Schouten-Van Meeteren AYN *et al.*: Second primary tumors in hereditary retinoblastoma: A register-based study, 1945–1997: Is there an age effect on radiation-related risk? *Ophthalmology* 108:979, 2001

Murphree AL: Intraocular retinoblastoma: the case for a new group classification. *Ophthalmol Clin North Am* 18:41, 2005

Palazzi MA, Yunes JA, Cardinalli IA *et al.*: Detection of oncogenic human papillomavirus in sporadic retinoblastoma. *Acta Ophthalmol Scand* 81:396, 2003

Sawan A, Randall B, Angus B *et al.*: Retinoblastoma and p53 gene expression related to relapse and survival in human breast cancer: An immunohistochemical study. *J Pathol* 168:23, 1992

Schocket LS, Beaverson KL, Rollins IS *et al.*: Bilateral retinoblastoma, microphthalmia, and colobomas in the 13q deletion syndrome. *Arch Ophthalmol* 121:916, 2003

Shields CL, Mashayekhi A, Au AK *et al.*: The International Classification of Retinoblastoma predicts chemoreduction success. *Ophthalmology* 113:2276, 2006

Shields CL, Mashayekhi A, Demirci H *et al.*: Practical approach to management of retinoblastoma. *Arch Ophthalmol* 122.729, 2004

Shields CL, Shields JA, Shah P: Retinoblastoma in older children. *Ophthalmology* 98:395, 1991

Smith JH, Murray TG, Fulton L *et al.*: Siblings of retinoblastoma patients: Are we underestimating their risk? *Am J Ophthalmol* 129:396, 2000

Tamboli A, Podgor MJ, Horm JW: The incidence of retinoblastoma in the United States: 1974 through 1985. *Arch Ophthalmol* 108:128, 1990

Wilson GA, Devaux A, Aroichane M: Retinoblastoma, microphthalmia and the chromosome 13q deletion syndrome. *Clin Exp Ophthalmol* 32:101, 2004

Heredity

Belt PJ, Smithers M, Elston T: The triad of bilateral retinoblastoma, dysplastic naevus syndrome and multiple cutaneous malignant melanomas: a case report and review of the literature. *Melanoma Res* 12:179, 2002

Bojinova RI, Schorderet DF, Addor MC *et al.*: Further delineation of the facial 13q14 deletion syndrome in 13 retinoblastoma patients. *Ophthalmic Genet* 22:11, 2001

Brichard B, Heusterspreute M, De PP *et al.*: Unilateral retinoblastoma, lack of familial history and older age does not exclude germline RB1 gene mutation. *Eur J Cancer* 42:65, 2006

Bunin GR, Emanuel BS, Meadows AT *et al.*: Frequency of 13q abnormalities among 203 patients with retinoblastoma. *J Natl Cancer Inst* 81:370, 1989

Cibis GW, Freeman AI, Pang V *et al.*: Bilateral choroidal neonatal neuroblastoma. *Am J Ophthalmol* 109:445, 1990

Corson TW, Huang A, Tsao MS *et al.*: KIF14 is a candidate oncogene in the 1q minimal region of genomic gain in multiple cancers. *Oncogene* 24:4741, 2005

de Jong PT, Mooy CM, Stoter G *et al.*: Late-onset retinoblastoma in a well-functioning fellow eye. *Ophthalmology* 113:1040, 2006

Harbour JW: Overview of RB gene mutations in patients with retinoblastoma: Implications for clinical genetic screening. *Ophthalmology* 105:1442, 1998

Harbour JW, Lai S-L, Whang-Peng J *et al.*: Abnormalities in structure and expression of the human retinoblastoma gene in SCLC. *Science* 241:353, 1988

Keith CG, Webb GC: Retinoblastoma and retinoma occurring in a child with a translocation and deletion of the long arm of chromosome 13. *Arch Ophthalmol* 103:941, 1985

Lavanchy L, Munier FL, Cousin P *et al.*: Molecular characterization of the deletion in retinoblastoma patients with 13q14 cytogenetic anomalies. *Ophthalmic Genet* 22:1, 2001

Lee W-H, Bookstein R, Hong F et al.: Human retinoblastoma susceptibility gene: Cloning, identification, and sequence. *Science* 235:1394, 1987

Lemieux J, Milot J, Barsoum-Homsy M et al.: First cytogenetic evidence of homozygosity for the retinoblastoma deletion in chromosome 13. *Cancer Genet Cytogenet* 43:73, 1989

mare Kadam PS, Ghule P, Jose J et al.: Constitutional genomic instability, chromosome aberrations in tumor cells and retinoblastoma. *Cancer Genet Cytogenet* 150:33, 2004

Marx J: Oncogenes reach a milestone. *Science* 266:1942, 1994

Naumova A, Sapienza C: The genetics of retinoblastoma, revisited. *Am J Hum Genet* 54:264, 1994

Naumova A, Hansen M, Strong L et al.: Concordance between parental origin of chromosome 13q loss and chromosome 6p duplication in sporadic retinoblastoma. *Am J Hum Genet* 54:274, 1994

Notis CM, Niksarli K, Abramson DH et al.: Parents with unilateral retinoblastoma: Their affected children. *Br J Ophthalmol* 80:197, 1996

Roarty JD, McLean IW, Zimmerman LE: Incidence of second neoplasms in patients with bilateral retinoblastoma. *Ophthalmology* 95:1583, 1988

Scheffer H, te Meerman GJ, Kruize GJ et al.: Linkage analysis of families with hereditary retinoblastoma: Nonpenetrance of mutation, revealed by combined use of markers within and flanking the RBI gene. *Am J Hum Genet* 45:252, 1989

Schwartz IV, Felix TM, Riegel M et al.: Atypical macrocephaly-cutis marmorata telangiectatica congenita with retinoblastoma. *Clin Dysmorphol* 11:199, 2002

Simpson JL, Carson SA, Cisneros P: Preimplantation genetic diagnosis (PGD) for heritable neoplasia. *J Natl Cancer Inst Monogr* 87, 2005

T'Ang A, Varley JM, Chakraborty S et al.: Structural rearrangement of the retinoblastoma gene in human breast carcinoma. *Science* 242:263, 1988

Tsai T, Gombos D, Fulton L et al.: Retinoblastoma and hypochondroplasia: a case report of two germline mutations arising simultaneously. *Ophthalmic Genet* 26:107, 2005

Tucker T, Friedman JM: Pathogenesis of hereditary tumors: beyond the "two-hit" hypothesis. *Clin Genet* 62:345, 2002

Wiggs DL, Dryja TP: Predicting the risk of hereditary retinoblastoma. *Am J Ophthalmol* 106:346, 1988

Wiggs J, Nordenskjold M, Yandell D et al.: Prediction of the risk of hereditary retinoblastoma using DNA polymorphisms within the retinoblastoma gene. *N Engl J Med* 318:151, 1988

Yandell DW, Campbell TA, Dayton SH et al.: Oncogenic point mutations in the human retinoblastoma gene: their application to genetic counseling. *N Engl J Med* 321:1689, 1989

Zhu X, Dunn JM, Phillips RA et al.: Preferential germline mutation of the paternal allele in retinoblastoma. *Nature* 340:312, 1989

Clinical Features

Assegid A: Pattern of ophthalmic lesions at two histopathology centres in Ethiopia. *East Afr Med J* 78:250, 2001

Badhu B, Sah SP, Thakur SK et al.: Clinical presentation of retinoblastoma in Eastern Nepal. *Clin Exp Ophthalmol* 33:386, 2005

Benson WE, Cameron JD, Furgiuele FP et al.: Presumed spontaneously regressed retinoblastoma. *Ann Ophthalmol* 10:897, 1978

Biswas J, Das D, Krishnakumar S et al.: Histopathologic analysis of 232 eyes with retinoblastoma conducted in an Indian tertiary-care ophthalmic center. *J Pediatr Ophthalmol Strabismus* 40:265, 2003

de GP, Barkhof F, Moll AC et al.: Retinoblastoma: MR imaging parameters in detection of tumor extent. *Radiology* 235:197, 2005

Finger PT, Khoobehi A, Ponce-Contreras MR et al.: Three dimensional ultrasound of retinoblastoma: initial experience. *Br J Ophthalmol* 86:1136, 2002

Finger PT, Meskin SW, Wisnicki HJ et al.: High-frequency ultrasound of anterior segment retinoblastoma. *Am J Ophthalmol* 137:944, 2004

Gizewski ER, Wanke I, Jurklies C et al.: T1 Gd-enhanced compared with CISS sequences in retinoblastoma: superiority of T1 sequences in evaluation of tumour extension. *Neuroradiology* 47:56, 2005

Heinrich T, Messmer EP, Höpping W et al.: Das Metastasierungsrisiko beim Retinoblastom [the metastatic risk in retinoblastoma]. *Klin Monatsbl Augenheilkd* 199:319, 1991

Kao LY, Su WW, Lin YW: Retinoblastoma in Taiwan: survival and clinical characteristics 1978–2000. *Jpn J Ophthalmol* 46:577, 2002

Karcioglu ZA: Fine needle aspiration biopsy (FNAB) for retinoblastoma. *Retina* 22:707, 2002

Kramer TR, Watanabe TM, Miller JM et al.: Unilateral retinoblastoma presenting as acute secondary glaucoma with intraocular inflammation. *Ophthalmic Pract* 17:20, 1999

Materin MA, Shields CL, Shields JA et al.: Diffuse retinoblastoma simulating uveitis in a 7-year-old boy. *Arch Ophthalmol* 118:418, 2000

McCaffery S, Simon EM, Fischbein NJ et al.: Three-dimensional high-resolution magnetic resonance imaging of ocular and orbital malignancies. *Arch Ophthalmol* 120:747, 2002

Morgan KS, McLean IW: Retinoblastoma and persistent hyperplastic vitreous occurring in the same patient. *Ophthalmology* 88:1087, 1981

Mozorrutia-Alegria V, Bravo-Ortiz JC, Vazquez-Viveros J et al.: Epidemiological characteristics of retinoblastoma in children attending the Mexican Social Security Institute in Mexico City, 1990–94. *Paediatr Perinat Epidemiol* 16:370, 2002

Pe'er J, Neufeld M, Baras M et al.: Rubeosis iridis in retinoblastoma: Histologic findings and the possible role of vascular endothelial growth factor in its induction. *Ophthalmology* 104:1251, 1997

Puig JJ, Arrondo E, Garcia-Arumí J et al.: Multiple anterior chamber cystic lesions as the first sign of advanced retinoblastoma. *Arch Ophthalmol* 120:1385, 2002

Sanders BM, Draper GJ, Kingston JE: Retinoblastoma in Great Britain 1969–80: Incidence treatment, and survival. *Br J Ophthalmol* 72:576, 1988

Sang DN, Albert DM: Retinoblastoma: Clinical and histopathologic features. *Hum Pathol* 13:133, 1982

Shields CL, Shields JA, Pankajkumar S: Retinoblastoma in older children. *Ophthalmology* 98:395, 1991

Shields JA, Shields CL, Suvarnamani C et al.: Retinoblastoma manifesting as orbital cellulitis. *Am J Ophthalmol* 112:442, 1991

Stafford WR, Yanoff M, Parnell BL: Retinoblastoma initially misdiagnosed as primary ocular inflammations. *Arch Ophthalmol* 82:771, 1969

Takahashi T, Tamura S, Inoue M et al.: Retinoblastoma in a 26-year-old adult. *Ophthalmology* 90:179, 1983

Tamboli A, Podgor MJ, Horm JW: The incidence of retinoblastoma in the United States: 1974 through 1985. *Arch Ophthalmol* 108:128, 1990

Histology

Abramson DH, Greenfield DS, Ellsworth RM et al.: Neuron-specific enolase and retinoblastoma. *Retina* 9:148, 1989

Agarwal M, Biswas JSK, Shanmugam MP: Retinoblastoma presenting as orbital cellulitis: report of four cases with a review of the literature. *Orbit* 23:93, 2004

Antoneli CB, Steinhorst F, de Cassia Braga RK et al.: Extraocular retinoblastoma: a 13-year experience. *Cancer* 98:1292, 2003

Barr FG, Chatten J, D'Cruz CM et al.: Molecular assays for chromosomal translocations in the diagnosis of pediatric soft tissue sarcomas. *JAMA* 273:553, 1995

Bhatnagar R, Vine AK: Diffuse infiltrating retinoblastoma. *Ophthalmology* 98:1657, 1991

Burnier MN, McLean IW, Zimmerman LE et al.: Retinoblastoma. *Invest Ophthalmol Vis Sci* 31:2037, 1990

Detrick B, Evans CH, Chader G et al.: Cytokine-induced modulation of cellular proteins in retinoblastoma. *Invest Ophthalmol Vis Sci* 32:1714, 1991

Dyer MA, Bremner R: The search for the retinoblastoma cell of origin. *Nat Rev Cancer* 5:91, 2005

Eagle RC, Shields JA, Donoso L et al.: Malignant transformation of spontaneously regressed retinoblastoma, retinoma/retinocytoma variant. *Ophthalmology* 96:1389, 1989

Gass P, Frankfurter A, Katsetos CD et al.: Antigenic expression of neuron-associated class 111 beta-tubulin isotype (hB4) and microtubule-associated protein 2 (map2) by the human retinoblastoma cell line WERI-Rb1. *Ophthalmic Res* 22:57, 1990

Haik BG, Dunleavy SA, Cooke C et al.: Retinoblastoma with anterior chamber extension. *Ophthalmology* 94:367, 1987

He W, Hashimoto H, Tsuneyoshi M et al.: A reassessment of histologic classification and an immunohistochemical study of 88 retinoblastomas: A special reference to the advent of bipolar-like cells. *Cancer* 70:2901, 1992

Hogan MJ, Zimmerman LE, eds: *Ophthalmic Pathology: An Atlas and Text*, 2nd edn. Philadelphia, WB Saunders, 1962:519

Howard MLA, Dryja TP, Walton DS et al.: Identification and significance of multinucleate tumor cells in retinoblastoma. *Arch Ophthalmol* 107:1025, 1989

Katsetos CD, Herman MM, Frankfirter A et al.: Neuron-associated class 111 sB-tubulin isotype, microtubule-associated protein 2, and synaptophysin in human retinoblastomas in situ. *Lab Invest* 64:45, 1991

Korswagen LA, Moll AC, Imhof SM et al.: A second primary tumor in a patient with retinoma. *Ophthalmic Genet* 25:45, 2004

Leal-Leal CA, Rivera-Luna R, Flores-Rojo M et al.: Survival in extra-orbital metastatic retinoblastoma: treatment results. *Clin Transl Oncol* 8:39, 2006

Lin CCL, Tso MOM: An electron microscopic study of calcification of retinoblastoma. *Am J Ophthalmol* 96:765, 1983

Loeffler KU, McMenamin PG: An ultrastructural study of DNA precipitation in the anterior segment of eyes with retinoblastoma. *Ophthalmology* 94:1160, 1987

Marcus DM, Craft JL, Albert DM: Histopathologic verification of Verhoeff's 1918 irradiation cure of retinoblastoma. *Ophthalmology* 97:221, 1990

Nork TM, Millecchia LL, Poulsen G: Immunolocalization of the retinoblastoma protein in the human eye and in retinoblastoma. *Invest Ophthalmol Vis Sci* 35:2682, 1994

Nork TM, Schwartz TL, Doshi HM et al.: Retinoblastoma: Cell of origin. *Arch Ophthalmol* 113:791, 1995

Sawaguchi S, Peng Y, Wong F et al.: An immunopathologic study of retinoblastoma protein. *Trans Am Ophthalmol Soc* 88:51, 1990

Sawai J, Nakazato Y, Yamane Y et al.: Immunohistochemical localization of human pineal tissue antigens in normal retina and retinoblastomas. *Neuropathology* 23:119, 2003

Schouten-Van Meeteren AY, van d V, van der Linden HC et al.: Histopathologic features of retinoblastoma and its relation with in vitro drug resistance measured by means of the MTT assay. *Cancer* 92:2933, 2001

Shuler RK Jr, Hubbard GB III, Grossniklaus HE: Retinal neovascularization associated with retinoblastoma. *Am J Ophthalmol* 139:210, 2005

Singh AD, Santos MCM, Shields CL et al.: Observations on 17 patients with retinocytoma. *Arch Ophthalmol* 118:199, 2000

Skubitz APN, Grossman MD, McCarthy JB et al.: The decreased adhesion of Y79 retinoblastoma cells to extracellular matrix proteins is due to a deficit of integrin receptors. *Invest Ophthalmol Vis Sci* 35:2820, 1994

Tso MOM, Fine BS, Zimmerman LE: The Flexner–Wintersteiner rosettes in retinoblastoma. *Arch Pathol* 88:664, 1969

Tso MOM, Zimmerman LE, Fine BS: The nature of retinoblastoma: I. Photoreceptor differentiation. *Am J Ophthalmol* 69:339, 1970

Tso MOM, Fine BS, Zimmerman LE: The nature of retinoblastoma: II. An electron microscopic study. *Am J Ophthalmol* 69:350, 1970

Tsuji M, Goto M, Uehara F et al.: Photoreceptor cell differentiation in retinoblastoma demonstrated by a new immunohistochemical marker mucin-like glycoprotein associated with photoreceptor cells (MLGAPC). *Histopathology* 40:180, 2002

Tulvatana W, Adamian M, Berson EL et al.: Photoreceptor rosettes in autosomal dominant retinitis pigmentosa with reduced penetrance. *Arch Ophthalmol* 117:399, 1999

Wang AG, Lai CR, Hsu WM et al.: Clinicopathologic factors related to apoptosis in retinoblastoma. *J Pediatr Ophthalmol Strabismus* 38:295, 2001

Wright JH: Neurocytoma or neuroblastoma, a kind of tumor not generally recognized. *J Exp Med* 12:556, 1910

Yamashita N, Nishiuchi R, Oda M et al.: Molecular detection of metastatic retinoblastoma cells by reverse transcription polymerase reaction for interphotoreceptor retinoid-binding protein mRNA. *Cancer* 91:1568, 2001

Yanoff M: The rosettes of James Homer Wright (letter). *Arch Ophthalmol* 108:167, 1990

Prognosis

Abramson DH, Frank CM: Second nonocular tumors in survivors of bilateral retinoblastoma: A possible age effect on radiation-related risk. *Ophthalmology* 105:573, 1998

Bautista D, Emanuel JR, Granville C et al.: Identification of mutations in the K-ras gene in human retinoblastoma. *Invest Ophthalmol Vis Sci* 37:2313, 1996

Camassei FD, Cozza R, Acquaviva A et al.: Expression of the lipogenic enzyme fatty acid synthase (FAS) in retinoblastoma and its correlation with tumor aggressiveness. *Invest Ophthalmol Vis Sci* 44:2399, 2003

Eng C, Li FP, Abramson DH et al.: Mortality from second tumors among long-term survivors of retinoblastoma. *Cancer Inst* 85:1121, 1993

Finger PT, Harbour JW, Karcioglu ZA: Risk factors for metastasis in retinoblastoma. *Surv Ophthalmol* 47:1, 2002

Gatta G, Capocaccia R, Stiller C et al.: Childhood cancer survival trends in Europe: a EUROCARE Working Group study. *J Clin Oncol* 23:3742, 2005

Helton KJ, Fletcher BD, Kun LE et al.: Bone tumors other than osteosarcoma after retinoblastoma. *Cancer* 71:2847, 1993

Karatza EC, Shields CL, Flanders AE et al.: Pineal cyst simulating pinealoblastoma in 11 children with retinoblastoma. *Arch Ophthalmol* 124:595, 2006

Kerimogglu H, Kiratli H, Dincturk AA et al.: Quantitative analysis of proliferation, apoptosis, and angiogenesis in retinoblastoma and their association with the clinicopathologic parameters. *Jpn J Ophthalmol* 47:565, 2003

Khelfaoui F, Validire P, Auperin A et al.: Histopathologic risk factors in retinoblastoma: A retrospective study of 172 patients treated in a single institution. *Cancer* 77:1206, 1996

Kivela T, sko-Seljavaara S, Pihkala U et al.: Sebaceous carcinoma of the eyelid associated with retinoblastoma. *Ophthalmology* 108:1124, 2001

Kopelman JE, McLean IW, Rosenberg SH: Multivariate analysis of risk factors for metastasis in retinoblastoma treated by enucleation. *Ophthalmology* 94:371, 1987

Lam BL, Judisch GF, Sobol WM *et al.*: Visual prognosis in macular retinoblastomas. *Am J Ophthalmol* 110:229, 1990

Lueder GT, Judish GF, O'Gorman TW: Second nonocular tumors in survivors of heritable retinoblastoma. *Arch Ophthalmol* 104:372, 1986

Magramm I, Abramson DH, Ellsworth RM: Optic nerve involvement in retinoblastoma. *Ophthalmology* 96:217, 1989

Marback EF, Arias VE, Paranhos A Jr *et al.*: Tumour angiogenesis as a prognostic factor for disease dissemination in retinoblastoma. *Br J Ophthalmol* 87:1224, 2003

Mashayekhi A, Shields CL, Eagle RC Jr *et al.*: Cavitary changes in retinoblastoma: relationship to chemoresistance. *Ophthalmology* 112:1145, 2005

Mendoza AE, Shew JY, Lee E *et al.*: A case of synovial sarcoma with abnormal expression of the human retinoblastoma susceptibility gene. *Hum Pathol* 19:487, 1988

Messmer EP, Heinrich LT, Hopping W *et al.*: Risk factors for metastases in patients with retinoblastoma. *Ophthalmology* 98:136, 1991

Mohney BG, Robertson DM: Ancillary testing for metastasis in patients with newly diagnosed retinoblastoma. *Am J Ophthalmol* 118:707, 1994

Notis CM, Niksarli K, Abramson DH *et al.*: Parents with unilateral retinoblastoma: Their affected children. *Br J Ophthalmol* 80:197, 1996

Pinarli FG, Oguz A, Karadeniz C *et al.*: Second primary myogenic sarcoma in a patient with bilateral retinoblastoma. *Pediatr Hematol Oncol* 21:545, 2004

Roarty JD, McLean IW, Zimmerman LE: Incidence of second neoplasms in patients with bilateral retinoblastoma. *Ophthalmology* 95:1583, 1988

Rossler J, Dietrich T, Pavlakovic H *et al.*: Higher vessel densities in retinoblastoma with local invasive growth and metastasis. *Am J Pathol* 164:391, 2004

Shields CL, Shields JA, Baez KA *et al.*: Choroidal invasion of retinoblastoma: Metastatic potential and clinical risk factors. *Br J Ophthalmol* 77:544, 1993

Shields CL, Shields JA, Baez KA *et al.*: Optic nerve invasion of retinoblastoma: Metastatic potential and clinical risk factors. *Cancer* 73:692, 1994

T'Ang A, Varley JM, Chakraborty S *et al.*: Structural rearrangement of the retinoblastoma gene in human breast carcinoma. *Science* 242:263, 1988

Traboulsi EI, Zimmerman LE, Manz HJ: Cutaneous malignant melanoma in survivors of heritable retinoblastoma. *Arch Ophthalmol* 106:1059, 1988

Pseudoglioma

General Information

Guemes A, Wright KW, Humayun M *et al.*: Leukocoria caused by occult penetrating trauma in a child. *Am J Ophthalmol* 124:117, 1997

Paysee EA, Coats D, Chévez-Barrios P: An unusual case of leukocoria: Heterotopic brain arising from the retina. *Arch Ophthalmol* 121:119, 2003

Shields JA, Parsons HM, Shields CL *et al.*: Lesions simulating retinoblastoma. *J Pediatr Ophthalmol Strabismus* 28:338, 1991

Shields JA, Shields CL, Parsons HM: Differential diagnosis of retinoblastoma. *Retina* 11:232, 1991

Yanoff M: Pseudogliomas: differential diagnosis of retinoblastoma. *Ophthalmol Dig* 34:9, 1972

Leukokoria: Persistent Hyperplastic Primary Vitreous

Caudill JW, Streeten BW, Tso MOM: Phacoanaphylactoid reaction in persistent hyperplastic primary vitreous. *Ophthalmology* 92:1153, 1985

Chang BM, Liebmann JM, Ritch R: Angle closure in younger patients. *Trans Am Ophthalmol Soc* 100:201, 2002

Font RL, Yanoff M, Zimmerman LE: Intraocular adipose tissue and persistent hyperplastic primary vitreous. *Arch Ophthalmol* 82:43, 1969

Fryssira H, Papathanassiou M, Barbounaki J *et al.*: A male with polysyndactyly, linear skin defects and sclerocornea. Goltz syndrome versus MIDAS. *Clin Dysmorphol* 11:277, 2002

Fujita H, Yoshii A, Maeda J *et al.*: Genitourinary anomaly in congenital varicella syndrome: case report and review. *Pediatr Nephrol* 19:554, 2004

Goldberg MF: Persistent fetal vasculature (PFV): An integrated interpretation of signs and symptoms associated with persistent hyperplastic primary vitreous (PHPV). LIV Edward Jackson Memorial Lecture. *Am J Ophthalmol* 124:587, 1997

Guigis MF, White FV, Dunbar JA *et al.*: Optic nerve teratoma and odontogenic dermoid cyst in a neonate with persistent fetal vasculature. *Arch Ophthalmol* 120:1582, 2002

Hermsen VM, Conahan JB, Koops BL *et al.*: Persistent hyperplastic primary vitreous associated with protein C deficiency. *Am J Ophthalmol* 109:608, 1990

Khaliq S, Hameed A, Ismail M *et al.*: Locus for autosomal recessive nonsyndromic persistent hyperplastic primary vitreous. *Invest Ophthalmol Vis Sci* 42:2225, 2001

Khan AO: Buphthalmos in the setting of persistent hyperplastic primary vitreous cataract. *Am J Ophthalmol* 136:945, 2003

Lee SJ, Ling JX, Aaberg TM *et al.*: Lenticular fibroxanthomatous nodule. *Am J Ophthalmol* 135:229, 2003

Nguyen DQ, Chatterjee S, Bates R: Persistent hyperplastic primary vitreous in association with neurofibromatosis 2. *J Pediatr Ophthalmol Strabismus* 42:247, 2005

Pollard ZF: Persistent hyperplastic primary vitreous: Diagnosis, treatment and results. *Trans Am Ophthalmol Soc* 95:488, 1997

Sanghvi DA, Sanghvi CA, Purandare NC: Bilateral persistent hyperplastic primary vitreous. *Australas Radiol* 49:72, 2005

Suzuki K, Nakamura M, Amano E *et al.*: Case of chromosome 6p25 terminal deletion associated with Axenfeld–Rieger syndrome and persistent hyperplastic primary vitreous. *Am J Med Genet A* 140:503, 2006

Leukokoria: Retinal Dysplasia

Fulton AB, Craft JL, Howard RO *et al.*: Human retinal dysplasia. *Am J Ophthalmol* 85:690, 1978

Godel V, Romano A, Stein R *et al.*: Primary retinal dysplasia transmitted as X-chromosome-linked recessive disorder. *Am J Ophthalmol* 86:221, 1978

Hoepner J, Yanoff M: Spectrum of ocular abnormalities in trisomy 13–15. *Am J Ophthalmol* 74:729, 1972

Lahav M, Albert DM: Clinical and histopathologic classification of retinal dysplasia. *Am J Ophthalmol* 75:648, 1973

Leukokoria: Retinopathy of Prematurity

Chan-Ling T, Tour S, Hollander H *et al.*: Vascular changes and their mechanisms in the feline. *Invest Ophthalmol Vis Sci* 33:2128, 1992

Coats DK, Miller AM, Hussein MA *et al.*: Involution of retinopathy of prematurity after laser treatment: factors associated with development of retinal detachment. *Am J Ophthalmol* 140:214, 2005

Csak K, Szabo V, Szabo A *et al.*: Pathogenesis and genetic basis for retinopathy of prematurity. *Front Biosci* 11:908, 2006

Darlow BA, Horwood LJ, Clement RS: Retinopathy of prematurity: risk factors in a prospective population-based study. *Paediatr Perinat Epidemiol* 6:62, 1992

Fetter WP, van Duin VJ, Baerts W *et al.*: Visual acuity and visual field development after cryocoagulation in infants with retinopathy of prematurity. *Acta Paediatr* 81:25, 1992

Foos RY: Retinopathy of prematurity: Pathologic correlation of clinical stages. *Retina* 7:260, 1987

Garcia-Valenzuela E, Kaufman LM: High myopia associated with retinopathy of prematurity is primarily lenticular. *J AAPOS* 9:121, 2005

Hartnett ME, McColm JR: Retinal features predictive of progressive stage 4 retinopathy of prematurity. *Retina* 24:237, 2004

Keith CG, Doyle LW: Retinopathy of prematurity in infants weighing 1000–1499 g at birth. *Paediatr Child Health* 31:134, 1995

Kivlin JD, Biglan AW, Gordon RA *et al.*: Early retinal vessel development and iris vessel dilatation as factors in retinopathy of prematurity. *Arch Ophthalmol* 114:150, 1996

Palmer EA, Flynn JT, Hardy RJ *et al.*: Incidence and early course of retinopathy of prematurity. *Ophthalmology* 98:1628, 1991

Patz A: Observations on the retinopathy of prematurity. *Am J Ophthalmol* 100:164, 1985

Repka MX, Palmer EA, Tung B *et al.*: Involution of retinopathy of prematurity. *Arch Ophthalmol* 118:645, 2000

Reynolds JD, Dobson V, Quinn GE *et al.*: Evidence-based screening criteria for retinopathy of prematurity: natural history data from the CRYO-ROP and LIGHT-ROP studies. *Arch Ophthalmol* 120:1470, 2002

Rowlands E, Ionides AC, Chinn S *et al.*: Reduced incidence of retinopathy of prematurity. *Br J Ophthalmol* 85:933, 2001

Shah PK, Narendran V, Saravanan VR *et al.*: Fulminate retinopathy of prematurity—clinical characteristics and laser outcome. *Indian J Ophthalmol* 53:261, 2005

Sira IB, Nissenkorn I, Kremer I: Retinopathy of prematurity. *Surv Ophthalmol* 33:1, 1988

Steidl SM, Hirose T: Subretinal organization in stage 5 retinopathy of prematurity. *Graefes Arch Clin Exp Ophthalmol* 241:263, 2003

Stone J, Chan-Ling T, Pe'er J *et al.*: Roles of vascular endothelial growth factor and astrocyte degeneration in the genesis of retinopathy of prematurity. *Invest Ophthalmol Vis Sci* 37:290, 1996

Leukokoria: Coats' Disease

Alexandridou A, Stavrou P: Bilateral Coats' disease: long-term follow up. *Acta Ophthalmol Scand* 80:98, 2002

Anandan M, Porter NJ, Nemeth AH *et al.*: Coats-type retinal telangiectasia in case of Kabuki make-up syndrome (Niikawa–Uroki syndrome). *Ophthalmic Genet* 26:181, 2005

Beby F, Roche O, Burillon C *et al.*: Coats' disease and bilateral cataract in a child with Turner syndrome: a case report. *Graefes Arch Clin Exp Ophthalmol* 243:1291, 2005

Cahill M, O'Keefe M, Acheson R *et al.*: Classification of the spectrum of Coats' disease as subtypes of idiopathic retinal telangiectasis with exudation. *Acta Ophthalmol Scand* 79:596, 2001

Chang M, McLean IW, Merritt JC: Coats' disease. A study of 62 histologically confirmed cases. *J Pediatr Ophthalmol Strabismus* 21:163, 1984

Crow YJ, McMenamin J, Haenggeli CA *et al.*: Coats' plus: a progressive familial syndrome of bilateral Coats' disease, characteristic cerebral calcification, leukoencephalopathy, slow pre- and post-natal linear growth and defects of bone marrow and integument. *Neuropediatrics* 35:10, 2004

Eibschitz-Tsimhoni M, Johnson MW, Johnson TM *et al.*: Coats' syndrome as a cause of secondary open-angle glaucoma. *Ophthalmic Surg Lasers Imaging* 34:312, 2003

Galluzzi P, Venturi C, Cerase A *et al.*: Coats disease: smaller volume of the affected globe. *Radiology* 221:64, 2001

Gass JD, Oyakawa RT: Idiopathic juxtafoveolar retinal telangiectasis. *Arch Ophthalmol* 100:769, 1982

Haik BG: Advanced Coats' disease. *Trans Am Ophthalmol Soc* 89:371, 1991

Khurana RN, Samuel MA, Murphree AL *et al.*: Subfoveal nodule in Coats' disease. *Clin Exp Ophthalmol* 33:301, 2005

Maruoka K, Yamamoto M, Fujita H *et al.*: A case of Coats' disease in a low-birth-weight infant. *Ophthalmologica* 219:401, 2005

Paunescu LA, Ko TH, Duker JS *et al.*: Idiopathic juxtafoveal retinal telangiectasis: new findings by ultrahigh-resolution optical coherence tomography. *Ophthalmology* 113:48, 2006

Pe'er J: Calcification in Coats' disease. *Am J Ophthalmol* 106:742, 1988

Senft SH, Hidayat AA, Cavender JC: Atypical Coats' disease. *Retina* 14:36, 1994

Shields JA, Fammartino J, Shields CL: Coats' disease as a cause of anterior chamber cholesterolosis. *Arch Ophthalmol* 113:975, 1995

Shields JA, Shields CL, Honavar SG *et al.*: Classification and management of Coats disease: The 2000 Proctor Lecture. *Am J Ophthalmol* 131:572, 2001

Shields JA, Shields CL, Honavar SG *et al.*: Clinical variations and complications of Coats' disease in 150 cases. The 2000 Sanford Gifford Memorial Lecture. *Am J Ophthalmol* 131:561, 2001

Smithen LM, Spaide RF: Photodynamic therapy and intravitreal triamcinolone for a subretinal neovascularization in bilateral idiopathic juxtafoveal telangiectasis. *Am J Ophthalmol* 138:884, 2004

Smithen LM, Brown GC, Brucker AJ *et al.*: Coats' disease diagnosed in adulthood. *Ophthalmology* 112:1072, 2005

Watzke RC, Klein ML, Folk JC *et al.*: Long-term juxtafoveal retinal telangiectasia. *Retina* 25:727, 2005

Leukokoria: Norrie's Disease

Bateman JB, Kojis TL, Cantor RM *et al.*: Linkage analysis of Norrie disease with an X-chromosomal ornithine aminotransferase locus. *Trans Am Ophthalmol Soc* 91:299, 1993

Chen ZY, Battinelli EM, Fielder A *et al.*: A mutation in the Norrie disease gene (NDP) associated with X-linked familial exudative vitreoretinopathy. *Nat Genet* 5:180, 1993

Chynn EW, Walton DS, Hahn L *et al.*: Norrie disease: Diagnosis of a simplex case by DNA analysis. *Arch Ophthalmol* 114:1136, 1996

Clement F, Beckford CA, Corral A *et al.*: X-linked familial exudative vitreoretinopathy: Report of one family. *Retina* 15:141, 1995

Dryja TP: Bilateral leukocoria (Norrie's disease) in a newborn. Presented at the Verhoeff Society meeting, 1994

Enyedi LB, de Juan E, Gaitan A: Ultrastructural study of Norrie's disease. *Am J Ophthalmol* 111:439, 1991

Luhmann UF, Lin J, Acar N *et al.*: Role of the Norrie disease pseudoglioma gene in sprouting angiogenesis during development of the retinal vasculature. *Invest Ophthalmol Vis Sci* 46:3372, 2005

Ohlmann A, Scholz M, Goldwich A *et al.*: Ectopic norrin induces growth of ocular capillaries and restores normal retinal angiogenesis in Norrie disease mutant mice. *J Neurosci* 25:1701, 2005

Rehm HL, Zhang DS, Brown MC *et al.*: Vascular defects and sensorineural deafness in a mouse model of Norrie disease. *J Neurosci* 22:4286, 2002

Royer G, Hanein S, Raclin V *et al.*: NDP gene mutations in 14 French families with Norrie disease. *Hum Mutat* 22:499, 2003

Ruether K, van de Pol D, Jaissle G *et al.*: Retinoschisis alterations in the mouse eye caused by gene targeting of the Norrie disease gene. *Invest Ophthalmol Vis Sci* 38:710, 1997

Shastry BS, Pendergast SD, Hartzer MK *et al.*: Identification of missense mutations in the Norrie disease gene associated with advanced retinopathy of prematurity. *Arch Ophthalmol* 115:651, 1997

Sims KB, Irvine AR, Good WV: Norrie disease in a family with a manifesting female carrier. *Arch Ophthalmol* 115:517, 1997

Wong F, Goldberg MF, Hao Y: Identification of a nonsense mutation at codon 128 of the Norrie's disease gene in a male infant. *Arch Ophthalmol* 111:1553, 1993

Xu Q, Wang Y, Dabdoub A *et al.*: Vascular development in the retina and inner ear: control by Norrin and Frizzled-4, a high-affinity ligand-receptor pair. *Cell* 116:883, 2004

Leukokoria: Incontinentia Pigmenti

Aradhya S, Bardaro T, Galgoczy P *et al.*: Multiple pathogenic and benign genomic rearrangements occur at a 35 kb duplication involving the NEMO and LAGE2 genes. *Hum Mol Genet* 10:2557, 2001

Berlin AL, Paller AS, Chan LS: Incontinentia pigmenti: a review and update on the molecular basis of pathophysiology. *J Am Acad Dermatol* 47:169, 2002

Bodak N, Hadj-Rabia S, Hamel-Teillac D *et al.*: Late recurrence of inflammatory first-stage lesions in incontinentia pigmenti: an unusual phenomenon and a fascinating pathologic mechanism. *Arch Dermatol* 139:201, 2003

Catalano RA: Incontinentia pigmenti. *Am J Ophthalmol* 110:696, 1990

Chan YC, Happle R, Giam YC: Whorled scarring alopecia: a rare phenomenon in incontinentia pigmenti? *J Am Acad Dermatol* 49:929, 2003

Cox JJ, Holden ST, Dee S *et al.*: Identification of a 650 kb duplication at the X chromosome breakpoint in a patient with 46,X,t(X;8)(q28;q12) and non-syndromic mental retardation. *J Med Genet* 40:169, 2003

Ferreira RC, Ferreira LC, Forstat L *et al.*: Corneal abnormalities associated with incontinentia pigmenti. *Am J Ophthalmol* 123:549, 1997

Fowell SM, Greenwald MJ, Prendiville JS *et al.*: Ocular findings of incontinentia pigmenti in a male infant with Klinefelter syndrome. *J Pediatr Ophthalmol Strabismus* 29:180, 1992

Goldberg MF: The blinding mechanisms of incontinentia pigmenti. *Trans Am Ophthalmol Soc* 92:167, 1994

Goldberg MF, Custis PH: Retinal and other manifestations of incontinentia pigmenti (Bloch–Sulzberger syndrome). *Ophthalmology* 100:1645, 1993

Jean-Baptiste S, O'Toole EA, Chen M *et al.*: Expression of eotaxin, an eosinophil-selective chemokine, parallels eosinophil accumulation in the vesiculobullous stage of incontinentia pigmenti. *Clin Exp Immunol* 127:470, 2002

Kenwrick S, Woffendin H, Jakins T *et al.*: Survival of male patients with incontinentia pigmenti carrying a lethal mutation can be explained by somatic mosaicism or Klinefelter syndrome. *Am J Hum Genet* 69:1210, 2001

Martinez-Pomar N, Munoz-Saa I, Heine-Suner D *et al.*: A new mutation in exon 7 of NEMO gene: late skewed X-chromosome inactivation in an incontinentia pigmenti female patient with immunodeficiency. *Hum Genet* 118:458, 2005

Montes CM, Maize JC, Guerry-Force ML: Incontinentia pigmenti with painful subungual tumors: a two-generation study. *J Am Acad Dermatol* 50:S45, 2004

Porksen G, Pfeiffer C, Hahn G *et al.*: Neonatal seizures in two sisters with incontinentia pigmenti. *Neuropediatrics* 35:139, 2004

Renas-Sordo ML, Vallejo-Vega B, Hernandez-Zamora E *et al.*: Incontinentia pigmenti (IP2): familial case report with affected men. Literature review. *Med Oral Patol Oral Cir Bucal* 10(Suppl. 2):E122, 2005

Shields CL, Eagle RC Jr, Shah RM *et al.*: Multifocal hypopigmented retinal pigment epithelial lesions in incontinentia pigmenti. *Retina* 26:328, 2006

Wald KJ, Mehta MC, Katsumi O *et al.*: Retinal detachments in incontinentia pigmenti. *Arch Ophthalmol* 111:614, 1993

Wu HP, Wang YL, Chang HH *et al.*: Dental anomalies in two patients with incontinentia pigmenti. *J Formos Med Assoc* 104:427, 2005

Yanoff M: Incontinentia pigmenti (letter). *Arch Ophthalmol* 94:1631, 1976

Leukokoria: Other Causes

Bekibele CO, Ogunbiyi JO: Inflammatory orbital pseudotumor simulating retinoblastoma in a one year old girl. *West Afr J Med* 21:77, 2002

Bhende P, Babu K, Kumari P *et al.*: Solitary retinal astrocytoma in an infant. *J Pediatr Ophthalmol Strabismus* 41:305, 2004

Freitag SK, Eagle RC Jr, Shields JA *et al.*: Melanogenic neuroectodermal tumor of the retina (primary malignant melanoma of the retina). *Arch Ophthalmol* 115:1581, 1997

Imhof SM, Moll AC, van d V *et al.*: Retinoblastoma and retinal astrocytoma: unusual double tumour in one eye. *Br J Ophthalmol* 86:1441, 2002

Lev D, Binson I, Foldes AJ *et al.*: Decreased bone density in carriers and patients of an Israeli family with the osteoporosis-pseudoglioma syndrome. *Isr Med Assoc J* 5:419, 2003

Patel S, Dondey J, Chan HS *et al.*: Leukocoria caused by intraocular heterotopic brain tissue. *Arch Ophthalmol* 122:390, 2004

Reese AB: Massive retinal fibrosis in children. *Am J Ophthalmol* 19:576, 1936

Shields JA, Shields CL, Eagle RC Jr *et al.*: Endogenous endophthalmitis simulating retinoblastoma. *Retina* 15:213, 1995

Shields CL, Shields JA, Eagle RC Jr *et al.*: Progressive enlargement of acquired retinal astrocytoma in 2 cases. *Ophthalmology* 111:363, 2004

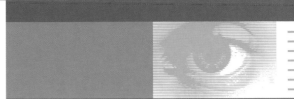

Index